SAMOUR & KING'S

Pediatric Nutrition

in Clinical Care FIFTH EDITION

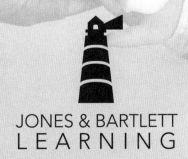

Susan Konek, MA, RDN, CSP, LD, FAND
Clinical Nutrition Management Consultant
Pediatric Nutrition Partners, LLC - Partner
Dayton, Ohio

Patricia Becker, MS, RDN, CSP, CNSC
Pediatric Nutrition Specialist
Owner: KidsRD.com/PediatricMalnutrition.com
Dayton Childrens Hospital Medical Center
Dayton, Ohio

JONES & BARTLETT
LEARNING

World Headquarters
Jones & Bartlett Learning
5 Wall Street
Burlington, MA 01803
978-443-5000
info@jblearning.com
www.jblearning.com

Jones & Bartlett Learning books and products are available through most bookstores and online booksellers. To contact Jones & Bartlett Learning directly, call 800-832-0034, fax 978-443-8000, or visit our website, www.jblearning.com.

Production Credits
VP, Product Management: Amanda Martin
Director of Product Management: Cathy L. Esperti
Product Manager: Sean Fabery
Product Specialist: Rachael Souza
Project Specialist: Lori Mortimer
Digital Products Supervisor: Jordan McKenzie
Digital Products Specialist: Rachel Reyes
Director of Marketing: Andrea DeFronzo
VP, Manufacturing and Inventory Control: Therese Connell

Composition & Project Management: Exela Technologies
Cover Design: Kristin E. Parker
Text Design: Kristin E. Parker
Rights & Media Specialist: Maria Maimone
Media Development Editor: Shannon Sheehan
Cover Image (Title Page, Part Opener, Chapter Opener): © Gajus/istock/Getty Images
Printing and Binding: McNaughton & Gunn
Cover Printing: McNaughton & Gunn

Library of Congress Cataloging-in-Publication Data
Names: Konek, Susan, editor.
Title: Samour & King's pediatric nutrition in clinical care / [edited by]
   Susan Konek and Patricia Becker.
Other titles: Pediatric nutrition. | Samour and King's pediatric nutrition in
   clinical care | Pediatric nutrition in clinical care
Description: Fifth edition. | Burlington, MA : Jones & Bartlett Learning,
   [2020] | Revison of: Pediatric nutrition. c2012. 4th ed. | Includes
   bibliographical references and index.
Identifiers: LCCN 2018041765 | ISBN 9781284146394 (paperback)
Subjects: LCSH: Children–Nutrition–Handbooks, manuals, etc. |
   Infants–Nutrition–Handbooks, manuals, etc. |
   Children–Diseases–Nutritional aspects–Handbooks, manuals, etc. | BISAC:
   HEALTH & FITNESS / Nutrition.
Classification: LCC RJ206 .H23 2019 | DDC 618.92--dc23
LC record available at https://lccn.loc.gov/2018041765

6048

Printed in the United States of America
23 22 21 20 19   10 9 8 7 6 5 4 3 2 1

This edition is dedicated to pediatric nutrition practitioners, in all disciplines, who provide optimal nutrition care to infants, children, and adolescents. It is through their expertise and collaboration that our field has achieved a high standard in patient care. The development of this text has brought together an outstanding group of these experts to share this expertise with their fellow practitioners and with students learning about pediatric nutrition. I thank them!

—Susan Konek

This edition is dedicated to all the children who struggle with food and nutrition challenges, as well as the pediatric dietitians who care for them. Throughout my career, I have continued to be awed and inspired by this dedicated and remarkable group of individuals and the children they care for.

—Patricia Becker

Brief Contents

Contents

SECTION II Perinatal Nutrition   85

Chapter 5 Nutritional Implications of the Developing Fetus........ 87

Kristen Leavitt and *Nancy Nevin-Folino*

Chapter 6 Human Milk................. 103

Jacqueline J. Wessel

SECTION III Nutrition Throughout Childhood   121

Chapter 7 Nutrition for Premature Infants   123

Diane M. Anderson and *Marsha Dumm*

Chapter 8   Infant Nutrition 145

Stephanie Merlino Barr and *Sharon Groh-Wargo*

Chapter 9   Normal Nutrition through Childhood and Adolescence 175

Beth Ogata and *Sharon Feucht*

Chapter 13 Critical Care 313

Katelyn Ariagno, Nicolle Quinn and *Lori J. Bechard*

Chapter 14 Cardiology 325

Melanie Savoca and *Megan Horsley*

Chapter 15 Pulmonary Diseases 351

Laura Grande Padula, Emily Bingham and *Andrea Nepa*

Foreword

Pediatric Nutrition in Clinical Care (formerly *Pediatric Nutrition*) evolved over the last four editions to become the "go-to" resource for nutrition practitioners managing the nutritional care of pregnant women, infants, children, and adolescents. The intent was always to combine the best science and research with practical clinical experience, with chapters having been written by dietitians/nutritionists and physicians who are experts in their respective areas of clinical practice. This text was originally intended to cover a broad scope of practice settings, including public health, community, inpatient clinical, and ambulatory care; its scope covered traditional therapies as well as emerging integrative therapies.

This *Fifth Edition* has a more focused intent than prior editions. The two editors are well known and respected in pediatric nutrition. They have done a stellar job of lining up many former contributors as well as new chapter authors who are pediatric nutrition experts. We are proud that they will continue providing a cutting-edge text, continuing our legacy by ensuring a quality resource for those who provide nutrition care for our infants and children: Our future.

This text has always been considered the "go-to" reference, and we know it will continue to be the best for our pediatric nutrition practitioners.

Patt Samour & Kathy King

Preface

Commonly used by dietetic practitioners studying for pediatric specialty exams, this is the fifth edition of the most comprehensive text available that focuses on pediatric nutrition from the premature infant through the adolescent and on all pediatric disorders impacting nutrition. It is used widely in academic settings, as well as by pediatric nutrition clinicians. *Pediatric Nutrition in Clinical Care, Fifth Edition* is intended for use by healthcare professionals of all disciplines who are learning about pediatric nutrition and by practitioners managing the nutrition of pediatric groups and individuals. The emphasis is on clinical nutrition care.

With each chapter written by recognized experts in their practice area, the text can be used by dietetic practitioners and others specializing in pediatrics in all areas of practice (medical, nursing, as well as dietetics). Students in these areas of study will find this text to be a thorough yet readable review of all major topics in pediatric nutrition. The *Fifth Edition* has been expanded to 28 chapters, with nine returning chapter contributors or teams of contributors and 19 new contributors. There are eight new chapters. The book covers the latest clinical research, practical applications, alternative therapies, and studies of the normal child from fetal life through adolescence.

The chapters in this text are written to help the reader identify and apply key pediatric nutrition practices and principles. In addition to important updates in all major areas of pediatric nutrition, the *Fifth Edition* has been expanded to include evolving areas in pediatric nutrition. These include malnutrition related to undernutrition, the nutrition-focused physical exam, human milk and its use in the clinical setting, critical care nutrition, nutrition for the surgical patient, integrative medicine and nutrition, and measuring outcomes.

The goal for all infants and children is to grow and develop happily and in good health. Normal nutrition, as much as possible, is always the goal of nutrition care. As pediatric practitioners, we want to assess growth and nutritional intake and intervene as needed to maximize health status. This goal is the same for all infants and children regardless of when they are born (premature or full-term) and whether they have a disease or other condition affecting their nutritional status.

Growth, screening and assessment parameters, and routes of nutrition may change, but the desired outcomes are the same.

▶ Developing the *Fifth Edition*

This edition of *Pediatric Nutrition in Clinical Care* has been written by new authors, Susan Konek and Patricia Becker, building on the comprehensive resources provided in the *Fourth Edition*. We wanted to ensure that *Pediatric Nutrition in Clinical Care* continues to be available to practitioners and students of pediatric nutrition in the future. Long-time authors Patt Samour and Kathy King supported our proposal to write *Pediatric Nutrition in Clinical Care, Fifth Edition*, and we are pleased to have the opportunity to continue and expand this resource to reflect new science, new areas of interest, and current standards of practice.

The recent recognition of malnutrition related to undernutrition in pediatrics as well as nutrition-focused physical assessment to aid in identifying the malnourished child are examples of topics new to this text.

As pediatric nutrition practitioners with acute care experience, we have found value in an extensive survey by the publisher of academic users of *Pediatric Nutrition, Fourth Edition*, as we determined content essential to meet the curriculum requirements of students. Revisions of most *Fourth Edition* chapters have been included to meet these criteria. In addition to maintaining the wide variety of condition/disease-specific topics, we have added newly requested or expanded chapters, including those on human milk (including donor milk), nutrition for premature infants, gastrointestinal diseases, and feeding disorders.

▶ Features and Benefits

Students, instructors, and pediatric nutrition clinicians will benefit from many features provided in *Pediatric Nutrition in Clinical Care, Fifth Edition*. These include:

- Comprehensive coverage of all major areas of pediatric nutrition, from fetal life through childhood and adolescence, with important updates in all areas. This expert level of review provides exposure to current and developing nutrition care on all topics.

- Students and instructors will benefit from learning objectives, critical-thinking questions, and case studies in all appropriate chapters. Case studies, in particular, support learning as they provide examples of how practitioners use nutrition to identify, diagnose, and treat pediatric conditions through nutrition. The case studies include tools and standards of measure used in assessment of nutrition status.

- The Academy of Nutrition and Dietetics Nutrition Care Process (NCP) is utilized where appropriate in managing nutrition in all assessments, diagnoses, interventions, monitoring, and evaluation. The goal is to provide examples of actual nutrition management as seen in pediatric clinical nutrition practice.

- Written by recognized experts in their subspecialties, all chapters include a current review of literature. Although references support the content of the chapter, they also serve as starting points for more in-depth study of the chapter topics.

- Chapters new to the *Fifth Edition* expand the scope of this text to include a collection of topics reflecting evolution of the field of pediatric nutrition. These provide the student and the pediatric nutrition clinician with advanced knowledge of emerging subspecialty topics, including pediatric malnutrition and its treatment, pediatric nutrition-focused physical exam, use and management of human milk, critical care nutrition, nutrition considerations in pediatric surgery, and an evidence-based review of integrative medicine and nutrition.

- The latest research and best practice in major areas, conditions, and disorders of pediatrics are included. Neonatal nutrition, infant nutrition, normal nutrition throughout childhood, enteral and parenteral nutrition support, gastrointestinal disorders, cardiology, oncology and hematology, diabetes, renal/chronic kidney disease, and numerous other topics are presented for pediatric nutrition clinicians as well as students.

- Users of this text are provided thorough, yet succinct, overviews and updates on all topics.

- Comprehensive treatment of all pediatric topics makes this text the perfect review resource when studying for specialty exams for registered dietitians/nutritionists; physicians, including gastroenterologists, pediatricians, and fellows; and others practicing on pediatric nutrition-related teams (such as critical care, gastroenterology, eating and feeding disorders, cardiology, pulmonary, surgery, and oncology/hematology).

- Comprehensive coverage of pediatric nutrition topics that require special management of nutrition, including obesity and weight management, eating and feeding disorders, sports nutrition, food sensitivities and intolerance, and genetic screening/inborn errors of metabolism. Evidence-based behavioral approaches, as appropriate, are important components of these chapters.

- Integrative medicine and nutrition is covered in a new chapter reflecting the rapid growth in the use of complementary and alternative medicine and nutrition to treat pediatric conditions. This chapter provides an evidence-based review of this growing approach to pediatric medicine through nutrition. Students and clinicians will benefit from this review based on current science.

▸ Overview of the Text

This text is organized with the recognition of how pediatric nutrition practitioners practice.

It begins with fundamental techniques—nutrition assessment, growth and growth assessment, nutrition-focused physical exam, and malnutrition related to undernutrition—all utilized at the starting point in the nutrition status evaluation of infants, children, and adolescents.

Chapter topics move into the care of the developing fetus, the neonate, and infant nutrition. New to this edition is a chapter on human milk, its properties, use, and donor milk. Normal nutrition through childhood completes the introductory chapters of this edition.

Advanced modalities that support nutrition are addressed in comprehensive chapters on enteral and parenteral nutrition, both utilizing updated guidelines from the Academy of Nutrition and Dietetics (AND) and the American Society of Enteral and Parenteral Nutrition (ASPEN). These foundational chapters support the nutrition care for all diseases and conditions with nutritional considerations. Included are all subspecialty areas: Gastrointestinal disorders, critical care, cardiology, pulmonary, oncology and hematology, surgery, renal disease, burns, diabetes, food sensitivities and intolerance, genetic screening, and inborn errors of metabolism. Chapters on conditions and disorders requiring behavioral interventions are included in the next group of chapters. These include obesity and weight management, eating and feeding disorders, sports nutrition for children, and children with special needs.

Chapters that reflect new areas of focus in the work of pediatric nutrition include integrative medicine and measuring outcomes—how we evaluate the impact of our pediatric nutrition interventions.

To ensure consistency across chapters, the majority of the chapters include the following features:

- Learning Objectives
- Introduction
- Case Studies
- Conclusion
- Review Questions
- References

Reference chapters—including those on nutrition assessment, human milk, and the nutrition-focused physical assessment—will not include case studies, while the chapter on measuring outcomes has an outcomes research example instead.

▶ Organization of the Text

Because *Pediatric Nutrition, Fourth Edition* was published in 2012, contributors to the *Fifth Edition* were charged with completing a comprehensive review of the literature and including new science and practice in their writing. All chapters have been written to focus on this goal, providing content that is current and that reflects evolving science and practice.

Chapter 1, "Nutrition Assessment," focuses on the standardized methods to evaluate children for nutritional risk, as well as the first step in the NCP. This chapter serves as a reference for all of the later chapters in the text, including common information such as Resting Energy Equations and Dietary Reference Intake data. This chapter will be most useful to students and dietitians new to the practice of pediatric nutrition.

Chapter 2, "Growth and Maturation," provides a concise overview of the process of physical growth and maturation over the course of childhood. This includes clear explanations of the timing of changes that occur in various tissues of the body as

children age. Growth charts (WHO and CDC) and the standards for their use support an understanding of these important tools that are used for ongoing nutrition status and growth assessment. The chapter evaluates the strengths and weaknesses of the different growth reference charts and provides guidance for their use in real-world assessment and monitoring of childhood growth. Case studies are provided to support understanding of the use of growth charts. This may be of particular benefit to students.

Chapter 3, "Nutrition-focused Physical Exam," provides a thorough review of nutrition-focused physical assessment as an important tool in the assessment of children and adolescents. This chapter is new to this edition, reflecting the expansion of this method of assessment into pediatrics. Experts in this field share this evolving practice.

Chapter 4, "Malnutrition Related to Undernutrition," provides a comprehensive review of this important initiative to standardize the diagnosis and treatment of malnutrition in children, including criteria for defining illness-related and non-illness-related pediatric malnutrition. The reader will learn how to identify pediatric malnutrition utilizing the recommended indicators. Emphasis on the best-practice use of z-scores to assess growth in the pediatric population covers the recent innovation in the development of criteria for pediatric malnutrition.

Chapter 5, "Nutrition Implications of the Developing Fetus," returns with updates on how nutrition affects the fetus and provides guidelines for those caring for pregnant women and their developing fetuses. The chapter provides detailed information on the effects of specific micronutrients on fetal development, nutrition therapy for mothers, and information on the impact of endocrine abnormalities on fetal development.

Chapter 6, "Human Milk," is a comprehensive review of human milk, including the numerous advantages of the use of breast milk to babies preterm and term gestation. It includes a complete description of the unique properties of human milk including those that make them critically important to preterm infants and those fragile due to complications. The role for adequately fortified donor milk (banked milk) as the next best choice is discussed. The American Academy of Pediatrics' recommendation for illicit drugs and the use of human milk is also included.

Chapter 7, "Nutrition for Premature Infants," provides an extensive review of the nutrition for these most fragile of pediatric patients. All nutrition modalities needed to support growth and development are reviewed in full, including human milk and new products for parenteral nutrition support. Nutrition management from birth, early parenteral support, and transition to enteral nutrition are detailed.

Chapter 8, "Infant Nutrition," addresses the current recommended feeding practices for healthy full-term infants and common feeding problems encountered during the first year of life. These recommendations may apply to all infants and as a starting point for those with conditions addressed in subsequent chapters.

Chapter 9, "Normal Nutrition Through Childhood and Adolescence," focuses on the nutritional needs and issues of normal, healthy children during the growth years through adolescence. This chapter provides information on nutrition and physical activity, school nutrition, adolescent nutrition, and dental nutrition. There is new information on age-based feeding guidelines and age-based vitamin–mineral recommendations for children.

Chapters 10, "Enteral Nutrition," and 11, "Parenteral Nutrition," provide extensive updates and all details needed to manage the nutritional status for infants and children who cannot be nourished and grow on an oral diet. The use of these modalities may be short-term in the acute care setting, or long-term, spanning years. Updated standards of practice, products, and innovation for managing children on enteral nutrition are described in detail.

Chapter 12, "Gastrointestinal Disorders," provides current science and practice in managing the wide range of conditions occurring within this subspecialty. This chapter incorporates the extensive use of the NCP to explain how to assess, diagnose, and manage conditions such as celiac disease, lactose intolerance, inflammatory bowel disease, and pancreatitis. The management of short gut syndrome and intestinal transplant are included in detail. The unique challenges to handling children with these disorders are addressed in order to achieve the goal of growth and optimal health. A discussion of normal digestion and absorption of the gastrointestinal tract is included.

Chapter 13, "Critical Care," addresses the expanding science and practice in the subspecialty of nutrition for children in critical care situations. The chapter identifies the key elements of the cascade of critical illness, describes relationships between critical

illness and nutritional status, explains how to assess signs and symptoms of critical illness that impact nutrition interventions and delivery, and describes the development of a nutrition care plan for the acute phase of pediatric critical illness.

Chapter 14, "Cardiology," expands on the growing science of caring for infants and children with congenital heart defects and optimal nutrition to support their progress. An overview of the anatomy of congenital heart disease and other cardiac diseases and associated nutrition problems contributing to malnutrition is provided. The nutritional challenges that result in malnutrition and growth disruption are addressed in detail. Current modalities of nutrition care for children with extracorporeal membrane oxygenation (ECMO), cardiomyopathy, pulmonary hypertension, lymphatic disorders, and hyperlipidemias are discussed.

Chapter 15, "Pulmonary Diseases," provides a comprehensive review of the role of nutrition in pediatric pulmonary diseases, including cystic fibrosis, bronchopulmonary dysplasia, and asthma. The nutritional complications of these diseases are discussed. In particular, those occurring in cystic fibrosis, pancreatic insufficiency, micronutrient deficiencies, and CF-related diabetes are covered. The challenges of meeting increased nutrient needs in the BPD population are discussed. The role of nutrition in risk of developing asthma and other asthma related nutrition issues are reviewed.

Chapter 16, "Hematology and Oncology," presents an extensive review of current nutrition support and management for children with cancer. The authors explain nutrition assessment and monitoring parameters for pediatric oncology patients. The chapter reviews appropriate nutrition support practices related to pediatric oncology, including enteral and parenteral nutrition. Nutrition management of children with cancer undergoing oncologic therapy is described at length, as is the long-term nutritional sequelae associated with pediatric malignancies. An overview of sickle cell disease and its nutritional complications are included.

Chapter 17, "Pediatric Surgical Nutrition: Principles and Techniques," is new to the *Fifth Edition*, reflecting the expanding understanding of the importance of nutrition in the care of children undergoing surgery. The authors examine the role of nutrition in infants and children with surgical correction of congenital surgical anomalies and other pediatric surgeries, including fundoplication. Lengthy consideration of the calorie and protein needs of the pediatric surgical patient is provided. A discussion of nutritional additives that may benefit a pediatric surgical patient is also included.

Chapter 18, "Chronic Kidney Disease," addresses all nutrition care components of the infant or child before and during dialysis and after kidney transplant. The specific nutrients of concern in this disease, combined with the challenges for growth are covered. This chapter provides additional information on fluid and electrolyte balance and bone health in this population.

Chapter 19, "Nutrition for Burned Pediatric Patients," addresses the metabolic changes and physiologic challenges of providing adequate nutrition to the infant or child in this stressed state. Ongoing evaluation of energy requirements is emphasized, as is the use of all nutrition support modalities used in acute care and for rehabilitation post-burn.

Chapter 20, "Diabetes," provides a comprehensive review of current science and practice in the nutrition care of children with diabetes. This discussion reflects advances in medical treatment that have brought change to the nutritional management needed to control this disease. Increased incidence of type II diabetes is discussed. The role of the registered dietitian/nutritionist to support the family's efforts to maintain diabetes control for their child and help promote healthy eating habits is discussed. Issues discussed include dyslipidemias, weight control, disordered eating, and use of the glycemic index. As seen with medical advances in diabetes care, new research and technologies continue, as do approaches to nutritional care.

Chapter 21, "Obesity and Weight Management," addresses obesity and the many factors that contribute to obesity, as well as key issues such as prevalence and trends, screening, assessment, and medical complications. The use of BMI in assessment, bariatric surgery for adolescents, and intervention programs are detailed.

Chapter 22, "Eating and Feeding Disorders," expands on the information presented in the *Fourth Edition,* with this content having now been broken out from the chapter on weight management. Eating disorders can affect a wide range of ages and are thus covered in detail; however, this chapter distinguishes itself by addressing feeding disorders, including food aversion, an inability to advance in oral feeding found in a population of young children, and the diagnosis of avoidant-restrictive food intake disorder. In addition to nutritional support of children with these conditions, the chapter considers behavioral, social, and medical interventions provided through specialized teams and family-based care.

Chapter 23, "Pediatric Sports Nutrition," provides an overview of the nutritional needs of children with high levels of physical activity, including hydration, and energy and protein needs. Information on optimizing performance and body composition for specific sports is provided. This chapter also contains information for the vegetarian and vegan child athlete. There is a section on areas of nutrition risk for the child athlete that should be considered. Case Studies are included to help the reader apply the information in the chapter to the practice of sports nutrition.

Chapter 24, "Children with Special Needs," addresses many of the more common types of disabilities and their nutritional challenges and concerns. Topics such as performing a nutritional assessment on a child with cerebral palsy and use of the ketogenic diet to control seizures are included. Current evidence on using nutritional intervention to treat attention deficit disorders is discussed.

Chapter 25, "Food Allergy," deals with the pathophysiology, diagnosis, and treatment of infants and children with food sensitivity. The chapter is essential for the practitioner working with infants and/or children with food allergies. It details such issues as food challenges, elimination diet, and the importance of label reading. Advances in the prevention and management of food allergies, specifically peanut allergies and evidence-based recommendations regarding these changes, are an important addition to the *Fifth Edition.*

Chapter 26, "Nutrition Management in Inborn Errors of Metabolism," is a detailed resource for the practitioner having to manage the nutrition care of infants and children with inborn errors of metabolism (IEM). Included in the chapter are newborn screening of IEMS and the principles and practical considerations in nutrition support of IEMS. Discussions cover the nutrition management of disorders of amino acid, nitrogen, carbohydrate, and fatty acid metabolism. Sample formula calculations for diet prescription are included, which can help the RD less familiar with special medical foods determine accurate measurements on appropriate feedings for the infant or child with an IEM.

Chapter 27, "Measuring Outcomes," focuses on the advances in quality improvement (QI) in healthcare, and specifically in nutrition and dietetics. Outcomes related to quality improvement in healthcare are defined. Terms, tools, and resources for conducting quality improvement research are provided. Examples of how to develop QI studies in nutrition are included.

Chapter 28, "Integrative Medicine and Nutrition," is a new addition, reflecting the rapid growth in the use of complementary and alternative medicine and nutrition to treat pediatric conditions. This chapter provides an evidence-based review of this growing approach to pediatric medicine through nutrition. Students and clinicians will benefit from this review based on current science.

▶ Online Resources

Readers can access a collection of relevant web links at http://health.jbpub.com/PediatricNutrition5e.

▶ Instructor Resources

We are pleased to support classroom instruction by offering the following to qualified instructors:

- A comprehensive Test Bank, supporting exam development and highlighting key takeaways from each chapter
- Slides in PowerPoint format, covering key points in each chapter

Susan Konek
Patricia Becker

About the Authors

Susan Konek, MA, RDN, CSP, LD, FAND

Susan Konek has worked in the field of pediatric nutrition for the past 30 years, with clinical experiences in nutrition support, cystic fibrosis, and critical care nutrition. She is a board-certified specialist in pediatric nutrition. Clinical nutrition management has also been a primary focus for much of this time.

Before her retirement from full-time work in 2015, her position as Director of Clinical Nutrition at the Children's Hospital of Philadelphia provided an opportunity to support the development of an outstanding clinical nutrition program and a large team of pediatric registered dietitians. Support for clinical nutrition departments through consultation and project specific employment has extended Sue's experience and collaboration with pediatric nutrition practitioners. Sue has been recognized for her achievement in clinical nutrition leadership through the 2017 Academy of Nutrition and Dietetics Excellence in Practice Management Award.

In addition to her professional experiences, Sue has taken an active role in the Academy of Nutrition and Dietetics as a leader at the state (President of the Delaware Academy of Nutrition and Dietetics), dietetic practice group (Pediatric Nutrition Practice Group Chair), and Academy (House of Delegates representative and Quality Management Committee member) level. This involvement has provided opportunities to collaborate with pediatric nutrition practitioners throughout the U.S.

Sue is currently a member of the National Quality Forum Standing Committee for Pediatric Measures. Contributions to publications as an author, reviewer, and editor have allowed Sue to develop a love for pediatric nutrition literature and experience to support this expertise.

Patricia Becker, MS, RDN, CSP, CNSC

Patricia Becker is a board-certified specialist in pediatric nutrition and nutrition support. She has had a wide range of experience as a dietitian. For the past 20 years Pat has worked in a variety of settings including Dayton Children's Hospital Medical Center, Cincinnati Children's Hospital and Medical Center, The University of North Carolina Children's Hospital, and her private practice KidsRD.com as a pediatric dietitian taking care of children from conception to adulthood, specializing in pediatric undernutrition.

She has served as chair of the Academy of Nutrition and Dietetics Evidence Analysis Library Pediatric Nutrition Screening Project, chair of the Pediatric Nutrition Practice Group DPG, author of the Pediatric Malnutrition Section of the *Pediatric Nutrition Care Manual*, member of the Academy of Nutrition and Dietetics/ASPEN Pediatric Malnutrition Work group, and lead author of the Consensus statement for ASPEN/AND pediatric malnutrition. She is also the author of "Identifying Malnutrition in Preterm and Neonatal Populations: Recommended Indicators," chair of the PNPG Malnutrition Committee, member of the ASPEN Malnutrition Committee, and a part of the ASPEN malnutrition "state of the science" paper author group.

Contributors

Diane M. Anderson, PhD, RD, LD
Associate Professor of Pediatrics
Baylor College of Medicine
Houston, Texas

Katelyn Ariagno, RD, LDN, CNSC
Clinical Nutrition Specialist III
GI Center for Nutrition
Boston Children's Hospital
Boston, Massachusetts

Jennifer Autodore, MPH, RDN, SCP, LDN
Pediatric Clinical Dietitian
Policy & Procedure System Specialist
Children's Hospital of Philadelphia
Philadelphia, Pennsylvania

Stephanie Merlino Barr, MS, RDN, LD
Neonatal Nutritionist
MetroHealth Medical Center
Cleveland, Ohio

Lori J. Bechard, PhD, MEd, RD
Clinical Research Manager, Pediatric Critical Care
 Nutrition
Boston Children's Hospital
Boston, Massachusetts

Patricia Becker, MS RDN, CSP, CNSC
Pediatric Nutrition Specialist
Owner, KidsRD.com/RDIII
Dayton Children's Hospital Medical Center
Dayton, Ohio

Rashelle Berry, MPH, MS, RDN, LD
Nutrition Manager, Children's Feeding Program
Children's Healthcare of Atlanta
Atlanta, Georgia

Emily Bingham, RD-AP, CNSC, LDN
Neonatal Dietitian
Children's Hospital of Philadelphia
Philadelphia, Pennsylvania

Thane Blinman, MD
Associate Professor of Surgery
General, Thoracic, and Fetal Surgery
Children's Hospital of Philadelphia
Philadelphia, Pennsylvania

Alison Cassin, MS, RD, CSP, LD
Registered Dietitian
Cincinnati Children's Hospital and Medical Center
Cincinnati, Ohio

Audrey C. Choh, PhD
Assistant Professor of Epidemiology
Department of Epidemiology, Human Genetics,
 and Environmental Sciences
School of Public Health
University of Texas Health Science Center
 at Houston
Houston, Texas

Harriet Holt Cloud, MS, RD, FAND
Owner
Nutrition Matters
Birmingham, Alabama

Amy Coen, RD, LD
Pediatric Dietitian
Dayton Children's Hospital
Dayton, Ohio

Robin C. Cook, MS, RD, CSP, LDN
Pediatric Surgical/Trauma Dietitian
The Children's Hospital of Philadelphia
Philadelphia, Pennsylvania

Stefan A. Czerwinski, PhD
Professor
Department of Epidemiology, Human Genetics
 and Environmental Sciences
School of Public Health
University of Texas Health Science Center
 at Houston
Brownsville, Texas

Julie Cooper, MS, RD, LDN
Outpatient Nutrition Manager
Children's Hospital of Philadelphia
Philadelphia, Pennsylvania

Kelly Green Corkins, MS, RD, LDN, CNSC
Clinical Dietitian III
LeBonheur Children's Hospital
Memphis, Tennessee

Julia Driggers, RD, CNSC, LDN
Pediatric Dietitian
The Children's Hospital of Philadelphia
Philadelphia, Pennsylvania

Marsha Dumm, MS, RDN
Neonatal Nutritionist
Pediatric Nutrition Partners, LLC
Circleville, Ohio

Sharon Feucht, MA, RDN, CD
Nutritionist—LEND Program
Editor, *Nutrition Focus*
Center on Human Development and Disability
   (CHDD)
Clinical Instructor
University of Washington
Seattle, Washington

Andrea Gilbaugh, RD, CNSC
Clinical Dietitian
Lucile Packard Children's Hospital
Palo Alto, California

Susan L. Goolsby, MS, RD, CEDRD, LD
Assistant Director Clinical Nutrition
Arkansas Children's Hospital
Little Rock, Arkansas

Michele Morath Gottschlich, PhD, RD, LD, CSP, CCRP
Clinical Research Investigator/Pediatric Nutrition
   Specialist
Shriners Hospital for Children
Adjunct Associate Professor
Department of Surgery
University of Cincinnati
Cincinnati, Ohio

Sharon Groh-Wargo, PhD, RD, LD
Professor of Pediatrics and Nutrition
Case Western Reserve University School of Medicine
Neonatal Nutritionist Department of Pediatrics
MetroHealth Medical Center
Cleveland, Ohio

Christine Hall, MS, RD, CSP, LDN
Metabolic Dietitian
UNC Health Care
Chapel Hill, North Carolina

Kerri Heckert, MS, RD, LDN
Clinical Dietitian - Eating Disorder Assessment
   and Treatment Program
Children's Hospital of Philadelphia
Philadelphia, Pennsylvania

Megan Horsley, RD, LD, CSP, CNSC
Clinical Registered Dietitian III
Cincinnati Children's Hospital and Medical Center
Cincinnati, Ohio

Kathryn L. Hunt RDN, CD
Clinical Pediatric Oncology Dietitian
Seattle Children's Hospital
Seattle, Washington

Susan Konek, MA, RDN, CSP, LD, FAND
Clinical Nutrition Management Consultant
Pediatric Nutrition Partners, LLC
Dayton, Ohio

Kristen Leavitt, RD, CSP, LD
Registered Dietitian II
Cincinnati Children's Hospital and Medical Center
Cincinnati, Ohio

Miryoung Lee, PhD, CPH
Associate Professor
Department of Epidemiology, Human Genetics,
   and Environmental Sciences
School of Public Health
The University of Texas Health and Science Center
   at Houston
Brownsville, Texas

Paula Charuhas Macris, MS, RD, CSO, FAND, CD
Nutrition Education Coordinator and Pediatric
   Nutrition Specialist
Seattle Cancer Care Alliance
Seattle, Washington

Maria Mascarenhas, MBBS
Department of GI, Hepatology, and Nutrition
Children's Hospital of Philadelphia
Philadelphia, Pennsylvania

Kasey M. Metz, MS, RD, LD
Pediatric Dietitian
Dayton Children's Hospital
Dayton, Ohio

Mary Mullens, MS, RD, LDN
Registered Dietitian/Nutritionist
Rush University Medical Center
Chicago, Illinois

Nancy Nevin-Folino, MEd, RD, CSP, LD, FADA
Neonatal Nutrition Specialist
Dayton Children's Hospital
Dayton, Ohio

Andrea Nepa, MS, RD
Clinical Dietitian
The Children's Hospital of Philadelphia
Philadelphia, Pennsylvania

Christine O'Connor, RD, CSR, LD
Renal Dietitian
Cincinnati Children's Hospital and Medical Center
Cincinnati, Ohio

Beth Ogata, MS, RDN, CSP
Nutritionist
Center on Human Development and Disability
University of Washington
Seattle, Washington

Laura Grande Padula, MS, RD, LDN
Clinical Dietitian III
Cystic Fibrosis Center
The Children's Hospital of Philadelphia
Philadelphia, Pennsylvania

Kristy Paley, MS, RD, LDN, CNSC
Duke University Hospital
Durham, North Carolina

Jennifer Panganiban, MD
Department of GI, Hepatology, and Nutrition
Children's Hospital of Philadelphia
Philadelphia, Pennsylvania

Nicolle Quinn, MS, RD, LDN
Clinical Nutrition Specialist
Boston Children's Hospital
Boston, Massachusetts

Megan Robinson, MS, RD, CDE, CSSD, LDN
Advanced Practice Dietitian
The Children's Hospital of Philadelphia
Philadelphia, Pennsylvania

Alison Ruffin, RD, LD, CNSC
Manager, Clinical Nutrition
Dayton Children's Hospital
Dayton, Ohio

Melanie Savoca, MS, RD, CNSC, LDN
Pediatric Clinical Dietitian
Children's Hospital of Philadelphia
Philadelphia, Pennsylvania

Britt Schuman-Humbert, RD, CSP, CSSD, LDN, CNSC
Clinical Dietitian
University of North Carolina Healthcare
Chapel Hill, North Carolina

Christina A. Sunderman, MS, RD, LD, CNSC
Lead Clinical Dietitian
Shriner's Hospital for Children
Cincinnati, Ohio

Ama Tettey-Fio, MD
Cooper Medical School of Rowan University
Camden, New Jersey

Susan Tulley, MPH, RD, CSP, LD
Registered Dietitian II
Nephrology
Cincinnati Children's Hospital and Medical Center
Cincinnati, Ohio

Holly A. Van Poots, RDN, CSP, FAND
Be Balanced Nutrition, LLC
Harrisonburg, VA

Sarah Vermilyea, MS, RD, CSP, LD, CNSC
Registered Dietitian
St. Joseph Home
Cincinnati, Ohio

Jacqueline J. Wessel, RD, MEd, CNSC, CDE, CSP
Neonatal Nutritionist
Cincinnati Children's Hospital and Medical Center
Cincinnati, Ohio

Rebecca Wilhelm, MS, RD, LD, CNSC
Clinical Dietitian II
Division of Gastroenterology, Hepatology
    and Nutrition
Cincinnati Children's Hospital and Medical Center
Cincinnati, Ohio

Reviewers

Jennifer Colson, RD
Professor
Department of Human Sciences
Middle Tennessee University
Murfreesboro, Tennessee

Matthew Edwards, RD, CSP, CD
Clinical Dietitian Specialist
Children's Hospital of Wisconsin
Milwaukee, Wisconsin

Nicole Fabus, RD, CD, CNSC
Clinical Dietitian Specialist
Children's Hospital of Wisconsin
Milwaukee, Wisconsin

Heather Fortin, RD, CD, CDE
Clinical Dietitian Specialist
Children's Hospital of Wisconsin
Milwaukee, Wisconsin

Melissa Froh, MS, RD, CD, CNSC
Clinical Dietitian Specialist
Children's Hospital of Wisconsin
Milwaukee, Wisconsin

Tracy L. Gidden, MSN, APRN, PPCNP-BC, CNE
Senior Lecturer
College of Nursing
Kent State University
Kent, Ohio

Becky Heisler, RD, CNSC, CD
Clinical Dietitian Specialist
Children's Hospital of Wisconsin
Milwaukee, Wisconsin

Linda Heller, MS, RD, CSP, CLC, FAND
Manager of Clinical Nutrition and Lactation
Children's Hospital Los Angeles
Los Angeles, California

Kyndal Hettich, RD, CSP, CD
Clinical Dietitian Specialist
Children's Hospital of Wisconsin
Milwaukee, Wisconsin

Kristine Jordan, PhD, MPH, RD
Director, Coordinated Master's Program in Nutrition
    and Dietetics
Associate Professor
Department of Nutrition and Integrative Physiology
University of Utah
Salt Lake City, Utah

Catherine A. Karls, MS, RD, CD, CNSC
Advanced Practice Dietitian
Children's Hospital of Wisconsin
Milwaukee, Wisconsin

Haley Lynn, MS, RD, CD
Clinical Dietitian
Children's Hospital of Wisconsin
Milwaukee, Wisconsin

Lauren Matschull, MBA, RD, CD, CNSC
Clinical Dietitian Specialist
Children's Hospital of Wisconsin
Milwaukee, Wisconsin

Julie Metos, PhD, MPH, RDN
Associate Chair and Assistant Professor
Department of Nutrition and Integrative Physiology
University of Utah
Salt Lake City, Utah

Malki Miller, MS, RD, CNSC
Adjunct Lecturer
Department of Health and Nutrition Sciences
Brooklyn College
Brooklyn, New York

Paul Moore, MBA, MS, RD, CSSD, LDN, CSCS, NSCA-CPT
Lecturer and Dietetic Internship Director
Department of Nutrition and Health Care
    Management
Appalachian State University
Boone, North Carolina

Anita M. Nucci, PhD, RD, LD
Associate Professor
Department of Nutrition
Georgia State University
Atlanta, Georgia

Elizabeth Polzin, MBA, RD, CD, CNSC
Clinical Dietitian Specialist
Children's Hospital of Wisconsin
Milwaukee, Wisconsin

Kimberly Powell, PhD, RD, LDN
Assistant Professor
Department of Human Sciences
North Carolina Central University
Cary, North Carolina

Ashleigh Spitza, RD, CD
Clinical Dietitian Specialist
Children's Hospital of Wisconsin
Milwaukee, Wisconsin

Karen Steitz, MS, RD, CSP, LD
Adjunct Faculty
Doisy College of Health Sciences
Saint Louis University
Frontenac, Missouri

Elizabeth Tenison, MS, RD, CSP, CNSC
Director, Dietetic Internship Program
Department of Nutrition
University of Saint Joseph
West Hartford, Connecticut

Jennifer L. Thorpe, MBA, RD, LDN, FAND
Director of Clinical Nutrition
Department of Clinical Nutrition
The Children's Hospital of Philadelphia
Philadelphia, Pennsylvania

Julie Thurlow, DrPH, RD, CD
Lecturer
Department of Nutritional Sciences
University of Wisconsin—Madison
Madison, Wisconsin

Megan Van Hoorn, MS, RD, CD, CNSC
Clinical Dietitian Specialist
Children's Hospital of Wisconsin
Milwaukee, Wisconsin

Bridget Wardley, MS, RDN, CSP
Adjunct Faculty
Department of Nutrition and Food Studies
New York University
New York City, New York

L. Hope Wills, MA, RD, CSP, IBCLC
Program Director, USC UCEDD Dietitian Internship
Clinical Dietitian
Children's Hospital Los Angeles
Los Angeles, California

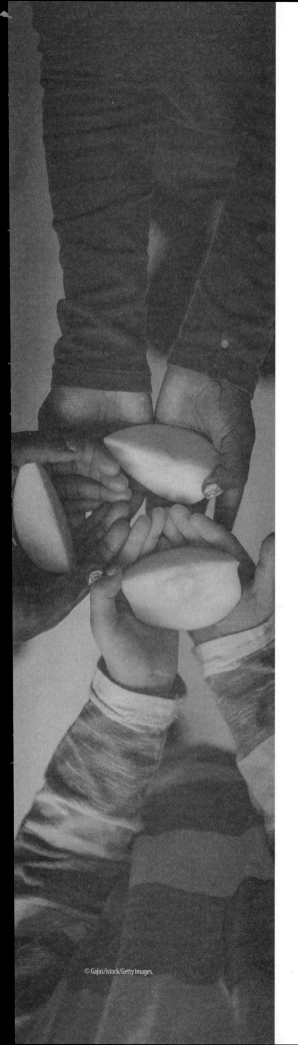

SECTION I

Assessment of Nutritional Status

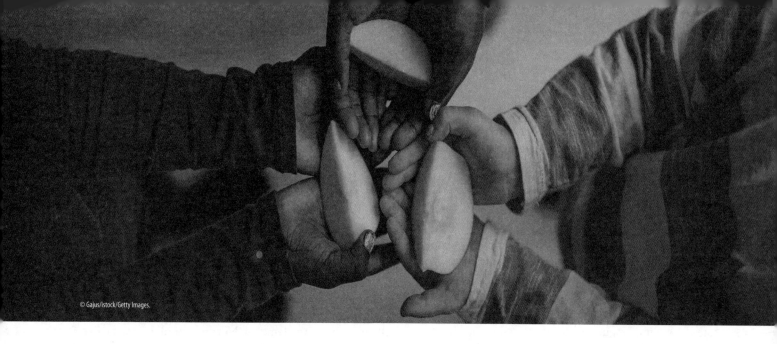

© Gajus/istock/Getty Images.

CHAPTER 1

Nutritional Assessment

Patricia J. Becker and Sarah Vermilyea

LEARNING OBJECTIVES

- Identify the key components of a pediatric nutrition assessment.
- Describe the elements of each component.

▶ Introduction

The purpose of nutrition assessment is to gather, verify, and assess information about a child that will help identify nutrition-related problems, their causes and their impact on the child's growth and development. Nutrition assessment is not a single act but an ongoing process of data collection and evaluation in comparison to nutrition criteria.[1]

A nutrition assessment is the first step in the **Nutrition Care Process** (NCP). And while a nutrition screen is performed before the assessment, it is not part of the NCP. However, it remains a critical component and the step that starts the process. The purpose of the nutrition screen is to identify children who may benefit from nutrition assessment by a **registered dietitian/nutritionist** (RDN). The nutrition screen is commonly performed by a healthcare provider other than the RDN. If the screen identifies the child to be

at risk for a nutrition-related problem, the child is referred to the RDN and a consult for nutrition assessment is initiated.[2,3]

▶ Screening

The completion of in-depth nutrition assessments on all children served by a healthcare system is neither practical nor essential for providing quality nutrition care. Well-designed nutrition screening performed by trained personnel is effective for identifying children who are at nutrition risk and, therefore, may require a nutrition assessment.[4,5] Health risk screens that help identify nutrition-related problems and nutrition referral in the community are one type of nutrition screen.[6] This can include referral for such things as hypercholesterolemia, declining renal function, or prediabetes, which are discovered at routine medical visits.[7–9]

Screening for risk of malnutrition in the acute care setting, which requires a systemic approach by the healthcare team and the use of pediatric nutrition screening tools, is a second type of nutrition screening process. The information gathered for screening includes nutrition care indicators routinely collected during scheduled healthcare appointments or upon admission to a healthcare facility.

Nutrition screening has been defined as "the process of identifying patients, clients, or groups who may have a nutrition diagnosis and benefit from nutrition assessment and intervention by a registered dietitian/nutritionist," and/or "as a process to identify an individual who is malnourished or is at risk for malnutrition to determine if a detailed nutrition assessment is indicated."[10,11] Simply put, nutrition screening is the step that initiates the nutrition care process and the nutrition assessment, the diagnosis of a nutrition problem, and the nutrition intervention.

Nutrition screening should be quick, simple, population sensitive and specific, reliable among those who perform the screen and done for all patients.[12] There are a number of pediatric screening tools for identifying risk of malnutrition that have been devised and validated but are not in general use. These include the **Nutrition Risk Score** (NRS), the **Pediatric Nutrition Risk Score** (PNRS), the **Screening Tool for the Assessment of Malnutrition in Pediatrics** (STAMP), the **Pediatric Yorkhill Malnutrition Score** (PYMS), the **Screening Tool for Risk of Impaired Nutritional Status and Growth** (STRONGkids), and the **Pediatric Nutrition Screening Tool** (PNST). These validated tools utilize a combination of obtained anthropometric measurements and questions answered by caregivers related to food intake and weight, recent growth, and weight changes.[13,14] An example of the tools is available in **TABLE 1.1**. Additional information on pediatric nutrition screening is available through the Academy of Nutrition and Dietetics Evidence Analysis Library at https://www.andeal.org.

Subjective Global Assessment

A **Subjective Global Assessment** (SGA) collects information provided by the patient/family about the patient's

TABLE 1.1 STRONGkids		
Screening Risk of Malnutrition: One Time Per Week	**Score**	**Points**
Is there illness with risk for malnutrition (see list*) or pending major surgery?	**No = 0**	**Yes = 2**
Is the child in poor nutrition status based on clinical observation?	**No = 0**	**Yes = 1**

Does the child have:
  excessive loose stool (>5/day) vomiting (>3/day)?
  reduced food intake for >3 days?
  preexisting nutrition intervention?
  unable to consume adequate nutrient intake due to pain?
	No = 0	**Yes = 1**

Has there been loss of weight or failure to gain weight in a child under 2 years in the last few months?	**No = 0**	**Yes = 1**
Risk for Malnutrition and Need for Intervention		
Consult pediatric registered dietitian/nutritionist for nutrition assessment, nutrition diagnosis, and nutrition intervention.	4–5 points	High Risk
Rescreen at weekly intervals. Consult pediatric registered dietitian/nutritionist for determination of nutrition risk if there is an increase in risk screen score.	1–3 points	Moderate Risk
No intervention needed. Rescreen at admission day 14 or per policy.	0 points	Low Risk

* Anorexia nervosa - burns - bronchopulmonary dysplasia - celiac disease - cystic fibrosis - history of preterm birth - congenital heart defect - IBD - liver failure - short gut - critical illness - trauma - CKD - cancer

Data from Hulst J, Zwart H, Hop W, Joosten K. Dutch national survey to test STRONGkids nutritional risk screening tool in hospitalized children. *Clin Nutr*. 2010. 29(1):106–111.[14]

nutritional status and observations made by the clinician, and evaluates this information using clinical judgment. The adult SGA method has been modified and validated for use in some pediatric populations and is called the **Pediatric Subjective Global Nutritional Assessment** (SGNA).[15-20]

Objective measures of nutritional status may be inaccurate or inadequate in the formulation of a complete nutrition assessment.[16] Some example scenarios include: specific nutrition related lab values may be skewed by illness; measurement of height in a child without lower extremities; or lack of access to appropriate weighing scales.

SGNA is designed to be used as part of an initial nutrition assessment.[16] It is not a screen to decide if RDN intervention is needed, nor is it responsive enough to be used as a reassessment tool in most cases.[16] It encompasses ten assessment areas as illustrated in **FIGURE 1.1** (later in this chapter) and includes a structured questionnaire, medical history review, and nutrition–focused physical assessment.[16] An overall normal/moderate/or severe malnutrition rating is assigned to the child which then helps guide nutrition interventions.

Nutritional Assessment

As part of the nutrition assessment the pediatric RDN determines if a nutrition problem or diagnosis exists and if nutrition intervention is indicated. The pediatric RDN would also determine the need for additional data. Data sources for nutritional assessment can include two sources:

- The health record: biochemical data, medical/surgical history, vital signs, medical procedures/consultations, medication
- Data created during the assessment: client interview, nutrient intake data, anthropometric measurements, physical assessment

For children, additional information including birth history, feeding history, developmental history, and achievement of developmental milestones as well as social and family environment may be essential in the determination of the nutrition diagnosis.

Medical History

Approximately 10–15% of children in the United States have special healthcare needs and are defined as "having or being at risk for congenital or acquired conditions that affect physical and/or cognitive growth and development."[21] These children may be at risk for associated nutrition problems. There are many conditions in children that affect nutritional status that are part of a child's medical history. **TABLE 1.2** lists some of the conditions that affect the nutritional status of children.[22]

Feeding History

For children under the age of two who have been found to be at nutritional risk, a review of their feeding history may be pertinent. Identifying if they were bottle or breast fed, what infant formulas were provided, when complementary foods were introduced and how that transition went, and how new food textures are tolerated can be valuable in assessing food intake and nutrient impact on growth.

For older children, a review of feeding behavior as part of the nutrition history should be obtained. When asked, more than 50% of parents report that at least one of their children eats poorly, suggesting the 20–30% of children have some level of feeding difficulty.[23] Of the 20–30% of children identified by parents as having feeding difficulty, only 3–10% of children have true feeding disorders; however 40–70% of children with complex medical histories meet the criteria for a feeding disorder.[24-27] **TABLE 1.3** provides information on signs and symptoms of feeding difficulties in children.

Anthropometric Data

Age-appropriate growth is the hallmark of adequate nutrition. Although other factors play a role in growth, nutrition is the major determinant. Anthropometric data include obtaining weight and measuring length/height, head and mid-upper arm circumference. With these data, several analysis calculations can be computed including weight for length in children ages 0 to 24 months, **body mass index** (BMI) in children over the age of 2 years, and weight gain velocity assessment in children up to 59 months of age.

Weight, Length, Height, and Head Circumference

Monitoring growth by measuring weight, length/height, and head circumference in children three years of age or less is a routine practice in pediatrics and is essential for assessing nutritional status.

It is also essential that measurements are done accurately and at regular intervals. The **World Health Organization** (WHO) and the **Centers for Disease Control and Prevention** (CDC) are sources for training information for techniques for accurate measurement of children. The CDC Division of Nutrition, Physical Activity and Obesity has guidelines for "Measuring Children's Height and Weight Accurately at Home".[28] The WHO child growth standards include a series of training modules including module B: measuring growth.[29]

These guides instruct healthcare providers in methods for the accurate measurement of children and

PEDIATRIC SGNA RATING FORM

Consider severity and duration of changes, as well as recent progression when rating each item.

NUTRITION-FOCUSED MEDICAL HISTORY	SGNA SCORE		
	Normal	**Moderate**	**Severe**
Appropriateness of Current Height for Age (stunting) a) Height percentile: _____ □ ≥ 3rd centile □ just below 3rd centile □ far below 3rd centile			
b) Appropriate considering mid-parental height[a]?: □ yes □ no			
c) Serial growth[b]: □ following centiles □ moving upwards on centiles □ moving downwards on centiles (gradually or quickly)			
Appropriateness of Current Weight for Height (wasting) Ideal Body Weight = _____ kg Percent Ideal Body Weight: __ __ __ % □ >90% □ 75-90% □ <75%			
Unintentional Changes in Body Weight a) Serial weight[b]: □ following centiles □ crossed ≥ 1 centile upwards □ crossed ≥ 1 centile downwards			
b) Weight loss: □ < 5% usual body weight □ 5-10% usual body weight □ >10% usual body weight			
c) Change in past 2 weeks: □ no change □ increased □ decreased			
Adequacy of Dietary Intake a) Intake is: □ adequate □ inadequate - hypocaloric □ inadequate - starvation (ie, taking little of anything)			
b) Current intake versus usual: □ no change □ increased □ decreased			
c) Duration of change: □ < 2 weeks □ ≥ 2 weeks			
Gastrointestinal Symptoms a) □ no symptoms □ one or more symptoms; not daily □ some or all symptoms; daily			
b) Duration of symptoms: □ < 2 weeks □ ≥ 2 weeks			
Functional Capacity (nutritionally related) a) □ no impairment, energetic, able to perform age-appropriate activity □ restricted in physically strenuous activity, but able to perform play and/or school activities in a light or sedentary nature; less energy; tired more often □ little or no play or activities, confined to bed or chair > 50% of waking time; no energy; sleeps often			
b) Function in past 2 weeks: □ no change □ increased □ decreased			
Metabolic Stress of Disease □ no stress □ moderate stress □ severe stress			

[a]Mid-parental height: Girls: subtract 13 cm from the father's height and average with the mother's height. Boys: add 13 cm to the mother's height and average with the father's height. Thirteen cm is the average difference in height of women and men. For both girls and boys, 8.5 cm on either side of this calculated value (target height) represents the 3rd to 97th percentiles for anticipated adult height. (29)

[b]30% of healthy term infants cross one major percentile and 23% cross two major percentiles during the first 2 years of life, typically towards the 50th percentile rather than away from it. This is normal seeking of the growth channel.

FIGURE 1.1 Pediatric Subjective Global Nutritional Assessment (SGNA) rating form. (continued on next page)

PHYSICAL EXAM	SGNA SCORE		
	Normal	**Moderate**	**Severe**
Loss of subcutaneous fat ☐ no loss in most or all areas ☐ loss in some but not all areas ☐ severe loss in most or all areas			
Muscle Wasting ☐ no wasting in most or all areas ☐ wasting in some but not all areas ☐ severe wasting in most or all areas			
Edema (nutrition-related) ☐ no edema ☐ moderate ☐ severe			

GUIDELINES FOR AGGREGATING ITEMS INTO GLOBAL SCORE

In assigning an overall global score, consider all items in the context of each other. Give the most consideration to changes in weight gain and growth, intake, and physical signs of loss of fat or muscle mass. Use the other items to support or strengthen these ratings. Take recent changes in context with the patient's usual/chronic status. Was the patient starting off in a normal or nutritionally-compromised state?

Normal/Well nourished
This patient is growing and gaining weight normally, has a grossly adequate intake without gastrointestinal symptoms, shows no or few physical signs of wasting, and exhibits normal functional capacity. Normal ratings in most or all categories, or significant, sustained improvement from a questionable or moderately malnourished state. It is possible to rate a patient as well nourished in spite of some reductions in muscle mass, fat stores, weight and intake. This is based on recent improvement in signs that are mild and inconsistent.

Moderately malnourished
This patient has definite signs of a decrease in weight and/or growth, and intake and may or may not have signs of diminished fat stores, muscle mass and functional capacity. This patient is experiencing a downward trend, but started with normal nutritional status. Moderate ratings in most or all categories, with the potential to progress to a severely malnourished state.

Severely malnourished
This patient has progressive malnutrition with a downward trend in most or all categories. There are significant physical signs of malnutrition—loss of fat stores, muscle wasting, weight loss >10%—as well as decreased intake, excessive gastrointestinal losses and/or acute metabolic stress, and definite loss of functional capacity. Severe ratings in most or all categories with little or no sign of improvement.

	Normal	**Moderate**	**Severe**
OVERALL SGNA RANKING			

FIGURE 1.1 (continued)

the correct equipment to be used for obtaining those measurements. Once accurate measurements have been obtained, growth should be assessed against an established/accepted reference standard.

Weight, recumbent length for children under 24 months of age, height for children 2 years and older, and head circumference for children up to age three years are plotted on growth charts according to age for comparison with the growth of a reference population of healthy, normal infants/children. The recommendations for growth charts used in the United States are the CDC growth charts for children ages 2 to 19 years and the WHO growth charts for children ages zero to 24 months of age.

The WHO charts are available in percentile and z-score charts for ages zero to 59 months. The CDC charts are available in percentile chart, with z-score tables available for older children. Z-score calculations for older children are available through the website www.Peditools.org. In US pediatric medical practices, percentile charts are most commonly used. However, z-scores are a more accurate measure and method to assess and interpret growth in children.

Z-scores are better than percentiles for interpreting growth for children because z-scores, or standard deviation scores, are a mathematical calculation of the deviation from the norm/median/mean. The z-score scale is linear and, therefore, a fixed interval. The

TABLE 1.2 Conditions that Put Children at Nutritional Risk

	Growth			Diet			Medical	
	Under-weight	Over-weight	Short Stature	Low Energy Needs	High Energy Needs	Feeding Difficulty	Malnutrition	Medications that Impact Nutrition
Autism	✓					✓	✓	✓
Bronchopulmonary dysplasia	✓		✓		✓	✓	✓	✓
Cerebral palsy	✓	✓	✓	✓	✓	✓	✓	✓
Chronic kidney failure	✓	✓	✓	✓		✓	✓	✓
Cystic fibrosis	✓		✓		✓	✓	✓	✓
Down syndrome	✓	✓	✓	✓		✓		✓
Neonatal abstinence syndrome	✓	✓	✓	✓	✓	✓	✓	✓
Heart disease (congenital)	✓		✓		✓	✓	✓	✓
Eating disorders	✓		✓		✓	✓	✓	
Liver failure	✓		✓		✓	✓	✓	✓
Prader-Willi syndrome	✓	✓	✓	✓		✓	✓	
Premature birth	✓		✓		✓	✓	✓	✓
Seizure disorder			✓					✓
Short bowel syndrome	✓		✓		✓	✓	✓	✓
Irritable Bowel disease	✓	✓	✓	✓	✓	✓	✓	✓

Data from Kyle U, Shekerdemian L, Coss-Bu, J. Growth failure and nutrition considerations in chronic childhood wasting diseases. *NCP*. 2015;30(2):227–238.[22]

z-scores have the same fixed interval for height difference in centimeters or weight difference in kilograms for all children of the same age. This is not true for percentiles. Z-scores have the same statistical distribution around the mean/median at all ages, so that the results are comparable across age groups and indicators. For this reason, z-scores are used in research. The pediatric RDN should use z-scores for discussion with children and families because using z-scores allows for calculating a discrete number that can identify changes in growth in the short term and interpreting growth beyond the curves, outside the lines.

TABLE 1.3 Presenting Features of Feeding Difficulties

Signs & Symptoms	Medical Problems	Behavior Problems
Prolonged meal times	Dysphagia/difficulty chewing	Food fixation
Food refusal > one month	Aspiration	Force feeding
Disruptive/stressful mealtimes	Pain with eating	Abrupt cessation of feeding after triggered event
Lack of appropriate self-feeding	Vomiting/diarrhea	Anticipatory gagging
Need for distraction to allow for intake	Developmental delay/ low muscle tone	Self-induced gagging/vomiting
Prolonged bottle or breast feeding	Food allergy/intolerance/GERD	Growth failure
Failure to advance textures	Growth failure	Delayed introduction

Data from Kerzner B. Clinical investigation of feeding difficulty in young children: a practical approach. *Clin Peds.* 2009;48(9):960–965.[25]

Percentiles are intended to be stated as intervals such as when a plotted point falls between the fifth percentile and the tenth percentile. Although current electronic charting methods will provide a percentile number other than the interval, these numbers are not mathematically accurate.

Information from the WHO about z-scores can be helpful for RDNs, staff, and parents in understanding how a child's growth compares with the reference standard. The WHO training modules, which are available on the WHO website, describe how to plot growth on the z-score chart in clear language.

The following description from the WHO training module might be shared with families or staff to describe the use of z-scores:

Interpret plotted points for growth indicators: The curved lines printed on the growth charts will help interpret the plotted points that represent a child's growth status. The line labeled "0" on each chart represents the median, which is, generally speaking, the average. The other curved lines are the z-scores, which indicate distance from the average. The median and the z-score lines on each growth chart were derived from measurements of children in the WHO Multicentre Growth Reference Study who were fed and raised in environments that favored optimal growth.

Z-score lines on the growth charts are numbered positively (1, 2, 3) or negatively (1, 2, 3). Generally, a plotted point that is far from the median in either direction (for example, close to the 3 or -3 z-score line) may represent a growth problem, although other factors must be considered, such as the growth trend, the health condition of the child, and the height of the parents.

Identify growth problems from plotted points. Read points as follows:

A point between the z-score lines -2 and -3 is "below 2."

A point between the z-score lines 2 and 3 is "above 2."[29]

Mid-Upper Arm Circumference

Mid-Upper Arm Circumference (MUAC) is the circumference of the upper arm, measured at the midpoint between the tip of the shoulder and the tip of the elbow (olecranon process and the acromion). MUAC is used to assess nutritional status. It is a good predictor of mortality, and in many studies, MUAC predicted mortality in children better than any other anthropometric indicator. The MUAC measurement requires little equipment and is easy to perform even on the most debilitated individuals. Although it is important to train healthcare providers in how to take the measurement, the correct technique can be readily taught to minimally trained health workers and community-based volunteers.[30–32] The RDN may choose to measure the left or the right arm but must continue to measure that same arm on subsequent visits.

The Consensus Statement of the Academy of Nutrition and Dietetics/American Society of Parenteral and

Enteral Nutrition: Indicators Recommended for the Identification and Documentation of Pediatric Malnutrition (undernutrition) recommend the use of MUAC in the assessment of all ages of children.[33]

The major determinants of MUAC, arm muscle, and subcutaneous fat are both important determinants of survival in individuals with malnutrition. MUAC is less affected than weight or BMI by edema or ascites and is a more sensitive indication of fat and muscle loss than low body weight. It is also useful for assessing acute energy deficiency during starvation and it is relatively independent of height and body shape.[30-32] Growth Charts for MUAC in both percentile and z-scores are available from the WHO for children ages 0 to 59 months. Recent work by several groups has provided MUAC growth curves in both percentile and z-scores for children ages 5 to 18 years. Given that MUAC has been proven to be highly predictive for both morbidity and mortality, and performing better than BMI for age and weight for height z-scores, these tools are highly recommended to the pediatric RDN as an essential hands-on assessment tool.[34-36]

Weight for Length

Children who are under 24 months of age generally have a recumbent length measurement taken verses a standing height measurement. Therefore, the index used to determine body proportion is weight for length. The child's weight and length is then plotted on the WHO 2006 Weight for Length growth curve in order to determine the z-score/percentile, which is used to assess growth status.[37] BMI for age weight status categories, in children 2 to 19, are based on expert committee recommendations for the American Academy of Pediatrics and the Consensus Statement of the Academy of Nutrition and Dietetics/American Society for Parenteral and Enteral Nutrition for the identification of pediatric malnutrition (undernutrition).[33]

Body Mass Index

The most widely used index to evaluate adiposity and proportionality is the **body mass index** (BMI). The BMI, also known as the Quetelet Index,[38] is derived by dividing weight in kilograms by height in meters squared (wt/ht^2). For example, the BMI of a 14-year-old female who is 5′1″ (1.54 meters) and 110 pounds (50 kilograms.) is $50/(1.54)^2$ or 21 kg/m^2. BMI can also be calculated using pounds and inches by dividing the weight in pounds by the square of height in inches, multiplied by 703 ($lbs/in^2 \times 703$). In children, the calculated BMI is then plotted on the CDC 2000 BMI for age growth curve in order to determine the BMI for age z-score/percentile, which is used to assess growth status.[39] BMI for age weight status categories are based on expert committee recommendations from the American Academy of Pediatrics and the Consensus Statement of the Academy of Nutrition and Dietetics/American Society for Parenteral and Enteral Nutrition for the identification of pediatric malnutrition (undernutrition).[33] Z-scores and percentiles both describe weight status and growth in children. **TABLE 1.4** compares z-score and percentile ranges and nutritional status categories for children.

TABLE 1.4 Z-score/Percentile Ranges for Under and Over Weight

Weight Status Category	Z-Score Range	Percentile Range
Severe malnutrition	−3 or below	0.2%
Moderate malnutrition	−2 to −2.99	2%
Mild malnutrition	−1 to −1.99	10% − 2%
Normal range	0	50%
Overweight	+1.04	85%
Overweight	+1.64	95%
Obese	+2	98%
Obese	+3	>99%

Data from Becker P, Carney L, Corkins M, et al. Consensus Statement of the Academy of Nutrition and Dietetics/American Society for Parenteral and Enteral Nutrition: Indicators recommended for the identification and documentation of pediatric malnutrition (undernutrition). *J Acad Nutr Diet*. 2014;114(12):1988–1995.[33]

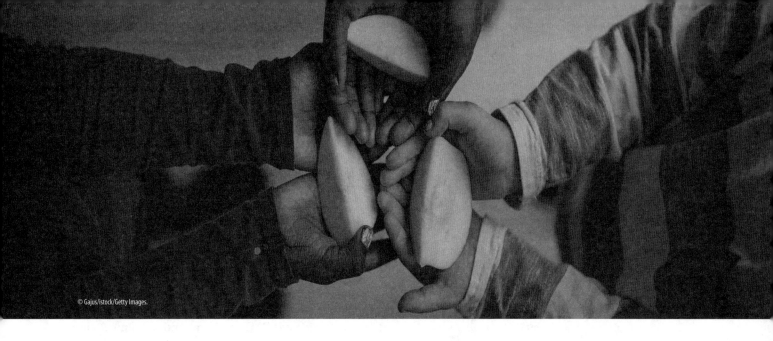

© Gajus/istock/Getty Images.

CHAPTER 2

Growth and Maturation

Stefan A. Czerwinski, Audrey C. Choh, and Miryoung Lee

LEARNING OBJECTIVES

- Discuss the processs of physical growth and maturation over the course of childhood.
- Explain the timing of changes that occur in various tissues of the body as children age.
- Evaluate the strengths and weaknesses of the different growth reference charts and apply this knowledge in the real world assessment and monitoring of childhood growth.

▶ Introduction

The objective of this chapter is to provide an overview of the process of physical growth and maturation. This chapter discusses the measurement of growth, the changes that occur over childhood in various tissues of the body, and the use of growth references for assessing and monitoring growth.

What is Growth?

Physical growth is the increase in body size that occurs as a newborn child becomes an adult. Adequate nutrition and exercise are necessary for optimal growth and maturation. Most normal, healthy children grow and mature with few, if any, problems. Proper evaluation of growth is important for assessing a child's health status. Growth assessment can provide useful information on a variety of conditions during childhood including overweight/ obesity, genetic disorders, social/environmental stress and/or malnutrition.[1-3] This chapter summarizes the processes of growth and maturation, as well as methods for their assessment. It is also illustrated by a case study and a brief discussion of abnormal growth.

How is Growth Measured?

Accurate and reliable measurements of body size provide a broad description of a child's growth status. The most useful measurements are recumbent length from birth to around 2 years of age, stature after age 2 years, head circumference from birth to age 3 years (see **FIGURES 2.1**, **2.2**, and **2.3**, respectively), and weight at every age.[4] Additionally, the indices of weight-for-length (for infants under 2 years of age) and **body mass index** (BMI) (for children older than 2 years, when

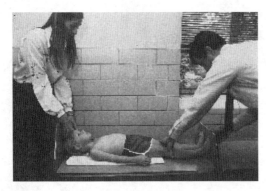

FIGURE 2.1 Measuring a Child's Recumbent Length

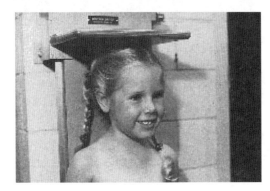

FIGURE 2.2 Measuring a Child's Stature

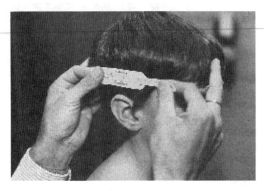

FIGURE 2.3 Measuring a Child's Head Circumference

stature measurements are possible) are useful indicators for determining whether a child is overweight. Descriptions and protocols for these measurements are available in various formats from the **Centers for Disease Control and Prevention** (CDC, http://www.cdc.gov/growthcharts)/**National Center for Health Statistics** (NCHS), and **World Health Organization** (WHO, http://www.who.int/childgrowth/training/en). These websites demonstrate standardized measurement techniques similar to those in the *Anthropometric Standardization Reference Manual.*[4]

Recumbent length and stature describe linear growth, while weight is a measure of the mass of all body tissues. Weight indexed for stature can describe levels of

overweight or obesity, but this measure of adiposity is most accurate when applied to groups rather than individuals. BMI is the most common stature-standardized weight indicator for overweight or obesity in children.[2,5] BMI is computed as weight (in kilograms) divided by stature (in meters squared), (kg/m²). Additionally, less commonly used measurements related to body fatness are limb and trunk circumferences, and skinfold thicknesses. Midarm circumference is an index of the underlying fat and muscle tissue; abdominal circumference is an indicator of abdominal fatness; while skinfolds measure subcutaneous adipose tissue thickness. Two common skinfold sites are the triceps on the back of the arm over the triceps muscle and the subscapular measured just below the scapula. Values at the high end of the distribution for BMI, midarm, and abdominal circumferences and triceps and subscapular skinfolds are positively correlated with increases in total and percent body fat in children.[6–8]

It is important to assess a child's level of fatness because obesity is the most prevalent health problem of childhood. More children are obese today than in the past, and there are greater levels of obesity than 10 to 20 years ago.[9,10] Today, a "large" child (i.e., one who exceeds expected stature and weight standards for a given age) is likely overweight or obese rather than just healthy. Childhood obesity is frequently linked with asthma, type 2 diabetes, fatty liver disease, muscular skeletal disease, dyslipidemia, hypertension, and increased risk for atherosclerosis and other measures of subclinical cardiovascular disease among children. The childhood incidence of overweight, obesity, and cardiovascular disease track with high predictability into adulthood, which increases concern for future health.[5,15,16] It is also important to measure bone mineral content (BMC) and bone mineral density (BMD) in children in order to identify those with low levels (due to low calcium, vitamin D, and/or protein intake) who are at risk for low bone mass and osteoporosis in adulthood.[17–19] Measuring a child's body composition can identify risk factors for some chronic adult diseases at an early point in time when treatment or intervention may be most effective.

Periods and Patterns of Growth

A child's growth pattern can be divided into four general periods. These periods overlap to some extent but can be defined according to growth processes that occur during each period. And they may differ somewhat from standard clinical definitions. These growth periods are:

■ Infancy (from birth to 2 years of age)
■ Preschool years (from about 3 to 6 years of age)
■ Middle childhood (from about 7 to 10 years of age)
■ Adolescence (from about 11 to 18 years of age)

Growth patterns and levels of maturation differ among children during these periods and overlap occurs because children's growth and maturation varies. A child's growth and size are related to his or her level of maturity and also reflect his or her genetic potential. At the same age, early-maturing children are taller and heavier than late-maturing children; tall parents tend to have taller children and short parents tend to have shorter children. Weight has a strong genetic component that explains the familial aspects of obesity, but epigenetic and environmental factors also influence the development of obesity.[20,21]

Infancy: Birth through 2 years

Infancy is distinguished by very rapid growth. Body size and dimensions increase faster than at any other time in postnatal life. Many healthy infants lose weight shortly after birth but regain their birth weight after about a week.[22] Most normal infants approximately double their birth weight in about 5 months and triple it by one year of age. During the first year of life, weight, on average, increases approximately 280%, while body length increases ~150%, and head circumference grows ~130%. Similar changes occur in the trunk, arms, and legs. Between one and two years of age, the average infant grows about 12 cm in length and gains about 2.5 kg in weight.[23,24]

An infant's head is disproportionately large compared with the dimensions of other body parts. At birth, its diameter exceeds that of the chest, and its length is about a quarter of the body's total length. Head circumference increases from an average of about 34 cm at birth to an average of about 45 cm at 1 year of age.[25] Measures of head circumference reflect brain growth, and the brain doubles its birth weight by 1 year of age.[26] Head circumference is a useful clinical measurement that can be plotted on growth charts to determine whether a child's brain is growing too fast or too slow. This information may indicate the presence of nutritional issues, microcepahaly, or other disorders.

Preschool Years: 3 to 6 Years of Age

During the preschool years, the rate of growth slows, and it stabilizes by about 4 to 5 years of age. Between the ages of 3 and 6 years, the average increase in stature and weight is about 6–9 centimeters/year and about 1.9–2.5 kilograms/year, respectively.[24,25] Head circumference remains an important measurement during the preschool years because the brain more than triples its birth weight by 3 years of age and is approximately 85% of its final adult size.[24] Sex differences in size and weight during the preschool years are small. Sex differences in body measures (i.e., sexual dimorphism) begin to occur in body composition, and girls accrue greater amounts of adipose tissue compared with boys at around 6 years of age.[27,28] This is also a critical period for the development of overweight and the onset of obesity in boys and girls, and the risk increases for subsequent obesity later in childhood and adulthood. During this period, overweight children should be monitored closely for increases in their BMI percentiles, patterns of dietary intake, and physical activity.[5,12,29,30]

Middle Childhood: 7 to 10 Years of Age

During middle childhood, children grow at a steady rate. The average child at age 7 years grows about 5 to 7 centimeters/year in stature and about 2 kilograms/year in weight, but the increase in weight is about 4 kilograms/year by age 10 years.[31] During this period, the increasing maturity of the average girl causes her to grow more per year in stature and weight than the average boy, which contributes, in part, to the larger size of girls at the start of adolescence. At 7 years of age, boys are, on average, heavier and taller than girls. By 10 years of age, the average girl is approximatly 0.30 centimeters taller and 0.3 kilograms heavier.[31] Middle childhood is again a critical period of increased risk for the development of subsequent obesity. Based on their BMI percentiles, overweight and obese children during this period are at an increased risk for being obese in adulthood.[5]

Adolescence: 11 to 18 Years of Age

Adolescence starts before puberty and spans the years until growth and maturation are mostly completed, which is around 16 to 18 years of age in girls and 18 to 21 years of age in boys.[32] This final increase in body size, shape, and weight transforms a child into an adult. Most girls have their pubescent growth spurts between 11 and 14 years of age, and, on average, are taller than boys who are the same age.[33] Typically, girls reach their final adult height around 2 years after first menstruation or menarche. Boys, on average, enter their pubescent growth spurts about 2 years after girls, so they have an additional 2 years of prepubertal growth. Additionally, the pubescent growth spurt lasts longer in boys than girls, and the associated amount of growth is larger in boys.[34,35] The average peak height velocity (i.e., the maximum rate of growth in stature during the growth spurt) in boys is estimated to be about 9.5–10.3 centimeters/year with an average age at peak height velocity, while in girls the maximum velocity is about 7.9–8.3 centimeters/year.[24,34–36] These sex differences result in men having a larger average body size than women. During adolescence, girls add more body fat than boys, but boys develop considerably more skeletal muscle tissue. These result in the sex difference in adult body size and shape and, to a large extent, the increased muscle mass of the average boy.[37]

Assessing Growth Status

Recumbent length, stature, and weight along with head circumference and BMI are the most common terms used to describe a child's growth status. These measures should be collected at regular intervals and plotted on growth charts.[31] In the first three years of life, growth assessment should be conducted at well-child visits (e.g, at 2-, 4-, 6- and 9-month visits) and afterwards at annual physical examinations. Growth charts present an assessment or comparison of the stature or length, weight, head circumference, and BMI of an infant, child, or adolescent with the percentile distribution of a reference population of other children at the same ages. The CDC/NCHS and the WHO each produce growth charts, both of which are recommended for use with US children.[31,38,39] Recently; however, the CDC recommended that healthcare practitioners use the WHO growth standard charts for assessing US children from birth to 2 years of age, for reasons described later in this chapter.[39] Copies of these charts can be downloaded from the CDC (https://www.cdc.gov/growthcharts/index.htm) and WHO (http://www.who.int/childgrowth) websites.

CDC 2000 Growth Charts

In 2000, the CDC/NCHS revised the 1977 US growth charts.[31,40] This revision combined national data from infants and children in the 1977 NCHS charts[40] with additional data from the **National Health and Nutrition Examination Survey** (NHANES) II and III for a sample of over 64,000 US children measured between 1960 and 1994. These charts are for infants and children from birth to 36 months of age and for children from 2 to 20 years of age.[41] The data represented on these revised charts include a greater proportion of non-Hispanic black and Hispanic children than the earlier 1977 national charts. The infants and children in this revised sample had feeding patterns common in the United States at the time the data were collected, and approximately 25% reportedly received some breastfeeding. The 2- to 20-year charts do not include any body weight data from the NHANES III conducted from 1988 to 1994 because the obesity epidemic affecting the United States' (and the rest of the world's) pediatric population was already evident in these data. Using these data would have resulted in spuriously higher weights of children in this reference sample. At this time, the first BMI-for-age charts were also released and replaced the previous weight-for-stature charts used in the 1977 growth charts.

WHO Growth Charts

WHO Growth Standards for 0 to 2 Years Old and 2 to 5 Years Old Scientists in the Department of Nutrition for Health and Development at the WHO and their international collaborators[25,38] developed a new set of growth charts in 2006 based on longitudinal and cross-sectional data from infants and children from ages 0 to 60 months who were observed between 1997 and 2003 as part of the WHO **Multicentre Growth Reference Study** (MGRS). The healthy infants and children used to construct these WHO child growth standards were recruited from non-smoking families in urban, middle-class communities in Brazil, Ghana, Oman, Norway, India, and the United States (California). The more than 800 infants in the longitudinal sample were enrolled at birth and observed in their homes at 1, 2, 4, and 6 weeks, then monthly until 12 months, and then bimonthly until 24 months. These infants were either exclusively or predominantly breastfed for the first 3 to 4 months of life with complete weaning occurring after their first birthday. For these reasons, these data serve as a "growth standard" because they are based on healthy children living under excellent environmental conditions that favor optimal growth and achievement of one's genetic potential in growth. The WHO charts are divided into two sets; one for infants from birth to 24 months of age (https://www.cdc.gov/growthcharts/who_charts.htm), and the second for children from 2 to 5 years of age.[25] The cross-sectional sample of almost 7000 children for the 2- to 5-year-old charts was drawn from similar urban middle-class communities in the six countries mentioned. These children reportedly received some breastfeeding for at least 3 months. The infants and children in the longitudinal and cross-sectional groups comprised samples of convenience within their geographic locations.

WHO Growth Reference for 5 to 19 Years Old In 2007, the WHO developed an additional set of growth charts for children and adolescents between the ages of 5 and 19 years.[42] These WHO charts use a combination of data from the cross-sectional WHO 2- to 5-year-old growth charts[25] and data for US children from 2 to 19 years of age from the 1977 NCHS US growth charts.[40] These charts are considered a growth reference (as opposed to a growth standard) and represent "healthy" weights and BMI values. Data from children who were directly part of the obesity epidemic were specifically excluded from the reference sample.

Using the CDC or the WHO Growth Charts

The CDC and WHO growth charts were created by using large samples of children at all ages, and the data were statistically smoothed to minimize age-to-age variations,[43] even though these charts are designed to be used clinically for a single infant or child. The primary clinical utility of growth charts is to help identify an infant or a child who is not growing normally (i.e., whose age- and sex-standardized percentile value for head circumference, recumbent length, weight, stature, or BMI indicates some possible clinical concern or health risk). To assist in screening for obesity and other growth disorders, the CDC and WHO charts are available at their respective websites. The standard set for both has percentile lines on all charts from the 5th to the 95th percentiles. The other set has percentile lines on all charts from the 3rd to the 97th percentiles, which improves discrimination of children at the extremes of the distributions for head circumference, recumbent length, weight, height, and BMI. The WHO infant and child growth charts are also available in different age groupings, resulting in differing widths between the lines from the 3rd to the 97th percentiles. This also facilitates the plotting of children at different ages or with possible growth disorders, in order to provide a clearer clinical interpretation.

Plotting a child's growth values on either the CDC or WHO growth chart indicates that at a particular time and age, the child has a normal value (between the 15th and 85th percentiles), which represents 70% of the population. It can also indicate that additional information is needed to determine the validity of a possibly unusual value (below the 15th or above the 85th percentiles), which represents the remaining 30% of the population who are either above or below these percentiles. Additional health information is needed to determine the reason for a child's unusual percentile value location. For example, a child whose height is above the 85th or below the 15th percentile may have very tall or short parents, respectively, or may have a clinical growth deficiency or hormonal abnormality. The WHO charts are also available as z-score charts, where zero represents the median and a positive or negative z-score is one standard deviation (SD) above or below the median. These charts may not be readily understandable to parents but are of great utility for clinical assessment and research purposes compared with the percentile charts.

BMI Growth Charts

To help address the current pediatric obesity epidemic, the CDC and WHO growth charts from 2 to 20 years of age now contain charts to plot a child's BMI percentile or standardized score (z-score), two useful, recommended indices of overweight and obesity. The CDC classifies overweight in children as a BMI for age between the 85th and 95th percentile and obesity as greater than the 95th percentile. The WHO BMI charts are like the CDC charts, but the WHO defines overweight and obesity separately for children under 5 years of age and above 5 years. For children who are under 5 years of age, overweight is defined as weight-for-stature between 2 SD (i.e., z-score) and less than 3 SD above the age- and sex-specific median, while obesity is weight-for-stature greater than or equal to 3 SD above the median. For children between the ages of 5 and 19 years, overweight in children is defined as a BMI for age greater than or equal to 1 SD above the age- and sex-specific median in the WHO reference and obesity is defined as greater than or equal to 2 SD above the age- and sex-specific median.

Race/Ethnicity

There are growth and maturational differences among black, white, and Mexican American children, but mostly these differences, on average, are small.[41] There are also small differences in the growth and maturation of healthy Chinese American, Japanese American, and other racial or ethnic American children when compared with white, black, and Mexican American children represented in the current CDC growth charts. These differences are also the case for the WHO growth charts.[44,45] Similar race/ethnicity differences are reported by clinicians in other countries who also use the CDC and WHO charts. Despite these differences, the CDC indicates that one set of growth charts should be used for

---

🔍 CASE STUDY

Demonstrating the Use of the CDC Growth Charts

In this example, a boy is observed for a regular checkup at 10, 11, and 12 years of age. At each visit, his weight and stature are measured and plotted on the CDC growth chart (**FIGURE 2.4**). His weight at 10 years was 37 kilograms, 45 kilograms at age 11, and 54 kilograms at age 12. His stature was 143 centimeters at 10 years, 150 centimeters at 11 years, and 156 centimeters at 12 years. Plotting these values on his growth chart indicates that this boy had a weight at the 75th percentile at 10 years of age, however, his weight progressed to the 90th percentile by 12 years of age. His stature was at the 75th percentile at 10 years of age also, and it has risen slightly above the 75th percentile at 11 and 12 years of age. Based on these data, it is reasonable to assume that this boy, whose weight and stature were within normal values at age 10 years, is possibly entering his adolescent growth spurt early. However, no corresponding increase in stature accompanies his increase in weight, which limits this assumption.

To clarify these data, the boy's BMI was calculated and plotted on the CDC BMI growth chart (**FIGURE 2.5**). At age 10 years, his BMI of 18.1 kg/m² was at the 75th percentile, which would be normal, but by age 12, his BMI had increased to 22.2 kg/m² at the 90th percentile. The additional BMI plotted data lend support to the reasonable possibility that this

(continues)

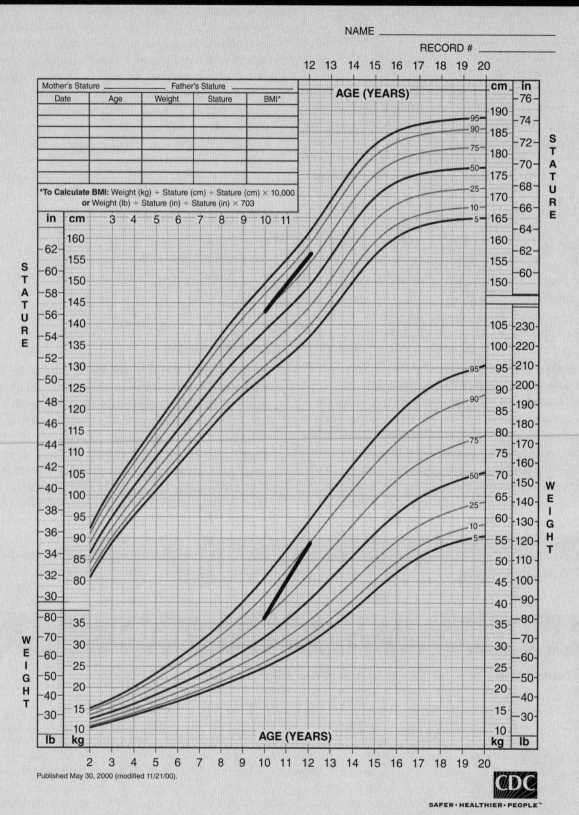

FIGURE 2.4 CDC Growth Chart for Boys

Data from Developed by the National Center for Health Statistics in collaboration with the National Center for Chronic Disease Prevention and Health Promotion (2000). Available at: http://www.cdc.gov/growthcharts.

NAME _____

RECORD # _____

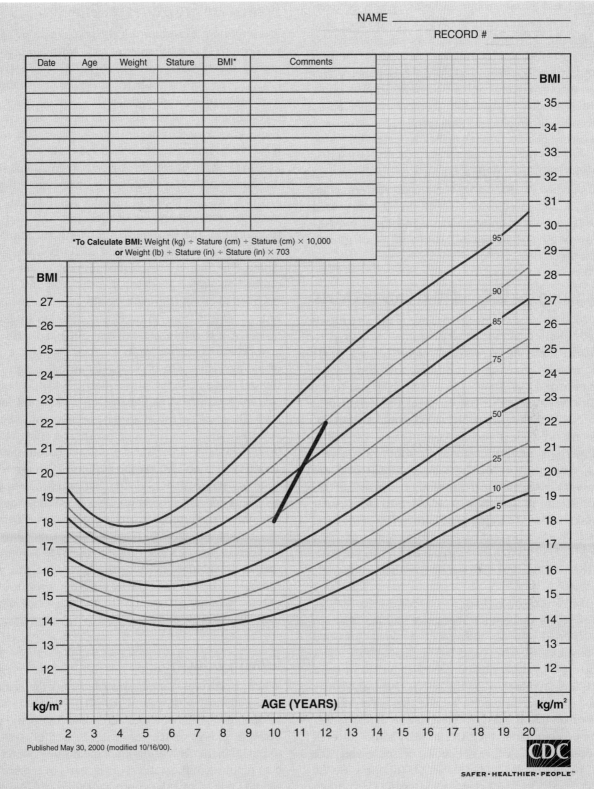

Date	Age	Weight	Stature	BMI*	Comments

*To Calculate BMI: Weight (kg) ÷ Stature (cm) ÷ Stature (cm) × 10,000
or Weight (lb) ÷ Stature (in) ÷ Stature (in) × 703

Published May 30, 2000 (modified 10/16/00).

SAFER·HEALTHIER·PEOPLE™

FIGURE 2.5 CDC BMI Chart for Boys

boy has progressed from a normal weight to an overweight category either based on the CDC criteria or on the WHO category (> 1 SD above the median). This change from a normal weight to overweight places this boy by 12 years of age at risk for obesity in adolescence and later in adulthood. Dietary intervention along with increased physical activity should be considered as possible treatments after further health information is obtained.

all racial and ethnic groups as the differences between groups are likely due more to environmental rather than true genetic differences (https://www.cdc.gov/nccdphp /dnpao/growthcharts/training/overview/page4.html).

Additionally, when a child reaches puberty and progresses through his or her adolescent growth spurt, the individuality of that child creates large percentile differences during these adolescent years compared with earlier positions that usually dissipate with maturity. The percentile position on the growth chart of that infant or child is, in part, a function of the differences in his or her genetic background and environmental exposure compared with that of the children used to construct these growth charts, and these individual disparities occur regardless of the set of growth charts used.

Comparing the CDC and WHO Growth Charts

The 2000 CDC growth charts have flaws (as do all growth charts). Because the combined data used to construct these charts were not collected in a single study over a defined period of time, the changes that have occurred over time, which have given rise to the obesity epidemic, limit the utility of the weight data from many of the earlier NHANES samples. Further, there are differences and improvements in the statistical methods used to create and smooth the percentiles.[41] The majority of the cross-sectional data are from very large national probability samples of US children, and these data were adjusted to reflect their complex national sampling structure. The 2000 CDC growth charts represent national data from the largest sample of US children ever assembled for this purpose, and they are the best national data of their kind available today.

The WHO growth charts reflect the growth of breastfed infants for the first few months of life, and there are well-reported growth differences between breastfed and formula-fed infants and their potential subsequent health effects.[25,38] After infancy, the diet and nutrition of the children represented on the WHO charts, which may be above average in quality because they were selected from urban middle class families, may be similar to that of the US children on the CDC growth charts. However, this information is either not known or unavailable. The CDC recommends that healthcare practitioners use the WHO growth standard charts for assessing US children from birth to 2 years of age, and use CDC growth charts for US children age 2 years and above.[39] This recommendation is due to several methodological advantages of the newer WHO standard from birth to 2 years. These advantages include important aspects of sampling and focuses on evaluating children against a reference reflective of optimal conditions (ie., non-smoking, breastfed, and access to healthcare).

Premature Growth/Fetal Growth

It is important to account for the gestational age of premature infants or those small at birth when plotting their growth on the current WHO or CDC/NCHS growth charts.[46] The amount of prematurity can be subtracted from an infant's chronologic age (e.g., for an infant with a gestational age of 28 weeks, there is a correction of 12 weeks or 3 months of chronological age). This adjustment for prematurity is utilized for evaluating growth over the first 2 years of life. A recent international study, the Intergrowth-21st Study (http://www.intergrowth21 .org.uk), was conducted to produce new fetal and prematurity growth charts for all children.[47] This study was sponsored by the University of Oxford and the WHO with funding from the Bill and Melinda Gates Foundation. The Intergrowth-21st Study was a multicenter, multiethnic project modeled after the WHO-MGRS and designed to examine growth, health, nutrition, and neurodevelopment from <14weeks of gestation to 2 years of age. It was conducted between 2009 and 2014 with a worldwide sampling from 8 urban geographic areas including: Pelotas, Brazil; Shunyi County, Beijing, China; Central Nagpur, India; Turin, Italy; Parklands Suburb, Nairobi, Kenya; Muscat, Oman; Oxford, UK; and Seattle, USA. The results of this study have been recently released and are available on the Intergrowth-21st Study website (http://www.intergrowth21.org.uk). The website includes a variety of tools and resources (https://intergrowth21 .tghn.org/standards-tools/) for practioners and researchers. These scientifically robust clinical tools may be used to monitor and evaluate maternal and fetal wellbeing as well as infant health and nutrition at an individual and population level.[48] More recently, the WHO published new multinational fetal growth charts. The data were collected as part of the WHO-MGRS and provide longitudinal ultrasound measures for a variety of biometrics including estimated fetal weight.[49]

Growth Velocity

When growth is measured at repeated visits, the change in a measurement or the rate of growth per unit of time can be quantified. This provides additional information; for example, growth velocity can describe a child's response to nutritional intervention. Increment growth reference data supplement the status growth charts by indicating if a child's rate of growth is normal or unusual. The WHO has developed increment (or rate) charts with percentiles reflecting the tempo of growth for children between 1 and 5 years of age using the longitudinal data from the breastfed infants in the WHO-MGRS (http://www.who .int/childgrowth/standards/en/). There have been similar increment charts for US children[50,51], but these are almost 30 years old. Recently, new incremental charts for BMI have been published[29] using data from mostly white children from the Fels Longitudinal Study.[52] These incremental charts provide reference values for changes in BMI over 6-month and 1-year intervals.[29] Generally, incremental charts aid in the short-term growth assessment in children and may also be useful in monitoring the effectiveness of nutritional therapy or interventions.

▶ Maturation

The central nervous system integrates the activities of the endocrine system, coordinating both growth and sexual maturation. Before puberty, the central nervous system inhibits hormone production, but this inhibition decreases near puberty when the sex hormones reach adult concentrations. Endocrine and adrenal androgens influence growth, sexual maturation, and the development of secondary sex characteristics. The reproductive system matures at puberty, making sexual reproduction possible. Puberty is identified in girls by the onset of menarche, but there is no similar marker in boys. The ages of individual children at the onset and completion of growth and sexual maturation are highly variable.

The progression of sexual maturation is assessed using Tanner stages[34,35] as indicators of the development of breasts in girls, genitals in boys, and pubic hair in each sex. Breast buds in girls (Tanner stage B-2) and genital enlargement in boys (Tanner stage G-2) indicate the onset of sexual maturation, which is then followed by the appearance of pubic hair (Tanner stage PH-2) in both sexes. In girls, the 25th to 75th percentiles for the age at onset of sexual maturation, Tanner stage B-2, range from 8.5 to 10.5 years in non-Hispanic blacks, 8.6 to 11.2 years in Mexican Americans, and 9.5 to 11 years for non-Hispanic whites.[53] The 25th to the 75th percentiles for the age at onset of sexual maturation, Tanner stage G-2 for boys, range from 7.5 to 10.9 years in non-Hispanic blacks, 8.9 to 11.7 years in Mexican Americans, and 8.6 to 11.4 years for non-Hispanic whites. The onset of sexual maturation is significantly earlier in non-Hispanic black girls and boys than in non-Hispanic white and Mexican American girls and boys.[53]

The sequence of Tanner stages between paired indicators is concordant for about 60% of white, black, and Mexican American children. However, about 30% of these children are discordant (i.e., they enter or are in a stage for one indicator and at the same time enter or are in earlier or later stages for the other indicator), and this discordance affects their growth. Boys whose pubic hair stages are more advanced than their genital stages and girls whose breast development stages are more advanced than their pubic hair stages are heavier and have higher BMI percentiles than concordant children.[54] Children with the opposite discordance weigh less and have lower BMI percentiles than concordant children. This variation in weight and BMI among concordant and discordant children is greater than that among early and late maturing children.[54]

A girl attains menarche or starts to menstruate about 2 years after her breasts start to grow and about 12 to 18 months after her peak height velocity.[55] Approximately 80% of non-Hispanic white girls start to menstruate between about 11.3 and 13.8 years of age, with a median age of 12.6 years, while 80% of non-Hispanic black girls start to menstruate between about 10.5 and 13.6 years of age, with a median age of 12.1 years, and 80% of Mexican American girls start to menstruate between about 10.8 and 13.7 years of age, with a median age of 12.2 years.[55] The ages at menarche for 50% of non-Hispanic black girls and 25% of Mexican American girls are significantly earlier than those of white girls, but there are no significant differences between the black girls and Mexican American girls in their ages at menarche. Girls who attain menarche before 10.5–11.0 years are relatively "early" and those who attain menarche after 13.8 years are relatively "late." Although peak height velocity (the age for most rapid growth in stature) occurs in girls about a year or two before it does in boys, sex difference in age between sexual maturity stages can be less than half a year.

Some reports have indicated that the onset of puberty was possibly occurring earlier among US children than in the past several decades[56] based on the prevalence of Tanner stage 2 breast and/or pubic hair development. Despite slight declines over the past two decades, there is currently no conclusive evidence of a significantly earlier age at menarche among non-Hispanic white and black girls.[57-59] Analysis of US national health survey data indicates that sexual maturation among US children also has not started significantly earlier, but additional survey data are needed to examine this trend and answer this important health concern.[58]

Body Composition

Muscle, adipose tissue, and bone are the primary body tissues that change during growth. These tissues are frequently quantified into **fat** (FM) and **fat-free** (FFM) components. **Lean body mass** (LBM) is metabolically active and differs from FFM in that it is composed of muscle tissue, the internal organs, and the skeleton and contains a small amount of fat (from the bone marrow). In contrast, FFM is LBM without any fat. The density of fat varies little at any age, but the density of lean tissue varies depending upon its hydration and the relative proportions of muscle and bone, which vary among children based on age, sex, race, level of maturation, exercise, and nutritional status.[60] Accurate body composition estimates are calculated from a model that measures body density, bone density, and the volume of total body water and accounts for differences among growing children in their levels of fatness, muscle mass, age, ethnicity, and sex.[61] There are numerous methods for estimating body composition, but **dual energy x-ray absorptiometry** (DXA) is the most accurate, precise, and easiest method for children and even infants. There is a growing reference literature on the body composition of children and adolescents including FFM, **total body fat** (TBF), and **percent body fat** (%BF),[61,62] but body composition references for infants and very young children remain limited.[63,64] NHANES national reference data for body composition from DXA are available for US children.[61,65–67] Reference averages for lean mass index (kg/m², lean mass divided by stature squared) and %BF estimates[61] are presented in **FIGURES 2.6** and **2.7**, respectively. There are differences in median values between non-Hispanic white and non-Hispanic black and Mexican American children for FFM and %BF.

Growth of Muscle

Growth in FFM and LBM is primarily due to an increase in skeletal muscle mass, which is the largest single tissue component of the body, the major constituent of which is water. At birth, 20% of body weight is skeletal muscle, and this increases to about 35% to 40% of body weight at adulthood.[68,69] FFM, LBM, and skeletal muscle mass are positively associated with stature (i.e., a tall child has a greater amount of these than a shorter child at the same level of maturity). Skeletal muscle mass increases in boys and girls during childhood and is roughly equal and parallel[61] between them until about 13 to 14 years of age (Figure 2.6). In girls, muscle continues to grow into adolescence, but slows down around 16 years of age. In boys, skeletal muscle grows rapidly after 13 years of age and well into late adolescence. This growth period in boys is about twice as long as in girls, and as a result, boys have several times as much skeletal muscle as girls, which is located primarily in the shoulders and arms. At maturity, boys have greater absolute amounts of FFM or LBM than girls, irrespective of stature.

Growth of Body Fat

Body fat stores energy. In children, the majority of the body's fat is subcutaneous, but adipose tissue is also deposited in the visceral parts of the body. From infancy up to adolescence, the growth of body fat or adipose tissue is fairly steady, although not at the same levels in boys and girls.[24,61] Adipose tissue thickness on the arms, legs, and trunk increases during childhood in both sexes but

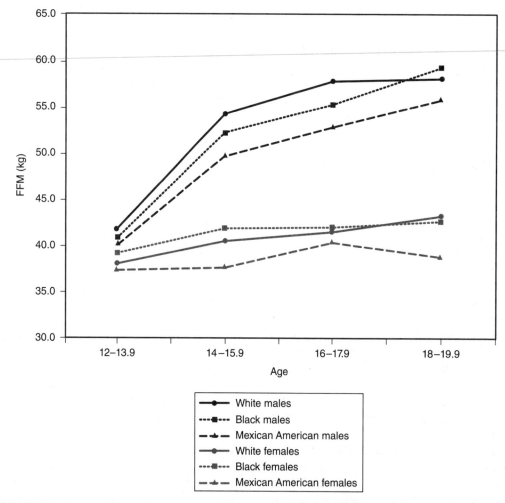

FIGURE 2.6 NHANES Lean Mass Index

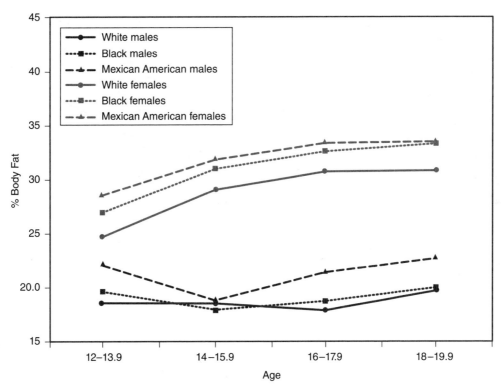

FIGURE 2.7 NHANES Percent Body Fat Index

slightly more so in girls, so that by about age 10, girls have about 20% more body fat than boys.[61] Body fatness continues to increase during adolescence (Figure 2.7) in girls, but in boys decreases after about 13 years of age because the underlying skeletal muscle and bone grow at a greater rate at this time. Boys and girls also differ in the deposition and patterning of adipose tissue during adolescence. Both sexes deposit adipose tissue on the torso, but adolescent girls add adipose tissue to breasts, buttocks, thighs, and across the back of the arms, which accentuates the adult sex differences in body shape.[69] Differences in the deposition of abdominal visceral fat between the sexes begin at 12 years.[70] The majority of TBF growth among obese children is subcutaneous, but recently, internal adipose tissue deposition (i.e., deposition of abdominal visceral fat) similar to that of middle-aged adults, is starting to appear in obese children.[71]

Skeletal Growth

Skeletal growth is a continuous process. The bones of the legs and the vertebrae are the major locations of growth in stature, which reflects growth in bone length. Bone growth in length is rather steady until the adolescent growth spurt but slows afterward. At around 16 years of age for girls and 19 years of age for boys, the epiphyses or growth plates at the ends of long bones have fused to the shaft or diaphysis and the skeleton is mature.[72] Assessing skeletal maturation from radiographs of the hand/wrist or knee is an index of a child's biological age and is known as *skeletal age*. Two children of the same chronological age may have different levels of skeletal maturation or

skeletal ages, just as they may also have different levels of sexual maturation.

The skeleton is the body's reserve of calcium and an important aspect of skeletal growth is the building of this calcium reserve. In children, the importance of this reserve is that those who end growth with a low bone mass are at an increased risk for developing adult osteoporosis and fracture. Peak bone mass is the maximum mineral mass attained by the skeleton. This peak may be achieved in the late-middle part of the third decade of life depending on the skeletal site.[17,18] Bone mineral acquisition throughout the adolescent growth spurt and puberty shows growth patterns different from growth patterns of bone length. Peak rates of mineral acquisition in the whole body lag about 0.8 to 1.2 years in girls and about 0.6 to 0.9 years behind age of peak height velocity in boys. The age at peak velocity of bone mineral accrual differs by various skeletal sites; the age at peak velocity for femoral neck BMC acquisition is about 11.4 years while at the ultradistal radius it is about 13.0 in African American girls.[17] There are also sex and racial/ethnic differences in the timing of maximal growth and the magnitude of skeletal growth.[17,73,74]

Reference data for BMC and BMD are now available for children[75] and national data are available from the current NHANES[61] (see **FIGURE 2.8**) and the Bone Mineral Density in Childhood Study.[19,65] These reference data based on DXA provide a means for monitoring skeletal growth. This information can be useful in identifying children with low bone mass and density in order to intervene and improve peak bone mass and reduce future risk of osteoporosis.

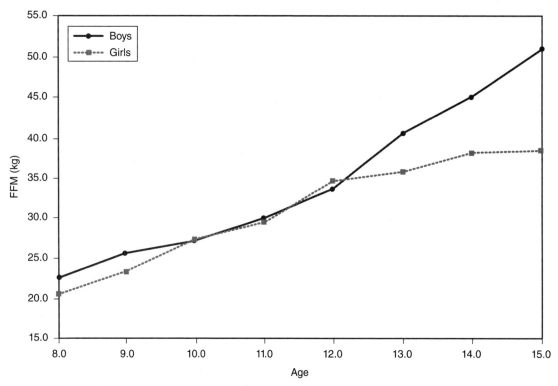

FIGURE 2.8 NHANES Total Body BMD

Children with Special Healthcare Needs

Assessing the growth status of children with Down's syndrome, cerebral palsy, contractures, braces, mental retardation, and similar conditions can be difficult. The heterogeneity of these conditions limits recommended standard methodology and there is limited reference data.[76,77] If the child can stand, standard methods can be used. If the child is non-ambulatory, then recumbent length assessment is recommended. If recumbent length is not possible, using other anthropometric indicators, such as segmental lengths, is preferred. Reference data from the NCHS need to be interpolated, depending upon the condition of the child in question.

In the growth assessment of a handicapped child, one measurement is probably not sufficient. It may be necessary to take several measurements, especially for more difficult measurements or for uncooperative children. Accurate records are important, and the CDC/NCHS growth charts can be used. A child may be at the third percentile or less, but these growth charts can still provide information about a child's status, especially over time. For children with some specific conditions, such as Trisomy 21, several websites provide useful information, including the Down Syndrome Growing Up Study (DSGS, https://www.cdc.gov/ncbddd/birthdefects/downsyndrome/growth-charts.html).[76,78] For other children, such as those with cerebral palsy, specific growth charts continue to be developed.[79]

▶ Summary

The objective of this chapter is to provide an overview of the process of physical growth and maturation. This chapter discusses measuring growth, the changes that occur over childhood in various tissues of the body, and the use of growth references for assessing and monitoring of growth.

Suggested Readings

Cameron N, Bogin B. *Human Growth and Development*. 2nd. ed. London, UK: Elsevier/Academic Press; 2012.

Roche AF, Sun SS. *Human Growth Assessment and Interpretation*. Cambridge, UK: Cambridge University Press; 2003.

World Health Organization. *WHO Child Growth Standards Length/Height-for-Age, Weight-for-Length, Weight-for-Height and Body Mass Index-for-Age, Methods and Development*. Geneva, Switzerland: World Health Organization; 2006. Available at: http://www.who.int/childgrowth/standards/technical_report/en/index.html

Review Questions

1. What can growth assessment be used for?

2. At what age is stature measured?

3. What growth charts are the most appropriate for US children under 2 years of age, and why?

4. What are the most important indices used for determining overweight/obesity status in children?

5. What physical changes occur over the course of puberty?

6. Why is the assessment of head circumference important in early childhood?

References

1. Dietz WH, Economos CD. Progress in the control of childhood obesity. *Pediatrics.* 2015;135(3):e559–e561.

2. Ogden CL, Carroll MD, Lawman HG, et al. Trends in obesity prevalence among children and adolescents in the United States, 1988–1994 through 2013–2014. *JAMA.* 2016;315(21):2292–2299.

3. Camhi SM, Katzmarzyk PT. Tracking of cardiometabolic risk factor clustering from childhood to adulthood. *Int J Pediatr Obes.* 2010;5(2):122–129.

4. Lohman TG, Roche AF, Martorell R. *Anthropometric Standardization Reference Manual.* Champaign, IL: Human Kinetics Books; 1988.

5. Guo SS, Wu W, Chumlea WC, Roche AF. Predicting overweight and obesity in adulthood from body mass index values in childhood and adolescence. *Am J Clin Nutr.* 2002;76(3):653–658.

6. Addo OY, Himes JH. Reference curves for triceps and subscapular skinfold thicknesses in U.S. children and adolescents. *Am J Clin Nutr.* 2010;91(3):635–642.

7. Liem ET, De Lucia Rolfe E, L'Abee C, Sauer PJ, Ong KK, Stolk RP. Measuring abdominal adiposity in 6 to 7-year-old children. *Eur J Clin Nutr.* 2009;63(7):835–841.

8. Roche AF, Sievogel RM, Chumlea WC, Webb P. Grading body fatness from limited anthropometric data. *Am J Clin Nutr.* 1981;34(12):2831–2838.

9. Ogden CL, Carroll MD, Lawman HG, et al. Trends in obesity prevalence among children and adolescents in the United States, 1988–1994 through 2013–2014. *JAMA.* 2016;315:2292–2299.

10. Johnson W, Soloway LE, Erickson D, et al. A changing pattern of childhood BMI growth during the 20th century: 70 y of data from the Fels Longitudinal Study. *Am J Clin Nutr.* 2012;95:1136–1143.

11. Fitzgerald DA. The weighty issue of obesity in paediatric respiratory medicine. *Paediatr Respir Rev.* 2017;24:4–7.

12. Force USPST, Grossman DC, Bibbins-Domingo K, et al. Screening for obesity in children and adolescents: U.S. Preventive Services Task Force recommendation statement. *JAMA.* 2017;317(23):2417–2426.

13. Krebs NF, Jacobson MS, American Academy of Pediatrics Committee on N. Prevention of pediatric overweight and obesity. *Pediatrics.* 2003;112(2):424–430.

14. McGill HC, McMahan CA, Edward HE, Gray MT, Richard TE, Strong JP. Origin of atherosclerosis in childhood and adolescence. *Am J Clin Nutr.* 2000:1307–1315.

15. Zhang H, Zhang T, Li S, et al. Long-term impact of childhood adiposity on adult metabolic syndrome is modified by insulin resistance: The Bogalusa Heart Study. *Sci Rep.* 2015;5:17885.

16. Freedman DS, Ogden CL, Kit BK. Interrelationships between BMI, skinfold thicknesses, percent body fat, and cardiovascular disease risk factors among U.S. children and adolescents. *BMC Pediatr.* 2015;15:188.

17. McCormack SE, Cousminer DL, Chesi A, et al. Association between linear growth and bone accrual in a diverse cohort of children and adolescents. *JAMA Pediatr.* 2017;171(9):e171769.

18. Lu J, Shin Y, Yen MS, Sun SS. Peak bone mass and patterns of change in total bone mineral density and bone mineral contents from childhood into young adulthood. *J Clin Densitom.* 2016;19(2):180–191.

19. Kalkwarf HJ, Gilsanz V, Lappe JM, et al. Tracking of bone mass and density during childhood and adolescence. *J Clin Endocrinol Metab.* 2010;95(4):1690–1698.

20. Rzehak P, Covic M, Saffery R, et al. DNA-methylation and body composition in preschool children: epigenome-wide-analysis in the European Childhood Obesity Project (CHOP)-study. *Sci Rep.* 2017;7(1):14349.

21. Khalil N, Chen A, Lee M. Endocrine disruptive compounds and cardio-metabolic risk factors in children. *Curr Opinion Pharmacol.* 2014;19C:120–124.

22. Moore WM, Roche AF. *Pediatric Anthropometry.* 3rd ed. Columbus, OH: Ross Laboratories; 1987.

23. Tanner JM. *Fetus into Man: Physical Growth from Conception to Maturity.* Revised and enlarged ed. Cambridge, Massachusetts: Harvard University Press; 1990.

24. Rogol AD, Roemmich JN, Clark PA. Growth at puberty. *J Adolesc Health.* 2002;31(6 suppl):192–200.

25. WHO Multicentre Growth Reference Study Group. *WHO Child Growth Standards: Length/height-for-age, weight-for-age, weight-for-length, weight-for-height and body mass index-for-age: Methods and development.* Geneva: World Health Organization;2006.

26. Dekaban AS. Changes in brain weights during the span of human life: relation of brain weights to body heights and body weights. *Ann Neurol.* 1978;4(4):345–356.

27. Fomon SJ, Haschke F, Ziegler EE, Nelson SE. Body composition of reference children from birth to age 10 years. *Am J Clin Nutr.* 1982;35(5 suppl):1169–1175.

28. Wells JC, Williams JE, Chomtho S, et al. Pediatric reference data for lean tissue properties: density and hydration from age 5 to 20 y. *Am J Clin Nutr.* 2010;91(3):610–618.

29. von Hippel PT, Nahhas RW, Czerwinski SA. How much do children's body mass indices change over intervals of 6–12 months? Statistics from before and after the obesity epidemic. *Pediatr Obes.* 2015;10(6):468–475.

30. Whitaker RC, Wright JA, Pepe MS, Seidel KD, Dietz WH. Predicting obesity in young adulthood from childhood and parental obesity. *N Engl J Med.* 1997;337(13):869–873.

31. Kuczmarski RJ, Ogden CL, Grummer-Strawn LM, et al. CDC growth charts: United States. *Adv Data.* 2000;8(314): 1–27.

32. Roche AF, Davila GH. Late adolescent growth in stature. *Pediatrics.* 1972;50(6):874–880.

33. Tanner JM, Whitehouse RH, Marshall WA, Carter BS. Prediction of adult height from height, bone age, and occurrence of menarche, at ages 4 to 16 with allowance for midparent height. *Arch Dis Child.* 1975;50(1):14–26.

34. Marshall WA, Tanner JM. Variations in pattern of pubertal changes in girls. *Arch Dis Child.* 1969;44(235):291–303.

35. Marshall WA, Tanner JM. Variations in the pattern of pubertal changes in boys. *Arch Dis Child.* 1970; 45(239):13–23.

36. Abbassi V. Growth and normal puberty. *Pediatrics.* 1998; 102(2 Pt 3):507–511.

37. Flanagan SD, Dunn-Lewis C, Hatfield DL, et al. Developmental differences between boys and girls result in sex-specific physical fitness changes from fourth to fifth grade. *J Strength Cond Res.* 2015;29(1):175–180.

38. de Onis M, Onyango AW, Van den Broeck J, Chumlea WC, Martorell R. Measurement and standardization protocols for anthropometry used in the construction of a new international growth reference. *Food Nutr Bull.* 2004;25 (1 suppl):S27–S36.

39. Grummer-Strawn LM, Reinold C, Krebs NF, Centers for Disease Control and, Prevention. Use of World Health Organization and CDC growth charts for children aged 0–59 months in the United States. *MMWR Recomm Rep.* 2010;59 (RR-9):1–15.

40. Hamill PVV. NCHS growth curves for children : birth-18 years, United States. *Vital and Health Statistics : Series 11, Data from the National Health Survey no 165.* Hyattsville, Md.: U.S. Dept. of Health, Education, and Welfare, Public Health Service U.S. Govt. Printing Office; 1977:iv, 74 p.

41. Kuczmarski RJ, Ogden CL, Guo SS, et al. 2000 CDC growth charts for the United States: methods and development. *Vital Health Stat 11.* 2002(246):1–190.

42. de Onis M, Onyango AW, Borghi E, Siyam A, Nishida C, Siekmann J. Development of a WHO growth reference for school-aged children and adolescents. *Bull World Health Organ.* 2007;85(9):660–667.

43. Chumlea WC. Which growth charts are the best for children today? *Nutr Today.* 2007;42(4):148.

44. Oshiro CE, Novotny R, Grove JS, Hurwitz EL. Race/Ethnic differences in birth size, infant growth, and body mass index at age five years in children in Hawaii. *Child Obes.* 2015;11(6):683–690.

45. Natale V, Rajagopalan A. Worldwide variation in human growth and the World Health Organization growth standards: a systematic review. *BMJ Open.* 2014;4(1):e003735.

46. Cameron N, Bogin B. *Human Growth and Development.* 2nd ed. London, UK: Elsevier/Academic Press; 2012.

47. Villar J, Altman DG, Purwar M, et al. The objectives, design and implementation of the INTERGROWTH-21st Project. *BJOG.* 2013;120 Suppl 2:9–26, v.

48. Villar J, Cheikh Ismail L, Victora CG, et al. International standards for newborn weight, length, and head circumference by gestational age and sex: the Newborn Cross-Sectional Study of the INTERGROWTH-21st Project. *Lancet.* 2014;384(9946):857–868.

49. Kiserud T, Piaggio G, Carroli G, et al. The World Health Organization Fetal Growth Charts: A Multinational Longitudinal Study of Ultrasound Biometric Measurements and Estimated Fetal Weight. *PLoS Med.* 2017;14(1):e1002220.

50. Baumgartner RN, Roche AF, Himes JH. Incremental growth tables: supplementary to previously published charts. *Am J Clin Nutr.* 1986;43(5):711–722.

51. Roche AF, Himes JH. Incremental growth charts. *Am J Clin Nutr.* 1980;33(9):2041–2052.

52. Roche AF. *Growth, Maturation, and Body Composition: the Fels Longitudinal Study, 1929-1991.* Cambridge ; New York, NY: Cambridge University Press; 1992.

53. Sun SS, Schubert CM, Chumlea WC, et al. National estimates of the timing of sexual maturation and racial differences among U.S. children. *Pediatrics.* 2002;110(5):911–919.

54. Schubert CM, Chumlea WC, Kulin HE, Lee PA, Himes JH, Sun SS. Concordant and discordant sexual maturation among U.S. children in relation to body weight and BMI. *J Adolesc Health.* 2005;37(5):356–362.

55. Chumlea WC, Schubert CM, Roche AF, et al. Age at menarche and racial comparisons in U.S. girls. *Pediatrics.* 2003;111(1):110–113.

56. Herman-Giddens ME, Slora EJ, Wasserman RC, et al. Secondary sexual characteristics and menses in young girls seen in office practice: a study from the Pediatric Research in Office Settings network. *Pediatrics.* 1997;99(4):505–512.

57. Sun SS, Schubert CM, Liang R, et al. Is sexual maturity occurring earlier among U.S. children? *J Adolesc Health.* 2005;37(5):345–355.

58. Cabrera SM, Bright GM, Frane JW, Blethen SL, Lee PA. Age of thelarche and menarche in contemporary U.S. females: a cross-sectional analysis. *J Pediatr Endocrinol Metab.* 2014;27(1–2):47–51.

59. Rosenfield RL, Bachrach LK, Chernausek SD, et al. Current age of onset of puberty. *Pediatrics.* 2000;106(3):622–623.

60. Lohman TG. Applicability of body composition techniques and constants for children and youths. *Exerc Sport Sci Rev.* 1986;14:325–357.

61. Kelly TL, Wilson KE, Heymsfield SB. Dual energy X-Ray absorptiometry body composition reference values from NHANES. *PLoS One.* 2009;4(9):e7038.

62. Weber DR, Leonard MB, Zemel BS. Body composition analysis in the pediatric population. *Pediatr Endocrinol Rev.* 2012;10(1):130–139.

63. Gallo S, Vanstone CA, Weiler HA. Normative data for bone mass in healthy term infants from birth to 1 year of age. *J Osteoporos.* 2012;2012:672403.

64. Koo WW, Walters JC, Hockman EM. Body composition in human infants at birth and postnatally. *J Nutr.* 2000;130(9):2188–2194.

65. Zemel BS, Kalkwarf HJ, Gilsanz V, et al. Revised reference curves for bone mineral content and areal bone mineral density according to age and sex for black and non-black children: results of the bone mineral density in childhood study. *J Clin Endocrinol Metab.* 2011;96(10):3160–3169.

66. Baxter-Jones AD, Burrows M, Bachrach LK, et al. International longitudinal pediatric reference standards for bone mineral content. *Bone.* 2010;46(1):208–216.

67. Ogden CL, Li Y, Freedman DS, Borrud LG, Flegal KM. Smoothed percentage body fat percentiles for U.S. children and adolescents, 1999-2004. *Natl Health Stat Report.* 2011(43):1–7.

68. Holliday MA. Body composition and energy needs during growth. In: Falkner F, Tanner JM, eds. *Human Growth.* Vol 2. 2 ed. New York Plenum; 1986:101–117.

69. Katch VL, Campaigne B, Freedson P, Sady S, Katch FI, Behnke AR. Contribution of breast volume and weight to body fat distribution in females. *Am J Phys Anthropol.* 1980;53(1):93–100.

70. Shen W, Punyanitya M, Silva AM, et al. Sexual dimorphism of adipose tissue distribution across the lifespan: a cross-sectional whole-body magnetic resonance imaging study. *Nutr Metab (Lond).* 2009;6:17.

71. Katzmarzyk PT, Shen W, Baxter-Jones A, et al. Adiposity in children and adolescents: correlates and clinical consequences of fat stored in specific body depots. *Pediatr Obes.* 2012;7(5):e42–e61.

72. Crowder C, Austin D. Age ranges of epiphyseal fusion in the distal tibia and fibula of contemporary males and females. *J Forensic Sci.* 2005;50(5):1001–1007.

73. Bachrach LK, Hastie T, Wang MC, Narasimhan B, Marcus R. Bone mineral acquisition in healthy Asian, Hispanic, Black, and Caucasian youth: a longitudinal study. *J Clin Endocrinol Metab.* 1999;84(12):4702–4712.

74. Gilsanz V, Skaggs DL, Kovanlikaya A, et al. Differential effect of race on the axial and appendicular skeletons of children. *J Clin Endocrinol Metab.* 1998;83(5): 1420–1427.

75. Maynard LM, Guo SS, Chumlea WC, et al. Total-body and regional bone mineral content and areal bone mineral density in children aged 8–18 y: the Fels Longitudinal Study. *Am J Clin Nutr.* 1998;68(5):1111–1117.

76. Zemel BS, Pipan M, Stallings VA, et al. Growth charts for children with down syndrome in the United States. *Pediatrics.* 2015;136(5):e1204–e1211.

77. Zemel BS. Influence of complex childhood diseases on variation in growth and skeletal development. *Am J Hum Biol.* 2017;29(2).

78. Cronk C, Crocker AC, Pueschel SM, et al. Growth charts for children with Down syndrome: 1 month to 18 years of age. *Pediatrics.* 1988;81(1):102–110.

79. Brooks J, Day S, Shavelle R, Strauss D. Low weight, morbidity, and mortality in children with cerebral palsy: new clinical growth charts. *Pediatrics.* 2011;128(2):e299–e307.

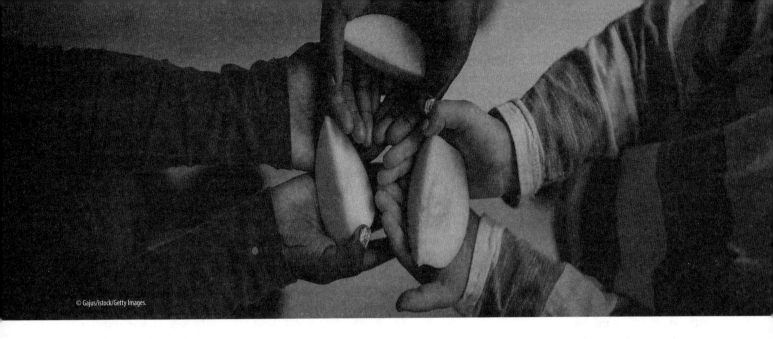

© Gajus/istock/Getty Images.

CHAPTER 3

Nutrition-Focused Physical Examination

Kelly Green Corkins and Holly A. Van Poots

LEARNING OBJECTIVES

- Discuss why nutrition-focused physical examination is an important element of a comprehensive nutrition assessment.
- Identify components of a head-to-toe nutrition-focused physical examination for pediatric patients with emphasis on the impact of growth and development.
- Describe signs and symptoms of muscle wasting, subcutaneous fat depletion, and micronutrient deficiencies.
- Describe how to physically assess hydration status.

▶ Introduction

Nutrition-focused physical examination (NFPE) is an important step in the nutrition care process as defined by the Academy of Nutrition and Dietetics.[1] The goal of the NFPE is to identify signs and clinical symptoms of malnutrition, and the NFPE should be incorporated into a complete nutrition assessment along with a medical record review and interview.[2,3] The examination is a subjective assessment compared with anthropometric measurements or laboratory values that are objective assessments.[4] It is important to note that no one objective parameter or value provides a complete nutrition assessment, and information gained through NFPE can strengthen a nutrition diagnosis.[2,5,6]

The recommended indicators for identifying pediatric malnutrition do not include any subjective parameters, as the adult malnutrition clinical characteristics do.[7,8] This is not to say that subjective parameters have no place in assessing malnutrition in pediatric patients. Subjective Global Nutritional Assessment, which utilizes both objective and subjective parameters, has been validated as a nutrition assessment tool with pediatric patients.[4,6] There are issues with relying solely on objective measures.[6]

Laboratory values are often unreliable.[9] Anthropometric measurements are often difficult to obtain in a healthcare setting. Measurements may be impaired by improper technique, uncalibrated or improperly functioning devices, physical impairment of the child, or edema.[4,7,10,11] Some professionals argue that physical examination and touching your patient more accurately confirms nutrition issues and is less subjective than other nutrition assessment tools such as asking a parent to recall what his or her child has eaten recently.[12,13] Incorporating NFPE into the assessment can help identify problems with the anthropometric measurements and prompt new measurements when appropriate, confirm information gained through the medical record review and gain additional information to complete the nutrition assessment, and ultimately provide better nutrition care of the patient.[2,3]

A significant disadvantage of using subjective parameters during the nutritional assessment of a patient is that these parameters are slow to change and, therefore, make it difficult to evaluate the immediate effectiveness of nutrition interventions.[14] This is not to say that reassessment is not necessary. Instead, routine reassessment is necessary to note changes, but a longer time interval for reassessment may be more appropriate.[12]

▶ Techniques

NFPE is relatively easy to learn but its techniques do require mastering.[12,15] Inspection, palpation, percussion, and auscultation are the physical assessment techniques used in NFPE.[3,16] See **TABLE 3.1** for definitions and tools needed for each technique. Physicians and nurses use these physical assessment techniques regularly, but usually their focus is not nutrition-related. Because of their mastery in these assessment techniques, physicians and nurses can aid dietitians and other nutrition

professionals who are learning NFPE, and the dietitian can enlighten other healthcare professionals on the nutrition-focused aspects.[9] Most of the information on NFPE is adult-based; and though the techniques are the same, children are growing, and the body composition changes during growth, so knowledge on growth and development of children is important.[17] Additionally, individuals must be responsible for their own competence in order to assure that these subjective assessments are consistent.[18]

Before the Examination

Before the examination starts, the practitioner should be familiar with the patient's history and understand why the patient is at nutrition risk. A thorough medical record review can guide the practitioner on how to focus the physical examination or what issues may prevent a complete physical examination (such as being unable to move a trauma patient to complete the exam).[3,15,16] Objective data from the medical record includes diagnosis (with emphasis on those with nutrition implications), admitting diagnosis, anthropometric measurements, biochemical values, surgical history, medications, and use of any vitamin, mineral, or herbal supplements. In children less than 3 years of age, prenatal and birth history is useful. Tanner Stage is useful for preteens and teens in order to assess development.[4,17] The information gathered during the medical record review can be verified during the interview and physical examination.[3]

Before entering the room, be sure to have collected any tools you might need. Most commonly used tools are: penlight, tongue depressor, tape measure, and skin calipers.[2,17] If the patient is in the hospital, check with the bedside nurse to make sure the child has not just fallen asleep and that it is a good time to do the examination. The relationship with the patient should be established

TABLE 3.1 Techniques and Tools for NFPE			
Technique	**Definition**	**What Is Being Assessed**	**Tools**
Inspection	Visual assessment	Color, shape, texture, and symmetry	Penlight, tongue depressor, gloves
Palpation	Assessing by touch	Texture, temperature, muscle rigidity, tenderness, hydration of skin	Gloves
Percussion	Tapping to produce sound	Determining fluids, solids, and gas; determining the borders and position of organs	Gloves
Auscultation	Listening	Sounds produced by percussion; bowel sounds	Stethoscope

Data from Pogatshnik C, Hamilton C. Nutrition-focused physical examination: skin, nails, hair, eyes, and oral cavity. *Support Line*. 2011;33(2):7–13.[3]
Esper DH. Utilization of nutrition-focused physical assessment in identifying micronutrient deficiencies. *Nutr Clin Pract*. 2015;30(2):194–202. doi:10.1177/0884533615573054[9]

before starting the examination. The clinician should introduce him/herself and explain the reason for the examination. Ask permission of the patient and/or the parent, wash or sanitize hands, and put on gloves.[2]

Beginning the Examination

Start with a general overall inspection. This general inspection reveals if the patient is over- or underweight, and any generalized edema can be noted. The examination then proceeds, usually in a head-to-toe order.[2,3,9,15] Both sides of the body should be examined in order to determine if the findings are bilateral.[2] Specific to pediatrics is growth and development and the changes in body composition associated with it. Children have increased fat deposition just before a growth spurt. The increased adiposity is not obesity but energy reserves to support the increased growth. Decreased adiposity or malnutrition could hinder growth.[17]

▶ Nutrition Assessment

Subcutaneous Fat Loss

Body composition varies during normal childhood development, and differences between males and females are observed at all ages. During infancy, body fat peaks at around 3 to 6 months at approximately 32% for females and 29% for males. **Body mass index** (BMI), although commonly used as a screening tool for both undernutrition and overweight/obesity, does not differentiate between fat mass and fat-free mass.[19] BMI-for-age peaks at around 6 to 7 months for both male and female infants[20] and reaches a nadir at between 4 and 7 years of age with

the median age being 5 to 6 years. BMI then increases throughout adolescence and into adulthood.[19,21] While BMI increases for both sexes throughout adolescence, body composition changes become more pronounced with greater lean body mass and less fat mass in males than in age-matched females.[19]

When assessing for subcutaneous fat loss during an NFPE, the clinician must have an understanding of normal variations in body composition during growth and development and take these patterns into account when evaluating changes. Obtaining a baseline during the initial nutrition assessment is helpful for future comparisons when monitoring and evaluating the effectiveness of the nutrition care plan.

The face (eyes and cheeks), upper arms, and torso/buttocks are examined in the assessment of subcutaneous fat loss in pediatric populations (See **TABLE 3.2**). Inspection and palpation are used to identify bony prominences, muscular outlines, loose or hanging skin, as well as to assess the fat pads under the skin.[14] Fat loss may be evident in the orbital fat pads, the buccal fat pads, the triceps skinfold, and around the ribcage.[14,22] In infants and children, the buttocks may also appear wasted, flat, or baggy in cases of severe malnutrition.[14]

Orbital Fat Pads

The fat pads in the area around the eye socket should be gently palpated with the fingertips in a circular motion. Slightly bulged fat pads are normal, while slightly dark circles may be observed with mild to moderate malnutrition; and hollow, depressed dark circles may be seen with severe malnutrition. Loose skin, a prominent brow bone, and a "hollow-eye" appearance may also be seen.[22]

TABLE 3.2 Assessment of Subcutaneous Fat Loss

NFPE Region	Anatomical Landmarks	NFPE Technique(s)
Orbital fat pads (eyes)	Orbital bones/eye socket and brow bone (supraorbital ridge)	Inspection and palpation
Buccal fat pads (cheeks)	Cheek bones (zygomatic or malar bones) and upper lip	Inspection and palpation
Triceps (upper arm)	Back of upper arm midway between elbow and armpit when shoulder and elbow are flexed to 90°	Inspection and palpation
Torso/Trunk (Ribcage, Lower Back, Pelvis)	Costal arch and intercostal spaces of front ribs, midaxillary line, thoracic and lumbar vertebrae, iliac crest of pelvis; buttocks (infants and children)	Inspection and palpation

Data from Secker DJ, Jeejeebhoy KN. How to perform subjective global nutritional assessment in children. *J Acad Nutr Diet.* 2012;112(3):424–431.e6. doi:10.1016/j.jada.2011.08.039.[6]
Mordarski B, Wolff J, eds. *Pediatric Nutrition Focused Physical Exam Pocket Guide.* Chicago, IL: Academy of Nutrition and Dietetics; 2015.[22]
OpenStax. *Anatomy & Physiology.* OpenStax CNX. Available at: http://cnx.org/contents/14fb4ad7-39a1-4eee-ab6e-3ef2482e3e22@8.108. Published August 1, 2017. Accessed January 21, 2018.[24]

Buccal Fat Pads

The buccal fat pads lie in the deep layers of tissue in the center of the cheek at the level of the upper lip and above. The buccal fat is continuous with the deep fat of the temple area.[23] Full, round, filled out cheeks are normal. Flat cheeks may indicate mild to moderate malnutrition. A hollow, sunken, or narrow face may be seen with severe malnutrition.[14]

Triceps

The back of the upper arm is assessed with the arm bent at a 90° angle in either the sagittal or coronal plane. Pinch the fat between the thumb and fingers and roll down to separate muscle from fat. A thick fat fold between the fingers is a normal finding. Some space between the fingers is consistent with mild to moderate malnutrition. Severe malnutrition may be indicated by a minimal space between the fingers with the fingers almost touching.[14,22]

Ribs/Midaxillary Line

The anatomical landmarks for assessing fat loss in the trunk include the front ribs, the iliac crest, the midaxillary line, and the ribs at the lower back. When facing the patient, if the ribs do not show in the front of the body, this is a normal finding. If ribs are apparent with slight depressions in the intercostal spaces, this may be indicative of mild to moderate malnutrition. Very apparent depressions between ribs in the intercostal spaces and around the costal margin are consistent with severe malnutrition. The iliac crest may be apparent in some adolescents as a normal finding, but prominent protrusion may also indicate fat loss in the abdominal region. Ribs can also be viewed and palpated at the midaxillary line. Skinfold thickness at the midaxillary line in the waist area, below the ribs and above the iliac crest, may reveal fat loss. When the patient is facing away from the clinician, the ribcage at the lower back can be viewed. If the patient pushes against an object, a better view of the back can be obtained. As with the front ribs, the clinician is looking for apparent ribs with depressions in the intercostal spaces.[12,14,22]

Mid-Upper Arm Circumference (MUAC)

Mid-upper arm circumference (MUAC) is an additional objective anthropometric measurement that may be particularly useful in assessing children whose weights may be skewed by overhydration/fluid retention, edema, ascites, or steroid use.[25] Comparative standards are available for ages 3 months to 5 years from the **World Health Organization** (WHO) **Multicenter Growth Reference Study** (MGRS) data[26] while -zscores for ages 2 months to 18 years have been generated from NHANES MUAC data from 1999–2012.[27] Both sets of reference values can generate

MUAC z-scores with the web-based Peditools calculator available at www.peditools.org.[28] Of note, NHANES MUAC measurements were obtained using the right arm[29] while WHO MGRS measurements used the left arm.[30]

To measure MUAC, the child should stand facing away from the clinician with his/her elbow flexed to a 90° angle in the sagittal plane and the palm facing up. The acromion process of the shoulder should be located by palpation, and the distance from the posterior aspect to the olecranon process of the elbow is then measured. Average the two measurements, mark the midpoint, and have the child relax the marked arm at his/her side. A non-stretchable flexible tape is used to measure around the arm at the midpoint with the circumference being measured to the nearest tenth of a centimeter.[29,31]

Consistent use of the same arm for serial MUAC measurements is important for evaluating any trends. Noting which arm was measured can be helpful when multiple clinicians are caring for the same child. If a child is neurologically impaired, the unaffected arm should be chosen for measurement. In other cases, the arm chosen may be selected based on the reference standards used for comparison (left arm for WHO, right arm for CDC NHANES). In acute care settings, access to the arm or the presence of intravenous lines may influence selection of which side to use.

Bilateral Muscle Wasting

The temples, chest, shoulders, back, thighs, knees, and calves are examined when assessing muscle wasting in pediatric populations (See **TABLE 3.3**). Inspection and palpation are used to identify prominent bone structures and flat or hollowed muscles since these are signs of muscular wasting. Note that the lower body is less sensitive to change than the upper body, so loss of muscle mass in the temples, chest, shoulders, and back may be seen before wasting is evident in the thighs and calves. Other than malnutrition, low muscle mass may result from neurodegenerative conditions or muscular disorders.[14]

Temporalis (Temples)

Muscle wasting can be observed in the temporalis region. Palpate the temporalis muscle horizontally and vertically to assess for muscle tone. Ask the patient to chew to help locate the muscle. Normal findings are a well-defined muscle, while a slight depression can be seen or felt with mild to moderate wasting. A hollowing or scooping depression is observed in cases of severe malnutrition.[12,14,22]

Pectoralis (Chest)

The clavicle is the anatomical landmark for assessing the muscle tone of the pectoralis major muscle.[14,22] The pectoralis major muscle has two parts—the clavicular

TABLE 3.3 Assessment of Bilateral Muscle Wasting

NFPE Region (Muscle)	Anatomical Landmarks	NFPE Technique(s)
Temples (Temporalis)	Temporalis muscle	Inspection and palpation
Chest (Pectoralis Major)	Clavicle	Inspection and palpation
Shoulders (Deltoid)	Acromion process	Inspection and palpation
Back (Trapezius, Supraspinatus, Infraspinatus)	Scapula	Inspection and palpation
Anterior Thigh and Knee (Quadriceps)	Patella	Inspection and palpation
Calf (Gastrocnemius)	Posterior calf	Inspection and palpation

Data from Secker DJ, Jeejeebhoy KN. How to perform subjective global nutritional assessment in children. *J Acad Nutr Diet.* 2012;112(3):424–431.[14]

Mordarski B, Wolff J, eds. *Pediatric Nutrition Focused Physical Exam Pocket Guide.* Chicago, IL: Academy of Nutrition and Dietetics; 2015.[22]

OpenStax. *Anatomy & Physiology.* OpenStax CNX. Available at: http://cnx.org/contents/14fb4ad7-39a1-4eee-ab6e-3ef2482e3e22@8.108. Published August 1, 2017. Accessed January 21, 2018.[24]

head and the sternal head. The clavicular head originates on the medial aspect of the clavicle and inserts on the humerus. It is responsible for flexion of the upper arm, horizontal adduction of the arm, and internal rotation at the shoulder joint.[32] Muscle tone of the clavicular head of the pectoralis major is palpated below the clavicle bone and may be easiest to assess during a muscular contraction. The fingers should not slide under the clavicle when good muscle tone is present. In a well-nourished individual, the clavicle may be visible but not prominent, while a prominent clavicle may be a normal finding in some females. In cases of mild to moderate malnutrition, some protrusion of the clavicle is evident. Findings of severe malnutrition include a protruding, prominent clavicle.[12,14,22,31]

Deltoid (Shoulders)

With the arms at the patient's sides, observe the shape of the shoulder and look for prominent bones including the acromion process. Palpate by grasping the muscle at the shoulder joint.[14,22] The deltoid muscle has three parts with the anterior origin on the lateral part of the clavicle,[33] the lateral origin on the acromion,[34] and the posterior origin on the spine of the scapula.[35] All three heads of the deltoid insert on the humerus. The deltoid muscle flexes the shoulder in the sagittal and coronal planes.[33–35] Normal findings include a rounded, curved junction between the shoulders and neck. Mild to moderate wasting is indicated by a slight protrusion of the acromion process with the shoulders not square. Severe malnutrition is indicated by square shoulders with prominent bones.[14,22]

Trapezius, Supraspinatus, Infraspinatus (Upper Back)

Inspect and palpate the scapula for muscle tone of the trapezius, supraspinatus, and infraspinatus. Muscle tone can be observed while the patient is pushing on an object. A well-nourished individual will not have prominent scapula bones or evident depressions around the scapular borders. Mild to moderate malnutrition is indicated by some areas of the scapula being evident. Severe malnutrition is indicated by a prominent scapula with depressions above, between, and below the scapula.[12,14,22] Muscle wasting of the latissimus dorsi muscle may also be noticeable below the scapula in the area of the thoracic vertebrae.

Quadriceps (Knee and Thigh)

While the patient is in a seated position with his/her leg propped and knee bent, observe and palpate for muscle tone around the knee joint. Both right and left legs should be observed for symmetry. The quadriceps muscles protrude and bones are not prominent in a well-nourished individual. The knee bone may be noticeable with little muscle mass when mild to moderate malnutrition is present. In severe malnutrition, a square, prominent knee is evident with no muscle mass.[12,14,22]

The quadriceps muscle has four heads. The rectus femoris originates on the ilium and inserts on the tibial tuberosity. It is responsible for knee extension and hip flexion. The remaining three heads originate on the femur and insert on the tibia. These muscles are responsible for knee flexion.[36] The quadriceps can be grasped while the patient is in a seated position with the leg propped, and the muscle can be differentiated from fat. Normal findings are a well-rounded muscle without depressions. The muscle should not be able to be reduced. With mild to moderate malnutrition, a slight depression along the inner thigh is apparent. In severe malnutrition, the clinician can significantly reduce the quadriceps muscle with an obvious depression along the inner thigh.[14,22]

Gastrocnemius (Calf)

The gastrocnemius is a bulb-shaped muscle of the posterior calf. Well-developed muscles are firm. With mild to moderate malnutrition, there is some shape and firmness while with severe malnutrition, a thin, flat muscle without definition is observed. Grasp the muscle to determine the amount of tissue.[14,22] Ask the patient to point and flex the toes to engage the muscle.

Assessment of Hydration Status

Hydration status is assessed by reviewing vital signs, laboratory findings, and findings from the physical exam.

Over Hydration/Edema

To test for dependent edema, press on the middle to distal surface of the foot for 5 seconds and observe it for pitting. In non-ambulatory individuals, the sacral area over the posterior pelvis should be palpated. No fluid accumulation is a normal finding. Moderately deep pitting (2–4 mm) that persists for up to 30 seconds may be indicative of moderate malnutrition. Severe malnutrition may be indicated by deep pitting (4–8 mm) lasting greater than 30 seconds. If edema is due to a medical problem rather than a nutritional deficit, this should be noted as it may affect evaluation of anthropometrics.[14,22]

When overhydration is suspected, laboratory findings such as changes in sodium, chloride, **blood urea nitrogen** (BUN), creatinine, decreased serum osmolality, and decreased urine specific gravity may also be observed. Clinical findings of hypertension or elevated central venous pressure along with physical findings of weight gain, puffy eyes, light-colored urine, moist skin, anasarca, dyspnea, and lung crackles may also be apparent.[37]

Dehydration

Delayed capillary refill and poor skin turgor may indicate dehydration. Alterations in laboratory findings, clinical findings, and physical findings may also be apparent. Increased sodium and chloride, BUN and creatinine, serum osmolality, and urine specific gravity are possible along with hypotension and tachycardia. Weight loss, sunken eyes, dark urine or decreased urine output, dry mucous membranes, thick saliva, clammy skin, and cracked lips may be observed. Vital signs should be evaluated for parameters that are outside of normal ranges.[37]

Assessment of Functional Status

Usual energy and activity levels should be assessed as part of the NFPE. The severity of dysfunction, worsening impairment, and any changes in function over the previous two weeks should be noted. Any changes should be compared with the child's own baseline rather than comparing parameters with age-matched children.[14]

Developmental Milestones

An understanding of typical developmental milestones during early childhood is helpful in assessing functional status (See **TABLE 3.4**). Developmental delays should be noted, however, changes in activity level or a regression in skills from a child's own baseline are used to evaluate functional impairment.[14] Collaboration with physical therapy, occupational therapy, and/or speech-language pathology may provide additional insight into a child's developmental level and skills.

Handgrip Strength

Handgrip strength (HGS) measured with a hand dynamometer is a simple, noninvasive method that can be used to objectively assess functional status in individuals 6 years of age or older.[25] HGS has been used both in hospital and ambulatory settings as a marker of muscle function in children, and a positive correlation has been observed between HGS and both BMI-for-age and MUAC z-scores.[6,39,40] Studies in adult populations have found that HGS may indicate an earlier response to nutritional changes than either labs or anthropometrics.[41] Comparative standards for both absolute and normalized (grip strength [kilograms]/ weight [kilograms]) grip strength in the form of reference percentiles were published in 2015 for ages 6 to 80 years and were based on NHANES 2011–2012 data.[42] Note that HGS does not quantify malnutrition; however, changes over time for an individual can suggest either improvement or deterioration of nutrition status. Calibrated equipment, clinicians trained in measurement protocol (described elsewhere[43,44]), the ability of patient to follow directions, and the use of age and sex-specific reference data are necessary for accurate HGS measurement.[25]

Micronutrient Exam

Micronutrient deficiencies can occur even in the absence of protein-calorie malnutrition.[9] Micronutrient deficiencies are caused by inadequate intake,

TABLE 3.4	Developmental Milestones
Age	**Developmental Skill**
6 months	Mimics sounds; looks at self in mirror; rolls from front to back and back to front; begins to sit unsupported; likes to interact with others; responds to name; babbles vowel sounds (ah, eh, oh); begins to say consonant sounds (m, b); shows curiosity
12 months	Uses and copies simple gestures (shaking head no, waving goodbye); responds to simple spoken requests; can say "mama" and "dada"; pulls to stand; may walk holding onto furniture or stand alone; may show stranger anxiety; has favorite things and people
18 months	Walks independently; drinks from a cup; eats with a spoon; identifies common objects and their uses (phone, spoon); speaks several single words; points to show interest; plays pretend such as feeding a doll; may have temper tantrums; scribbles
2 years	Speaks 2–4 word sentences; shows excitement around other children; follows simple instructions; can kick a ball and stand on tiptoe; identifies objects or pictures by pointing when named; might use one hand more than the other; may show defiant behavior
3 years	Mimics actions of others; converses using 2–3 sentences at a time; climbs; runs; plays make-believe; shows affection; dresses and undresses self; may get upset with changes in routine
4 years	Hops and stands on one foot for up to 2 seconds; pours; cuts with supervision and mashes own food; tells stories; sings songs; recites simple rhymes; uses "he" and "she" correctly; enjoys playing with other children and can play cooperatively; draws a stick figure; uses scissors
5 years	Speaks clearly; knows name and address; understands real and make-believe; counts 10 or more things; can print some letters or numbers; copies geometric shapes; uses a fork and spoon; can use the bathroom on his/her own; swings and climbs; hops or skips

Data from Milestone checklists [fact sheet]. Atlanta, GA: Centers for Disease Control and Prevention. https://www.cdc.gov/ncbddd/actearly/pdf/checklists/all_checklists.pdf. Accessed January 21, 2018.[38]

malabsorption, losses in stools, losses in urine, increased nutrient requirements, wound losses, and disease process.[9] Various disease states such as Crohn's, cystic fibrosis, and organ failure are associated with micronutrient deficiencies related to the disease process.[9,45] Chronic disease states require medications, and these medications may interfere with micronutrient availability and activity.[9,45] See **TABLE 3.5** for potential deficiencies related to diseases or conditions.

Physical signs of micronutrient deficiencies are at many times non-specific, but they are the best way to determine micronutrient deficiencies since biochemical tests do not always accurately assess total body stores.[9,45,48] Areas examined for signs of micronutrient deficiencies include the skin (specifically on the face and extremities), hair, eyes, and oral cavity.[2,9,48] The clinician can start with a general inspection of the skin on the face and upper extremities. Skin should be uniform in color and smooth, soft and even in texture. The clinician inspects for color, texture, lesions, ulcers, rashes, wounds, and bruises. During the inspection, the clinician can palpate for moisture, temperature, and texture.[2,3,5,9] Turgor and mobility are assessed by gently pinching a small section of skin on the forearm and then releasing.[5] See **TABLE 3.6** for examples of abnormal skin findings related to specific nutritional deficiencies.

Following along with the head-to-toe guideline, the clinician starts at the top of the head with the hair and scalp. The clinician inspects the scalp, which should appear normal in color.[5] In toddlers 1–2 years old, palpate the anterior fontanelle. This usually closes at around 18 months of age.[15,17] Hair is inspected for pigmentation, texture, quantity, distribution, and shine.[3,9,15] Hair should appear smooth, uniformly thick, and evenly distributed.[2,5,9] The clinician loosely grasps a small section of hair and tugs gently.[2] Hair should not be easily pluckable.[2,5,9] See **TABLE 3.7** for examples of abnormal hair and scalp findings related to specific nutritional deficiencies.

The clinician inspects the eyes for color of the conjunctiva and sclera. The conjunctiva is the transparent mucous membrane that lines the eyelids and covers the

TABLE 3.5 Potential Deficiencies Associated With Certain Diseases or Conditions

Disease or Condition	Potential Deficiencies	Potential Etiology
Cystic fibrosis, pancreatic insufficiency	Fat-soluble vitamins (A, D, E, K), zinc, essential fatty acids	Fat malabsorption
Biliary disease	Fat-soluble vitamins (A, D, E, K)	Fat malabsorption
Liver disease	Vitamin K, essential fatty acids	Malabsorption
Celiac disease	Vitamin A, vitamin D, vitamin K, essential fatty acids, zinc, copper, niacin, folate, riboflavin, vitamin B_{12}	Malabsorption
Inflammatory bowel disease, Crohn's disease	Vitamin A, vitamin D, vitamin K, niacin, essential fatty acids, zinc, iron, folate, selenium, calcium, vitamin B_{12}	Malabsorption, medication interactions, impaired absorption
Chronic diarrhea	Zinc, vitamin A, folate, copper, magnesium, vitamin B_{12}	Malabsorption
Intestinal failure	Zinc, calcium, magnesium; duodenal involvement: iron, folate	Malabsorption
Renal disease	Zinc, copper, iron, magnesium	Increased elimination
Dialysis	Water-soluble vitamins, especially vitamin C	Filtered out in dialysis
Prematurity	Vitamin D, calcium, essential fatty acids, if receiving human milk: iron	Decreased stores
Burns	Vitamin A, vitamin C, zinc	Increased elimination
Chylothorax	Essential fatty acids	Malabsorption
Post–solid organ transplantation	Magnesium	Medication interaction
Seizure disorder	Vitamin D, folate, biotin	Medication interaction
Vegetarians	Zinc, iron, calcium; vegans (and breastfed infants of vegans): vitamin B_{12}	Decreased intake
Long-term parenteral nutrition	Iron, zinc, biotin	Decreased intake

Data from Jen M, Yan AC. Syndromes associated with nutritional deficiency and excess. *Clin Dermatol.* 2010;28:669–685.[46]
Leonberg B, ed. *Pediatric Nutrition Care Manual.* Chicago, IL: Academy of Nutrition and Dietetics; 2013.[47]

sclera (white of the eye). Ask about changes in vision and palpate for dryness and cracks.[9] Eyes should be bright and clear with a smooth cornea and membranes should be pink and moist.[2] To perform a full eye exam the patient must be able to understand and follow directions, so the exam may be limited by the developmental stage of the patient. The clinician asks the patient to open his/her eyes wide and to look to the right and to the left. With younger children, point in the direction you want the child to look versus using "right" and "left." While the patient is looking from side to side, the clinician shines a light across, not into, the eye in order to inspect the cornea. Inspect the lower eyelid by gently pulling just below the eye.[2] See **TABLE 3.8** for examples of abnormal eye findings related to specific nutritional deficiencies.

TABLE 3.6 Skin Findings Related to Nutritional Deficiencies

Abnormal Findings	Potential Deficiencies
Pallor	Iron, B vitamins, copper
Petechiae	Vitamin C
Ecchymosis (bruising)	Vitamin K
Seborrheic dermatitis, scaly, rough, dry	Vitamin A, essential fatty acids, B vitamins
Red scaly rash on face, neck, hands	Zinc
Non-healing wounds	Vitamin C, zinc, vitamin A

Data from Kilde K, Nitzsche L. Nutrition-focused physical examination: a head-to-toe approach with a focus on micronutrient deficiencies. *Support Line.* 2016;38(4):3–9.[2]
Pogatshnik C, Hamilton C. Nutrition-focused physical examination: skin, nails, hair, eyes, and oral cavity. *Support Line.* 2011;33(2):7–13.[3]
Esper DH. Utilization of nutrition-focused physical assessment in identifying micronutrient deficiencies. *Nutr Clin Pract.* 2015;30(2):194–202.[9]

TABLE 3.7 Hair and Scalp Findings Related to Nutritional Deficiencies

Abnormal Findings	Potential Deficiencies
Alopecia, dull, lackluster, thin, sparse hair	Protein, iron, zinc, essential fatty acids, biotin
Corkscrew, coiled hair	Vitamin C
Alopecia, fine, sparse hair	Zinc, biotin, essential fatty acids, selenium, iron
Hypopigmentation	Selenium, zinc
Open anterior fontanelle >18 months of age	Vitamin D
Scaly, flaky scalp	Essential fatty acids

Data from Kilde K, Nitzsche L. Nutrition-focused physical examination: a head-to-toe approach with a focus on micronutrient deficiencies. *Support Line.* 2016;38(4):3–9.[2]
Pogatshnik C, Hamilton C. Nutrition-focused physical examination: skin, nails, hair, eyes, and oral cavity. *Support Line.* 2011;33(2):7–13.[3]
Esper DH. Utilization of nutrition-focused physical assessment in identifying micronutrient deficiencies. *Nutr Clin Pract.* 2015;30(2):194–202.[9]
Goldberg LJ, Lenzy Y. Nutrition and hair. *Clin Dermatol.* 2010;28:412–419.[49]

The examination of the oral cavity should include the lips, the mucous membranes, the gums, the teeth, and the tongue.[2,3,9,48] A Speech-Language Pathologist may be a resource when assessing the oral cavity. When assessing the oral cavity, ask the patient or the parents about any problems with changes in taste or difficulty chewing.[5,48] Children may have loose teeth that may interfere with eating. Inflamed gums may occur just before tooth eruption in infants and during the early childhood years.[17] Mouth lesions that are painful, whether nutritional in origin or not, can compound malnutrition because intake might be decreased.[5] The cells in the oral cavity rapidly turn over (~3–5 days), so the oral cavity is a good place to assess any recent changes in nutrient intake.[2,9,48] A recent diet history is useful to support the examination findings. Additionally, a follow-up examination of the oral cavity is useful in order to assess the effectiveness of nutritional interventions.[48] A penlight, tongue depressors, and disposable gloves are useful during the oral cavity examination.[48]

First inspect the lips for symmetry, color, edema, and surface abnormalities.[2,5,48] Lips should be smooth, moist, and without sores.[2,48] Ask the patient to open his/her mouth or gently open the patient's mouth with a gloved hand. Using the penlight and tongue depressor or your finger, inspect the mucous membranes of the oral cavity. The mucous membranes should be pinkish-red, smooth, and moist.[5,48] Inspect the gums which should be slightly stippled, light pink to dark

TABLE 3.8 Eye Findings Related to Nutritional Deficiencies

Abnormal Findings	Potential Deficiencies
Itching, burning, corneal inflammation	Riboflavin, niacin
Night blindness, foamy spots on eyes (Bitot's spots)	Vitamin A
Pale conjunctiva	Iron, folate, vitamin B_{12}
Abnormal dryness	Vitamin A
Conjunctival inflammation	Riboflavin

Data from Kilde K, Nitzsche L. Nutrition-focused physical examination: a head-to-toe approach with a focus on micronutrient deficiencies. *Support Line.* 2016;38(4):3–9.[2]
Pogatshnik C, Hamilton C. Nutrition-focused physical examination: skin, nails, hair, eyes, and oral cavity. *Support Line.* 2011;33(2):7–13.[3]
Collins N, Harris C. The physical assessment revisited: inclusion of the nutrition-focused physical exam. *Ostomy Wound Manage.* 2010;56(11):18–22.[5]
Esper DH. Utilization of nutrition-focused physical assessment in identifying micronutrient deficiencies. *Nutr Clin Pract.* 2015;30(2):194–202.[9]

pink, and follow a curved line around each tooth.[2,5] The gums should not bleed easily.[48] Ask the patient to stick out his/her tongue.[48] Inspect the tongue for swelling, color, coating, ulcerations, and size.[5,48] The tongue will be moist, appear a dull red color, and appear rough (due to papillae).[2,5,48] See **TABLE 3.9** for examples of abnormal oral cavity findings related to specific nutritional deficiencies.

Nail Assessment

When inspecting the nail plates, look for color, length, shape, symmetry, and texture.[2,3,9] Also look for the presence or absence of lunulae, the white crescent-shaped area on the proximal nail plate.[50] Rub a finger across the nail plate to assess the shape and texture of it, and then apply light pressure to the tips of the nails and note any color changes.[2] Nail plates should be smooth, hard, securely attached to the nail bed, and appear symmetrical.[2,3] Nail plates should blanch when light pressure is applied and then return to their usual pink color.[2] If an inconsistency is noted on just one or two nails, it is most likely related to an injury and not nutritionally related. See **TABLE 3.10** for examples of abnormal nail findings related to specific nutritional deficiencies.

TABLE 3.9 Oral Cavity Findings Related to Nutritional Deficiencies

Abnormal Findings	Potential Deficiencies
Dry, cracked lips	Dehydration
Cheilosis and angular stomatitis	Riboflavin, pyridoxine, niacin
Bleeding gums	Vitamin C, riboflavin
Bright red marginal discoloration of gums	Vitamin A
Pallor of the mucous membranes	Iron, folate, vitamin B_{12}, biotin
Smooth red tongue	Niacin, vitamin B_{12}
Glossitis	Riboflavin, niacin, folic acid, vitamin B_{12}, pyridoxine
Reddened tongue	Niacin, pyridoxine, folate, vitamin B_{12}, biotin
Magenta tongue	Advanced riboflavin
Tongue edema	Niacin
Dry mouth	Zinc
Thrush	Vitamin C, iron

Data from Kilde K, Nitzsche L. Nutrition-focused physical examination: a head-to-toe approach with a focus on micronutrient deficiencies. *Support Line*. 2016;38(4):3–9.[2]
Pogatshnik C, Hamilton C. Nutrition-focused physical examination: skin, nails, hair, eyes, and oral cavity. *Support Line*. 2011;33(2):7–13.[3]
Collins N, Harris C. The physical assessment revisited: inclusion of the nutrition-focused physical exam. *Ostomy Wound Manage*. 2010;56(11):18–22.[5]
Esper DH. Utilization of nutrition-focused physical assessment in identifying micronutrient deficiencies. *Nutr Clin Pract*. 2015;30(2):194–202.[9]
Radler DR, Lister T. Nutrition deficiencies associated with nutrition-focused physical findings of the oral cavity. *Nutr Clin Pract*. 2013;28(6):710–721.[48]

TABLE 3.10 Nail Findings Related to Nutritional Deficiencies

Abnormal Findings	Potential Deficiencies
Beau's lines (transverse grooves)	Protein, zinc, niacin
Koilonychia (spoon-shaped nails)	Protein, iron
Splinter hemorrhages	Vitamin C
Pallor of the nail plate	Iron
Blanches poorly	Vitamin A, vitamin C
Soft nails	Vitamin A, pyridoxine, vitamin C, vitamin D
Brittle thin nails	Magnesium, selenium, vitamin A

Data from Kilde K, Nitzsche L. Nutrition-focused physical examination: a head-to-toe approach with a focus on micronutrient deficiencies. *Support Line*. 2016;38(4):3–9.[2]
Pogatshnik C, Hamilton C. Nutrition-focused physical examination: skin, nails, hair, eyes, and oral cavity. *Support Line*. 2011;33(2):7–13.[3]
Collins N, Harris C. The physical assessment revisited: inclusion of the nutrition-focused physical exam. *Ostomy Wound Manage*. 2010;56(11):18–22.[5]
Esper DH. Utilization of nutrition-focused physical assessment in identifying micronutrient deficiencies. *Nutr Clin Pract*. 2015;30(2):194–202.[9]
Cashman MW, Sloan SB. Nutrition and nail disease. *Clin Dermatol*. 2010;28:420–425.[50]

🔍 CASE STUDY

Assessment

C.W. is a 12-year-old male with a history of dilated cardiomyopathy who has been admitted to the surgical ward of a pediatric hospital for ventricular assist device (VAD) placement. Poor wound healing is noted postoperatively. Admission weight is 40 kilograms (44th percentile, z = –0.16), height is 59 inches (49th percentile, z = –0.03), BMI = 17.8 (48th percentile, z = –0.04). No weight loss was reported before admission, and his weight remains stable 1 week after surgery. MUAC = 21.2 centimeters (14th percentile, z = –1.10). Normalized HGS at preoperative evaluation was 0.45 (~25th percentile using Peterson 2015 reference curves). C.W.'s diet history reveals fair to good appetite with intakes meeting 85%–100% minimum estimated needs. Frequent consumption of processed and convenience foods includes dry cereal, peanut butter crackers, pretzels, rice, and sports drinks. NFPE findings were remarkable for generalized edema, redness at surgical incision with tenderness reported by the nursing staff, tiny white foamy patches seen in the conjunctiva of the eye, and splinter hemorrhages seen in the fingernails on both hands. In addition, C.W. reports worsening vision in low light areas.

Diagnosis

Mild, chronic, illness-related malnutrition related to increased nutrient needs and an inadequate intake of nutrient-dense foods as evidenced by a MUAC z-score of –1.1, diet history with adequate kcal and protein intake but inadequate in vitamins and minerals, poor wound healing, and signs of possible vitamin A and C deficiency on NFPE.

Intervention

Nutrition education: stress the importance of consuming nutrient-dense foods to promote wound healing and recovery; collaboration and referral of nutrition care: NFPE findings discussed in patient care rounds, pediatric ophthalmology referral recommended, and labs to be checked with next blood draw including vitamin C, vitamin A, and zinc.

Monitoring and Evaluation

Food and Nutrient Intake: intakes need to be adequate to meet minimum estimated needs for calories, protein, fluid, and micronutrients; Anthropometric Measurements: minimize weight change/loss of lean body mass; Biochemical Data: follow up on lab results for vitamin C, vitamin A, and zinc and replete as indicated.

Discussion

C.W.'s weight and BMI on admission fell within normal ranges since his calorie and protein intakes were likely adequate despite inadequate micronutrient intakes. A z-score below –1 for MUAC is consistent with mild malnutrition and may indicate some loss of lean body mass despite a stable weight, which may have been skewed due to the presence of generalized edema. Vitamin A, vitamin C, and zinc deficiencies are likely, given the presence of poor wound healing and signs and symptoms of deficiencies such as Bitot's spots and splinter hemorrhages. Lab values and subspecialist involvement are needed to confirm. Therapeutic supplementation will be needed, depending on the degree of deficiency. Tolerance to supplementation and response to treatment should be monitored closely. Since a baseline HGS measurement is available before surgery, a repeat measurement may be helpful for evaluating changes in muscle function during the hospitalization.

Review Questions

1. During the examination for micronutrient deficiencies, which area is the best place to note recent changes in nutrient status and follow up on changes once a nutrition intervention has been initiated?
   A. Hair/Scalp
   B. Eyes
   C. Oral Cavity
   D. Nails

2. Which two techniques are the most commonly used in NFPE?
   A. Palpation and Auscultation
   B. Palpation and Inspection
   C. Percussion and Auscultation
   D. Percussion and Inspection

3. Why should NFPE be included in the nutrition assessment of pediatric patients if the malnutrition definition does not include these subjective parameters?

4. Biochemical values are the most reliable way to assess micronutrient status. True or False?

5. Assessment of subcutaneous fat loss includes examination of which of the following?
   A. Eyes, upper arms, scapula, and thigh
   B. Cheeks, hands, posterior calf, and pelvis
   C. Face, upper arms, ribs, and lower back
   D. Temples, triceps, scapula, and pelvis

6. Prominent scapular borders with depressions above, between, and below the scapula is indicative of severe malnutrition. True or False?

7. Handgrip strength is a useful tool to quantify malnutrition in pediatric populations. True or False?

8. List at least five physical findings that may be seen with dehydration.

References

1. Academy of Nutrition and Dietetics. Nutrition care process. Available at: http://www.eatrightpro.org/resources /practice/practice-resources/nutrition-care-process. Accessed January 15, 2018.

2. Kilde K, Nitzsche L. Nutrition-focused physical examination: a head-to-toe approach with a focus on micronutrient deficiencies. *Support Line.* 2016;38(4):3–9.

3. Pogatshnik C, Hamilton C. Nutrition-focused physical examination: skin, nails, hair, eyes, and oral cavity. *Support Line.* 2011;33(2):7–13.

4. Vermilyea S, Slicker J, El-Chammas K, et al. Subjective global nutritional assessment in critically ill children. *J Parenter Enteral Nutr.* 2013;37:659–666.

5. Collins N, Harris C. The physical assessment revisited: inclusion of the nutrition-focused physical exam. *Ostomy Wound Manage.* 2010;56(11):18–22.

6. Secker DJ, Jeejeebhoy KN. Subjective global nutritional assessment for children. *Am J Clin Nutr.* 2007;85: 1083–1089.

7. Mehta NM, Corkins MR, Lyman B, et al. Defining pediatric malnutrition: a paradigm shift toward etiology-related definitions. *J Parenter Enteral Nutr.* 2013;37(4):460–481.

8. White JV, Guenter P, Jensen G, et al. Consensus statement of the Academy of Nutrition and Dietetics/American Society for Parenteral and Enteral Nutrition: characteristics recommended for the identification and documentation of adult malnutrition (undernutrition). *J Acad Nutr Diet.* 2012;112(5):730–738.

9. Esper DH. Utilization of nutrition-focused physical assessment in identifying micronutrient deficiencies. *Nutr Clin Pract.* 2015;30(2):194–202.

10. Corkins MR, Lewis P, Cruse W, Gupta S, Fitzgerald J. Accuracy of infant admission lengths. *Pediatrics.* 2002; 109(6):1108–1111.

11. Wood AJ, Raynes-Greenow CH, Carberry AE, Jeffery HE. Neonatal length inaccuracies in clinical practice and related percentile discrepancies by simple length-board. *J Paediatr Child Health.* 2013;49:199–203.

12. Fischer M, JeVenn A, Hipskind P. Evaluation of muscle and fat loss as diagnostic criteria for malnutrition. *Nutr Clin Pract.* 2015;30(7):239–248.

13. Bouma S. Diagnosing pediatric malnutrition: paradigm shifts of etiology-related definitions and appraisal of the indicators. *Nutr Clin Pract.* 2017;32(1):52–67.

14. Secker DJ, Jeejeebhoy KN. How to perform subjective global nutritional assessment in children. *J Acad Nutr Diet.* 2012;112(3):424–431.

15. Hammond K. The nutritional dimension of physical assessment. *Nutrition.* 1999;15(5):411–419.

16. Moccia L, DeChicco R. Abdominal examinations: a guide for dietitians. *Support Line.* 2011;33(2):16–21.

17. Green Corkins K. Nutrition-focused physical examination in pediatric patients. *Nutr Clin Pract.* 2015;30(2):203–209.

18. The Academy Quality Management Committee. Academy of Nutrition and Dietetics: Revised 2017 scope of practice for the Registered Dietitian Nutritionist. *J Acad Nutr Diet.* 2018;118(1):141–165.

19. Weber DR, Leonard MB, Zemel BS. Body composition analysis in the pediatric population. *Pediatr Endocrinol Rev.* 2012;10(1):130–139.

20. World Health Organization. Child growth standards BMI-for-age. Available at: http://www.who.int/childgrowth /standards/bmi_for_age/en. Accessed January 21, 2018.

21. Centers for Disease Control and Prevention. Clinical growth charts. Available at: https://www.cdc.gov /growthcharts/clinical_charts.htm. Updated June 16, 2017. Accessed January 21, 2018.

22. Mordarski B, Wolff J, eds. *Pediatric Nutrition Focused Physical Exam Pocket Guide.* Chicago, IL: Academy of Nutrition and Dietetics; 2015.

23. Tostevin PM, Ellis H. The buccal pad of fat: a review. *Clin Anat.* 1995;8(6):403–406.

24. OpenStax. *Anatomy & Physiology.* OpenStax CNX. Available at: http://cnx.org/contents/14fb4ad7-39a1-4eee-ab6e -3ef2482e3e22@8.108. Published August 1, 2017. Accessed January 21, 2018.

25. Becker PJ, Carney LN, Corkins MR, et al. Consensus statement of the Academy of Nutrition and Dietetics/American Society for Parenteral and Enteral Nutrition: indicators recommended for the identification and documentation of pediatric malnutrition (undernutrition). *J Acad Nutr Diet.* 2014;114(12):1988–2000.

26. World Health Organization. Child growth standards arm circumference-for-age. Available at: http://www.who.int /childgrowth/standards/ac_for_age/en. Accessed January 21, 2018.

27. Abdel-Rahman SM, Bi C, Thaete K. Construction of lambda, mu, sigma values for determining mid-upper arm circumference z scores in U.S. children aged 2 months through 18 years. *Nutr Clin Pract.* 2017;32(1):68–76.

28. PediTools. Available at: www.peditools.org. Accessed January 21, 2018.

29. Centers for Disease Control and Prevention. National Health and Nutrition Examination Survey (NHANES) anthropometry procedures manual. Available at: https:// wwwn.cdc.gov/nchs/data/nhanes/2017–2018/manuals /2017_Anthropometry_Procedures_Manual.pdf. Accessed January 21, 2018.

30. De Onis M, Onyango AW, Van den Broeck J, Chumlea WC, Martorell R. Measurement and standardization protocols for anthropometry used in the construction of a new international growth reference. *Food Nutr Bull.* 2004;25 (suppl 1):S27–S36.

31. Corkins KG, Teague EE. Pediatric nutrition assessment: anthropometrics to zinc. *Nutr Clin Pract.* 2017;32(1): 40–51.

32. ExRx.net. Pectoralis major (clavicular head). Available at: http://www.exrx.net/Muscles/PectoralisClavicular.html. Accessed January 21, 2018.

33. ExRx.net. Deltoid (anterior). Available at: http://www.exrx.net/Muscles/DeltoidAnterior.html. Accessed January 21, 2018.

34. ExRx.net. Deltoid (lateral). Available at: http://www.exrx.net/Muscles/DeltoidLateral.html. Accessed January 21, 2018.

35. ExRx.net. Deltoid (posterior). Available at: http://www.exrx.net/Muscles/DeltoidPosterior.html. Accessed January 21, 2018.

36. ExRx.net. Quadriceps. Available at: http://www.exrx.net/Muscles/Quadriceps.html. Accessed January 21, 2018.

37. Litchford MD. Clinical: biochemical, physical, and functional assessment. In: Mahan LK, Raymond JL, eds. *Krause's Food & the Nutrition Care Process.* 14th ed. St. Louis, MO: Elsevier; 2017:98–121.

38. Centers for Disease Control and Prevention. Milestone checklists [fact sheet]. Available at: https://www.cdc.gov/ncbddd/actearly/pdf/checklists/all_checklists.pdf. Accessed January 21, 2018.

39. Jensen KC, Bellini SG, Derrick JW, Fullmer S, Eggett D. Handgrip strength and malnutrition (undernutrition) in hospitalized versus nonhospitalized children aged 6–14. *Nutr Clin Pract.* 2017;32(5):687–693.

40. Silva C, Amaral TF, Silva D, Oliveira BM, Guerra A. Handgrip strength and nutrition status in hospitalized pediatric patients. *Nutr Clin Pract.* 2014;29(3):380–385.

41. Norman K, Stobäus N, Gonzalez MC, Schulzke JD, Pirlich M. Hand grip strength: outcome predictor and marker of nutritional status. *Clin Nutr.* 2011;30(2):135–142.

42. Peterson MD, Krishnan C. Growth charts for muscular strength capacity with quantile regression. *Am J Prev Med.* 2015;49(6):935–938.

43. Scollard TM. Handgrip strength assessment: a skill to enhance diagnosis of disease-related malnutrition. *Support Line.* 2017;39(2):7–13.

44. Centers for Disease Control and Prevention. National Health and Nutrition Examination Survey (NHANES) muscle strength procedures manual. Available at: https://www.cdc.gov/nchs/data/nhanes/nhanes_11_12/Muscle_Strength_Proc_Manual.pdf. Published April 2011. Accessed January 21, 2018.

45. Fuhrman MP, Parker M. Micronutrient assessment. *Support Line.* 2004;26(1):17–24.

46. Jen M, Yan AC. Syndromes associated with nutritional deficiency and excess. *Clin Dermatol.* 2010;28:669–685.

47. Leonberg B, ed. *Pediatric Nutrition Care Manual.* Chicago, IL: Academy of Nutrition and Dietetics; 2013.

48. Radler DR, Lister T. Nutrition deficiencies associated with nutrition-focused physical findings of the oral cavity. *Nutr Clin Pract.* 2013;28(6):710–721.

49. Goldberg LJ, Lenzy Y. Nutrition and hair. *Clin Dermatol.* 2010;28:412–419.

50. Cashman MW, Sloan SB. Nutrition and nail disease. *Clin Dermatol.* 2010;28:420–425.

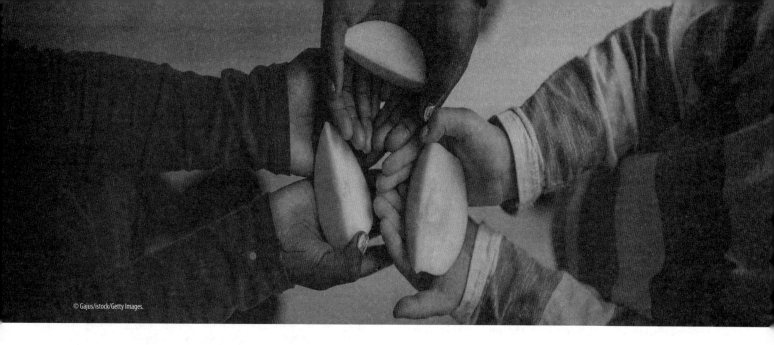

© Gajus/istock/Getty Images.

CHAPTER 4

Malnutrition Related to Undernutrition

Patricia J. Becker

LEARNING OBJECTIVES

- Define illness related and non-illness related pediatric malnutrition.
- Identify pediatric malnutrition utilizing the recommended indicators.
- State the best practice use of z-scores to assess growth in the pediatric population.
- Develop a nutrition care plan for the treatment of mild to moderate and severe malnutrition.

▶ Introduction

When confronted with illness, injury, or trauma, it is understood that well-nourished children have better outcomes than malnourished children. This statement makes it clear that identifying, documenting, and treating malnutrition is essential in the care and treatment of children.

"Malnutrition is at times inevitable. It should not however, be a consequence of inattention from clinicians. The absence of timely nutrition assessment, diagnosis, and implementation of a nutrition care plan for pediatric patients with mild-moderate-severe malnutrition should be a never event."[1]

Defining Pediatric Malnutrition

Over the years, the terms used to describe pediatric malnutrition related to undernutrition have varied and the parameters have been different depending on the author's definition. Historically, these terms have included kwashiorkor, marasmus, underweight, stunting, wasting, and failure to thrive.

The term kwashiorkor was first introduced by Jamaican pediatrician Cicely Williams in her 1935 *Lancet* article and has been used to identify malnutrition that is characterized by severe protein-undernutrition.[2] The terms marasmus and failure to thrive have a more general use and describe undernutrition due to starvation and faltering weight to indicate insufficient weight gain or inappropriate weight loss. The **World Health Organization (WHO)** has defined the terms under-weight, wasting, and stunting.

Other definitions have been proposed and used in practice to varying degrees. Other commonly used definitions include the Waterlow Criteria and the WHO growth indicators, but many others have been proposed.[3,4]

The American Society for Parenteral and Enteral Nutrition defines Pediatric malnutrition related to under-nutrition as an imbalance between nutrient requirement and nutrient intake resulting in a cumulative deficit of energy, protein, or micronutrients that negatively impact growth, development, and relevant outcome.[5]

The Academy of Nutrition and Dietetics uses the **International Dietetics and Nutrition Terminology** (IDNT) definition: Nutrition Diagnostic Terminology. Malnutrition falls into the clinical domain.

The definitions stated in the Nutrition Terminology Reference Manual or eNCPT for Pediatric malnutri-tion are presented in **FIGURES 4.1** and **4.2**. Definitions include both illness-related and non–illness-related mal-nutrition, which is consistent with language used in the Consensus Statement of the Academy of Nutrition and Dietetics/American Society of Enteral and Parenteral Nutrition: Indicators Recommended for the Identifi-cation and Documentation of Pediatric Malnutrition (undernutrition).[6] **TABLE 4.1** describes the recommended

Definition: Nutrient deficit or imbalance due to disease or injury, which may negatively affect growth, development, and/or other outcomes.

Etiology: (cause/contributing risk factors) Factors gathered during the nutrition assessment process that contribute to the existence or the maintenance of pathophysiological, psychosocial, situational, developmental, cultural, and/or environmental problems.

Physiological causes increasing nutrient needs due to prematurity, genetic/congenital disorders, illness, injury, trauma. Inadequate intake related to anorexia or feeding intolerance. Alteration in gastrointestinal structure or function. Alterations in nutrient utilization. Food and nutrition knowledge deficit and other psychological causes such as depression or disease.

Signs/Symptoms: Defining characteristics. A typical cluster of subjective and objective signs and symptoms gathered during the nutrition assessment process that provide evidence that a problem exists; quantify the problem and describe its severity.[7]

Modified from Academy of Nutrition and Dietetics. Terminology Reference Manual (eNCPT). Dietetics language for nutrition care. Illness/non-illness related pediatric malnutrition (undernutrition). Available at: *NCPT.webauthor.com*. Accessed December 10, 2017.[8]

FIGURE 4.2 Illness-Related Pediatric Malnutrition (Undernutrition) (NC-4.1.5)[7]

indictors for the identification and diagnosis of pediatric malnutrition related to undernutrition.

This information and the definitions can be helpful in making the diagnosis of malnutrition.

Acute vs. Chronic

It is important to consider the duration of malnutri-tion in its identification, documentation, and treat-ment. Acute conditions are generally considered to be 3 months' duration or fewer while chronic conditions are 3 months or more. Acute malnutrition, such as that seen in the critical care setting, can have high incidence of mortality in children if left untreated.[9] Chronic mal-nutrition can lead to lifelong deficits in height, health, and cognitive function.

Classification and Characterization of Pediatric Malnutrition

In 2012, The Academy of Nutrition and Dietetics Malnutrition Work Group and the **American Society for Parenteral and Enteral Nutrition** (A.S.P.E.N.) Malnutrition Task Force have recommended defin-ing characteristics for identifying and documenting adult undernutrition.[10] These recommendations include etiology-based definitions and characteristics for diag-nosing moderate and severe malnutrition.

Definition: Inadequate nutrient intake due to environmental or behavioral factors, which may negatively affect growth, development, and/or other outcomes.

Etiology: (cause/contributing risk factors) Factors gathered during the nutrition assessment process that contribute to the existence or the maintenance of pathophysiological, psychosocial, situational, developmental, cultural, and or environmental problems, such as lack of or limited access to food, eg, economic constraints, restricting food/feedings given to children, neglect or abuse, adoption/immigration/refugee from or in poorly resourced or conflict-torn countries. Interruption or intolerance to feedings. Social, economic, behavioral, cultural, or religious practices that affect access to food.

Signs/Symptoms: Defining characteristics. A typical cluster of subjective and objective signs and symptoms gathered during the nutrition assessment process that provide evidence that a problem exists; quantify the problem and describe its severity.

Modified from Academy of Nutrition and Dietetics. Terminology Reference Manual (eNCPT). Dietetics language for nutrition care. Illness/non-illness related pediatric malnutrition (undernutrition). Available at: *NCPT.webauthor.com*. Accessed December 10, 2017.[8]

FIGURE 4.1 Non–illness-Related Pediatric Malnutrition (Undernutrition) (NC-4.1.4)[7]

TABLE 4.1 Potential Indicators of Malnutrition Diagnosis

Nutrition Assessment Category	Potential Indicator of this Nutrition Diagnosis
Anthropometric measurements	When a single data point is available **Mild malnutrition** −1 to −1.99 wt. for length/BMI for age z-score/MUAC z-score **Moderate malnutrition** −2 to −2.99 wt. for length/BMI for age z-score/MUAC z-score **Severe malnutrition** −3 or below wt. for length z-score/BMI for age z-score/MUAC z-score/length or height for age z-score When 2 or more data points are available **Mild malnutrition** 75%–51% of the norm wt. gain velocity in children 24 mo. or younger 5% loss usual body weight ages 2 to 18 years Decline of one standard deviation (z-score) in weight for length or BMI for age **Moderate malnutrition** 50%–26% of the norm wt. gain velocity in children 24 mo. or younger 7.5% loss usual body weight ages 2 to 18 years Decline of two standard deviation (z-score) in wt. for length or BMI for age **Severe malnutrition** 25% < of the norm wt. gain velocity in children 24 mo. or younger 10% or greater loss usual body weight ages 2 to 18 years Decline of three standard deviation (z-score) in wt. for length or BMI for age
Nutrition-focused physical findings	Stagnation in Tanner Stages or other developmental milestones **Moderate malnutrition** Mild loss of Sub Q fat: orbital, triceps, fat on ribs. Mild muscle loss, wasting at temples (temporalis muscle) clavicles (pectoralis & deltoids) shoulders (deltoids) interosseous muscles, scapula, thigh, calf. Mild, localized edema or generalized fluid accumulation. **Severe malnutrition** Severe loss of Sub Q at: eg, orbital, triceps, fat on ribs. Severe muscle loss, eg, wasting of the temples, clavicles, shoulders, interosseous muscles, scapula, thigh, calf. Severe, localized edema or generalized fluids accumulation.
Food/nutrition related history	Reports or observations of: changes in functional indicators: handgrip strength, hours of play, nap time, or other measures of physical activity or strength. Norms for handgrip strength for children ages 6+ yrs are available. **Mild malnutrition** 75%–51% of estimated energy/protein need **Moderate malnutrition** 50%–26% of estimated energy/protein need **Severe malnutrition** 25% or less of estimated energy/protein need
Client history	Report or observation of: Diagnosis that limits food intake: such as Anorexia Nervosa, avoidant restrictive food intake disorder, abuse, neglect, existing diagnosis of malnutrition or failure to thrive.

Modified from Academy of Nutrition and Dietetics. Terminology Reference Manual (eNCPT). Dietetics language for nutrition care. Illness/non-illness related pediatric malnutrition (undernutrition). Available at: *NCPT.webauthor.com*. Accessed December 10, 2017.[8]

These etiology-based malnutrition definitions included three types: starvation-related malnutrition, chronic disease-related malnutrition, and acute disease/injury-related malnutrition. There are six characteristics recommended for diagnosis, which include the following:

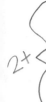

- Insufficient energy intake
- Weight loss
- Loss of muscle mass
- Loss of subcutaneous fat
- Localized or overall fluid accumulation, which may mask weight loss
- Diminished functional capacity measured by hand grip strength

These criteria, depending on the extent, can quantify the severity of the malnutrition. Given that no single parameter is definitive for adult malnutrition, the presence of two or more of these characteristics is recommended for diagnosis. For growing children, the characteristics recommended for diagnosis must be different from those recommended for adults.[11]

For children, the A.S.P.E.N. Pediatric Malnutrition Definition Workgroup summarized the definition of malnutrition as an imbalance between nutrient requirements and intake that results in cumulative deficits of energy, protein, or micronutrients that may negatively affect growth, development, and other relevant outcomes. The workgroup also made recommendations for defining, identifying, and documenting pediatric malnutrition that include five criteria domains consisting of anthropometric variables, growth, chronicity of malnutrition, etiology of malnutrition, and the impact of malnutrition on functional status. As with the adult definitions, the pediatric definitions contain criteria related to severity and the presence of illness or non–illness-related factors.

1. Illness-related
   a. Definition: disease- or trauma-specific caused by nutrient imbalance and associated with negative outcome(s)
   b. Etiology: the specific cause of illness-related malnutrition
   c. Severity: based on the deterioration of markers of growth and development
   d. Chronicity: should be identified as either acute (<3 months) or chronic (>3 months)
2. Non–illness-related
   a. Definition: malnutrition related to environmental or behavioral factors caused by nutrient imbalance and associated with negative outcomes
   b. Severity: based on the deterioration of markers of growth and development
   c. Chronicity: should be identified as either acute (being of short duration, <3 months), or chronic (being of long duration, >3 months)

Using the recommendations of the A.S.P.E.N. work group, the pediatric dietitian can employ several indicators to identify and document pediatric malnutrition.[5]

▶ Anatomy, Physiology, and Pathology of Condition

The impact of malnutrition on the health of children is significant. It affects every organ and system of the body, it can have a prolonged duration, and, in some cases, such as with stunting, it can be permanent and lifelong.

Impact of Malnutrition on Critical Illness

In a study reported in the *Journal of Parenteral and Enteral Nutrition*, malnourished children in intensive care were reported to be at greater risk of poor outcomes when compared with well-nourished children. Malnourished children with hyperglycemia were at a greater risk of mortality, independent of clinical severity. Hypoglycemia was shown to be associated with mortality, longer length of ICU stay, and fewer ventilator-free days only in malnourished children.[12]

Impact of Malnutrition on Cardiac Disease

Children with heart defects, who are also malnourished, experience longer lengths of stay both in the hospital and in the ICU. One study found the prevalence of acute protein-energy malnutrition and chronic protein-energy malnutrition to be as high as 51.2% and 40.5%, respectively. The median hospital stay for mild, moderate, and severe chronic protein-energy malnutrition was 31, 20, and 22.5 days, vs. a normal 15 days. Malnourished cardiac patients also required longer periods of time to achieve nutrient intake goals. The average number of children whose energy and protein requirement goals were met by day 7 were 68 ± 27% and 68 ± 40%, respectively.

Nearly half of the patients were malnourished during their admission and during their admission, only two-thirds of their recommended caloric and protein requirements were provided within the first 7 days of admission.[13]

Impact of Malnutrition on Cognitive Function

In a study of preschool children, chronic and acute malnutrition were associated with stunting, selenium deficiency, and poor cognitive performance in the population studied compared with controls.[14]

Impact of Malnutrition on Quality of Life, Hospital Length of Stay, and Disease Complication

In a prospective, multicenter study, children with BMI for age z-scores -2 or below had longer lengths of stay, increased incidence of gastrointestinal and infectious complications, and reduced quality of life.[15]

▶ Condition-Specific Nutrition Screening

Nutrition screening is the first step in identifying the child who is at risk of malnutrition. The nutrition screen can be performed by any healthcare provider and is intended to be a quick and simple tool to trigger a further assessment. Stated simply, screening determines the risk of malnutrition where assessment determines the presence of malnutrition.

A screening tool should be quick and easy to administer and meet the goals of the organization, whether that is to determine malnutrition risk or the presence of malnutrition, or to improve outcomes such as reducing a length of stay.

Presently, there are several nutrition screening tools for children, including the **Nutrition Risk Score** (NRS)[16], the **Pediatric Nutrition Risk Score** (PNRS), the **Screening Tool for the Assessment of Malnutrition in Pediatrics** (STAMP), the **Pediatric York Malnutrition Score** (PYMS)[17], and the **Screening Tool for Risk Of Impaired Nutritional Status and Growth** (STRONGKIDS).[18,19,20]

The criteria to determine malnutrition varies somewhat among the tools, although they have some criteria in common. **TABLE 4.2** lists the criteria for malnutrition used in several nutrition screening tools for children.

For more in-depth information related to pediatric nutrition screening tools, a systemic review is available on the Academy of Nutrition and Dietetics Evidence Analysis Library on the Topic List under Nutrition Screening Pediatric. (http://www.andeal.org)

▶ Nutrition Assessment

As part of the nutrition assessment for the child with malnutrition, the following parameters should be assessed: illness and non–illness-related conditions, anthropometrics, nutrient intake, functional status, and growth and development.

Illness and Non–illness Related Conditions

Malnutrition can be illness or non-illness related. Some of the factors that may put a child at risk for malnutrition are listed in **TABLE 4.3**.

Anthropometrics

When assessing malnutrition, accurate anthropometric data are essential. Accurate weight and length/height should be obtained by using calibrated equipment by trained staff each time the child presents in the healthcare setting. This vital information, which is easy to obtain, can provide those who care for children with valuable information to improve the outcome of the care provided. Accurate weights and lengths for children under age 2 and heights for children over age 2 at first visit and upon subsequent visits can reduce risk and occurrence of pediatric malnutrition.

TABLE 4.2 Criteria for Malnutrition					
	NRS	**PNRS**	**STAMP**	**PYMS**	**STRONG**
Criteria					
Anthropometrics	X	X		X	X
Weight loss	X	X		X	X
Reduced intake	X	X	X	X	X
Illness/condition severity	X	X	X	X	X
Other		Pain assessment			

TABLE 4.3 Risk Factors for Pediatric Malnutrition

Bone Marrow Transplant	Congenital Heart Defect	Congenital Renal Defects/Anomalies
Solid tumor cancer	Heart failure	Kidney failure
Treatment side effects	Preterm birth	Genetic Anomalies
Third-degree burns	Malabsorption syndrome	Behavioral disorders
Major trauma	Inflammatory bowel disease	Homelessness/food insecurity
Critical Illness	Short bowel syndrome	Neglect
Spinal muscular atrophy	Congenital gastrointestinal anomalies	Famine
Feeding Disorders	Cystic fibrosis	Abuse

Measuring Weight, Length, Height, and Mid-upper Arm Circumference

Accuracy of anthropometric measurements is essential for assessing a child's nutritional status and identifying pediatric malnutrition. Healthcare providers must employ consistent, accurate, and precise techniques when obtaining anthropometric measurements.

The procedures in **TABLE 4.4** for obtaining growth parameters have been recommended by the WHO and the American Academy of Pediatrics.

Nutrient Intake

Assessing a child's nutrient intake includes determining what is eaten orally, as well as what is provided parenterally and enterally by feeding tube. Oral intake can be assessed by obtaining information from caregivers. Oral, enteral, and parenteral intake information may be available in the child's medical records. Daily food records or food diaries, calorie counts, and food frequency questionnaires may also be used to obtain nutrient intake information.

TABLE 4.4 Measuring Weight, Length, Height, and Mid-upper Arm Circumference

Measurement	Equipment	Procedure
Seated weight: measure of infants and small children (as able) who are unable to stand.	Flatbed scale that allows child to sit or recline	1. Undress child, preferably without diaper. If this is not possible, change child to a dry diaper that has been weighed and subtract weight of dry diaper from weight measurement. 2. Place a clean paper liner on scale tray. 3. Calibrate the scale to zero. 4. Place the infant on the scale tray. 5. Ensure that the infant is not touching objects beyond the scale tray. 6. Note the measurement and record to the nearest 0.1 kilogram.
Standing weight: measure the child ≥2 years of age who can stand unassisted.	Digital scale that records in pounds or kilograms.	1. Ensure child is in light clothing without shoes, preferably in underclothes. 2. Calibrate scale to zero. 3. Place child on scale.

Measurement	Equipment	Procedure
		4. Ensure that the child is in the center of the scale, feet together, heels touching, standing erect with arms at sides. 5. Activate digital scale for measurement. Read and record weight to the nearest 0.1 kilogram.
Recumbent length: for children, up to 24 months of age or in older children who are unable to stand. Two attendants are required, one to hold the child and one to perform the measurement.	Length board with a fixed headboard and moveable footboard positioned perpendicular to the base with a ruler along one side.	1. Ensure child is dressed in light clothing without shoes. 2. Place the child on the board lying on his or her back. 3. Hold the crown of the head and bring it into contact with the fixed head board. 4. While the head remains in contact with the headboard, the second attendant grasps the legs at the ankles to extend the legs. 5. Move the footboard to rest firmly against the heels, making sure the toes point upwards and the knees are flat against the base. 6. Read and record the value of the measurement on the ruler at the side of the base and record the value to the nearest 0.1 centimeter.
Standing height: measure the child ≥2 years of age who can stand unassisted.	Fixed ruler/ measure device attached to a wall, block squared at right angles or moveable head projection attached at right angles to the device. A stadiometer is a good example of such a device.	1. In stockings or bare feet, the child should stand with his or her back to the wall, with heels together. Back straight; arms at sides; heels, head, back, and shoulders touching the wall or vertical surface of the device. Assistance from another adult to ensure knees and ankles are steady may be needed. The child's line of vision should be horizontal. 2. Place the head projection upon the crown of the child's head. 3. Hold the block/bar steady and have the child step away from the device. 4. Note the measurement and record to the nearest 0.1 centimeter. 5. Repeat this measurement three times to ensure accuracy.
MUAC: the charts for normal values for MUAC use the right arm. The left arm may be used if it is the dominant arm or if the right arm has an IV line or port-a-cath. Consistent use of the same arm is the most important factor.	Firm, non-stretch measuring tape.	1. Remove clothing from the arm to be measured. 2. Place the child in a seated position, facing forward. Infants may be held by an adult on the lap. 3. Place the child's right arm with the right hand on the right hip at a right (90°) angle. 4. Measure the length of the arm from the acronium process of the scapula to the olecranon (elbow tip). Note the mid-point. Mark with sticker. 5. Measure around the arm at the level of the mark with firm contact, without compression of the soft tissue. 6. Note the measurement. Record to the nearest 0.1 centimeter.

Data from Wonoputri N, Djais J, Rosalina I. Validity of nutritional screening tools for hospitalized children. *J Nutr Metab*. 2014. Epub 2014 Sep 2014.[20]

Duggan MB. 2010. Anthropometry as a tool for measuring malnutrition: impact of the new WHO growth standards and references. *Ann Trop Paediatr*. 2010;30:1–7.[21]

Height and Weight Measurement. Child Guidelines. Available at: www.ihs.gov/hwm/index.cfm?module=dsp_hwm_child_guidelines. Accessed May 2017.[22]

Centers for Disease Control and Prevention. Measuring children's height and weight accurately. Available at: www.cdc.gov/healthyweight/assessing/bmi/childrens_bmi/measuring_children.html. Accessed May 2017.[23]

World Health Organization. Job aid: weighing and measuring a child. Available at: www.who.int/childgrowth/training/jobaid_weighing_measuring.pdf. Accessed May 2017.[24]

▶ Growth and Development

Developmental Milestones

Malnutrition may impact the timing when a child achieves developmental milestones. Muscle weakness, lethargy, and growth retardation may impact a child's ability to sit, stand, crawl, and walk at age appropriate time periods. Assessing developmental milestones should be part of a comprehensive nutrition assessment of a child. (WHO growth standards) **FIGURE 4.3** shows the developmental milestones by age.

Growth Charts

Anthropometric measures should be recorded and assessed in relation to population standards by using standardized growth charts.

Growth charts are an essential tool when assessing growth. They allow the practitioner to assess the degree to which the infant or child's nutritional needs are being met to support adequate growth.

The WHO charts, released in 2006, are based on data collected by the WHO **Multicenter Growth Reference Study** (MGRS). This study was designed to produce a standard that defines how a child should grow and any deviations from the standard are evidence of abnormal growth.[25]

The MGRS data are based on healthy children living under conditions favorable to achieving their full genetic growth potential. It included data gathered between 1997 and 2003 from a diverse sample from six countries including the United States. Children in the study were followed from birth to 71 months of age who were exclusively breastfed until at least 4 months of age and the initiation of complimentary food was deferred until 6 months of age.[25,26]

As the data from the MGRS did not include older children, it is recommended that the CDC 2 to 20 years' growth chart be used for children greater than 24 months

of age. The Centers for Disease Control and Prevention, the American Academy of Pediatrics, the American Academy of Nutrition and Dietetics, and the Department of Health and Human Services recommend using the WHO growth charts for ages 0–24 months and the CDC growth charts for ages 2 to 20 years of age.[27,28] The WHO growth chart can be found at: http://www.who.int/childgrowth/standards/en/ while the CDC growth charts can be found at: http://www.cdc.gov/growthcharts/zscore.htm.

Mid-Upper Arm Circumference (muAc)

In parts of the world where obtaining anthropometric measurements for children has been difficult, MUAC has been a valuable tool in identifying pediatric malnutrition due to undernutrition. MUAC tapes are portable and inexpensive compared with scales and stadiometers.

In the past, a fixed cut-off value of 12.5–13 cm has been used to identify malnutrition in children less than 5 years of age. However, this did not accurately identify malnutrition in infants, very young children, and older children. Recent data show that MUAC z-scores that adjust for differences of age and sex are a more useful indicator than a fixed cut-off value. Differences according to age can be striking. The WHO found that the fixed cut-off value identified a much lower rate of malnutrition in children compared with the use of age- and gender-specific z-score charts.[29]

MUAC also has relevant use in ambulatory and acute care settings. Other anthropometric measures can be inaccurate or skewed due to a variety of factors. Height may be difficult to obtain in children with developmental disorders, such as cerebral palsy. Weight may be skewed by fluid retention, peritoneal dialysate, casts, or other medical devices. Identifying malnutrition with MUAC using z-score tables will allow the pediatric dietitian to diagnose undernutrition and assess the effectiveness of nutrition interventions in children with medical conditions.[30, 31]

Age in months	4	6	8	10	12	14	16	18
	Sits without support							
		Stands with assistance						
		Crawls						
			Stands alone					
				Walks alone				

FIGURE 4.3 Child Developmental Milestones

Several tools are available for measuring MUAC that can help to facilitate more accurate measurement. Some tools even include a hand grip with a retractable tape that measures MUAC using a single hand, allowing the clinician to help hold the child's arm at a right angle for a more accurate measurement. MUAC measuring tapes are available through the **United Nations Children's Fund** (UNICEF) supply division. A new standard MUAC tape was made available in May 2009 when the WHO and UNICEF issued a joint statement on WHO child growth standards and the identification of severe acute malnutrition in infants and children.

z-scores

The definition of a z-score line on a growth chart is a score that indicates how far a measurement is from the median score, which is zero. Also, known as a standard deviation score, the reference lines on the chart are called z-score lines.

Why z-scores Are Best

The advantages of using z-scores to describe growth status in children include:

- Percentiles are intended to be stated as intervals. For example, if a child's weight for length is between the 10th percentile and the 25th percentile, it must be stated as such. It should not be stated as the 18th percentile even though that number may be suggested by the electronic health record system.
- z-scores allow for the statement of a precise and discrete number. This is of particular value if a child falls below the percentiles (such as below the 5th percentile). As improvement or decline is difficult to express.
- z-scores outside of +2 and −2 are more likely to be abnormal.
- The z-score scale is linear. Therefore, a fixed interval of z-scores has a fixed height difference in centimeters or weight difference in kilograms for all children of the same age. This means that the number of centimeters between z-score limits is the same number, whether it is between −1 and −2 or between a z-score of zero and a z-score of +1. This allows for comparison and statistical analysis.
- z-scores have the same statistical relationship to the distribution around the mean at all ages, so the results are comparable across age groups and indicators.
- The use of z-scores can help determine a precise score for children who might fall above the 97th percentile or below the 3rd percentile on a standard growth chart.
- z-scores are widely recognized as the best system for analysis and presentation of anthropometric data because a group of z-scores can be subjected to summary statistics such as mean and standard deviation.

Using z-score growth charts is very much like using growth charts that have percentiles. When plotting body mass index- (BMI-) for-age for a girl who is 12 years old, you would plot the point of intersection for her age and her BMI. For example, a 12-year-old girl with a BMI of 18 would plot with a z-score of zero. Given that a z-score of zero is at the median for her age, this is considered ideal, as would a BMI-for-age at the 50th percentile. Also, as with growth charts that use percentiles, when using z-score growth charts, the practitioner can assess a single data point in relation to the median or zero z-score line. With multiple data points, the practitioner can assess growth trends. A diagnosis of malnutrition can only be determined using z-scores.

Children who are growing well will follow a trend (or track) that is parallel to the median and z-score lines. Indications that there are issues with growth can include plotted points that cross z-score lines. This can present as a sharp incline or decline in the child's track or when the child's growth trend stagnates (eg, remains flat on the growth chart) due to no gain in weight or stature.

A trend of plotted anthropometric measurement points that cross z-score lines suggests possible nutrition risk. When the trend is toward the median or the zero z-score line, this generally indicates a positive trend and that the child is growing appropriately. However, when the growth track for the child trends away from the median z-score line, a problem with growth might be present.

Growth Velocity
Growth Velocity Charts

Growth and the standards for rates of growth are based on the WHO's Multi-Center Growth Reference Study (MGRS) Child Growth Standards. Growth velocity based charts for weight and height or length are available in monthly increments. Normal rates of growth, gains in weight and in height for children who can stand to be measured, or in length for children who are measured in the recumbent position are referred to as weight and height gain velocity. The WHO, as part of the MGRS, established child growth standards that included weight and length/height velocity charts for both girls and boys at birth, at one month of age, at 2 months, at 4 months, and at 6 months of age intervals.

▶ Nutrition Diagnosis

Recommended indictors for identifying and documenting malnutrition in children are available to allow for the standardization of definition and diagnosis. The indicators include weight for length for children ages

TABLE 4.5 Primary Indicators when Only a Single Data Point is Available for Use as a Criterion for Identifying and Diagnosing Malnutrition Related to Undernutrition

Primary Indicator	Mild Malnutrition	Moderate Malnutrition	Severe Malnutrition
Weight for length/height z-score	−1 to −1.9 z-score	−2 to −2.9 z-score	−3 or greater z-score
BMI for age z-score	−1 to −1.9 z-score	−2 to −2.9 z-score	−3 or greater z-score
Length/height z-score	No data	No data	−3 or greater z-score
Mid-upper arm circumference	−1 to −1.9 z-score	−2 to −2.9 z-score	−3 or greater z-score

Reproduced from Becker PJ, et al. Consensus statement of the Academy of Nutrition and Dietetics/American Society for Parenteral and Enteral Nutrition: Indicators recommended for the identification and documentation of pediatric malnutrition (undernutrition) JAND Dec 2014. 114(12):1988–2000. Reprinted with permission.[33]

1 to 24 months of age, BMI for age for children 2 to 18 years of age, length/height for age z-score, mid-upper arm circumference when only a single data point is available or weight gain velocity percentage of the norm, weight loss percentage of usual body weight, decline in weight for length or BMI for age z-score, and inadequate intake when two or more data points are available.[6] The purpose of the recommended indictors is to assist with identifying, diagnosing, and documenting pediatric malnutrition.

Intended Population

The population for whom the recommended indictors are intended include term infants who are 1 month old and children through the 18th year of life. Newborns are not included in the intended population due to the weight loss and regain of birth weight that occurs within the first month of life.

The intended population includes term infants. The definition of term infants is an infant born at 37 weeks postmenstrual age[32] who are day of life 30 or greater. This would include infants who may be admitted to **Neonatal Intensive Care Units** (NICUs) including preterm infants who are of an age corrected to term. The intended population also includes children up to and including the 18th year of life.

Recommended Indicators

Weight for Length/BMI for Age/Height for Age/Mid-upper Arm Circumference

The purpose of growth charts is to identify growth problems. Growth charts for Weight for length/BMI for

age/and Mid-upper arm circumference are available in z-scores for mild, moderate, and severe malnutrition and Height for age z-score for severe malnutrition are presented in **TABLE 4.5**.

When more information about the child is available, a more in-depth assessment is possible and additional indicators may be used. Weight gain velocity is a short-term indictor of poor growth in young children, as is inadequate intake. Weight loss and deceleration in weight for length or BMI for age in older children can also be a sign of growth problems.

Inadequate Energy - Protein Intake Percentage of Estimated Need

Energy needs can be either calculated or estimated by using indirect calorimetry or standard equations. Measured energy calculations are preferred, although it is not always possible. Equations for children include the WHO equation,[34] the Schofield Equation,[35] the 1989 RDA[36] (IOM 2000), and the 2005 DRI.[37]

Weight Loss Percentage of Usual Body Weight

Determining "usual body weight" in a growing child can be problematic. For older children, the child's most recent stable weight can be used; for a young child, the child's highest ever weight can be used.

Primary indicators that are used when there are two or more data points available for use as criteria for identifying and diagnosing malnutrition related to undernutrition are described in **TABLE 4.6**.

TABLE 4.6 Primary Indicators When Two or More Data Points Are Available for Use as a Criterion for Identifying and Diagnosing Malnutrition Related to Undernutrition

Primary Indicator	Mild Malnutrition	Moderate Malnutrition	Severe Malnutrition
Weight gain velocity (<2 years of age)	<75% of the norm for expected weight gain	<50% of the norm for expected weight gain	<25% of the norm for expected weight gain
Weight loss (2 to 20 years of age)	5% usual body weight	7.5% usual body weight	10% usual body weight
Deceleration in weight for length/height or BMI for age	Decline of 1 z-score	Decline across 2 z-score lines	Decline across 3 z-score lines
Inadequate nutrient intake	51%–75% of estimated energy-protein need	26%–50% of estimated energy-protein need	≤25% of estimated energy-protein need

Reproduced from Becker PJ, et al. Consensus statement of the Academy of Nutrition and Dietetics/American Society for Parenteral and Enteral Nutrition: Indicators recommended for the identification and documentation of pediatric malnutrition (undernutrition) JAND Dec 2014. 114(12):1988–2000. Reprinted with permission.[33]

▶ Nutrition Intervention

Once the nutrition diagnosis has been made, a nutrition intervention should be prescribed and implemented. Regarding the malnutrition diagnosis, it means taking into consideration the degree of the child's malnutrition. Development of the intervention includes consulting practice guidelines or other sources of nutrition care recommendations such as feeding protocols.[38]

The benefits of nutrition care protocols are that they standardize care and automate the process of nutrition care rather than leaving them to individuals to plan and initiate the intervention, advance the care, and make modifications.[39]

The development of nutrition care protocols should be evidence-informed and/or based on expert consensus. Nutrition care and feeding protocols are associated with significant improvements in nutrition practice and delivery of nutrition interventions to children.[40]

Feeding protocols include common elements, such as determining protein and energy goals and advancing guidelines to those goals. In a study of nutritional practices and their relationship to clinical outcomes in critically ill children, those for whom feeding protocols were employed had lower rates of infection, independent of severity of illness. Children with the lowest energy intakes, less than 33% of estimated need and an indicator of severe malnutrition, had the highest mortality rates. Children with an energy intake from 33%–66% of estimated need, had a significantly decreased risk of death.

Feeding protocols have been shown to increase both energy and protein intake.[41]

For children diagnosed with severe malnutrition, suboptimal intake has been shown to result in inadequate energy and protein intake resulting in weight loss and reduced weight gain velocity in young children.[42]

Provision of oral nutritional supplements (ONS) is a frequent intervention for a child with mild to moderate malnutrition. In a retrospective analysis of 557,348 hospitalizations of children ages 2–8 years, the use of ONS on length of stay (LOS) and episode cost was assessed. Of the 6066 children prescribed ONS, those hospitalizations with ONS had a lower LOS and a lower episode cost.[43]

In a study of pre-school aged children at risk of malnutrition with BMI for age indicating mild malnutrition and a history of picky eating behavior, ONS plus dietary counseling over a 3-month period led to significantly greater improvement in BMI for age, weight for age, and height for age indicators compared with counseling alone.[44]

Children receiving ONS were found to have higher energy intakes than children who did not receive ONS[45] and children undergoing cancer treatment who consumed ONS were less likely to experience weight loss than children who did not.[46]

One way to ensure the provision and administration of ONS to a hospitalized child is by adding nutritional products to the medication order set and to the medication administration record or MAR. In a quality improvement project, the process of delivery and administration of ONS was examined, revised, and the outcome noted. The result was that 86% more patients received their ONS than before the change.[47]

Nutrition protocols have been shown to improve nutrient intake in the pediatric population. Standardizing care to ensure that optimal nutrient profiles are provided ensures that all of a child's needs are provided for. Implementing a protocol once a diagnosis is made helps the child meet their nutrient goals in the timeliest manner. Medical nutrition therapy for treating malnutrition includes providing a high-calorie, high-protein diet, nutrient-dense foods, frequent meals and snacks, and oral nutritional supplements.

Therefore, the recommendations for feeding protocols for mild and moderate malnutrition include the recommended **medical nutrition therapy** (MNT).[48]

Mild Malnutrition Therapy Protocol

A nutrition protocol for diagnosing mild malnutrition could include recommending a high calorie, high protein diet[48] (1.25–1.5 times estimated protein and/or energy needs), providing oral nutritional supplements[49] and/or education on increasing the child's intake of high calorie, high protein foods, and ingredients added to foods in order to increase the energy and protein content of foods. It is also recommended that an analysis of nutrient intake/calorie count/food record be obtained in order to assess if the child's food intake is meeting his or her needs.

Moderate Malnutrition Nutrition Therapy Protocol

A nutrition protocol for diagnosing moderate malnutrition would include the medical nutrition therapy recommended for treating mild malnutrition. Then, if there is no improvement in the child's nutritional status or if child does not meet nutrition care goals, the protocol guideline would recommend providing appropriate enteral/parenteral nutrition support for up to 50% of nutrient needs until nutrition care goals are met.[50–52]

Severe Malnutrition Nutrition Therapy Protocol

For children with a diagnosis of severe malnutrition, the recommendation of the protocol would be to provide 100% of the child's nutrient needs by oral, enteral, or parenteral nutrition support until the child improves and meets nutrition care goals, growth goals, or moderate malnutrition criteria, at which time a moderate malnutrition therapy protocol may be implemented.[53,54]

▶ Nutrition Monitoring and Evaluation

The purpose of nutrition monitoring and evaluation is to determine if the nutrition intervention is effective, to measure the amount of progress made, and to assess if goals are being achieved.

What to Monitor

In monitoring for improvement or recovery from malnutrition, a review or reassessment of the following indicators should be completed:

- Weight and weight for age z-score
- Height or length and height or length for age z-score
- Mid-upper arm circumference
- Weight gain velocity
- Height or length gain velocity
- Energy–protein intake percentage of estimated need
- Deceleration or acceleration of weight for length or BMI for age z-score

A review of the nutrition care plan/interventions should be assessed for effectiveness, tolerance, acceptability, and need for modification or advancement. Changes and modifications to the interventions and goals should be made as needed to the nutrition care plan in order to ensure that continued progress to recovery is made.

How Often to Monitor

Currently, there are no set standards for how frequently children with malnutrition should be monitored, although it stands to reason that the more severe the malnutrition, the more frequently the child should be assessed. The healthcare setting to which the child presents will also impact the frequency of assessment and evaluation. A child with a diagnosis of malnutrition who is in the hospital will receive more frequent monitoring than a child in a community setting would.

Suggestions for frequency of monitoring/follow-up are presented in **TABLE 4.7**

Identifying Malnutrition in Preterm and Neonatal Populations

The preterm infant is at high risk for malnutrition. This risk is related to reduced nutrient stores at birth, immature organ systems for nutrient absorption and utilization, delayed advancement of parenteral and enteral feeds, and dependence on the healthcare provider to identify and meet nutritional needs during a period of rapid growth and development.[55] Malnutrition in the preterm infant and neonate can have a lifelong negative impact.

TABLE 4.7 Recommended Timeframes for Monitoring of Pediatric Malnutrition			
Mild Malnutrition	Inpatient: one time per week	Outpatient: one time per month	Community: monthly
Moderate Malnutrition	Inpatient: 1–2 times per week	Outpatient: one time per week	Community: weekly
Severe Malnutrition	Inpatient: every 1–3 days	Outpatient: one time per week	Community: weekly

In early 2018, *The Journal of the Academy of Nutrition and Dietetics* published recommended indicators for identifying malnutrition in preterm infants and neonates. These suggested criteria were authored by an expert panel of Neonatal Registered Dietitians from the Pediatric Nutrition Practice Group. These recommended indictors were evidence informed and consensus driven.[56]

The data used to assess for the presence of malnutrition of the preterm infant or neonate is similar to those used for the pediatric population. Evaluating nutrient intake, anthropometric measurements, and growth velocity are used in order to determine if an infant is malnourished. The 2013 Fenton preterm growth chart or the 2010 Olsen intrauterine growth curves are the reference standard and should be used for infants born at 36 weeks and 6/7 weeks or earlier.[57,58] The WHO child growth standards should be used for infants born at 37 0/7 weeks' gestation and older.

Growth assessment begins at birth by identifying whether an infant is **small for gestational age** (SGA), **appropriate for gestational age** (AGA), or **large for gestational age** (LGA) or has experienced **intrauterine growth restriction** (IUGR). SGA is defined as a *z*-score below −1.25 (less than the 10th percentile) for gestational age, AGA is a *z*-score between −1.25 and 1.25 (10th to 90th percentile). IUGR is defined as a pathological process that causes weight to be less than the genetically predicted weight. IUGR is diagnosed by intrauterine growth failure with normal head circumference.[59]

Regain of birth weight: Most infants, both term and preterm, demonstrate an initial postnatal weight loss. This usually results in a loss of 7%–10% of birth weight during the first few days of life. It is generally expected that infants will regain birth weight by 7 to 14 days of age.[60] When used in conjunction with adequate nutrient intake, the length of time required for the infant to regain birth weight when longer than usual suggests malnutrition.

Weight gain velocity: The growth goal for the infant to maintain a weight gain velocity that will allow them to improve or maintain stability of their weight for age *z*-score/percentile ranges from 15 grams to 30 grams per day.[61] As with older children, weight gain velocity that is less than the weight gain needed to maintain stable growth is an indicator of malnutrition.[56]

The rate of weight gain velocity needed to maintain a stable weight for age *z*-score varies with weight, age, and gender; therefore, weight gain velocity goals need to be adjusted frequently.[61] Weight gain goals can be established using preterm growth charts or a preterm growth calculator program or application.

Change in weight for age z-score: Faltering growth as indicated by a decline in weight for age z-score is one of the recommended indicators for identifying malnutrition in the preterm/neonatal population.

The indicator for decline in weight for age z-score is based on the study by Rochow and colleagues.[62]

This large, international, longitudinal, observational study reported that infants with uncomplicated postnatal adaptation transitioned to a weight gain trajectory 0.8 SD below birth at day of life 21. The cutoffs for mild, moderate, and severe malnutrition also reflect the very rapid expected rate of weight gain of preterm infants and neonates.

Length: The indicators related to length include less than expected linear growth velocity and decline in length for age z-score.

Linear growth is dependent on fat-free mass accretion and adequate protein and micronutrient intake. Therefore, assessment of linear growth may be used in conjunction with nutrient intake in identifying malnutrition.[56,63,64]

Criteria for identifying malnutrition in the preterm infant are described in **TABLE 4.8**.

▶ Conclusion

The goal of this chapter is to provide the pediatric nutrition professional with the tools needed to identify, document, and treat malnutrition in children from birth into adulthood. In recent years, pediatric nutrition professional organizations have begun working together in order to standardize the definition of pediatric malnutrition and

TABLE 4.8 Recommended Indicators of Preterm/Neonatal Infant Malnutrition

Primary Indicator	Mild Malnutrition	Moderate Malnutrition	Severe Malnutrition	Use of Indicator
Days to regain birth weight	15–18 days	19–21 days	>21 days	Use in conjunction with nutrient intake
Weight gain velocity Not appropriate for first 2 weeks of life	<75% of expected rate of weight gain to maintain growth rate	<50% of expected rate of weight gain to maintain growth rate	<25% of expected rate of weight gain to maintain growth rate	
Decline in weight of z-score Not appropriate for first 2 weeks of life	Decline of 0.8–1.2 in z-score	Decline of >1.2–2 in z-score	Decline of >2 z-score	
Linear growth velocity	<75% of expected rate of weight gain to maintain growth rate	<50% of expected rate of weight gain to maintain expected growth rate	<25% of expected rate of weight gain to maintain expected growth rate	May be deferred until day of life 14 and in critically ill unstable infants Use in conjunction with another indicator when accurate length measurement available
Decline in length of z-score Not appropriate for first two weeks of life	Decline of 0.8–1.2 in z-score	Decline of >1.2–2 in z-score	Decline of >2 in z-score	May be deferred until day of life 14 and in critically ill, unstable infants Use in conjunction with another indicator when accurate length measurement available
Nutrient Intake The best indicator during the first 2 weeks of life	≥ 3–5 Consecutive days of protein/energy intake ≤75% of estimated needs	≥ 5–7 consecutive days of protein/energy intake ≤ 75% of estimated needs	>7 consecutive days of protein/energy intake ≤ 75% of estimated needs	

adopt common recommended indicators to identify and document its diagnosis and care.

Although the prevalence of pediatric malnutrition remains unknown at this time, those who care for children continue to work to identify, diagnose, and treat malnutrition at all ages. The causes of malnutrition are many and are not addressed in this chapter. Other chapters provide information on diseases and conditions that put children at risk for malnutrition, as well as offer nutrition therapy recommendations for treatment.

🔍 CASE STUDIES

Case Study 1–24 months
Patient History
Sara, a 20-month-old female, was admitted to the children's hospital with a diagnosis of acute pancreatitis. Her previous medical history included a history of preterm birth at 30 weeks' gestational age, short bowel syndrome, feeding intolerance, gastrostomy tube feeding, and developmental delay.

Her admission weight was 9.21 kg. Her previous weights were: 1 month prior: 9.39 kg/3 months prior: 9.5 kg. Her length at admission was 89 centimeters.

Her caregiver reported that she had been having a lot of vomiting and diarrhea prior to her admission, so her feedings had been diluted to half strength. Her formula intake at admission was 3 cans Pediatric Compleat plus 3 cans water/60 milliliters per hour for 24 hours per day. Providing 720 calories per day/24 grams of protein per day.

Assessment
Age: 20 months
Sex: female
Weight: 9.21 kg
Length: 89 cm.
Weight for age z-score: −1.20
Length for age z-score: 2.10
Weight for length z-score: −3.36
Weight gain velocity percentage of the norm: 0%
Estimated nutrient intake: 720 calories per day. (based on the DRI/74% of estimated need)
24 grams per day (2.6 gm/kg/day)

Estimated nutrient need:
Energy:
RDA: $102 \times 9.21 = 939.4$ calories
DRI: $\{(89 \times 9.21) - 100 + 20\} \times 1.31 = 969$ calories
Schofield: $\{(16.252 \times 9.21) + (10.232 \times 89) - 413.5\} = 646.9 \times$ activity factor $1.3 = 841$ calories WHO: $(61.9 \times 9.21) - 54 = 570 \times$ activity factor $1.3 = 741$ calories.

Protein:
RDA: 1.2 gm/kg/day
DRI: 1.05 gm/kg/day
ASPEN Clinical Care Guidelines: Nutrition Support of the Critically Ill Child: 1.5 – 2 gm/kg/day[38]
Percentage of nutrient intake of estimated need: Energy intake based on DRI = 74% of estimated need. Protein intake based on DRI = 250% estimated need. Based on ASPEN guidelines: 130%.

Diagnosis
Severe malnutrition related to acute pancreatitis, short bowel syndrome as evidenced by weight for length z-score below the −3 and weight gain velocity percentage of the norm less than 25%.

Intervention
A combination of parenteral - enteral nutrition support is ordered to provide 100% nutrient needs should be provided until Sarah is able to tolerate full strength feedings that will support weight gain velocity goals and acceleration of weight for length trajectory on the growth chart. Recovery from malnutrition and tolerance to nutrition therapy will dictate the need for modifying the nutrition interventions of the nutrition care plan.

Monitoring and Evaluation
Weight gain velocity – adequacy of nutrient intake compared with nutrient need and changes in weight for length z-scores should be monitored for change. In children with severe malnutrition, frequent monitoring for tolerance of nutrition intervention is essential. Reassessment every 2–3 days is warranted.

Discussion Questions
1. What micronutrient(s) are of concern in children with short bowel syndrome and malabsorption?
2. What are Sara's weight gain velocity goals?
3. Describe Sara's nutritional parameters that would need to improve and how they would need to improve to correct her severe malnutrition.

Case Study 2–18 years

History

Aiden is a 16-year-old male with a history of autism, developmental delay, and liver failure that required transplant that resulted in a complicated course. He was admitted to the hospital with loose stools and poor oral intake for the past 2 weeks. He was diagnosed with cytomegaloviremia.

Caregivers report that Aiden, who is a picky eater, was only eating crackers and drinking sports drinks for the past 5–7 days. The dietitian estimated his intake to be 600-700 calories per day. Protein intake approximately 16 grams per day. In the past, Aiden has accepted several types of ONS, prefers chocolate, and had taken sips of some ONS over the past few days.

Assessment

Age: 16 years old
Sex: male
Weight: 47.8 kg.
Length: 164 cm.
Usual Body weight: 53 kg.
Weight for age z-score: −2.64
Height for age z-score: −1.71
BMI for age z-score: −2.00
Weight loss percentage usual body weight: 9.8%

Estimated nutrient intake: 650 calories per day. 16 gm protein. (.33 gm/kg/day)

Estimated nutrient need:
RDA: TEE/2151
DRI: TEE/2597
Schofield: TEE/1820–2428
WHO: REE 1336 calories x stress factor of 1.2–1.6 = TEE/1603–2138 calories
Protein: RDA 0.9 gm/kg/day DRI 0.85 gm/kg/day
ASPEN Clinical Care Guidelines: Nutrition Support of the Critically Ill Child: 1.5 gm/kg./day [38]
Percentage of nutrient intake of estimated need: based on DRI: 25% estimated energy need. 22% of estimated protein needs based on ASPEN guidelines.

Diagnosis

Severe malnutrition related to acute infection by cytomegalovirus as evidenced by inadequate nutrient intake less than 25% of estimated nutrient need.

Discussion

This child has several positive indicators of malnutrition. His BMI for age -score which is a −2.00 indicates moderate malnutrition according to the recommended indicators. He also has had some weight loss, so there is evidence of a weight loss percentage of usual body weight of 9.8%, which would meet the criteria for moderate malnutrition for the indicator, of weight loss of 7.5% but less than 10% usual body weight. However, when assessing the whole child, it is important to select the indicator for malnutrition with the highest acuity/severity. This ensures that the highest level of care is assigned to the care and coverage of the child.[39]

Intervention

Combined high calorie/high protein oral diet – enteral nutrition support – oral nutritional supplement with initiation of analysis of nutrient intake and audit of enteral nutrition support intake.

Monitoring and Evaluation

Weight gain velocity – adequacy of nutrient intake compared with nutrient need and changes in BMI for age z-scores should be monitored for change. In children with severe malnutrition, frequent monitoring for tolerance of nutrition intervention is essential. Reassessment every 2–3 days is warranted.

Discussion Questions

1. What would Aiden's short-term nutrition goals be?
2. What would his long-term nutrition goals be? Should his long-term plan include continued oral nutrition supplementation?
3. What is his goal weight and calorie intake?

Review Questions

1. Why is the identification of malnutrition related to undernutrition important in the care of children? How many reasons can you find?

2. How does malnutrition affect outcomes for children?

3. What is the definition of illness related malnutrition?

4. What is the definition of non-illness related malnutrition?

5. List the single data point recommended indicators for malnutrition?

6. List the multiple data point recommended indicators for malnutrition?

7. Identify the statement that is **NOT** correct.
   a. z-scores outside of +2 and −2 are more likely to be normal
   b. z-scores allow for the statement of a precise and discrete number.
   c. The z-score scale is linear.
   d. The use of z-scores allows for the determination of a precise score for children who might fall above the 97th percentile or below the 3rd percentile on a standard growth chart.

8. Acute malnutrition is of 3 months' duration or greater. True or false?

9. Weight gain velocity is plotted on growth charts that are based on standards that include 2 months, 4 months, and 6 months of age intervals. True or False?

10. Nutrient intake percentage of estimated need (predictive equations vs measured). Mild malnutrition can be diagnosed by a nutrient intake of that is 51%–75% of estimated energy-protein need. True or False?

11. Monitoring and evaluating a patient with malnutrition should include
    a. Height gain velocity
    b. Fluid intake and output
    c. Daily weights
    d. Recorded blood glucose

References

1. Guenter P, Jensen G, Patel V, et al. Addressing disease related malnutrition in hospitalized patients: a call for a national goal. *Joint Comm J Qual Pt Saf.* 2015;41(10):469–473.

2. Williams, CD. Kwashiorkor. *Lancet.* 1935; 226(5855): 1151.

3. Waterlow JC. Classification and definition of protein-calorie malnutrition. *BMJ.* 1972;3(5826):566–569.

4. de Onis M, Blossner M. *WHO Global Database on Child Growth and Malnutrition.* World Health Organization Publication. WHO/Nut/97.4;1997.

5. Mehta NM, Corkins MR, Lyman B, et al. American Society for Parenteral and Enteral Nutrition (A.S.P.E.N.) Board of Directors. Defining pediatric malnutrition: a paradigm shift towards etiology-related definitions. *J Parenter Enteral Nutr.* 2013;37(4):460–481.

6. Becker P, Carney LN, Corkins MR, et al. Consensus statement of the Academy of Nutrition and Dietetics/American Society for Parenteral and Enteral Nutrition: indicators recommended for the identification and documentation of pediatric malnutrition. *J Academy Nutr Diet.* 2014.114(12):1988–2000.

7. Academy of Nutrition and Dietetics. Nutrition terminology reference manual (eNCPT): Dietetics language for nutrition care. Illness/non-illness related pediatric malnutrition (undernutrition). Available at: *NCPT.webauthor. com.* Accessed December 10, 2017.

8. Academy of Nutrition and Dietetics. Terminology Reference Manual (eNCPT). Dietetics language for nutrition care. Illness/non-illness related pediatric malnutrition (undernutrition). Available at: *NCPT. webauthor.com.* Accessed December 10, 2017.

9. Mikhailov T, Kuhn E, Manzi J. et al. Early enteral nutrition is associated with lower mortality in critically ill children. *JPEN.* 2014;38(4):459–466.

10. White JV, Guenter P, Jensen G, et al. Consensus statement of the Academy of Nutrition and Dietetics/American Society for Parenteral and Enteral Nutrition: Characteristics recommended for the identification and documentation of adult malnutrition – undernutrition. *J Parenter Enteral Nutr.* 2012;36(2):275–283.

11. Malone A, Hamilton C. The Academy of Nutrition and Dietetics/The American Society for Parenteral and Enteral Nutrition consensus malnutrition characteristics: application in practice. *Nutr Clin Prac.* 2013;28(6):639–650.

12. Leite HP, de Lima LF, de Oliveira Iglesias SB, Pacheco JC, de Carvalho WB. Malnutrition may worsen the prognosis of critically ill children with hyperglycemia and hypoglycemia. *JPEN.* 2013;37(3):335–341.

13. Toole BJ, Toole LE, Kyle UG, Cabrera AG, Orellana RA, Coss-Bu JA. Perioperative nutritional support and malnutrition in infants and children with congenital heart disease. *Congenit Heart Dis.* 2014;9(1):15–25.

14. Gashu D, Stoecker B, Bougma K, et al. Stunting, selenium deficiency and anemia are associated with poor cognitive performance in preschool children from rural Ethiopia. *Nutr J.* 2016;15(38):2–8.

15. Hecht C, Weber M, Grote V, Daskalou E. Disease associated malnutrition correlates with length of hospital stay in children. *Clin Nutr.* 2015;Feb;34(1):53–59.

16. Sermet-Gaudelus I, Poisson-Salomon A, Colomb V, et al. Simple pediatric nutrition risk score to identify children at risk of malnutrition. *Am J Clin Nutr.* 2000;72:64–70.

17. Gerasimidis K, Keane O, Macleod I, Flynn D, Wright C. A four stage evaluation of the Pediatric Yorkhill Malnutrition Score in a tertiary pediatric hospital and a district general hospital. *Br J Nutr.* 2010;104:751–756.

18. Hartman C, Shamir R, Hecht C, Koletzko B. Malnutrition screening tools for hospitalized children. *Curr Opinions.* 2012;15(3):303–309.

19. Joosten K, Hulst J. Nutrtional screening tools for hospitalized children: methodological considerations. *Clin Nutr.* 2014;33:1–5.

20. Wonoputri N, Djais J, Rosalina I. Validity of nutritional screening tools for hospitalized children. *J Nutr Metab.* 2014;143649.

21. Duggan MB. 2010. Anthropometry as a tool for measuring malnutrition: impact of the new WHO growth standards and references. *Ann Trop Paediatr.* 2010;30:1–7.

22. Height and Weight Measurement. Child Guidelines. Available at: www.ihs.gov/hwm/index.cfm?module=dsp_hwm _child_guidelines. Accessed May 2017.

23. Centers for Disease Control and Prevention. Measuring children's height and weight accurately. Available at: www .cdc.gov/healthyweight/assessing/bmi/childrens_bmi /measuring_children.html. Accessed May 2017.

24. World Health Organization. Job aid: weighing and measuring a child. Available at: www.who.int/childgrowth/training /jobaid_weighing_measuring.pdf. Accessed May 2017.

25. Onyango AW, de Onis M. *Training Course on Child Growth Assessment. WHO Child Growth Standards. Interpreting Growth Indicators.* 2008 World Health Organization, pub. ISBN: 978 92 4 1595070.

26. Cole TJ, Flegal KM, Nicholls D, Jackson AA. Body mass index cut offs to define thinness in children and adolescents: International Survey. *BMJ.*2007;335:194–200.

27. de Onis M, Garza C, Onyango AW. Comparison of the WHO Child Standards and the CDC 2000 Growth Charts. *J Nutr.* 2007;137(1):144–148.

28. Tanner JM, Goldstein H, Whitehouse RH. Standards for children's height at ages 2–9 years allowing for heights of parents. *Arch Dis Child.* 1970;l45(244):755–762.

29. de Onis M, Yip R, Mei Z. *The Development of MUAC-for-age Reference Data Recommended by a WHO Expert Panel.* Bulletin of the World Health Organization. 1997;75(1):11–18.

30. Barr R, Collins L, Nayiager T, et al. Nutritional status at diagnosis in children with cancer. An assessment by arm anthropometry. *J Ped Hematol Oncol.* 2011;33(3):101–104.

31. Jelliffe DB, Jelliffe EFP. The arm circumference as a public health index of protein calorie malnutrition in early childhood. *J Trop Pediatr.* 1969;15:177–260.

32. Clark SL, Fleischman AR. Term Pregnancy: Time for a Redefinition. *Clin Perinatol.* 2011; 38(3):557–564.

33. Becker PJ, Carney, LN, Corkins, MR, et al. Consensus statement of the Academy of Nutrition and Dietetics/ American Society for Parenteral and Enteral Nutrition: Indicators recommended for the identification and documentation of pediatric malnutrition (undernutrition) *Nutr Clin Pract.* 2016;30(1):147–161.

34. World Health Organization. Energy and protein requirements. WHO Technical Report Series no. 724. Geneva, Switzerland: WHO; 1985.

35. Schofield WN. Predicting basal metabolic rate: new standards and review of previous work. *Clin Nutr.* 1985;39c(1s):5–42.

36. Institute of Medicine, Food and Nutrition Board. *Dietary Reference Intakes Applications in Dietary Assessment. A Report of the Subcommittee on Interpretation and Use of DRIs.* Washington, D.C.: National Academy Press; 2000.

37. Institute of Medicine, Food and Nutrition Board. *Dietary Reference Intakes for Energy, Carbohydrate, Fiber, Fat, Fatty Acids, Cholesterol, Protein and Amino Acids.* Prepub ed. Washington, DC: National Academies Press; 2005.

38. Skillman H, Mehta N. Nutrition therapy in the critically ill child. *Curr Opinions.* 2012;18(2):192–198.

39. Academy of Nutrition and Dietetics. Nutrition terminology reference manual (eNCPT) dietetics language for nutrition care. NCP Step 3: nutrition intervention. Available at: https://ncpt.webauthor.com. Accessed February 1, 2018.

40. Deriver N, Dowsett D, Gleeson E, Carr S, Cornish C. Evaluation of over and underfeeding following the introduction of a protocol for weaning from parenteral to enteral nutrition in the intensive care unit. *NCP.* 2012;27(6):781–787.

41. Heyland DK, Cahill N, Dahaliwal R, et al. Impact of enteral feeding protocols on enteral nutrition delivery: results of a multicenter observational study. *JPEN.* 2010;34(6):675–684.

42. Mehta N, Bechard L, Cahill N, et al. Nutritional practices and their relationship to clinical outcomes in critically ill children – An international multicenter cohort study. *Crit Care Med.* 2012;40(7):2204–2211.

43. Mehta N. Bechard L, Leavitt K, et al. Cumulative energy imbalance in the pediatric intensive care unit: Role of targeted indirect calorimetry. *JPEN.* 2009;33(2)336–344.

44. Lakdawalla D, Mascarenhas M, Jena AB, et al. Impact of oral nutritional supplements on hospital outcomes in pediatric patients *JPEN.* 2014;38 (supp 2):42s–49s.

45. Huynh DT, Estorninos E, Capeding R, et al. Longitudinal growth and health outcomes in nutritionally-at-risk children who received long-term nutritional intervention. *J Hum Nutr Diet.* 2015;28(6):623–635.

46. Francis DK, Smith J, Saljuqi T, Watling RM. Oral protein calorie supplementation for children with chronic disease. *Cochrane Database Syst Rev.* 2015;27;(5):CD001914.

47. Gurlek-Gokcebay D, Emir S, Bayhan T, Demir HA, Gunduz M, Tunc B. Assessment of nutrition status in children with cancer and effectiveness of oral nutritional supplements. *Ped Hematol Onc.* 2015;32(6):423–432.

48. Citty SW, Kamel A, Garvan C, et al. Optimizing the electronic health record to standardize administration and documentation of nutritional supplements. *BMJ Qual Improv Rep.* 2017;6(1):u212176.w4867.

49. Kleinman RE, Greer FR, eds. Failure to Thrive. In: *Pediatric Nutrition.* 7th ed. Elk Grove Village, IL: Am. Academy Ped. Publisher.; 2014: 663–700.

50. Koen FM, Joosten MD, Hulst JM. Malnutrition in pediatric hospitalized patients: current Issues. *Nutrition.* 2011;27:133–137.

51. Yoshimura S, Miyazu M, Yoshizawa S, et al. Efficacy of an enteral feeding protocol for providing nutrition support after pediatric cardiac surgery. *Anaesth Intensive Care.* 2015;43(5):587–593.

52. Kyle U, Lucas L, Mackey G, et al. Implementation of nutrition support guidelines may affect energy and protein intake in the pediatric intensive care unit. *J Acad Nutr Diet.* 2016;116(5):844–850.

53. Mikhailov T, Kuhn E, Mani J, et al. Early enteral nutrition is associated with lower mortality in critically ill children. *JPEN.* 2014;38(4):459–466.

54. Mehta N, Skillman H, Irving S, et al. Guidelines for the provision and assessment of nutrition support therapy in the pediatric critically ill patient. Society of Critical Care Medicine & American Society for Parenteral and Enteral Nutrition. *Pediatr Crit Care Med.* 2017; 18(7):675–715.

55. Gentles E, Mara J, Diamantidi K, et al. Delivery of enteral nutrition after the introduction of practice guidelines and participation of dietitians in pediatric critical care clinical teams. *J Acad Nutr Diet.* 2014;114(12);1974–1981.

56. Neu, J. Gastrointestinal development and meeting the nutritional needs of premature infants. *Am J Clinc Nutr.* 2007;85(suppl):629s–634s.

57. Goldeberg D, Becker P, Brigham K, et al. Identifying malnutrition in preterm and neonatal populations: Recommended indicators. *J Acad Nutr Diet.* 2018; pii: S2212-2672(17)31629-5.

58. Fenton TR, Kim JH. A systematic review and meta-analysis to revise the Fenton growth chart for preterm infants. *BMC Pediatr.* 2013;13:59.

59. Olsen IE, Groveman SA, Lawson ML, Clark RH, Zemel BS. New intrauterine growth curves based on United States data. *Pediatrics.* 2010;125(2):e214–e224.

60. IUGR citation: Victora CG, Villar J, Barros FC, et al. Anthropometric characterization of impaired fetal growth: risk factors for and prognosis of newborns with stunting or wasting. *JAMA Pediatr.* 2015;169(7):e151431.

61. Rochow N, Fusch G, Mühlinghaus A, et al. A nutritional program to improve outcome of very low birth weight infants. *Clin Nutr.* 2012;31(1):124–131.

62. Martin CR, Brown YF, Ehrenkranz RA, et al. Nutritional practices and growth velocity in the first month of life in extremely premature infants. *Pediatrics.* 2009;124(2):649–657

63. Rochow N, Raja P, Liu K, et al. Physiological adjustment to postnatal growth trajectories in healthy preterm infants. *Pediatr Res.* 2016;79(6):870–879.

64. Olsen IE, Harris CL, Lawson ML, Berseth CL. Higher protein intake improves length, not weight, z scores in preterm infants. *J Pediatr Gastroenterol Nutr.* 2014;58(4):409–416.

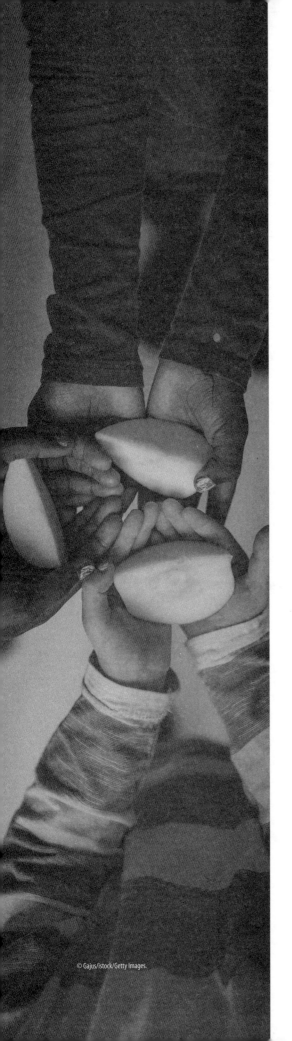

SECTION II
Perinatal Nutrition

© Gajus/istock/Getty Images.

85

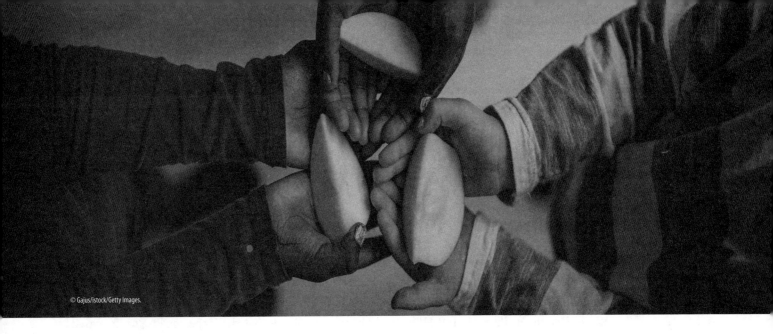

© Gajus/istock/Getty Images.

CHAPTER 5

Nutritional Implications of the Developing Fetus

Kristen Leavitt and Nancy Nevin-Folino

LEARNING OBJECTIVES

- Discuss the effects of maternal nutrition on the developing fetus.
- Discuss what micronutrients are important to meet the needs of the developing fetus and what stage of the pregnancy is relevant/affected by excess/deficiency.
- Identify what supplements are beneficial for the mother to take preconception and prenatally.
- Describe the impact of maternal endocrine/metabolic abnormality on fetal development.

▶ Introduction

Nutrition during pregnancy and early postnatal life is one of the most important factors that determines microbiological, metabolic, and immunologic development. The nutrient intake of the mother has a direct impact on the developing fetus. The fetus undergoes rapid growth and development; therefore, it is important that the macronutrient and micronutrient needs of the baby are met. More studies are showing that the inadequate or excess intake of certain nutrients can have an adverse effect on the outcomes of pregnancy. Additional evidence indicates that there is a greater risk of metabolic abnormalities including type 2 diabetes, hypertension, and cardiovascular disease in the setting of certain nutritional aberrations/deficits in pregnancy.[1,2] Also, micronutrient needs can vary greatly throughout pregnancy and in different areas of the world[3,4] Micronutrient assessment should be evaluated at several stages of the pregnancy and nutritional modifications should be a priority for improving maternal health in an effort to improve perinatal health and outcomes.

▶ Macronutrients

Energy

Energy requirements for the developing fetus are estimated to increase throughout the pregnancy. Additional energy is needed for growth and maintenance of the fetus, placenta, and maternal tissues.[5,6] The basal metabolism increases throughout the pregnancy but varies among women.[5,6] Based on theoretical calculations and individual assessment, it is recommended that women increase their energy intake by a mean of 85 calories per day in the first trimester and an additional 300–450 calories are recommended for women of normal weight during the second and third trimesters respectively.[5,7] **The World Health Organization** (WHO) recommends that pregnant women get an additional 300 calories per day and an additional 10–15 grams of protein per day.[6] For each additional fetus, a factor of approximately two should be used. For example, an additional 300 calories per day will be needed for each fetus that is being carried. Epidemiologic data have shown that women who have no economic constraints and eat to appetite do not need to increase their dietary intake during pregnancy and lactation.[6] However, the nutritional state of the mother, whether it is over- or undernutrition, has an impact on the outcome of the baby. If the energy intake did not increase during pregnancy in chronically undernourished women, the tissue growth of the fetus and mother can be limited and can have a negative impact on the mother and fetus[5,6] Some studies have found that infants who are underweight when born have a greater risk of becoming obese in their lifetime.[1,8,9] There is evidence that infants are more likely to develop insulin resistance, type 2 diabetes, and obesity later in life if the mother had poor nutritional status, specifically poor dietary intakes of energy, protein, and micronutrients during the first trimester of pregnancy.[8–11] Female offspring appear to be more vulnerable to these effects when maternal nutrition is insufficient compared with the male offspring.[10]

Supplementing food, protein, and energy during pregnancy is an intervention that has been proven to benefit birth outcomes, especially in women who are malnourished prior to pregnancy.[5,6,12,13] In malnourished women, a significant increase in birthweight has been seen when they were given protein and energy supplementation; there was also a decrease in **low birth weight** (LBW) and **small for gestational age** (SGA) birth due to this supplementation.[5,6,12,13] Even though dietary supplements throughout pregnancy are the most effective in improving maternal and fetal nutrition, food supplementation was found to be very beneficial when it was given over shorter periods during any trimester of the pregnancy.[6] There is also evidence that food supplementation during pregnancy and during the first 2 years of life in the child has positive effects on cognition.[12]

Undernutrition and Fetal Growth

Maternal undernutrition is a risk factor for adverse birth outcomes and fetal growth restriction.[13,14] The Barker hypothesis is a phenomenon that shows an association between low birth weight and an increased likelihood for metabolic and other chronic diseases later in life.[9,11,14,15] Evidence shows that when a fetus or infant is exposed to a challenge, there is a physiological adaptation that happens that might have long lasting effects.[5,9,11,16] Additionally, the elements that maintain the intrauterine environment can modify fetus development when there is some sort of external challenge, leading to increased risk for chronic illnesses later in life.[5,9,16]

Undernutrition in each trimester appears to have different increased disease risks later in life. The Dutch Famine studies were the result of a famine that occurred in 1944 when pregnant women had only 400–800 kcal/day.[15] In this study it was found that at 19 years of age, the risk of obesity was significantly higher for those born to a mother who was exposed to the Dutch Hunger winter famine during the first half of the pregnancy compared with mothers who were not exposed to the famine.[10] Additionally, these offspring were also at greater risk for schizophrenia, accelerated cognitive aging, metabolic, cardiovascular, and other chronic diseases.[15,17] There is evidence of epigenetic modifications where the detrimental effects of the famine can be transmitted to subsequent generations.[17] The offspring of women who were exposed to the famine in utero during the second trimester had offspring with increased risk of impaired renal function as adults, and those exposed in the third trimester of pregnancy had a lower risk of obesity but a greater prevalence of glucose intolerance and type 2 diabetes.[10,16,17] These same offspring with mothers exposed to famine in the first trimester had a greater prevalence of coronary heart disease, hyperlipidemia, increased concentrations of blood clotting factors, and obesity.[10,16,17]

Fetal growth has been found to be directly related to the placental size and function when supplying nutrients to the developing fetus.[1,16] Animal studies measured restricted growth of the placenta, restricted food intake, and gave low-calorie and protein diets found lower placental weight and suboptimal placental efficiency, which led to lower birthweight and IUGR.[1] Maternal undernutrition has been found to affect outcomes of the pregnancy and is likely due to suboptimal energy provision to the developing fetus.[1,10,12,14,16] The adverse outcomes associated with maternal undernutrition include **low birth weight** (LBW), preterm birth, and **small for gestational age** (SGA).[10,12,14] There is a strong correlation with inadequate maternal nutrition and the increased risk for overweight and obesity later in life for the offspring.[1,10,14] There is also a higher risk of metabolic syndrome in offspring born with low birthweight.[10] This is believed to happen because suboptimal maternal nutrition can influence adipocyte metabolism and the fat mass of the fetus, which then may lead to obesity later in its life.[1] Low birthweight is associated with inadequate nutrition in the pregnant mother, as well as rate of post natal catch-up growth that has been found to lead to insulin resistance later in life.[10,14] This has also been associated with "reduced fat mass and lean mass, poor cognition in childhood, and increased risk for type 2 diabetes and high blood pressure in adulthood."[1,10,16] Lower birthweight has been associated with an increased risk of cardiac mortality, including heart disease, increased blood pressure and stroke, metabolic syndrome, and central obesity.[10,15,16] Markers of disease are increased in children born with low birth weights.[15,16] Additionally, poor developmental outcomes in infancy and early childhood have been associated with fetal growth restriction that led to low birth weight.[12] Compared with these low birthweight outcomes, normal birthweight offspring had higher BMI as adults, but this was associated with lower fat mass and higher fat-free mass.[10]

Thinness at birth has been found to be inversely related to type 2 diabetes risk and glucose intolerance.[16] Additionally, if BMI is elevated in childhood, those born thinner at birth were also found to have an increased risk of coronary heart disease mortality, type 2 diabetes, and metabolic syndrome.[16] These data suggest that if growth in utero is affected negatively, that there is a programming effect on the developing fetus that permanently affects function of the organs during the aging process later in life.[16]

Overnutrition and Fetal Growth

Due to the recent increase in overweight and obesity, it has been found that overnutrition can also affect the outcomes of the pregnancy. Epidemiological studies have found that there is an increased risk for fetal macrosomia and **large for gestation age** (LGA) in the setting of maternal overweight (BMI of ≥25 kg/m^2).[1,18] It is thought to be due to the fetus being exposed to more energy than it needs. This has been found to have long-term consequences for the offspring later in life.[1,15,17] Offspring of women who gained excessive weight during pregnancy have been found to have an increased risk of obesity in childhood and later in life.[1,14,16] Studies in Australia and New Zealand found that compared with normal weight, obesity is an independent risk factor for SGA infants.[1] A study in Canada found that while a maternal BMI >40 kg/m^2 was protective against LBW, this level of obesity was not protective against SGA and had an increased risk of LGA and birthweights >4000 grams.[1]

Over the past few decades in the middle and upper income groups of women, there has been a reduction in physical activity level and an increase in the consumption of high-calorie food items due to affordable cost and increasing availability. Because of this there has been increased energy intake resulting in increased obesity in this population of women.[6] These women tend to be very well educated and believe (from mass media hype) that they should decrease activity levels and increase nutritional intake during pregnancy. Despite being well nourished, these women will often increase their energy intake during pregnancy, which results in excessive weight gain and obesity postpartum.[6] An alternative for this group of women is to encourage physical activeness and not increase their energy intake beyond what is needed to satiate their appetite. This practice would help prevent the long-term effects of maternal overnutrition on their offspring as they grow.

Chronic inflammation and oxidative stress are created in both pregnancy and obesity.[1,17,18] Additionally, lower serum micronutrient levels are seen in obese pregnant women compared with normal weight pregnant women, even when taking the same prenatal vitamin.[18] When the pregnant woman consumes a high-fat diet, the offspring's appetite regulating system is genetically altered, leading to a preference for energy-dense foods later in life, adiposity, and leptin resistance.[1,19] Additionally, the increased inflammation of the mother can predispose the offspring to various vascular diseases later in life.[17] A maternal high-saturated-fat diet has been shown to increase inflammation pathways in the offspring.[17] In pregnancies with maternal obesity, proinflammatory cytokines are elevated compared with normal pregnancies, leading to an increased risk of complications for the fetus and fetal infections.[1,18] The inflammation caused by obesity and metabolic dysregulation has been shown to increase the risk of inflammatory diseases as an adult in the offspring, including asthma, cardiovascular diseases, and atherosclerosis.[17]

Oxidative stress of the placenta can also occur as the result of maternal obesity, which may lead to impaired placental function and may impact fetal metabolism.[1,9,18] Because the placenta is involved with nutrient delivery to the fetus, this has an impact on the growth and development of the fetus.[1] Fetal development is impacted when the placenta is too small or is not delivering the needed nutrients, resulting in IUGR and SGA. Inflammation of the placenta, which is a characteristic of maternal obesity, comes with an increased risk of obesity in the offspring.[9] Adverse pregnancy outcomes, including early pregnancy loss, congenital malformation, poor fetal growth, and preeclampsia, put the fetus at risk for IUGR and preterm deliveries, as well as oxidative stress.[18]

In industrialized countries, 10%–20% of pregnancies are complicated by gestational diabetes mellitus or maternal obesity.[15] In gestational diabetes, increased levels of glucose, free fatty acids, and amino acids, which the fetus is exposed to, can lead to increased fetal insulin production. The epigenetic changes of hyperinsulinism and hyperglycemia, which occur as a result of maternal obesity/diabetes, can predispose the offspring for metabolic disease later in life.[15] Additionally, the fetus can have a higher gestational weight and adiposity when exposed to maternal obesity and gestational diabetes that can lead to other problems.[15]

Higher birthweights, which can result from maternal overnutrition, are also associated with a higher BMI later in life.[10] A large proportion of these infants exposed to overnutrition do not experience hunger and have difficulty orally consuming intake for progressive growth secondary to the glucose/glucagon altered metabolism. This leads to increased hospital cost and often surgical placement of a gastrostomy tube in order to be discharged from an intensive care unit because hunger does not occur metabolically.

An effective treatment for morbid obesity and diabetes is bariatric surgery. Studies that looked at siblings who were conceived before and after bariatric surgery of the mother showed that the sibling who was not exposed to maternal obesity had decreased risk of developing obesity, improved insulin sensitivity, metabolic status, and lipid profiles.[15] When the genome was analyzed before and after maternal weight loss, the gene expression and methylation differences were seen in ~5000 genes.[15] Improvements were seen in genes that influence glucose metabolism, diabetes signaling, inflammation, and autoimmune disease.[15]

In summary, higher prepregnancy BMI is associated with adverse perinatal outcomes due to increased placental weight and size; maternal obesity is associated with increased oxidative stress, lower serum micronutrient levels, and placental insufficiency, which are associated with IUGR.[1,18] Maternal and fetal undernutrition have also been associated with maternal obesity, which may lead to IUGR and change the epigenetic programming, which has been linked to chronic diseases in the offspring later in life.[1] While the mechanisms in which the fetus copes with excessive fuels during development are unknown, there is enough evidence that shows that high BMI can alter the in utero environment, leading to short- and long-term consequences in the offspring.[1,18]

Fetal Insulin Hypothesis

It has been proposed that the adult insulin resistance, which is seen when an infant is born with low birthweight, is genetically determined.[20] This insulin resistance that is believed to be genetically mediated may result in low birth weight, insulin resistance throughout life, and outcomes that may include glucose intolerance, diabetes, and hypertension. The hypothesis is that all of these issues come from the same insulin-resistant

genotype.[20] The main concept is that the fetal genetic factor, which is responsible for regulating the sensitivity of the fetal tissues to the effects of the insulin or the sensitivity of the fetal tissues to the insulin, affects fetal growth; this is secondary to fetal insulin secretion and is a key part of fetal growth.[20]

Maternal blood glucose concentrations in the third trimester have a direct correlation with the birthweight of the fetus. It has been proposed that macrosomia results from increased fetal insulin secretion in response to maternal high blood glucose levels rather than an increase of nutrients that are transferred to the fetus.[20] This hypothesis proposes that fetal growth is influenced not only by maternal high blood glucose levels but also by the fetal genetic factors described above. It is this genetic predisposition to insulin resistance that is believed to result in the adverse development of the vascular system and distribution of body fat that results in an increased risk of cardiovascular disease.[20] This hypothesis may be part of the explanation for the varying fetal weights and lifelong health sequelae.

Protein

Populations in the world who are considered poor or have a low **socioeconomic status** (SES) have diets that are based mostly on cereals, which are their main source of protein,[5] resulting in lower amounts of protein than is ideal/sufficient. Additionally, lysine, an amino acid that is a primary limiting amino acid in cereal protein, is, therefore, needed in greater amounts due to its critical role in protein synthesis.[5] Abu-Saad et al found that when flour was fortified with lysine in these populations with wheat-based diets, the growth among children was significantly higher than those who did not have access to the lysine fortified flour.[5] When getting protein from dairy sources, maternal protein intake, both prior to conception and very early in pregnancy, was associated with increased birthweight.[5]

In a study of chronically undernourished Indian women with very little or no intake of protein from animal sources, Abu-Saad et al found that intake from dairy products every other day in early pregnancy showed significantly higher birthweights.[5] Abu-Saad et al found another study in Guatemala that offered pregnant women either a protein-rich supplement or an energy-rich supplement. Those who had the high-protein supplement had offspring with significantly improved growth (born heavier, gained more height), lower plasma glucose levels, and improved intellectual development than the mothers in the non-protein group.[5,10] This same study found that the higher birthweight was associated with less adiposity in the offspring as adults.[10]

In a cohort study done in the United Kingdom, Abu-Saad et al found that maternal protein and fat intake were significantly associated with the fat and protein intake of the offspring, which was also positively associated with their fat mass.[10] However, with regard to maternal dietary intake and their offspring's fat mass or fat-free mass, there was no significant association.[10]

Very low protein intake has been associated with a greater risk of obesity among offspring.[10] A protein-restricted diet in animal studies has been associated with impaired immune response, increased sensitivity to oxidative stress, metabolic abnormalities, and unstable glucose levels.[17]

During pregnancy, approximately one kilogram (1000 gm) of protein is used by the fetus and placenta, with the largest need for the protein in the second and third trimesters.[3] The Institute of Medicine recommends that a pregnant woman consume at least 1.1 g/kg/day of protein using the prepregnancy weight.[21] Lean meats, low-fat dairy, and a diet containing whole foods like fruits and vegetables during pregnancy are good for appropriate birthweight.[1]

Essential Fatty Acids

Fatty acids, omega-3 and omega-6, are essential nutrients for fetal growth[5,17,22] and must be obtained from the diet as the body is unable to synthesize these nutrients. Fatty acids are an important part of the structure of cell membranes and play an essential role in the formation of tissues.[5] Inadequate intake of long chain polyunsaturated fatty acids leads to abnormal DNA methylation patterns, which can have detrimental effects on fetal programming, leading to increased risk of cardiovascular diseases later in life.[17] Trials of supplementation of omega-3 fatty acids have had mixed results. Some evidence has shown that increased maternal intakes of omega-3 fatty acids may improve fetal growth and increase the length of gestation; however, there is not enough evidence at this time that shows a reduction in risk of low birth weight when the pregnant mother supplements her diet with omega-3 fatty acids.[1,5]

Populations who have high seafood intakes compared with populations with low seafood intakes have better birth outcomes with the higher seafood intakes.[5] Studies have concluded that there are maternal and fetal benefits with omega-3 fatty acid intake, but excess intake could have negative effects due to contaminants from seafood.[5]

One of the fatty acids that plays an important role in central nervous development and fetal growth is **docosahexaenoic acid** (DHA). It is estimated that the DHA in utero accretion rate is 43 mg/kg/day.[1] The most important time for the fetus to receive DHA is during the third trimester, since this is when the fetus starts accumulating fat.[1] If there are insufficient amounts of DHA available to the fetus during this time, the areas of the brain that produce dopamine and serotonin may experience an irreversible, detrimental effect.[1]

During the second half of pregnancy, DHA accumulates in the neural cortex tissues and retinal membrane synapses, and as a result, has been positively associated with cognitive and visual abilities in the offspring.[23]

Because it is unknown how much DHA is synthesized or released from adipose stores, it is believed that DHA in the maternal diet is important for the developing fetus.[23] Observational studies have found positive associations between maternal DHA intake and improved cognitive and visual abilities; however, these studies were unable to establish causality.[23] Omega-3 supplementation may be a good strategy to improve outcomes in the next generation, but based on some reviews, the evidence is not conclusive that this supplementation definitely improves cognitive or visual development in the offspring.[23]

▶ Socioeconomic Status (SES) and Fetal Development

There is a strong association between socioeconomic factors and adverse birth outcomes.[5] Low birth weight, preterm birth, and IUGR are seen more frequently in developing countries compared with developed countries; in developed countries, these adverse birth outcomes are seen most often in low-SES groups.[5] While there is no direct effect on fetal growth due to low SES, it is the unhealthy exposures that are associated with SES that increase the risk of poor birth outcomes. These exposures include maternal nutrition; physically demanding work; lack of access to prenatal care; psychosocial factors like stress, anxiety, and depression; substance use/abuse; and living areas that contain industrial pollution.[5] Additionally, the educational level of any population has been the most consistent predictor of health with regard to SES.[5] Education and employment are both predictors of the quality of the diet and nutrient intake; among rural Indian women, the intake of dairy products had a strong association with birth size and SES.[5]

Several studies have observed that to achieve better nutritional outcomes in low SES or in developing countries, the interventions should include improving the socioeconomic circumstances of the family as well as encouraging maternal lifestyle changes.[5] Abu-Saad et al concluded that

> *"It may not be possible to eliminate the higher risks of IUGR and preterm birth among the poor without eliminating poverty itself."*[5]

It was observed that in countries that were able to achieve the lowest poor birth outcome rates, they had done so by reducing the prevalence of socioeconomic disadvantage rather than through healthcare interventions alone.[5] In summary, to improve outcomes in these low SES populations, avocation for improvements to the issues of poverty in addition to promoting proven nutritional interventions be made feasible in resource-poor countries and populations.[5]

▶ Micronutrients

Micronutrients, or vitamins and minerals, are very important to growth, overall wellbeing, and illness prevention. Small exogenous amounts must be consumed from the diet, even though small amounts often are all that are required. These vitamins and minerals help the body produce hormones, enzymes, and other nutrients, which are needed for growth and development.[24] Evidence shows that a poor maternal diet, which is lacking in appropriate micronutrients, could affect fetal programming since micronutrients have a role in DNA methylation.[11] The daily micronutrient requirements during pregnancy are higher due to the increased nutritional needs of the pregnancy and the rapidly growing fetus. As stated before, nutrient deficiencies are typically found in lower socioeconomic status populations and often involve multiple deficiencies.[5] The different micronutrients and their roles in the developing fetus will be discussed as well as the benefits of multiple micronutrient supplementations.

Zinc

Zinc is an essential nutrient for fetal growth and development. Zinc plays a role in protein and carbohydrate metabolism, antioxidant functions, and nucleic acid synthesis.[17,25] It is recommended that pregnant women in the United States get 11 mg/day of zinc in their diet daily. A deficiency of zinc is believed to effect the fetus through decreased protein synthesis, decreased cell generation, and/or reduced rates of tubulin polymerization (this action plays a role in the structure of the cell).[1,17] In some cases, zinc deficiency has been found to be teratogenic since it can interfere with embryonic development and increase the risks of malformation of the fetus.[1] Immune dysregulation from deficiency of zinc may also lead to chronic inflammatory disease and increased cardiovascular disease risk.[17] Some animal studies have found that zinc supplementation during pregnancy leads to lower DNA methylation in the intestinal cells, which possibly have an anti-inflammatory effect on the gut mucosa.[17] Other trials have found no negative effects of antenatal zinc supplementation on child cognitive or motor development.[12] Supplementation of zinc during pregnancy has been found to decrease the risk of preterm birth by 14%. Unfortunately, the birth size was not affected.[4,12] Other studies have found that supplementation of zinc has had significant beneficial increase in birth weight and head circumference.[26] However, a Cochrane review of 15,000 women and their babies showed that zinc supplementation, when compared with placebo, did not have an effect on reducing the risk of low birth weight or SGA.[26] The evidence is insufficient to say that maternal zinc deficiency is related to birthweight in babies or that it is teratogenic.[1]

Zinc deficiency can interfere with fetal development and can compromise immune function.[12,24] Global estimates of zinc deficiency in pregnancy are not available, but studies that are population based in South Asia have shown zinc deficiencies that vary from 15%–74%.[4]

Iron

Iron is needed to transport oxygen in the red blood cells and to support the growth and development of the placenta and the fetus.[24] Iron is transferred to the fetus throughout pregnancy, but the largest accumulation of iron in the fetus occurs during the third trimester. The iron that is stored in the fetus during this last trimester is the primary source of iron for the infant in the first 6 months of life.[4] When a fetus is born prematurely, he or she is born with minimal iron stores and is at the greatest risk for anemia. The risk of developing iron-deficiency anemia is at its highest during pregnancy because maternal iron requirements are higher than the average absorbable iron intakes.[5]

It is estimated that the worldwide prevalence of iron deficiency anemia, a hemoglobin of <110 g/L, in pregnancy is 15%–20%.[4] The WHO estimates that, on average, 18% of pregnant women in developed countries are anemic and 56% of pregnant women in developing countries are anemic.[5]

During fetal development, iron plays a role in the developing hippocampus, therefore, deficiency may lead to an alteration in brain energy metabolism, neurotransmitters, and myelination.[4,12] Iron deficiency in the first trimester of pregnancy has been found to cause significant reduction in fetal growth and is more damaging to fetal outcome than iron deficiency in the second and third trimesters.[5]

The WHO recommends perinatal and antenatal use of iron in order to reduce the risk of iron deficiency anemia and risk of low birth weight in the fetus.[4,5,12,13,24,27] In a Cochrane review of daily iron supplementation during pregnancy, there was a 70% reduction in anemia at term, a 67% reduction in iron deficiency anemia, and a 19% reduction in low birthweight.[13]

The WHO recommends a daily dosage of 30–60 grams of elemental iron starting as early as possible in pregnancy. Ideally, maternal iron status should be improved before pregnancy.[5] Iron exposure to the fetus has been associated with improved cognitive function, but in more developed, high-income countries, iron supplementation has not been shown to improve mental and cognitive development; however, some benefit was seen in psychomotor tests.[4] In Nepal, a country with high levels of iron deficiency, Gernand et al found that children at the age of 7–9 years old had improved intellectual, motor, and executive scores in mothers who received iron and folic acid supplementation during pregnancy vs. a placebo.[4] Iron and folic supplementation during pregnancy greatly improved facets of general intelligence, executive functioning, and fine motor function in early school-age children.[12]

Folate

Folate plays an important role in the developing fetus. It is needed for DNA and RNA metabolism as well as for amino acid metabolism.[5,11,17,24] Additionally, early in the development of the embryo (2–8 weeks of gestation), the neural tube and crest undergo rapid cell division where the number of cells may double as quickly as every 5 hours, leading to a high need for folate.[4,17]

Folate is also the only micronutrient that has proven to be effective at reducing the risk of congenital anomalies, specifically neural tube defects.[4,11] Many trials have shown that folate given before conception reduces the risk of neural tube defects by 72%.[4,13,24] Supplementation of folic acid during pregnancy showed an improved mean birthweight and a 79% reduction in megaloblastic anemia.[13] This led to fortification of grain products with folate in the United States starting in the 1990s and the incidence of neural tube defects decreased as a result. While not as obvious as the benefits in preventing neural tube defects, adequate folate status may also prevent some birth defects like cleft lip, cleft palate, and limb malformations.[24] Inadequate maternal folate intake has also been associated with low birth weight, IUGR, and preterm birth.[5] Cellular growth in the fetus and placenta can be impaired when maternal folate intake is suboptimal.[5] Several large studies found that a low folate intake from preconception to mid-pregnancy was associated with at least a 2- to 4-fold increase in the risk of preterm birth and low birthweight, especially in low-income populations.[5] Vanes et al showed an association with high-dose folic acid (≥5 mg folic acid/day) and increased neurodevelopment, which resulted in improved vocabulary development, communication skills, and verbal comprehension at 18 months of age when given in early pregnancy.[11] However, in another study, Vanes et al found that when folic acid was given later in pregnancy, there was more of an association seen with childhood asthma and wheezing than when given early in pregnancy; these data are controversial, however, and need further study.[11] A Cochrane review that looked at folic acid supplementation alone or with other macronutrients when compared with no folic acid showed that the mean difference in birthweight was significantly greater in the folic acid groups, but with regard to low birth weight.[28]

Global estimates of folate deficiency in pregnancy are not available, but studies that are population based in South Asia have shown deficiencies of folate that vary from 0–26%.[4] However, in women of reproductive age in West Africa, folate deficiency has been reported as high as 86%.[4]

The WHO recommends 400 μg of folic acid daily with iron for antenatal use in order to reduce risk of iron deficiency anemia in pregnant women and birth defects (if started before conception) in the fetus.[4,29]

Calcium

Calcium supplementation has been recommended for pregnant women in areas where dietary calcium intake is low since it has been shown to help prevent pre-eclampsia.[12] The impact this could have on the developing fetus is possible prevention of IUGR, which has been associated with pre-eclampsia. Calcium supplementation has a significant protective benefit in preventing pre-eclampsia and improves mean infant birth weight when supplemented during pregnancy.[29] In populations with risk of low calcium intake, a Cochrane review found that maternal calcium supplementation reduced gestational hypertension by 35%, pre-eclampsia by 55%, and preterm births by 24%.[13] Langley-Evans et al showed reduced blood pressure in 6-month-old infants when mothers were supplemented with calcium.[16]

The third trimester is when the fetus needs the greatest amount of calcium. Calcium has several roles in the developing fetus including development of the skeleton.[1] A Cochrane review showed that low birth weight and IUGR were not affected by calcium supplementation, even in high-dose supplementation (>1000 mg/day).[1] However, higher birthweights were seen when calcium was supplemented when compared with placebo.[1]

The WHO recommends supplementing the mother's diet with 1.5–2 g of calcium daily.[12]

Vitamin D

Vitamin D deficiency has not been well estimated in pregnancy but is seen in many countries, including high-income countries like the United States.[4] Infants born to mothers who are vitamin D deficient will also be deficient and are at risk of developing rickets and poor skeletal growth and mineralization as well as poor infant tooth mineralization.[24] Deficiency occurs in the fetus because of the suboptimal transfer of 25(OH)D during pregnancy, and the minimal amounts in breastmilk.[1,4] However, there is currently no recommendation to increase vitamin D during pregnancy.[1]

Vitamin D supplementation to the fetus has been shown to reduce the risk of low birth weight by 60% and also reduce preterm birth risk by 64%.[4,29,30] A meta-analysis by Per Grieger et al, showed that during pregnancy, a 25(OH)D insufficiency (<37.5 nmol/L) led to an increased risk for SGA infants compared with pregnant women with higher 25(OH)D levels.[1] This review also found that pregnant women with 25 (OH) D insufficiencies had lower birth weight infants compared with infants born to mothers with higher levels.[1] Langley-Evans et al showed an association between higher vitamin D intake during pregnancy and a decreased risk of asthma in 3-year-old children.[16]

Vitamin D treatment alone was found to be borderline significant in decreasing risk for SGA and reducing the risk of premature birth when compared with a placebo or no supplementation at all per a Cochrane review.[1,30] Vitamin D supplementation alone also seems to increase the head circumference and the length of the newborn.[30] However, there is not enough evidence to support promoting using Vitamin D supplementation during pregnancy in order to reduce low birth weight.[1,30] Per the Institute of Medicine, the current estimated requirement is 800 mg/day of calcium and 400 IU/day of vitamin D.[1]

Iodine

An essential nutrient for creating thyroid hormones, iodine is an important part of normal growth and development. Fetal hypothyroidism and goiter can result from iodine deficiency.[12,31] Additionally, cretinism, a severe stunting in mental and physical growth, and brain damage are found in offspring born to women with severe iodine deficiency during pregnancy.[2,12,24,31] Because of this, one of the most common preventable causes of delayed mental development is iodine deficiency.[2,4,24] There is strong evidence that iodine in the antenatal period will improve cognition in the developing fetus. Before the fetal thyroid gland is able to function independently, thyroxine, a thyroid hormone that contains iodine, is required for developing the fetal brain during the first two trimesters.[4] Risk of cretinism is greatly reduced when deficient mothers are supplemented with iodine before conception.[2,4,24] Mild iodine deficiency has been linked with an increased risk of cognitive impairments in several observational studies, and supplementation of iodine may help prevent this.[2,4,12,24,31] Several randomized trials looked at maternal iodized oil supplementation in iodine-deficient populations and there was a 73% reduction in cretinism and a 10%–20% increase in developmental scores of the offspring.[13]

However, there is evidence that routine supplementation of iodine in pregnancy may come with some risk. The upper limit of iodine supplementation is unknown at this time since the fetal thyroid is also susceptible to an excess of iodine.[2] Pregnant women who were supplemented with too much iodine were found to have offspring with congenital hypothyroidism.[2] Shao et al showed that poorer mental and psychomotor development is associated with the supplementation of ≥150 μg/day of iodine.[2,31] Because of the uncertainty of supplementation in areas with mild to moderate iodine deficiency, there are RCTs that are investigating whether the supplementation benefits the pregnant mother and improves neonatal outcomes.[2]

The WHO recommends using iodized salt, or supplementation of 250 μg of iodine per day in countries with minimal access to iodized salt.[4,13,24,31] However, it is advised to take no more than 500 μg per day in pregnancy due to an increased risk of subclinical hypothyroidism.[31]

Selenium

Selenium is an essential trace element that plays a role in antioxidant defense in order to protect the cellular membranes of the body. It also acts as a catalyst for the production of thyroid hormones.[25,32] Selenium deficiency has been found to have reproductive complications, including SGA in infants.[24,25,32] It has been shown that plasma concentrations of selenium fall during pregnancy, causing an increased need for selenium due to the rapidly growing fetus.[25] However, low plasma selenium concentrations have also increased the risk for SGA in infants, with a concomitant possible increased risk of cardiovascular disease later in life.[24,25] It is postulated that the low concentrations of selenium may affect the antioxidant properties of this element, causing compromised protection against the oxidative stress of the placenta, which in turn may affect fetal growth.[25]

Mao et al conducted a study that supplemented pregnant mothers with selenium. The study found that supplementation of selenium altered thyroid function by reducing free T4 levels. The authors concluded that additional research is needed on selenium supplementation during pregnancy and that routinely supplementing selenium during pregnancy is not recommended at this time.[33]

Choline

Choline is a water-soluble vitamin that is an integral part of cell walls. It ensures the integrity of the cell wall and allows the cells to communicate with each other. The role of choline in fetal development is in neural tube development, influencing stem-cell proliferation and apoptosis of midline structures of the fetus.[17,34] Choline is necessary for the closure of the neural tube and then during the last trimester it plays a role in developing the hippocampus.[34] During pregnancy, the need for choline is high and maternal levels can be depleted easily due to rapid transfer of this vitamin from the mother to the fetus and also from alcohol use/excess.[34] Currently, one of the leading causes of choline deficiency is due to alcohol intake during pregnancy.[34] The Institute of Medicine recommends a daily intake of 450 mg/day of choline during pregnancy.[34] Choline is available in foods like eggs (two eggs contain 400 mg of choline), chicken, milk, broccoli, and cauliflower.[34] Choline is available in some prenatal vitamins, but not all, and in lesser amounts than the current recommendations.[34]

Copper

Copper is a trace mineral that is present in all body tissues and plays an essential role in forming red blood cells, as well as forming the organs and tissues of the body. It is a cofactor for several enzymes that are involved in metabolic reactions, the development of new blood vessels, antioxidant protection, and oxygen transport.[24,25] Plasma copper concentrations have been found to increase significantly during pregnancy, and return to normal levels after delivery.[25] There have been reports that lower plasma levels in the placenta are associated with SGA births, but the data surrounding this are very limited.[25] Currently, there is no recommendation for additional copper supplementation during pregnancy.

Vitamin A

Vitamin A, as well as vitamins E and K, have roles in immunity and inflammation.[35] Vitamin A, and the retinoids associated with it, play an important role in growth, homeostasis, and development.[11,24,35] Early in the life of the developing fetus, vitamin A plays a role in embryonic development. In animal models, almost every tissue that has been studied, including the eye, heart, bones, respiratory system, nervous system, pancreas and ear structure, and the retinoic acid receptors, have reinforced the importance of vitamin A early in fetal life.[4,11,24] A clinical trial in Nepal showed that supplementation of vitamin A improved lung function.[35]

A low serum retinol of <0.70 μmol/L defines vitamin A deficiency, often seen in low-income countries, and affects an estimated 15% of women who are pregnant.[4] It is estimated that between 1% and 5% of all pregnant women have some signs and symptoms of vitamin A deficiency.[6] In up to 8% of women, the deficiency of vitamin A is severe enough that it leads to night blindness.[4] A deficiency of vitamin A during fetal development, in addition to other micronutrients, may lead to changes in the structure of the kidney, pancreas, and vasculature, possibly predisposing the child to cardiac and metabolic disease as an adult.[4] Vitamin A deficiency may also make iron-deficiency anemia worse, and it has been found that vitamin A supplementation with iron may be more beneficial in helping iron-deficiency anemia than supplementing either micronutrient alone.[24]

The children born to women supplemented with vitamin A in rural settings were found to have higher levels of circulating natural antibodies, which is evidence of innate immunity as well as expanded lung capacity.[4] The mothers of these children were randomly assigned to receive the equivalent of the RDA of supplemental vitamin A or a placebo before, during, and after pregnancy. Vitamin A supplementation did not show effects on blood pressure or microalbuminuria.[4]

The WHO recommends vitamin A supplementation of up to 10,000 IU per day or 25,000 IU per week in countries where vitamin A deficiency is prevalent to prevent night blindness in the pregnant mother.[4]

Despite the strong need for vitamin A during pregnancy, too much preformed vitamin A in pregnancy has resulted in birth defects. It is recommended that a pregnant woman consume no more than 5,000 IU in supplementation per day.[24]

Lutein

Lutein is a carotenoid that has anti-inflammatory and antioxidant properties.[36] It has been found to regulate inflammatory processes and overcome oxidants.[36] The fetus has an impaired antioxidant system abetting oxidative stress, which causes cellular damage and interferes with the development of organs and tissues[36] The fetus has oxidative stress because of the immaturity of the developing organs, increased aerobic metabolism due to rapid growth and energy demand, and an environment that leads to increased free iron levels with high free radical production.[36] Because lutein can effectively neutralize oxidants, it can have protective effects on oxidative injuries.[36] However, the body is unable to make lutein; therefore, the intake of lutein is dependent on the maternal diet. Lutein is abundant in foods like dark green leafy vegetables, kale, and spinach, for example, and eggs. While lutein supplementation in the neonatal period has been found to increase antioxidant capacities and decrease plasma biomarkers of oxidative stress in the first few days of life, there is little information available on supplementation during pregnancy[36]; therefore, there is no recommended supplementation at this time of lutein during pregnancy.

Vitamin B$_{12}$

Vitamin B$_{12}$ is important in pregnancy because it has a role in DNA methylation.[17,19,24] Elevated homocysteine levels occur in vitamin B$_{12}$ deficiency leading to adverse pregnancy outcomes that include preeclampsia, preterm birth, low and very low birthweight, neural tube defects, and still birth.[24] Global estimates of vitamin B$_{12}$ deficiency in pregnancy are not available, but population-based studies in South Asia have shown deficiencies of B$_{12}$ that vary from 19%–74%.[4] Vanhees et al showed that offspring of mothers with high folic acid levels and low vitamin B$_{12}$ levels had higher body fat percentage, higher abdominal fat, and were insulin resistant at 6 years of age, increasing their risk of developing type 2 diabetes.[11] There is some evidence that folic acid supplementation during pregnancy may mask the signs of vitamin B$_{12}$ deficiency.[24] Because vitamin B$_{12}$ is only found in foods of animal origin, it is important that a vegetarian pregnant mother be supplemented with vitamin B$_{12}$. The recommendation in pregnancy is 2.6 mcg/day of vitamin B$_{12}$.[24]

Vitamin E

Vitamin E has been found to have anti-inflammatory properties, which include free radical-scavenging activities and playing a role in immune system function and development.[35] Studies have found that the oxidative stress that is caused by free radicals can be part of the etiology of preeclampsia.[24] A study by Kumar et al was conducted that supplemented pregnant women with vitamin C and vitamin E and there was a 76% reduction in preeclampsia and a 21% decrease in indicators of placental dysfunction.[24] This is important because preeclampsia is associated with IUGR and preventing this is beneficial for fetal growth. Global estimates of vitamin E deficiency in pregnancy are not available, but studies that are population based in South Asia have shown deficiencies of vitamin E that vary from 50%–70%.[4] Currently, there is not enough evidence to show that vitamin E supplementation will benefit or harm the developing fetus or the pregnancy.

Role of Other Micronutrients

Chromium is involved in glucose and fat metabolism. When studied in rats with maternal induced chromium restriction, there was increased body fat in the offspring.[11] This same outcome was seen in chronic maternal restriction of magnesium, iron, zinc, and calcium.[11] When zinc was restricted in rats during gestation, there was increased body weight in the offspring but no difference in birth weight. These same offspring had increased blood glucose levels and lower sensitivity to insulin and stimulation of glucose.[11] This increased body weight and insulin sensitivity was only seen in the offspring of rats that received less prenatal zinc but had adequate nutrition postnatally.[11] Since micronutrients can have the role of an antioxidant, there is a belief that micronutrients can have an effect on antioxidant systems. When there are deficiencies in antioxidants during pregnancy there may be damage done to organs and embryonic development may be impaired.[11,18] While many of these studies were done in animals, there is enough evidence to conclude that exposure in utero to micronutrients that act as antioxidants can have a positive, long-lasting effect on the offspring's antioxidant defense system.[11]

Micronutrient Supplementation

Currently, the only recommended universal supplementation in pregnancy is for iron and folic acid. However, many physicians in developed countries are recommending multiple vitamin and mineral supplementation during pregnancy in order to prevent micronutrient deficiencies.[14] Supplementation of multiple micronutrients (multivitamin-mineral) in the antenatal period is becoming an important public health intervention in low-income countries and has been found to improve birth outcomes over IFA or multivitamin supplementation alone.[4,5,12,13,27,29,37] Antenatal multiple micronutrient supplementation has been shown in several randomized trials to lower the risk of preterm birth and increase birth weight more than iron and folic acid supplementation alone, showing an average reduction in low birth weight of 12%.[4,5,12,13,27,29,37] When used in the preconception and prenatal periods, multivitamin use has been associated with a slower rate of growth in the percent fat mass of the offspring in the first 5 months of life.[14] Additionally, there was a reduction of SGA births and a head circumference that was larger in those infants who were exposed to multiple micronutrient supplementation when compared with those on iron and folic acid supplementation alone, multivitamin supplements, or placebo.[4,29,37] These same children also had improved linear growth and cognitive development with smaller skinfold thickness.[4,37] In an impoverished population, maternal multiple micronutrient supplementation had a positive effect on the fetus that continued into childhood, where an increase was observed in both weight and body size.[29] Unfortunately, regarding micronutrient supplementation and its effects on long-term outcomes of blood pressure, kidney function, and insulin resistance, evidence from childhood studies are inconclusive.[4]

When looking at cognitive or motor development, there is not enough evidence to support the benefits of iron, zinc, or multiple micronutrient supplementation. However, there is some benefit of supplementation in high-risk groups, like malnourished mothers or mothers who have HIV infection.[4] There is enough evidence to support multiple micronutrient supplementations during pregnancy when compared with iron and folic acid alone, especially in low-income and middle-income countries.[4,27,37]

The ideal way to prevent micronutrient deficiencies in pregnancy and the developing fetus is through a varied diet. However, this diet is difficult to obtain in many areas of the world and can be expensive. It has been concluded that multiple micronutrient supplementation is beneficial in preventing poor birth outcomes for both the mother and the neonate, even into childhood.[28,37] While the risk of preterm birth, SGA infants, and neonatal mortality appears to be decreased due to multiple micronutrient supplementation, more studies are needed in order to determine proper dosage and combinations of micronutrient supplements, especially in areas with high amounts of malnutrition.[29]

The WHO recommends micronutrient supplementation for pregnant women in populations with a large amount of maternal nutritional deficiencies but does not currently universally recommend multiple micronutrient supplementations.[4,27] **TABLE 5.1** provides information on micronutrient supplementation for pregnant women with low income or in food emergency settings.

TABLE 5.1 Recommended Micronutrient Supplementation for Pregnant and Lactating Women in Food Insecure or Emergency Settings

Micronutrient	Dose
Vitamin A	800 μg
Vitamin D	5 μg
Vitamin E	15 mg
Vitamin C	55 mg
Thiamine	1.4 mg
Riboflavin	1.4 mg
Niacin	18 mg
Vitamin B$_6$	1.9 mg
Vitamin B$_{12}$	2.6 μg
Folic acid	600 μg
Iron	27 mg
Zinc	10 mg
Copper	1.15 mg
Selenium	30 μg
Iodine	250 μg

Data from Gernand A, Schulze K, Stewart C, et al. Micronutrient deficiencies in pregnancy worldwide: health effects and prevention. *Nat Rev Endocrinol.* 2016;12(5):274–289;[4] and WHO/UNICEF/WFP. Preventing and controlling micronutrient deficiencies in populations affected by an emergency: multiple vitamin and mineral supplements for pregnant and lactating women, and for children aged 6 to 59 months. Available at: www.who.int/nutrition/publications/WHO_WFP_UNICEFstatement.pdf.[38]

▶ Preconception Nutrition

Many countries are starting interventions in the period leading up to conception because this can have a large impact on the health and outcome of the fetus. Fortifying flour with folic acid is one example. Other potential interventions being considered are fortifying salt with iron and iodine, iron-fortified flour, and bio-fortification of foods like rice and maize.[4]

However, data on the health outcomes of these types of interventions are either not available or not instituted at this time. While multiple micronutrient supplementation appears to be beneficial, there are other interventions that should be considered in order to maintain optimal maternal nutritional status and give the best nutrition to the developing fetus. These interventions include reducing the burden of infection, providing fortified food supplements, and reducing household food insecurity.[5]

Epigenetics

Any change in the phenotype or gene expression caused by some type of exposure or modification is what defines epigenetics.[9] The developmental programming hypothesis is that during critical periods of development and growth, the influences of the fetal environment can cause lifelong effects on the health and well-being of the offspring.[9,17,19] Some of these influences include the nutritional status of the mother and fetus (both over- and undernutrition), pollutant exposure, metabolic disturbances, placental insufficiency, and the composition of the microbiota.[9,17] Specifically, the nutritional environment that the fetus develops in can increase the risk of metabolic disorders later in life, as discussed previously. More evidence suggests that this is the result of epigenetic (environmental) programming, which can have multigenerational effects.[9,17,19] Some of the changes that occur include permanent changes to the organ structure, gene expression changes that are caused by epigenetic modifications and permanent changes to cellular aging, as well as an increased risk of chronic diseases later in life.[17,19]

There is also evidence that the gut microbiome composition is significantly correlated with epigenetic changes in genes that are related to immunological, neurological, and metabolic development and functions.[9,17] The microbiota of the mother is an important source of intestinal bacteria for the developing fetus.[9] Microbial contact in the prenatal period is an important part of developing the microbiota and, therefore, establishing the metabolic and immune response in the infant, possibly impacting the disease risk later in life.[9,17] Recent evidence shows that the fetus is exposed to microorganisms in utero, which helps with the colonization process of the microbiota.[9] Observational studies suggest an association between the composition of the gut microbiota during pregnancy and body weight and metabolic biomarkers of the infant.[9] Other studies have shown that weight gain during pregnancy also has an effect on the microbiota of the infant.[9] Regarding the supplementation of bacteria, there has been a reduction in the incidence of atopic dermatitis when there was maternal and infant supplementation of probiotics in the last weeks of pregnancy until the infant was 6 months old; this effect was still noticeable at 7 years of age.[17]

The development of the immune system can be affected by events or exposures during pregnancy as epigenetic mechanisms can modify the gene expression and, therefore, determine the functionality of the immune system.[9] At birth, there are differences in the immune response that are already detectable, which suggests in utero exposures can have an impact on the set point of the immune system at birth.[9] With the rise in immune-mediated disease, this shows how changes in our environment, including the intrauterine environment, can impact immune development.[9]

As discussed previously, there is an epidemic of obesity that is increasing every year concomitantly, resulting in increased rates of metabolic diseases. This supports that the increase in metabolic diseases and obesity may be due to epigenetic (environmental) effects.[17,19] Specifically, the Developmental Origins of Health and Disease hypothesis surmises that there are predictive adaptations that the fetus makes in response to certain cues from the intrauterine environment; these changes cause permanent adjustments in the homeostatic systems, which helps the fetus survive and improve its success in a difficult postnatal environment.[19] It is these adaptations that are believed to cause an increased risk of chronic disease later in life or transmit risk factors across generations.[17,19] It has been found that from the preconception period into postnatal life (the first 1000 days of life) is when most of the epigenetic changes are likely made.[17,19] However, the effect of these modifications during development may not be seen until later in life.[17,19] Babies who are born prematurely may experience metabolic alterations possibly secondary to exposure in the intrauterine environment. Changes in the epigenetics of the offspring are seen in maternal obesity and early life overnutrition.[19] There is also evidence that paternal obesity can alter DNA methylation, suggesting that the developing sperm are also susceptible to environmental insults.[19]

Currently, the evidence shows that developmental programming may be a multigenerational problem, which can be inherited from either the mother or the father.[17,19] It is assumed that these adaptive gene programs occurring in the parent can become part of the next generation as well; the hypothesis is that this allows the future offspring to live better in a possible suboptimal environment.[17,19] It appears that these early life exposures, including poor early life nutrition, can result in epigenetic changes in the parent that are then passed to the offspring.[17,19]

▶ Prematurity

A preterm infant's outcome is significantly interconnected to maternal health. Causation of preterm birth could be related to the mother/infant or both. Maternal health conditions can lead to preterm birth. The lower the gestational age of a preterm infant when born, the higher the risk for morbidity and mortality.

Etiology and function of a preterm infant depends on a myriad of intrauterine metabolism and exposure.

Maternal disease exposure in utero can lead to overall life-altering metabolic dysfunction. With premature infants surviving at 22–24 weeks gestational age, the alteration in body function, response to treatment, and growth post birth is emerging almost in an individualized metabolic adaptation with unknown life outcomes.

Nutrition needs are "estimated" but with each infant in the intrauterine environment and mother's health as well as the maturity for age of the infant necessitates individual consideration and monitoring of parenteral and enteral delivery. Two approaches to nutrition have changed premature infants' long-term outcomes significantly in the last decade and a half.

The first is to start enteral nutrition delivery as soon as possible, either in the delivery room at a maternity facility with a **neonatal intensive care unit** (NICU), or at free-standing neonatal care units. Nutrition/trophic feeds (colostrum/transitional human milk) are started as soon as possible in lower **gestational age** (GA)/birth weight as minimal drip/mouth care.[39] This has been shown to improve immune function and gut maturation.

The other intervention is to use human milk as the sole source of enteral feeding until a determined gestational age/weight is reached as a priority medical treatment.[40] Human milk supports the infant's immune system and development. Fortifying milk for low GA premature infants is standard protocol in order to provide nutrients at a level as equal as possible to delivery of nutrients in utero. Every effort is made to support the mother in delivery, using every drop (milliliter) expressed. Although not mother/baby dyad specific, donor milk is becoming a second alternative to mother's milk if the mother is unable to pump, or the medical condition of either the mother or the infant precludes breastmilk delivery. The donor milk is usually a blend of many mothers' milk in order to reduce specific nutrient deficiencies. This donor breastmilk nonspecific (not from the baby's mother) to a premature infant results in lower growth, but is generally tolerated with fewer feed stops or intolerance. In the past 5 or so years, donor milk has become standard medical practice if the infant's mother is incapable or decides not to provide milk. The addition of specifically created fortification products improves weight gain and brings the levels of nutrients needed by the preterm infant closer to needs for growth ex-utero.[41] The medical team accepts lower weight gain for higher tolerance to the delivery of donor milk. Ongoing research on outcomes of an all human milk diet is being conducted. Presently, most of the research is of donor milk vs. preterm formula on growth. With an overwhelming increase of human and donor milk in the premature population over the last 4 to 5 years, this may also improve outcomes for infants born to mothers who experienced severe maternal health problems.

If maternal disease is present as mentioned in this chapter, an infant born premature is not only at high risk medically with prematurity in and of itself but also with concomitant exposure to altered conditions/metabolism in utero. The above mentioned medical nutrition interventions of early and exclusive human milk feeds helps to reduce the severity of the maternal nutrition sequelae.

Boghossian et al[42] studied extremely preterm (22 to 28 weeks GA) infants born to insulin-dependent diabetic mothers and found that premature infants born to mothers who had insulin use before pregnancy (IBP) had higher risks for necrotizing enterocolitis, sepsis, and small head circumference compared with those who started insulin use during the pregnancy. There was also indication of higher in-hospital mortality risk among these infants as well. The surviving infants of this segment (IBP) evaluated at 18–22 months corrected age had lower average head circumference *z*-scores when compared with mothers without insulin-dependent diabetes mellitus.

Ono et al[43] studied neonatal outcome in chronically hypertensive mothers. The researchers found that uncontrolled chronic severe hypertension in the later part of gestation results in poor neonatal outcome. There were three study groups, which were divided into three groups with perinatal and neonatal outcomes compared. Groups were: (1 SP) preeclampsia superimposed on chronic hypertension; (2 uCH) chronic hypertension with severe hypertension uncontrolled in spite of intravenous or multiple oral antihypertensive medications in the latter part of pregnancy and (3 cCH) chronic hypertension with controlled mild hypertension with or without medication. The investigators found that preterm birth rate was significantly increased in the first two groups. Birth weights: low birth weight, very low birth weight, and extremely low birth weight decreased in order equal to the highest weights in the SP category.

Par-Miron et al[44] evaluated the effect of **borderline personality disorder** (BPI) on obstetrical and neonatal outcomes and found that the disorder was associated with several adverse outcomes including premature rupture of membranes and preterm birth. The authors recommended monitoring from a multi-disciplinary healthcare team before and after pregnancies for these women in order to decrease the incidence of poor outcomes both prenatally and postnatally.

In an older study, a Swedish research group conducted research[45] on birth size distribution in infants born to mothers with Type 1 Diabetes. LGA was described as >2 standard deviations above the mean. The group found that preterm infants in the study had significantly larger mean body weight and length than term. The proportion of LGA preterm infants was larger in total number in preterm infants than those born at term in the study comparisons. The study also unexpectedly found that there were significantly higher values of birth weight of term and preterm female infants born to diabetic mothers.

Perinatal substance abuse is a rising critical public health crisis.[46] The most common used substances in pregnancy are nicotine, followed by alcohol, marijuana, and cocaine. The rate of opiate use increase has been phenomenal. Between 2000 and 2009, the United States saw a five fold increase in opiate use as well as an epidemic of opiate prescription abuse. Adverse effects during pregnancy include premature rupture of membranes, placental abruption, preterm birth, low birth weight, and SGA infants. Methamphetamine use/abuse is linked to short gestation, lower birth weight, fetal loss, developmental and behavioral defects, preeclampsia, gestational hypertension, and intrauterine fetal death. Also, there is a concomitant, undesirable consequence of prenatal substance use of coexisting substance abuse and comorbid psychiatric illness. The women in this situation also experience inadequate prenatal care, poor nutrition, chronic medical problems, poverty, and domestic violence. All of this combined could lead to maternal-infant bonding dysfunction, spiraling into a long-term health crisis.

Breastfeeding has the potential for reducing/stopping substance abuse in the postpartum period. This is the only available intervention shown to lower the **neonatal abstinence syndrome** (NAS).

Neonatal research is ongoing and expanding to help define and identify specific nutrient delivery/modality to preterm infants exposed in utero to maternal disease, to decrease post birth morbidity, and to increase positive neonatal growth.

▶ Conclusion

Ensuring that the pregnant mother has adequate and balanced energy, protein, and micronutrient intakes may help to prevent obesity. Improving the nutritional status of women before and during pregnancy can reduce the risk of low birthweight. Overall, offspring with lower birthweights have lower BMI and less lean body mass but have an increased risk for cardiovascular and other chronic diseases due to greater fat mass.[10]

While micronutrients may play a role in helping with fetal growth and better birth weights, it has not been established what the mechanism the micronutrients use in utero in order to achieve the expected developmental outcome. Deficiencies in nutrients like folate, vitamin B_{12}, and zinc may predispose the fetus to chronic diseases later in life; these diseases include obesity, dyslipidemia, and insulin resistance.[4] However, the data are from animal models; therefore, data from humans are limited and need to be studied in vitro.

Assessing specific outcomes based on individual nutrients can be difficult because outcomes can be related to so many different dietary and environmental exposures. Looking at whole foods, rather than specific nutrients, may be the optimal way to assess nutrition for the developing fetus.

The Auckland Birthweight Collaborative study looked at whole foods and the effects on the developing fetus.

The *traditional* food pattern, which is a diet with fruit, vegetables, yogurt, and lean meat, in early stages of pregnancy had a decreased risk of SGA.[1] The *Western* food pattern, which is a diet that consisted of high-fat dairy, processed meat, refined grains, beer, and sweets, was divided into two categories but had similar results. There was a 26%–32% reduced risk for SGA in those who had a higher intake of vegetables, fruits, poultry, and breakfast cereals, which was referred to as the *health conscious* food pattern.[1] The other category, the *intermediate* food pattern, which had low-fat dairy and fruit but also included red meat, dairy, and vegetables, had similar results.[1]

A study in the Netherlands looked at the Mediterranean diet in the first trimester of pregnancy; those who were considered to have a low and medium adherence to the diet in the first trimester of pregnancy were associated with lower birthweight.[1] In a cohort study in Spain, higher birthweights with reduced risk of IUGR were associated with higher intakes of legumes, fish, and dairy products; however, intakes of fruits, cereal, and nuts did not show a relationship with birthweight.[1] Overall, it was seen that higher intakes of Mediterranean foods decreased the risk of preterm birth.[1]

The studies that look at whole foods in pregnancy propose that eating whole foods such as low-fat dairy, lean meats, fruits, and vegetables during pregnancy may help reduce the risk for LBW babies, but it cannot be determined if healthy food choices during a certain trimester are ideal.[1,5]

While more studies are always beneficial, it has been found that maternal multiple micronutrient supplements with iron have beneficial effects and that iron-folic acid as part of micronutrient supplements provide even better benefits than iron-folic acid alone.[27] Multiple micronutrient supplements were also found to have improved female neonate survival and provided improved birth outcomes for infants that were born to undernourished and anemic pregnant women in low- and middle-income countries.[27] It is most beneficial when supplementation is started early in pregnancy and the pregnant woman adheres to multiple micronutrient supplementation daily.[27]

Additionally, taking maternal nutrition and micronutrient status into account, optimal nutritional status should be ideally achieved before conception and continued through more than one pregnancy and reproduction cycle.[5] While many women in developed countries are taking a multivitamin and mineral supplement when they may not need it, it has been found that this extra supplementation does not have a harmful effect on the body size of the offspring and overall rate of growth; however, it appears that there may be a protective effect from this supplementation regarding the relative growth in adiposity.[14]

Epidemiologic studies show that the nutritional environment can have a large impact on the modification of the genome.[9] From conception until the neonatal stage, the quality and quantity of nutrition has a large impact on the development of chronic diseases later in life. Additionally, the nutritional environment can play a key role in developmental programming that not only affects the offspring but can also be transferred to future generations.

In conclusion, a diet that is unbalanced or lacking in both the mother and father can have long-term effects on the offspring's overall health. Associations with maternal diet and the onset of diabetes, obesity, cancer, and colitis have been shown to increase oxidative stress.[11] Exposure to oxidative stress, combined with impaired antioxidant defenses in pregnancy, may contribute to poor outcomes in the fetus as well as the pregnant woman.[18] There is evidence that flavonoids may be beneficial and protect against reactive oxygen species and environmental carcinogens at an adult age.[11] Finally, vitamins and minerals perform a very important role in the function of organ systems later in life. Antioxidants are vital in helping the offspring cope with the chronic diseases that are seen as an adult as the result of oxidative stress.[11] It is important to avoid over supplementing micronutrients since this can be as harmful as inadequate micronutrient intake. While the optimal diet for pregnant women and future fathers is not yet established, evidence is showing that an unbalanced micronutrient intake can have long-lasting consequences for the health of the offspring.

References

1. Grieger, J, Clifton, V. A review of the impact of dietary intakes in human pregnancy on infant birthweight. *Nutrients*. 2015;7:153–178.

2. Shao J, Anderson A, Gibson R, Makrides M. Effect of iodine supplementation in pregnancy on child development and other clinical outcomes: a systematic review of randomized controlled trials. *Am J Clin Nutr*. 2013;98:1241–1254.

3. Garner C, Lockwood C, Barss V. Nutrition in pregnancy. UpToDate. Waltham, MA: UpToDate Inc. Available at: http://www.uptodate.com. Accessed December 15, 2017.

4. Gernand A, Schulze K, Stewart C, et al. Micronutrient deficiencies in pregnancy worldwide: health effects and prevention. *Nat Rev Endocrinol*. 2016 May;12(5):274–289.

5. Abu-Saad K, Fraser D. Maternal nutrition and birth outcomes. *Epidemiol Rev*. 2010;32:5–25.

6. Ramachandran P. Maternal nutrition – effect on fetal growth and outcome of pregnancy. *Nutr Rev*. 2002;60(5): S26–S34.

7. Academy of Nutrition and Dietetics. Healthy weight during pregnancy. Available at: http://www.eatright.org/resource/health/pregnancy/prenatal-wellness/healthy-weight-during-pregnancy. Accessed November 2017.

8. Ellis B, Giannetti L, Fagan J. The effects of maternal nutrition on the developing fetus later in life. Available at: https://pdfs.semanticscholar.org/4bd1/60cae6186145938f32bae77f3d50adf5a503.pdf. Accessed November 2017.

9. Nauta AJ, Ben Amor K, Knol J, et al. Relevance of pre- and postnatal nutrition to development and interplay between the microbiota and metabolic and immune systems. *Am J Clin Nutr.* 2013;98(suppl):586S–593S.

10. Yang Z, Huffman SL. Nutrition in pregnancy and early childhood and associations with obesity in developing countries. *Maternal and Child Nutr.* 2013;9:105–119.

11. Vanhees K, Vonhogen IG, van Schooten F, Godschalk RW. You are what you eat, and so are your children: the impact of micronutrients on the epigenetic programming of offspring. *Cell Mol Life Sci.* 2014;71:271–285.

12. Christian, P, Mullany L, Hurley K, et al. Nutrition and maternal, neonatal and child health. *Semin Perinatol.* 2015;39:361–372.

13. Bhutta ZA, Das JK, Rizvi A, et al. Evidence-based interventions for improvement of maternal and child nutrition: what can be done and at what cost? *Lancet.* 2013;382:452–477.

14. Sauder KA, Starling AP, Shapiro AL, et al. Exploring the association between maternal prenatal vitamin use and early infant growth: the healthy heart study. *Pediatr Obes.* 2015;11:434–441.

15. Hajj NE, Schneider E, Lehnen H, Haaf T. Epigenetics and life-long consequences of an adverse nutritional and diabetic intrauterine environment. *Reproduction.* 2014; 148:R111–R120.

16. Langley-Evans S. Nutrition in early life and the programming of adult disease: a review. *J Hum Nutr Diet.* 2015;2 (suppl. 1):1–14.

17. Indrio F, Martini S, Francavilla R, et al. Epigenetic matters: the link between early nutrition, microbiome, and long-term health development. *Front Pediatr.* 2017;5:178.

18. Sen S, Lyer C, Meydani SN. Obesity during pregnancy alters maternal oxidant balance and micronutrient status. *J Perinatol.* 2014;34:105–111.

19. Vickers MH. Early life nutrition, epigenetics and programming of later life disease. *Nutrients.* 2014;6:2165–2178.

20. Hattersley A, Tooke J. The fetal insulin hypothesis: an alternative explanation of the association of low birthweight with diabetes and vascular disease. *Lancet.* 1999;353:1789–1792.

21. Institute of Medicine. *Dietary Reference Intakes: The Essential Guide to Nutrient Requirements.* Washington, DC: National Academies Press; 2006.

22. Cetin, I, Alvino, G, Cardellicchio, M. Long chain fatty acids and dietary fats in fetal nutrition. *J Physiol.* 2009;587:3441–3451.

23. Gould JF, Smithers LG, Makrides M. The effect of maternal omega-3 (n-3) LCPUFA supplementation during pregnancy on early childhood cognitive and visual development: a systematic review and meta-analysis of randomized controlled trials. *Am J Clin Nutr.* 2013;97:531–544.

24. Kumar A, Bhatnagar G. Micronutrients in pregnancy. *Indian Obst Gynecol.* 2016;6:21–26.

25. Mistry HD, Kurlak LO, Young SD, et al. Maternal selenium, copper and zinc concentrations in pregnancy associated with small-for-gestational age infants. *Maternal and Child Nutr.* 2014;10:327–334.

26. Mori R, Ota E, Middleton P, Tobe-Gai R, et al. Zinc supplementation for improving pregnancy and infant outcome. *Cochrane Database Syst Rev* 2012;7:CD000230.

27. Smith ER, Shankar AH, Wu SF, et al. Modifiers of the effect of maternal multiple micronutrient supplementation on stillbirth, birth outcomes, and infant mortality: a meta-analysis of individual patient data from 17 randomized trials in low-income and middle-income countries. *Lancet.* 2017;5:e1090–e1100.

28. Lassi Z, Salam R, Haider B, Bhutta Z. Folic acid supplementation during pregnancy for maternal health and pregnancy outcomes. *Cochrane Database Syst Rev* 2013;3:CD006896.

29. Zerfu TA, Ayele HT. Micronutrients and pregnancy: effect of supplementation on pregnancy and pregnancy outcomes: a systematic review. *Nutr J.* 2013;12:20.

30. Neto CM. Vitamin D supplementation for women during pregnancy. *Sao Paulo Med J.* 2016;134(3):274–275.

31. Taylor P, Vaidya B. Iodine supplementation in pregnancy – is it time? *Clin Endocrinol.* 2016;85:10–14.

32. Piecynska J, Grajeta H. The role of selenium in human conception and pregnancy. *J Trace Elements Med Biol.* 2015;29:31–38.

33. Mao J Pop VJ, Bath SC, Vader HL, Redman CW, Rayman MP. et al. Effect of low-dose selenium on thyroid autoimmunity and thyroid function in UK pregnant women with mild-to-moderate iodine deficiency. *Eur J Nutr.* 2014;8:6–7.

34. Bell CC, Aujla J. Prenatal vitamins deficient in recommended choline intake for pregnant women. *J Fam Med Dis Prev.* 2016;2:048.

35. Maslova E, Hansen S, Strom M, et al. Maternal intake of vitamins A, E and K in pregnancy and child allergic disease: a longitudinal study from the Danish Birth Cohort. *Brit J Nutr.* 2014;111:1096–1108.

36. Buonocore G, Tei M, Perrine S. Lutein as protective agent against neonatal oxidative stress. *J Pediatr Neonat Individual Med.* 2014;3(2):e030244.

37. Asemi Z, Samimi M, Tabassi Z, Ahmad E. Multivitamin versus multivitamin-mineral supplementation and pregnancy outcomes: a single-blind randomized clinical trial. *Int J Prev Med.* 2014;5(4):439–446.

38. WHO/UNICEF/WFP. Preventing and controlling micronutrient deficiencies in populations affected by an emergency: multiple vitamin and mineral supplements for pregnant and lactating women, and for children aged 6 to 59 months. Available at: www.who.int/nutrition/publications/WHO _WFP_UNICEFstatement.pdf. Accessed September 30, 2018.

39. Tudehope D. Human milk and the nutritional needs or preterm infants. *J Pediat.* 2013;162(3 suppl):S17–S25.

40. Meier PP, Engstrom J, Patel AL, Jegier BJ, Bruns NE. Improving the use of human milk during and after the NICU stay. *Clin Perinatal.* 2010;37(1):217–245.

41. Underwood, MA. Human Milk for the premature infant. *Pediatr Clin North AM.* 2013;60(1):189–207.

42. Boghossian NS, Hanson NI, Bell EF, et al. Outcomes of extremely preterm infants born to insulin-dependent diabetic mothers. *Pediatrics.* 2016;137(6) e20153424.

43. Ono Y, Takagi K, Seki H, et al. Neonatal outcomes in infants of chronically hypertensive mothers. *J Obstet Gynaecol Res.* 2013;39(6):1142–1146.

44. Pare-Miron V, Czuzoj-Shulman, Oddy L, et al. Effects of borderline personality disorder on obstetrical and neonatal outcomes. *Women's Health Issues.* 2016; 26(2):190–195.

45. Pearson M, Hanson U, Pasupathy D, Norman M. Birth size distribution in 3,705 infants born to mothers with type 1 diabetes. *Diabetes Care.* 2011;34:1145–1149.

46. Forray A. Substance abuse during pregnancy. *F1000RES.* 2016; 13(5):F1000 Faculty Rev-887.

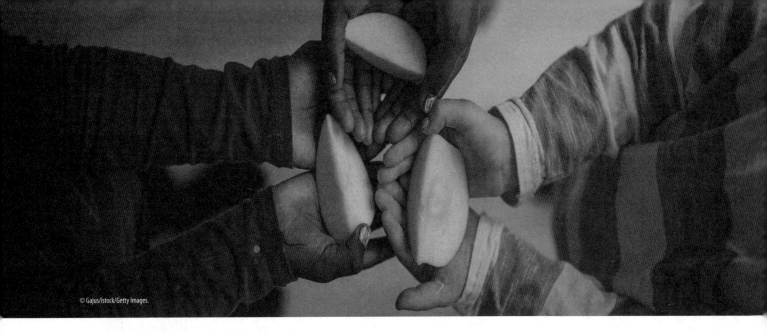

CHAPTER 6

Human Milk

Jacqueline J. Wessel

LEARNING OBJECTIVES

- Describe the unique properties of human milk.
- State the American Academy of Pediatrics recommendation for illicit drugs and the use of human milk.
- Identify two components of maternal diet that can alter human milk content.
- State two differences between maternal and donor human milk.

▶ Introduction

Using human milk for infants has been advocated by the American Academy of Pediatrics as well as numerous other medical societies.[1–8] The United States Healthy People 2020 goals are for 81.9% of infants to have ever breastfeed (see **TABLE 6.1**).[7] Fortunately, the latest results from 2014 show that this goal is currently being met, with a steady increase in breastfeeding since 2002.[7] A 2017 quote from the Surgeon General describes the problems and inequities still found: *"Rates of breastfeeding in the United States vary widely because of the multiple and complex barriers mothers face when starting and continuing to breastfeed."*[8] Rates of ever breastfeeding are still the lowest for black infants (68%) compared with the conglomerate national average at 82.5% in the 2014 Center for Disease Control and Prevention survey.[8]

TABLE 6.1 Healthy People 2020 Objectives[8]	
MATERNAL AND CHILD HEALTH 21 Increase the Proportion of Infants Who Are Breastfed	
MICH 21.1 Ever	81.9%
MICH 21.2 at 6 months	60.6%
MICH 21.3 at 12 months	34.1%
MICH 21.4 Exclusively through 3 months	46.2%
MICH 21.5 Exclusively through 6 months	25.5%

Data from Surgeon General. Surgeon General call to action support of breastfeeding. Available at: www.surgeongeneral.gov/breastfeeding. Accessed Dec 1, 2017.[8]

▶ Breastmilk

The numerous advantages of using breast milk are often discussed in terms of nutritional, immunological, psychosocial, and economic/societal.[9] See **TABLE 6.2**. Most of these benefits are well known; probably the latest additions are those concerning maternal cardiovascular health. There are several proposed mechanisms for these changes. That with the caloric cost, an average of 480 calories/day[10] and the results on postpartum weight change are inconclusive, breastfeeding may lower fat stores accumulated during pregnancy. Breastfeeding also may have a favorable effect on glucose and lipid metabolism through the "Reset Hypothesis." This hypothesis suggests that breastfeeding resets the maternal metabolism from what it was set for in pregnancy, so that it reverses fat accumulation and increases in lipid and triglyceride

levels as well as insulin resistance.[11] The hormones of breastfeeding, oxytocin, and prolactin may also have an effect on maternal blood pressure.[12] Most of the maternal advantages of breastfeeding are based on a cumulative breastfeeding duration of ~24 months, some are 12 to 24 months in total duration.

Colostrum to Mature Milk

This is the first human milk produced by mothers after delivery. It is limited in volume and is thought by many to have a primary immunological purpose since it is high in secretory IgA, lactoferrin, leukocytes, and epidermal growth factor. It is low in lactose, potassium, and calcium; and high in sodium, chloride, and magnesium. These levels change with the evolution to transitional milk.[48–50]

TABLE 6.2 Benefits of Breastfeeding

Mother	Improved mother-infant bonding[1]
	More rapid uterine involution[1]
	Postpartum weight loss[9,13]
	Decreased incidence of premenopausal breast cancer[14–16]
	Decreased incidence of ovarian cancer[14,15]
	May protect against development of rheumatoid arthritis[17]
	May have an decreased risk for osteoarthritis[18]
	Decreasing metabolic risk factors[19]
	Decreasing prevalence, incidence, and mortality from cardiovascular disease[11,19]
	Decreasing hypertension[11,12]
Infant	Decreases the incidence of and severity of a wide range of infectious diseases including:
	Diarrhea[12]
	Bacteremia[11]
	Respiratory tract infections[20]
	Bacterial meningitis[20]
	Necrotizing enterocolitis[24,25]
	Otitis media[20,26]
	Urinary tract infections (with one negative article)[27,28]
	Decrease post-neonatal infant mortality rate in the United States by 21%[7]
	Decreased rate of sudden infant death syndrome[14,15,29]
	Reduction in incidence of type 1 and type 2 diabetes[20,30–32]
	Overweight and obesity[32–34]
	Hypercholesterolemia[20]
	Lymphoma, leukemia, and Hodgkin disease[20,35,36]
	Inflammatory bowel disease[37]
	Celiac disease[38,39]
	Reduction of atopic disease in the first 3-4 months; not clear after that time concerning the introduction of foods[40–43]
	Enhanced performance on cognitive development tests[44,45]
	Repeat exposure to flavors from maternal diet[46]
Society	Reduced time off work for mothers of breastfed infants for infant's illness[1]
	Reduced healthcare costs[1,47]

Transitional milk is the next stage and the levels of lactose are higher while the levels of electrolytes alter with lower sodium and higher potassium. This transition goes from approximately 5 days to 2 weeks, but by approximately 1-month, milk is considered fully mature with much less fluctuation. With that said, human milk changes over time, over a day, and over a feeding.[51] The gold standard for milk composition studies is to sample several 24-hour collections from the same donor instead of from spot collections. Many studies take an analysis from donations to a milk bank, which may not reveal a true representation of nutrient composition.

The protein content from the milk of mothers who deliver preterm is generally considered to be higher in most, but not all, mothers.[52] Estimates from some research studies as to macronutrient content is included in **TABLE 6.3**. For all mothers, irrespective of the preterm or term delivery, the protein content of human milk decreases over the first 4 to 6 weeks or more of life.[46,51,53] Protein content in human milk is not influenced by maternal diet but increases with increased maternal weight for height. Mothers who are high producers have been found to have lower protein and fat content in their milk but have higher amounts of lactose.[53] The protein in human milk is divided into the whey and casein constituents, and there is a significant nonprotein nitrogen, which includes nucleotides, amino acids, urea, uric acid, creatine, and creatinine.[10]

The fat component of human milk is a major source of calories with a mean of 44%.[54] The fat component can be variable within a day; with one study finding the lowest fat concentration in night and morning feedings compared with afternoon and evening feedings.[55] The lipid component is highest in the latter part of a feeding, the hindmilk. The fat content of hind milk can be 2 to 3 times the content of the foremilk[10] or the earliest part of the feeding, which sometimes is almost blueish in color compared with the yellowish tint of hindmilk. Paula Meier has done extensive work on "lacto engineering" human milk to improve outcomes in preterm infants.[56] By dividing the pumping session into two parts, hindmilk can be collected and given to infants in order to enhance caloric intake. This does not obviate the need for fortification, since this is mainly changing the fat, and, therefore, the caloric intake of the feed.[57]

As noted, there can be a significant difference in the fat content of individual feedings throughout the day. Feedings early in the morning and at night can be lower in fat than afternoon and evening feedings.[48] For the term breastfed infant who gets all of these feedings, it evens out. For infants who may get only part of the 24-hour feedings, this could have an impact.

The **long chain polyunsaturated fats** (LC PUFAs), including omega 6 **arachidonic acid** (ARA) and omega 3 **docosahexaenoic acid** (DHA), have received a lot of attention. The fat content of the maternal diet can influence the fat content of human milk.[58-60] This is clear from the approximate 3-fold increase of linoleic acid content in mature human milk in the United States since the mid 1940s with the increase of dietary vegetable oil and linoleic content of the diet. Linolenic acid content has been stable through this period.[61] The average Western diet away from coastal areas is high in Omega 6 fat. Because of the dietary change, the average omega 6 to 3 ratio in human milk has increased 3-fold.[61] Stable isotope studies have enabled researchers to conclude that 90% of human milk ARA comes from maternal lipid stores, whereas dietary DHA is the main determinant of human milk DHA content.[62] For breastfeeding women to reach a DHA content of at least 0.3% or 100 mg DHA/day, the dietary intake of the mother would need to be at least 200 mg/day.[59,63] A systematic review of human studies with the Early Nutrition Academy has made this intake recommendation for breastfeeding women.[63]

Milk fat globule membrane (MFGM), another component of human milk, has also received attention. MFGM has a high density of bioactive components and has been a recent addition to infant formula. The studies of adding bovine MFGM and/or the complex lipids provided with the addition of MFGM have suggested that this has important roles in developing the immune and nervous system functions.[64]

The major carbohydrate of human milk is lactose. This component does not vary as much as the other macronutrients, other than it is higher in high-volume milk producers.[53]

The macronutrient composition of human milk is described in Table 6.3.

Human Milk Oligosaccharides

The third largest components in human milk, which have generated a great deal of research interest, are **Human Milk Oligosaccharides** (HMOs). These compounds are 3 to 32 sugars in size and are not broken down to provide nutrition to the infant.[48] They survive the lower pH of the infant's stomach, the higher pH of the upper small intestine, and reach the colon intact and then are excreted in the infant's feces. They are neither affected by human milk pasteurization nor freeze drying.[66] HMOs are part of the bioactive components of human milk. A bioactive component of food *"has an effect on biological processes or substrates and hence has an impact on body function or condition or ultimately health."*[67] See **TABLE 6.4**.

Human milk is not sterile and contains microbes that vary with maternal characteristics and length of lactation.[48] The first function elucidated for HMOs was that of prebiotics to feed beneficial bacteria in the infant's gastrointestinal tract.[68] Their function has now been found to be much more than that, since they can function as antiadhesive antimicrobials that act as decoy receptors and thus prevent the adhesion of pathogens to the

TABLE 6.3 Macronutrient Composition of Human Milk*	
Nutrient	**Amount**
Protein Term Infants	0.9–1.2 g/dl
Protein Preterm Infants	11 gm/dl ± 0.37 (0.2–2.2 g) range
Protein, Donor Milk	0.6 to 1.4 g/dl
Fat, Term Infant	3.2 to 3.6 g/dl
Fat, Preterm	3.2 ± 0.85 g/dl (1.1–6.1 g) range
Fat, Donor Milk	1.8 to 8.9 g/dl
Lactose	6.7 to 7.8 g/dl
Lactose, Preterm	6.6 ± 0.34 g/dl (5.5–8.0 g) range
Lactose, Donor Milk	6.4 to 7.6 g/dl
Kcal/100 ml	65 to 70 kcal/dl
Kcal/100 ml Preterm	60 ± 1.1 kcal/dl (39–94) range
Kcal/100 ml, Donor Milk	50–115 kcal/dl

Data from Ballard O, Morrow AL. Human milk composition: nutrients and bioactive factors. *Pediatr Clin North Am.* 2013;60:49–74.[48]

Kreissl A, Zwiauer V, Repa A, et al. Human Milk Analyzer shows that the lactation period affects protein levels in preterm breastmilk. *Acta Paediatr.* 2016;105:635–640.[65]

*Sampled from a 24-hour collection, analyzed by MIRIS analyzer.

infant's GI tract's mucosal surface. Through that mechanism, HMOs can lower the risk of viral, bacterial, and protozoan infections in the infant.[68] They also may modulate immune responses, lower the risk of **necrotizing enterocolitis (NEC)**, and provide sialic acid, which may be essential for brain development and cognition.[68] Additionally, there is research that shows that differences in HMO composition may affect infant growth and body composition.[69] Mothers vary as to their HMO profile in type and amounts as part of their genetic profile similar to Lewis blood types, secretor status (secretor vs. nonsecretor) and where they are in stages and over the lactation period.[70] Unlike the normal response to blood types, there is no incompatibility seen. It is thought that the differences may be pathogen specific in order to help with

survival in a certain area. A recent international observational HMO study from urban and rural areas of the United States, Europe, South America, and sub Saharan Africa indicated that there were effects on the individual cohort on almost all of the HMOs, showing a geographical as well as an environmental difference.[71]

HMOs are thought to be an integral part of the protection that human milk confers upon infants compared with infants who are fed formula.[48,68] An example of this is in the case of premature infants who acquire NEC. From recent literature, we now know that the fetus is not in a sterile environment.[72–74] The infant is exposed to microbes in the amniotic fluid and, as the fetus ingests up to 150 ml/kg of fluid per day, microbes enter its gastrointestinal tract.[74] Premature infants receiving their own mother's milk are much less likely to acquire NEC, a potentially devastating disease that can kill the intestine. Many factors in human milk may be responsible for this difference including lactoferrin, immunoglobulins, the microbes present, but also the HMOs, which increase the growth of *Bifidobacteria* and protect against infection.[68,74–77]

Researchers have looked at the fecal microbes using 16s rRNA sequencing in stool sampling in order to determine how the infant goes through different colonization as he or she matures.[74–82] There is evidence that premature infants have different colonization for those who later develop NEC and those who do not.[74–82] There is a steady increase in the phylum *Proteobacteria* compared with *Firmicutes*, *Bacteroides*, and *Negatvicutes*, with less diversity seen in those who develop NEC. This has been seen now by multiple research labs. The HMOs not only play a role as prebiotics but also as a decoy to bind potentially harmful pathogens so they do not adhere to the surface of the intestine.[48,74–84] Anything that disturbs the infant's microbiota such as empiric use of antibiotics or H2 blockers, appears to put the infant at greater risk for NEC.[85–87] The contribution of HMOs is considerable, but there are many other bioactive components that together make human milk such a valuable feeding for infants.

Relationship of Maternal Diet to Breastmilk

Human milk is a dynamic fluid.[88] The impact of maternal diet on human milk has been explored in an extensive review by Keikha et al.[89] Maternal dietary intake does alter breast milk composition in terms of fatty acid content, vitamins A, D, B_1 B_2, B_3, B_6 B_{12}, and iodine,[90] but for many other components, diet does not seem to change composition. It is recommended that vitamin D and vitamin K be supplemented to breastfed infants.[90] It is also recommended that mothers who are breastfeeding take a multivitamin supplement as maternal diet is not always optimal.[48,91,92]

TABLE 6.4 Major Bioactive Factors in Human Milk

Component	Function	Reference
Cells		
Macrophages	Protection against infection, T-cellactivation	Jarvinen, 2002; Yagi, 2010; Ichikawa, 2003
Stem cells	Regeneration and repair	Indumathi, 2012
Immunoglobulins		
IgA/sIgA	Pathogen-binding inhibition	Van de Perre, 2003; Cianga, 1999; Brandtzaeg, 2010; Kadaoui, 2007; Corthësy, 2009; Hurley, 2011; Agarwal, 2010; Castellote, 2011
IgG	Anti-microbial, activation of phagocytosis (IgG1, IgG2, IgG3); anti-inflammatory, response to allergens (IgG4)	Cianga, 1999; Agarwal, 2010
IgM	Agglutination, complement activation	Brandtzaeg, 2010; Van de Perre, 1993; Agarwal, 2010
Cytokines		
IL-6	Stimulation of the acute phase response, B cell activation, pro-inflammatory	Ustundag, 2005; Meki, 2003; Mizuno, 2012; Agarwal, 2010; Castellote, 2011
IL-7	Increased thymic size and output	Aspinall, 2011; Ngom, 2004
IL-8	Recruitment of neutrophils, pro-inflammatory	Claud, 2003; Ustundag, 2005; Meki, 2003; Maheshwari, 2002; Maheshwari, 2003; Maheshwari, 2004; Hunt, 2012; Agarwal, 2010; Castellote, 2011; Mehta, 2011
IL-10	Repressing Th1-type inflammation, induction of antibody production, facilitation of tolerance	Meki, 2003; Agarwal, 2010; Castellote, 2011; Mehta, 2011
IFNγ	Pro-inflammatory, stimulates Th1 response	Hrdý, 2012; Agarwal, 2010
TGFβ	Anti-inflammatory, stimulation of T cell phenotype switch	Penttila, 2010; Kalliomäki, 1999; Saito, 1993; Nakamura, 2009; Letterio, 1994; Ando, 2007; Ozawa, 2009; Donnet-Hughes, 2000; Verhasselt, 2008; Verhasselt, 2010; Penttila, 2003; Mosconi, 2010; Okamoto, 2005; Penttila, 2006; Peroni, 2009; McPherson, 2001; Ewaschuk, 2011; Castellote, 2011
TNFα	Stimulates inflammatory immune activation	Rudloff, 1992; Ustundag, 2005; Erbağci, 2005; Meki, 2003; Agarwal, 2010; Castellote, 2011

(continues)

TABLE 6.4 Major Bioactive Factors in Human Milk *(continued)*

Component	Function	Reference
Chemokines		
G-CSF	Trophic factor in intestines	Gilmore, 1994; Gersting, 2003; Calhoun, 2003; Gersting, 2004;
MIF	Macrophage Migratory Inhibitory Factor: prevents macrophage movement, increases anti-pathogen activity of macrophages	Magi, 2002; Vigh, 2011
Cytokine Inhibitors		
TNFRI and II	Inhibition of TNFα, anti-inflammatory	Buescher, 1998; Buescher, 1996; Meki, 2003; Castellote, 2011
Growth Factors		
EGF	Stimulation of cell proliferation and maturation	Patki, 2012; Kobata, 2008; Hirai, 2002; Wagner, 2008; Dvorak, 2003; Dvorak, 2004; Chang, 2002; Khailova, 2009; Coursodon, 2012; Clark, 2004; Castellote, 2011; Untalan, 2009
HB-EGF	Protective against damage from hypoxia and ischemia	Radulescu, 2011
VEGF	Promotion of angiogenesis and tissue repair	Loui, 2012; Ozgurtas, 2011
NGF	Promotion of neuron growth and maturation	Rodrigues, 2011; Boesmans 2008; Sánchez 1996; Fichter, 2011;
IGF	Stimulation of growth and development, increased RBCs and hemoglobin	Chellakooty, 2006; Blum, 2002; Burrin, 1997; Philipps, 2002; Milsom, 2008; Prosser, 1996; Elmlinger, 2007; Peterson, 2000; Murali, 2005; Corpeleijn, 2008; Baregamian, 2006; Baregamian, 2012; Büyükkayhan, 2003; Philipps, 2000; Kling, 2006;
Erythropoietin	Erythropoiesis, intestinal development	Carbonell-Estrany 2000; Juul, 2003; Kling, 2008; Miller-Gilbert, 2001; Pasha, 2008; Soubasi, 1995; Shiou, 2011; Arsenault, 2010; Miller, 2002; Untalan, 2009
Hormones		
Calcitonin	Development of enteric neurons	Struck, 2002; Wookey, 2012
Somatostatin	Regulation of gastric epithelial growth	Chen, 1999; Rao, 1999; Gama, 1996

Component	Function	Reference
Anti-microbial		
Lactoferrin	Acute phase protein, chelates iron, anti-bacterial, anti-oxidant	Adamkin, 2012; Sherman, 2004; Manzoni, 2009; Hirotani, 2008; Buccigrossi, 2007; Velona, 1999
Lactadherin/MFG E8	Anti-viral, prevents inflammation by enhancing phagocytosis of apoptotic cells	Stubbs, 1990; Kusunoki, 2012; Aziz, 2011; Shi, 2004; Chogle, 2011; Baghdadi, 2012; Peterson, 1998; Newburg, 1998; Shah, 2012; Miksa, 2006; Komura, 2009; Miksa, 2009; Wu, 2012; Matsuda, 2011; Silvestre, 2005
Metabolic Hormones		
Adiponectin	Reduction of infant BMI and weight, anti-inflammatory	Martin, 2006; Newburg, 2010; Woo, 2009; Woo, 2012; Ley, 2011; Dundar 2010; Ozarda, 2012; Savino, 2008; Weyerman, 2006
Leptin	Regulation of energy conversion and infant BMI, appetite regulation	Savino, 2008; Savino, 2012a; Savino 2012b; Palou, 2009; Weyermann, 2006
Ghrelin	Regulation of energy conversion and infant BMI	Savino, 2008; Savino, 2012; Dundar 2010
Oligosaccharides & Glycans		
HMOS	Prebiotic, stimulating beneficial colonization and reducing colonization with pathogens; reduced inflammation	Newburg, 2005; Morrow, 2005; DeLeoz, 2012; Marcoba, 2012; Kunz, 2012; Ruhaak, 2012; Bode, 2012
Gangliosides	Brain development; anti-infectious	Wang B, 2012
Glycosaminoglycans	Anti-infectious	Coppa, 2012; Coppa 2011
Mucins		
MUC1	Block infection by viruses and bacteria	Ruvoen-Clouet, 2006; Liu, 2012; Sando, 2009; Saeland, 2009; Yolken, 1992
MUC4	Block infection by viruses and bacteria	Ruvoen-Clouet, 2006; Liu, 2012; Chaturvedi, 2008

Reproduced from Ballard O, Morrow AL. Human milk composition: nutrients and bioactive factors. *Pediatr Clin North Am.* 2013;60:49–74.[48]

Vitamin Supplementation

Since the American Academy of Pediatrics recommendation in 1961, term infants in the United States. have been receiving a shot of 1 mg intramuscular vitamin K shortly after birth to prevent **vitamin K deficiency bleeding** (VKDB). Preterm infants weighing less than 1500 grams receive 0.5 mg.[1]

Research shows that human milk is low in ergocalciferol, vitamin D2; cholecalciferol, vitamin 3; and 25 hydroxy-vitamin D in fore- and hindmilk during the first 9 months of lactation. It was found that without direct sunlight exposure (as recommended) that exclusively breastfed infants received (77 IU) < 20% of the recommended vitamin D dose of 400 IU.[93]

Researchers have found that breast milk concentration of vitamin D is correlated with maternal plasma concentrations, with those mothers taking vitamin D supplements having higher concentrations in their breast milk but still having a mean concentration of 77 IU. Hindmilk is higher in vitamin D than foremilk. The American Academy of Pediatrics guideline and the Global Consensus recommendation is that all breastfed infants and those infants taking less than 1 liter of formula have a supplement of 400 IU beginning soon after birth.[94,95] There is research regarding super supplementing mothers with 4000 IU[96] and 6400 IU vitamin D[97] in order to enrich the content of their breast milk as well as their vitamin D levels; and that was equivalent to supplementing infants with oral vitamin D. Additional research is ongoing.

Canadian guidelines are that all healthy breastfed infants receive 400 I.U.; however, those living in the northern latitudes, north of 55 degrees, which is about the level of Edmonton, Alberta, should take 800 IU. Those with other risk factors such as darker skin, and living between the 40th and 55th parallel, should also supplement with 800 IU/day between October and April.[98,99]

Drug Use and Human Milk

The role of prescribed maternal medications and their effect on human milk is a concern for all clinicians. The AAP's guidance on weighing the risks and benefits of medications given to mother while she is lactating include the following factors:

a. The need of the drug by the mother
b. The potential effects of the drug on milk production
c. The amount of the drug excreted into human milk
d. The extent of oral absorption by the breastfeeding infant
e. The potential adverse effects on the breastfeeding infant; as well as considering
f. The age of the infant[100]

The AAP Clinical Report on the transfer of drugs is an excellent resource for the clinician.

Hale's Medications and Mother's Milk, now in its 17th edition (2017), compiles the known data on medications and is updated regularly.[101] It is also available in an online version as Medications and www.medsmilk.com Mothers Milk Online 2018.[102] Another on line resource is Lactmed, which is part of the National Library of Medicine's Toxicology Data Network and is a database of drugs and dietary supplements that may affect breastfeeding.[103] As with the Hale reference, the data are from the scientific body of literature and is fully referenced.[103] The Academy of Breastfeeding Medicine

has clinical protocols on Galactogogues,[104] Analgesia and Anesthesia for the Breastfeeding Mother,[105] Use of Antidepressants for Nursing Mothers,[106] and for Substance Abuse and Breastfeeding.[107] They are available at www.bfmed.org. These protocols are also well researched and referenced; they are also professionally translated and available in several languages on their website.

A special problem is the mother who plans to breastfeed but who also admits to abusing drugs. Adequately nourished mothers who have had consistent prenatal care with no other contraindications (such as HIV), who are narcotic dependent but enrolled and active in a treatment program are supported in their choice to breastfeed their infant.[107] There is obviously concern about the neurodevelopmental and medical implications for a baby who has been exposed prenatally to drugs of abuse. The hope is that the beneficial effects of human milk can help these infants. This remains an area needing further research.

The drug that often causes the most controversy, especially now that the use is legal in some states, is marijuana. The psychoactive component of marijuana, **delta-9-tetrahydrocannabinol** (THC), attaches to fat and is present in human milk up to eight times that of maternal plasma[107] and is present in infant feces as well, meaning that it is absorbed by the infant.[108] Another concern is that exposure to secondhand smoke of marijuana has been associated with independent two times possible risk of **sudden infant death syndrome (SIDS)**.[109] There is research that exposure during critical periods of brain development could induce subtle and long-lasting alterations in brain function.[110] In a convenience sampling of participants in a lactation conference in New England, 41% recommended continuing breastfeeding as the benefit was thought to outweigh the harm. Fifteen percent thought women should not breastfeed if they cannot stop using marijuana. Forty-four percent said it depended on factors such as severity of maternal use.[111] A recent review of the literature noted large gaps in the literature and that studies need to focus on the short- and long-term consequences of maternal use of marijuana. Until this is done, it was recommended that practitioners need to weigh the benefits of breastfeeding for mother and child, with the potential of marijuana on infant development when making the determination regarding feeding.[112] The Committee on Obstetric Practice Opinion 2017 discourages the use of marijuana during breastfeeding.[113]

Contraindications for the Use of Human Milk

There are very few absolute contraindications for using human milk but there are some. Various inborn errors of metabolism limit nutrients that the infant cannot metabolize completely. Sometimes, a small amount of human milk may be permitted with the specialty diet under the guidance of a metabolic dietitian.

In the United States, although the recommendation is not to breastfeed if the mother is HIV positive, in countries where the risk of formula feeding is considerable, the WHO is recommending exclusive breastfeeding for the first six months. This was outlined in a 2010 Bulletin, which also revised drug therapy guidelines to include treatment with antiretrovirals for the mother or baby during lactation and until the infant is 12 months of age.[114] Central to their decision were the results of two studies that showed, with the use of antiretrovirals and exclusive breastfeeding, that the risk of HIV transfer from mother to infant dropped by 42% in the Bora study and dramatically, in the Malawi study to 1.8%.[114]

Donor Human Milk

Maternal breastmilk is the best choice for infants; however, the next best feeding would be donor milk from a milk bank. The **Human Milk Banking Association of North America (HMBANA)** has published guidelines for the methodology of milk banking.[115] HMBANA also has guidelines for collecting and storing human milk.[116] The donation process starts with a telephone interview, then an intensive questionnaire, and includes blood sampling from the prospective donor mother for HIV, hepatitis B and C, human T-lymphocytic virus (HTLV), and Syphilis at the milk bank's expense. Donors are volunteers. There has been an increase in the number of milk banks opening over the past several years as more Newborn Intensive Care Units are using donor milk for **very low birth weight (VLBW)** preterm infants. There are now 26 HMBANA-associated milk banks in the United States and Canada with four more in development.[117]

There are other commercial donor milk products available now as well from Prolacta®[118] and Medolac®.[119] These companies also screen mothers and have rigorous standards for safe handling of human milk.

Buying milk from the Internet is not advised for a number of reasons. There is a report from researchers who analyzed purchased milk[120] and found the samples, at times, contain not all human milk, had high bacterial counts,[121,122] or had nicotine metabolites in milk that was advertised as coming from a nonsmoking mother.[123] Casual sharing of milk between mothers is done but potentially carries the risk of transmission of disease without rigorous testing.

One of the issues with using donor milk is that the donor might be from a different stage of lactation.[48,124] As discussed earlier, protein declines over time as does zinc content.[52,124,125] Two studies analyzed milk donations to milk banks and reported a mean of 0.85[126] and 0.9 g/dl[127]

protein. See Table 6.3. There is also wide variability in fat concentrations.[124] Some mothers donate as their term infants get older and are eating more supplemental food. This milk would be perfect for their infant but may be significantly lower in protein from what is needed for a premature infant. DHA levels were often found to be low, often less than the US mean DHA concentration.[124,127]

There is also the customization of an infant's mother's milk, with the mother making antibodies to the antigens in her and the baby's environment.[128] Thus, the immune profile may not be perfectly in sync with the needs of the infant receiving donor milk.

Colaizy has provided a thorough discussion of the research regarding the benefit of using donor human milk in terms of lowering infection rates.[124] More research needs to be done in looking at the most common use of donor milk, that as a bridge when maternal milk is insufficient and additionally fortified.

Growth has been an issue when using donor milk, with earlier reports of slower growth.[129] Newer studies with augmented supplementation show equivalent growth.[130]

Effects of Pasteurization

There are now several studies looking at the effect of Holder pasteurization on the bioactive components of human milk. Akinbi et al found that lysozyme, lactoferrin, lactoperoxidase, and secretory immunoglobulin A were reduced by 50% to 82% in pasteurized donor milk compared with freshly expressed maternal milk. Bacterial proliferation in pasteurized donor milk were increased 1.8- to 4.6-fold when compared with fresh or frozen maternal milk.[131]

Others have found that despite a decrease in some of the bioactive factors, the use of donor milk still reduces the risk of infection including NEC.[132]

This is why there are special considerations for the care and handling of donor milk since it does not have the same ability to fight infection as nonpasteurized milk. Pasteurization is important to guarantee the safety of donor milk, but it also has drawbacks. Other forms of sterilizations are being investigated.

Human Milk Used for Infants With Chylothorax

Occasionally after cardiac surgery, an infant will develop chylothorax, which requires chest tube placement. Treatment algorithms suggest a diet that is low in long chain fat and higher in medium chain triglycerides.[129] To avoid essential fatty acid deficiency, the diet must contain some long chain fats or be given these through intravenous fat infusion.

A high medium chain triglyceride formula can be used, but researchers have devised several strategies for defatting human milk so it can be used for these infants.[130] Initially, a centrifuge method was used,[131] then a method using 24-hour refrigeration. With both methods, a syringe is used to carefully remove the fat layer, and that has shown to be more effective than using a spoon.[132]

Some studies have shown slower growth,[133] while some studies have shown improved growth (Fogg) when compared with the growth on a high MCT-containing formula.[134] The use of defatted breast milk has been shown to be effective for treating chylothorax (chest tube output has not increased).[131] A recent study compared three methods using refrigeration, refrigerated centrifuge, and regular centrifuge. Using the refrigerator method resulted in less loss of IGa and protein but had somewhat more residual fat compared with the centrifuge methods.[135] The centrifuge methods had greater fat removal but also had greater protein and IgA loss.[135]

▶ Conclusion

Human milk is the preferred milk for infants. When that cannot be provided, adequately fortified donor milk is the next best choice followed by the appropriate choice for gestational age formula.[136–139] Efforts should be continued to assist women with the resources needed, including access to trained lactation consultants in order to provide milk for their infants.

Review Questions

1. Which fat component in human milk comes predominately from that in fat stores, not daily diet?
   A. DHA
   B. ARA

2. Protein can be increased in breast milk with additional protein in the diet.
   A. True
   B. False

3. Which macronutrient gradually declines over the period of lactation?
   A. Carbohydrate
   B. Protein
   C. Lipid

4. Human milk oligosaccharides contribute to the following except for:
   A. Immune function
   B. Changing the bacterial flora in the GI tract
   C. Lower incidence of diarrhea
   D. Increased visual acuity

5. Human milk contains human milk oligosaccharides, which, as a carbohydrate, contribute:
   A. 4 kcal/gm
   B. 9 kcal/gm
   C. 2 kcal/gm
   D. 0 kcal/gm

6. The energy cost of lactation averages:
   A. 300 kcal/day
   B. 480 kcal/day
   C. 600 kcal/day
   D. 720 kcal/day

7. Vitamins that must be supplemented in human milk include:
   A. Vitamin D and C
   B. Vitamin B_1 and Vitamin B_{12}
   C. Vitamin D and K
   D. Vitamin D and B_{12}

8. It is recommended by the Early Nutrition Academy that a breastfeeding mother take in at least 200 mg/day of DHA.
   A. True
   B. False

9. The goal for DHA intake for an infant is @ 100 mg/day of DHA.
   A. True
   B. False

10. Donor human milk and maternal human milk have the same protein content.
    A. True
    B. False

References

1. Section on Breastfeeding. Breastfeeding and the use of human milk. *Pediatrics*. 2012;129(3):e827-e841.
2. Critch J, Canadian Paediatric Society, Nutrition Gastroenterology Committee. Nutrition for healthy term infants, birth to six months: an overview. *Paediatr Child Health*. 2013;18:206–207.
3. Critch J, Canadian Paediatric Society, Nutrition Gastroenterology Committee. Nutrition for healthy term infants, 6 to 24 months: an overview. *Paediatr Child Health*. 2014;19(10):547–552.
4. Carlo, A, Braegger C, Decsi T, et al. Breast-feeding: a commentary by the ESPGHAN Committee on Nutrition. *J Pediatr Gastro Enterol Nutr*. 2009;49:112–125.
5. Fewtrell M, Bronsky J, Domellöf M, et al. Complementary feeding: a position paper by the ESPGHAN Committee on Nutrition. *J Pediatr Gastroenterol Nutr*. 2017;64:119–132.

6. WHO Statement. Exclusive breastfeeding for six months best for babies everywhere. Available at: www.WHO.int. Accessed Dec 1, 2017.

7. U.S. Department of Health and Human Services. Healthy People 2020: Breastfeeding Objectives. Available at: www.Healthypeople.gov. Accessed Dec 1, 2017.

8. Surgeon General. Surgeon General call to action support of breastfeeding. Available at: www.surgeongeneral.gov /breastfeeding. Accessed Dec 1, 2017.

9. Chowdury R, Sinha B, Sankar MJ, et al. Breastfeeding and maternal health outcomes: a systematic review and meta-analysis. *Acta Pediatric.* 2015;104:96–113.

10. Butte NF, Wong WW, Hopkinson JM. Energy requirements of lactating women derived from doubly labeled water and milk energy output. *J Nutr.* 2001;131:53–58.

11. Stuebe AM, Rich-Edwards JW. The reset hypothesis: lactation and maternal metabolism. *Am J Perinatol.* 2009;26:81–88.

12. Schwarz EB, Ray RM, Stuebe AM, et al. Duration of lactation and risk factors for maternal cardiovascular disease. *Obstet Gynecol.* 2009;113:974–982.

13. Neville CE, McKinley MC, Holmes VA, et al. The relationship between breastfeeding and postpartum weight change—a systematic review and critical evaluation. *Int J Obes.* 2014;38:577–590.

14. Ip S, Chung M, Raman G, et al. Tufts-New England Medical Center Evidence Based Practice Center: breastfeeding and maternal and infant health outcomes in developed countries. *Evid RepTechnol Assess.* 2007;153:1–186.

15. Ip S, Chung M, Raman G, Trikalinos TA, Lau J. A summary of the Agency for Healthcare Research and Quality's evidence report on breastfeeding in developed countries. *Breastfeed Med.* 2009;4(suppl 1):S17–S30.

16. Stuebe AM, Willett WC, Xue F, et al. Lactation and incidence of premenopausal breast cancer: a longitudinal study. *Arch Intern Med.* 2009;169(15):1364–1371.

17. Karlson EW, Mandl LA, Hankinson SE, Grodstein F. Do breastfeeding and other reproductive factors influence future risk of rheumatoid arthritis? Results from the Nurses' home study. *Arthritis Rheum.* 2004;50:3458–3487.

18. Park CY. Breastfeeding for one month or longer is associated with higher risk of osteoarthritis in older adults: NHANES 1999-2012. *Clin Nutr Res.* 2017;6:277–284.

19. Nguyen B, Jin K, Ding D. Breastfeeding and maternal cardiovascular risk factors and outcomes: a systematic review. *PloS One.* 2017;12(11):e0187923.

20. Duijts L, Jaddoe VW, Hofman A, et al. Prolonged and exclusive breastfeeding reduces the risk of infectious diseases in infancy. *Pediatrics.* 2010;126:e18.

21. Quigley MA, Kely YJ, Sacker A. Breastfeeding and hospitalization for diarrheal and respiratory infection in the United Kingdom Millennium Cohort Study. *Pediatrics.* 2007;119(4):e837-e842.

22. Walker WA. Protection of the neonate by the immune system of developing gut and of human milk. *Pediatr Res.* 2007;61:2–8.

23. Walker A. Breast milk as the gold standard for protective nutrients. *J Pediatr.* 2010;156:S3–S7.

24. Sisk PM, Lovelady CA, Dillard RG, et al. Early human milk feeding is associated with a lower risk of necrotizing enterocolitis in very low birth weight infants. *J Perinatol.* 2007;27(7):428–433.

25. Meinzen-Derr J, Poindexter B, Wrage L, et al. Role of human milk in extremely low birth weight infants' risk of necrotizing enterocolitis or death. *J Perinatol.* 2009;29: 57–62.

26. Li R, Dee D, Li CM, et al. Breastfeeding and risk of infections at 6 years. *Pediatrics.* 2014;134(supp 9):S13-S20.

27. Kaktikaneni R, Ponnapakkam T, Ponnanapakkam A, et al. Breastfeeding does not protect against urinary tract infection in the first 3 months of life, but vitamin D supplementation increases the risk by 76%. *Clin Pediatr.* 2009;48:760–765.

28. Vennemann MM, Bajanowski T, Brinkman B, et al. Does breastfeeding reduce the risk of sudden infant death syndrome? *Pediatrics.* 2009;123:e406–e410.

29. Savilahti E, Saarinen KM. Early infant feeding and type I diabetes. *Eur J Nutr.* 2009;48(4):243–249.

30. Rosenbauer J, Herzig P, Giani G. Early infant feeding and risk of type I diabetes mellitus-a nationwide population-based case-control study in pre-school children. *Diabetes Med Res Rev.* 2008;24(3):211–222.

31. Das UN. Breastfeeding prevents type 2 diabetes mellitus but, how and why? *Am J Clin Nutr.* 2007;85:1436–1437.

32. Metzger MW, McDade TW. Breastfeeding as obesity prevention in the United States. A sibling difference model. *Am J Hum Biol.* 2010; 22:291–296.

33. Ventura AK. Does breastfeeding shape food preference? Links to obesity. *Ann Nutr Metab.* 2017;70(suppl 3):8–15.

34. Moore BF, Sauder KA, Starling KP, et al. Exposure to secondhand smoke, exclusive breastfeeding and infant adiposity at age 5 months in the Healthy Start Study. *Pediatr Obes.* 2017; 12(suppl 1):111–115.

35. Amitay EL, Dubnov Raz G, Keinan-Boker L. Breastfeeding. Other early life exposure and childhood leukemia and lymphoma. *Nutr Cancer.* 2016;68:968–977.

36. Amitay EL, Keinan-Boker L. Breastfeeding and childhood leukemia incidence: a meta-analysis and systematic review. *JAMA Pediatr.* 2015;169:e151025.

37. Viera Borba V, Sharif K, Shoenfeld Y. Breastfeeding and autoimmunity: Programming health from the beginning. *Am J Reprod Immun.* 2018;79.

38. Ivarsson A, Hernell O, Stenlund H, et al. Breastfeeding protects against celiac disease. *Am J Clin Nutr.* 2002;75:914–921.

39. Akobeng AK, Ramanan AV, Buchan I, Heller RF. Effect of breastfeeding on risk of coeliac disease: a systematic review and meta-analysis of observational studies. *Arch Dis Child.* 2006;91(1):39–43.

40. Saarinen IJM, Kajosaari M, Backnman A, et al. Prolonged breastfeeding as prophylaxis for atopic disease. *Lancet.* 1979;2:163–166.

41. Kramer MS. Does breastfeeding help protect against atopic disease? Biology, methodology and a golden jubilee of controversy. *J Pediatr.* 1988;112:181–190.

42. Thygarejan A, Burks AW. American Academy of Pediatrics recommendations on the effect of early nutritional interventions on the development of atopic disease. *Curr Opin Pediatr.* 2008;20:698–702.

43. Greer FR, Sicherer SH, Burks W, et al. Effects of nutritional interventions on the development of atopic disease in infants and children: the role of maternal diet restriction, timing of introduction of complementary foods, and hydrolyzed formulas. *Pediatrics.* 2008;121:183–190.

44. Kim JL, Kim BN, Kim JW, et al. Breastfeeding is associated with enhanced learning skills. *Child Adolesc Psychiatry Ment Health*. 2017;11:36.

45. Patra K, Hamilton M, Johnson TJ, et al. NICU Human milk dose and 20-month neurodevelopmental outcome in very low birth weight infants. *Neonatology*. 2017;112(4):330–336.

46. Forestell CA. Flavor perception and preference development in human infants. *Ann Nutr Metabol*. 2017;70(suppl 3): 17–25.

47. Ajetunmobi OM, Whyte B, Chalmers J, et al. Breastfeeding is associated with reduced childhood hospitalization: evidence from a Scottish Birth Cohort (1997-2009). *J Pediatr*. 2015;166:620–625.

48. Ballard O, Morrow AL. Human milk composition: nutrients and bioactive factors. *Pediatr Clin North Am*. 2013;60:49–74.

49. Hsu Y, Chen C, Lin M, et al. Changes in preterm breast milk nutrient content in the first month. *Pediatr Neonatol*. 2014;320:1–6.

50. Lawrence RA, Lawrence RM. *Breastfeeding: A Guide for the Medical Profession*. 8th ed. St. Louis, MO: Mosby; 2015.

51. Mitoulas LR, Kent JC, Cox DB, et al. Variation in fat, lactose, and protein in human milk over 24 h and throughout the first year of life. *Br J Nutr*. 2002;88:29–37.

52. Arslanoglu S, Moro GE, Ziegler EE. Preterm infants fed fortified human milk receive less protein than they need. *J Perinatol*. 2009;29:489–492.

53. Nommsen LA, Lovelady CA, Heinig MJ, Lönnerdal B, Dewey KG. Determinants of energy, protein, lipid, and lactose concentrations in human milk during the first 12-month of lactation: the DARLING Study. *Am J Clin Nutr*. 1991;53(2):457–465.

54. Grote V, Verduci E, Scaglioni S, et al. Breast milk composition and infant nutrient intakes during the first 12 months of life. *Eur J Clin Nutr*. 2016;70:250–256.

55. Kent JC, Mitoulas LR, Cregan MD, et al. Volume and frequency of breastfeeding and fat content of breast milk throughout the day. *Pediatrics*. 2006;117:e387–e395.

56. Meier PP, Engstrom JL, Patel AL, et al. Improving the use of human milk during and after the NICU stay. *Clin Perinatol*. 2010;37:217–245.

57. Adamkin D, Dreyer G, Gould JB, et al. *Neonatal Clinical Management Guidelines*, 9th ed. Pg. Available at: 10. www.UHC.com. Accessed December 10, 2017.

58. Bradbury J. Docosahexaenoic Acid (DHA): an ancient nutrient for the modern brain. *Nutrients*. 2011;3: 529–554.

59. Koletzko B. Human milk lipids. *Ann Nutr Metabol*. 2016;69(suppl 2):28–40.

60. Brenna JT, Varamini B, Jensen RG, et al. Docosahexaenoic and arachidonic concentrations in human breast milk worldwide. *Am J Clin Nutr*. 2007;85:1457–1464.

61. Allhaud G, Massiera F, Weill P, et al. Temporal changes in dietary fats: role of n-6 polyunsaturated fatty acids in excess adipose tissue development and relationship to obesity. *Prog Lipid Res*. 2006;45:203–236.

62. Del Prado M, Villalpando S, Elizondo A, et al. Contribution of dietary and newly formed arachidonic acid to human milk lipids in women eating a low fat diet. *Am J Clin Nutr*. 2001; 74(2):241–247.

63. Koletzko B, Boey CCM, Campoy C, et al. Current information and Asian perspectives on long chain polyunsaturated fatty acids in pregnancy, lactation, and infancy. Systematic review and practice recommendations from an early Nutrition Academy workshop. *Ann Nutr Metab*. 2014;65:49–80.

64. Hernell O, Timby N, Domellof M, et al. Clinical benefits of milk fat globulin membrane for infants and children. *J Pediatr*. 2016;173(suppl):560–565.

65. Kreissl A, Zwiauer V, Repa A, et al. Human milk analyzer shows that the lactation period affects protein levels in preterm breastmilk. *Acta Paediatr*. 2016;105:635–640.

66. Schrezenmeir J, Korhonen H, Williams C, et al. Foreword. *Br J Nutr*. 2000;84(suppl 1), S1.

67. Bode L. Human milk oligosaccharides: Every baby needs a sugar mama. *Glycobiology*. 2012;22:1147–1142.

68. Alderete TL, Autran C, Brekke BE, et al. Associations between human milk oligosaccharides and infant body composition in the first 6 months of life. *Am J Clin Nutr*. 2015;102:1381–1388.

69. Kunz C, Meyer C, Collado MC, et al. Influence of gestational age, secretor, and Lewis blood group status on the oligosaccharide content of human milk. *J Pediatr Gastroenterol Nutr*. 2017;64:789–798.

70. McGuire MK, Meehan CI, McGuire MA, et al. What's normal? Oligosarrharide concentrations and profiles in milk produced by healthy women vary geographically. *Am J Clin Nutr*. 2017;105:1086–1100.

71. DiGiulio DB, Romero B, Kusanovic JF, et al. Prevalence and diversity of microbes in the amniotic fluid, the fetal inflammatory response, and pregnancy outcome in women with preterm pre-labor rupture of membranes. *Am J Reprod Immunol*. 2010;64:38–57.

72. DiGiulio DB. Diversity of microbes in amniotic fluid. *Semin Fetal Neonatal Med*. 2012;64:2–11.

73. Neu J, Pammi M. Pathogenesis of NEC: Impact of an altered intestinal microbiome. *Sem Perinatol*. 2015;41:29–35.

74. Neu J. Necrotizing Enterocolitis. In: Koletzko B, Poindexter B, Uauy R, eds. *World Review of Nutrition and Dietetics Vol. 110: Nutritional Care of Preterm Infants*. Basel, Switzerland: Karger, 2014:253–263.

75. Good M, Sodhi CP, Yamaguchi Y, et al. The human milk oligosaccharide 2"—fucosyllactose attenuates the severity of experimental necrotizing enterocolitis by enhancing mesenteric blood perfusion in the neonatal intestine. *Br J Nutr*. 2016;116:1175–1187.

76. De Leoz ML, Kalenetra KM, Bokulich NA, et al. Human milk glycomics and gut microbial genomics in infant feces show a correlation between human milk oligosaccharides and gut microbiota: a proof of concept study. *J Proteome Res*. 2015;14:491–502.

77. Dobbler PT, Procianoy RS, Mai V, et al. Low microbial diversity and abnormal microbial succession is associated with necrotizing enterocolitis in preterm infants. *Frontiers Microbiol*. 2017;8:2243.

78. Patel RM, Denning PW. Intestinal microbiota and its relationship with necrotizing enterocolitis. *Pediatr Res*. 2015;78:232–238.

79. Wang Y, Hoenig JD, Malin KJ, et al. 16S rRNA gene-based analysis of fecal microbiota from preterm infants with and without necrotizing enterocolitis. *ISME J*. 2009; 3(8):944–954.

80. Warner BB, Deych E, Zhou Y, et al. Gut bacteria dybiosis and necrotizing enterocolitis in very low birthweight infants: a prospective case controlled study. *Lancet*. 2016; 387:1928–1936.

81. Mai V, Young CM, Ukhanova M, et al. Fecal microbiota in premature infants prior to necrotizing enterocolitis. *PLoS One*. 2011;6(6): e20647.

82. Morrow AL, Lagomarcino AJ, Schibler KR, et al. Early microbial and metabolomic signatures predict later onset of necrotizing enterocolitis in preterm infants. *Microbiome.* 2013;1(1):13.

83. Kuppala VS, Meinzen-Derr J, Morrow AL, et al. Prolonged empirical antibiotic treatment is associated with adverse outcomes in premature infants. *J Pediatr.* 2011;159:720–725.

84. Ting JY, Synnes A, Roberts A, et al. Association between antibiotic use and neonatal mortality and morbidities in very low birthweight infants without culture-proven sepsis or necrotizing entercolitis. *JAMA Pediatr.* 2016;170(12):1181–1187.

85. Greenwood C, Morrow AL, Lagomarcino AJ, et al. Early empiric antibiotics in preterm infants is associated with lower bacterial diversity and higher relative abundance of Enterobacter. *J Pediatr.* 2014;165(1):23–29.

86. Romaine A, Ye D, Ao Z, et al. Safety of histamine-2 receptor blockers in hospitalized VLBW infants. *Early Hum Dev.* 2016;99:27–30.

87. Kakulas F, Geddes DB. Breastmilk composition is dynamic: infant feeds, mother responds. International Milk Genomics Consortium. Available at: http://milkgenomics.org /breastmilk=composition-dynamic-infant-feeds-mother -responds/. Accessed December 15, 2017.

88. Keikha M., Bahreynian M, Saleki M, et al. Macronutrients and micronutrients of human milk composition: are they related to maternal diet? A comprehensive systematic review. *Breastfeed Med.* 2017,12:517–127.

89. Valentine CJ, Wagner CL. Nutritional management of the breastfeeding dyad. *Pediatr Clin N Am.* 2013;60:261–274.

90. Greer FR. Do breastfed infants need supplemental vitamins? *Pediatr Clinics N Amer.* 2001;48:415–423.

91. Allen LH. B vitamins in breast milk: relative importance of maternal status and intake, and effects on infants status and function. *Adv Nutr.* 2012;3:362–369.

92. vio Streym S, Højskov CS, Møller UK, et al. Vitamin D content in human breast milk: a 9-month follow-up study. *Am J Clin Nutr.* 2016;103(1):107–114.

93. Wagner CL, Greer FR, American Academy of Pediatrics Section on Breastfeeding, American Academy of Pediatrics Committee on Nutrition. Prevention of rickets and vitamin d deficiency in infants, children, and adolescents. *Pediatrics.* 2008;122(5):1142–1152.

94. Munns CF, Shaw N, Kiely M, et al. Global consensus recommendations on prevention and management of nutritional rickets. *J Clin Endocrinol Metab.* 2016;101:394–415.

95. Hollis BW, Wagner CL. Vitamin D requirements during lactation: high dose maternal supplementation as therapy to prevent hypovitaminosis D for both the mother and the nursing infant. *Am J Clin Nutr.* 2004;80(6 suppl): 1752S–1758S.

96. Wagner CL, Hulsey TC, Fanning D, Ebeling M, Hollis BW. High-dose vitamin D3 supplementation in a cohort of breastfeeding mothers and their infants: a 6-month follow-up pilot study. *Breastfeed Med.* 2006;1(2):59–70.

97. Ward LM. Vitamin D deficiency in the 21st century: a persistent problem among Canadian infants and mothers. *CMAJ.* 2005;172:769–770.

98. Godel JC, Canadian Paediatric Society. Vitamin D supplementation: recommendations for Canadian mothers and infants. *Paediatr Child Health.* 2007;12:583–589.

99. Sachs HC, Committee on Drugs. The Transfer of drugs and therapeutics into human breast milk: an update on selected topics. *Pediatrics.* 2012;132(3):e796–e809.

100. Hale T. *Medications and Mothers Milk 2017.* 17th ed. Amarillo, TX: Hale Publishing, LP; 2016.

101. Hale, T, Medications and Mothers Milk Online 2018. Available at: www.medsmilk.com. Accessed December 1, 2017.

102. National Library of Medicine, Toxicology Data Network. Lactmed. Available at: http://toxnet.nlm.nih.gov/cgi-bin /sis/htmigen?LACT. Accessed December 20, 2017.

103. Academy of Breastfeeding Medicine Protocol Committee. Academy of Breastfeeding Medicine Clinical Protocol #9. Use of galactogogues in initiating or augmenting the rate of maternal milk secretion. *Breastfeed Med.* 2011;6(1):41–49.

104. Reece-Stremtan S, Campos M, Kokajko L, Academy of Breastfeeding Medicine. ABM Clinical protocol #15: analgesia and anesthesia for the breastfeeding mother, revised 2017. *Breastfeed Med.* 2017;12(9):500–506.

105. Sriraman NK, Melvin K, Meltzer-Brody S, et al. ABM Clinical Protocol #18: Use of antidepressants in breastfeeding mothers. *Breastfeed Med.* 2015;10(6):290–299.

106. Reece-Stremtan S, Marinelli KA. Academy of Breastfeeding Medicine. ABM Clinical Protocol #21: Guidelines for breastfeeding and substance use or substance use disorder, revised 2015. *Breastfeed Med.* 2015;10(3):135–141.

107. Perez-Reyes M, Wall ME, Presence of delta 9-tetrahydrocannabinol in human milk. *N Engl J Med.* 1982;307:819–820.

108. Klonoff-Cohen H, Lam-Kruglick P. Maternal and paternal drug use and sudden infant death syndrome. *Arch Pediatric Adolesc Med.* 2001;155:765–770.

109. Campolongo P, Trezza V. Palmery M, et al. Developmental exposure to cannabinoids causes subtle and enduring neurofunctional alterations. *Int Rev Neurobiol.* 2009;85:117–133.

110. Bergeria CL, Heil SH. Surveying lactation professionals regarding marijuana use and breastfeeding. *Breastfeed Med.* 2015;10:377–380.

111. Mourh J, Rowe H. Marijuana and breastfeeding: applicability of the current literature to clinical practice. *Breastfeed Med.* 2017;12:582–596.

112. Committee on Obstetric Practice, Committee Opinion no. 722: Marijuana use during pregnancy and lactation. *Obstet Gynecol.* 2017;130:e205–e209.

113. Bulletin of the World Health Organization. 2010;88:1–80.

114. Human Milk Banking Association of North America. Guidelines for the Establishment and Operation of a Donor Human Milk Bank. 2015. Fort Worth, TX: HMBANA.

115. Human Milk Banking Association of North America. 2011 Best Practice for Expressing, Storing and Handling Human Milk in Hospitals, Homes, and Child Care Settings. Fort Worth, TX: HMBANA. 3rd Edition 2011.

116. www.hmbana.org (Accessed 12/12/17)

117. www.prolacta.com (Accessed 12/12/17)

118. www.medolac.com (Accessed 12/12/17)

119. Geraghty SR, McNamara KA, Dillon CE, et al. Buying human milk via the internet: just a click away. *Breastfeed Med.* 2013;8(6):474–478.

120. St-Onge M, Chaudhry S, Kpren G. Donated breast milk stored in banks versus breast milk purchased online. *Can Fam Physician.* 2015;61:143–148.

121. Keim SA, Hogan JS, McNamara KA, et al. Microbial contamination of human milk purchased via the internet. *Pediatrics.* 2013;132(5):e1227–e1235.

122. Geraghty SR, McNamara KA, Kwiek JJ, et al. Tobacco metabolites and caffeine in human milk purchased on the internet. *Breastfeed Med.* 2015;10:419–424.

123. Colaizy TT. Donor human milk for preterm infants. *Clin Perinatol*. 2014;41:437–450.

124. Songul Yalcin S, Yalcin S, Ihsan Gucus A. Zinc and copper concentrations in breast milk during the first nine months of lactation: a longitudinal study. *Pediatrics*. 2015;135(suppl 1).

125. Drulis JM, Ziegler EE. Donor human milk for premature infants, mother's milk of Iowa. Presented at the 14th ISRHML International Conference; January 2008; Perth, Australia.

126. Valentine CJ, Morrow G, Fernandez S, et al. Docosahexaenoic acid and amino acid contents in pasteurized donor milk are low for premature babies. *J Pediatr*. 2010;157:906–910.

127. Kleinman RE, Walker WA. The enteromammary immune system: an important new concept in breast milk host defense. *Dig Dis Sci*. 1979;24:876–882.

128. Committee on Nutrition, Section on Breastfeeding, Committee on Fetus and Newborn. Donor human milk for the high-risk infant: preparation, safety, and usage options in the United States. *Pediatrics*. 2017;139(1):e20163440.

129. Church JT, Antunez AG, Dean A, et al. Evidence-based management of chylothorax in infants. *J Pediatr Surg*. 2017;52(6):907–912.

130. DiLauro S, Unger S, Sloan D, et al. Human milk for ill and medically fragile infants: strategies and ongoing innovation. *J Parenter Enteral Nutr*. 2016;40:768–782.

131. Chan GM, Lechtenberg E. The use of fat-free human milk in infants with chylous pleural effusion. *J Perinatol*. 2007;27(7):434–436.

132. Drewniak MA, Lyon AW, Fenton TR. Evaluation of fat separation and removal methods to prepare low-fat breast milk for fat-intolerant infants with chylothorax. *Nutr Clin Pract*. 2013;28(5):599–602.

133. Kocel SL, Russell J, O'Connor DL. Fat-modified breast milk resolves chylous pleural effusion in infants with post-surgical chylothorax but is associated with slow growth. *J Parenter Enteral Nutr*. 2016;40(4):543–551.

134. Fogg KL, DellaValle DM, Buckly JR, Graham EM, Zyblewski SC. Feasibility and efficacy of defatted human milk in the treatment for chylothorax after cardiac surgery in infants. *Pediatr Cardiol*. 2016;37(6):1072–1077.

135. Drewniak M, Waterhouse CCM, Lyon AW, Fenton, TR. Immunoglobulin A and protein content of low-fat human milk prepared for the treatment of Chylothorax. *Nutr Clin Pract*. 2018;33(5):667–670.

136. Colaizy TT, Carlson SE, Saftlas AF, et al. Growth in VLBW infants fed predominately fortified maternal and donor human milk diets: a retrospective cohort study. *BMC Pediatr*. 2012;12:124.

137. Akinbi H, Meinzen-Derr J, Auer C, et al. Alterations in the host defense properties of human milk following prolonged storage or pasteurization. *J Pediatr Gastroenterol Nutr*. 2010; 51(3):347–352.

138. Quigley MA, McGuire W. Formula milk versus donor breast milk for feeding preterm or low birth weight infants. *Cochrane Database Syst Rev*. 2014;4:CD002971.

139. ESPGHAN Committee on Nutrition, Arslanoglu S, Corpeleijn W, et al. Donor human milk for preterm infants: current evidence and research directions. *J Pediatr Gastroenterol Nutr*. 2013;57(4):535–542.

References for Bioactive Components of Human Milk

1. Jarvinen KM, Suomalainen H. Leucocytes in human milk and lymphocyte subsets in cow's milk-allergic infants. *Pediatr Allergy Immunol*. 2002;13(4):243–254.

2. Yagi Y, Watanabe E, Watari E, et al. Inhibition of DC-SIGN-mediated transmission of human immunodeficiency virus type 1 by Toll-like receptor 3 signaling in breast milk macrophages. *Immunology*. 2010;130(4):597–607.

3. Ichikawa M, Sugita M, Takahashi M, et al. Breast milk macrophages spontaneously produce granulocyte-macrophage colony-stimulating factor and differentiate into dendritic cells in the presence of exogenous interleukin-4 alone. *Immunology*. 2003;108(2):189–195.

4. Indumathi S, Dhanasekaran M, Rajkumar JS, Sudarsanam D. Exploring the stem cell and non-stem cell constituents of human breast milk. *Cytotechnology*. 2013;65(3):385–393.

5. Van de Perre P. Transfer of antibody via mother's milk. *Vaccine*. 2003;21(24):3374–3376.

6. Cianga P, Medesan, Richardson JA, et al. Identification and function of neonatal Fc receptor in mammary gland of lactating mice. *Eur J Immunol*. 29: 2515–2523.

7. Brandtzaeg P. The mucosal immune system and its integration with the mammary glands. *J Pediatrics*. 2010;156 (2 suppl):S8–S15.

8. Kadaoui KA, Corthésy B. Secretory IgA mediates bacterial translocation to dendritic cells in mouse peyer's patches with restriction to mucosal compartment. *J Immunol*. 2007;179:7751–7757.

9. Corthésy B. Secretory immunoglobulin A: well beyond immune exclusion at mucosal surfaces. *Immunopharmacol Immunotoxicol*. 2009;31(2):174–179.

10. Hurley WL, Theil PK. Perspectives on immunoglobulins in colostrum and milk. *Nutrients*. 2011;3(4):442–474.

11. Agarwal S, Karmaus W, Davis S, Gangur V. Immune markers in breast milk and fetal and maternal body fluids: a systematic review of perinatal concentrations. *J Hum Lact*. 2011;27(2):171–186.

12. Castellote C, Casillas R, Ramirez-Santana C, et al. Premature delivery influences the immunological composition of colostrum and transitional and mature human milk. *J Nutr*. 2011;141(6):1181–1187.

13. Ustundag B, Yilmaz E, Dogan Y, et al. Levels of cytokines (IL-1beta, IL-2, IL-6, IL-8, TNF-alpha) and trace elements (Zn, Cu) in breast milk from mothers of preterm and term infants. *Mediators Inflamm*. 2005;2005(6):331–336.

14. Meki A-RMA, Saleem TH, Al-Ghazali MH, Sayed AA. Interleukins -6, -8 and -10 and tumor necrosis factor alpha and its soluble receptor I in human milk at different periods of lactation. *Nutr Res*. 2003;23:845–855.

15. Mizuno K, Hatsuno M, Aikawa K, et al. Mastitis is associated with IL-6 Levels and milk fat globule size in breast milk. *J Hum Lact*. 2012;28(4):529–534.

16. Aspinall R, Prentice AM, Ngom PT. Interleukin 7 from maternal milk crosses the intestinal barrier and modulates T-cell development in offspring. *PloS ONE*. 2011;6(6):e20812.

17. Ngom P, Collinson A, Pido-Lopez J, Henson S, Prentice A, Aspinall R. Improved thymic function in exclusively breastfed infants is associated with higher interleukin 7 concentrations in their mothers' breast milk. *Am J Clin Nutr*. 2004;80(3):722–728.

18. Claud EC, Savidge T, Walker WA. Modulation of human intestinal epithelial cell IL-8 secretion by human milk factors. *Pediatr Res*. 2003;53:419–425.

19. Maheshwari A, Lu W, Lacson A, et al. Effects of Interleukin-8 on the developing human intestine. *Cytokine*. 2002;20(6): 256–267.

20. Maheshwari A, Christensen RD, Calhoun DA. ELR+ CXC chemokines in human milk. *Cytokine*. 2003;24:91–102.

21. Maheshwari A, Lacson A, Lu W, et al. Interleukin-8/CXCL8 forms an autocrine loop in fetal intestinal mucosa. *Pediatr Res*. 2004;56(2):240–249.

22. Hunt KM, Williams JE, Shafii B, et al. Mastitis is associated with increased free acids, somatic cell count, and Interleukin-8 concentrations in human milk. *Breastfeed Med*. 2013;8(1):105–110.

23. Mehta R, Petrova A. Very preterm gestation and breast milk cytokine content during the first month of lactation. *Breastfeed Med*. 2011;6:21–24.

24. Hrdý J, Novotná O, Kocourková I, Prokešová L. Cytokine expression in the colostral cells of healthy and allergic mothers. *Folia Microbiologica*. 2012;57(3):215–219.

25. Pentilla I. Milk derived transforming growth factor beta and the infant immune response. *J Pediatr* 2010;156 (2 suppl):S21–S25.

26. Kalliomäki M, Ouwehand A, Arvilommi H, et al. Transforming growth factor-β in breast milk: a potential regulator of atopic disease at an early age. *J Allergy Clin Immunol*. 1999:1251–1257.

27. Saito S, Yoshida M, Ichijo M, et al. Transforming growth factor-beta (TGF-f) in human milk. *Clin Exp Immunol*. 1993;94:220–224.

28. Nakamura Y, Miyata M, Ando T, et al. The latent form of transforming growth factor-beta administered orally is activated by gastric acid in mice. *J Nutr*. 2009;139: 1463–1468.

29. Letterio JJ, Geiser AG, Kulkarni Ashok B, et al. Maternal rescue of transforming growth factor-b1 null mice. *Science*. 1994;264:1936–1938.

30. Ando T, Hatsushika K, Wako M, et al. Orally administered TGF-b is biologically active in the intestinal mucosa and enhances oral tolerance. *J Allergy Clin Immunol*. 2007;120:916–923.

31. Ozawa T, Miyata M, Nishimura M, et al. Transforming growth factor-b activity in commercially available pasteurized cow milk provides protection against inflammation in mice. *J Nutr*. 2009; 139:69–75.

32. Donnet-Hughes A, Duc N, Serrant P, Vidal K, Schiffrin EJ. Bioactive molecules in milk and their role in health and disease: The role of transforming growth factor-b. *Immunol Cell Biol*. 2000; 78:74–79.

33. Verhasselt V, Milcent V, Cazareth J, et al. Breast milk-mediated transfer of an antigen induces tolerance and protection from allergic asthma. *Nat Med*. 2008;14(2): 170–175.

34. Verhasselt V. Neonatal tolerance under breastfeeding influence: the presence of allergan and transforming growth factor-beta in breast milk protects the progeny from allergic asthma. *J Pediatr*. 2010;156(2 suppl):S16–S20.

35. Pentilla IA, Flasch IB, McCrie AL, et al. Maternal milk regulation of cell infiltration and interleukin 18 in the intestine of suckling rat pups. *Gut*. 2003;52:1579–1586.

36. Mosconi E, Rekima A, Seitz-Polski B, Kanda A, et al. Breast milk immune complexes are potent inducers of oral tolerance in neonates and prevent asthma development. *Mucosal Immunol*. 2010;3:461–474.

37. Okamoto A, Kawamura T, Kanbe K, et al. Supression of serum IgE response and systemic anaphylaxis in a food allergy model by orally administered high-dose TGF-beta. *Int Immunol*. 2005;17:705–712.

38. Penttila IA. Milk-derived transforming growth factor-b and the infant immune response. *J Pediatr*. 2010;156: S21–S25.

39. Peroni D, Piacentini G, Bodini A, Pigozzi R, Boner A. Transforming growth factor-b1 is elevated in unpasteurized cow's milk. *Pediatr Allergy Immunol*. 2009;20:42–44.

40. McPherson RJ, Wagner Cl. The effect of pasteurization on transforming growth factor alpha and transforming growth factor beta 2 concentrations in human milk. *Adv Exp Med Biol*. 2001;501:559–566.

41. Ewaschuk JB, Unger S, O'Connor DL, et al. Effect of pasteurization on selected immune components of donated human breast milk. *J Perinatol*. 2011;31(9):593–598.

42. Rudloff HE, Schmalstieg FC Jr, Mushtaha AA, et al. Tumor necrosis factor-alpha in human milk. *Pediatr Res*. 1992;31(1):29–33.

43. Erbağci A, Cekmen M, Balat O, et al. Persistency of high proinflammatory cytokine levels from colostrum to mature milk in preeclampsia. *Clin Biochem*. 2005;38(8):712–716.

44. Gilmore W, McKelvey-Martin V, Rutherford S, et al. Human milk contains granulocyte colony-stimulating factor. *Eur J Clin Nutr*. 1994;48(3):222–224.

45. Gersting JA, Kotto-Komeb CA, Dua Y, et al. Bioavailability of granulocyte colony-stimulating factor administered enterally to suckling mice. *Pharmacol Res*. 2003;48: 643–647.

46. Calhoun DA, Maheshwari A, Christensen RD. Recombinant Granulocyte Colony-Stimulating Factor administered enterally to neonates is not absorbed. *Pediatrics*. 2003;112(2):421–423.

47. Gersting JA, Christensen RD, Calhoun DA. Effects of enterally administering granulocyte colony-stimulating factor to suckling mice. *Pediatr Res*. 2004;55(5):802–806.

48. Magi B, Ietta F, Romagnoli R, et al. Presence of macrophage migration inhibitory factor in human milk: evidence in the aqueous phase and milk fat globules. *Pediatr Res*. 2001; 51:619–624.

49. Vigh E, Bodis J, Garai J. Longitudinal changes in macrophage migration inhibitory factor in breast milk during the first three months of lactation. *J Reprod Immunol*. 2011; 89:92–94.

50. Buescher E, Malinowska I. Soluble receptors and cytokine antagonists in human milk. *Pediatr Res*. 1996;40(6): 839–844.

51. Buescher ES, McWilliams-Koeppen P. Soluble Tumor necrosis factor-α (TNF-α) receptors in human colostrum and milk bind to TNF-α and neutralize TNF-α bioactivity. *Pediatr Res*. 1998;44:37–42.

52. Patki S, Patki U, Patil R, et al. Comparison of the levels of the growth factors in umbilical cord serum and human milk and its clinical significance. *Cytokine*. 2012;59(2):305–308.

53. Kobata R, Tsukahara H, Ohshima Y, et al. High levels of growth factors in human breast milk. *Early Human Dev.* 2008;84(1):67–69.

54. Hirai C, Ichiba H, Saito M, et al. Trophic effect of multiple growth factors in amniotic fluid or human milk on cultured human fetal small intestinal cells. *JPGN.* 2002;34:524–528.

55. Wagner CL, Taylor SN, Johnson D. Host factors in amniotic fluid and breast milk that contribute to gut maturation. *Clinic Rev Allerg Immunol.* 2008;34:191–204.

56. Dvorak B, Fituch CC, Williams CS, et al. Increased epidermal growth factor levels in human milk of mothers with extremely premature infants. *Pediatr Res.* 2003;54(1):15–19.

57. Dvorak B, Fituch CC, Williams CS, et al. Concentrations of epidermal growth factor and transforming growth factor-alpha in preterm milk. In: al. Pe., editor. *Protecting Infants Through Human Milk.* Kluwer Academic/Plenum Publishers; 2004:407–409.

58. Chang C-Y, Chao JC-J. Effect of human milk and epidermal growth factor on growth of human intestinal caco-2 cells. *JPGN.* 2002;34:394–401.

59. Khailova L, Dvorak K, Arganbright KM, et al. Changes in hepatic cell junctions structure during experimental necrotizing enterocolitis: effect of EGF treatment. *Pediatr Res.* 2009;66(2):140–144.

60. Coursodon CF, Dvorak R. Epidermal growth factor and necrotizing enterocolitis. *Curr Opin Pediatr.* 2012;24:160–164.

61. Clark JA, Lane RH, MacLennan NK, et al. Epidermal growth factor reduces intestinal apoptosis in an experimental model of necrotizing enterocolitis. *Am J Physiol Gastrointest Liver Physiol.* 2005;288:755–762.

62. Untalan PB Keeney SE, Palkowetz KH, et al. Heat susceptibility of interleukin -10 and other cytokines in donor human milk. *Breastfeed Med.* 2009; 4:137–144.

63. Radulescu A, Zhang H-Y, Chen C-L, et al. Heparin-binding EGF-like growth factor promotes intestinal anastomotic healing. *J Surg Res.* 2011;171:540–550.

64. Loui A, Eilers E, Strauss E, et al. Vascular endothelial growth factor (VEGF) and soluble VEGF Receptor 1 (Sflt-1) levels in early and mature human milk from mothers of preterm versus term infants. *J Hum Lact.* 2012;28(4):522–528.

65. Ozgurtas T, Aydin I, Turan D, et al. Soluble vascular endothelial growth factor receptor in human breast milk. *Horm Res Paediatr.* 2011;76:17–21.

66. Rodrigues D, Li A, Nair D, Blennerhassett M. Glial cell line-derived neurotrophic factor is a key neurotrophin in the postnatal enteric nervous system. *Neurogastroenterol. Motil.* 2011;23:e44–e56.

67. Boesmans W, Gomes P, Janssens J, et al. Brain-derived neurotrophic factor amplifies neurotransmitter responses and promotes synaptic communication in the enteric nervous system. *Gut.* 2008;57:314–322.

68. Sánchez M, Silos-Santiago I, Frisén J, et al. Renal agenesis and the absence of enteric neurons in mice lacking GDNF. *Nature.* 1996;382(6586):70–73.

69. Fichter M, Klotz M, Hirschberg DL, et al. Breast milk contains relevant neurotrophic factors and cytokines for enteric nervous system development. *Mol Nutr Food Res.* 2011;55:1592–1596.

70. Chellakooty M, Boisen KA, Damgaard IN, et al. A prospective study of serum insulin-like growth factor I (IGF-1) and IGF-binding protein-3 in 942 healthy infants: associations with birth weight, gender, growth velocity, and breastfeeding. *J Clin Endocriniol Metab.* 2006;91:820–826.

71. Blum JW, Baumrucker CR. Colostral and milk insulin-like growth factors and related substances: mammary gland and neonatal (intestinal and systemic) targets. *Dom Anim Endocrin.* 2002;23:101–110.

72. Burrin DG. Is milk-borne insulin-like growth factor-1 essential for neonatal development? *J Nutr.* 1997;127(suppl 5):975S–979S.

73. Philipps AF, Kling PJ, Grille JG, et al. Intestinal transport of insulin-like growth factor-I (IGF-I) in the suckling rat. *JPGN.* 2002;35:539–544.

74. Milsom SR, Blum WF, Gunn AJ. Temporal changes in insulin-like growth factors I and II and in insulin-like growth factor binding proteins 1, 2, and 3 in human milk. *Horm Res.* 2008;69:307–311.

75. Prosser CG. Insulin-like growth factors in milk and mammary gland. *J Mammary Gland Biol & Neoplas.* 1996;1(3):297–306.

76. Elmlinger MW, Hochhaus F, Loui A, et al. Insulin-like growth factors and binding proteins in early milk from mothers of preterm and term infants. *Horm Res.* 2007;68:124–131.

77. Peterson CA, Gillingham MB, Mohapatra NK, et al. Enterotrophic effect of insulin-like growth factor-I but not growth hormone and localized expression of insulin-like growth factor-I, insulin-like growth factor binding protein-3 and -5 mRNAs in jejunum of parenterally fed rats. *JPEN.* 2000;24(5):288–295.

78. Murali SG, Nelson DW, Draxler AK, et al. Insulin-like growth factor-I (IGF-I) attenuates jejunal atrophy in association with increased expression of IGF-I binding protein-5 in parenterally fed mice. *J Nutr.* 2005;135(11):2553–2559.

79. Corpeleijn WE, Vliet IV, Dana-Anne H, et al. Effect of enteral IGF-1 supplementation on feeding tolerance, growth, and gut permeability in enterally fed premature neonates. *JPGN.* 2008;46:184–190.

80. Baregamian N, Song J, Jeschke MG, et al. IGF-1 protects intestinal epithelial cells from oxidative stress-induced apoptosis. *J Surg Res.* 2006;136:31–37.

81. Baregamian N, Song J, Chung DH. Effects of oxidative stress on intestinal type I insulin like growth factor receptor expression. *Eur J Pediatr Surg.* 2012, 22:97–104.

82. Büyükkayhan D, Tanzer F, Erselcan T, et al. Umbilical serum insulin-like growth factor 1 (IGF-1) in newborns: effects of gestational age, postnatal age, and nutrition. *Int J Vitam Nutr Res.* 2003;73(5):343–346.

83. Philipps AF, Dvorak B, Kling PJ, et al. Absorption of milk-borne insulin-like growth factor-I into portal blood of suckling rats. *JPGN.* 2000;31:128–135.

84. Kling PJ, Taing KM, Dvorak B, et al. Insulin-like growth factor-I stimulates erythropoiesis when administered enterally. *Growth Factors.* 2006;24(3):218–223.

85. Carbonell-Estrany X, Figueras-Aloy J, Alvarez E. Erythropoietin and prematurity – where do we stand? *J Perinat Med.* 2005;33:277–286.

86. Juul SE. Enterally dosed recombinant human erythropoietin does not stimulate erythropoiesis in neonates. *J Pediatr.* 2003;143:321–326.

87. Kling PJ, Willeitner A, Dvorak B, Blohowiak SE. Enteral erythropoietin and iron stimulate erythropoiesis in suckling rats. *JPGN.* 2008;46:202–207.

88. Miller-Gilbert AL, Dubuque SH, Dvorak B, et al. Enteral absorption of erythropoietin in the suckling rat. *Pediatr Res.* 2001;50:261–267.

89. Pasha YZ, Ahmadpour-Kacho M, Hajiahmadi M, et al. Enteral erythropoietin increases plasma erythropoietin level in preterm infants: a randomized controlled trial. *Indian Pediatr.* 2008;45:25–28.

90. Soubasi V, Kremenopoulos G, Diamanti E, et al. Follow-up of very low birth weight infants after erythropoietin treatment to prevent anemia of prematurity. *J Pediatr.* 1995;127:291–297.

91. Shiou S-R, Yu Y, Chen S, et al. Erythropoietin protects intestinal epithelial barrier function and lowers the incidence of experimental neonatal necrotizing enterocolitis. *J Biol Chem.* 2011;286(14):12123–12132.

92. Arsenault JE, Webb AL, Koulinska IN, Aboud S, Fawzi WW, Villamor E. Association between breast milk erythropoietin and reduced risk of mother-to-child transmission of HIV. *JID.* 2010;202(3):370–373.

93. Miller M, Iliff P, Stolzfus RJ, et al. Breastmilk erythropoietin and mother to child HIV transmission through breastmilk. *Lancet.* 2002;360:1246–1248.

94. Untalan PB, Keeney SE, Palkowetz PB, et al. Host susceptibility of interleukin 10 and other cytokines in donor human milk. *Breastfeed Med.* 2003;4:137–144.

95. Struck J, Almeida PD, Bergmann A, Morgenthaler NG. High concentrations of procalcitonin but not mature calcitonin in normal human milk. *Horm Metab Res.* 2002;34:460–465.

96. Wookey PJ, Turner K, Furness JB. Transient expression of the calcitonin receptor by enteric neurons of the embryonic and early post-natal mouse. *Cell Tissue Res.* 2012;347:311–317.

97. Chen A, Laskar-Levy O, Koch Y. Selective expression of neuropeptides in the rat mammary gland: somatostatin gene is expressed during lactation. *Endocrinology.* 1999;140:5915–5921.

98. Streym S, Hojskov C, Miller U, et al. Vitamin D content in human breast milk: a 9-month follow-up study. *Am J Clin Nutr.* 2016;103:107–114.

99. Rao RK, Davis TP, Williams C, et al. Effect of milk on somatostatin degradation in suckling rat jejunum in vivo. *JPGN.* 1999;28(1):84–94.

100. Gama P, Alvares EP. LHRH and somatostatin effects on the cell proliferation of the gastric epithelium of suckling and weaning rats. *Reg Peptides.* 1996;63:73–78.

101. Adamkin DH. Mother's milk, feeding strategies, and lactoferrin to prevent necrotizing enterocolitis. *JPEN.* 2012:36.

102. Sherman MP, Bennett SH, Hwang FF, Yu C. Neonatal small bowel epithelia: enhancing anti-bacterial defense with lactoferrin and Lactobacillus GG. *Biometals.* 2004;17(3):285–289.

103. Manzoni P, Rinaldi M, Cattani S, et al. Bovine lactoferrin supplementation for prevention of late-onset sepsis in very-low-birth-weight neonates: a randomized trial. *JAMA.* 2009;302(13):1421–1428.

104. Hirotani Y, Ikeda K, Kato K, et al. Protective effects of lactoferrin against intestinal mucosal damage induced by liposaccharide in human intestinal Caco-2 cells. *Yakugaku Zasshi.* 2008;128:1363–1368.

105. Buccrossi V, de Marco G, Bruzzese E, et al. Lactoferrin induces concentration dependent functional modulation of intestinal proliferation and differentiation. *Pediatr Res.* 2007;61:410–414.

106. Velona T, Abbiati L, Beretta B, et al.. Protein profiles in breast milk from mothers delivering term and preterm babies. *Pediatr Res.* 1999;45(5):658–663.

107. Stubbs J, Lekutis C, Singer K, et al. cDNA cloning of a mouse mammary epithelial cell surface protein reveals the existence of epidermal growth factor-like domains linked to factor VIII-like sequence. *PNAS.* 1990;87:8417–8421.

108. Kusunoki R, Ishihara S, Aziz M, et al. Roles of milk fat globule epidermal growth factor 8 in intestinal inflammation. *Digestion.* 2012;85:103–107.

109. Aziz M, Jacob A, Matsuda A, et al. Review: milk fat globule-EGF factor 8 expression, function, and plausible signal transmission in resolving inflammation. *Apoptosis.* 2011;16:1077–1086.

110. Shi J, Hoegaard CW, Rasmussen JT, et al. Lactadherin binds selectively to membranes containing phosphatidyl-1-serine and increased curvature. *Biochim Biophys Acta.* 2004;1667:82–90.

111. Chogle A, Bu H-F, Wang X, Brown JB, Chou PM, Tan XD. Milk fat globule-EGF factor 8 is a critical protein for healing of dextran sodium sulfate-induced colitis in mice. *Mol Med.* 2011;17(5–6):502–507.

112. Baghdadi M, Chiba S, Yamashina T, et al. MFG-E8 regulates the immunologenic potential of dendritic cells primed with necrotic cell-mediated inflammatory signals. *PloS ONE.* 2012; 7(6):e396D7.

113. Peterson JA, Hamosh M, Scailan CD, et al. Milk fat globule glycoproteins in human milk and in gastric aspirates of mother's milk-fed preterm infants. *Pediatr Res.* 1998;44:499–506.

114. Newburg DS, Peterson JA, Ruiz-Palacios GM, et al. Role of human milk lactadherin in protection against symptomatic rotavirus infection. *Lancet.* 1998;351:1160–1164.

115. Shah KG, WU R, Jacob A, et al. Recombinant human milk fat globule-EGF factor 8 produces dose-dependent benefits in sepsis. *Intensive Care Med.* 2012;38:128–136.

116. Miksa M, Wu R, Dong W, et al. Dendritic cell-derived exosomes containing milk fat globule epidermal growth factor-factor VIII attenuate proinflammatory responses in sepsis. *Shock.* 2006;25:586–593.

117. Komura H, Miksa M, Wu R, et al. Milk fat globule epidermal growth factor-factor VIII is down regulated in sepsis via the lipopolysaccharide-CD14 pathway. *J Immunol.* 2009;182:581–587.

118. Miksa M, Wu R, Dong W, et al. Immature dendritic cell derived exosomes rescue septic animals via milk fat globule epidermal growth factor-factor VIII [corrected]. *J Immunol.* 2009;183:5983–5990.

119. Wu R, Dong W, Wang Z, et al. Enhancing apoptotic cell clearance mitigats bacterial translocation and promotes tissue repair after gut ischemia-reperfusion injury. *Int J Mol Med.* 2012;30:593–598.

120. Matsuda A, Jacob A, Wu r, et al. Milk fat globule EGF factor VIII in sepsis and ischemia reperfusion injury. *Mol Med.* 2011;17:126–133.

121. Silvestre JS, Thery C, Harnard G, et al. Lactadherin promotes VEGF-dependent neovascularization. *Nat Med.* 2005;11:499–506.

122. Martin LJ, Woo JG, Geraghty SR, et al. Adiponectin is present in human milk and is associated with maternal factors. *Am J Clin Nutr.* 2006;83:1106–1111.

123. Newburg DS, Woo JG, Morrow AL. Characteristics and potential functions of human milk adiponectin. *J Pediatr.* 2010;156:S41–S46.

124. Woo JG, Guerro ML, Altaya M, et al. Human milk adiponectin is associated with infant growth in two independent cohorts. *Breastfeed Med.* 2009;4:101–109.

125. Woo JG, Guerrero ML, Guo F, et al. Human milk adiponectin affects infant weight trajectory during the second year of life. *J Pediatr Gastroenterol Nutr.* 2012;54(4):532–539.

126. Ley SH, Hanley AJ, Stone D, et al. Effects of pasteurization on adiponectin and insulin concentrations in donor human milk. *Pediatr Res.* 2011;70:278–281.

127. Dündar NO, Dündar B, Cesur G, et al. Ghrelin and adiponectin levels in colostrum, cord blood and maternal serum. *Pediatr Int.* 2010;52:622–625.

128. Ozarda Y, Gunes Y, Tuncer GO. The concentration of adiponectin in breast milk is related to maternal hormonal and inflammatory status during 6 months of lactation. *Clin Chem Lab Med.* 2012;50:911–917.

129. Savino F, Liguori SA. Update on breast milk hormones: leptin, ghrelin and adiponectin. *Clin Nutr.* 2008;27: 42–47.

130. Weyermann M, Beerman C, Brenner H, et al. Adiponectin and leptin in maternal serum, cord blood, and breast milk. *Clin Chem.* 2006;52:2095–2102.

131. Savino F, Sorrenti M, Benetti S, Lupica MM, Liguori SA, Oggero R. Resistin and leptin in breast milk and infants in early life. *Early Hum Devel.* 2012a;88:779–782.

132. Savino F, Rossi L, Benetti S, et al. Serum reference values for leptin in healthy infants. *PLoS ONE.* 2012b;9:e113024.

133. Dundar NO, Dundar B, Cesur G, et al. Ghrelin and adiponectin levels in colostrum, cord blood, and maternal serum. *Pediatr Int.* 2010;52:622–625.

134. Newburg DS, Ruiz-Palacios GM, Morrow AL. Human milk glycans protect infants against enteric pathogens. *Ann Rev Nutr.* 2005;25:37–58.

135. Morrow AL, Ruiz-Palacios GM, Jiang X, et al. Human-milk glycans that inhibit pathogen binding protect breast-feeding infants against infectious diarrhea. *J Nutr.* 2005;135(5):1304–1307.

136. De Leoz ML, Gaerlan SC, Strum JS, et al. Lacto-N-tetraose, fucosylation, and secretor status are highly variable in human milk oligosaccharides from women delivering preterm. *J Proteome Res.* 2012;11(9):4662–4672.

137. Marcobal A, Sonnenburg JL. Human milk oligosaccharide consumption by intestinal microbiota. *Clin Microbiol Infect.* 2012;18(suppl 4):12–15.

138. Kunz C. Historical aspects of human milk oligosaccharides. *Adv Nutr.* 2012;3:430S–439S.

139. Ruhaak LR, Lebrilla CR. Analysis and role of oligosaccharides in milk. *BMB Rep.* 2012; 45:442–451.

140. Bode L, Kuhn L, Kim HY, et al. Human milk oligosaccharide concentration and risk of postnatal transmission of HIV through breastfeeding. *Amer J Clin Nutr.* 2012;96:831–839.

141. Wang B. Molecular mechanism underlying sialic acid as an essential nutrient for brain development and cognition. *Adv Nutr.* 2012;3:465S–472S.

142. Coppa GV, Gabrielli O, Zampini L, et al. Glycosaminoglycan content in term and preterm milk during the first month of lactation. *Neonatology.* 2012;101:74–76.

143. Coppa GV, Gabrielli O, Zampini L, et al. Oligosaccharides in 4 different milk groups: bifidobacteria, and Ruminococcus obeum. *J Pediatr Gastroenterol Nutr.* 2011;53:80–87.

144. Ruvoen-Clouet N, Mas E, Mariounneau S, et al. Bile-salt-stimulated lipase and mucins from milk of 'secretor' mothers inhibit the binding of Norwalk virus capsids to their carbohydrate ligands. *Biochem J.* 2006;393:627–634.

145. Liu B, Yu Z, Chen C, et al. Human milk mucin 1 and mucin 4 inhibit Salmonella enterica serovar typhimurium invasion of human intestinal epithelial cells in vitro. *J Nutr.* 2012;142:1504–1509.

146. Sando L, Pearson R, Gray C, et al. Bovine MUC1 is a highly polymorphic gene encoding an extensively glycosylated mucin that binds bacteria. *J Dairy Sci.* 2009;92:5276–5291.

147. Saeland E, de Jong MA, Nabatov AA, et al. MUC1 in human milk blocks transmission of human immunodeficiency virus from dendritic cells to T cells. *Mol Immunol.* 2009;46(11–12):2309–2316.

148. Yolken RH, Peterson JA, Vonderfecht SL, et al. Human milk mucin inhibits rotavirus replication and prevents experimental gastroenteritis. *J Clin Invest.* 1992;90: 1984–1987.

149. Chaturvedi P, Singh AP, Batra SK. Structure, evolution, and biology of the MUC4 mucin. *FASEB J.* 2008;22(4): 966–981.

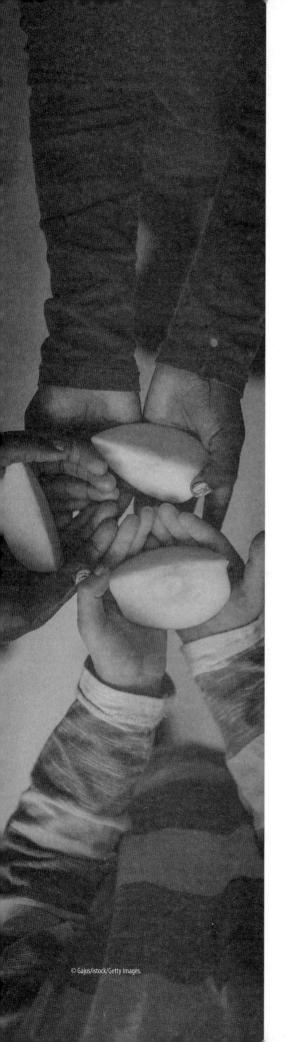

SECTION III

Nutrition Throughout Childhood

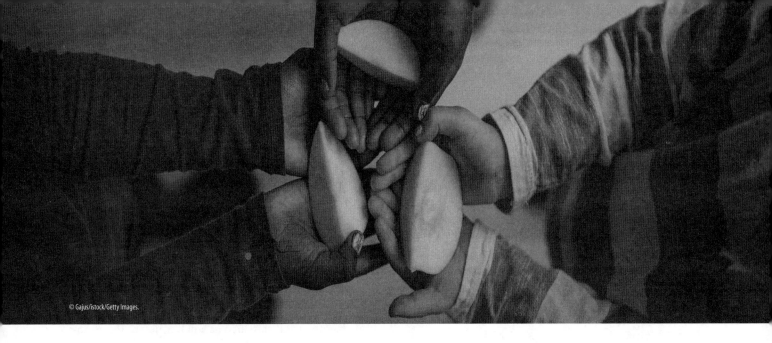

© Gajus/istock/Getty Images.

CHAPTER 7

Nutrition for Premature Infants

Diane M. Anderson and Marsha Dumm

LEARNING OBJECTIVES

- Readers will be able to identify the unique nutritional challenges and risks associated with an infant born before 37 weeks' gestation.
- Readers will identify optimal timing for initiation of parenteral nutrition and the stepwise progression to goal.
- Readers will describe the benefits of human milk feedings and a standardized feeding schedule to improve feeding tolerance and decrease the risk of necrotizing enterocolitis.
- Readers will be able to identify the elements of assessing nutritional adequacy and growth.

▶ Introduction

Premature infants are defined as infants born before 37 weeks' gestation compared with full-term infants born from 37 to 41 weeks and 6 days.[1] The physiologic immaturity of premature infants renders them susceptible to a number of problems (see **TABLE 7.1**), many of which imperil their nutrition and growth (see **TABLE 7.2**). **Low birth weight** (LBW) refers to infants with a birth weight of less than 2500 g (5 pounds, 8 ounces); **very low birth weight** (VLBW) infants weigh less than 1500 g (3 pounds, 5 ounces), and **extremely low birth weight** (ELBW) infants weigh less than 1000 g (2 pounds, 3 ounces).[1] Infants can be LBW but still be full term due to poor intrauterine growth.

Assessing intrauterine growth is determined by plotting the infant's birth weight by gestational age on growth charts. On the Fenton or Olsen growth chart, **small-for-gestational-age (SGA)** infants have a birth weight of less than the 10th percentile.[3,6,7] **Large-for-gestational-age (LGA)** infants have a birth weight greater than the 90th percentile.[3,6,7] **Appropriate-for-gestational-age** (AGA) infants are between the 10th and 90th percentiles. On the Fenton and Olsen charts, SGA and LGA can also be defined as two standard deviations from the mean birth weight (approximately the 3rd and the 97th percentiles, respectively).[3] The Fenton chart may be downloaded from http://ucalgary.ca/fenton while the Olsen chart can be downloaded from https://www.aap.org/en-us/Documents/GrowthCurves.pdf

TABLE 7.1 Potential Problems of the Premature Infant

- Undernutrition
- Poor growth
- Glucose instability
- Hypocalcemia
- Fat malabsorption
- Decreased gastric motility
- Uncoordinated sucking, swallowing, and breathing
- Perinatal depression
- Respiratory distress syndrome
- Hypotension
- Poor temperature control
- Patent ductus arteriosus

- Apnea
- Infection
- Hyperbilirubinemia
- Immature renal function
- Necrotizing enterocolitis
- Osteopenia
- Intraventricular hemorrhage
- Periventricular leukomalacia
- Bronchopulmonary dysplasia
- Retinopathy of prematurity
- Anemia

Data from American Academy of Pediatrics Committee on Nutrition. Nutritional needs of the preterm infant. In: Kleinman RE, Greer FR, eds. *Pediatric Nutrition Handbook*. 7th ed. Elk Grove Village, IL: American Academy of Pediatrics; 2014:83–121.[2]
Smith VC. The high-risk newborn: anticipation, evaluation, management and outcome. In: Eichenwald EC, Hansen AR, Martin CR, Stark AR, eds. *Cloherty; and Stark's Manual of Neonatal Care*. 8th ed. Philadelphia, PA: Wolters Kluwer/Lippincott Williams & Wilkins; 2017:76–93.[3]

TABLE 7.3 lists the etiologies for SGA, and **TABLE 7.4** lists the factors associated with LGA infants. These assessments are used to anticipate medical and nutritional problems and manage the needs of the infant (see **TABLE 7.5**). For example, consider a female infant born at 34 weeks gestation whose birth weight is 1200 g. This infant is premature because the gestational age is less than 37 weeks. On these two intrauterine growth charts, she is SGA because birth weight is less than the 10th percentile or less than two standard deviations from the mean birth weight.[3,6,7]

SGA infants are further classified by their body length and head circumference as symmetrically or asymmetrically growth restricted.[3] The symmetrically SGA infant's birth weight, head circumference, and body length are all classified as small, whereas the asymmetrically SGA infant has a small body weight but an appropriate head circumference and body length. Infants who experience asymmetrical growth restriction usually stand a better chance for catch-up growth.[3,11] The potential for catch-up growth is determined by the etiology of the poor fetal growth.[11] Those infants who have the insult late in gestation due to placental insufficiency or uterine restrictions will grow when provided appropriate nutrition.[11] Those infants who had an early perinatal insult related to congenital infection or genetic disorders remain small in physical size.[11]

TABLE 7.2 Premature Infant's Risk Factors for Nutritional Deficiencies

1. Decreased nutrient stores
   - Premature infants are born before anticipated quantities of nutrients are deposited.
   - Low stores include glycogen, fat, protein, fat-soluble vitamins, calcium, phosphorus, magnesium, iron and trace minerals.

2. Rapid growth
   - Depletes small body nutrient stores.
   - With rapid growth, energy and nutrient needs will be increased.

3. Immature physiological systems
   - Digestion and absorption capabilities are decreased due to low concentrations of lactase, pancreatic lipase, and bile salts.
   - Gastrointestinal motility and stomach capacity are decreased, which limits gastric emptying and feeding volume.
   - A coordinated suck, swallow, and breathing pattern is not developed until 32–34 weeks' gestation.
   - Hepatic enzymes are deceased, which may make specific amino acids conditionally essential (cysteine) or toxic (phenylalanine), due to the inability to synthesize or degrade.
   - Immature renal function limits the infant's ability to control fluid, electrolytes, and acid/base status.

4. Cold stress results in energy expenditure for heat production instead of growth.

5. Illnesses
   - Respiratory distress syndrome will decrease gastrointestinal motility. Trophic feedings, which are small-volume feedings, will frequently be introduced.
   - Patent ductus arteriosus may require fluid restriction, which limits caloric and nutrient intake. If the infant is treated with indomethacin or ibuprofen, feedings may be limited to trophic volumes.

- Necrotizing enterocolitis forces nutrition management to parenteral nutrition for bowel rest. With refeeding, human milk is used but an elemental infant formula may be indicated. Some infants may develop short-gut syndrome as a complication and require extensive nutritional management for malabsorption.
- Bronchopulmonary dysplasia can lead to an increased energy demand with fluid restriction. Nutrient-dense milks are often utilized. Chronic diuretic use will create electrolyte depletion.
- Hyperbilirubinemia may be treated by phototherapy, which may increase the infant's insensible water loss and fluid requirement.
- Sepsis may result in withholding all enteral fluids until it is established that the infant is stable.

Data from American Academy of Pediatrics Committee on Nutrition. Nutritional needs of the preterm infant. In: Kleinman RE, Greer FR, eds. *Pediatric Nutrition Handbook*. 7th ed. Elk Grove Village, IL: American Academy of Pediatrics; 2014:83–121.[2]

Anderson DM, Poindexter BB, Martin CR. Nutrition. In: Eichenwald EC, Hansen AR, Martin CR, Stark AR, eds. *Cloherty and Stark's Manual of Neonatal Care*. 8th ed. Philadelphia, PA: Wolters Kluwer/Lippincott Williams & Wilkins; 2017:248–284.[4]

Clyman R, Wickremasinghe A, Jhaveri N, et al. Enteral feeding during indomethacin and ibuprofen treatment of a patent ductus arteriosus. *J Pediatr*. 2013;163(2):406–411.[5]

TABLE 7.3 Etiologic Factors for SGA Births

Genetic size	High altitude
Pregnancy-induced hypertension	Maternal age young or advanced
Chronic hypertension	Multiple gestation
Chronic renal disease	Congenital malformations
Diabetes with vascular complications	Chromosomal abnormalities
Intrauterine infection	Placental insufficiency
Poor gestation weight gain	Twin-to-twin transfusion
Cigarette smoking	Placental and cord defects
Drug or alcohol abuse	Short interpregnancy interval

Data from Smith VC. The high-risk newborn:anticipation, evaluation, management and outcome. In: Eichenwald EC, Hansen AR, Martin CR, Stark AR, eds. *Cloherty; and Stark's Manual of Neonatal Care*. 8th ed. Philadelphia, PA: Wolters Kluwer/Lippincott Williams & Wilkins; 2017:76–93.[3]

Calkings KL, Devaskar SU. Intrauterine growth restriction. In: Martin RJ, Fanaroff AA, Walsh MC, eds. *Fanaroff and Martin's Neonatal-Perinatal Medicine Diseases of the Fetus and Infant*. 10th ed. Philadelphia, PA: Elsevier/Saunders; 2015:227–235.[8]

TABLE 7.4 Factors Associated With LGA Births

Infant of diabetic mother	Genetic predisposition
Beckwith-Wiedemann Syndrome	Maternal obesity prior to pregnancy
Some post-term infants	High gestation weight gain

Data from Smith VC. The high-risk newborn:anticipation, evaluation, management and outcome. In: Eichenwald EC, Hansen AR, Martin CR, Stark AR, eds. *Clohert ;and Stark's Manual of Neonatal Care*. 8th ed. Philadelphia, PA: Wolters Kluwer/Lippincott Williams & Wilkins; 2017:76–93.[3]

Stang J, Huffman LG. Position of the Academy of Nutrition and Dietetics: Obesity, Reproduction, and Pregnancy Outcomes. *J Acad Nutr Diet*. 2016; 116:677–691.[9]

8 months of age has been independently associated with decreased intellectual quotients, cognitive functioning skills, and behavior problems at school age.[9] Many premature infants remain smaller than infants born with normal birth weight or at term gestation.[13]

Premature infants represent a heterogeneous population for nutrition management. Intrauterine growth establishes nutritional status at birth, and gestational age determines the nutrient need and the feeding modality employed. As the infant matures, postnatal nutrient needs and feeding modality will vary. Finally, the infant's clinical condition can acutely change and alter nutrition care. Due to these factors, their nutrition management is a day-to-day decision-making process regarding what to feed, what volume and nutrient density to provide, and how to administer nourishment. The goal is to provide nutrition for optimal growth and development to take place. The intrauterine growth rate and weight gain composition without metabolic complications has been advocated as the goal for premature infant nutrition.[2]

Catch-up growth for premature infants continues until adulthood for weight and length.[12,13] Head circumference catch-up is limited to the first 6 to 12 months of life.[14] A suboptimal head circumference measurement at

TABLE 7.5 Anticipated Problems for SGA and LGA Infants

Problems	Issues
Small for Gestational Age	
Hypoglycemia	Caused by Low glycogen stores Decreased gluconeogenesis Decreased glycogenolysis Decreased fat stores Hyperinsulinemia
Increased energy demand	Caused by Increased growth rate Increased energy cost of growth
Heat loss	Caused by Large surface area Decreased subcutaneous fat
Large for Gestational Age	
Birth trauma	Shoulder dystocia, fractured clavicle, brachial plexus injury, perinatal depression
Hypoglycemia	Caused by hyperinsulinism

Data from Smith VC. The high-risk newborn:anticipation, evaluation, management and outcome. In: Eichenwald EC, Hansen AR, Martin CR, Stark AR, eds. *Cloherty, and Stark's Manual of Neonatal Care*. 8th ed. Philadelphia, PA: Wolters Kluwer/Lippincott Williams & Wilkins; 2017:76–93.[3]
Calkings KL, Devaskar SU. Intrauterine growth restriction. In: Martin RJ, Fanaroff AA, Walsh MC, eds. *Fanaroff and Martin's Neonatal-Perinatal Medicine Diseases of the Fetus and Infant*. 10th ed. Philadelphia, PA: Elsevier/Saunders; 2015:227–235.[8]
Stang J, Huffman LG. Position of the Academy of Nutrition and Dietetics: Obesity, Reproduction, and Pregnancy Outcomes. *J Acad Nutr Diet*. 2016; 116:677–691.[9]
Poindexter BB, Ehrenkranz RA. Nutrition requirements and provision of nutrition support in the preterm newborn. In: Martin RJ, Fanaroff AA, Walsh MC, eds. *Fanaroff and Martin's Neonatal-Perinatal Medicine Diseases of the Fetus and Infant*. 10th ed. Philadelphia, PA: Elsevier/Saunders; 2015:592–612.[10]

Infants lose weight after birth and will follow a lower intrauterine weight curve than the one established at birth.[16] After regaining birthweight, infants can grow at the intrauterine growth rate of 15 g/kg/day, but their weight curve may fall below the 10th percentile for their postmenstrual age.[16] AGA premature infants can become SGA before hospital discharge due to illness and inadequate nutrition intake.[2] Extrauterine growth restriction (EUGR) has decreased in recent years due to changes in medical management and nutrition practices.[17] However, the time and rate for catch up growth to occur with premature infants for optimal neurodevelopment and the prevention of adult onset diseases is not known.[2]

▶ Parenteral Nutrition

Parenteral nutrition (PN) is often indicated and initiated in the first day of life to allow the premature infant to adapt to the extrauterine environment and to supplement the small-volume enteral feedings initiated. Enteral feedings are often slowly advanced, because premature infants have decreased enteral feeding tolerance and small gastric capacities, which limit volume intakes and advancements. Premature infants are at risk for **necrotizing enterocolitis** (NEC), and enteral feedings will be cautiously advanced.[2,18,19] For the VLBW infant, PN should be initiated within the first 2 hours of life in order to promote energy intake and glucose homeostasis, establish nitrogen balance, and prevent essential fatty acid deficiency.[20,21] The provision of amino acids, as part of PN within the first 24 hours of life, has been associated with positive nitrogen balance, improved glucose tolerance, which facilitates greater glucose administration, increased protein synthesis, normal plasma amino acid levels, and growth.[20,21] Starter solutions that contain glucose, protein, and perhaps calcium are kept in stock in order to facilitate early parenteral protein nutrition delivery for the VLBW infant. These starter solutions can be ordered with a separate order of intravenous fat. Nitrogen balance is improved with the addition of lipids.[22] As soon as possible, PN can be ordered to meet each infant's individual nutritional needs.

TABLES 7.6 and **7.7** give suggested guidelines for parenteral administration of specific nutrients. **TABLE 7.8** briefly describes a protocol for parenteral nutrition management.

Peripheral lines can be used for short-term intervals in order to provide parenteral nutrition, but they are limited by the nutrition concentration that can safely be provided. During the first week of life, umbilical venous catheters are utilized to provide parenteral nutrition. A central venous catheter is needed for the infant who requires prolonged parenteral nutrition, has limited venous access, is fluid restricted, or has an increased nutrient demand that cannot be met by peripheral nutrition. **Peripheral inserted central venous catheters** (PICC) are frequently used with premature infants because the PICC line can be placed at an infant's bedside. A PICC line can reduce the stress to the infant caused by repeated insertion of peripheral lines and can facilitate the delivery of concentrated parenteral nutrients.[27] A tunneled, central venous catheter is placed when a PICC line cannot be inserted.

TABLE 7.6 Parenteral Nutrition Guidelines: Energy, Protein, and Minerals per Day

Nutrient	Unit/kg
Energy (kcal)	90–100
Glucose (mg/kg/min)	11–12
Fat (g)	1–3
Protein (g)	2.7–4
Sodium (mEq)	2–4
Potassium (mEq)	1.5–2
Chloride (mEq)	2–4
Calcium (mg)	60–80
Phosphorus (mg)	39–67
Magnesium (mg)	4.3–7.2
Zinc (µg)	400
Copper (µg)	20
Chromium (µg)	0.0006
Manganese (µg)	1
Selenium (µg)	2.0
Iodide (µg)	1

Data from American Academy of Pediatrics Committee on Nutrition. Nutritional needs of preterm infants. In: Kleinman RE, Greer FR, eds. *Pediatric Nutrition Handbook*. 7th ed. Elk Grove Village, IL: American Academy of Pediatrics; 2014:83–121.[2]
Vanek VW. Review of trace mineral requirements for preterm infants: what are the current recommendations for clinical practice? *NCP*. 2015;30(5):720–721.[23]
Vanek VW, et al. ASPEN position paper: recommendations for changes in commercially available parenteral multivitamin and multi-trace element products. *NCP*. 2012;27(4):440–491.[24]

TABLE 7.7 Parenteral Vitamin Guidelines per Day

Vitamin	Dose/kg	Maximum Dose per Day*
Vitamin A (IU)	920	2300
Vitamin E (IU)	2.8	7
Vitamin K (µg)	80	200
Vitamin D (IU)	160	400
Vitamin C (mg)	32	80
Thiamin (mg)	0.48	1.2
Riboflavin (mg)	0.56	1.4
Niacin (mg)	6.8	17
Vitamin B_6 (mg)	0.4	1
Folate (µg)	56	140
Vitamin B_{12} (µg)	0.4	1
Biotin (µg)	8	20
Pantothenic acid (mg)	2	5

*Preterm infants receive 40% of the daily dose MVI Pediatric (Hospira) or INFUVITE Pediatric (Baxter) per kg until the maximum daily dose is achieved at 2.5 kg.
Data from American Academy of Pediatrics Committee on Nutrition. Nutritional needs of preterm infants. In: Kleinman RE, Greer FR, eds. *Pediatric Nutrition Handbook*. 7th ed. Elk Grove Village, IL: American Academy of Pediatrics; 2014:83–121.[2]
Greene HL, Hambidge KM, Schanler R, Tsang RC. Guidelines for the use of vitamins, trace elements, calcium, magnesium, and phosphorus in infants and children receiving total parenteral nutrition: report of the Subcommittee on Pediatric Parenteral Nutrient Requirements from the Committee on Clinical Practice Issues of the American Society for Clinical Nutrition. *Am J Clin Nutr*. 1988;48:1324–1342.[25]

Management Concerns and Medical Problems

Fluid management is very individualized for the preterm infant. Insensible water losses will be high, and the infant's renal function and neuroendocrine control will be immature.[28] Fluid volume may be limited to prevent or treat **patent ductus arteriosus** (PDA) and bronchopulmonary dysplasia (BPD).[29,30] **TABLE 7.9** presents laboratory parameters that should be observed in guiding PN therapy.

Insensible fluid losses are high for many reasons.[28] First, the premature infant has a large surface area related to total weight, which facilitates easy heat and water losses. Second, the premature infant's skin offers little protection from evaporative losses. There is a high water content and the epidermis is thin and highly permeable. Finally, environmental factors in the newborn intensive care unit; such as using radiant warmers, phototherapy, and high or low ambient temperature; increase insensible fluid losses.[29] These losses can be decreased by the use of humidified incubators, plastic shields, and plastic wraps or clothing.

TABLE 7.8 Parenteral Nutrition Progression

	DOL to Begin	Beginning Quantity	Increase	Maximum or Goal	Considerations
Fluid (mL/kg/day)	1	80–100	10–20	140–160	■ Fluid needs will vary by birth weight, gestational age, postnatal age, and environmental conditions. ■ Humidified incubators decrease insensible water loss and fluid requirement. ■ Fluids should be provided to keep the infant in normal hydration status. Refer to Table 7.9 for monitoring guidelines.
Glucose (mg/kg/min)	1	4.5–6	1–2	11–12	■ Begin on DOL 1 to prevent hypoglycemia. ■ Decrease glucose load for hyperglycemia. Glucose homeostasis will usually improve in 1–2 days. ■ Insulin infusions should be avoided. Insulin usage may result in unstable blood glucose levels, hypoglycemia, and acidosis.
Protein (g/kg/day)	1	2–3	—	2.7–4.0	■ Begin on DOL 1. advance protein to meet needs. There is no documentation that gradual protein advancement is needed.
Lipids (g/kg/day)	1	1–2	1	3	■ Provide over a 24 hour period. ■ The 20% intralipid is preferred over the 10% emulsion. Serum levels of cholesterol, triglycerides, and phospholipids are lower with use of the 20% emulsion.
Sodium chloride (mEq/kg/day)	2–3	1–3	—	2–4	■ Allow diuresis to occur the first few days of life to decrease extracellular blood volume. ■ Start sodium to prevent hyponatremia.
Potassium (mEq/kg/day)	2	1.5–2	—	2–3	■ Add potassium after urine flow is established and serum potassium level is normal.
Magnesium (mg/kg/day)	1	4.3–7.2	—	4.3–7.2	■ May remove magnesium from initial parenteral nutrition when mother has received magnesium.
Vitamins and trace minerals	1				

Abbreviations: DOL, day of life; ELBW, extremely low birth weight.

Parenteral nutrition progression may be slowed with fluid and electrolyte imbalance, glucose imbalance, renal failure, the anticipation of enteral feedings, or the initiation and tolerance of enteral feedings.

Data from American Academy of Pediatrics Committee on Nutrition. Nutritional needs of the preterm infant. In: Kleinman RE, Greer FR, eds. *Pediatric Nutrition Handbook*. 7th ed. Elk Grove Village, IL: American Academy of Pediatrics; 2014; 83–121.[2]

Anderson DM, Poindexter BB, Martin CR. Nutrition. In: Eichewald EC, Hansen AR, Martin CR, and Stark AR., eds. *Cloherty and Stark's . Manual of Neonatal Care*. 8th ed. Philadelphia, PA: Wolters Kluwer 2017:248–284.[4]

Thureen PJ, Melara D, Fennessey PV, et al. Effect of low versus high intravenous amino acid intake on very low birth weight infants in the early neonatal period. *Pediatr Res*. 2003;53:24–32.[26]

TABLE 7.9 Fluid and Electrolyte Monitoring Parameters

Fluid intake	80–150 mL/kg*
Urine output	1–3 mL/kg/hour
Daily body weights	10–15% maximum total weight loss
Serum sodium	133–146 mmol/L
Serum potassium	3.2–6 mmol/L
Serum chloride	97–110 mmol/L
Serum creatinine	0.3–0.9 mg/dL
Blood urea nitrogen	3–25 mg/dL

*The critically ill premature infant has highly variable fluid needs. This range represents the usual volume of fluid administered. To prevent over- or underhydration, fluids should be provided so as to keep the other monitoring parameters within normal levels. Serum sodium levels are most helpful.

Data from Stanley FL. Reference ranges for laboratory test and procedures. In: Kliegman RM, Stanton BF, StGeme JW, Schor NF, eds. *Nelson Textbook of Pediatrics.* 20th ed. Philadelphia, PA: Elsevier; 2015:3464–3473.[31]

Dell KM, Fluid, electrolyte, and acid base homeostasis. In: Martin RJ, Fanaroff AA, Walsh MC, eds. *Fanaroff and Martin's Neonatal-Perinatal Medicine Diseases of the Fetus and Infant.* 10th ed. Philadelphia, PA: Elsevier/Saunders; 2015:613–629.[32]

Intralipid® is the intravenous fat emulsion used in the United States. Preterm infants have a limited ability to hydrolyze triglycerides. Elevated serum triglyceride levels are more frequently found with lower birthweight, younger birth gestational age, infection, surgical stress, malnutrition, and with the SGA infant.[18,33] It is recommended that serum triglyceride levels be kept under 200 mg/dL,[2] but there are a lack of data to support this level.[34] Although the free fatty acids from Intralipid® compete with indirect bilirubin for binding onto albumin, Intralipid® may be provided during hyperbilirubinemia at the present recommended intakes. Intralipid® should be administered at a maximum of 3 g/kg over a 24-hour infusion.[2,35] The concern is that free bilirubin may cross the blood–brain barrier and cause kernicterus. At this level of intake and rate of infusion; however, it appears to be safe.[35]

There are two additional lipid emulsions being used with neonates and these are produced by Fresenius Kabi in Germany. The first is Omegaven®, a fish oil-based lipid emulsion used to treat **parenteral nutrition associated liver disease** (PNALD). Omegaven®'s composition helps treat cholestasis with its anti-inflammatory properties of omega 3 fatty acids and vitamin E, and the absence of phytosterols that are contained in soy-based lipids.[36] The soy-based lipids (Intralipid®) are omega 6 fatty acids, which are inflammatory and the phytosterols, which are present decrease bile acid synthesis and bile flow. The use of fish oil-based lipid emulsions in the United States had required compassionate use approval from the United States **Food and Drug Administration** (FDA) to treat PNALD.[37] As of July 27, 2018, the FDA has approved the use of Omegaven to treat pediatric patients with PNALD. One gram of Omegaven per kilogram per day is the recommended dose. Information is available at the FDA website https://www.accessdata.fda.gov/scripts/cder/daf/index.cfm?event=overview.process&ApplNo=210589. SMOFlipid® (soy oil, medium chain triglycerides, olive oil, and fish oil) is the second emulsion. SMOFlipid® has been approved for adult use by the FDA and is used off labeled for neonates. Since SMOFlipid® is a blend of oils, it may offer different advantages/disadvantages with the prevention and treatment of PNALD. Current research results have been mixed regarding the benefits of SMOFlipid® in order to prevent and/or treat cholestasis.[36] Current studies are being conducted to examine the growth and prevention of PNALD in infants provided SMOFlipid®.[38]

Several amino acid parenteral solutions are formulated for the pediatric patient.[39] These solutions contain a larger percentage of total nitrogen as essential amino acids and branch chain amino acids, and they have a balanced pattern of nonessential amino acids instead of a single amino acid concentration.[39] Using a pediatric amino acid solution, compared with an adult product, results in plasma amino acid levels that are similar to the breastfed infant and improve weight gain and nitrogen balance.[40] The addition of cystine to TrophAmine®, one of the pediatric amino acid solutions, may improve nitrogen balance.[41] The addition of cysteine hydrochloride decreases the pH of the solution, which allows greater levels of calcium and phosphorus to be added.[18,39]

Transitioning to Enteral Feedings

Transitioning from parenteral to enteral feedings is a slow process that is necessary in order to facilitate feeding tolerance and prevent the development of NEC.[2,18,42] Enteral feedings are gradually increased in volume and strength as parenteral fluids are decreased at a similar volume.

The two fluid types are coordinated in order to provide appropriate fluid and nutrients. Parenteral fluids are discontinued when enteral feedings reach approximately 100 mL/kg/day.

▶ Enteral Nutrition

Oral care with the mother's own colostrum and milk can be provided to aid in the development of the infant's oral microbiota and the infant's immune development.[43,44] Administration to the infant begins as soon as colostrum is available by swabbing the oropharyngeal mucosa or injecting by syringe into the buccal pouch of the oral cavity. The dosing frequency and duration of oral care and the benefits of oral care require further investigation.[44]

Premature infants are at risk for NEC and feeding intolerance, so enteral feedings are slowly introduced and advanced.[39,45] Trophic feedings have been advocated for the first week of life to facilitate gut development and have not been associated with increasing the incidence of NEC.[2,46] Trophic feedings are small volumes of feedings given to nourish the gut but do not serve as a major source of nutrition. Volumes of 1 mL/kg to 25 mL/kg have been studied.[2] Individual study benefits are listed in **TABLE 7.10**. Trophic feedings should consist of the preferred human milk diet (mom's or pasteurized donors') provided at 10–20 mL/kg/day for 3 to 7 days.[39] Premature infant formula may be used if human milk is not available.[45] The use of umbilical artery catheters should not be a contraindication for starting trophic feedings.[2,45,47] For the healthy premature infant, feedings can be initiated and advanced during the first week of life. Feeding advancement for the VLBW infant is often limited to 20 mL/kg/day or less because rapid feeding advancement has been associated with NEC.[19,48] In one study, the enteral feeding advancement of 35 mL/kg/day and 15 mL/kg/day were both tolerated.[49] A higher volume rate results in a shorter time to achieve full enteral feedings, a shorter time to regain birthweight, and less infection[50] Each infant must be evaluated daily for feeding advancement. Using a standardized feeding schedule, which includes time to initiate feeds, feed volume advancement, and the use of human milk has been associated with a decreased incidence of NEC.[51,52]

The use of human milk has been linked to a decreased incidence of NEC.[54] Pasteurized donor human milk is frequently used when mother's milk is unavailable or to supplement mother's own milk in order to provide this protection.[55] A recent study demonstrated that the use of human milk and liquid pasteurized donor milk fortifier decreased the incidence of NEC.[56] The type of milk selected depends on individual factors and can sometimes involve complex decisions. **TABLE 7.11** lists factors that must be considered. Whatever milk is chosen, it should provide appropriate amounts of energy, protein, minerals, and vitamins (see **TABLE 7.12**). The goal is to promote growth and to prepare the infant for hospital discharge. In **TABLE 7.13**, selected nutrients are compared (at 150 ml/kg of milk). This value represents the average volume intake for a premature infant on full enteral feedings. Fortified human milk or premature infant formulas will meet the needs of most premature infants.

The FDA has recommended that powder infant formulas not be fed to premature infants or other immunized compromised infants unless there is no alternative.[2] Powder infant formula is not sterile and carries the risk of Enterobacter sakazakii infection. The FDA link is www.fda.gov/iceci/enforcementactions/enforcementstory/enforcementstoryarchive/ucm105959.htm

Infant and pediatric feedings: Guidelines for preparation of human milk and formula in healthcare facilities, 3rd Ed. (eBook) are published by the Academy of Nutrition and Dietetics (www.eatright.org). These guidelines address the physical facilities, equipment, personnel, formula and milk preparations, infection control, and quality control to ensure the feeding of a safe milk to the infant.

The premature infant's vitamin needs will be met by using concentrated liquid and powdered bovine-fortified human milk or premature infant formula; no additional supplementation is indicated.[2] Low-iron formulas are no longer available in the United States because low-iron stores may result in long-term neurodevelopmental outcomes. Commercial donor milk fortifiers are not vitamin fortified, so multiple vitamin supplementation is recommended. Iron needs will be met by consuming 120 kcal/kg of an iron-fortified premature infant formula, because this will provide 2 mg/kg of iron, which is the goal.[2] For the infant receiving human milk, iron supplementation

---

TABLE 7.10 Benefits of Trophic Feedings

- Feeding
  - Improved feeding tolerance
  - Achieve full feedings sooner
  - Achieve full per os PO sooner

- Gastrointestinal
  - Increased plasma gastrin
  - Decreased intestinal transit time
  - More mature intestinal motor pattern
  - Increased calcium, copper, and phosphorus retention

- Clinical
  - Decreased serum bilirubin and days of phototherapy
  - Decreased incidence of cholestasis
  - Lower serum alkaline phosphatase activity levels

- Decreased length of stay

Data from American Academy of Pediatrics Committee on Nutrition. Nutritional needs of preterm infants. In: Kleinman RE, Greer FR. eds. *Pediatric Nutrition Handbook*. 7th ed. Elk Grove Village, IL: American Academy of Pediatrics; 2014:83–121.[2]
Ziegler EE. Human milk and human milk fortifiers. In: Koletzko B, Poindexter B, Uauy R, eds. *Nutritional Care of Preterm Infants: Scientific Basis and Practical Guidelines*. Basel, Karger, 2014:215–227.[53]

TABLE 7.11 Milk and Formula Selection Indications and Concerns

Milk	Indications	Concerns
Human milk	▪ Nutrients are readily absorbed. ▪ Anti-infective factors are present. ▪ Incidence of NEC and sepsis is decreased. ▪ Nutrient composition is unique. ▪ Maternal–infant attachment is enhanced. ▪ Maternal emotional support by family and healthcare team is indicated to facilitate lactation. ▪ Full enteral feedings are achieved earlier vs. premature infant formula. ▪ Infants have slower weight gain, but earlier discharge on fortified human milk feedings vs. premature infant formula.	▪ Milk from mothers who deliver prematurely will often contain a higher protein concentration than that found in the milk from mothers who deliver at term. This elevated protein concentration decreased by 28 days of lactation and may not meet the protein needs of the rapidly growing premature infant. ▪ The concentration of protein, calcium, phosphorous, and sodium are too low to meet the needs of many premature infants. To increase nutrient density, human milk fortifiers should be added to the milk. ▪ Iron supplementation at 2–4 mg/kg is needed for those infants receiving the low iron–containing fortifier. For those who are provided the fortifier with iron, no iron supplementation is needed. ▪ Milk volume production may be inadequate to nourish the infant.
Formulas for premature infants	▪ Glucose polymers comprise 50%–60% of the carbohydrate calories, which decreases the lactose load presented to the premature infant for digestion. ▪ Glucose polymers also decrease the osmolality of the formula. ▪ Lactose comprises 40%–50% of the carbohydrate calories. ▪ Medium chain triglycerides (MCTs) are 40%–50% of the fat calories. MCTs do not require pancreatic lipase or bile salts for digestion and absorption. ▪ Protein is at a higher concentration than that incorporated into standard infant formula to meet the increased protein needs of the preterm infant. ▪ The protein is a 60/40 or 100/0 whey/casein ratio compared with the 18/82 ratio found in bovine milk. This whey predominance prevents the elevation of plasma phenylalanine and tyrosine levels. ▪ Calcium and phosphorous are two to three times the concentration found in standard infant formulas. These levels will maintain normal serum calcium and phosphorous levels, prevent osteopenia, and promote calcium and phosphorous accretion at the fetal rate. ▪ Sodium, potassium, and chloride concentrations are greater than in standard infant formulas to meet the increased electrolyte needs of the premature infant. ▪ Vitamins, trace minerals, and additional minerals are incorporated into these formulas at high concentration to meet the infant's increased nutrient need while facilitating a limited volume intake. ▪ Iron-fortified formulas are available, which eliminates the need for iron supplementation. ▪ Formula osmolality is within the physiologic range at 235–300 mOsm/kg water for the 20–24 kcal/ounce, which facilitates formula tolerances and decreases the risk of NEC. ▪ A 30 kcal/ounce formula is available for the infant who needs fluid restriction to support growth, such as the infant with BPD. The osmolality is 325 mOsm/kg water.	▪ Feeding volumes should be advanced slowly with the very-low-birth weight infant. ▪ Vitamin and iron supplements are not indicated for the infant receiving iron-fortified premature infant formula.

(continues)

TABLE 7.11 Milk and Formula Selection Indications and Concerns *(continued)*

Milk	Indications	Concerns
	▪ Premature formulas can be used until the infant reaches 2.5–3.6 kg, depending on the formula vitamin concentration and volume intake.	
Premature discharge formulas (transition formulas)	▪ Transition formulas are designed for the premature infant at discharge. The infant should weigh at least 1.8 kg when this formula is provided. ▪ Formula should be initiated at least 3 days before discharge to document formula tolerance and weight gain. ▪ Formulas have a nutrient composition between the concentrated premature formulas and the standard infant formulas. ▪ Glucose polymers comprise 50%–60% of the carbohydrate calories, and lactose comprises 40%–50%. ▪ Medium Chain Triglycerides (MCTs) are 20%–25% of the fat calories. ▪ The protein is either a 60/40 or 50/50 whey/casein ratio. ▪ Improved bone mineral concentration and greater weight and length gains were documented with premature infants fed a transition formula for the first 9 months of life.	▪ Indications for this formula are not clearly defined. There is no consensus as to which premature infants should receive this formula nor the length of time they should remain on this formula. One suggestion is that the premature infant should remain on this formula until weight for length is between the 25th and 50th percentiles. ▪ Transitional formulas can be provided up to 1 year of corrected age if needed. The greatest effect is during the first 3 to 6 months of corrected age. ▪ Formulas are iron fortified and vitamin dense such that nutrient supplementation may not be needed. To meet the term infant guideline of 400 IU/day for vitamin D, a vitamin D supplement may be needed. ▪ Formulas are available as a powder and can be concentrated to meet the needs of the infant with bronchopulmonary dysplasia. This formula can be provided in the nursery and in the home setting.
Standard infant formulas	▪ Can be used at discharge for larger premature infants who can gain 20–30 g/day while consuming at least 180 mL/kg/day of this formula.	▪ Nutrient content is inadequate for the premature infant during the neonatal period. ▪ During the early neonatal period, these formulas may not be tolerated well. Lactose is the sole carbohydrate source, and only long chain fatty acids are incorporated into these formulas.
Elemental infant formula	▪ Infants who are recovering or suffering from gastrointestinal disorders can benefit from elemental infant formula. ▪ Casein hydrolysates and amino acid formulas are available. ▪ MCTs are a component of some of these formulas. ▪ Glucose or glucose and sucrose are the carbohydrate sources.	▪ Nutrient content is inadequate for the premature infant, with special reference to calcium and phosphorus levels. ▪ The time to switch to a premature formula must always be considered to improve nutrient intake. Depending on the infant's feeding history, the formulas can be switched or the premature infant formula can be provided as one feed per day and advanced by one additional feed per day as tolerated.
Soy formulas		▪ These formulas are not indicated for premature infants. ▪ The premature infant is at risk for osteopenia. The phytates in the formula bind phosphorous and make it unavailable for absorption. ▪ Nutrient absorption and utilization are not documented.

Data from American Academy of Pediatrics Committee on Nutrition. Nutritional needs of preterm infants. In: Kleinman RE, Greer FR, eds. *Pediatric Nutrition Handbook*. 7th ed. Elk Grove Village, IL: American Academy of Pediatrics 2014:83–121.[2]
Schanler RJ, Anderson D. The low birth weight infant. Inpatient care. In: Duggan C, Watkins JB, Walker WA, ed. *Nutrition in Pediatrics: Basic Science Clinical Applications*. 4th ed. Hamilton, Ontario, Canada: BC Decker; 2008:377–394.[39]
American Academy of Pediatrics Committee on Nutrition. Failure to thrive. In: Kleinman RE, Greer FR, eds. *Pediatric Nutrition Handbook*. 7th ed. Elk Grove Village, IL: American Academy of Pediatrics; 2014:601–636.[11]
Abbott Nutrition. Our products. Available at: www.abbottnutrition.com/our-products/for-professionals.nutrition.html. Accessed February 26, 2018.[57]
Mead Johnson Nutrition. Healthcare professional resource center product information. Available at: www.meadjohnson.com/pediatrics/us-en/products.information. Accessed February 26, 20118.[58]

TABLE 7.12   Enteral Nutrient Guidelines per kg/day

Nutrient	Amount	Nutrient	Amount
Energy (kcal)	110–130[1],105–130[2]	Molybdenum (µg)	0.3–5[1]
Protein (g)	3.5–4.5[1], 3.5–4[2]	Iodine (µg)	10–55[1]
Carbohydrate (g)	11.6–13.2[1]	Vitamin A (IU)	1332–3663[1]
Fat (g)	4.8–6.6[1]	Vitamin D (IU)	400–1000[1] 200–400[2] *
Sodium (mEq)	3–5[1]	Vitamin E (mg α-TE)	2.2–11[1]
Potassium (mEq)	2–5[1]	Vitamin K (µg)	4.4–28[1]
Chloride (mEq)	3–5[1]	Vitamin C (mg)	20–55[1]
Calcium (mg)	120–200[1], 100–220[2]	Thiamin (µg)	140–300[1]
Phosphorus (mg)	60–140[1]	Riboflavin (µg)	200–400[1]
Magnesium (mg)	8–15[1]	Niacin (mg)	1–5.5[1]
Iron (mg)	2-3 [1],2–4[2]	Vitamin B_6 (µg)	50–300[1]
Zinc (µg)	1400–2500[1]	Folate (µg)	35–100[1]
Copper (ug)	100–230[1]	Vitamin B_{12} (µg)	0.1–0.8[1]
Chromium (ng)	30–2250[1]	Biotin (µg)	1.7–16.5[1]
Manganese (µg)	1–15[1]	Pantothenic acid (mg)	0.5–2.1[1]
Selenium (µg)	5–10[1]		

*Maximum of 400 IU/day & 1000 IU/day of Vitamin D

Data from American Academy of Pediatrics Committee on Nutrition. Nutritional needs of preterm infants. In: Kleinman RE, Greer FR. eds. *Pediatric Nutrition Handbook*. 7th ed. Elk Grove Village, IL: American Academy of Pediatrics; 2014:83–121.[2]

Koletzko B. Poindexter B, Uauy R. (eds.) Recommended nutrient intake levels for stable, fully enterally fed very low birth weight infants. In: *Nutrition Care of Preterm Infants: Scientific Basis and Practical Guidelines*. Basel, Switzerland: Karger. 2014:297–299.[59]

can be initiated at 2 to 4 mg/kg/day once full-volume feedings have been achieved or after 2 weeks of age.[2] The fortifiers vary in their iron content, and extra iron supplements should be limited to those who have low iron content. When erythropoietin therapy is employed, iron supplementation at 6 mg/kg/day to facilitate red cell production is recommended.[2]

Pharmacological dosage of vitamin E (50 to 100 mg/kg/day) for premature infants in order to prevent retinopathy of prematurity, BPD, or intraventricular hemorrhage is not recommended.[2] Although vitamin E is an antioxidant, it has not consistently prevented these illnesses; complications associated with its pharmacological dosing

include NEC, sepsis, intraventricular hemorrhage, and death.[61]

To prevent BPD in the ELBW infant, vitamin A supplementation has been suggested due to its role in cell differentiation and tissue repair.[62] Providing 5000 IU of vitamin A intramuscularly (IM) three times per week for the first month of life will lower oxygen requirements at 36 weeks' gestation.[62] Developmental follow-up scores at 18 months corrected age demonstrated no difference from premature infants who had not received extra vitamin A.[63] It is recommended that physicians decide whether to use vitamin A supplementation in their nurseries.[2] Considerations include the variation in the incidence of BPD

TABLE 7.13 Milk Comparison for the Premature Infant at 150 mL/kg

Guideline (per kg)	EBM + HMF 24 kcal/oz (powder bovine)	EBM + HMF 24 kcal/oz (liquid bovine)	EBM + HMF 24 kcal/oz (liquid donor milk)	Premature Infant Formula 24 kcal/oz	Premature Discharge Formula 22 kcal/oz
105–130 kcal	120	120	123	120	110
3.5–4 g protein	2.9–3	3.5	3.45	3.6–4	3.1–3.2
100–220 mg calcium	169–209	206	185	197–219	117–132
2–4 mg iron	0.5–2.3	0.7	0.3	2.2	2
1–3 mg zinc	1.38–1.8	1.95	1.46	1.56–1.8	1.33–1.38
150–400 IU vitamin D	180–225	177	41	183–288	77–88

Abbreviations: EBM, expressed breast milk; HMF, human milk fortifier; term human milk nutrient concentrations used for calculations.

Data from American Academy of Pediatrics Committee on Nutrition. Nutritional needs of preterm infants. In: Kleinman RE, Greer FR, eds. *Pediatric Nutrition Handbook*. 7th ed. Elk Grove Village, IL: American Academy of Pediatrics; 20014:83–121.[2]

Abbott Nutrition. Product guides. Available at: www.abbottnutrition.com/our-products/for-professionals/nutrition.html. Accessed February 26, 2018.[57]

MeadJohnson Nutrition. Healthcare professional resource center product information. Available at:www.meadjohnson.com/pediatrics/us-en/products-information. Accessed February 26, 2018.[58]

Prolacta 1 H2MF™. Nutrient Values. Prolacta Bioscience MKT-0180 Rev-1. 20014.[60]

among nurseries, the lack of additional benefits of vitamin A supplementation, and the acceptance of IM therapy.[2,64] Additional factors associated with the occurrence of BPD are antenatal steroids, exogenous surfactant, mode of ventilation, and postnatal steroids. The criteria used to prescribe oxygen varies among **Newborn Intensive Care Unit** (NICU) practices, which will alter the incidence of BPD by the definition of BPD being the oxygen requirement at 36 weeks **postmenstrual age (PMA)**.[64]

Metabolic bone disease (MBD) is commonly reported for premature infants when the intake of calcium and phosphorus is inadequate, and this is in addition to their poor nutrient stores at birth.[65] Risk factors include prolonged PN, dexamethasone, cholestasis and/or diets of unfortified human milk.[66,67] A diet of fortified human milk or premature infant formula will meet the infant's needs.[67] Vitamin D intake at 200 to 400 IU per day with the calcium- and phosphorus-enriched premature formula is adequate.[66,68] Chronic diuretic use can increase urinary calcium losses.[65,66]

Premature infants are at risk for trace mineral deficiency due to their poor nutrient stores at birth, rapid growth, and their dependence on adequate intake. By using today's PN guidelines, premature infant formula, or fortified human milk, deficiencies should be uncommon.[69] Infants who have excessive losses via an ileostomy drainage or high urine output related to renal failure may need two to three times the recommended guidelines for zinc.[39,70] Additional case reports of zinc deficiency have

been reported when the mother's milk had an extremely low zinc content or the infant had been provided with copper and/or iron supplements that compete with zinc for absorption.[69,71]

The two long chain polyunsaturated fatty acids, docosahexaenoic acid and arachidonic acid, are present in human milk and have been added to infant formulas. However, study results on the addition of these two fatty acids to the premature infant's diet have been mixed for physical growth, visual function, and neurodevelopment.[72]

The feeding method employed will depend on the infant's gestational age, clinical condition, and nursery staff experience.[2] **TABLE 7.14** describes the methods in use, and **TABLE 7.15** provides guidelines for the amounts and rates of feedings. Due to the infant's constantly changing clinical condition and development, several methods will be used. Both continuous and bolus infusions are used with gavage feedings.[2] A recent study demonstrated improved weight gain and feeding tolerance with the use of bolus vs. continuous infusion.[73] The use of transpyloric feedings dictates using continuous infusion in order to prevent an osmotic load from being presented to the intestine and dumping from occurring.[39] The delivery of nutrients to the infant is decreased with continuous infusions.[2,74] Specifically, human milk fat and fat additives and minerals in the human milk fortifier adhere to or precipitate in the delivery system.[74] A bolus feeding or a feeding given over 30 to 120 minutes on a pump can decrease the nutrient loss.[2,74]

TABLE 7.14 Methods of Feeding

Type	Considerations
Breast/ bottle	Most physiological methods
	Infant at least 32–34 weeks' gestation
	Infant medically stable
	Infant's respiratory rate less than 60 breaths per minute
Gavage	Supplement to breast/bottle feedings
	Suggested for infants less than 32 weeks' gestation
	Use for intubated infant
	Use for neurologically impaired neonate
Transpyloric	Employ when gavage feedings not tolerated
	Use when the infant is at risk for milk aspiration
	Use for the infant with decreased gut motility
	Use for the infant with anatomic abnormality of the gastrointestinal tract
	Infant intubated
	Tube is placed under guided fluoroscopy
	Complications include dumping syndrome, nutrient malabsorption, and perforation of intestine
	Continuous infusions indicated
Gastrostomy	Gastrointestinal malformation Infant neurologically impaired

Data from American Academy of Pediatrics Committee on Nutrition. Nutritional needs of preterm infants. In: Kleinman RE, Greer FR, ed. *Pediatric Nutrition Handbook.* 7th ed. Elk Grove Village, IL: American Academy of Pediatrics; 2014:83–121.[2]
Schanler RJ, Anderson D. The low birth weight infant. Inpatient care. In: Duggan C, Watkins JB, Walker WA, eds. *Nutrition in Pediatrics: Basic Science Clinical Applications.* 4th ed. Hamilton, Ontario, Canada: BC Decker; 2008:377–394.[39]
Sapsford A, Smith C. Enteral nutrition. In: Pediatric Nutrition Practice Group, Groh-Wargo S, Thompson M, Cox JH, eds. *AND Pocket Guide to Neonatal Nutrition.* Chicago: American Dietetic Association; 2016:76–124.[75]
Anderson DM, Poindexter BB, Martin CR. Nutrition. In: Eichenwald EC, Hansen AR, Martin CR, Stark AR, eds. *Cloherty and Stark's Manual of Neonatal Care.* 8th ed. Philadelphia, PA: Wolters Kluwer/Lippincott Williams & Wilkins; 2017:248–284.[76]

TABLE 7.15 Feeding Guidelines

Trophic feedings*	Provide to infants < 1250 g BW
	Give for 3 days, up to 5 days ≤ 750 g BW
	10–20 mL/kg/day
	Human milk
	Bolus feedings
Feeds initiation and advancement	< 1250 g BW
	10–20 mL/kg/day
	1251–1500 g BW
	20 mL/kg/day
	1501–2000 g BW
	Initiate at 20 mL/kg/day and advance by 20–40 mL/kg/day
	2001–2500 g BW
	Initiate at 25–30 mL/kg/day and advance by 25–40 mL/kg/day to ab libitum (ab lib) depending on clinical status of infant
	> 2500 g BW
	Start at 50 mL/kg/day or ab lib with minimum and advance by 25–40 mL/kg/day
Milk selection	< 1800–2000 g BW or < 34 weeks PMA
	• Human milk; fortify with four packs human milk fortifier/100 mL milk when 100 mL/kg feeds achieved.
	• Liquid donor milk fortifier added at 40–100 mL/kg/day of human milk
	• Premature infant formula ≥ 2000 g BW or > 34 weeks PMA
	• Human milk
	• Standard infant formula

* Trophic feedings should begin on day 1 or 2 for the medically stable infant. The infant should have a physiologic range blood pressure while receiving 5 µg/kg/min or less of dopamine.
Abbreviations: BW, birthweight; PMA, postmenstrual age.
Data from Chan SW, Hair A, Enteral Nutrition. In: Fernandes CJ, Pammi M, Katakam L , eds. *Guidelines for Acute Care of the Neonate.* 25th ed. Houston, TX: Section of Neonatology Department of Pediatrics, Baylor College of Medicine; 2017–2018:167–178.[77]

Breastfeeding

Human milk is the preferred feeding for nearly all infants, but mothers who want to breastfeed their premature infant must usually express their milk. During the infant's prolonged hospitalization, it will be difficult for the mother to be available for 24-hour breastfeeding. Further, the infants are too premature and/or sick to nurse. The infant will not be able to feed orally until 32–34 weeks' gestation. Family members, friends, and nursery staff must provide support for these women in order to enable them to be successful in providing milk during this stressful period (see **TABLE 7.16**). Early expression of milk within the first hour

TABLE 7.16 Steps to Support Lactating Women

1. Instruction
   - Provision of evidence-based instruction material
   - Methods and timing of milk expression
   - Sterilization of expression equipment
   - Storage and transport of milk
   - Diet for lactation
   - Tips for relaxation

2. Tips to help with let down before expression
   - Showering
   - Hand massaging of the breasts
   - Applying warm washcloths to the breasts
   - Consuming warm beverages
   - Visiting the infant
   - Talking to the infant's nurse by phone
   - Placing the infant's picture on the pump   *cute*

3. Nursery staff and nursery support
   - Availability of lactation consultant for mothers and staff
   - Education of nursery staff on milk expression and breastfeeding
   - Electric pump and pumping room conveniently available to the nursery
   - Electric pumps available for rental and hand pumps for purchase
   - Hospital grade storage containers provided by the hospital
   - Mother's milk used to feed the infant whenever it is available
   - Help mother with the initiation of nursing
   - Promote kangaroo care for skin-to-skin contact

4. Initiation of breastfeeding
   - Wake baby up
   - Express a little milk prior to nursing so nipple is easier to grasp by the small infant
   - Position infant so mother and infant are stomach to stomach
   - Allow mother to room in with baby prior to discharge to establish breastfeeding pattern

Data from American Academy of Pediatrics Committee on Nutrition. Nutritional needs of preterm infants. In: Kleinman RE, Greer FR, eds. *Pediatric Nutrition Handbook*. 7th ed. Elk Grove Village, IL: American Academy of Pediatrics; 2014:83–121.[2]
Parker LA, Sullivan S, Krueger C, et al. Effect of early breast milk expression on milk volume and timing of lactogenesis stage II among mothers of very low birth weight infants: a pilot study. *J Perinatol*. 2012;32:205–209.[78]
Meier PP, Johnson TJ, Patel AL, Rossman B. Evidence-based methods that promote human milk feeding of preterm infants: An expert review. *Clin Perinatol*. 2017;44:1–22.[81]

after delivery has been associated with increased maternal milk volume over several months.[78] Kangaroo care (skin-to-skin contact between the parent and the infant) will facilitate parent–infant bonding and has been linked to an increase in maternal milk volume and a longer period of lactation by the mother who delivers prematurely.[79,80]

Nutritional Assessment

Nutrition assessment is a continual process for the premature infant that can ensure optimal nutritional intakes. Dietary considerations, anthropometric measurements, feeding tolerance, and laboratory indices will need to be monitored.

Dietary Considerations

Daily assessment is necessary to determine the need for changing feeding volume, solution strength, or feeding method. Intake is evaluated against nutrient guidelines. Finally, feeding technique needs to be advanced to the most physiological method possible for the infant. Breast or bottle feedings are introduced as the infant's coordination of sucking, swallowing, and breathing is developed at 32–34 weeks' gestation.[2] The initiation of oral feedings may be guided by an infant-driven feeding readiness scale that can evaluate whether the infant is awake, alert, and ready to feed.[82] There is some evidence to suggest that the advance of oral feedings, based on infant cues and the demonstration of successful feeding, may allow the infant to achieve full oral feedings faster.[83] Enteral feedings may be limited to 20 minutes per feeding period in order to prevent fatigue and excessive energy expenditure.[84]

Anthropometric Measurements

Anthropometric measurements are difficult to perform on premature infants, principally because of an infant's small size and clinical condition. Medical equipment can interfere with measuring or can add to the recorded weight. Also, the infant is at risk for cold stress during these procedures, which diverts energy from growth to heat production. The new high humidity hybrid incubators contain bed scales that enable infants to be weighed without removing them from their humidity- and temperature-controlled environment.[30]

Preterm infants are weighed daily, and weekly weights, lengths, and head circumferences are plotted on intrauterine growth charts in order to track longitudinal growth and to assess whether the infant is growing at the intrauterine growth rate. Most premature infants will parallel their birth curve and demonstrate catch-up growth later in life. Initial weight loss that reflects the loss of extracellular fluid ranges from 10%–15% of birth weight during the first week of life.[32] After regaining birth weight, the weight gain goal is 15–20 g/kg/day for infants who have a gestational age of 23–36 weeks.[85] When the infant weighs 2 kg or more, a weight gain of 20 to 30 g/day has been used.[39] Head circumferences should increase by 0.9 cm/wk and length measurements should increase by 1.0 cm/wk.[84] Daily weights and weekly lengths and head circumferences can be plotted on postnatal premature infant growth charts.[16] These charts reflect the growth of a population of premature infants after birth. The infant's growth is assessed against a group of their peer premature infants and demonstrates how the infant is growing compared with other premature infants. These charts profile the initial weight loss seen with infants at week 1 of life. Intrauterine growth, which is the goal, cannot be assessed by these postnatal growth charts. The Fenton and the Olsen intrauterine growth charts can be used to monitor the premature infant's growth.[6,7] The Fenton chart can be downloaded from http://ucalgary.ca/fenton and the Olsen chart can be downloaded from https://www.aap.org/en-us/us/Documents/GrowthCurves.pdf

Weights will be influenced by the medical equipment attached to the infant, the use of different scales, the infant's hydration status, and total nutrient intake. Weights taken at the same time each day will avoid recording diurnal variations. Alterations in the head circumference measurement will occur from birth to week 1 of life due to head molding or edema. Length board measurements should be used to obtain accurate length measurements.

Skinfolds and mid-arm circumference measurements do not change rapidly enough to be more helpful than weight measurements for diet changes. These measurements are generally not employed for routine clinical care but are indicated for growth studies. There are limited standards.[86,87]

Assessing Inadequate Weight Gain

When a series of daily or weekly measurements indicates inadequate growth, a search must be made for the cause. **TABLE 7.17** outlines areas to check.

TABLE 7.17 Possible Etiologies for Inadequate Weight Gain

1. Nutrient calculations are incorrect.

2. Parenteral nutrition is not optimized.

3. Infant just achieved full enteral feedings meeting guidelines.

4. Infant is not receiving ordered diet.
   - Intravenous fluid administration has been interrupted to give blood or drugs, or the intravenous line has become infiltrated.
   - Infant is unable to consume what is ordered by bottle, and no gavage supplements were provided.
   - Feedings were held because the infant's respiratory rate increased or body temperature instability developed.
   - Feedings were held for clinical tests.

5. Infant does not tolerate given formula.

6. Calculated nutrient guidelines are inadequate for the infant due to illness.

7. Infant is cold stressed.

8. Infant has outgrown previous diet order.

9. Nutrition solution was not prepared correctly.

10. Incorrect formula was provided to infant.

11. Human milk issues
    - Continuous infusion will lead to fat separation in feeding syringe. Switch to bolus feedings or put over a pump for 30 to 90 minutes.
    - Ensure correct number of fortifier packets were added to milk.
    - Ensure infant is not receiving only the foremilk, which is low in fat.

12. Metabolic issues
    - Acidosis
    - Electrolyte abnormality

13. Low hemoglobin

14. Ostomy output

Data from Anderson DM. Nutritional assessment and therapeutic interventions for the preterm infant. *Clin Peri.* 2002;29:313–326.[88]
Anderson DM. Nutrition for premature infants. In: Samour PQ, King K, eds. *Pediatric Nutrition.* 4th ed. Boston, MA: Jones and Bartlett Publishers; 2010:63–65.[89]

Assessment of Feeding Tolerance

Feeding intolerance and clinical compromise are common for the premature infant, so constant surveillance is required to detect early signs of feeding intolerance, sepsis, or NEC.[39,45] Depending on the findings, feedings may be held, decreased, diluted, discontinued, or their frequency may be changed. Feedings will often be held due to signs of illness, including persistent apnea and bradycardia, temperature instability, or lethargy. There are no universally agreed upon criteria for feeding assessment.[39] Residuals are often present and may be due to immature intestinal motor activity because they are seen before the initiation of feeds.[39,45] Selective evaluation of gastric residuals may be used in assessing a clinically unstable infant. However, there are no clear standards regarding what constitutes acceptable residual volumes and residuals are not a consistent marker of feeding intolerance. Recent studies suggest that routine evaluations of gastric residuals are not reliable. When routine checks were eliminated, stable infants had fewer days of PN, fewer days of central access, fewer days to full enteral feeds, and shorter length of stay compared with those with routine evaluations based on the volume of the residual. No increase in the incidence of sepsis, PNALD or NEC was reported.[90,91]

The tonicity of the abdomen should be observed. Increases will occur with air swallowing, feeding intolerance, infrequent stooling, or NEC. When the abdomen is distended and/or tender, an evaluation to rule out bowel obstruction is done.[92] A workup for sepsis and NEC may be considered with other signs of feeding intolerance or when an increase in abdominal tone is noted. Visible loops of bowel may indicate illness.

Blood in the stool or residual is a concern and should be evaluated. Blood may be a sign of illness, feeding-tube irritation of the intestine, anal fissure, swallowed blood during delivery, cow's milk protein allergy, or NEC.

Assessing Nutrient Adequacy and Tolerance: Both the specific clinical signs of nutrient deficiency/toxicity and the associated laboratory values should be assessed regularly. Vitamin and trace mineral assays should be performed when a deficiency is suspected.[69,93] Serial plasma trace mineral levels may be more helpful than one plasma level when assessing a trace mineral deficiency.[39] There are several reviews on clinical signs.[69,93,94] Acceptable standards for laboratory values are difficult to establish because premature infants differ by their physical maturity, clinical condition, and nutrient stores. For example, serum proteins will vary by the infant's hepatic maturity, energy, and protein intake, vitamin and mineral nutritional status, and clinical condition. Blood urea nitrogen does not correlate to parenteral protein intake the first week of life but may be helpful for the premature infant fed human milk in order to determine protein supplementation needs.[95,96]

During the first week of life, serum electrolytes, glucose, creatinine, and urea nitrogen are monitored daily, or more frequently when values are abnormal. Since these blood parameters stabilize, they can be examined as clinically indicated.[39] Serum electrolytes are assessed for those infants receiving diuretics or for those with a history of abnormal values until values are normal. Additional parameters monitored when PN is being administered include serum triglycerides to check lipid tolerance, direct bilirubin to detect cholestasis, and **serum alanine aminotransferase** (AL-T) and **serum glutamic-pyruvic transaminase** (SGP-T) in order to evaluate hepatic function.[39] Serum calcium, phosphorus, and alkaline phosphatase levels may be monitored to detect osteopenia in the premature infant.[39] Hematocrit and hemoglobin levels are checked as needed.[39]

▶ Discharge Concerns

The premature infant is ready for discharge from the hospital when body temperature can be maintained, breastfeeding or bottle feeding supports growth, and cardiorespiratory function is mature and stable.[97] Most importantly, the caretaker must be ready to care for the high-risk infant. Family-centered care, 24-hour visitation, and rooming-in allow the parents to participate in the care of their infant and empowers them to care for their infant after discharge.[98,99]

The infant should be evaluated for participation in the Special Supplemental Nutrition Program for **Women, Infants, and Children** (WIC), early intervention programs, and a developmental follow-up program for premature infants. The follow-up program should monitor the infant's growth and development, offer aid with chronic illness management, provide early detection of problems, make referrals to specialized services as indicated, and give the parents support and guidance in caring for their prematurely born infant. These clinics not only aid with the early detection of problems but also evaluate the care that newborn intensive care units provide. A primary care physician must be identified in order to provide well-baby and sick care, and an appointment should be established before discharge to home.[97] Infants born prematurely may not have achieved optimal growth while in the hospital and may continue to face growth challenges after discharge.[100,101] Infants will be discharged home on human milk, preterm post-discharge (transition) formula, standard term formula, or combination of milks.[2] The breastfed infant may be given some feedings of fortified pumped milk or preterm post-discharge formula to enrich nutrient intake and support growth. Infants with a birthweight of less than 1250 grams or premature infants who have experienced intrauterine or extrauterine growth restriction should be considered for supplementation.[2] WIC is administered by each state and some states provide human milk fortifier or supplemental formula powder for fortification for the most vulnerable infants. The breastfed infant should also receive a daily multiple vitamin containing 400 IU of vitamin D and 2 mg/kg iron supplement.[2,102] The formula-fed infant will not require additional iron supplementation. Infants receiving the premature discharge formula will not require extra vitamins, and the premature infant receiving term formula should receive a multivitamin.[2] There is no evidence-based guideline as to which infants should be provided with the preterm post-discharge formula or how long it should be given. Two studies reported improved growth when infants were fed preterm discharge formulas.[103,104] However, a recent meta-analysis of 16 trials found no significant differences in growth between the post-discharge and standard-term, formula-fed infants.[105] Despite these findings, it is recommended that formula-fed premature infants be evaluated for post-discharge formula in order to optimize growth during the first year of life.[2] Periodic assessment of growth will help determine the length of time that post-discharge formula should be provided.[2] Infants who do not meet growth goals or have other co-morbidities may need nutrient-dense feedings and pumped milk can be fortified or premature discharge formula can be concentrated to 24 or 27 kcal/fl oz.

▶ Conclusion

Although premature infants begin life in a compromised nutritional state, nutrition and medical therapies continue to evolve that enhance the infant's potential for optimal growth and neurodevelopmental outcomes.[2] Daily nutrition evaluation in the NICU and follow-up after discharge are necessary to ensure that appropriate nutrition therapy is provided.

🔍 CASE STUDY

Nutrition Assessment

Patient history: A 980-gram female infant was born at 27 weeks' gestation and classified as an appropriate for gestational age premature infant on the Fenton growth chart. Length was 36 cm and head circumference was 25 cm. Today, the patient is 21 days old or 30 weeks' **postmenstrual age** (PMA). Patient had respiratory distress syndrome, which required intubation and surfactant therapy. Patient is now on room air.

Nutrition history: Patient was on parenteral nutrition, but is now on total enteral feedings of human milk from her mother at 160 mL/kg.

Anthropometric Measurements

Weight: 1085 g
Length: 38 cm
Head circumference: 27 cm

Nutrition Problem

Nutrient intake is inadequate for the premature infant.

Nutrition Interventions

As discussed on team rounds, concentrated liquid bovine human milk fortifier will be added to human milk to provide 24 kcal/oz milk. At 160 mL/kg the infant will receive 128 kcal/kg and 3.5 g protein/kg. The fortifier will bring the nutrient content up to meet the guidelines for prematurity.

Monitoring and Evaluation

The infant's weekly rate of weight, head circumference and length will be calculated and measurements recorded on the Fenton Growth Chart.

Questions for the Reader

1. How did weight, length, and head circumference plot at birth and at 3 weeks or 30 weeks' gestation on the Fenton growth chart?
2. What are the kilocalorie and protein goals per kg for this infant?
3. What milk is recommended for the premature infant?
4. What would the feed volume be per feed for feeding every 3 hours at 160 mL/kg?
5. Write one PES.
6. Calculate energy and protein intakes on fortified human milk with powdered bovine fortifier at 160 mL/kg.
7. What should be monitored on a weekly basis in this infant before discharge?

Review Questions

1. An infant is born at 30 weeks and is classified as SGA. Identify the nutrition risks for this infant and appropriate nutrient interventions?

2. What are the benefits and risks of the elements of parenteral nutrition?

3. What is the ideal feeding for nearly all infants and what would be your recommendation for administration?

4. Which vitamins and minerals should be supplemented if the infant is on full enteral feeds of human milk or preterm infant formula?

5. What nutrient interventions would reduce the risk of metabolic bone disease?

6. What parameters would be monitored to evaluate nutritional adequacy at discharge?

References

1. American Academy of Pediatrics, American College of Obstetricians and Gynecologists. *Guidelines for Perinatal Care.* 8th ed. Elk Grove, IL: American Academy of Pediatrics; 2017.

2. American Academy of Pediatrics Committee on Nutrition. Nutritional needs of preterm infants. In: Kleinman RE, Greer FR, eds. *Pediatric Nutrition Handbook.* 7th ed. Elk Grove Village, IL: American Academy of Pediatrics; 2014:83–121.

3. Smith VC. The high-risk newborn: anticipation, evaluation, management and outcome. In: Eichenwald EC, Hansen AR, Martin CR, Stark AR, eds. *Cloherty and Stark's Manual of Neonatal Care.* 8th ed. Philadelphia, PA: Wolters Kluwer/Lippincott Williams & Wilkins; 2017:76–93.

4. Anderson DM, Poindexter BB, Martin CR. Nutrition. In: Eichenwald EC, Hansen AR, Martin CR, Stark AR, eds. *Cloherty and Stark's Manual of Neonatal Care.* 8th ed. Philadelphia, PA: Wolters Kluwer/Lippincott Williams & Wilkins; 2017:248–284.

5. Clyman R, Wickremasinghe A, Jhaveri N, et al. Enteral feeding during indomethacin and ibuprofen treatment of a patent ductus arteriosus. *J Pediatr.* 2013;163(2):406–411.

6. Fenton TR, Kim JH. A systematic review and meta-analysis to revise the Fenton growth chart for preterm infants. *BMC Pediatrics.* 2013;13:59.

7. Olsen IE, Groveman SA, Lawson ML, et al. New intrauterine growth curves based on United States data. *Pediatrics.* 2010;125:e214–e224.

8. Calkings KL, Devaskar SU. Intrauterine growth restriction. In: Martin RJ, Fanaroff AA, Walsh MC, eds. *Fanaroff and Martin's Neonatal-Perinatal Medicine Diseases of the Fetus and Infant.* 10th ed. Philadelphia, PA: Elsevier/Saunders; 2015:227–235.

9. Stang J, Huffman LG. Position of the Academy of Nutrition and Dietetics: Obesity, Reproduction, and Pregnancy Outcomes. *J Acad Nutr Diet.* 2016; 116:677–691.

10. Poindexter BB, Ehrenkranz RA. Nutrition requirements and provision of nutrition support in the preterm newborn. In: Martin RJ, Fanaroff AA, Walsh MC, eds. *Fanaroff and Martin's Neonatal-Perinatal Medicine Diseases of the Fetus and Infant.* 10th ed. Philadelphia, PA: Elsevier/Saunders; 2015:592–612.

11. American Academy of Pediatrics Committee on Nutrition. Failure to thrive. In: Kleinman RE, Greer FR, eds. *Pediatric Nutrition Handbook.* 7th ed. Elk Grove Village, IL: American Academy of Pediatrics; 2014:663–700.

12. Hack M, Schluchter M, Cartar L, et al. Growth of very low birth weight infants to age 20 years. *Pediatrics.* 2003;112:e30–e38.

13. Hack M. Young adult outcomes of very-low-birth-weight children. *Semin Fetal Neonat Med.* 2006;11:127–137.

14. Wilson-Costello DE, Payne AH. Early childhood neurodevelopment outcome of high-risk neonates. In: Martin RJ, Fanaroff AA, Walsh MC, eds. *Fanaroff and Martin's Neonatal-Perinatal Medicine Diseases of the Fetus and Infant.* 10th ed. Philadelphia, PA: Elsevier; 2015:1018–1031.

15. Hack M, Breslau N, Weissman B, et al. Effect of very low birth weight and subnormal head size on cognitive abilities at school age. *N Engl J Med.* 1991;325:231–237.

16. Ehrenkranz RA, Younes N, Lemons JA, et al. Longitudinal growth of hospitalized very low birth weight infants. *Pediatrics.* 1999;104:280–289.

17. Horbar JD, Ehrenkranz RA, Badger GJ et al. Weight growth velocity and postnatal growth failure in infants 501 to 1500 grams: 2000 – 2013. *Pediatrics.* 2015;136:e84–e92.

18. American Academy of Pediatrics Committee on Nutrition. Parenteral nutrition. In: Kleinman RE, Greer FR, eds. *Pediatric Nutrition Handbook.* 7th ed. Elk Grove Village, IL: American Academy of Pediatrics; 2014:571–590.

19. Talavera MM, Bixler G, Cozzi C, et al. Quality improvement initiative to reduce the necrotizing enterocolitis rate in premature infants. *Pediatrics.* 2016;137(5):e20151119.

20. Thureen PJ, Melara D, Fennessey PV, et al. Effect of low versus high intravenous amino acid intake on very low birth weight infants in the early neonatal period. *Pediatr Res.* 2003;53:24–32.

21. Te Braake FWJ, Van Den Akker CHP, Wattimena DJL, et al. Amino acid administration to premature infants directly after birth. *J Pediatr.* 2005;147:457–461.

22. Vlaardingerbroek H, Vermeulen MJ, Rook D, et al. Safety and efficacy of early parenteral lipid and high-dose amino acid administration to very low birth weight infants. *J Pediatr.* 2013;163:638–44.

23. Vanek VW. Review of trace mineral requirements for preterm infants: what are the current recommendations for clinical practice? *NCP.* 2015;30(5):720–721.

24. Vanek VW, Borum P, Buchman A. ASPEN position paper: recommendations for changes in commercially available parenteral multivitamin and multi-trace element products. *NCP.* 2012;27(4):440–491.

25. Greene HL, Hambidge KM, Schanler R, Tsang RC. Guidelines for the use of vitamins, trace elements, calcium, magnesium, and phosphorus in infants and children receiving total parenteral nutrition: report of the Subcommittee on Pediatric Parenteral Nutrient Requirements from the Committee on Clinical Practice Issues of the American Society for Clinical Nutrition. *Am J Clin Nutr.* 1988;48:1324–1342.

26. Thureen PJ, Melara D, Fennessey PV, et al. Effect of low versus high intravenous amino acid intake on very low birth weight infants in the early neonatal period. *Pediatr Res.* 2003;53:24–32.

27. Carlson SJ, Kavars AM. Parenteral nutrition. In: Pediatric Nutrition Practice Group, Groh-Wargo S, Thompson M, Cox JH, eds. *AND Pocket Guide to Neonatal Nutrition.* 2nd ed. Chicago, IL: American Dietetic Association; 2016:32–75.

28. Doherty EG. Fluid and electrolyte management. In: Eichenwald EC, Hansen, AR, Martin CR, Stark AR, eds. *Cloherty and Stark's Manual of Neonatal Care.* 8th ed. Philadelphia: Wolters Kluwer; 2017:296–311.

29. Stephens BE, Gargus RA, Walden RV, et al. Fluid regimens in the first week of life may increase risk of patent ductus arteriosus in extremely low birth weight infants. *J Perinatol.* 2008; 28:123–128.

30. Kim SM, Lee EY, Chen J, et al. Improved care and growth outcomes by using hybrid humidified incubators in very preterm infants. *Pediatrics.* 2010;125:e137–e145.

31. Stanley FL. Reference ranges for laboratory test and procedures. In: Kliegman RM, Stanton BF, StGeme JW, Schor NF, eds. *Nelson Textbook of Pediatrics.* 20th ed. Philadelphia, PA: Elsevier; 2015:3464–3473.

32. Dell KM. Fluid, electrolyte, and acid base homeostasis. In: Martin RJ, Fanaroff AA, Walsh MC, eds. *Fanaroff and Martin's Neonatal-Perinatal Medicine Diseases of the Fetus and Infant.* 10th ed. Philadelphia, PA: Elsevier/Saunders; 2015:613–629.

33. Shulman RJ, Phillips S. Parenteral nutrition in infants and children. *J Pediatr Gastroenterol Nutr.* 2003; 36:587–607.

34. Neu J. Is it time to stop starving premature infants? *J Perinatol.* 2009;29:399–400.

35. Putet G. Lipid metabolism of the micropremie. *Clin Perinatol.* 2000;27:57–69.

36. Hojsak I, Colomb V, Braegger C, et al. ESPGHAN committee on nutrition position paper. Intravenous lipid emulsions and risk of hepatotoxicity in infants and children: a systematic review and meta-analysis. *J Pediatr Gastroenerol Nutr.* 2016;62:776–792.

37. Premkumar MH, Carter B, Hawthorne KM, et al. Fish-oil-based lipid emulsions in the treatment of parenteral nutrition-associated liver disease: an ongoing positive experience. *Adv Nutr.* 2014;5:65–70.

38. National Institutes of Health. Phase 3 study to compare safety and efficacy of Smoflipid 20% to Intralipid 20% in hospitalized neonates and infants. Available at www.clinicaltrials.gov Enter NCT number 02579265. Accessed September 19, 2018

39. Schanler RJ, Anderson D. The low birth weight infant. Inpatient care. In: Duggan C, Watkins JB, Walker WA, eds. *Nutrition in Pediatrics: Basic Science Clinical Applications.* 4th ed. Hamilton, Ontario, Canada: BC Decker; 2008:377–394.

40. Helms RA, Christensen ML, Mauer EC, et al. Comparison of pediatric versus standard amino acid formulation in preterm neonates requiring parenteral nutrition. *J Pediatr.* 1987;110:466–472.

41. Rivera A, Bell EF, Stegink LD, Ziegler EE. Plasma amino acid profiles during the first three days of life in infants with respiratory distress syndrome: effect of parenteral amino acid supplementation. *J Pediatr.* 1989;115:464–468.

42. Poindexter BB, Ehrenkranz RA. Nutrient requirements and provision of nutritional support in the premature neonate. In: Martin RJ, Fanaroff AA, Walsh MC eds. *Fanaroff and Martin's Neonatal-PerinatalMedicine: Diseases of the Fetus and Infant. 10* ed. Philadelphia, PA: Elsevier; 2015:592–612.

43. Soh K, Kalanetra KM, Mills DA, et al. Buccal administration of human colostrum: impact on the oral microbiota or premature infants. *J Perinatol.* 2016;36:106–111.

44. Gephart SM, Weller M. Colostrum as oral immune therapy to promote neonatal health. *Adv Neonatal Care.* 2014;14:44–51.

45. Senterre T. Practice of enteral nutrition in very low birth weight and extremely low birth weigh infants. In: *Nutritional Care of Preterm Infants. Scientific Basis and Practical Guidelines.* Koletzko B, Poindexter B, Uauy R. eds. Basel, Switzerland: Karger; 2014:201–214.

46. Dunn L, Hulman S, Weiner J, Kliegman R. Beneficial effects of early hypocaloric enteral feeding on neonatal gastrointestinal function: preliminary report of a randomized trial. *J Pediatr.* 1988;112:622–629.

47. Davey AM, Wagner CL, Cox C, et al. Feeding premature infants while low umbilical artery catheters are in place: a prospective, randomized trial. *J Pediatr.* 1994;124:795–799.

48. Jesse N, New J. Necrotizing enterocolitis: relationship to innate immunity, clinical features, and strategies for prevention. *NeoReviews.* 2006;7:e143–e150.

49. Rayyis SF, Ambalavanan N, Wright L, et al. Randomized trial of "slow" versus "fast" feed advancements on the incidence of necrotizing enterocolitis in very low birth weight infants. *J Pediatr.* 1999;134:293–297.

50. Oddie SJ, Young L, and McGuire. Slow advancement of enteral feed volumes to prevent necrotizing enterocolitis in very low birth weight infants. *Cochrane Database Syst Rev.* 2017;Aug 30(8) : CD001241. doi: 10.1002/14651858. CD001241 pub7.

51. Stefanescu BM, Gillam-Krakauer M, Stefanescu AR et al. Very low birth weight infant care: adherence to a new nutrition protocol improves growth outcomes and reduces infectious risk. *Ear Hum Devlop.* 2016;94:25–30.

52. Jasani B, Patole S. Standardized feeding regimen for reducing necrotizing enterocolitis in preterm infants: an updated systematic review. *J Perinatol.* 2017;37:827–833.

53. Ziegler EE. Human milk and human milk fortifiers. In: Koletzko B, Poindexter B, Uauy R, eds. *Nutritional Care of Preterm Infants: Scientific Basis and Practical Guidelines.* Basel, Karger, 2014:215–227.

54. Schanler RJ, Shulman RJ, Lau C. Feeding strategies for premature infants: beneficial outcomes of feeding fortified human milk versus preterm formula. *Pediatrics.* 1999;103:1150–1157.

55. Morales Y, Schanler RJ. Human milk and clinical outcomes in VLBW infants: how compelling is the evidence of benefit? *Sem Perinatol.* 2007;31:83–88.

56. Sullivan S, Schanler RJ, Kim JH, et al. An exclusively human milk-based diet is associated with a lower rate of necrotizing enterocolitis than a diet of human milk and bovine milk-based products. *J Pediatr.* 2010;156:562–574.

57. Abbott Nutrition. Our products. Available at: www.abbottnutrition.com/our-products/for-professionals.nutrition,html. Accessed February 26, 2018.

58. MeadJohnson Nutrition. Healthcare professional resource center product information. Available at: www.meadjohnson.com/pediatrics/us-en/products.information. Accessed February 26, 20118.

59. Koletzko B. Poindexter B, Uauy R. (eds.) Recommended nutrient intake levels for stable, fully enterally fed very low birth weight infants. In: *Nutrition Care of Preterm Infants: Scientific Basis and Practical Guidelines.* Basel, Switzerland: Karger. 2014:297–299.

60. Prolacta 1 H²MF™. Nutrient Values. Prolacta Bioscience MKT-0180 Rev-1. 20014.

61. Institute of Medicine. *Dietary Reference Intakes for Vitamin C, Vitamin E, Selenium and Carotenoids.* Washington, DC: National Academies Press; 2000.

62. Tyson JE, Wright LL, Oh W, et al. Vitamin A supplementation for extremely-low-birth-weight infants. *N Eng J Med.* 1999;340:1962–1968.

63. Ambalavanan N, Tyson JE, Kennedy KA, et al. Vitamin A supplementation for extremely low birth weight infants: outcome at 18 to 22 months. *Pediatrics.* 2005;115:e249–e254.

64. Darlow BA, Graham PJ, Rojas-Reyes MX. Vitamin A supplementation to prevent mortality and short- and long-term morbidity in very low birthweight infants (Review). *Cochrane Database Syst Rev.* 2016;Aug 22 (8):CD000501. doi: 10.1002/14651858.CD000501.pub4.

65. Mitchell SM, Rogers S, Hicks PD, et al. High frequencies of elevated alkaline phosphatase activity and rickets exist in extremely low birth weight infants despite current nutritional support. *BMC Pediatr.* 2009; 9(47): doi:10.1186/1471-2431-9-47.

66. Abrams AA and Committee on Nutrition. Calcium and vitamin D requirements of enterally fed preterm infant. *Pediatrics.* 2013;131:e1676–e1683.

67. Ukarapong S, Venkatarayappa SKB, Navarette C, Berkovitz G. Risk factors of metabolic bone disease of prematurity. *Early Hum Dev.* 2017;112:29–34.

68. Koo WWK, Krug-Wispe S, Neylan M, et al. Effect of three levels of vitamin D intake in preterm infants receiving high mineral containing milk. *J Pediatr Gastroenterol Nutr.* 1995;21:182–189.

69. Domellof M. Nutritional care of premature infants: Microminerals. In: Koletzko B, Poindexter B, Uauy R. eds. *Nutritional Care of Preterm Infants. Scientific Basis and Practical Guidelines.* Basel, Switzerland: Karger, 2014:121–139.

70. Shulman RJ. Zinc and copper balance studies in infants receiving total parenteral nutrition. *Am J Clin Nutr.* 1989;49:879–883.

71. American Academy of Pediatrics Committee on Nutrition. Trace Elements. In: Kleinman RE, Greer FR, eds. *Pediatric Nutrition Handbook,* 7th ed. Elk Grove Village, IL: American Academy of Pediatrics; 2014:467–494.

72. Delphanque B, Gibson R, Koletzko B, et al. Lipid quality in infant nutrition: Current knowledge and future opportunities. *JPGN.* 2015;61:8–17.

73. Schanler RJ, Shulman RJ, Lau C, et al. Feeding strategies for premature infants: randomized trial of gastrointestinal priming and tube-feeding method. *Pediatrics.* 1999;103:434–439.

74. Rogers S, Hicks PD, Hamzo M, et al. Continuous feedings of fortified human milk lead to nutrient losses of fat, calcium and phosphorous. *Nutrients.* 2010;2(3):230–240.

75. Sapsford A, Smith C. Enteral nutrition. In: Pediatric Nutrition Practice Group, Groh-Wargo S, Thompson M, Cox JH, eds. *AND Pocket Guide to Neonatal Nutrition.* Chicago: American Dietetic Association; 2016:76–124.

76. Anderson DM, Poindexter BB, Martin CR. Nutrition. In: Eichenwald EC, Hansen AR, Martin CR, Stark AR, eds. *Cloherty and Stark's Manual of Neonatal Care.* 8th ed. Philadelphia, PA: Wolters Kluwer/Lippincott Williams & Wilkins; 2017:248–284.

77. Chan SW, Hair A. Enteral Nutrition. In: Fernandes CJ, Pammi M, Katakam L, eds. *Guidelines for Acute Care of the Neonate.* 25th ed. Houston, TX: Section of Neonatology Department of Pediatrics, Baylor College of Medicine; 2017–2018:167–178.

78. Parker LA, Sullivan S, Krueger C, et al. Effect of early breast milk expression on milk volume and timing of lactogenesis stage II among mothers of very low birth weight infants: a pilot study. *J Perinatol.* 2012;32:205–209.

79. Hurst NM, Valentine CJ, Renfro L, et al. Skin-to-skin holding in the neonatal intensive care unit influences maternal milk volume. *J Perinatol.* 1997;17:213–217.

80. Parker LA, Sullivan S, Krueger C, et al. Strategies to increase milk volume in mothers of VLBW infants. *MCN Am J Matern Child Nurs.* 2013;38(6):385–390.

81. Meier PP, Johnson TJ, Patel AL, Rossman B. Evidence-based methods that promote human milk feeding of preterm infants: An expert review. *Clin Perinatol.* 2017;44:1–22.

82. Ganni ML, Sannino P, Bezze E, et al. Usefulness of the infant driven scale in the early identification of preterm infants at risk for delayed oral feeding independency. *Early Hum Dev.* 2017;115:18–22.

83. Watson J, McGuire W. Responsive versus scheduled feeding for preterm infants. *Cochrane Database Syst Rev.* 2016 Aug 31;(8):CD005255.

84. Adamkin DH, Radmacher PG, Lewis S. Nutrition for the High-Risk Neonate. In: Fanaroff AA, Fanaroff JM, eds. *Klaus & Fanaroff's Care of the High-Risk Neonate.* 6th ed. Philadelphia, PA: Elsevier Saunders; 2013:151–184.

85. Fenton TR, Anderson D, Groh-Wargo S, et al. An attempt to standardize the calculation of growth velocity of preterm infants—Evaluation of practical bedside methods. *J Pediatr.* 2018;196:77–83.

86. Vaucher YE, Harrison GG, Udall JN, Morrow G. Skinfold thickness in North American infants 24–41 weeks gestation. *Hum Biol.* 1984;56:713–731.

87. Sasanow SR, Georgieff MK, Pereira GR. Mid-arm circumference and mid-arm/head circumference ratios: standard curves for anthropometric assessment of the neonatal nutritional status. *J Pediatr.* 1986;109:311–315.

88. Anderson DM. Nutritional assessment and therapeutic interventions for the preterm infant. *Clin Peri.* 2002;29:313–326.

89. Anderson DM. Nutrition for premature infants. In: Samour PQ, King K, eds. *Pediatric Nutrition.* 4th ed. Boston, MA: Jones and Bartlett Publishers; 2010:63–65.

90. Torrazza RM, Parker LA, Li Y, et al. The value of routine evaluation of gastric residuals in very low birth weight infants. *J Perinatol.* 2015;35:57–60.

91. Riskin A, Cohen K, Kugelman A, et al. The impact of routine evaluation of gastric residual volumes on the time to achieve full enteral feeding in preterm infants. *J Pediatr.* 2017;189:128–134.

92. Parker L, Torazza RM, Li Y, et al. Aspiration and evaluation of gastric residuals in the neonatal intensive care unit. *J Perinatal Neonatal Nurs.* 2015;29:51–58.

93. Leaf A, Lansdowne A. Vitamins – Conventional uses and new insights. In: Koletzko B, Poindexter B, Uauy R. eds. *Nutritional Care of Preterm Infants. Scientific Basis and Practical Guidelines*. Basel Switzerland: Karger; 2014: 152–166.

94. Benson Szekely LJ, Thompson M. Nutrition assessment In: Pediatric Nutrition Practice Group, Groh-Wargo S, Thompson M, Cox JH, eds. *AND Pocket Guide to Neonatal Nutrition*. 2nd ed. Chicago, IL: American Dietetic Association; 2016:1–31.

95. Ridout E, Melara D, Rottinghaus S, et al. Blood urea nitrogen concentration as a marker of amino-acid intolerance in neonates with birthweight less than 1250 g. *J Perinatol*. 2005;25:130–133.

96. Arslanoglu S. IV. Individualized fortification of human milk: Adjustable fortification. *JPGN*. 2015;61:S4–S5.

97. American Academy of Pediatrics Committee on Fetus and Newborn. Hospital discharge of the high-risk neonate. *Pediatrics*. 2008;122:1119–1126.

98. American Academy of Pediatrics Committee on Hospital Care and Institute for Patient- and Family Centered Care. Patient- and family-centered care and the pediatrician's role. *Pediatrics*. 2012;129:394–404. Reaffirmed February 2018.

99. Discenza D. Providing equal family centered care in every NICU. *Neonatal Netw*. 2018;37:45–49.

100. McKenzie BL, Edmonds L, Thomson R, et al. Nutrition practices and predictors of postnatal growth in preterm infants during hospitalization: A longitudinal study. *J Pediatr Gastroenterol Nutr*. 2018;66:312–317.

101. Franz AR, Pohlandt F, Bode H. Intrauterine, early neonatal, and postdischarge growth and neurodevelopmental outcome at 5.4 years in extremely preterm infants after intensive neonatal nutrition support. *Pediatrics*. 2009;123:101–109.

102. Golden NH, Abrams SA and Committee on Nutrition. Optimizing bone health in children and adolescents. *Pediatrics*. 2014;134:e1229–e1243.

103. Carver JD, Wu PYK, Hall R, et al. Growth of preterm infants fed nutrient-enriched or term formula after hospital discharge. *Pediatrics*. 2001;107:683–689.

104. Lucas A, Fewtrell MS, Morley R, et al. Randomized trial of nutrient-enriched formula versus standard formula for postdischarge preterm infants. *Pediatrics*. 2001;108:703–711.

105. Young L, Embleton ND, McGuire W. Nutrient-enriched formula versus standard formula for preterm infants following hospital discharge. *Cochrane Database Syst Rev*. 2016;12: CD004696.

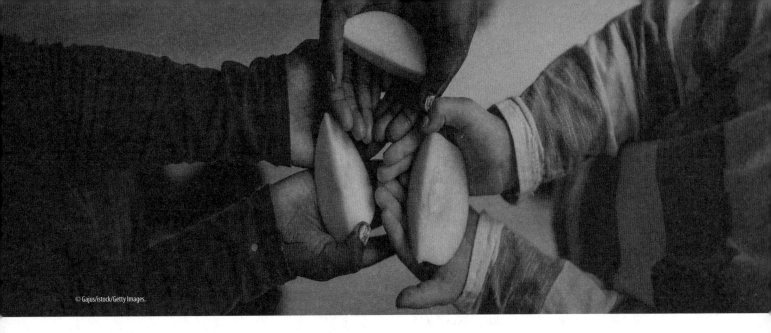

© Gajus/istock/Getty Images.

CHAPTER 8

Infant Nutrition

Stephanie Merlino Barr and Sharon Groh-Wargo

LEARNING OBJECTIVES

- List nutrient requirements of healthy infants.
- Review initiation and management of breastfeeding.
- Identify infant formula choices and bottle-feeding methods.
- State vitamin and mineral supplement needs.
- Review the introduction of solid foods and the feeding progressions of the first year.
- Discuss strategies for managing common feeding problems in infancy.

▶ Introduction

Nutrition delivery during infancy is the most important time of the lifecycle for health, growth, and development. Ideal feeding experiences are those that meet nutrient demands while focusing on the individual infant's developmental readiness. The objectives of this chapter are to discuss recommended feeding practices for healthy, full-term infants and to discuss common feeding problems encountered during the first year.

▶ Nutrition Issues at Birth

Newborn infants are born with a relatively poor vitamin K status due to low placental transfer of vitamin K, decreased gastrointestinal vitamin K synthesis, and the low content of vitamin K in breast milk. Therefore, newborns are at risk for vitamin K deficiency bleeding, including gastrointestinal bleeding, as well as bleeding at the umbilicus and the site of circumcision. A one-time intramuscular injection of 1 mg vitamin K is recommended for all newborn infants at birth.[1] There is a more thorough discussion of vitamin K later in the section titled "Supplementation."

All states in the United States now mandate that newborn infants be screened for congenital disorders.[2] Each year, approximately 4 million infants are screened leading to the diagnosis and treatment of over 12,000 infants.[3] The test is performed by taking small droplets of blood and placing them onto a screening card. State laboratories then analyze them using tandem mass spectrometry. Actual test procedures and the various

145

disorders screened are state specific. Most states screen for a core panel of 32 conditions, with some screening for up to an additional 25 secondary conditions.[2]

The goal of newborn screening is to identify congenital disorders such as in-born errors in metabolism, endocrine disorders, hemoglobinopathies, and perinatally acquired infectious diseases before symptoms occur. Some of these disorders, such as phenylketonuria and maple syrup urine disease, are treatable with alterations in nutrition. It is the responsibility of the primary care physician to make sure newborn screening is done in the appropriate time frame. The dietitian's role is to help determine the appropriate method of feeding when a congenital disease is diagnosed. Links to state-specific education, fact sheets and support can be accessed through the **National Newborn Screening and Global Resource Center** (NNSGRC): http://genes-r-us.uthscsa.edu/resources/consumer/statemap.htm

▶ Nutrient Needs

Most newborns can obtain all necessary nutrient requirements from human milk or infant formula alone. Vitamin D is the most likely exception. As the infant reaches 4 to 6 months, nutrient needs become greater than human milk or formula alone can provide. Solid foods become necessary for adequate satiety. Supplemental iron and fluoride also may become necessary. Adding solid foods to the diet may alter the distribution of nutrients. This is a significant factor when deciding on the type and amount of solids to add to the diet. (See "Supplementation" and "Weaning and Feeding Progression" later in this chapter.)

Dietary reference intakes (DRIs) for infants are expressed as **adequate intakes** (AI) and are available online from the Institute of Medicine of the National Academies at: http://nationalacademies.org/HMD/Activities/Nutrition/SummaryDRIs/DRI-Tables.aspx. Fluid needs are estimated at 700 mL per day for 0- to 6-month-old infants and 800 mL per day for 7- to 12-month-old infants. Average estimated daily energy requirements (kcal/kg) based on reference body weights for 0–6 months (6 kg) and 7–12 months (9 kg) of age are 90 kcal/kg and 80 kcal/kg, respectively, with a range of 80–110 kcal/kg. Specific energy needs can be estimated with the equations in **FIGURE 8.1**. An online calorie calculator is available through the **United States Department of Agriculture** (USDA) National Agriculture Library's Food and Nutrition Information Center at: https://www.nal.usda.gov/fnic/interactiveDRI/dri_results.php

Mean daily protein needs are estimated at 9.1 g and 11 g for 0–6-month-old and 7–12-month-old infants, respectively.

0–3 months: $(89 \times \text{weight [kg]} - 100) + 175$ kcal
4–6 months: $(89 \times \text{weight [kg]} - 100) + 56$ kcal
7–12 months: $(89 \times \text{weight [kg]} - 100) + 22$ kcal

Data from Institute of Medicine. *Dietary Reference Intakes for Energy, Carbohydrate, Fiber, Fat, Fatty Acids, Cholesterol, Protein, and Amino Acids (Macronutrients)*. Washington, DC: National Academies Press; 2005.[4]

FIGURE 8.1 Equations for Calculating Energy Needs of Infant

▶ Breastfeeding

Breastfeeding is the recommended method of feeding for virtually all infants.[1,5–7] Both the **American Academy of Pediatrics** (AAP) and the **Academy of Nutrition and Dietetics** (AND) strongly suggest exclusive breastfeeding for the first 6 months of life followed by continued breastfeeding with appropriate complementary foods until 1 year of age or longer.[5,6] Despite these long-standing recommendations, the overall initiation rate of breastfeeding in the US is 75%, which is less than the Healthy People 2020 target for breastfeeding initiation of 81.9%.[8] The distribution of women who choose to breastfeed varies among different cultures, ethnic backgrounds, education levels, and ages. Statistically, those with the lowest initiation rates for breastfeeding are African Americans, the poor, the less educated, those younger than 20 years of age, and those women participating in the Special Supplemental Nutrition Program for **Women, Infants, and Children** (WIC).[5] Education and support can help these groups make informed choices. Although there have been modest gains in the rate of "any breastfeeding" at 6 month, the 60.5% Healthy People 2020 target has not been met. Rates of exclusive breastfeeding at 3 and 6 months are even farther from Healthy People 2020 targets. The average rates of exclusive breastfeeding at 3 and 6 are 33% and 14%, respectively, and are lower than the Healthy People 2020 goals of 44% and 24%, respectively.[5] Health professionals need to be knowledgeable about both the science and art of breastfeeding, as well as understand the general nutrition needs of their patients.[6]

Breastfeeding research is complicated by methodological challenges related to both the inability to ethically conduct randomized clinical trials as well as the effects of confounding demographic factors including as socio-economic status.[5] Despite these research challenges, there are many nutritional and health advantages associated with breastfeeding and human milk that appear to improve outcomes for mothers and babies. Many studies find dose-response relationships and outcomes related to breastfeeding duration. Here are some commonly listed advantages for human milk and breastfeeding:

Infant Protections:[5,6]

■ Decreased incidence of respiratory and gastrointestinal infections and otitis media

- Decreased incidence of sudden infant death syndrome (SIDS)
- Decreased incidence of atopic dermatitis, eczema, and asthma
- Reduction in the risk of obesity, diabetes, childhood leukemia and lymphoma, celiac disease, and inflammatory bowel disease, especially in infants breastfed for 6 months or longer
- Possible improvements in long-term neurodevelopmental outcomes

Maternal Outcomes: [5,6]

- Less postpartum hemorrhage
- Delayed ovulation
- Decrease in postpartum depression
- Lower rates of hypertension, hyperlipidemia, diabetes, cardiovascular disease, and some cancers, especially when the mother accumulates a significant lactation history

Breastfeeding also offers economic benefits[4] and, after breastfeeding is well established, most mothers find breastfeeding significantly more convenient than formula feeding. There are very few true contraindications to breastfeeding. They include infants diagnosed with galactosemia, and mothers who are positive for human T-cell lymphotrophic virus type I or II or untreated brucellosis. In the developed world, including the US, it is not recommended that HIV-positive mothers breastfeed.[5] Some conditions may require that the mother and baby be separated and/or only be given pump milk.[5]

Human Milk Composition

Human milk offers superior nutritional composition and numerous immunological, anti-microbial, hormonal, and enzymatic compoments.[6] Human milk is not a uniform body of fluids but a secretion of the mammary gland that has a changing composition.[7] The composition of human milk varies from individual to individual, and also with the stage of lactation, the time of day, the time into feeding, and the maternal diet.[7] The four stages of human milk expression are colostrum, transitional milk, mature milk, and extended lactation, each containing its own significant biochemical components and properties.

Management of Lactation

Successful lactation is greatly influenced by the motivation and confidence of the mother, and by support from family and friends, especially the spouse or partner, and from medical professionals. The ability to lactate is a natural characteristic of all mammals, and infants have the capability to suckle even in utero.

Infant suckling stimulates the release of the hormones prolactin, responsible for milk production; and oxytocin, responsible for milk release from the pituitary.[6] Therefore, in order to establish and sustain lactation, it is necessary to allow the baby access to the breast on demand. The more a mother nurses, the more milk she will produce.

The **World Health Organization/United Nations Children's Fund** (WHO/UNICEF) suggests "Ten Steps to Successful Breastfeeding" for use during the initial hospital stay (See **TABLE 8.1**). Scoring systems such as LATCH (**L**atch, **A**udible swallowing, **T**ype of nipple,

TABLE 8.1	WHO/UNICEF Ten Steps to Successful Breastfeeding
1.	Have a written breastfeeding policy that is routinely communicated to all health care staff.
2.	Train all health care staff in the skills necessary to implement this policy.
3.	Inform all pregnant women about the benefits and management of breastfeeding.
4.	Help mothers initiate breastfeeding within the first hour of birth.
5.	Show mothers how to breastfeed and how to maintain lactation even if they are separated from their infants.
6.	Give newborn infants no food or drink other than breast milk, unless medically indicated.
7.	Practice rooming-in (allow mothers and infants to remain together) 24 hours a day
8.	Encourage breastfeeding on demand
9.	Give no artificial nipples or pacifiers to breastfeeding infants*
10.	Foster the establishment of breastfeeding support groups and refer mothers to them on discharge from the hospital.

*The American Academy of Pediatrics does not support a categorical ban on pacifiers because of their role in SIDS reduction and their analgesic benefit during painful procedures. Mother of healthy term breastfed infants should be instructed to delay pacifier use until breastfeeding is well-established, usually about 3–4 weeks.[5]
Data from World Health Organization. *Evidence for the Ten Steps to Successful Breastfeeding.* Geneva, Switzerland: World Health Organization; 1998.[12]

Comfort, Hold/positioning) can objectively assess attachment and milk transfer.[9] A normogram is available for use following vaginal and cesarean deliveries in order to insure appropriate weight loss over the first 3–4 days postpartum.[10] Although formula supplements are not recommended unless medically necessary, there is some evidence that newborns with high early weight loss (≥5%) may benefit from limited volumes of formula during the birth hospitalization. A small study found that early limited formula by syringe (10 ml following each breastfeeding until mature milk came in) actually reduced longer-term formula use and increased breastfeeding at 3 months.[11]

The following list offers some tips for ensuring breastfeeding success[5,7]:

- *Initial breastfeeding:* This should take place as soon after delivery as possible, ideally within the first hour of life. Direct skin-to-skin contact is strongly encouraged.
- *Positioning:* The mother should find a comfortable position either lying down or sitting up. Pillows can support the baby's body and the mother's back and arms. She should change the position of the baby with every feeding during the first few weeks so that pressure on the mother's nipple is rotated, allowing complete emptying of all milk ducts. The mother should use one hand to support and guide her breast and the other hand around the baby's back, cupping the infant's bottom to support and move the baby.
- *Latching on:* The mother can stimulate the rooting reflex by touching the baby's closest cheek. When the mouth is open wide, she pulls the baby close. Be sure that most of the mother's areola is in the baby's mouth, the baby's lower lip is turned out, and the tongue is under the mother's nipple. Rapid sucking, followed by slower, rhythmic sucking and swallowing, will stimulate the **milk ejection reflex** (MER), or the actual release of milk. Signs that let-down has occurred include rapid swallowing by the infant, tingling in the breast, tightening in the uterus, milk around the baby's mouth, or milk dripping from the other breast. The mother can insert her finger in the side of the baby's mouth to break the suction before moving the baby off the breast.
- *Timing:* During the first few weeks, the baby should be nursed 8 to 12 times a day, or about every 2–3 hours. The feedings will become less frequent after breastfeeding is established. It is more important to completely empty the first breast and get adequate hind milk than it is to breastfeed from both sides. Alternating breasts from feeding to feeding establishes good milk supply on both sides. The baby should dictate the duration of feeding. No supplements including

water, glucose water, infant formula, or other fluids are offered unless medically indicated.

- *Assessing adequacy (or "How do I know if my baby is getting enough?"):* A newborn who is receiving adequate fluid and calories will (1) have at least six to eight thoroughly wet diapers a day (maybe only four to five heavy wet diapers if they are disposable); (2) have a bowel movement with most feedings; (3) nurse 8 to 12 times a day; (4) seem satisfied after nursing; and (5) gain approximately 1 oz a day in the first 3 months of life.

A number of situations arise during the early weeks of breastfeeding that, if unanticipated and poorly managed, can jeopardize a successful nursing experience. **TABLE 8.2** points out the most frequent complaints from breastfeeding mothers and possible treatments. Many new mothers return to work or school after their babies are born. They can continue to breastfeed by:

- Arranging to go to the baby or having the baby brought to them
- Pumping and saving the milk in a refrigerator for use within 48 hours or a freezer for up to 3 months
- Discontinuing the feeding(s) when they are away but continuing to nurse at other times

Mothers of hospitalized, high-risk newborns face special challenges with establishing and maintaining lactation. This is the result of long-term separation from their babies and the immature and delayed suck-swallow-breathe coordination due to prematurity.

Two recent practices around breastfeeding deserve special mention: bottle-feeding of breast milk and milk sharing. Some mothers are unsuccessful in getting the baby to latch or are not interested in putting their babies to breast. They may choose to express some or all of the milk needed to meet nutritional requirements and then bottle feed it to the baby. This practice is not ideal since the baby does not get the benefit of the change in milk composition over the course of the feeding or the contact with the mother's skin flora. Evidence suggests that babies who take breast milk from a bottle rather than from the breast actually have an eating and weight gain pattern closer to formula fed babies than breastfed babies.[14,15] The baby, however, still benefits from the superior nutritional content and digestibility of human milk and most of its anti-infective qualities, unless the milk is stored for long-periods of time.

Some mothers produce inadequate quantities of human milk and may seek expressed breastmilk from friends and family through informal milk-sharing. This practice is not recommended by the Academy of Breastfeeding Medicine, the AAP, or the **Food and Drug Administration** (FDA).[16–18] Risks are significantly more serious when babies are fed milk purchased on the internet. This practice is common in some communities and

TABLE 8.2 Most Frequent Complaints from Breastfeeding Mothers

Problem	Description	Treatment
Sore nipples	These are most often the result of improper positioning.	Involves nursing on the least sore nipple first and changing the position of the baby's mouth on the mother's nipple.
Engorgement	This painful swelling of the breast can occur as mature milk production begins and is accompanied by an increase in blood flow and fluid accumulation.	Frequent nursing may help to minimize the discomfort until the breast adjusts. Expressing more milk than is necessary to relieve the pressure will only result in increased milk production and should be discouraged.
Jaundice	In the newborn, this is associated with an elevated bilirubin level and is often the result of inadequate feeding.[2]	Early and frequent feedings will facilitate a good milk supply and stimulate increased gut motility, thus decreasing the absorption of bilirubin.
Poor milk supply	This is probably more a theoretical concern than an actual problem because many mothers are insecure with their ability to successfully provide adequate nutrition without tangible evidence of consumption. Overuse of pacifiers may deter the mother from offering the breast as comfort.	Information about assessing adequacy should be presented in a positive and supportive manner. Frequent feedings and adequate rest will do more to promote milk production than forcing fluids or increasing calories in the mother, unless the diet is severely restricted.

Data from Lawrence, RA, Lawrence RM. *Breastfeeding: A Guide for the Medical Professions,* 8th ed. Philadelphia, PA: Elsevier; 2016.[7]
American Academy of Pediatrics, American College of Obstetricians and Gynecologists. *Breastfeeding Handbook for Physicians,* 2nd ed. Washington, DC: American Academy of Pediatrics Department of Marketing and Publications; 2014.[13]

should be very strongly discouraged since milk purchased on the internet has been shown to arrive at temperatures outside those recommended to preserve quality and may contain contaminants including infectious microbes, cows milk, and other diluting fluids.[19–21]

Human milk provides numerous nutritional, physiological, and personal benefits to mothers, babies and communities. Many resources for breastfeeding are available online including:

The La Leche League: https://www.lllusa.org/

The Centers for Disease Control and Prevention: https://www.cdc.gov/breastfeeding/index.htm

USDA and WIC: https://www.fns.usda.gov/wic/breastfeeding-priority-wic-program

USDA and My Plate: https://www.choosemyplate.gov/moms-breastfeeding-nutritional-needs

LactMed NIH Drugs and Lactation Database: https://toxnet.nlm.nih.gov/newtoxnet/lactmed.htm

▶ Formula Feeding

Breast milk composition continues to be the gold standard by which infant formulas are modeled. However, when breastfeeding is not chosen, is unsuccessful, or is stopped before 1 year of age, bottle-feeding with a commercially prepared iron-fortified infant formula is the recommended alternative.[1] The infant formula market continues to expand and offers a wide variety of products.

Infant Formula Composition

The AAP[1] and the **Food and Drug Administration** (FDA)[22] have identified the importance of regulating the composition and safety of infant formulas. The Infant Formula Act of 1980 was reviewed and updated by an expert panel within the **Life Science Research Office** (LSRO) and focused on the minimums and maximums of nutrients present in infant formulas.[22] Desirable ranges for each nutrient must remain at optimal bioavailable levels throughout the shelf life of each product and provide complete nutrition for the first 4 to 6 months of life.[1] Formulas can be grouped by the following categories: standard, soy, protein hydrolysate, elemental or amino acid, and follow-up formulas. Recent reviews are available.[23,24] The formulas described in this chapter meet all the nutritional needs of term infants assuming appropriate vitamin D and fluoride supplements are given.

See **FIGURE 8.2** for an overview of infant formula products. Updated product information and detailed

Standard milk protein-based formulas:

- Ready-to-feed liquid; liquid concentrate; powder
- Examples: Enfamil Infant; Gerber Good Start Gentle; Similac Advance
- Indications: Infants birth to one year
- Carbohydrate: Lactose
- Protein: Cow's milk protein (intact or partially hydrolyzed)
- Fat: Variety of vegetable oils

Tolerance formulas – Fussiness:

- Ready-to-feed liquid; liquid concentrate; powder
- Examples: Enfamil Gentlease; Gerber Good Start Soothe; Similac Sensitive
- Indications: Infants birth to one year with extreme fussiness and/or gas
- Carbohydrate: Corn syrup solids and/or maltodextrin and/or sucrose; lactose (0–30%)
- Protein: Cow's milk protein (intact or partially hydrolyzed)
- Fat: Variety of vegetable oils

Tolerance formulas – Spitting up:

- Ready-to-feed liquid; powder
- Examples: Enfamil A.R.; Similac for Spit-Up
- Indications: Infants birth to one year with frequent spitting up
- Carbohydrate: Corn syrup solids and/or maltodextrin and/or lactose and/or sucrose; rice starch for thickening
- Protein: Cow's milk protein
- Fat: Variety of vegetable oils

Soy protein-based formulas:

- Ready-to-feed liquid; liquid concentrate; powder
- Examples: Enfamil ProSobee; Gerber Good Start Soy; Similac Soy Isomil
- Indications: Infants birth to one year with IgE-associated allergy or sensitivity to cow milk protein; galactosemia or congenital lactase deficiency; vegetarian family
- Carbohydrate: Corn syrup solids and/or maltodextrin and/or sucrose; lactose-free
- Protein: Soy protein isolate (intact or partially hydrolyzed) with L-methionine
- Fat: Variety of vegetable oils

Protein hydrolysate formulas:

- Ready-to-feed liquid; liquid concentrate; powder
- Examples: Enfamil Nutramigen; Enfamil Pregestimil Gerber Extensive HA; Similac Alimentum
- Indications: Hypoallergenic formula for infants from birth to one year with significant cow milk or soy-protein allergy or sensitivity; protein maldigestion
- Carbohydrate: Variety of sources; lactose-free
- Protein: Extensively hydrolyzed casein or whey protein
- Fat: Variety of vegetable oils; medium chain triglycerides (MCT) (0–55%)

Amino acid-based formulas:

- Powder
- Examples: EleCare for Infants; Neocate; PurAmino
- Indications: Amino acid-based formula for infants birth to one year with severe cow milk or soy-protein allergy; allergy associated with short bowel syndrome; eosinophilic esophagitis (EoE), maldigestion and/or malabsorption
- Carbohydrate: Corn syrup solids; lactose-free
- Protein: Free amino acids
- Fat: Variety of vegetable oils; medium chain triglycerides (MCT) (33%)

Note: Product information is subject to change. Please consult manufacturer websites, product handbooks, and product labels for specific information on nutritional content and ingredients.

FIGURE 8.2 Overview of Infant Formula Products

nutrient composition is available at company websites including:

http://abbottnutrition.com (Abbott Nutrition/Similac products)

https://medical.gerber.com/ (Gerber/Nestle Good Start products)

http://www.meadjohnson.com (Mead Johnson/Enfamil products)

http://www.nutricia-na.com/hcp.html (Nutricia/Neocate products)

http://www.perrigonutritionals.com (store brand)

Standard Formulas

The most common human milk substitute is standard infant formula. These formulas are made from cow's milk by decreasing the protein, removing the butterfat, adding vegetable oils, and adjusting the vitamins and minerals, and are appropriate for most healthy full term infants. Approximately 40–50% of energy provided by standard formula comes from fat. Human milk contains **long-chain polyunsaturated fatty acids** (LC-PUFAs), including **arachidonic acid** (ARA) and **docosahexaenoic acid** (DHA), and these fats are associated with many immune, cognitive, visual, and motor benefits in infants.[21] Most infant formulas now contain DHA and ARA and supplementation has been shown to increase DHA in the brain.[25,26] Palm olein oils as a source of fat in infant formulas has been found to decrease the absorption of calcium in infants.[27] Recent studies suggest that the protein content of some standard infant formulas may be associated with excess weight gain in infancy and that a lower protein density could decrease obesity later in childhood although this remains controversial.[28,29] Several standard cow's milk-based standard formulas on the market are labeled "organic." These formulas meet all the standards of the Infant Formula Act and must comply with the Organic Foods Production Act regulated by the USDA, however, no health benefits have been associated with their use and there are no significant differences in nutritional composition between the organic and regular versions of the products.[23] No differences in hormone levels or the presence of antibiotics between organic and regular infant formulas have been found.[30] A final sub-category of standard infant formulas are products labeled "for breastfeeding supplementation." There is very limited information that these products offer any benefit over regular versions of infant formula to supplement breastfeeding.[23]

Tolerance Formulas

Tolerance formulas include a group of products that can be roughly divided into two groups - those for "fussiness and gas" and those for "spitting up." While marketing claims are managed by the Regulatory Affairs of the FDA, the claims do not require scientific evidence of benefit but rather must meet the somewhat lower bar of "truthful and not misleading."[31]

Formulas for "fussiness and gas" are milk-based but are either lactose-free or contain decreased amounts of lactose compared with standard milk-based formulas, and/or may contain partially hydrolyzed casein or whey protein. Lactose is the primary carbohydrate in breast milk and full term babies are born with mature levels of intestinal lactase.[23] Congenital lactase deficiency is very rare although temporary lactase deficiency can occur following acute gastroenteritis.[23] Reduced-lactose or lactose-free formulas may shorten the course of diarrhea, however, in most cases infants with diarrhea can remain on breastmilk or the formula they were on before their illness.[32] Although parents often report improved feeding tolerance in their babies with a change from full lactose to reduced lactose formula, there is no strong scientific evidence to support this experience. Milk-based reduced-lactose or lactose-free formulas are not appropriate for infants with galactosemia.

Formulas for "spitting up" contain partially hydrolyzed casein or whey protein, and added rice starch. **Gastroesophageal reflux** (GER) is common in infancy. If weight gain is good, treatment in formula fed infants with uncomplicated GER may include non-pharmaceutical interventions such as changes in positioning, feeding schedules, or the caloric density of the formula. One common modification is changing the viscosity of the formula. Adding dry rice cereal to thicken formula displaces nutrients, increases the caloric density, and slows gastric emptying time which may exacerbate reflux.[33,34] Formulas with added rice starch that thicken in the low pH environment of the stomach are a better choice and may reduce the regurgitation and chocking/coughing in infants with uncomplicated GER.[34–36]

Soy Formulas

In the 1960s, soy formulas were developed for infants who could not tolerate cow's milk protein or lactose. Soy formulas can also be useful for infants with galactosemia, those with congenital lactase deficiency, or those who are born to families practicing vegetarianism.[32,37] Recent studies have discouraged the use of soy formulas for infants with **cow's milk protein** (CMP) allergy. About 10–14% of infants with CMP allergy will also have a soy allergy.[38,39] Infants with CMP allergy, or infants with CMP-induced enteropathy or enterocolitis, should be fed protein hydrolysates or amino acid–based formulas. The routine use of soy formula has no proven value in preventing or managing infantile colic or fussiness.[37]

Soy formulas contain methionine-, carnitine-, and taurine-fortified soy protein isolate.[23] The protein content of soy formula is higher than that of standard formula because the biologic value of soy protein is lower than cow's milk protein. Most soy formulas are supplemented with ARA and DHA. Though all soy formulas are lactose free, some are also sucrose free or corn free. Soy phytates and fiber oligosaccharides contained in soy formulas have been found to interfere with the absorption of calcium, phosphorous, zinc, and iron. For this reason, calcium and phosphorous levels in soy formulas have been increased by 20% over those of cow's milk–based formulas and are fortified with zinc and iron.[37,40] These formulas meet all requirements for vitamins and minerals established by the AAP and FDA.[37]

There is no evidence that dietary soy isoflavones are associated with adverse effects on development, reproduction, or endocrine function.[37] Overall, studies have confirmed that soy formulas promote normal growth and development when fed to full-term, healthy infants. Soy formulas are not recommended for premature infants.[37]

Protein Hydrolysates

Indications for using hydrolyzed protein formulas include CMP allergy, soy allergy, or significant nutritional challenges related to a variety of gastrointestinal or liver diseases.[32,39] CMP allergy is usually diagnosed in infants with a strong family history of allergy and can present with any combination of cutaneous (e.g., atopic dermatitis), respiratory (e.g., asthma), and gastrointestinal complaints such as blood in the stool, a classic symptom.[24,39] The estimated prevalence of cow milk allergy that presents in the first year is somewhere between 2 and 7%.[41,42] Both partially hydrolyzed and extensively hydrolyzed formulas are available. Extensively hydrolyzed formulas contain some free amino acids and small peptides that have a molecular weight of less than 3000 D and are considered truly hypoallergenic.[39] Data support using extensively hydrolyzed formulas during the first year of life for infants who are at risk for atopic disease when exclusive breastfeeding for 4–6 months is not possible or for infants who are formula fed.[39,43] Sources of carbohydrate and fat vary among the protein hydrolysate formulas and should be considered when they are fed for indications other than protein allergy or hypersensitivity. The AAP takes no position on using hypoallergenic formulas for treating colic or irritability. Hydrolyzed formulas supplemented with probiotics appear to be well-tolerated in healthy infants.[44] Extensively hydrolyzed formulas are significantly more expensive than milk- or soy-based formulas.[33]

Differentiating between IgE-associated and non-IgE associated allergy can be difficult. Symptoms may overlap although, in general, non-IgE associated allergy mainly affects the gastrointestinal system and is characterized by a delayed onset of hours to days after cow milk consumption. IgE-associated allergy can cause symptoms in the GI tract as well but may also involve the skin and respiratory system. Symptoms may appear immediately and, in severe cases, cause systemic anaphylactic reactions.[24] Most infants with either type of allergy generally respond to extensively hydrolyzed formulas but if symptoms persist, a change to an amino acid-based formula is indicated.

Amino Acid–Based Formulas

Amino acid-based formulas provide all protein in the form of free amino acids with no pepetides.[24] Infants with severe protein hypersensitivity and persistence of symptoms on other formulas can be switched to amino acid–based formulas.[23,32] Besides severe allergy, amino-acid based formulas are indicated for dietary management of protein maldigestion, malabsorption, GI tract impairment, short bowel syndrome, and eosinophilic GI disorders.[33,45] Using amino acid–based formulas for preventing atopic disease has not been studied.[39] Amino acid–based formulas are extremely expensive and may be difficult for families to obtain. WIC provides these formulas to participants in some states; other families must pay out of pocket or apply for insurance coverage.

Other Products Fed to Infants and Young Toddlers

Two additional categories of formula products are available. One category is store brand products. "Generic" versions of infant formulas exist in most product categories. They must meet nutritional and quality standards established by the Infant Formula Act. Their lower price is related to the choice of their source ingredients, packaging, lack of a national sales force, and the limited research and development investment. Approximately 1 in 6 families report stretching, diluting, of infant formula to make it last.[46] Currently these store brand products are marketed through Perrigo Nutritionals. More information can be found at https://www.storebrandformula.com/. Secondly, a variety of infant formula products from smaller manufacturers are available. Examples of product names include Earth's Best (Boulder, CO; www.earthsbest.com), Honest Co. Organic (Santa Monica, CA; www.honest.com) and HiPP and Holle Organic Formulas (European locations; https://organicstart.com/). These products are marketed as alternatives to standard commercial infant formulas marketed in the US European infant formula powders may have reconstitution instructions that are different from the "1 scoop powder plus 2 oz water" recipe that is common for US infant formula brands.

There is a growing demand for goat's milk-derived infant formulas from families seeking alternative formula options. Currently, no infant goat's milk-based formulas are available for commercial purchase in the United States, but these are commonly sold in Europe and Oceania. Goat's milk-based formula should never be used as an alternative to cow's milk-based formula for infants with cow's milk protein allergy. While research has shown growth and nutritional adequacy of goat's milk-based infant formula, infants on goat's milk-based formulas in the published literature have had more frequent stooling and more episodes of blood-stained stools compared with infants receiving cow's milk-based formulas.[47,48] Goat's milk should not be given to infants less than one year of age and will be discussed later in this chapter (See: "Other Products Fed to Infants).

"Follow-up formulas" are designed for older infants and toddlers who are taking solid foods but not enough to meet all essential nutrients needed for optimal growth and development.[32] The AAP has stated that although nutritionally adequate, these formulas offer no clearly established superiority over traditional formulas or breast milk for infants. They may be appropriate as a beverage for a toddler whose diet is consistently poor.[1] In general, follow-up formulas cost less than standard infant formula but more than cow's milk, and are higher in iron than cow's milk. There is no evidence of a growth or developmental advantage over whole milk.[32]

Functional Ingredients

Contemporary commercial infant formulas contain a variety of functional ingredients that are added to design infant formulas that make them closer to human milk. Common ones include nucleotides and, pre- and probiotics. Nucleotides are nonprotein nitrogenous compounds considered "conditionally essential" in infancy. They perform a variety of important biological functions. And supplementation in infant formulas has been shown to promote growth, benefit the GI tract and immune function, and enhance mucosal recovery after intestinal injury.[49] Probiotics are live microorganisms that alter host microflora and interfere with the adherence of pathogenic bacteria.[23] Probiotics in human milk enhance both passive and active immunity, consequently, some manufacturers have added them to infant formula.[50] Probiotics may reduce the incidence and severity of diarrhea in infants.[51] Evidence on using probiotic Lactobacillus reuteri for treating infantile colic is mixed.[52] Further study is needed to produce evidence-based guidelines for using probiotics in infancy. Prebiotics are indigestible carbohydrates that stimulate the proliferation of healthy probiotic bacteria in the colon producing positive effects on mucosal immune system development.[23,53] Human milk contains high concentrations of a wide variety of oligosaccharides that are the third most abundant component of human milk and that function as prebiotics in the GI tract of breastfed infants.[24,54] Studies suggest that infants fed formulas supplemented with probiotics may have more bifidobacteria and lactobacillus in their colons than infants fed formula without supplemental probiotics. The supplemented infants have softer stools, and may benefit from protection against development of allergies and infections.[55–58] It is now possible to synthesize oligosaccharides that are chemically identical to human milk oligosaccharides.[59] Infants fed these supplemented formulas have lower markers of inflammation.[60]

Management of Formula Feedings

Pediatric professionals should not assume that caregivers are familiar with how to purchase or prepare infant formulas. The Infant Formula Act requires packaging to provide instructions for preparation, including pictorials.[1] Bottle-feeding parents need assistance from their healthcare professionals on appropriate volumes required to meet nutrient needs and the addition of age-appropriate solids.

Infant formulas come packaged in three ways: ready-to-feed, concentrated liquid, and powder. Ready-to-feed formulas provide sterile feedings of known caloric concentration for those who like the convenience or do not have the capability of preparing formulas at the time of a feeding (e.g., while traveling). Ready-to-feed formulas do not contain fluoride. They are generally the most expensive form of formula. Concentrated liquid formulas are readily available and mix easily by combining with water in a 1:1 ratio. Powder is ideal if only a small amount of formula is desired, and it may be the cheapest type of formula. Powder formula is popular among breastfeeding mothers who may want to occasionally offer a bottle feeding. Powder formula is generally prepared by mixing one level scoop of powder with 2 ounces of water. It is important to use the scoop provided in the can of powder because scoop sizes vary across different formula powders.

The source of water is important to consider. Both powder and concentrated liquid formula can be the source of fluoride for the infant if reconstituted with fluoridated water. This is especially important when the infant reaches 6 months of life and needs a source of dietary fluoride. At least initially, sterile water is used for formula preparation. The FDA recommends mixing infant formula "using ordinary cold tap water that's brought to a boil and then boiled for 1 minute and cooled."[61] Boiling longer than 1 minute may concentrate the minerals in the water to an undesirable degree. Infants older than 3 months of age start to develop their own immunological protection, so water no longer needs to be boiled, and formula prepared with water directly from the tap is satisfactory.[62] Bottled waters, including distilled and spring water, cannot be assumed to be sterile unless specifically labeled as such.[63] Bottled "nursery" water is sold near infant formula in many stores and is often labeled as sterile.

Hands should be washed thoroughly before mixing and feeding formula. Equipment is cleaned in a dishwasher or washed by hand in soapy water.[61,64] Bottles made of polycarbonate plastic contain bisphenol A, an environmental toxin. Infants may experience low-dose exposure to bisphenol A due to leaching from the bottle, especially if the plastic is scratched or worn. Long-term consequences from bisphenol A exposure are uncertain.[65,66]

Most prepared formulas can be kept in the refrigerator for 24 to 48 hours; however, it is safest to consume formula within 24 hours. Open cans of powder have a 30-day shelf life. Powdered formulas are not sterile and may contain the bacterium *Enterobacter sakazakii*.[67] Safe handling practices are especially important for reconstituting powders for very young infants. Mixing the smallest batch of formula that is practical and limiting storage periods decreases the time a potential pathogen has to proliferate.

There is currently no evidence that babies prefer warmed milk; however, most caregivers do not feed cold bottles from the refrigerator. Warming is best done by putting the unopened bottle in a bowl of warm water for 5–10 minutes before feeding.[61] Microwave heating is not advised because it is difficult to monitor the actual temperature of formula in the center of the bottle. Additionally, steam building within the bottle can result in an explosion and spraying of hot liquid. Overheating formula can cause serious harm to a baby and reports have associated facial and palatal burns of babies with the heating of bottles in a microwave.[61,68,69]

An update on infant formula from the FDA is available.[61]

Feeding Techniques and Schedules

The interaction between caregiver and infant should be intimate and focused during feeding. Good bottle-feeding technique includes: holding the infant in a semi-upright position, maximizing face-to-face contact, tilting the bottle so that the nipple is filled with milk, and holding the bottle so that the caregiver may react to the infant's feeding cues. Bottles should never be propped, as this practice removes the socialization aspect of feeding and causes a higher risk of choking and dental caries. Adding sugar to infant formula or feeding sucrose-containing fluids via bottle is also not recommended due to the risk of dental caries.[1] Please refer to the "Dental Caries in Infancy" section for more information. Breast- or bottle-feeding in the supine position is associated with an increased risk of ear infections.[70] Adding solids, such as cereal, to the bottle also is not recommended unless under medical supervision; this practice will be discussed in the "Gastroesophageal Reflux" section.

Most infants can finish a bottle in 15 to 30 minutes. If most feedings exceed this time frame, it is recommended that a pediatric feeding specialist evaluate the infant to rule out any severe oral or motor delays or dysfunction. Other possible reasons for slow feeding include having a nipple that is too small, clogged, or collapsed. Burping is usually done midway and at the end of the feeding. Partially used bottles should be discarded after the feeding and not saved for the next feeding time due to the risk of bacterial growth and contamination. **TABLE 8.3** gives a suggested bottle-feeding schedule for infants.

▶ Supplementation

Humans have evolved over the centuries on an infant diet of human milk alone, raising the argument that no routine supplementation should be necessary. There are several nutrients, however, for which this may not be entirely true. **TABLE 8.4** summarizes the most up-to-date vitamin and mineral supplementation recommendations for vitamin K, vitamin D, iron, and fluoride.[1] **TABLE 8.5** gives the composition of selected infant vitamin and mineral drops.

Vitamin K. A one-time intramuscular dose of vitamin K at birth (0.5–1.0 mg) protects against **vitamin K deficiency bleeding** (VKDB) in infants and is recommended for all newborns.[1] The diagnosis of VKDB is broken down into three categories: early (first 24 hours of life), classical (day of life 2–7), and late (2–12 weeks of life). Early VKDB is most commonly caused by pharmaceutical inhibition of vitamin K activity due to placental transfer of maternal drugs. Classical VKDB is most often due to low vitamin K intake, and presents as gastrointestinal or umbilical bleeding. Late VKDB is typically caused by malabsorption due to impaired hepatic function or inadequate intake, presenting typically with intracranial bleeding, a condition with significant risk for morbidity and mortality.[77] The risk of VKDB is greatest in exclusively breastfed infants due to breastmilk's low vitamin K concentration. Globally, there has been an increase in parental refusal of vitamin K prophylaxis at birth, resulting in an increase of VKDB. In the United States, the population that refuses vitamin K prophylaxis often overlaps with those who are against standard vaccinations; parents often refuse due to the belief that vitamin K prophylaxis is unnecessary or a desire for a natural birthing process.[78] This movement was fueled by research published by Golding et al in the 1990s that showed an association between vitamin K prophylaxis and childhood leukemias.[79,80] These findings have not been reproducible and have been refuted by all major health organizations, including the AAP.

Vitamin D. The AAP recommends supplementing all newborn infants with 400 IU vitamin D per day within the first few days of life to meet the Institute of Medicine's Daily Recommended Intake.[81,82] Supplementation should continue until at least 1 liter per day of vitamin D–fortified milk is consumed. Vitamin D is vital for bone health and is also helps protect against infection.[74,83] Rickets continues to be a major global public health problem, with vitamin D deficiency remaining as the leading cause of rickets.[81] Infants at highest risk for vitamin D deficiency are those who are exclusively breastfed, have limited sun exposure, and have skin with a greater concentration of melanin pigmentation. Consideration should be given to supplementing these high-risk infants with up to 800 IU vitamin D per day.[74] One mL per day of a poly-vitamin, tri-vitamin, or D-Vi-Sol (Mead Johnson) provides 400 IU vitamin D.

Vitamin A. The concentration of vitamin A in infant vitamins varies significantly between products. While 1500 IU per 1 mL was the standard, some supplements

TABLE 8.3 Guidelines for Progression of Infant Feeding

Age in Months	Feeding Skills	Physical Skills	Oral Motor Skills	Types of Food	Bottle Feeding Feed/day	Bottle Feeding Oz/Feed	Suggested Activities
Birth–4	Coordinated suck-swallow-breathe Able to swallow liquids and use tongue to suck	Poor control of head, neck, and trunk; requires support Brings hands to mouth around 3 months	Rooting reflex Sucking reflex Swallowing reflex Extrusion reflex	Breast milk Infant formula	8–12	2–6	Breast feeding Bottle-feeding
5	Able to grasp objects voluntarily Learning to reach mouth with hands	Good head control and able to sit with support Continues to grasp objects using palmer grasp reflex	Disappearance of extrusion reflex	Breast milk Infant formula	3–5	7–8	Possible introduction of thinned cereal
6	Ready for high chair Able to take spoonful of pureed or strained foods, swallow without choking	Able to recognize spoon and will hold mouth open when spoon approaches	Transfers food from front of tongue to back Closes lips around spoon	Breast milk Infant formula Infant cereal Strained fruit Strained vegetables	3–5	7–8	Prepare cereal with formula or breast milk to a semi-liquid texture Use spoon Feed from a dish Advance to $1/3$–$1/2$ cup cereal before adding fruits and vegetables

(continues)

TABLE 8.3 Guidelines for Progression of Infant Feeding *(continued)*

Age in Months	Feeding Skills	Physical Skills	Oral Motor Skills	Types of Food	Bottle Feeding Feed/day	Bottle Feeding Oz/Feed	Suggested Activities
7	Improved grasp Drinks from cup with help Begin to feed self with hands Easily eats from a spoon	Begin to sit alone unsupported Tracks food with eyes Transfers food between hands Grasps at foods with all fingers and pulls into palm	Mashes food with lateral movements of jaw Learns side-to-side or "rotary" chewing	Breast milk Infant formula Infant cereal Strained to junior texture of fruits, vegetables, and meats	3–5	7–8	Thicken texture to lumpier texture Sit child in high chair with feet supported Introduce cup
8–10	Holds bottle without help Drinks from cup without spilling Decreases fluid intake and increases solids	Sits alone easily Coordinates hand-to-mouth movement; self-feeds finger foods Uses pincer-grasp to pick up objects	Swallows with closed mouth	Breast milk Infant formula Soft, mashed, or minced table foods	3–4	7–8	Begin finger foods Do not add salt, sugar, or fats to foods Present soft foods in chunks ready for finger feeding
10–12	Feeds self with fingers and spoon Holds cup without help	Demands to spoon feed self Good eye-hand-mouth coordination	Tooth eruption Improved ability to bite and chew	Breast milk Infant formula Soft, chopped table foods	3–4	7–8	Provide meals in pattern similar to rest of family Use cup at meals

Data from Fomon SJ. *Nutrition of Normal Infants*. St. Louis, MO: Mosby; 1993.[71]

Butte N, Cobb K, Duyer J, Graney L, Heird W, Rickard K. The start healthy feeding guidelines for infants and toddlers. *J Amer Diet Assoc.* 2004;104:442–484.[72]

Hinton S, Kerwin D. *Maternal and Child Nutrition*. Chapel Hill, NC: Health Sciences Consortium Corporation; 1981.[73]

Misra M, Pacaud D, Petryk A, et al. Vitamin D deficiency in children and its management: review of current knowledge and recommendations. *Pediatrics.* 2008;122:398–417.[74]

United States Department of Agriculture. WIC infant feeding guide. 2017. Available at: https://wicworks.fns.usda.gov/infants/infant-feeding-guide. Accessed January 14, 2018.[75]

TABLE 8.4 Suggested Vitamin and Mineral Supplementation for Full-Term Infants (0–12 Months)

Product	Initiated at	Infants Fed Human Milk	Infants Fed Infant Formula
Vitamin K	Birth	Single dose 0.5–1 mg IM OR 2 mg oral dose 3 times (birth, 1–2 weeks, and 4 weeks of age)	Single dose 0.5–1 mg IM OR 2 mg oral dose 3 times (birth, 1–2 weeks, and 4 weeks of age)
Vitamin D	First days of life	400 IU/day	400 IU/day until 1 L/day of vitamin D–fortified milk is consumed
Iron	4–6 months	1 mg/kg/day from iron-fortified foods or iron supplement	At least 11 mg/day as iron-fortified formula (12 mg/qt)
Fluoride	6 months	0.25 mg/day if exclusively breastfed OR is partially breastfed AND local water has < 0.3 ppm fluoride	0.25 mg/day if using ready-to-feed formula OR local water has < 0.3 ppm fluoride

Abbreviations: IM, intramuscular; ppm, parts per million.

Data from Formula feeding in the term infant. In Kleinman R. *Pediatric Nutrition Handbook*, 7th ed. Elk Grove Village, IL: American Academy of Pediatrics; 2014.61–82.[1]

have reduced their concentrations to 750 IU per 1 mL drop. This reduction was done due to the increased risk of hypervitaminosis A with supplementation at higher levels. The UL of vitamin A is 2000 IU for 0–12 month olds.[84] Vitamin A toxicity most commonly presents as a bulging fontanel or other skeletal abnormalities in infants. Special attention should be paid to the type of multivitamin infants are receiving if clinical symptoms of hypervitaminosis A are present.

Iron. Term infants usually have adequate iron stores for the first 4–6 months of life.[1] Although the amount of iron in human milk is minimal, its bioavailability is approximately five times greater than bovine milk.[1] By 6 months of age, exclusively breastfed infants require additional iron (1 mg/kg/day) either as a supplement or through the introduction of sufficient iron-fortified infant cereal and/or meat.[1,85] For example, an average of two servings of iron fortified dry cereal, at ½ oz or 15 g per serving, is needed to meet the daily iron requirement. The AAP supports the use of iron-fortified formulas (12 mg iron/quart) as the preferred alternative to feeding infants if breastfeeding is not chosen.[1] Iron-fortified formula provides approximately 2 mg/kg per day of iron when fed at about

TABLE 8.5 Composition of Selected Infant Vitamin and Mineral Drops (1 mL)

Product	Brand Name and Manufacturer	Vitamin D (IU)	Vitamin C (mg)	Vitamin A (IU)	Iron (mg)
Tri-Vitamin	Tri-Vi-Sol (Mead Johnson)	400	35	1500/750	
Multi-Vitamin	Poly-Vi-Sol (Mead Johnson)	400	35	750	
Multi-Vitamin with Iron	Poly-Vi-Sol with Fe (Mead Johnson)	400	35	750	10
Vitamin D	D-Vi-Sol (Mead Johnson)	400			
Iron	Fer-In-Sol (Mead Johnson)				15

Data from Mead Johnson. Table data retrieved from manufacturers' websites. Available at: http://www.meadjohnson.com. Accessed January 10, 2018.[76]

120 kcal/kg per day. Several well-designed studies have shown that iron-fortified formulas are as well tolerated as low-iron formulas.[1] These interventions will decrease the risk of iron-deficiency anemia and its irreversible association with cognitive and motor impairments.[1]

Fluoride. A source of dietary fluoride is recommended for infants after 6 months of age. Commercial formulas do not contain fluoride, but if they are mixed with fluoridated water, no supplement is needed. Of note, bottled nursery or baby waters contain varying levels of fluoride, and are not necessarily fluoridated. Fluoride supplements are recommended until 16 years of age in children who do not have access to fluoridated water. The AAP recommends daily supplements of 0.25 mg fluoride for the following groups of infants:[1]

- Infants over 6 months of age living in areas where tap or well water supplies contain less than 0.3 ppm of fluoride
- Infants who consume ready-to-feed formula or formula reconstituted with nonfluoridated bottled water
- Exclusively breastfed infants

Diets of breastfeeding mothers should be assessed for adequacy of vitamin B_{12} if the mother is following an animal protein–restricted diet, especially those who comply with vegan guidelines.[1] When the mother takes a limited diet in any nutrient, supplementation is indicated for both the mother and infant.

▶ Physical and Developmental Readiness for Solids

Physical readiness includes gross motor and oral motor development. Before four months of age, infants have poor head control, uncoordinated lip closure, and an extrusion reflux that permits them to only swallow liquids.[86] During this phase, there is limited or no interest in oral feeding other than at breast or via bottle. From four to six months of age, infants learn oral and gross motor skills that help them accept solid foods. Oral motor skills evolve from the reflexive suck to the ability to swallow nonliquid foods and transfer contents from the front of the tongue to the back of the mouth. Gross motor development includes sitting independently and maintaining balance while using hands to reach and grasp for objects.[83,86] As head control improves, an infant is ready to sit in a high chair and grasp pieces of food. Infants will begin to turn toward food or watch others eating but still lack the hand-to-mouth coordination necessary to feed themselves and need assistance from caregivers.[87] At this stage of development, infants should be encouraged to sit in high chairs by themselves. It is important that they start developing independence with feeding and join the family around the table.

Independent eating behaviors are encouraged as infants advance from reflexive and imitative behaviors to more independent and exploratory behaviors. This transitional milestone occurs some time during the fourth month of life.[88] By six months, infants can indicate a desire for food by opening their mouth, leaning forward to indicate hunger, and leaning back and turning away to show disinterest or satiety. However, until an infant can express these feelings, feeding of solids will probably represent a type of forced feeding, potentially leading to overfeeding and risk of obesity or general anxiety around eating for the infant.

In addition to determining the quantity of feedings, infants should be encouraged to develop more independence with feeding in the following ways:

- Self-feeding of soft finger foods
- Sipping from a cup by six to eight months of age[88]
- Holding the bottle or cup independently
- Controlling the timing of feeds in order to promote self-regulation of hunger and satiety[89]

A variety of foods should be experienced throughout infancy. The introduction of unfamiliar foods is noteworthy because it allows the infant to gain experience with various tastes and textures, promoting successful weaning to the family diet. The importance of diversifying the diet at specific intervals during the infant's psychological development can be observed in deprived environments where the eating pattern is unvaried and monotonous, or where weaning is delayed. Both situations fail to stimulate interest in solid foods or self-feeding.[89] Caregivers who find it difficult to give freedom or control to infants with self-feeding often promote frustration and insecurity around eating for infants. Food refusal and failure to thrive often result from this negative feeding environment.

▶ Weaning and Feeding Progression

During infancy, the most important source of nutrition for growth and development is breast milk or iron-fortified infant formulas. During the second half of infancy, the addition of infant cereal and solid foods is vital for both continued nutritional adequacy of the infant's diet and the progression of normal infant development. The optimal timing and type of "complementary" foods introduced has been questioned for decades. The current foremost recommendation by the AAP, WHO, and UNICEF is that exclusive breastfeeding for the first six months of life is the ideal diet for infants. It is widely acknowledged that there is no nutritional nor developmental benefit to introducing solids before four months of life. Despite this, an analysis using data from the National Health and Nutritional Examination Survey (NHANES) database found that an estimated 16.3% of US infants are given solid foods before four months of life.[90] Early introduction of solid foods is most likely to occur in formula fed infants or when parents perceive their infant as fussy or unsatiated by bottle feeding. Timely initiation of solid foods is particularly important for exclusively breastfed infants. At around six months of age, breastfed infants may be at risk for iron deficiency anemia and should receive an additional dietary iron source such as iron-fortified cereals or meats.[1]

Readiness to start solid foods generally occurs around six months of life. Observations of individual physical and psychological developments are better determinants of readiness for starting complementary foods than age alone. All infants develop at different rates, which caregivers need to keep in mind when initiating spoon feeding and new textures. Awareness of the infant's hunger and satiety cues with spoon feeding is just as important as feeding cues during breast- and bottle-feeding. Infants who turn away during a feeding are usually indicating that they are satisfied and want the feeding to stop. Infants' self-regulating instinct can be affected by factors such as coercive feeding, overly restrictive feeding, or the feeding environment. Encouraging infants to establish a healthy self-confidence regarding satiety and hunger is one of the most important aspects of infant feeding. The main goals of solid food introduction during infancy are to provide adequate nutrition, balance nutrient needs with a variety of foods and textures, and encourage development of independent feeding skills.

Baby-led weaning is a practice growing in popularity, where infants are allowed to feed themselves as an alternative to the parent spoon feeding pureed foods. Caregivers provide age-appropriate and wholesome foods, and allow the infant to consume at their own pace. The practice is driven by beliefs that this may allow infants to accept a wider variety of foods, help avoid picky eating, and improve the infant's relationship with food. There are also claims that it may reduce the risk of overweight and obesity later in life, but this has been unsubstantiated in the published literature.[91] The risk of choking does not appear to be significantly different in baby-led weaning feeding mechanisms compared with traditional feeding methods.[92] Refer to **TABLE 8.6** to review choking precautions to follow if baby-led weaning is being practiced.

When considering introducing complementary foods, caregivers should consider the individual readiness of the infant along with the following potential concerns:

- Energy requirements and growth of the infant
- Iron and zinc status of the infant and foods being introduced

TABLE 8.6 Minimize Risk of Choking in Baby-Led Weaning
General Principles
1. Ensure foods are soft enough to mash with tongue on the roof of the mouth, or are large and fibrous enough that small pieces do not break off when sucked/chewed (e.g. meat)
2. Avoid foods that crumble in the mouth
3. Ensure foods offered are at least as long as the child's fist, on at least one side of the food
4. Ensure that the infant is always sitting upright while eating
5. Always monitor the infant while eating
6. Never let anyone but the infant put food in their mouth, the infant must eat at their own pace and under their own control
Foods to Avoid When Introducing Solids
1. Foods that can't be mashed with the tongue on the roof of the mouth
2. Very small foods including: nuts, grapes, and fruits that contain stones
3. Raw vegetables
4. Raw apples (whole or sliced)
5. Under ripe or hard fruit
6. Unpeeled citrus fruits
7. Whole nuts
8. Popcorn
9. Sausages, carrots, or other foods cut into rounds or "coins"

Data from Fangupo LJ, Heath ALM, Williams SM, et al. A baby-led approach to eating solids and risk of choking. *Pediatrics*. 2016;138(4):e20160772.[92]

- Risk of morbidities related to sanitation and water quality of the infant's environment
- Potential risk of atopic disease if there is a personal or family history of severe allergy
- Long-term impact on neurocognitive development and behavior

▶ Complementary Foods

As complementary foods begin to displace breast milk or formula in the diet, vitamin and mineral intake is affected. Foods selected for infant feeding should be nutrient-rich items. Some studies have encouraged introducing meats between 4 and 6 months in order to help prevent iron or zinc deficiency, especially for exclusively breastfed infants.[1] Introducing solids should not mislead caregivers into thinking consuming breast milk or infant formula is any less significant. Optimal volumes of breast milk and/or iron-fortified infant formula are still essential to meet the majority of the infant's nutrient needs. The **Feeding Infants and Toddlers Study** (FITS) from 2002 reported dramatic decreases in energy intake from breast milk and/or formula with the introduction of solid foods. The most significant decrease in breast milk or formula volume occurs from about four to five months of age to six to eight months of age, with a total energy decrease from 88% to 66% of total intake.[93]

Review infant formula composition in Figure 8.2. For more information on infant foods and infant feeding, the following online resources are available:

- http://www.gerber.com
- http://www.heinzbaby.com
- http://www.beechnut.com
- http://www.healthychildren.org (an AAP-sponsored site)

▶ First Foods

Commercial infant cereal, thinned to a semi-liquid consistency with breast milk or infant formula, is generally recommended as an infant's first food. This has become customary due to both the need for an additional source of dietary iron at this stage and because cereals are typically well tolerated by infants.[85] Avoidance of rice cereal is now recommended due to the risk of inorganic arsenic exposure and its negative impact on infant development.[94] Cereal should be spoon fed and not added to the infant's bottle. Resistance to initial spoon-feeding is common due to the infant's unfamiliarity with the spoon as a dispenser of nutrition. Holding the infant rather than sitting them in a high chair may relieve some of the initial apprehension. Each new food item introduced in the infant's diet should be fed for two to three days while examining the infant for symptoms of intolerance. Signs of potential intolerance may include skin rashes, vomiting, diarrhea, or wheezing. In the absence of such symptoms, the quantity, frequency, and consistency of the food item can be increased, and a second food can be presented. Once a variety of single ingredients have been introduced and tolerated, a combination of these ingredients can be offered.

Refer to Table 8.3 for further recommendations regarding the guidelines for progression of infant feeding.

A gag reflex of varying degrees is apparent until about seven to nine months of age, when most infants are beginning to chew and tolerate smooth to chunky foods. A normal gag reflex should be developing at this point. Choking indicates that the infant is not ready for transitioning to solid foods, regardless of their chronological age. It is not unusual for caregivers to be overly cautious about this natural gag reflex and mistake it for choking. Providers must be attentive to situations where infant feeding and solid texture progression is being delayed due to caregiver anxiety. Infants will pick up on this anxiety around feeding and begin to develop insecurity around the feeding environment. Parental support, encouragement, and even a feeding demonstration while at a medical visit can reduce feeding anxieties.

Many commercial baby food products are available on the market today. Virtually all are prepared without added sodium and many without added sugar. Juices are generally enriched with vitamin C. Cereals are enriched with iron, thiamine, riboflavin, niacin, calcium, and phosphorus. Those advertised as "first foods" are single-ingredient foods, in contrast to "dinners," baked goods, "graduates," "junior foods," and other items that contain a combination of ingredients. Textures from strained to chunky are available, along with foods designed for teething. Baby food manufacturers use various descriptors to identify the different textures. Words such as "stage," "first," "second," or "graduate" can tell a parent or caregiver approximately when in infancy the baby might be ready to handle the texture of the food. Commercial baby foods are a time-efficient means of providing an infant with solids, and if chosen wisely, can supply a nutrient-rich diet. Certain items will provide more nutrients than seemingly comparable choices. For example, plain meats contain from 220% to 250% of the protein and up to 200% of the iron of "meat dinners." The nutrient contents of selected commercial baby foods are listed in **TABLE 8.7**. Providers and caregivers can use the Nutrient Data Laboratory Website to view a nutrient analysis of commercial baby foods. The site is at https://ndb.nal.usda.gov/ndb/. Analysis includes macro and micronutrients as well as amino acid profiles of various serving sizes.

▶ Home Preparation of Baby Foods

Home-prepared baby foods are an alternative to commercially prepared foods. They are economical and allow greater flexibility in altering food consistency, but preparation can be time consuming. Home-prepared foods should focus on providing safe and adequate nutrition. Infant diets should have a variety of nutrient-dense foods. Foods should be easy to hold and vary in texture and temperature. Families should not be encouraged to make their own baby foods from their own meals if they lack variety in their diet. Caution should also be expressed if families lack refrigeration or have poor sanitation in their homes. Infants from developing countries are at a greater risk of food contamination or foodborne illness related to poor sanitation and unsafe water supplies. Homegrown foods should not be prepared for infants if the lead concentration of soil in residential areas is excessive.[95]

Infants can experience different tastes from maternal diets via amniotic fluid and breast milk.[96] For this reason, it is reasonable to consider that infants can handle a

TABLE 8.7 Nutrient Composition of Selected Commercial Baby Food Products

Food		Amount	Calories	Protein	Carbohydrates	Fat	Sodium	Sugar	Fiber
Instant Cereal	Single grain oatmeal	¼ cup (15 g)	60	2	10	1	0	2	<1
Stage 1 Vegetable	Carrots G	1 tub	30	0	5	0	20	4	1
	Carrots H	1 jar	35	1	8	0.2	60	4	3
Stage 1 Fruit	Bananas G	1 tub	60	<1	15	0	5	13	<1
	Bananas H	1 pouch	130	1	29	0	10	26	3
Stage 2 Vegetable	Pea Carrot Spinach G	1 tub	45	2	7	0	30	4	2
	Pea Pear Broccoli H	1 pouch	90	4	17	0.3	65	7	4
Stage 2 Fruit	Pear Apple Berry G	1 tub	90	0	21	0	5	16	2
	Apple Strawberry Raspberry H	1 pouch	60	0.2	15	0.1	1	11	2
Stage 2 Dinner	Sweet Potato Turkey G	1 tub	90	2	13	3	20	6	1
	Sweet Potato Turkey H	1 jar	100	5	19	0.2	15	7	1
Lil' Bits	Herb Vegetable Pasta Chicken	1 tub	120	4	16	4.5	60	4	1
Stage 3 Dinner	Chicken and Vegetable Paella	1 jar	140	9	20	3	85	3	3

Abbreviations: G, Gerber; H, Heinz.
Note: Values derived from http://www.gerber.com and http://www.heinzbaby.com. Accessed January 2018.

variety of flavors in their foods. Families should progress to multiple ingredient foods and spices after the infant has shown tolerance for all the items individually without adverse reaction. Exposing infants to an array of flavors and food textures is important, as it can help initiate lifelong healthy eating habits. **TABLE 8.8** provides detailed instructions for the home preparation of baby foods.

The diets of family members and caregivers play a significant role in influencing the types of foods infants eat. The FITS data showed that 18%–33% of infants and toddlers over 6 months of age consumed no fruits and vegetables.[100] This low level of produce intake can continue into childhood and adolescence, leading to long-term unhealthy eating habits. The primary influence of this reduction in produce consumption may be the poor example from parents, caregivers, and other children in the home. The final phase of infant feeding, between the 10th and 12th months, is a combination of mimicry and increasing independence with self-feeding. The caregiver and child interactions around eating are significant at this point and help establish healthy eating relationships that will extend into childhood and adulthood.

See the following websites for suggestions on making baby foods and recipes:

- http://www.cookinglight.com/food/baby-food-recipes
- https://www.parents.com/recipes/baby-food/

▶ Risk for Obesity

The global epidemic of childhood obesity has continued to grow in its prevalence and complexity as a public health crisis. Globally, the number of overweight or obese infants and children have increased from 32 million in 1990 to 41 million in 2016.[101] The rate of increase of childhood obesity in developing nations is 30% higher than in developed countries.[101] The WHO projects that the world will have 70 million overweight or obese 0 to 5-year olds by 2025 if no significant change to combat this global epidemic is made.[101] The United States continues to have a dangerously high childhood obesity rate, estimated at 17% from 2011–2014.[102] However, in the same timeframe, US infants enrolled in WIC showed a decline in high weight-for-length measurements, from 14.5% in 2010 to 12.5% in 2014.[103] Analysis has shown that there is significant risk for obesity later in life if weight-for-length measurements are greater than two standard deviations above the age-specific median set by the WHO growth standards. This documented trend among WIC enrolled infants may indicate a potential decrease in the risk for childhood obesity within this group, but it should not be interpreted as the beginning of the end of childhood obesity. Research continues to focus on when the initial risk for childhood overweight or obesity begins and who is at greatest risk.

Initial risk factors for infants and children becoming overweight or obese occur at preconception. Mothers who are overweight or obese, smoke, or gain excessive weight during pregnancy have a greater risk of having an infant and/or child who will be overweight at some point during childhood.[104] The greatest risk factor for overweight or obesity in infancy or childhood was having an overweight parent.

From birth, studies have looked at the possible influence of various infant feeding methods on the

TABLE 8.8 Steps in the Home Preparation of Baby Foods

1. Choosing appropriate foods:
   ■ Use fresh or unsalted frozen foods. Do not use canned foods because they may contribute excessive sodium to the infant's diet.
   ■ Spinach, carrots, broccoli, and beets should not be pureed at home because they may contain sufficient nitrite to cause methemoglobinemia in young infants.

2. Preparing fruits and vegetables:
   ■ Thaw frozen vegetables; wash fresh produce.
   ■ Remove peels, cores, and seeds.
   ■ Steam or boil.
   ■ Puree in blender or food processor to desired consistency. Use liquid from cooking to preserve nutrients otherwise lost in cooking. Do not over-blend because this may cause excessive oxidation of nutrients.

3. Preparing meats:
   ■ Bake, broil, or stew meat.
   ■ Remove all skins.
   ■ Chop into small pieces.
   ■ Puree in blender to desired consistency.

4. Storing prepared foods:
   ■ Keep refrigerated in a covered container. Use refrigerated foods within 48 hours.
   ■ Freeze in 2-tablespoon portions by pouring pureed food into an ice cube tray. Thaw desired portions in refrigerator before using.

Data from Kleinman R. *Pediatric Nutrition Handbook*, 7th ed. American Academy of Pediatrics; 2014.[1]
Hinton S, Kerwin D. *Maternal and Child Nutrition*. Chapel Hill, NC: Health Sciences Consortium Corporation; 1981.[97]
American Academy of Pediatrics, Committee on Nutrition. Infant methemoglobinemia: the role of dietary nitrate. *Pediatrics*. 1970;46:475–478.[98]
Kerr C, Reisinger K, Plankey F. Sodium concentration of homemade baby foods. *Pediatrics*. 1978;62:331–335.[99]

risk of childhood overweight and obesity. Researchers comparing breastfeeding and formula-feeding initially believed that breastfeeding had a protective effect against childhood obesity. Comparison studies revealed that formula-fed infants started to outgrow breastfed infants by as early as 2–3 months of age.[105] Research has found that being breastfed and the duration of breastfeeding appears to be inversely related to fat mass at 4 years of age.[106] However, the many confounding variables common with choosing whether to breastfeed make it difficult to declare breastfeeding as more protective against overweight and obesity.

One of the biggest confounders is that obese mothers are less likely to initiate and sustain breastfeeding than their non-obese counterparts. This is due to a multitude of factors. Obese women have higher rates of cesarean delivery, which is associated with lower rates of initiation and maintaining breastfeeding throughout the first six months of life.[107] Obesity also creates physiological changes that may negatively impact breastfeeding such as delaying the onset of lactogenesis II and a lesser breastmilk supply.[108,109] Breastmilk produced by obese mothers has higher concentrations of obesogenic factors and pro-inflammatory markers, like C-reactive protein, but its effect on obesity in infants is unknown.[110] The current published research does not support obesity as a contraindication to breastfeeding. All mothers should be encouraged to breastfeed their infant exclusively for the first 6 months of life.[110] Overweight and obese mothers should be provided additional social and healthcare support to meet this goal.

Methods of feeding significantly affect eating behaviors and may affect obesity risk. Infants put to breast learn how to self-regulate their intake of nutrition I order to meet individual satiety. Formula-fed infants are often given standard amounts of formula, and parents and caregivers may not be as attentive to feeding cues. This subtle difference in feeding environment may be enough to teach self-regulation with eating for years to come. In solid food introduction, both early (before four months) and late (seven months or later) introduction of solid foods have been associated with a risk of increased BMI or obesity later in life.[111,112] However, the evidence on this association is inconsistent between studied populations and experimental designs.[113] Greater consumption of fruits and vegetables in infancy is correlated with increased intake of these items later in childhood, which has a subsequent effect on body composition.[114] Infants who are fed more fruits, vegetables, and home-prepared foods were also leaner at 4 years.[106] There are many components that significantly impact an infant's long term risk for obesity, but initiating healthy habits early may improve long-term outcomes.

The earlier an infant or child is identified as overweight, the better predictability of life-long overweight.

The following goals have been established for infant feeding in order to prevent childhood overweight or obesity:[115]

- Breastfeed exclusively for 6 months
- Avoid sweet beverages
- Respect infant self-regulation during feeding (breast-, formula-, or solid food feedings)
- Avoid using food for comfort
- Introduce and offer a variety of fruits and vegetables as complementary feeds

▶ Dental Caries in Infancy

Tooth decay is one of the most common chronic disease of childhood.[1] **Baby bottle tooth decay** (BBTD) is an oral health disorder characterized by rampant dental caries associated with inappropriate infant feeding practices. Dental caries occur when carbohydrate-containing fluids contact teeth for a prolonged period of time. This gives plaque-forming bacteria, like *Streptococcus mutans*, an ideal environment to flourish. Bacteria will metabolize the carbohydrates and create acid as a byproduct, which demineralizes the tooth enamel, eventually resulting in a cavity.[116]

The disorder affects the primary teeth of infants and young children, particularly those who are permitted to fall asleep with a bottle filled with juice or other fermentable liquid.[1] Nursing caries, similar to tooth decay caused by BBTD from formulas, can also occur with prolonged or inappropriate breastfeeding at naptime or too frequently throughout the day. The 1999–2004 NHANES data set showed a significant increase in dental caries in primary teeth in children, with 42% of children aged 2–11 reporting tooth decay.[117] This is a reversal of the declining trend of tooth decay in children from the 1970s to the 1990s. Children have a 32 times greater chance of having caries by 3 years of age if they come from a low socioeconomic background, eat sugary foods, and have a mother with a low education level.[1]

Certain feeding practices can be altered to prevent BBTD. The **American Academy of Pediatric Dentistry** (AAPD) recommends the cessation of ad lib breast- or bottle-feeding with the initial eruption of teeth. Providing liquids concentrated in mono- and disaccharides, such as juice and sweetened beverages, is the leading cause of BBTD, and should be avoided. An infant sleeping with a bottle in their mouth has a decrease in salivary flow, causing a pooling of liquid around the teeth. Another contributing factor for tooth decay is the early introduction of juice. By the age of 1 year, nearly 90% of all infants in the United States have been introduced to juice; 25% before the age of 6 months.[1]

Receiving regular dental care is important for oral health. A recent study by the Medical Expenditure Panel Survey found that only 1.5% of infants and one-year olds had a dental visit. Appropriate fluoride exposure is also important for infants and children over six months of age. Fluoride works to reduce demineralization and promote remineralization while also inhibiting acid production by bacteria.[116] Infants who refuse cold foods or grimace when chewing should be examined for BBTD. Those afflicted will have tooth discoloration varying from yellow to black. Preventive measures include:

- Exposing teeth to fluoride
- Feeding only infant formula or water from a bottle
- Practicing good oral hygiene by cleaning the infant's teeth and gums with a damp washcloth or gauze pad after each feeding
- Avoiding juices in the first year; if given, offer in a cup rather than a bottle
- Filling bedtime bottles with water, if necessary
- Minimize exposure to sugar-rich foods and beverages
- Receiving regular dental care

▶ Whole Cow's Milk

In order to maintain optimal nutrition status, the AAP Committee on Nutrition recommends that infants should be provided breast milk, with the only alternative being iron-fortified formulas during the first 12 months of life.[1] As mentioned earlier, potential detrimental effects of the early introduction of whole cow's milk in the diet of infants include excessive renal solute load, gastrointestinal blood loss, poor iron delivery, and overall poor nutritional status of the infant.[1] More current studies have expanded this list of medical concerns to include chronic constipation and possibly an increased risk for type 1 diabetes.[1]

The incidence of cow's milk protein allergy in the first year is between 2 and 7%.[41,42] However, a 2010 study based in Israel found that only 0.5% of the studied cohort presented with an IgE-mediated cow's milk protein allergy.[118] This suggests that the prevalence of cow's milk protein allergy may be less common than typically reported in some populations. Previously, it was believed that the early introduction of cow's milk increased the risk of developing an allergy to milk protein. Current research has suggested that, apart from high-risk cases, early exposure to cow milk protein in infant formula may promote tolerance.[118,119] The impact of early exposure versus prolonged avoidance of major food allergens on incident of food allergy will be discussed later in this chapter.

Risks of iron deficiency anemia and other micronutrient deficiencies remain a problem when cow's milk replaces breast milk or formula before 12 months of age. Lower concentration and bioavailability of iron in cow's milk predisposes infants to iron deficiency anemia.[120] Cow's milk is also a poor source of vitamin C, vitamin E, and **essential fatty acids** (EFAs).

Lastly, the additional protein and electrolytes in cow's milk increases the renal solute load and places the infant at risk for dehydration during periods of vomiting, diarrhea, or exposure to dry heat in winter or to the sun in the summer. For these reasons, it is best to delay the introduction of cow's milk until the infant is one year old. Despite these recommendations and negative medical consequences, the FITS study found that nearly one third of infants were introduced to cow's milk and were consuming it daily within the first year of life.[100] When the infant's diet is changed to cow's milk after the first year, it should be whole cow's milk in order to provide essential fat and calories.

▶ Other Products Fed to Infants

Goat's milk is not recommended for infants less than one year of age. If fed to older infants in place of whole cow's milk, goat's milk must be supplemented with folic acid.[121] Soy (e.g., Silk), rice (e.g., Rice Dream), almond (e.g., Blue Diamond Almond Breeze), or other "milks" are not nutritionally adequate for infants and should not be fed during the first year of life. Please refer to **TABLE 8.9** for an overview of different milk compositions.

▶ Water in First Year

Additional water is not necessary during the first year if infants are receiving adequate amounts of breast milk or formula in order to sustain adequate weight gain. Even during hot months, infants can obtain adequate amounts of free water from breast milk or iron-fortified formula. Caregivers often feel thirsty or hot themselves and offer water to infants. Unfortunately, the free water usually displaces nutrient- and calorie-dense breast milk or infant formula, putting the infant at increased risk for electrolyte imbalance and weight loss. The only exception to this rule is if the caregiver observes the infant having a reduction in urine output or urine appears to be dark in color.[1] Caregivers should be advised that 6 or more wet diapers a day are the adequate number to ensure the infant's proper hydration status.

▶ Juice Consumption During Infancy

There has been debate in the past among healthcare providers regarding the benefit of consuming fruit juices during infancy. Juice had been suggested in the second half of infancy to treat hard stools; however, too often, infants were consuming excessive amounts, leading to inappropriate growth and malabsorption during

TABLE 8.9 Milk Product Compositions

	Cow's Milk	Soy	Almond	Coconut	Rice
Calories and Nutrients Per 1 Cup Serving					
Calories	149	120	29	46	113
Protein (g)	7.7	7	0.7	0	0.7
Total Fat (g)	7.9	4	2.3	4.5	2.3
Total Carbohydrates (g)	11.7	14	1.5	2	22
Calcium (mg)	276	350	444	101	283
Phosphorus (mg)	205	151	22	N/A	134
Potassium (mg)	322	360	178	41	65
Vitamin B-12 (ug)	1.1	3.1	N/A	3	1.5
Vitamin A (IU)	395	506	408	499	499
Vitamin D (IU)	124	101	103	120	101

Data from United States Department of Agriculture- USDA food composition databases. Available at: https://ndb.nal.usda.gov/ndb/search/list. Accessed January 15, 2018.[122]

infancy. Today, the AAP strongly encourages avoiding juices for the first 6 months of life. There is concern that any amount of juice intake will put the infant at risk of displacing nutrient-dense breast milk or formula with high-sugar and low-nutrient juices.[123]

If an infant is experiencing harder stools, small amounts of juice can be tried on an as-needed basis only. The carbohydrate source in fruit juice is primarily from a combination of fructose, glucose, and sorbitol. See **TABLE 8.10** for the carbohydrate sources in various fruit juices.[71] Studies summarized by Fomon suggest

that infants better absorb and have greater tolerance to juices containing fructose when they are combined with sucrose and glucose.[71,124] Fruit juices containing these sugars appear to have beneficial effects similar to those of fiber for infants suffering from constipation. Juices containing the greatest amounts of fructose and sorbitol include apple and pear juice.[125,126]

Excessive juice intake puts infants and children at risk for dental caries, failure to thrive, and short stature.[128] The role of juice in childhood obesity is still being debated. A 2017 meta-analysis by Auerbach et al found that small

TABLE 8.10 Carbohydrate Sources in Select Juices (g/100 g of food) (mOsm/kg H_2O)

Juice	Fructose	Glucose	Sucrose	Sorbitol	Osmolality
Apple	6.0	2.4	2.5	0.5	638
Pear	6.6	2.0	3.7	2.2	764
White grape	7.5	7.1	0.6		1030

Values may vary depending on the dilution of the juice and type of fruit used.
Data from Fomon SJ. *Nutrition of Normal Infants.* St. Louis, MO: Mosby; 1993.[71]
Smith MM, Davis M, Chasalow FI, et al. Carbohydrate absorption from fruit juice in young children. *Pediatrics.* 1995;95:340–344.[125]
Hyams JS, Etienne NL, Leichtner AM, et al. Carbohydrate malabsorption following fruit juice ingestion in young children. *Pediatrics.* 1988;82:64–68.[127]

amounts of 100% fruit juice are not directly causal of childhood obesity; however, the question of "how much is too much?" has not been fully determined.[129] The FITS Study revealed that more than 20% of infants ages 4–6 months were already having small amounts of juice in their diets daily.[100,130] If an infant has poor weight gain, it is very important to obtain a thorough diet history with specific inquiry into juice or water consumption.

▶ Feeding Problems

Formula intolerance, constipation, acute diarrhea, and food refusal are common feeding problems encountered during infancy. These problems can usually be resolved through simple measures. If ignored, the problems may become exacerbated and cause detrimental effects to an infant's nutritional status and growth.

Food Allergy in Infancy

Childhood food allergies remain a significant health problem in the United States. Approximately four out of every 100 US children are diagnosed with a food allergy.[131] Understanding how food allergies develop is rapidly changing within current pediatric research. Since 2006, the **Food Allergen Labeling Consumer Protection Act** (FALCPA) has mandated the clear labeling of the eight major food allergens in all products regulated by the FDA. The most common allergens are: milk, soy, egg, fish, crustacean shellfish, wheat, tree nuts, and peanuts.

Cow's milk protein allergy is the most common allergy reported in infancy, with as many as 5–15% of infants presenting with symptoms suggestive of allergy.[132] This allergy is usually identified within the first four months of infancy. The onset of cow's milk protein allergy is due to the immaturity of both the gastrointestinal tract and the immune system. In early infancy, the gastrointestinal tract adapts to the extrauterine environment, protecting against the penetration of harmful substances such as bacteria, toxins, and antigens within the intestinal lumen.[133] Mechanisms act to control and maintain the epithelium as an impermeable barrier to the uptake of such antigens as β-lactoglobulin and α-lactalbumin found in cow's milk. Intolerance to lactose must not be confused with milk protein allergy. Lactose intolerance is not common in infancy and has an enzymatic etiology, whereas milk allergy is based on immunologic mechanisms. Gastrointestinal disturbance is common to both disorders. Diarrhea is frequently observed in both, but vomiting is exclusive to milk allergy. Milk allergies also can present with dermatologic, respiratory, and possibly systemic reactions, such as anaphylactic shock, although this is rare.[134]

Most infants appear to outgrow cow's milk protein allergy as they go through the toddler years. However, some reactions can be severe or even life threatening and never outgrown. The fear of potentially life-threatening allergic reactions may cause caregivers to be overly sensitive to their infant's reactions to formulas. It is not unusual to interview caregivers who have changed their infant's formula several times because of perceived intolerances. Formula changes should be done methodically in order to assess for a true allergy or intolerance. If an infant is being exclusively breastfed and presenting with symptoms suggestive of an allergy or intolerance, mothers can be advised to eliminate major allergens from their diet. Most commonly, eliminating all dairy is sufficient to alleviate the infant's symptoms. If supplementation is needed, consider hypoallergenic or less allergenic formulas, which have been discussed previously.[135,136] The presence of milk protein allergy may correlate with allergies to other foods. Other potential risk factors for food allergies include exposure to tobacco smoke, alcohol, and medications.

Over the past 10–15 years, incidence of allergy in infants and children appears to be rising in both developed and developing countries; the World Allergy Organization predicts that the incidence of food allergy in preschoolers may be as high as 7–10%.[137] In the US prevalence of reported childhood food allergy increased 18% from 1997–2007.[131] The common practice and medical advice for years was restriction of all major allergens in pregnancy, infancy, and early childhood in order to avoid food allergy development. The past decade has shown an upheaval in childhood allergy research, as early exposure rather than avoidance has been postulated to help prevent the development of food allergies. This hypothesis began with a 2008 study by Du Toit et al. observing that rates of peanut allergies were significantly lower among Israeli children than Jewish children living in the United Kingdom. There were no significant differences between the studied populations except that the Israeli children commonly consumed peanut protein in high quantities in the first year of life, while UK infants were typically provided a diet void of peanuts.[138] This led to the development of the **Learning Early About Peanut Study** (LEAP), where children labeled "high risk" for peanut protein allergy development were randomized into either peanut protein exposure or avoidance groups until 60 months of age. This study found that the early introduction of peanut protein significantly reduced the incidence of peanut allergy development among high risk infants.[139] Now, infants who are not at high risk for food allergy development should be exposed to common allergens at around 6 months of life.[140] For infants deemed high-risk for food allergies, a monitored plan for allergen exposure should be created by the medical team and family.

Constipation and Stool Characteristics

Constipation is defined by timing and consistency of the stool compared with the usual number of bowel movements. Constipation in infancy is defined as significant spacing between bowel movements and defecation that is extremely dry, hard, or painful.[141] Caregivers may fail to understand that different types of infant feedings are expected to produce variations in stool patterns. "Normal" stooling patterns vary from infant to infant and with differences in dietary intake.

After passing meconium, ideally within the first 24 hours of life, the number of stools gradually decreases from over four times a day to one to two a day by the end of the first year.[142] Infants being breastfed or receiving hydrolyzed protein formulas typically experience between 1 and 12 bowel movements a day.[142] This can be at least twice as many stools as infants consuming cow's-milk-based or soy-based formulas.[143] Infants fed soy-based formulas tend to have more stools, which are hard and firm.[143] Infants who consume formulas with added prebiotics tend to have softer stools and increased stool frequency.

Stool color also varies with protein source in milk or formula. Breast milk–fed infants typically have stools that look loose to pasty and are yellowish in color. Constipation is rare in breastfed infants; however, infants may have days when they do not have a bowel movement due to enhanced absorption of nutrients from breast milk. Formulas with soy, whey, or casein hydrolyzed protein sources may produce stools that range from yellow to green or brownish in color.[142] Behaviors characteristic during infant stooling that might alarm parents or caregivers include flushing, grunting, and change in stool color with a change in diet.[141] These behaviors are actually normal and should decrease over time.

Treating nonanatomic constipation requires dietary intervention. Five measures can be taken in the following sequence:

1. Verify constipation through a family interview
2. Ensure the proper diet, including free fluid intake versus fluid losses
3. Ensure accurate preparation of formula if infant is bottle-fed
4. Feed two additional ounces of water after each feeding
5. Provide a maximum of two ounces of pear or apple juice per day

If there is no relief from these recommendations and the infant appears to be in pain or cramping, a physician should be notified.

Acute Diarrhea

Acute infantile diarrhea is defined as the sudden onset of increased stool frequency, volume, and water content with greater than three stools in a 24-hour period.[144] There are many causes for acute diarrhea including: viral infection, excessive juice intake, and antibiotic-associated diarrhea. Globally, most cases occur in areas where there is poor sanitation and limited availability of clean water supplies. Persistent diarrhea is defined as lasting greater than 14 days. Infants with persistent diarrhea are usually malnourished and have repetitive cycles of infection and malabsorption.

Diarrhea lasting more than four days or resulting in greater than 10% dehydration may require intravenous fluid therapy. However, bottle-fed infants suffering from mild to moderate diarrhea can be rehydrated with an oral rehydration solution for 4–6 hours (refer to **TABLE 8.11**).

TABLE 8.11 Nutrient Comparisons of Clear Liquids and Rehydration Solutions						
Product	**Na (mEq/L)**	**K (mEq/L)**	**Cl (mEq/L)**	**Sugar (g/L)**	**Starch (g/L)**	**Osmolality (mOsm/L)**
Cola	1.7	0.1–0.6	—	53–58.5	—	750
Apple Juice	4.6	26	1.1	39.5	—	747
Gatorade	20–23	2.5–3	23	25–28	—	330–365
Chicken Broth	250	8	—	—	—	500
Enfalyte	50	25	45	25	—	167
Pedialyte	45	20	35	25	—	270

Data from Swedberg J, Steiner J. Oral rehydration therapy in diarrhea: not just for Third World children. *Postgrad Med*. 1983;74:335–341.[145]

Synder J. Oral rehydration therapy for acute diarrhea. *Semin Pediatr Gastroenterol Nutr*. 1990;1:8. Product information provided by Abbott Nutrition and Mead Johnson Nutritionals.[146]

After dehydration status is assessed and resolved, reintroducing age-appropriate foods and liquids should occur as soon as possible. Studies revealed that this approach did not worsen stool output and helped maintain nutritional status.[144] Beverages such as juice, broth, carbonated beverages, or sport drinks should not be provided because their high osmolality may induce osmotic diarrhea, exacerbating the initial problem.[142] Continued breastfeeding is beneficial, despite controversial concerns related to secondary lactose intolerance during acute diarrhea. Lactose-free formulas could be considered in infants who are malnourished or have severe dehydration with persistent diarrhea.[144]

Gastroesophageal Reflux

Gastroesophageal reflux (GER), or chalasia, affects many infants. GER is otherwise referred to as regurgitation or spitting up. A clinical definition is the presence of gastric contents in the esophagus. When complications arise from recurrent reflux, the condition is called GERD, or **gastroesophageal reflux disease**.[147] All infants experience some degree of GER. Most infants have no significant complications associated with it, whereas others may develop irritability, poor weight gain, failure to thrive, or pulmonary aspiration with pneumonia.[147] Mild GER may be treated by modifying feeding positions and dietary regimens. More severe GERD may require pharmaceutical or surgical interventions.

An upright position during feeding may prevent GER. In this position, gravity aids in gastric emptying. When an infant is placed in the semi-upright position of an infant seat, however, reduced truncal tone, common in early infancy, may result in slumping.[148] Slumping submerges the infant's posterior gastroesophageal junction into the stomach, increasing abdominal pressure and GER. A truly upright position is most reliable in preventing GER.[149] Regardless of the presence of GER, infants should sleep in supine position in order to reduce the risk of **sudden infant death syndrome** (SIDS).[147]

Thickening formula with cereal has been a routine practice in preventing GER. Thickening formula with infant cereals or providing a commercially prepared formula with added starch can reduce regurgitation and vomiting. However, it does not decrease the number of reflux episodes.[150] Clinicians should also be aware that cereal increases the caloric concentration of formula, alters the protein:carbohydrate:fat ratio, and can interfere with breastfeeding, and possibly delay gastric emptying.

Milk protein intolerance can be a cause of reflux or vomiting in infants. If the feeding regimens suggested above do not improve symptoms, mothers can be counseled to eliminate dairy from their diet if breastfeeding, or trialing a hydrolyzed protein or amino acid based formula. If GER continues to persist or interferes with appropriate growth, medical and pharmacological interventions may be necessary.

Food Refusal

Two important feeding milestones occur during infancy: self-feeding and developing a positive relationship with food and eating. If these do not occur, a spiral effect of food refusal and poor nutrient intake can ensue. Food refusal can occur in infancy because of physical or emotional stress. This is more typically classified as organic, indicating a medical or functional etiology, caused by environmental influences. Illness and an unfavorable atmosphere for feeding are typical contributors to food refusal. Prolonged food refusal with inadequate oral intake may result in a failure to thrive.

During illness infants may become irritable due to fever, congestion, or lack of sleep. At these times, food refusal is inevitable. The encouragement of oral fluid intake, and in severe cases administrating parenteral fluids, is necessary in order to prevent or treat dehydration. Although food refusal of this nature can still cause significant weight loss and deplete nutrient stores, if identified early, it is usually self-limited.

Food refusal originating from excessive or deficient stimulation is more difficult to discern. Commotion and overly aggressive or restrictive caregivers can cause development of negative associations with feeding. Routine negative interactions at mealtime can keep an infant from wanting to explore and advance with the normal self-feeding progression. As the stages of eating advance from liquid and dependence as a newborn to table foods as a toddler, parents need to be attuned to their child's developmental transition with eating.[151] The caregiver may restrict the infant's exploration of food and/or rush through a meal, disrupting the feeding pace. Under these circumstances, it is not uncommon for an infant to begin to refuse food entirely. Concerned that the infant is feeding poorly or losing weight, caregivers become tense. This tension only exacerbates the reluctance to feed.

The most effective means of treating feeding disorders after identification is increasing appropriate behavior and decreasing maladaptive behavior between the infant and caregiver and between the infant and the feeding experience.[152] As infants get closer to their first birthday, their interest in self-feeding and encouragement of self-regulation with food intake should be promoted. Most literature related to feeding disorders promotes a calm, interactive, and supportive environment, and encourages the most positive relationship with infant feeding.

Suggested Websites

http://www.mypyramid.gov
http://www.aap.org
http://www.eatright.org
http://www.babycenter.com
http://www.keepkidshealthy.com
http://www.healthychildren.org
http://www.gerber.com
http://www.heinzbaby.com

▶ Conclusion

Issues related to breastfeeding, bottle-feeding, vitamin and mineral supplementation, the introduction and progression of solids, and common feeding problems have all been discussed in this chapter. Translating this scientific information into practical suggestions for parents and caregivers is necessary. Infancy is a time for developing healthy eating habits and family relationships around mealtimes. As early as infancy, pediatric healthcare professions have a responsibility for identifying those at greatest risk for developing feeding and nutrition problems and providing appropriate education and intervention as soon as possible.

References

1. Formula feeding in the term infant. In: Kleinman RE and Greer FR, eds. *Pediatric Nutrition Handbook*, 7th ed. Elk Grove Village, IL: American Academy of Pediatrics; 2014. 61–82.
2. Therrell BL, Padilla CD, Loeber JG, Kneisser I, Saadallah A, Borrajo GJC, Adams J. Current status of newborn screening worldwide: 2015. *Semins Perinatol*. 2015;39:171–187.
3. Boyle CA, Bocchini JA, Kelly J. Reflections on 50 years of newborn screening. *Pediatrics*. 2014;133(6):961–963.
4. Institute of Medicine. *Dietary Reference Intakes for Energy, Carbohydrate, Fiber, Fat, Fatty Acids, Cholesterol, Protein, and Amino Acids (Macronutrients)*. Washington, DC: National Academies Press; 2005.
5. American Academy of Pediatrics. Breastfeeding and the use of human milk. *Pediatrics*. 2012;129(3):e827–e841.
6. Position of the Academy of Nutrition and Dietetics: Promoting and supporting breast-feeding. *J Acad Nutr Diet*. 2015;115:444–449.
7. Lawrence RA, Lawrence RM. *Breastfeeding: A Guide for the Medical Profession*, 8th ed. Philadelphia, PA: Elsevier; 2016.
8. U.S. Department of Health and Human Services. Maternal, Infant, and Child Health. Healthy People 2020. Available at: https://www.healthypeople.gov/2020/topics-objectives/topic/maternal-infant-and-child-health. Accessed January 8, 2018.
9. Jensen D, Wallace S, Kelsay P. LATCH: A breastfeeding charting system and documentation tool. *J Obstet Gynecol Neonatal Nurs*. 1994; 23(1):27–32.
10. Flaherman VJ, Schaefer EW, Kuzniewicz MW, et al. Early weight loss nomograms for exclusively breastfed newborns. *Pediatrics* 2015;135(1):e16–e23.
11. Flaherman VJ, Aby J, Burgos AE, et al. Effect of early limited formula on duration and exclusivity of breastfeeding in at-risk infants: An RCT. *Pediatrics*. 2013;131(6):1059–1065.
12. World Health Organization. *Evidence for the Ten Steps to Successful Breastfeeding*. Geneva, Switzerland: World Health Organization; 1998.
13. American Academy of Pediatrics, American College of Obstetricians and Gynecologists. *Breastfeeding Handbook for Physicians,* 2nd ed. Washington, DC: American Academy of Pediatrics Department of Marketing and Publications; 2014.
14. Li R, Fein SB, Grummer-Strawn LM. Do infants fed from bottles lack self-regulation of milk intake compared with directly breastfed infants? *Pediatrics*. 2010;125: e1386–e1393.
15. Li R, Magadia J, Fein SB. Grummer-Strawn LM. Risk of bottle-feeding for rapid weight gain during the first year of life. *Arch Pediatr Adolesc Med*. 2012;166(5):431–436.
16. Sriraman NK, Evans AE, Lawrence R, Noble L, and the Academy of Breast Feeding Medicine's Board of Directors. Academy of Breastfeeding Medicine's 2017 Position Statement on informal breast milk sharing for the term health infant. *Breastfeeding Med*. 2017;13(1):1–3.
17. AAP Committee on Nutrition, Section on Breastfeeding, Committee on Fetus and Newborn. Donor human milk for the high-risk infant: Preparation, safety, and usage options in the United States. *Pediatrics*. 2017;139(1): e20163440.
18. U.S. Food and Drug Administration. Use of Donor Human Milk - FDA warning. Available at: http://www.fda.gov/ScienceResearch/SpecialTopics/PediatricTherapeutics Research/ucm235203.htm. Accessed January 8, 2017.
19. Geraghty SR, McNamara KA, Dillon CE et al. Buying human milk via the internet: Just a click away. *Breastfeeding Med*. 2013;8(6):474–478.
20. Keim SA, Hogan JS, McNamara KA et al. Microbial contamination of human milk purchased via the internet. *Pediatrics*. 2013;132(5):e1227–e1235.
21. Keim SA, Kulkarni MM, McNamara KA et al. Cow's milk contamination of human milk purchased via the internet. *Pediatrics*. 2015;135(5):e1157–e1162.
22. Life Science Research Office. LSRO report: assessment of nutrient requirements for infant formulas. *J Nutr*. 1998;128:2059–2078.
23. Corkins KG and Shurley T. What's in the bottle? A review of infant formulas. *Nutr Clin Prac*. 2016;31(6):723–729.
24. Martin CR, Ling P-R, Blackburn GL. Review of infant feeding: Key features of breast milk and infant formula. *Nutrients*. 2016;8(5): doi:10.3390/nu8050279.
25. Martinez M. Tissue levels of polyunsaturated fatty acids during early human development. *J Pediatr*. 1992;120:s129–s138.

26. Simmer K, Patole SK, Rao SC. Longchain polyunsaturated fatty acid supplementation in infants born at term. *Cochrane Database Syst Rev.* 2008;(1):CD000376.

27. Koo W, Hammami M, Margeson D, et al. Reduced bone mineralization in infants fed palm olein-containing formula: a randomized, double-blinded, prospective trial. *Pediatrics.* 2003;111:1017–1023.

28. Greer FR, Kleinman RE. Editorial: an infant formula with decreased weight gain and higher IQ: are we there yet? *Am J Clin Nutr.* 2014;99:757–758.

29. Michaelsen KF, Greer FR. Protein needs early in life and long-term health. *Am J Clin Nutr.* 2014;99:718S–722S.

30. Vincini J, Etherton T, Kris-Etherton P et al. Survey of retail milk composition as affected by label claims regarding farm-management practices. *J Am Diet Assoc.* 2007;108:1198–1203.

31. Belamarich PF, Bochner RE, Racine AD. A critical review of the marketing claims of infant formula products in the United States. *Clin Pediatr.* 2016;55(5):437–442.

32. O'Connor NR. Infant formula. *Am Fam Physician.* 2009;79(7):565–570.

33. Joeckel RJ, Phillips SK. Overview of infant and pediatric formulas. *Nutr Clin Prac.* 2009;24(3):356–362.

34. Vanderhoof JA, Moran JR, Harris CL, Merkel KL, Orenstein SR. Efficacy of pre-thickened infant formula: a multicenter, double-blind, randomized, placebo-controlled parallel group trial in 104 infants with symptomatic gastroesophageal reflux. *Clin Pediatr.* 2003;42(6):483–495.

35. Craig WR, Hanlo-Dearman A, Sinclair C, et al. Metoclopramide, thickened feedings, and positioning for gastro-oesophageal reflux in children under two years. *Cochrane Database Syst Rev.* 2004;(4):CD003502.

36. Moukarzel AA, Abdelnour H, Akatcherian C. Effects of a prethickened formula on esophageal pH and gastric emptying of infants with GER. *J Clin Gastroenterol.* 2007;41(9):823–829.

37. Bhatia J, Greer F, Committee on Nutrition. Use of soy protein-based formulas in infant feeding. *Pediatrics.* 2008;121:1062–1068.

38. Zeiger RS, Sampson HA, Bock SA, et al. Soy allergy in infants and children with IgE-associated cow's milk allergy. *J Pediatr.* 1999;134:614–622.

39. Greer FR, Sicherer SH, Burks AW, Committee on Nutrition and Section on Allergy and Immunology. Effects of early nutritional interventions on the development of atopic disease in infants and children: the role of maternal dietary restriction, breastfeeding, timing of introduction of complementary foods, and hydrolyzed formulas. *Pediatrics.* 2008;121:183–191.

40. American Academy of Pediatrics, Committee on Nutrition. Iron fortification of infant formulas. *Pediatrics.* 1999;104:119–123.

41. Luyt D, Ball H, Makwana N, et al. Standard of Care Committee (SOCC) of the British Society for Allergy and Clinical Immunology (BSACI). BSACI guideline for the diagnosis and management of cow's milk allergy. *Clin Exp Allergy.* 2014;44:642–672.

42. Turck D. Cow's milk and goat's milk. *World Rev Nutr Diet.* 2013;108:56–62.

43. Vanderplas Y, Bhatia J, Shamir R, et al. Hydrolyzed formulas for allergy prevention. *J Pediatr Gastroenterol Nutr.* 2014;58:549–552.

44. Scalabrin DM, Johnston WH, Hoffman DR, et al. Growth and tolerance of healthy term infants receiving hydrolyzed infant formulas supplemented with *Lactobacillus rhamnosus* GG: randomized, double-blind, controlled trial. *Clin Pediatr.* 2009;48(7):734–744.

45. Hill DJ, Murch SH, Rafferty K, et al. The efficacy of amino acid-based formulas in relieving symptoms of cow's milk allergy: a systematic review. *Clin Exp Allergy.* 2007;37:808–822.

46. Burkhardt MC, Beck AF, Kahn RS, Klein MD. Are our babies hungry? Food insecurity among infants in urban clinics. *Clin Pediatr.* 2012;51(3):238–243.

47. Zhou SJ, Sullivan T, Gibson RA, et al. Nutritional adequacy of goat milk infant formulas for term infants: a double-blind randomized controlled trial. *Brit J Nutr.* 2014;111:1641–1651.

48. Grant C, Rotherham B, Sharpe S, et al. Randomized, double-blind comparision of growth in infants receiving goat milk formula versus cow milk infant formula. *J Paediatr Child Health.* 2005;41:564–568.

49. Singhal A, Kennedy K, Lanigan J, et al. Dietary nucleotides and early growth in formula fed infants: a randomized controlled trial. *Pediatrics.* 2010;126:e946–e953.

50. Holscher HD, Czekies LA, Cekola P, et al. *Bifidobacterium lactis Bb12* enhances intestinal antibody response in formula-fed infants: a randomized, double-blind, controlled trial. *J Parenter Enteral Nutr.* 2012;36:106S–117S.

51. Chassard C, de Wouters T, Lacroix C. Probiotics tailored to the infant: A window of opportunity. *Curr Opin Biotechnol.* 2014;26:141–147.

52. Sung V, Hiscock H, Tang ML et al. Treating infant colic with the probiotic Lactobacillus reuteri: Double blind, placebo controlled randomised trial. *BMJ.* 2014;348:g2107.

53. Thomas DR, Greer FR. Clinical report – probiotics and prebiotics in pediatrics. *Pediatrics.* 2010;126(6):1217–1231.

54. Boehm G, Stahl B. Oligosaccharides from milk. *J Nutr.* 2007;137:847S–849S.

55. Fanaro S, Marten B, Bagna R, et al. Galacto-oligosaccharides are bifidogenic and safe at weaning: a double-blind randomized multicenter study. *J Pediatr Gastroenterol Nutr.* 2008;48:82–88.

56. Ziegler E, Vanderhoof JA, Petschow B, et al. Term infants fed formula supplemented with selected blends of prebiotics grow normally and have soft stools similar to those reported for breast-fed infants. *J Pediatr Gastroenterol Nutr.* 2007;44:359–364.

57. Moro G, Minoli I, Mosca M, et al. Dosage-related bifidogenic effects of galacto- and fructooligosaccharides in formula-fed term infants. *J Pediatr Gastroenterol Nutr.* 2002;34:291–295.

58. Arslanoglu S, Moro GE, Schmitt J, et al. Early dietary intervention with a mixture of prebiotic oligosaccharides reduces the incidence of allergic manifestations and infections during the first two years of life. *J Nutr.* 2008;138:1091–1095.

59. Coulet M, Phothirath P, Allais L, Schilter B. Pre-clinical safety evaluation of the synthetic human milk, nature-identical, oligosaccharide 2'-O-Fucosyllactose (2'FL). *Regul Toxicol Pharmacol.* 2014;68:59–69.

60. Goehring KC, Marriage BJ, Oliver JS et al., Similar to those who were breastfed, infants fed a formula containing 2'-Fucosyllactose have lower inflammatory cytokines in a randomized, controlled trial. *J Nutr.* 2016;146:2559–2566.

61. U.S. Food and Drug Administration. FDA takes final step on infant formula protections. Available at: http://www.fda.gov/ForConsumers/ConsumerUpdates/ucm048694.htm. Accessed January 10, 2018.

62. Insel RA, Looney RJ. The B-lymphocyte system. In: Stiehm ER, ed. *Immunologic Disorders in Infants and Children*. Philadelphia, PA: WB Saunders; 1996.

63. Robbins S, Meyers R. Formula preparation and handling. In: Robbins ST, Meyers R, Pediatric Nutrition Practice Group, eds. *Infant Feedings: Guidelines for Preparation of Human Milk and Formula in Health Care Facilities*. 2nd ed. Chicago, IL: American Dietetic Association; 2011:71–94.

64. Redmond EC, Grifith CJ. The importance of hygiene in the domestic kitchen: implications for preparation and storage of food and infant formula. *Perspect Public Health*. 2009;129(2):69.

65. Kang J, Kondo F, Katayama Y. Human exposure to bisphenol A. *Toxicology*. 2006;226:79–89.

66. Gillman MW, Barker D, Bier D, et al. Meeting report on the 3rd International Congress on Developmental Origins of Health and Disease (DOHaD). *Pediatr Res*. 2007;61:625–629.

67. Centers for Disease Control and Prevention. *Enterobacter sakazakii* infections associated with the use of powdered infant formula. *MMWR*. 2002;51:297–300.

68. Hibbard RA, Blevins R. Palatal burn due to bottle warming in a microwave oven. *Pediatrics*. 1988;82:382–384.

69. Puczynski M, Rademaker D, Gatson RL. Burn injury related to the improper use of a microwave oven. *Pediatrics*. 1983;72:714–715.

70. Tully SB, Bar-Halm Y, Bradley RL. Abnormal tympanography after supine bottle-feeding. *J Pediatr*. 1995;126:S105–S111.

71. Fomon SJ. *Nutrition of Normal Infants*. St. Louis, MO: Mosby; 1993.

72. Butte N, Cobb K, Duyer J, Graney L, Heird W, Rickard K. The start healthy feeding guidelines for infants and toddlers. *J Amer Diet Assoc*. 2004;104:442–484.

73. Hinton S, Kerwin D. *Maternal and Child Nutrition*. Chapel Hill, NC: Health Sciences Consortium Corporation; 1981.

74. Misra M, Pacaud D, Petryk A, et al. Vitamin D deficiency in children and its management: review of current knowledge and recommendations. *Pediatrics*. 2008;122:398–417.

75. United States Department of Agriculture. WIC infant feeding guide. 2017. Available at: https://wicworks.fns.usda.gov/infants/infant-feeding-guide. Accessed January 14, 2018.

76. Mead Johnson. Table data retrieved from manufacturers' websites. Available at: http://www.meadjohnson.com. Accessed January 10, 2018.

77. Sankar MJ, Chandrasekaran A, Kumar P, et al. Vitamin K prophylaxis for prevention of vitamin K deficiency bleeding: a systematic review. *J Perinatol*. 2016;36:S29–S34.

78. Marcewicz LH, Clayton J, Maenner M, et al. Parental refusal of vitamin K and neonatal preventive services: A need for surveillance. *Matern Child Health J*. 2017;21:1079–1084.

79. Golding J, Paterson M, Kinlen LJ. Factors associated with childhood cancer in a national cohort study. *Br J Cancer*. 1990;62:304–308.

80. Golding J, Greenwood R, Birmingham K, et al. Childhood cancer, intramuscular vitamin K, and pethidine given during labour. *BMJ*. 1992;305:341–346.

81. Wagner CL, Greer FR, Section on Breastfeeding and Committee on Nutrition. Prevention of rickets and vitamin D deficiency in infants, children, and adolescents. *Pediatrics*. 2008;122:1142–1152.

82. Institute of Medicine, Food and Nutrition Board. *Dietary Reference Intakes for Calcium and Vitamin D*. Washington, DC: National Academies Press; 2011.

83. Holick MF. Vitamin D deficiency. *N Engl J Med*. 2007;357:266–281.

84. Institute of Medicine, Food and Nutrition Board. *Dietary Reference Intakes for Vitamin A, Vitamin K, Arsenic, Boron, Chromium, Copper, Iodine, Iron, Manganese, Molybdenum, Nickel, Silicon, Vanadium, and Zinc*. Washington, DC: National Academy Press; 2001.

85. Fomon S. Feeding normal infants: rationale for recommendations. *J Am Diet Assoc*. 2001;101:1002–1005.

86. Lipsitt L, Crook C, Booth C. The transitional infant: behavioral development and feeding. *Am J Clin Nutr*. 1985;41:485–496.

87. Cloud H, Feeding problems of the child with special health care needs. In: Ekvall SW, ed. *Pediatric Nutrition in Chronic Diseases and Developmental Disorders: Prevention, Assessment, and Treatment*. New York, New York: Oxford University Press; 1993:203–218.

88. Chatoor I, Hirsch R, Persinger M. Facilitating internal regulation of eating: a treatment model of infantile anorexia. *Infants Young Child*. 1997;9(4):12–22.

89. Underwood B. Weaning practices in deprived environments: the weaning dilemma. *Pediatrics*. 1985;75(suppl):194–198.

90. Barrera CM, Hamner HC, Perrine CG, et al. Timing of introduction of complementary food to U.S. infants, National Health and Nutrition Examination Survey 2009-2014. *J Acad Nutr Diet*. 2018;17:S2212–S2672.

91. Taylor RW, Williams SM, Fangupo LJ, et al. Effect of a baby-led approach to complementary feeding on infant growth and overweight: a randomized clinical trial. *JAMA Pediatr*. 2017;171(9):838–846.

92. Fangupo LJ, Heath ALM, Williams SM, et al. A baby-led approach to eating solids and risk of choking. *Pediatrics*. 2016;138(4):e20160772.

93. Fox MK, Reidy K, Novak T, Ziegler P. Sources of energy and nutrients in the diets of infants and toddlers. *J Am Diet Assoc*. 2006;106:S28–S42.

94. Karagas MR, Punshon T, Sayarath V, et al. Association of rice and rice-product consumption with arsenic exposure early in life. *JAMA Pediatr*. 2016;170(6):609–616.

95. Oskarsson A. Exposure of Infants and Children to Lead. Working Document for the 30th meeting of the Joint FAO/WHO Expert Committee on food additives held in Rome, 2-11 June 1986. FAO *Food Nutr Pap*. 1989;45:1–55.

96. Blumberg S. Infant feeding: can we spice it up a bit? *J Am Diet Assoc*. 2006;106:504–505.

97. Hinton S, Kerwin D. *Maternal and Child Nutrition*. Chapel Hill, NC: Health Sciences Consortium Corporation; 1981.

98. American Academy of Pediatrics, Committee on Nutrition. Infant methemoglobinemia: the role of dietary nitrate. *Pediatrics*. 1970;46:475–478.

99. Kerr C, Reisinger K, Plankey F. Sodium concentration of homemade baby foods. *Pediatrics*. 1978;62:331–335.

100. Fox MK, Pac S, Devaney B, Jankowski L. Feeding infants and toddlers study: what foods are infants and toddlers eating? *J Am Diet Assoc*. 2004;104(suppl 1):S22–S30.

101. The World Health Organization. Report of the Commission on Ending Childhood Obesity. Geneva: WHO Document Production Services; 2016:1-50. Available at: http://www.who.int/end-childhood-obesity/publications/echo-report/en/. Accessed January 14, 2018.

102. Ogden CL, Carrol MD, Fryar CD, et al. Prevalence of obesity among adults and youth: United States, 2011-2014. *NCHS Data Brief.* 2015;219:1–8.

103. Freedman DS, Sharma AJ, Hamner HC, et al. Trends in weight-for-length among infants in WIC from 2000 to 2014. *Pediatrics.* 2017;139(1):e20162034.

104. Owen, CG, Martin RM, Whincup PH, et al. Effect of infant feeding on risk of obesity across the life course: a quantitative review of published evidence. *Pediatrics.* 2005;115:1367–1377.

105. Worobey J, Lopez MI, Hoffman D. Maternal behavior and infant weight gain in first year. *J Nutr Educ Behav.* 2009;41:169–175.

106. Robinson SM, Marriott LD, Crozier SR, et al. Variations in infant feeding practice are associated with body composition in childhood: a prospective cohort study. *J Clin Endocrinol Metab.* 2009;94:2799–2805.

107. Morillo AFC, Duque MD, López ABH, et al. A comparison of factors associated with cessation of exclusive breastfeeding at 3 and 6 months. *Breastfeeding Medicine.* 2017;12(7):430–435.

108. Hilson JA, Rasmussen KM, Kjolhede CL. High prepregnant body mass index is associated with poor lactation outcomes among white, rural women independent of psychosocial and deographic correlates. *J Hum Lact.* 2004;20(1):18–29.

109. Turcksin R, Bel S, Galjaard S, et al. Maternal obesity and breastfeeding intention, initiation, intensity, and duration: a systematic review. *Matern Child Nutr.* 2014;10(2):166–183.

110. Whitaker KM, Marino RC, Haapala JL, et al. Associations of maternal weight status before, during and after pregnancy with inflammatory markers in breast milk. *Obesity.* 2017;25(12):2092–2099.

111. Cong S, Foskey RJ, Allen KJ, et al. Impact of timing of introduction of solids on infant body mass index. *J Pediatr.* 2016;179:104–10.

112. Papoutsou S, Savva SC, Hunsberger M, et al. Timing of solid food introduction and association with late childhood overweight and obesity: The IDEFICS study. *Matern Child Nutr.* 2018;14:e12471.

113. Smith HA, Becker GE. Early additional food and fluids for healthy breastfed full-term infants. *Cochrane Database Syst Rev.* 2016;8:CD006462.

114. Rose CM, Birch LL, Savage JS. Dietary patterns in infancy are associated with child diet and weight outcomes at 6 years. *Int J Obesity.* 2017;41:783–788.

115. Murray R, Battista M. Managing the risk of childhood overweight and obesity in primary care practice. *Curr Probl Pediatr Adolesc Health Care.* 2009;39:145–166.

116. Clark MB, Slayton RL. Fluoride use in caries prevention in the primary care setting. *Pediatrics.* 2014;134(3):626–633.

117. National Institute of Dental and Craniofacial Research. Dental caries (tooth decay) in children (age 2 to 11). Available at: https://www.nidcr.nih.gov/DataStatistics/FindDataByTopic/DentalCaries/DentalCariesChildren2to11.htm. Accessed January 13, 2018.

118. Katz Y, Rajuan N, Goldberg MR, et al. Early exposure to cow's milk protein is protective against IgE-mediated cow's milk protein allergy. *J Allergy Clin Immunol.* 2010;126:77–82.

119. Snijders BEP, Thijs C, van Ree R, et al. Age at first introduction of cow milk products and other food products in relation to infant atopic manifestations in the first 2 years of life: the KOALA Birth Cohort Study. *Pediatrics.* 2008;122(1):e115–e122.

120. Walter T, DeAndraca I, Chadud P, et al. Iron deficiency anemia: adverse effects on infant psychomotor development. *Pediatrics.* 1989;84:7–17.

121. Basnet S, Schneider M, Gazit A, et al. Fresh goat's milk for infants: myths and realities: a review. *Pediatrics.* 2010;125(4):e973–e977.

122. United States Department of Agriculture- USDA food composition databases. Available at: https://ndb.nal.usda.gov/ndb/search/list. Accessed January 15, 2018.

123. American Academy of Pediatrics, Committee on Nutrition. The use and misuse of fruit juice in pediatrics. *Pediatrics.* 2001;107:1210–1213.

124. Hoekstra JH, van Kempen AA, Kneepkens CM. Apple juice malabsorption: fructose or sorbitol? *J Pediatr Gastroenterol Nutr.* 1993;16:39–42.

125. Smith MM, Davis M, Chasalow FI, et al. Carbohydrate absorption from fruit juice in young children. *Pediatrics.* 1995;95:340–344.

126. Lifschitz CH. Fruit juice [Letter to the editor]. *Pediatrics.* 1995;96:376.

127. Hyams JS, Etienne NL, Leichtner AM, et al. Carbohydrate malabsorption following fruit juice ingestion in young children. *Pediatrics.* 1988;82:64–68.

128. Levine AA. Excessive fruit juice consumption: how can something that causes failure to thrive be associated with obesity? [Selected summary]. *J Pediatr Gastroenterol Nutr.* 1997;25:554–555.

129. Auerbach B, Wolf F, Hikida A, et al. Fruit juice and change in body mass index: a meta-analysis. *Pediatrics.* 2017;139(4):e20162454.

130. Skinner JD, Ziegler P, Ponza M. Transitions in infants' and toddlers' beverage patterns. *J Am Diet Assoc.* 2004;104:S45–S50.

131. Branum AM, Lukacs SL. Food allergy among U.S. children: trends in prevalence and hospitalizations. *NCHS Data Brief.* 2008;10(10):1–8.

132. Høst A. Frequency of cow's milk allergy in childhood. *Ann Allergy Asthma Immunol.* 2002;89(6):33–37.

133. Walker A. Absorption of protein and protein fragments in the developing intestine: role in immunologic/allergic reactions. *Pediatrics.* 1985;75(suppl):167.

134. Wyllie R, Hyams JS. *Pediatric Gastrointestinal Diseases.* Philadelphia, PA: WB Saunders; 1993.

135. Pali-Scholl I, Renz H, Jensen-Jarolim E. Update on allergies in pregnancy, lactation, and early childhood. *J Allergy Clin Immunol.* 2009;123:1012–1021.

136. Sicherer SH, Burks AW. Maternal and infant diets for prevention of allergic diseases: understanding menu changes in 2008. *J Allergy Clin Immunol* 2008;122(1):29–33.

137. Prescott SL, Pawankar R, Allen KJ, et al. A global survey of changing patterns of food allergy burden in children. *World Allergy Organ J.* 2013;6:1–12.

138. Du Toit G, Katz Y, Sasieni P, et al. Early consumption of peanuts in infancy is associated with a low prevalence of peanut allergy. *J Allergy Clin Immunol.* 2008;122(5):984–991.

139. Du Toit G, Roberts G, Sayre PH, et al. Randomized trial of peanut consumption in infants at risk for peanut allergy. *N Engl J Med.* 2015;372:803–813.

140. Abrams EM, Greenhawt M, Fleischer DM, et al. Early solid food introduction: role in food allergy prevention and implications for breastfeeding. *J Pediatr.* 2017;184:13–18.

141. Montgomery DF, Navarro F. Management of constipation and encopresis in children. *J Pediatr Health Care.* 2008;22:199–204.

142. Hyams J, Treem WR, Etienne NL, et al. Effects of infant formula on stool characteristics of young infants. *Pediatrics.* 1995;95:50–54.

143. Hillemier C. Gastroesophageal reflux. *Pediatr Clin North Am.* 1996;43(1):197–212.

144. Grimwood K, Forbes D. Acute and persistent diarrhea. *Pediatr Clin N Am.* 2009;56:1343–1361.

145. Swedberg J, Steiner J. Oral rehydration therapy in diarrhea: not just for Third World children. *Postgrad Med.* 1983;74:335–341.

146. Synder J. Oral rehydration therapy for acute diarrhea. *Semin Pediatr Gastroenterol Nutr.* 1990;1:8.Product information provided by Abbott Nutrition and Mead Johnson Nutritionals.

147. Vandenplas Y, Rudolph C, Lorenzo CD, et al. Pediatric gastroesophageal reflux clinical practice guidelines: joint recommendations of the North American Society of Pediatric Gastroenterology, Hepatology, and Nutrition and the European Society of Pediatric Gastroenterology, Hepatology, and Nutrition. *J Pediatr Gastroenterol Nutr.* 2009;49:498–547.

148. Herbst J. Gastroesophageal reflux. *J Pediatr.* 1981;98:859–870.

149. Orenstein S, Whitington P. Positioning for prevention of infant gastroesophageal reflux. *J Pediatr.* 1983;103:534–537.

150. Horvath A, Dziechciarz P, Szajewska H. The effect of thickened-feed interventions on gastroesophageal reflux in infants: systematic review and meta-analysis of randomized, controlled trials. *Pediatrics.* 2008;122(6):e1268–e1277.

151. Couch SC, Falciglia GA. Improving the diets of the young: considerations for intervention design. *J Am Diet Assoc.* 2006;106:S10–S11.

152. Rudolph C, Link D. Feeding disorders in infants and children. *Pediatr Clin N Am.* 2002;49:97–112.

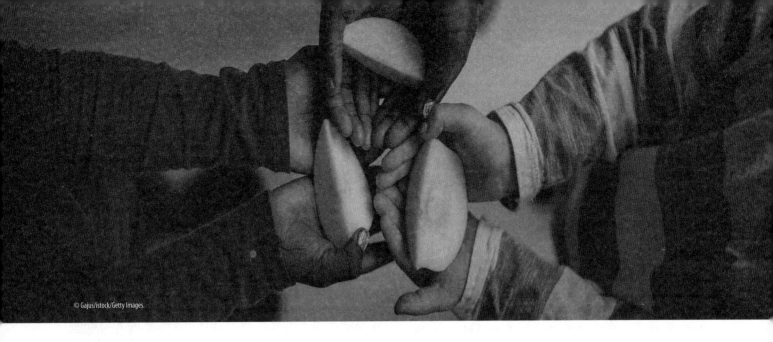

© Gajus/istock/Getty Images.

CHAPTER 9

Normal Nutrition through Childhood and Adolescence

Beth Ogata and Sharon Feucht

LEARNING OBJECTIVES

- Describe the influence of growth and development on nutrient needs and nutrition-related patterns of children and adolescents
- Identify nutrition-related issues and risk factors that are commonly screened for during childhood
- List factors that influence food patterns throughout childhood and adolescence
- Describe recommendations for nutrition (intake, patterns, habits) for healthy children and adolescents

▶ Introduction

From 1 year of age through adolescence, children experience enormous changes in physical, cognitive, and social-emotional growth. The 1-year-old toddler is taking his or her first steps into the bigger world, becoming more independent in self-help skills, and rapidly learning to communicate. At the other end of the spectrum, the 18-year-old is taking different steps into the world, becoming more independent and self-sufficient, and planning for their future. This chapter focuses on the nutritional needs and issues of normal, healthy children during these growing years.

▶ Anatomy, Physiology, Pathology of Condition

Progress in Growth and Development

After the rapid growth of infancy, there is a considerable slowing in physical growth during the preschool and school years. The elementary school years are often referred to as the *latent period* before the pubertal growth spurt of adolescence. Children have individual growth patterns, which may be erratic at times with spurts in height and weight followed by periods of little or no growth. These patterns usually correspond to similar changes in appetite and food intake in healthy children and teenagers. Parents and other caregivers need to realize that these changes are normal so they can avoid struggles over food and eating.

Developmental progress during the growing years influences many aspects of food and eating. The very young child prefers food that can be picked up or doesn't have to be chased across the plate. Food jags (periods of time when a child will eat only one food, or a small group of foods) may be more an expression of independence than of actual likes and dislikes. For older children, the influence of peers and of the media will affect snack choices. Teenagers want foods that fit into their lifestyles, are quick and easy to fix, and are inexpensive. Understanding the developmental characteristics and milestones at each age will help parents and professionals to set realistic expectations, support eating behavior and food decisions that are developmentally appropriate, and avoid unnecessary conflicts. Satter has described a "division of responsibility" in feeding that encourages parents to take the leadership role with the what, when, and where of feeding, with children of all ages having the responsibility of determining whether to eat and how much to eat of what is served. This feeding relationship between parents and children of all ages, incorporates developmental aspects.[1]

Note: Throughout the chapter, references to "family" and "parent" are made. The authors recognize that children and youth live and thrive in a variety of household settings, and in many instances, the primary food shopper, preparer, or influencer is not a biologic parent. For brevity, the terms "family" and "parent" are used.

▶ Condition Specific Nutrition Screening

Screening for nutrition-related conditions may be indicated when specific risk factors are identified. *Bright Futures in Practice: Nutrition* identifies nutrition-related issues and risk factors to address and/or screen for based on age and developmental stage.[2] Nutrition Questionnaires are available for children ages 1–10 years and adolescents ages 11–21. Questions focus on eating behaviors, food choices, food resources, weight and body image, physical activity, and lifestyle.

Obesity

The **United States Preventive Services Task Force** (USPSTF) suggests using **body mass index** (BMI) to screen for obesity among children age 6 years and older.[3] A clinical report from the **American Academy of Pediatrics** (AAP) provides recommendations and tools for health care professionals to use when addressing

obesity.[4] See chapter 21 "Obesity and Weight Management" for more information.

Iron Deficiency Anemia

The AAP recommends universal screening for iron deficiency for children ~1 year of age. Selective screening is recommended at any age, based on risk (including inadequate intake, feeding problems, and poor growth).[5] Guidelines for treatment and follow-up of iron deficiency anemia have been developed.[5,6] More information about iron deficiency anemia is included later in this chapter.

A heme profile (hemoglobin or hematocrit) is usually used to screen for anemia; however, other tests are more sensitive and can provide more information about an individual's iron status. The AAP suggests using hemoglobin along with serum ferritin and C-reactive protein or reticulocyte hemoglobin in order to identify iron deficiency. The combination of hemoglobin and serum transferrin receptor tests is also suggested, once standards for the latter are developed.[7]

Lipid and Cardiovascular Health

The AAP, **National Cholesterol Education Program** (NCEP), **National Heart, Lung, and Blood Institute** (NHLBI), and the American Heart Association have published recommendations for lipid screening and cardiovascular health in children.[8-11] Universal lipid screening (non-fasting total cholesterol, HDL cholesterol, and calculated non HDL cholesterol) is recommended for all children ages 9–11 years and 17–21 years. Screening is also recommended for children ages 9 years and older who have high risk medical conditions such as obesity, hypertension, diabetes, or concerning family histories such as premature cardiovascular disease.[11]

Recommendations for universal screening are somewhat controversial. The **US Preventive Services Task Force** (USPSTF) cites a lack of long-term randomized controlled trials that demonstrate effectiveness and identify risks associated with screening that includes over diagnosis and anxiety to the family as well as increased costs from follow-up testing and treatment in its recommendation.[12,13] Proponents for screening argue that there is evidence that modifying risk factors in children can decrease the risk of cardiovascular disease and note that the USPTSF's recommendation is a statement about the lack of evidence, not a recommendation against screening.[14,15]

In addition to dietary recommendations outlined later in this chapter, the groups suggest dietary intervention such as the use of low fat milk, based on risk factors (obesity and family history of obesity, dyslipidemia, and cardiovascular disease) as well as additional screening and intervention based on low-density lipoprotein (LDL) cholesterol categories.[8,10,11]

▶ Nutrition Assessment

A nutrition assessment is indicated when a nutrition risk is identified. Components of a complete nutrition assessment are described in chapter 1 and in the assessment sections of the condition-specific chapters. These components often include a comprehensive look at growth, intake, and other factors. A number of these factors are discussed below, based on general expectations for healthy children.

▶ Nutrient Needs

The primary factor in determining nutrient needs is usually a child's rate and stage of growth. Other factors include physical activity, body size, basal energy expenditure, and state of health. There is a wide range of actual needs based on individual characteristics. The **Dietary Reference Intakes** (DRIs), which include the **recommended dietary allowances** (RDAs) and **adequate intake** (AI), serve as a guide in order to prevent deficiency and/or to provide positive health benefits.[16] Many of the recommendations for children and adolescents, however, are extrapolated values. Because these guidelines provide a margin of safety greater than the physiologic requirements for most children in the United States, they are not meant to be marker goals for individual children. Intakes less than these guidelines do not presume inadequacies or adverse effects.

Energy

Energy needs are the most variable, due to individual differences in basal metabolism, growth, physical activity, onset of puberty, and body size. The DRIs include equations for **estimated energy requirements** (EERs) for children who are not overweight and weight maintenance **total energy expenditure** (TEE) for children who are overweight. Unlike previous guidelines for energy intake, the DRIs incorporate direct measures of energy expenditure using doubly labeled water studies. EER equations through age 2 years include allowing for age and weight. EER and TEE equations for children 3 years and older include allowing for age, sex, weight, height, and level of physical activity.[17] These references for energy intake in children and adolescents provide tools to both assess energy intake and develop nutrition care plans that incorporate the individual child's size, activity, and state of health.

Protein

Adequate protein intake is needed in order to provide for optimal growth in children and adolescents. National surveys have reported actual protein intakes to be in the range of 10–15% of energy for these ages.[18,19] This level assumes that enough energy is provided so that protein is spared for growth. Protein needs decrease as the growth rate slows after infancy, then increases again at puberty. Total protein intake increases steadily until about 12 years of age in girls and 16 years of age in boys.

In the United States, protein intakes usually exceed recommended allowances. Some children and adolescents, however, may be at risk for protein malnutrition if energy is inadequate so that protein is used for energy. Examples include those with inadequate energy intakes (extreme use of low-fat diets, limited access to food, dieting to lose weight, and athletes in training who limit food), those who are strict vegetarians, and some individuals with food allergies. Dietary evaluation of protein intake should include the growth rate, energy intake, and quality of the protein sources.

Minerals and Vitamins

Although clinical signs of vitamin or mineral deficiency are rare in the United States, dietary intake studies have reported that the nutrients most likely to be low or deficient in the diets of children and adolescents are calcium, vitamin D, magnesium, vitamin A, and vitamin E.[20-22] Certain populations of children, such as low-income, Native American, and other groups with limited food and health resources (e.g., the homeless) are more at risk for poor diet and nutrient deficiencies. Most of the recommended allowances for children and adolescents have been extrapolated from studies on infants and adults.

Calcium

Primarily needed for bone mineralization, calcium needs are determined by growth velocity, rates of absorption, and other nutrients, such as phosphorus, vitamin D, and protein. Because of individual variability, a child receiving less than the recommended allowance of calcium is not necessarily at risk. Approximately 100 mg of calcium per day is retained as bone in the preschool years. This doubles or triples for adolescents during peak growth periods.[23] Adolescence is a critical period for optimal calcium retention in order to achieve peak bone mass, especially for females who are at risk for osteoporosis in later years. Calcium intake, however, often decreases during the teen years. Balance studies indicate that young adolescent girls (younger than 16 years of age) may need to consume as much as 1600 mg per day to achieve maximum calcium intake and calcium balance.[23] The Food and Nutrition Board recommends an AI of 1300 mg of calcium per day for ages 9–18 years to support optimal bone mineralization.[24]

Those who consume none or only limited amounts of dairy products—the major source of calcium—are at risk for calcium deficiency. Some adolescents may also receive less calcium than needed because of rapid growth, dieting practices, and substituting carbonated beverages for milk. In assessing calcium status, vitamin D intake should be considered because of its major role in calcium metabolism. For children with limited sunshine exposure, dietary intake is critical. Vitamin D-fortified milk is the primary food source of this nutrient; other dairy products are not usually made with fortified milk. A child may be receiving adequate calcium from cheese and yogurt but taking very little fluid milk and, thus, receiving minimal dietary vitamin D. Younger children, especially, may be meeting calcium needs but not meeting vitamin D recommendations. **TABLE 9.1** contains a list of calcium food sources. Levels of physical activity also affect an individual's calcium needs for optimal bone development.

TABLE 9.1 Calcium Equivalents

1 cup milk* = approx. 300 mg calcium	1 cup (8 oz) yogurt[†]
	1 cup calcium-fortified orange juice
	1 cup calcium-fortified soy milk[‡]
	1 cup calcium-fortified rice milk or almond milk[‡,§]
²/₃ cup milk =	1 oz cheddar, jack, or Swiss cheese
	1 oz mozzarella or American cheese
½ cup milk =	2 oz canned sardines (with bones)
	2 oz canned salmon (with bones)
	½ cup cooked greens (mustard, collards, kale)
¼ cup milk =	½ cup custard or milk pudding
	½ cup cottage cheese
	½ cup ice cream
	¾ cup dried beans, cooked or canned

*Some low-fat or skim milks and some low-fat yogurts have additional nonfat dry milk (NFDM) solids added. Some labels will read "fortified." Such products will contain more calcium than indicated here.

[†]Most commercially prepared yogurt does not contain vitamin D.

[‡]The amount of calcium varies; not all milks are fortified with calcium and/or vitamin D.

[§]Rice and almond milks (and other nut milks) have significantly less protein than cow's milk and soy milk.

Data from US Department of Agriculture (USDA), Agricultural Research Service, Nutrient Data Laboratory. USDA National Nutrient Database for standard reference, legacy. Available at: http://www.ars.usda.gov/nutrientdata. Accessed May 1, 2018.[25]

Vitamin D

Vitamin D is increasingly recognized as an important nutrient for its role in bone health and for other potential roles, including preventing cancer, autoimmune disorders, cardiovascular disease, and infectious diseases. Serum 25-hydroxyvitamin D (25[OH]D) levels are used to measure deficiency and insufficiency; however, there is some controversy about the cut-off levels to indicate insufficiency; many experts feel the levels have been too low in the past. An analysis of **National Health and Nutrition Examination Survey** (NHANES) data indicated vitamin D deficiency in about 9% of children, and insufficiency in 61%.[26]

Iron

Requirements for iron are determined by the rate of growth, iron stores, increasing blood volumes, and the rate of absorption from food sources. Menstrual losses, as well as rapid growth, increase the need in adolescent females. To reach adulthood with an adequate storage of iron, recommended daily intakes are 7 mg for children ages 1–3 years, 10 mg for 4- to 8-year-olds, 11 mg for pubertal males, and 15 mg for pubertal females.[27] (See the iron deficiency anemia discussion later in this chapter.)

Vitamin–Mineral Supplements

Using supplements is a common practice in the United States. Almost 40% of preschool children take supplements, typically a multivitamin–mineral preparation. Supplement use declines among older children—29% for children ages 9–13 years and 26% among 14- to 18-year-olds.[28] Children taking supplements do not necessarily represent those who need them. Higher rates of use are found in families with higher incomes. However, the supplements may not be providing the marginal or deficient nutrients either; for example, a child may be taking a children's vitamin but may actually need extra calcium, not always provided in a supplement.

Except for fluoride supplementation in nonfluoridated areas, and vitamin D when intake is less than 600 IU per day, the AAP does not support routine supplementation for normal, healthy children.[7] It does, however, identify six groups at nutritional risk who might benefit from supplementation. These include children and adolescents:

1. With anorexia, inadequate appetite, or who consume fad diets
2. With chronic disease (e.g., cystic fibrosis, inflammatory bowel disease, hepatic disease)
3. From deprived families or those who are abused or neglected
4. Using a dietary program to manage obesity
5. Who do not consume adequate amounts of dairy products
6. With failure to thrive

Children with food allergies, those who omit entire food groups, and those with limited food acceptances will be likely candidates for supplementation. No risk is involved if parents wish to give their children a standard pediatric multivitamin. Megadose levels of nutrients should be discouraged and parents counseled regarding the dangers of toxicity, especially of fat-soluble vitamins. The DRIs include tolerable **upper intake levels** (UL), which can be used to determine excessive levels of vitamins and minerals from supplemental sources. Because many children's vitamins look and taste like candy, parents should be educated about keeping them out of the reach of children.

Use of other dietary supplements, including herbal preparations, is becoming more widespread. Although many supplements are harmless and may be beneficial, others may be dangerous and/or affect nutritional status by interacting with specific nutrients and/or medications. Evaluating dietary intake should include questions about the use of supplements.

Food Intake Patterns and Guidelines

Because appetite usually follows the rate of growth, food intake is not always smooth and consistent. After observing a good appetite in infancy, parents frequently describe their preschool children as having fair to poor appetites, a response to a slower growth rate. There is a wide variability in nutrient intake in healthy children. Daily energy intake of preschool children is surprisingly constant, despite a high variability from meal to meal. One classic longitudinal study found that the maximum intake of energy, carbohydrate, fat, and protein was two to three times the minimum intake, with bigger discrepancies for ascorbic acid and carotene.[29] With such variability being the norm for children, nutrition professionals need to use dietary assessment tools that include intake over time and not just a single day.

Just as there are changing trends of dietary patterns in the general public, similar patterns are seen in children. National dietary studies have shown decreased intakes of sugars and fats among children 2–19 years of age, although amounts consumed are still above recommendations. Whole grain consumption has increased slightly. For those 2–5 years of age, intake of oils increased. No changes were noted in fruit, vegetables, dairy and total meat, poultry, and seafood consumption.[30] When compared with national recommendations such as the US Dietary Guidelines, only the youngest children (ages 2–5 years) consume adequate fruit, whole grains, and dairy; all children's intake of vegetables is low.[31,32]

Children of all ages consume snacks and have increased the number of meals eaten away from home. Eighty-three percent of adolescents, 12–19 years of age, consume at least one snack per day, while almost one-quarter eat three or more snacks per day.[33] Foods, including sugar sweetened beverages, consumed away from home are associated with increased energy intake and lower diet quality, especially in teenagers. For teens, this association includes foods purchased at school. For younger children, ages 6–12 years, foods consumed at school do not differ in energy and nutrient intake from those consumed at home.[33]

Factors Influencing Food Intake

Food intake and habits are determined by numerous factors. For the child and/or adolescent, the additional influences from family, peers, and media and the concept of body image should be explored during the nutrition assessment.

Family

Family food choices and eating-related behaviors influence the types of foods children will accept.[34] Eating habits and food likes and dislikes are formed in the early years and often continue into adulthood. Parents and siblings are primary models for young children to imitate behavior. Mealtime atmosphere, both positive and negative, can influence how a child approaches and handles family meals. The positive effects of regular family meals can last into adulthood.[35]

The quality of dietary intake has been linked to family meals. School-aged children and adolescents who ate dinner with their families most often had higher consumptions of fruits and vegetables and nutrients including fiber, folate, calcium, iron, and vitamins B_6, B_{12}, C, and E. Intakes of saturated fat, soda, and fried foods were lower among individuals who ate with their families more often than among children with less frequent family meals.[35,36]

Children and adolescents who share family meals three or more times each week are more likely to be in a normal weight range and have healthier dietary and eating patterns, although this may vary by race, sex, and family education.[37,38] For teens and their parents, family meals can be a positive experience and benefit the adolescent's dietary intake and psychosocial health and decrease disordered eating behaviors and substance abuse.[39,40] The website, familydinnerproject.org, summarizes other benefits of family meals and offers guidance to families about successful family meals.

Media

Children of all ages are surrounded by media, both traditional (e.g., television, radio, and print) and new digital technologies. Newer technologies offer interactive and social options and children have immediate access to entertainment, information, and also the marketing of food.

Decreases in television viewing have been reported in children ages 2–11 years, but parents still reported two or more hours per day.[41] With consideration of all media, parents report that their children younger than 8 years of age spend an average of 2 hours, 19 minutes on screen media daily. Television averages 58 minutes per day, while mobile devices, DVDs, video games, and computers share the remaining time.[42] Tweens (8–12 years of age) and teenagers (13–18 years) report an average of six and nine hours, respectively, of media use daily, including television, online videos, games on video, computers or mobile devices, Internet access, social media contacts, reading, and listening to music.[42]

All media are a source of food marketing to this population. Television food advertising ranges from 11–29% of all ads on stations watched by children younger than 13 years. A child who watches only 2 hours of television per day will view 56–126 food advertisements weekly. In this global study, the US reported 5 advertisements per hour on children's' television, with 4 of the 5 ads for what is described as "noncore foods" (foods high in energy or undesirable nutrients as described by dietary standards). Thirty-two percent of US ads were for fast food products, the most frequently advertised items.[43] While advertisements for snack foods (sweet and savory foods) make up more than 40% of all food and beverage ads on television seen by children and teens ages 2–17 years, ads for cereals and sugary foods continue. In 2014, energy drinks and regular soda brands represent more than three-quarters of brands seen on various social media sites.[44]

Additionally, food products are marketed through cross-promotions with programs and characters and through fast-food restaurant promotions.[45]

The commercial messages are not based on nutrition but on an emotional/psychological appeal—fun, gives you energy, yummy taste. Younger children generally cannot discriminate between the regular program and commercial messages, frequently giving more attention to the latter because of their fast, attention-getting pace. The length of time watching television is associated with children gaining excess weight.[46] Other types of screen time may be associated with excess weight gain, but more research is needed. Screen time and low physical activity levels are related to overweight and obesity,[47] and television viewing has been inversely associated with fruit and vegetable intake.[47–50] In addition to encouraging inactivity, there is the steady presentation of food and eating cues.

Guidelines are available to health care professionals and families regarding media use and children. The AAP has updated policy statements with information for families.[51,52] For children younger than 18 months of age, media use (except for video chatting) is discouraged. If video media is introduced to children 18–24 months of age, programming should be high-quality and parents and children should watch together. For children 2–5 years, media use should be limited to one hour per day. For children 6 years and older, a family media use plan should be established, and media-free times should be designated.

Peers

As children move into the world, others influence their food choices. In preschool, the group snack time may encourage a child to try a new food. During school years, friends, rather than the menu, may decide participation in the school lunch program. Peer influence is particularly strong in adolescence since teenagers strive for more independence and eating becomes a more social activity outside the home. A chronic illness or disorder that requires diet modification, such as diabetes, phenylketonuria, or food allergies, can be a problem for children and teenagers when they want to be part of the group. These individuals need education regarding diet rationale appropriate to their developmental level, as well as problem-solving methods to explain it to their peers.

Body Image

Puberty is the period of greatest awareness of body image. It is normal for teens to be uncomfortable and dissatisfied with their changing bodies. The media and popular idols offer a standard that adolescents compare themselves with, no matter how unrealistic it may be. The average female store mannequin is representative of an underweight body size. Even pre-pubertal school-age girls have been increasingly preoccupied with body image and "dieting." To change their body image, they may try restrictive diets, purchase weight loss products, or in the case of males, try supplements or diets in the hope of increasing their muscles. Some of these dietary measures may put them at risk for poor nutritional status. The increasing prevalence of childhood overweight has also impacted the positive body image of growing children and adolescents.

▶ Nutrition Diagnosis

As children grow and develop, various nutrition-related issues or problems arise. These are not uncommon in otherwise healthy children, and they can be prevented or managed with minimal intervention. Other specific problems—obesity, allergies, and chronic diseases—are discussed in other chapters.

Problem, Etiology, Sign/Symptom statements used in the nutrition care process that are specific to children and appropriate for the nutrition diagnosis of children and adolescents include:

- NC 1.3   Breast feeding difficulty
- NC 3.3.1   Overweight pediatric
- NC 3.3.2   Obese pediatric
- NC 3.5   Growth rate below expected
- NC 3.3.2   Excessive growth rate
- NC 4.1.4   Non-illness related pediatric malnutrition
- NC 4.1.5   Illness related pediatric malnutrition

▶ Diet and Oral Health

Despite successful efforts in the past few decades, dental caries remain a common oral health disease in the pediatric population. In 2011–2012, approximately 23% of children aged 2–5 years and 56% of 6–8-year olds had caries in their primary teeth; 14% of 2–8-year-olds had untreated caries. About 21% of children aged 6–11 had caries in their permanent teeth, with about 6% having untreated caries. Among adolescents, 58% had caries, with the highest rates among 16–19-year-olds (67%).[53] Increased use of dental sealants have led to improved caries rates; however, oral health remains a significant problem in the United States.[53]

Nutrition and oral health are closely related. Inadequate intake of energy and protein can delay tooth eruption, affect tooth size, and cause salivary gland dysfunction. Micronutrients, calcium and vitamin D for mineralization, fluoride for enamel formation are also critical to the development and maintenance of oral structures.[54,55] A comparison of dietary quality and caries found lower rates of caries among young children who scored highest on the Healthy Eating Index, which is a measure of diet quality compared with federal dietary guidance.[56]

Poor oral health can negatively affect a child's nutritional status and has implications for overall health as well. Missing or decayed teeth may increase the risk of nutrient deficiency by preventing a child from eating certain foods. Pain or malformed teeth can contribute to problems with speech and communication, interfere with sleep, and negatively affect an individual's self-image, psychological status, and overall social function.

Dental caries develop in the presence of carbohydrate, bacteria, and a susceptible tooth. The process of decay begins with the interaction of the bacteria *Streptococcus mutans* and fermentable carbohydrate on the tooth surface. When the bacteria within the dental plaque (the gelatinous substance on the tooth surface) metabolize the carbohydrate, organic acids are produced. When the acid reduces the pH to 5.5 or less, demineralization of the tooth enamel occurs.[57] Some individuals seem to be more susceptible to caries than others, suggesting a hereditary influence.

Sucrose is the most common carbohydrate recognized in the caries process. Although starch is considered less cariogenic than sucrose, it can easily be broken down into fermentable carbohydrate by salivary amylase. Also, many foods high in starch often contain sucrose or other sugars, which may make the food more cariogenic than sugar alone because starch is retained longer in the mouth. Honey is just as cariogenic as sucrose.

The cariogenicity of specific foods depends not only on the type and amount of fermentable carbohydrate, but also on the retentiveness of foods to the tooth surface and the frequency of eating. Dental researchers believe that all of these factors influence the length of time the teeth are exposed to an acidic environment that leads to tooth decay.[57]

Some protein foods such as nuts, hard cheeses, eggs, and meats do not decrease plaque pH and are thought to have a protective effect against caries.[58] Eating these foods at the same time as high-sugar foods prevents a reduction in plaque pH. Why these foods are protective is not known, but theories include the presence of protein and lipids in these foods, the presence of calcium and phosphorus, and the stimulation of alkaline saliva.

Prevention of Caries

Because children of all ages eat frequently, snacks should emphasize foods that are low in sucrose, are not sticky, and stimulate saliva flow, thereby limiting acid production in the mouth (**TABLE 9.2**. Including protein foods such as cheese and nuts may provide nutritional as well as dental benefits. Desserts, when consumed, should be eaten with meals. School-age children and adolescents may benefit from chewing sugarless gum after snacks containing fermentable carbohydrate.

Good oral hygiene complements dietary efforts. In infancy, parents can clean the gums and teeth with a clean cloth. The toothbrush should be introduced in the toddler period. The key is to incorporate brushing and flossing as a regular, consistent routine, with parental supervision in the early years. If the water supply is not fluoridated, use of a fluoride supplement is recommended into the teen years. Topical fluoride applications are recommended based on assessment of caries risk. Varnishes, rinses, gels, and foams are also available to prevent caries and are often incorporated into local public health activities which include partnership with the public health department, schools, and early intervention program.

The AAP and **American Academy of Pediatric Dentistry** (AAPD) suggest establishing a dental home which is a primary dental care provider that provides or coordinates comprehensive care, including preventive oral health

TABLE 9.2 Foods that Make Nutritious Snacks

Protein Foods	Fruits#	Breads and Cereals#	Vegetables
Natural cheese	Apple wedges*	Whole-grain breads	Carrot sticks*
Milk	Bananas	Whole-grain, low-fat crackers	Celery*
Plain yogurt	Pears	Rice crackers	Green pepper strips*
Cooked turkey or beef	Berries	English muffins	Cucumber slices*
Unsalted nuts and seeds*	Melon	Bagels	Cabbage wedges*
Peanut butter*	Oranges and other citrus fruits	Tortillas	Tomatoes
Hard-cooked eggs	Grapes*	Pita bread	Jicama*
Cottage cheese	Unsweetened canned fruit	Popcorn*	Vegetable juices
Tuna	Unsweetened fruit juices		Cooked green beans
			Broccoli and cauliflower florets

*Foods that are hard, round, and do not easily dissolve can cause choking. Do not give to children under 3 years of age. (Peanut butter is more dangerous when eaten in chunks or spread thickly rather than thinly on crackers or bread.)

#Fruits, juices, and most cereal/bread products contain fermentable carbohydrate, which is a factor in the development of dental caries.

supervision and emergency care, with regular visits beginning in early childhood. The AAPD recommends a visit by 12 months of age or 6 months after the first tooth erupts.[59,60]

The US Surgeon General's Report on Oral Health identifies assessment and action by non-dental providers as critical to improving oral health. Screening (and appropriate referral) and anticipatory guidance are included in these actions.[61]

Early Childhood Caries

Children under 3 years of age are most likely to have **early childhood caries** (ECC). ECC is also known as baby bottle tooth decay, nursing caries, and nursing bottle caries. Depending on the definition of ECC (e.g., primary maxillary teeth only, all primary teeth, decayed and filled surfaces), the estimates of ECC prevalence range from 5–23% of 2–5 year olds. Prevalence is highest among poor and near-poor children.[53] Rampant caries develops on the primary upper front teeth (incisors) and often on the cheek surface of primary upper first molars. A history of ECC seems to increase the risk for future caries in permanent teeth.[59]

The primary cause of ECC is prolonged exposure of the teeth to a sweetened liquid such as formula, milk, juice, soda pop, or sweetened drinks. This occurs most often when the child is routinely given a nursing bottle at bedtime or during naps. During sleep, the liquid pools around the teeth, saliva flow decreases, and the child may continue to suck liquid over an extended period of time. Toddlers who hold their own bottles and have access to bottles or sippy cups with sweetened liquids anytime throughout the day are also at high risk. Dental treatment of ECC is expensive, often requires a general anesthetic, and may be traumatic for the child and family.

Education is the primary strategy to prevent ECC. Parents should be counseled about the disorder early in infancy and encouraged to avoid putting a baby to sleep with a bottle. Juices and liquids other than milk or formula should be offered in a cup. For typically developing infants, weaning from the bottle should begin at about 1 year of age. Child care providers and other caregivers should also be informed of the threat to oral health posed by use of the nursing bottle as a pacifier. For this educational approach to be successful, families often need help with positive parenting strategies and behavioral counseling.

▶ Iron Deficiency Anemia

Iron deficiency anemia is most common in children between 1 and 2 years of age, with a prevalence of about 7%.[62] Other high-risk groups are adolescent females, with deficiency noted among 9% of 12- to 15-year-olds and 16% of 16- to 19-year-olds.[63] Overweight children and adolescents have been identified as an at-risk group for iron deficiency.[64] Symptoms of iron deficiency anemia include pale skin/lips/nail beds, irritability, weakness, fatigue, shortness of breath, poor appetite, and frequent infections.

Over the past three decades, there has been an overall decrease in the prevalence of iron deficiency anemia, both in low-income and middle-class pediatric populations. Factors influencing this positive trend include increased and prolonged use of iron-fortified infant formulas, more breastfeeding, increased iron intake from other food sources, and the **Women, Infants, and Children** (WIC) food program. Despite the encouraging trends, some young children, especially those in low-income households, are at high risk for iron deficiency. Although the relationship between iron deficiency and cognitive/behavioral function has been debated for a long time, poorer cognitive performance and delayed psychomotor development have been reported in infants and preschool children with iron deficiency, compared with children without iron deficiency. Iron deficiency in infancy may have long-term consequences, as demonstrated by poorer performance on developmental tests in late childhood and early adolescence.[65,66] Children who are iron deficient are also at risk for increased lead absorption when exposed to sources of lead.

Dietary factors, as well as growth and physiologic needs, play a role in the development of anemia. Some toddlers consume a large volume of milk to the exclusion of solids; plain meats are often not well-accepted by preschool children because they require more chewing. For many of these children, most dietary iron comes from non-heme sources such as vegetables, grains, and cereals. Because the typical US diet contains approximately 6 mg iron per 1000 calories, adolescents dieting to lose weight will have minimal iron intake.

Absorption of iron from food depends on several factors. One is the iron status of the individual; those with low iron stores will have a higher absorption rate. There is a higher rate of absorption from heme iron (in meat, fish, and poultry) than from non-heme iron (in vegetables and grains). The absorption of non-heme iron can be increased by two enhancing factors: (1) ascorbic acid and (2) **meat, fish, or poultry** (MFP).[66] The presence of an ascorbic acid–rich food and/or MFP in a meal will increase the rate of non-heme-iron absorption. Other foods or compounds inhibit iron absorption. **TABLE 9.3** identifies good iron sources as well as absorption enhancers and inhibitors. Simple but conscientious menu planning can help improve iron availability to children and teenagers.

▶ Adolescent Pregnancy

Although pregnancy is a normal physiologic state, there are more risks and complications for pregnant teens compared with any other age group. They have higher rates of low-birth-weight infants, especially among those younger than 15 years old. In general, birth rates among adolescents have been declining since the 1990s. In 2015, the teen birth rate was 22.3 births per 1000 women.[67]

The nutritional status of the pregnant adolescent is influenced by both physiologic and environmental/social factors. There is evidence that young pregnant teenage girls are still growing, creating a maternal–fetal competition for nutrients, and thus indicating increased nutrient needs in addition to pregnancy.[68,69] Other risk factors include a low pre-pregnancy weight and minimal nutrient stores at the time of conception. Many social factors can also affect the health and nutritional status of the teen, including late or no prenatal care, little financial support, limited food resources, poor eating habits, family difficulties, and various other emotional stresses.

For a positive outcome of pregnancy, weight gain for the pregnant adolescent may need to be more than the usual 25 to 35 pounds. The Committee to Reexamine **Institute of Medicine** (IOM) Pregnancy Weight Guidelines of the Food and Nutrition Board released recommendations for weight gain based on BMI. The report recommends that pregnant teens follow the adult BMI cutoff points, recognizing that many adolescents will be categorized in a lighter group and advised to gain more weight.

TABLE 9.3 Food Sources of Iron

Food	Iron (mg)
Meat, Fish, and Poultry (1 oz)	
Chicken liver	3.7
Beef pot roast	0.9
Ground beef	0.7
Pork roast	0.4
Ham	0.2
Chicken breast	0.3
Chicken thigh	0.4
Tuna, canned	0.4
Hot dog	0.4
Salmon	0.3
Fish stick	0.3
Cereals, Grains, Vegetables, and Fruits	
Cooked cereals (½ cup)	0.7–1.8
Ready-to-eat cereals (¾ cup)	0.3–10.8
Whole-wheat bread, enriched bread (1 slice)	0.6–1.2
Legumes, cooked (½ cup)	
Greens (spinach, mustard, beet), cooked (½ cup)	1.5–2.0
Green peas, cooked (½ cup)	0.6–3.2
Dried apricots (5 pieces)	1.3
Nuts (2 Tbsp.)	1.1
Wheat germ (1 Tbsp.)	0.9–2.60.5
Molasses, light (1 Tbsp.)	0.9

*Heme iron sources (approximately 40% of the iron in these foods); well-absorbed.
#Nonheme sources; lower level of absorption; enhancers eaten at the same time will increase absorption.
Data from US Department of Agriculture (USDA), Agricultural Research Service, Nutrient Data Laboratory. USDA National Nutrient Database for standard reference, legacy. Available at: http://www.ars.usda.gov/nutrientdata. Accessed May 1, 2018.[25]

The committee also notes that younger adolescents often need to gain more to improve birth outcomes[70] and it may be more prudent to use pediatric cut-off ranges in order to estimate energy needs. The pattern of weight gain is important, with weight gain in the first and early second trimesters being related to improved birth weights.[68] Studies document that weight gain in adolescent pregnancy includes maternal weight gain and nutrient accretion (i.e., continued growth), in addition to the typical maternal weight and fetal weight gain that is expected during pregnancy in an adult.[71] Canadian recommendations call for a nutrition assessment for pregnant adolescents, including care to optimize weight gain and iron intake.[72]

Many adolescents do not have adequate intakes of calcium, folic acid, and/or iron and may, in fact, have iron deficiency anemia before pregnancy. These nutrients are of special concern, both to maintain good nutritional status of the mother and because of potential long-term effects on their children. A study of adolescent mothers found long-term effects of iron deficiency. At age 3, children of iron-deficient mothers were less active than children whose mothers had adequate iron status.[73] A U.K. study documented increased risk of **small-for-gestational-age** (SGA) births among adolescents with poor micronutrient (folate, iron, and vitamin D) intake and status.[71] Supplementation of iron, folate, and other micronutrients is often necessary.[72]

Education and counseling may be needed for the teen to accept the needed weight gain, plus the likelihood of a higher postpartum weight as part of a healthy pregnancy. An interdisciplinary healthcare team can best help pregnant teenagers to deal with their multiple health, psychosocial, and economic issues. This is most effective when provided as accessible prenatal care targeted to the teenage population in their own communities.[74,75] Education and resource referrals are also needed regarding infant care and feeding, continued schooling of the mother, parenting, and financial services.

▶ Substance Abuse

Alcohol, tobacco, and marijuana are the most widely used substances among teenagers. Inhalants and nonmedical use of prescription medications are also common.[76] Alcoholism in adolescence is a significant public health problem. A survey of 9th to 12th graders indicates that 17.2% of teens had some exposure to alcohol before the age of 13 years.[77] Sixty-three percent of this same group reported at least one drink by age 17 years, and binge drinking (five or more drinks in a few hours) is reported by 17.7% of this same group.[77] Any negative effect on nutritional status will depend on the frequency and amount of drinking as well as the usual food habits. For the female who consumes alcohol and becomes pregnant, there is the risk of fetal alcohol syndrome in her infant.

Smoking by adolescents has decreased slightly since 2002; 4.2% of 12–17-year olds report using cigarettes.[78] There may be an increased need for some nutrients such as ascorbic acid, and smoking during pregnancy can reduce infant birth weight. Not a benign substance, regular use is related to periodontal disease, oral cancer, dependence, and hypertension.

Illicit drugs are reported to be used by 8.8% of 12–17-year olds. This category includes marijuana and misuse of psychotherapeutic drugs (pain relievers, stimulants, tranquilizers, and sedatives); less than 1% use cocaine, heroin, and other drugs.[78]

The negative nutritional consequences of a substance user's habit will depend on factors such as lifestyle, available food, and money to buy food. During a nutrition evaluation, the areas of alcohol consumption, tobacco use, and illegal drug use should be explored. Information will most likely be shared if a matter-of-fact, nonthreatening approach is used. Depending on the individual's situation, nutrition education and counseling can focus on improving health and nutrition. Other teenagers will need comprehensive treatment programs that include a nutrition component.

▶ Nutrition Intervention

Nutrition interventions should be tailored to address the specific nutrition issue as well as what would work best for the individual child and family. Often food patterns are adjusted and/or nutrition education strategies are employed. Some general concepts related to these topics are discussed below.

Feeding the Toddler and Preschool Child

Parents often become concerned when their toddler refuses some favorite foods and appears to be disinterested in eating. These periods of food jags vary in intensity from child to child and may last a few days or years. At the same time, the child is practicing self-feeding skills, with frequent spills, and is often resorting to using their fingers. These changes and behaviors during the preschool years are a normal part of the development and maturation of young children. When parents understand this, they are more likely to avoid struggles, issues of control, and negative feedback around food and eating.

Portion sizes for young children are small by adult standards. **TABLE 9.4** provides a guide for foods and portion sizes. A long-standing rule of thumb is to initially offer 1 tablespoon of each food for every year of age for preschool children, with more provided according to appetite.

Because of smaller capacities and fluctuating appetites, most children eat four to six times a day. Snacks contribute significantly to the total day's nutrient

TABLE 9.4 Feeding Guide for Children

The following is a guide to a basic diet. Fats, sauces, desserts, and snack foods will provide additional energy to meet the growing child's needs. Foods can be selected from this pattern for both meals and snacks.

Food	2- to 3-Year-Olds Portion Size/ Servings		4- to 6-Year-Olds Portion Size/ Servings		7- to 12-Year-Olds Portion Size/ Servings		Comments
Milk and dairy products	½ cup (4 oz.)	4	½–¾ cup (4–6 oz.)	3–4	¾–1 cup (6–8 oz.)	3–4	The following may be substituted for ½ cup liquid milk: ½–¾ oz. cheese, ½ cup yogurt, 2 ½ Tbsp. nonfat dry milk.
Meat, fish, poultry, or equivalent	1–2 oz.	2	1–2 oz.	2	2 oz.	3–4	The following may be substituted for 1 oz. meat, fish, or poultry: 1 egg, 2 Tbsp. peanut butter, 4–5 Tbsp. cooked legumes.
Fruits and Vegetables							
Vegetables Cooked Raw*	 2–3 Tbsp. Few pieces	 4–5	 3–4 Tbsp. Few pieces	 4–5	5 ¼–½ cup Several pieces		Include one green leafy or yellow vegetable for vitamin A, such as carrots, spinach, broccoli, or winter squash.
Fruit Raw Canned Juice	 ½–1 small 2–4 Tbsp. 3–4 oz.		 ½–1 small 4–6 Tbsp. 4 oz.		 1 medium ¼–½ cup 4 oz.		Include one vitamin C–rich fruit, vegetable, or juice, such as citrus juices, orange, grapefruit, strawberries, melon, tomato, or broccoli.
Bread and grain products Whole-grain or enriched bread Cooked cereal Dry cereal	 ½–1 slice ¼–½ cup ½–1 cup	 3–4	 1 slice ½ cup 1 cup	 4–5	 1 slice ½–1 cup 1 cup	 5–6	The following may be substituted for 1 slice of bread: ½ cup spaghetti, macaroni, noodles, or rice; 5 saltines; ½ English muffin or bagel; 1 tortilla

*Do not give to young children until they can chew well.

Data from Lowenberg ME, Development of food patterns in young children. In: Pipes PL, ed. *Nutrition Infancy and Childhood*. 4th ed. W.B. Saunders; 1989.[79]

Note: This table is intended to provide a general idea of typical intakes of children and is not intended as a prescriptive guide. Nutrient needs and patterns of individual children will vary.

intake and should be planned accordingly. Foods that make nutritious snacks are listed in Table 9.2. Foods chosen for snacks should be those least likely to promote dental caries.

Parents of young children frequently become concerned about the adequacy of their children's intakes; plain meats are often refused because they are more difficult to chew, very little or too much milk may be consumed, and cooked vegetables are pushed away.

TABLE 9.5 offers nutrition solutions to these common, normal variations in eating behaviors.

Just as important as providing adequate nutrients to young children is supporting a positive feeding environment—both physically and emotionally—so that, as they grow, they acquire skills, develop positive attitudes, and have control over food decisions as appropriate for their developmental level. General guidance in this area is listed in **TABLE 9.6**.

TABLE 9.5 Common Feeding Concerns in Young Children

Common Concerns	Possible Solutions
Refuses meats	■ Offer small, bite-size pieces of moist, tender meat or poultry. ■ Incorporate into meatloaf, spaghetti sauce, stews, casseroles, burritos, or pizza. ■ Include legumes, eggs, and cheese. ■ Offer boneless fish (including canned tuna and salmon).
Drinks too little milk	■ Offer cheeses and yogurt, including cheese in cooking (e.g., macaroni and cheese, cheese sauce, pizza). Use milk to cook hot cereals. Offer cream soups and milk-based puddings and custards. ■ Allow child to pour milk from a pitcher and use a straw. ■ Include powdered milk in cooking and baking (e.g., biscuits, muffins, pancakes, meatloaf, casseroles)
Drinks too much milk	■ Offer water if thirsty between meals. ■ Limit milk to one serving with meals or offer at end of meal; offer water for seconds. ■ If bottle is still used, wean to cup.
Refuses vegetables and fruits	■ If child refuses vegetables, offer more fruits, and vice versa. ■ Prepare vegetables that are tender but not overcooked. ■ Steam vegetable strips (or offer raw if appropriate) and allow child to eat with fingers. ■ Offer sauces and dips (e.g., cheese sauce for cooked vegetables, dip for raw vegetables, yogurt to dip fruit). ■ Include vegetables in soups and casseroles. ■ Add fresh or dried fruit to cereals. ■ Prepare fruit in a variety of ways (e.g., fresh, cooked, juice, in gelatin, as a salad). ■ Continue to offer a variety of fruits and vegetables.
Eats too many sweets	■ Limit purchase and preparation of sweet foods in the home. ■ Avoid using as a bribe or reward. ■ Incorporate into meals instead of snacks for better dental health. ■ Reduce sugar by half in recipes for cookies, muffins, quick breads, and the like. ■ Work with staff of day care, preschools, and others to reduce use of sweets.

Children under age 4 are at greatest risk for choking on food. In some cases, this can lead to death from asphyxiation.[80] Foods most likely to cause choking are those that are round, hard, and do not readily dissolve in saliva, such as hot dogs, grapes, raw vegetables, popcorn, peanut butter, nuts, and hard candy. Other foods can also cause choking problems if too much is stuffed into the mouth, if the child is running while eating, or if the child is unsupervised. Choking episodes can be prevented by common-sense management of foods and the eating environment. **TABLE 9.7** outlines preventive approaches.

Fruit juice is a common beverage for children, usually replacing water and sometimes milk. Excessive fruit juice consumption has been linked to chronic diarrhea and failure to thrive, with improvement when juice is limited.[81] Consumption of 100% fruit juice by children 1–6 years was associated with a clinically insignificant weight gain; for those 7–18 years, no association was found. The intake of 100% fruit juice can improve nutrient intake, especially potassium, vitamin C, and magnesium.[82] The Dietary Guidelines state that one-half of fruit servings can be provided as 100% fruit juice, without

---

TABLE 9.6 Tips for a Happy Mealtime

Physical Setting

- Schedule meals at regular times.
- Avoid having a child get too hungry or too tired before mealtime.
- Snacks should be at least 1½ to 2 hours before meals.
- Child should be able to sit up to the table comfortably without reaching.
- Provide support for the legs and feet, such as a booster seat or stool.
- Use nonbreakable, sturdy dishes with sides to push food against.
- Spoons and forks should be blunt with broad, short handles.
- Use cups that are nonbreakable, broad based, and small.

Social-Emotional

- Serve a new food with familiar ones—don't be surprised by an initial rejection.
- Offer at least one food at a meal that you know your child will eat, but do not cater to his or her likes and dislikes.
- Avoid coaxing, nagging, bribing, or any other pressure to get your child to eat.
- Serve dessert (if any) with the meal—it becomes less important and cannot be used as a reward.
- Let children determine when they are full; amounts eaten will vary from child to child and day to day.
- Use the child's developmental stage to determine expectations for neatness and manners, but set limits on inappropriate behaviors (e.g., throwing food, playing).
- Attempt to have family meals be as pleasant as possible; avoid arguments and criticism.
- Allow children to help set the table or do part of the meal preparation.

---

added sugars, with portion sizes described equivalent to one serving of fruit.[83] The AAP suggests that fruit juice intake be limited to 4 ounces per day for children 1 to 3 years of age, 4–6 ounces per day for children 4 to 6 years of age, and 8 ounces per day for those 7 to 18 years of age.[84,85] One study compared intakes of fruit juice, milk, and sweetened beverages and adiposity. Intake of sugar sweetened beverages, but not milk or 100% fruit juice at age 5 years, was predictive of adiposity between ages 5 and 15 years.[86]

Feeding the School-Age Child

The years from 6 to 12 are a period of slow but steady growth, with increases in food intake as a result of appetite (see Table 9.4). Most food behavior problems from early childhood have been resolved except for extreme cases, but food dislikes may persist, especially if attention is given to them.

Because children are in school, they may eat fewer times in the day, but after-school snacks usually are a

---

TABLE 9.7 Guidelines for Feeding Safety: Preschool Children

- Have children sit while eating. It lets them concentrate on chewing and swallowing. While preschool-age children do have molars, they are still learning to chew effectively. Eating while walking or running may cause choking.
- An adult should supervise children at all times while they are eating.
- Children can be easily distracted, so meals and snacks should be presented in a calm atmosphere; overexcitement may cause choking.
- Offer well-cooked foods, modified if needed, so that the child can chew and swallow without difficulty.
- For children under age 3, avoid offering foods that can cause choking (e.g., hard candy, mini-marshmallows, popcorn, pretzels, chips, spoonfuls of peanut butter, nuts, seeds, large chunks of meat, hot dogs, raw carrots, raisins and other dried fruits, and whole grapes). For children between the ages of 3 and 5, modify these foods to make them safer (e.g., cut hot dogs in quarters lengthwise and into small pieces, cut whole grapes in half lengthwise, chop nuts finely, slice carrots into thin strips, spread peanut butter thinly on crackers or bread).
- Avoid eating in the car. If the child starts choking, it may be difficult to get to the side of the road safely and help the child.

Data from American Academy of Pediatrics Committee on Injury, Violence, and Poison Prevention. Prevention of choking among children. *Pediatrics*. 2010;125:601–607.[80]
Holt KA, ed. *Bright Futures in Practice: Nutrition*, 3rd ed. Elk Grove Village: American Academy of Pediatrics; 2011.[2]

routine. Skipping breakfast may begin in these years, with contributing factors such as time constraints, children left to get themselves off to school, and early school starts. With participation in organized sports, music programs, and other activities, sitting down to a family meal may be less frequent.

In the United States, some children not yet in their teens have responsibility for family shopping and cooking. Some children are frequently responsible for their own breakfasts, lunches, snacks, and even the dinner meal. They also do food shopping on a regular basis and influence the family food purchases. At the same time, increasingly sophisticated advertising is being aimed at these children.

Feeding the Adolescent

Adolescents in their rapid-growth period seem to eat all the time. Their appetites usually guide their intakes. As teenagers achieve more independence and spend a greater amount of time away from home, they have additional variable intakes and irregular eating patterns. Skipping meals is greatest in this age group, particularly for breakfast and lunch. On the other hand, snacking tends to be a common practice. Whether they are called snacks or meals, adolescents who eat less than three times a day have poorer diets than do those eating more often.

Although fast foods are popular with all segments of the population, they are especially appealing to teenagers. The food is inexpensive, well-accepted, and can be eaten informally without utensils or plates. Fast food restaurants are also socially acceptable and a common employer of adolescents. Generally, the menu items tend to be energy-dense, high in fat with some items provide more than 50% of energy as fat, high in sodium, and low in fiber, vitamin A, ascorbic acid, calcium, and folate. Although these establishments offer salads and lower-fat sandwiches, these foods are not necessarily chosen by teens. Negative impacts of fast foods on the diets of adolescents will depend on how frequently they are eaten and the choices made. About one-third of children and adolescents report consumption of fast food on a given day.[87]

▶ Nutrition Education

Children first learn about food and nutrition from their families in their own homes. This begins in an informal manner, with parental attitudes and foods commonly served; for example potatoes or tortillas may be served daily, okra or bok choy may never be served, and family opinions about what foods are good nutritionally. Later, more formal nutrition education occurs in preschools, Head Start programs, day care, schools, and clubs such as 4-H. Information is also assimilated from the media, advertising, written materials, the Internet, and peers.

A child's developmental level should be taken into account when teaching nutrition concepts. For example, Piaget's learning theory can be used to correlate developmental periods and cognitive characteristics with progress in feeding and nutrition. Younger children may do best with hands-on experience with food, not abstract nutrition concepts. A personal approach, such as using computer software to examine their own dietary profiles can be an appropriate activity for children and adolescents. Social marketing strategies including television, print, radio, and Internet media have been used to communicate health messages to children and parents.[88,89] Using an ecological model has been suggested in order to increase the understanding of eating behaviors, especially among adolescents. The ecological model examines the influences of individual (e.g., biologic), social environmental (e.g., peers), physical environmental (e.g., school), and macrosystem or societal (e.g., marketing) factors on behaviors.[90]

▶ Nutrition Monitoring and Evaluation

Nutrition monitoring will generally include evaluating growth parameters and nutrient intake, as well as factors specific to the identified nutrition-related problem. Consideration for how the intervention might affect other aspects of the family's life such as the feeding relationship is also important.

▶ Special Considerations

School Nutrition

Children and teens spend a lot of time in school and many participate in events outside the academic school day but still within the school setting. Most children eat at least one meal daily in the school environment; others may consume 2 meals and a snack. School lunches, school wellness policies, and food sources outside the cafeteria all have received attention with the goal to maximize health.

School Lunch Programs

Children usually participate in the school lunch program or bring a packed lunch from home. The **National School Lunch Program** (NSLP) and **School Breakfast Program** (SBP) are administered by the **US Department of Agriculture** (USDA) and supported by reimbursements and supplemental commodity foods. Lunches from home contained more sodium and fewer servings of fruit, vegetables, whole grains, and fluid milk. About 90% of lunches in this study contained desserts, chips, and sweetened beverages, which are not part of reimbursable school meals.[91]

The **Healthy, Hunger-Free Kids Act** (HHFKA) of 2010 revised nutrition standards for school meals, snacks, and beverages provided by the NSLP and SBP. These standards went into place in 2012. Besides guidelines to provide more fruits, vegetables, and whole grains and less sugar, salt, and fat, there are also age-specific guidelines for portion sizes and requirements for making water available during meals. Longitudinal data showed significant improvement in the nutritional quality of foods selected by students after implementing the HHFKA.[92,93] Since 2014, Smart Snacks requirements provide guidelines for foods that are sold ala carte in school stores and in vending machines.

Farm to school programs, fresh fruit and vegetable programs, and local school wellness programs are in place across the country as well all in an effort to promote a healthy school environment. Other efforts, such as recess before lunch and breakfast in the classroom, are implemented at district and local levels and have been shown to have positive impacts.[93]

The Academy of Nutrition and Dietetics, along with the Society for Nutrition Education and the School Nutrition Association call for the integration of school nutrition services with a coordinated, comprehensive school health program and school nutrition policy.[94]

Nutrition and Physical Activity

A child and adolescent's food intake contributes to growth, development, and overall health. In addition to nutrition, regular physical activity throughout life is important for maintaining a healthy body, enhancing psychological well-being, and preventing premature death.[95]

Current physical activity recommendations for those ages 6–17 years of age are:[96]

- Children and adolescents should do 1 hour or more of physical activity every day.
- Most of the 1 hour or more a day should be either moderate- or vigorous-intensity aerobic physical activity.
- As part of their daily physical activity, children and adolescents should do vigorous-intensity activity on at least 3 days per week. They also should do muscle-strengthening and bone-strengthening activity on at least 3 days per week.

The 2008 Physical Activity Guidelines for Americans contain information regarding activities that will meet these recommendations and are appropriate for children.[96] These guidelines are in the process of being updated.

Physical Activity in Children and Teens

Physical activity should be encouraged for all children and adolescents. Through physical activity, an individual's endurance, flexibility, and strength are improved.[96]

For those 5–17 years of age, strong evidence for the benefits from physical activity include improved muscular skeletal health and fitness, favorable body adiposity, and improvement in components of cardiovascular health. Moderate evidence suggests that activity may improve blood pressure, lipid profiles, and mental health.[97] Additionally, physical activity can help children and adolescents have fun, make new friends, and/or spend quality time with their families.[98]

The most recent youth surveillance survey of those in 9th to 12th grades reports that just under 50% (48.6) of students met recommended levels of physical activity. The survey standard was activity that increased the student's heart rate and made them breathe hard some of the time for a total of at least 60 minutes per day on 5 or more days. More than one-third of this same age group spends three or more hours a day on non-school-related computer activities and/or video games. Television watching time decreased slightly during the same time period.[77]

Others have found that for children 4–11 years of age, just over one-third have low levels of active play. Two-thirds of the sample had high screen time and approximately 25% of these children had both low activity levels of play and high screen time.[99]

Preschoolers' activity has also been examined; more research is needed in order to understand physical activity behavior in this age group. A review indicated that boys were more active than girls, children with active parents tended to be more active, and children who spent more time outdoors were more active than those spending less time outdoors.[100] A small increase in children's activity has been associated with family-based interventions, and methods to engage families are suggested.[101]

Sports Nutrition

Many children and adolescents participate in competitive sports, and they (or their parents and/or coaches) are interested in the effects of nutrition on athletic performance. It is important to ensure that an individual's energy and fluid intake is adequate to support growth and to meet the increased demands of physical activity. Children and adolescents who participate in sports may need to adjust their intakes pre-event, during long events, and/or post-event (for example, pregame snacks of foods with complex carbohydrates). Children with some medical conditions (e.g., diabetes) may require additional adjustments to food patterns and/or medications.

A large market exists for sports-focused nutritional supplements, and children and adolescents as well as parents and coaches are targeted by marketers. Evidence is not available to suggest that healthy athletes have increased needs beyond the recommended nutrition requirements for active individuals. Little evidence is available to support the use of dietary sports supplements in young athletes to enhance performance, lean muscle mass, or endurance.[102,103] Parents, coaches, and other youth sports organizations should encourage the young athlete to consume whole, nutritious foods for a balanced diet in addition to participating in appropriate physical training.

Health Promotion

Americans have been gradually altering their eating habits as a result of increased interest in their health and their concern about preventing heart disease, cancer, obesity, and hypertension. The federal government and nonprofit organizations have provided recommendations, such as the Dietary Guidelines, to promote healthy eating. To what degree, if any, should this advice be applied to growing children and adolescents?

For overall health promotion, moderation and common sense continue to be the best policy. Although prevention of obesity and other chronic conditions is a worthy goal, there are no conclusive data to support a massive change in the diets of growing children. For healthy, growing children, using low-fat dairy products and fewer high-fat foods is appropriate for those over 2 years of age. Limiting the intake of fermentable carbohydrate will enhance dental health. Increasing the intake of fruits, vegetables, whole-grain products, and legumes above the usual reported levels can have several benefits, including reducing the percentage of fat in the diet, increasing the fiber content, increasing the amount of beta-carotene and other dietary factors that may help prevent cancer, and making the total diet more nutrient dense. The more varied the diet, the more likely the child's nutrient needs will be met.

Heart Health

Recommendations for cardiovascular health in children have been published by the AAP and are very similar to guidelines recommended by the **National Cholesterol Education Program** (NCEP) and the American Heart Association.[8-11] These groups recommend that everyone over 2 years of age follow a diet that includes no more than 30% of energy as fat (7–10% from saturated fat), no more than 300 mg cholesterol per day, and limited amounts of trans fats. Population-based recommendations also include appropriate energy intake (which may include modifying sugar-sweetened beverage intake) to meet needs for growth and physical activity, limiting sodium intake, increasing access to fruits, vegetables, and dietary fiber. The American Heart Association suggests that the intake of added sugars be limited to 25 grams (6 teaspoons) per day, for children ages 2 years and older.[104] Dietary intervention should be tailored to the individual's needs and ongoing nutrition counseling is recommended to help families implement

recommendations for reducing cardiovascular risk and assuring adequate intake.[11]

For children identified by screening, the *Cardiovascular Health Integrated Lifestyle Diet* (CHILD 1) is suggested by the NHLBI expert recommendations.[11] This pattern emphasizes fat-free or low-fat dairy options and increased intake of fruits and vegetables and has been called a "DASH-style eating plan."

Fiber

National diet intake data have shown that children and adolescents consume a less-than-desirable intake of fiber and whole-grain foods, similar to the adult population.[105] An AI for fiber has been established as part of the DRIs. This is 14 grams of fiber per 1000 calories. This recommendation is significantly higher for children and adolescents than previous guidelines.[17] Increasing dietary fiber can help prevent constipation, protect against coronary heart disease, and often results in greater intake of fruits and vegetables.

Effect of Diet on Learning and Behavior

What impact does a child's diet have on his or her school performance and behavior? For decades, people have debated whether skipping breakfast affects classroom learning. Food additives, sugar, and allergies have been suggested as causes of hyperactivity in children. Although these are controversial issues, some scientific studies have examined them.

Diet and Learning Behavior

Although severe malnutrition early in life is known to negatively affect intellectual development, the impact of marginal malnutrition, skipping meals, or hunger has been more difficult to document. Experimental studies have used standardized tests to measure cognitive functions in healthy school-age children who were given either breakfast or no breakfast. A systematic review indicated that breakfast had short-term, positive effects on tasks that required attention, executive function, and memory.[106] The effects were greatest in children who were undernourished. Studies comparing healthy children to those stunted, those who suffered severe malnutrition early in life, and those currently wasted (low weight for height) showed even poorer results for the malnourished/undernourished children when they missed breakfast.[100,107]

The impact of diet and nutrition on a child's behavior has been a controversial topic for some time. Although malnourished children and those experiencing iron deficiency anemias often demonstrate decreased attention and responsiveness, less interest in their environment, and reduced problem-solving ability, the effects of periodic hunger or "food insecurity" is less clear. A report of families from a large **Community Childhood Hunger Identification Project** (CCHIP) found that the "hungry" children were three times more likely than "at-risk for hunger" children, and seven times more likely than "not hungry" children to have scores indicating irritability, anxiety, aggression, and oppositional behavior.[108] Data from NHANES III showed negative academic and psychosocial outcomes associated with food insufficiency. Children who were classified as food-insufficient had lower math scores and were more likely to have repeated a grade, to have seen a psychologist, and to have difficulty getting along with other children. Adolescents with food insufficiency were also more likely to have been suspended from school.[109] Although other unstudied factors could also be related to these negative behaviors, they could be tied to the family's food insecurity. Without broad policies to ensure children their basic needs, children and adolescents may suffer worsening behavioral and academic functioning.

Vegetarian Nutrition

Well-planned vegetarian diets are appropriate throughout the life cycle including childhood and adolescence.[110] Children, adolescents, and/or their families may practice vegetarian diet patterns for a variety of reasons including health benefits, economic issues, environmental concerns, religious beliefs, and animal rights. In 2014, 3% of 8- to 18-year olds in the United States said they never ate meat, poultry, fish, or seafood. In this same age group, 2 million are vegetarian, including vegan.[111]

Evidence indicates that those following a vegetarian pattern reduce their risk of ischemic heart disease, type 2 diabetes, hypertension, certain types of cancer, and obesity. Health benefits and risks of vegetarian food patterns were examined among 15–23-year olds as part of the Project EAT (Eating Among Teens)-II study. Benefits of vegetarian patterns included increased intake of fruits and vegetables. Current vegetarians were at increased risk for binge eating with loss of control, and former vegetarians were at increased risk for unhealthful weight control behaviors.[112]

By definition, a vegetarian diet does not contain meat, fish, or fowl or products containing these foods. However, vegetarian diet patterns cover a wide range, from lacto-ovo vegetarians (consume grains, vegetables, fruits, legumes, seeds, nuts, dairy products, and eggs), lacto vegetarians (no eggs consumed), ovo vegetarians (no dairy consumed), and vegans (exclude all products of animal origin) to food patterns that include only raw food or other specific food types. The more restrictive vegetarian food diets will most likely not meet the needs of growing children and adolescents.[7] Key nutrients to assess for infants, children, and adolescents following vegetarian food patterns include iron, zinc, vitamin B_{12}, and for some, calcium and vitamin D.[110] Levels of these nutrients should be assessed, and fortified foods and/or supplements used to meet the individual child's needs.

If a vegetarian lifestyle is reported a careful nutrition assessment will determine the actual intake and pattern used by the family or individual.

Families may choose to implement vegetarian food patterns throughout their child's development. Infants can be breastfed or receive soy formula (vegan) or cow's milk formula (lacto-). It is suggested that infants born prematurely not receive soy formula.[7] Solid foods should be introduced following recommended guidelines, based on developmental readiness. Depending on the type of vegetarian diet followed by the family, anticipatory guidance may include explaining the need for offering foods with appropriate textures, and foods that are energy- and nutrient-dense. Children consuming a well-planned and not overly restrictive diet grow and develop as their peers.[7] Adolescents with vegetarian food patterns may need guidance to ensure they consume a variety of foods to meet their needs. This guidance may also include use of vitamin and/or mineral supplements at appropriate levels.

▶ Resources

Resources related to pediatric nutrition are listed below.

Knowledge Path on Child and Adolescent Nutrition

https://www.ncemch.org/knowledge/childnutr.php

This extensive resource has information for professionals and families, with strategies for improving nutrition and eating behaviors within families, schools, and communities. There are resources on child care/early childhood, food safety, food marketing to children, food security and assistance programs, and school-based food and nutrition programs. Also included are many related nutrition Websites, electronic publications and newsletters, and many databases.

Bright Futures in Practice: Nutrition, 3rd Edition

https://brightfutures.aap.org/materials-and-tools/nutrition-and-pocket-guide/Pages/default.aspx

This nutrition guide emphasizes prevention and early recognition of nutrition concerns and provides developmentally appropriate nutrition supervision guidelines for infancy through adolescence. A PDF version is available for download, or print copies can be purchased. Additional resources, educational materials, and a pocket guide are also available.

Additional Bright Futures resources are listed on the Bright Futures at Georgetown University Website (http://www.brightfutures.org/georgetown.html). Links to educational materials, training materials, and other tools are listed, including those related to social and emotional development, mental health, oral health, and physical activity.

American Academy of Pediatrics

http://www.aap.org

The AAP Website features resources for professionals (e.g., policy statements, clinical practice guidelines, technical reports) and for families (e.g., educational materials, Health Topics, and Parenting Corner).

Food and Nutrition Information Center (FNIC)

https://www.nal.usda.gov/fnic

The FNIC site includes resources related to child nutrition and health, food allergies, food and nutrition education, food safety, and nutrition and food assistance. Click on "Lifecycle Nutrition" to find links to lists for specific lifestages (e.g., toddler nutrition, preschool nutrition, child nutrition, and teen nutrition).

National School Lunch Program (NSLP) and School Breakfast Program (SBP)

https://www.fns.usda.gov/nslp/national-school-lunch-program-nslp and https://www.fns.usda.gov/sbp/school-breakfast-program-sbp

The National School Lunch Program and School Breakfast Program are administered by the USDA and supported by reimbursements and supplemental commodity foods.

Physical Activity and Children and Adolescents Knowledge Path

https://www.ncemch.org/knowledge/phys-activity.php

This knowledge path offers a selection of recent, high-quality resources that analyze data, describe public health campaigns and other promotion programs, and report on research aimed at identifying promising strategies for improving physical activity levels within families, schools, and communities.

🔍 CASE STUDIES

Case Study #1: Kaylee

Kaylee
30 month old, female

Kaylee was born at term after an uncomplicated delivery. During her first year, there was some developmental concern by her healthcare providers based on "late" acquisition of crawling and independent walking. Currently, she is age-appropriate in terms of developmental milestones. She lives with her 22-year old mother and maternal grandparents. Her mother, Lila, attends school during the week. She plans on going to nursing school after graduation. Kaylee is cared for by her grandparents while Lila is at school. Her grandfather likes to take Kaylee for walks to the park. On the way back, he stops at the store and they each have a cookie. On weekends, Lila takes Kaylee to the park or swimming. Kaylee is learning to ride a tricycle.

Growth: Weight: 33 pounds, Height: 38.5 inches
Diet Information: Lila provided a 5-day food record, which "was typical."

	Sunday	Monday	Tuesday	Wednesday	Thursday
8 am	1 sausage Scrambled egg 4 oz orange juice	½ cup Cheerios 2 oz milk ½ banana 4 oz orange juice	Same as Monday	Same as Monday	1 pancake with butter and syrup 4 oz orange juice ¼ cup applesauce
10–11: Snack	2 oz yogurt ½ banana	Cookie and 4 oz chocolate milk with Grandpa	Same as Monday	Apple slices (1 apple) 15 goldfish crackers	Same as Monday

	Sunday	**Monday**	**Tuesday**	**Wednesday**	**Thursday**
12:30	½ Cup macaroni and cheese Sliced hot dog with ketchup 4 oz milk	½ PB sandwich, cup of juice (close to naptime, and tired, didn't want to eat much)	½ cup rice 2 chicken strips 1 slice cheese 4 oz juice	½ cup macaroni and cheese Sliced hot dog with ketchup 4 oz milk	½ PB sandwich 4 oz milk 10 grapes
5:30	½ cup lasagna ¼ cup green beans 2 oz milk	Meatloaf (1 slice with ketchup) ¼ cup noodles ¼ cup broccoli	½ cup tuna noodle casserole ¼ cup peas bite of tomato, bite of lettuce 4 oz milk	Spaghetti with meat sauce (½ cup) 1 slice bread 2 oz milk 1 bite salad	½ cup lasagna ¼ cup green beans 2 oz milk
6–8: Snack	2 oz milk 1 cookie	2 oz milk at storytime		A few bites of pie with Grandpa	Few bites of pear 2 oz juice

Questions

Answer the questions below. Indicate what additional information you might need for a more thorough response.

1. Plot and evaluate Kaylee's growth on the CDC chart. Calculate and plot BMI
2. Evaluate Kaylee's diet (nutrients you are concerned about, other aspects of her food pattern).
3. If Kaylee was being screened, are there any risk factors identified? Discuss risk factors and the potential impact on Kaylee's nutritional status.
4. Evaluate Kaylee's nutritional status and correlate with identified screening risks. Are any problems identified? Provide evidence.

Case Study #2: Brian

Brian is a 7-year, 4-month-old boy who gained 15 pounds during the past school year. His height is 50 ½ inches, and his weight is 75 pounds.

Brian moved to a new home and began a new school a year ago after his parents' divorce. After-school care has been provided by a retired neighbor who loves to bake for Brian. He has few friends in the neighborhood, and his main leisure activities have been watching television and playing video games. When he gets bored he often looks for a snack. His mother reports that they often rely on take-out and fast-food meals because of the time constraints of her full-time job, and she has gained weight herself. She recently started an aerobics class with a friend and is interested in developing healthier eating habits for herself and Brian.

After joint sessions with Brian and his mother, the following goals were identified by the family:

1. Explore after-school care at the local community center, which has a physical activity component
2. Alter grocery and menu selection to emphasize the MyPlate and low-fat choices while still meeting the family's time and resource constraints
3. Begin to incorporate physical activities (Brian identified swimming and bicycling as things he would like to do) on the weekends
4. Limit television and video games to no more than 2 hours daily

After 4 months, Brian has enrolled in the local community center's afterschool program and participates in organized soccer and "pick-up" basketball. Weekends are a challenge. Brian and his mother have not yet incorporated physical activity into their weekend routine, and Brian finds it tough to limit screen time to 2 hours on the weekends. Brian has lost 4 pounds and is taller; he is 51 inches tall and weighs 66 pounds.

7y 8m

Questions

1. Calculate and plot Brian's BMI over time using the CDC chart. Discuss the changes.
2. Write two nutrition diagnostic statements: one that would have been appropriate at his initial visit and one at the most recent follow-up visit
3. What other activities can Brian try to help him avoid or reduce the tendency to eat when he is not hungry?
4. What would you suggest to promote a positive feeding relationship between Brian and his mother, considering his age and level of development?
5. What recommendations can you make to decrease Brian's energy intake and make it more consistent with MyPlate recommendations? Consider ideas to alter Brian's favorite recipes (e.g., his favorite meal is fried chicken with gravy, mashed potatoes and ice cream), select healthy options from take-out or fast-food options, and modifications to snack options.
6. Are there any nutrient-related concerns because Brian's diet is being altered to help with weight management? Or because of his age? Or other factors?

References

1. Satter E. *How to Get Your Kid to Eat...But Not Too Much*. Palo Alto, CA:Bull Publishing Co.;1987.

2. Holt KA. *Bright futures: Nutrition*. 3rd ed. Elk Grove Village, Il:American Academy of Pediatrics; 2011.

3. U.S. Preventive Services Task Force. Agency for Healthcare Research and Quality. *Screening for obesity in children and adolescents*. Rockville, MD:2010.

4. Golden NH, Schneider M, Wood C, Committee on Nutrition, Committee on Adolescence, Committee on Obesity. Preventing Obesity and Eating Disorders in Adolescents. *Pediatrics*. 2016;138(3):e20161649.

5. Baker RD, Greer FR, American Academy of Pediatrics Committee on Nutrition. Diagnosis and prevention of iron deficiency and iron-deficiency anemia in infants and young children (0–3 years of age). *Pediatrics*. 2010;126(5):1040–1050.

6. Centers for Disease Control and Prevention. Iron deficiency—United States, 1999–2000. *JAMA*. 2002;288 (17):2114–2116.

7. American Academy of Pediatrics. *Pediatric Nutrition*, 7th ed. Elk Grove, IL: American Academy of Pediatrics; 2014.

8. Daniels SR, Greer FR, Nutrition Co. Lipid screening and cardiovascular health in childhood. *Pediatrics*. 2008;122(1): 198–208.

9. Lichtenstein AH, Appel LJ, Brands M, et al. Diet and lifestyle recommendations revision 2006: a scientific statement from the American Heart Association Nutrition Committee. *Circulation*. 2006;114(1):82–96.

10. Gidding SS, Dennison BA, Birch LL, et al. Dietary recommendations for children and adolescents: a guide for practitioners: consensus statement from the American Heart Association. *Circulation*. 2005;112(13):2061–2075.

11. Expert Panel on Integrated Guidelines for Cardiovascular Health and Risk Reduction in Children and Adolescents, National Heart Lung and Blood Institute. Expert panel on integrated guidelines for cardiovascular health and risk reduction in children and adolescents: summary report. *Pediatrics*. 2011;128(suppl 5):S213–S256.

12. Urbina EM, de Ferranti SD. Lipid screening in children and adolescents. *JAMA*. 2016;316(6):589–591.

13. Screening for lipid disorders in children and adolescents: recommendation statement. *Am Fam Physician*. 2016;94(12):Online.

14. Peterson AL, McBride PE. A review of guidelines for dyslipidemia in children and adolescents. *WMJ*. 2012;111(6):274–281.

15. Daniels SR. On the U.S. Preventive Services Task Force Statement on Screening for Lipid Disorders in Children and Adolescents: One Step Forward and 2 Steps Sideways. *JAMA Pediatr*. 2016;170(10):932–934.

16. Otten JJ, Hellwig JP, Meyers LD. *DRI, dietary reference intakes: the essential guide to nutrient requirements*. Washington, D.C.: National Academies Press; 2006.

17. Panel on Macronutrients, Panel on the Definition of Dietary Fiber, Subcommittee on Interpretation and Uses of Dietary Reference Intakes, and the Standing Committee on the Scientific Evaluation of Dietary Reference Intakes, Food and Nutrition Board. *Dietary reference intakes for energy, carbohydrate, fiber, fat, fatty acids, cholesterol, protein, and amino acids*. Washington, DC: National Academies Press; 2005.

18. Fulgoni VL. Current protein intake in America: analysis of the National Health and Nutrition Examination Survey, 2003–2004. *Am J Clin Nutr*. 2008;87(5):1554S–1557S.

19. Mathias KC, Almoosawi S, Karagounis LG. Protein and energy intakes are skewed toward the evening among children and adolescents in the United States: NHANES 2013–2014. *J Nutr*. 2017;147(6):1160–1166.

20. Moshfegh A, et al. What we eat in America, NHANES 2001–2002: usual nutrient intakes from food compared to dietary reference intakes. Washington, DC: U.S. Department of Agriculture, Agricultural Research Service; 2005.

21. Moshfegh A, Goldman J, Ahuja J, Rhodes D, LaComb R. What we eat in America, NHANES 2005–2006: usual nutrient intakes from food and water compared to 1997 dietary reference intakes for Vitamin D, Calcium, Phosphorus, and Magnesium. Washington, DC: U.S. Department of Agriculture, Agricultural Research Service; 2009.

22. Ahluwalia N, Herrick KA, Rossen LM, et al. Usual nutrient intakes of U.S. infants and toddlers generally meet or exceed Dietary Reference Intakes: findings from NHANES 2009–2012. *Am J Clin Nutr*. 2016;104(4):1167–1174.

23. Matkovic V, Fontana D, Tominac C, Goel P, Chesnut CH. Factors that influence peak bone mass formation: a study of calcium balance and the inheritance of bone mass in adolescent females. *Am J Clin Nutr*. 1990;52(5):878–888.

24. Ross AC, Institute of Medicine (U.S.). Committee to Review Dietary Reference Intakes for Vitamin D and Calcium. *Dietary reference intakes: calcium, vitamin D.* Washington, DC: National Academies Press; 2011.

25. U.S. Department of Agriculture (USDA), Agricultural Research Service, Nutrient Data Laboratory. USDA National Nutrient Database for standard reference, legacy. Available at: http://www.ars.usda.gov/nutrientdata. Accessed May 1, 2018.

26. Kumar J, Muntner P, Kaskel FJ, Hailpern SM, Melamed ML. Prevalence and associations of 25-hydroxyvitamin D deficiency in U.S. children: NHANES 2001–2004. *Pediatrics.* 2009;124(3):e362–e370.

27. Institute of Medicine (U.S.). Panel on Micronutrients. *DRI: Dietary Reference Intakes for Vitamin A, Vitamin K, Arsenic, Boron, Chromium, Copper, Iodine, Iron, Manganese, Molybdenum, Nickel, Silicon, Vanadium, and Zinc: a report of the Panel on Micronutrients ... and the Standing Committee on the Scientific Evaluation of Dietary Reference Intakes, Food and Nutrition Board, Institute of Medicine.* Washington, D.C.: National Academy Press; 2001.

28. Picciano MF, Dwyer JT, Radimer KL, et al. Dietary supplement use among infants, children, and adolescents in the United States, 1999–2002. *Arch Pediatr Adolesc Med.* 2007;161(10):978–985.

29. Beal VA. Dietary intake of individuals followed through infancy and childhood. *Am J Public Health Nations Health.* 1961;51:1107–1117.

30. Bowman S, Clemens J, Friday J, et al. Food Patterns Equivalents Intakes by Americans: What we Eat in America, NHANES 2003–04 and 2013–2014. Food Surveys Research Group. *Dietary Data Brief No. 17.* 2017.

31. Guenther PM, Casavale KO, Reedy J, et al. Update of the Healthy Eating Index: HEI-2010. *J Acad Nutr Diet.* 2013;113(4):569–580.

32. Banfield EC, Liu Y, Davis JS, Chang S, Frazier-Wood AC. Poor Adherence to U.S. Dietary Guidelines for Children and Adolescents in the National Health and Nutrition Examination Survey Population. *J Acad Nutr Diet.* 2016;116(1):21–27.

33. Mancino LT, Jessica E Guthrie, Joanne Lin, Biing-Hwan. *How Food Away From Home Affects Children's Diet Quality.* In: *ERR-104:* U.S. Dept. of Agriculture, Econ. Res. Serv; 2010.

34. Galloway AT, Lee Y, Birch LL. Predictors and consequences of food neophobia and pickiness in young girls. *J Am Diet Assoc.* 2003;103(6):692–698.

35. Larson NI, Neumark-Sztainer D, Hannan PJ, Story M. Family meals during adolescence are associated with higher diet quality and healthful meal patterns during young adulthood. *J Am Diet Assoc.* 2007;107(9):1502–1510.

36. Gillman MW, Rifas-Shiman SL, Frazier AL, et al. Family dinner and diet quality among older children and adolescents. *Arch Fam Med.* 2000;9(3):235–240.

37. Hammons AJ, Fiese BH. Is frequency of shared family meals related to the nutritional health of children and adolescents? *Pediatrics.* 2011;127(6):e1565–e1574.

38. Rollins BY, Belue RZ, Francis LA. The beneficial effect of family meals on obesity differs by race, sex, and household education: the national survey of children's health, 2003-2004. *J Am Diet Assoc.* 2010;110(9):1335–1339.

39. Neumark-Sztainer D, Larson NI, Fulkerson JA, Eisenberg ME, Story M. Family meals and adolescents: what have we learned from Project EAT (Eating Among Teens)? *Public Health Nutr.* 2010;13(7):1113–1121.

40. The National Center on Addiction and Substance Abuse at Columbia University. The importance of family dinners, VIII. Available at: http://www.casacolumbia.org/templates/Publications_Reports.aspx#r118. Accessed November 3, 2017.

41. Loprinzi PD, Davis RE. Secular trends in parent-reported television viewing among children in the United States, 2001–2012. *Child Care Health Dev.* 2016;42(2):288–291.

42. Rideout V. *The Common Sense census: Media use by kids age zero to eight.* San Francisco, CA: Common Sense Media; 2017.

43. Kelly B, Halford JC, Boyland EJ, et al. Television food advertising to children: a global perspective. *Am J Public Health.* 2010;100(9):1730–1736.

44. Harris J, Schwartz M, Shehan C, et al. Snack FACTS 2015 Evaluating snack food nutrition and marketing to youth. In: *UConn Rudd Center for Food Policy & Obesity*; November 2015, revised January 2016.

45. Bell RA, Cassady D, Culp J, Alcalay R. Frequency and types of foods advertised on Saturday morning and weekday afternoon English- and Spanish-language American television programs. *J Nutr Educ Behav.* 2009;41(6):406–413.

46. Danner FW. A national longitudinal study of the association between hours of TV viewing and the trajectory of BMI growth among U.S. children. *J Pediatr Psychol.* 2008;33(10):1100–1107.

47. Laurson KR, Eisenmann JC, Welk GJ, Wickel EE, Gentile DA, Walsh DA. Combined influence of physical activity and screen time recommendations on childhood overweight. *J Pediatr.* 2008;153(2):209–214.

48. American Public Health Association. Policy Statement 2003-17. Food marketing and advertising directed at children and adolescents: implications for overweight. Available at: https://www.apha.org/policies-and-advocacy/public-health-policy-statements/policy-database/2014/07/24/16/35/food-marketing-and-advertising-directed-at-children-and-adolescents-implications-for-overweight. Accessed November 3, 2017.

49. Boynton-Jarrett R, Thomas TN, Peterson KE, Wiecha J, Sobol AM, Gortmaker SL. Impact of television viewing patterns on fruit and vegetable consumption among adolescents. *Pediatrics.* 2003;112(6 Pt 1):1321–1326.

50. Harris JL, Bargh JA, Brownell KD. Priming effects of television food advertising on eating behavior. *Health Psychol.* 2009;28(4):404–413.

51. Council on Communications and Media. Media and young minds. *Pediatrics.* 2016;138(5):e20162591.

52. Hauk L. Use of media by school-aged children and adolescents: a policy statement from the AAP. *Am Fam Physician.* 2017;96(1):56–57.

53. Dye BA, Hsu KL, Afful J. Prevalence and measurement of dental caries in young children. *Pediatr Dent.* 2015;37(3):200–216.

54. Faine M. Nutrition and oral health. Paper presented at: Proceedings of Promoting Oral Health of Children with Neurodevelopmental Disabilities and Other Special Health Care Needs; May 2001; Seattle, WA.

55. Palmer CA. *Diet and nutrition in oral health.* 2nd ed. Upper Saddle River, N.J.: Pearson/Prentice Hall; 2007.

56. Nunn ME, Braunstein NS, Krall Kaye EA, Dietrich T, Garcia RI, Henshaw MM. Healthy eating index is a predictor of early childhood caries. *J Dent Res.* 2009;88(4):361–366.

57. White-Graves MV, Schiller MR. History of foods in the caries process. *J Am Diet Assoc.* 1986;86(2):241–245.

58. Navia JM. Carbohydrates and dental health. *Am J Clin Nutr.* 1994;59(suppl 3):719S–727S.

59. Policy on Early Childhood Caries (ECC): Classifications, Consequences, and Preventive Strategies. *Pediatr Dent.* 2016;38(6):52–54.

60. Section on Oral Health. Maintaining and improving the oral health of young children. *Pediatrics.* 2014;134(6):1224–1229.

61. U.S. Department of Health and Human Services. *Oral Health in America: A Report of the Surgeon General—Executive Summary.* Rockville, MD: U.S. Department of Health and Human Services, National Institute of Dental and Craniofacial Research, National Institutes of Health; 2000.

62. Gupta PM, Perrine CG, Mei Z, Scanlon KS. Iron, Anemia, and Iron Deficiency Anemia among Young Children in the United States. *Nutrients.* 2016;8(6):doi:10.3390/nu8060330.

63. Centers for Disease Control and Prevention (CDC). Iron deficiency—United States, 1999–2000. *MMWR Morb Mortal Wkly Rep.* 2002;51(40):897–899.

64. Nead KG, Halterman JS, Kaczorowski JM, Auinger P, Weitzman M. Overweight children and adolescents: a risk group for iron deficiency. *Pediatrics.* 2004;114(1):104–108.

65. Lozoff B, Beard J, Connor J, Barbara F, Georgieff M, Schallert T. Long-lasting neural and behavioral effects of iron deficiency in infancy. *Nutr Rev.* 2006;64(5 Pt 2):S34–S43.

66. Monsen ER, Hallberg L, Layrisse M, et al. Estimation of available dietary iron. *Am J Clin Nutr.* 1978;31(1):134–141.

67. Martin JA, Hamilton BE, Osterman MJ, Driscoll AK, Mathews TJ. Births: Final Data for 2015. *Natl Vital Stat Rep.* 2017;66(1):1.

68. Hediger ML, Scholl TO, Schall JI. Implications of the Camden Study of adolescent pregnancy: interactions among maternal growth, nutritional status, and body composition. *Ann N Y Acad Sci.* 1997;817:281–291.

69. Rees JM, Lederman SA, Kiely JL. Birth weight associated with lowest neonatal mortality: infants of adolescent and adult mothers. *Pediatrics.* 1996;98(6 Pt 1):1161–1166.

70. Rasmussen KM, Yaktine AL, Institute of Medicine (U.S.). Committee to Reexamine IOM Pregnancy Weight Guidelines. *Weight Gain During Pregnancy: Reexamining the Guidelines.* Washington, DC: National Academies Press; 2009.

71. Scholl TO, Hediger ML, Schall JI. Maternal growth and fetal growth: pregnancy course and outcome in the Camden Study. *Ann N Y Acad Sci.* 1997;817:292–301.

72. Fleming N, O'Driscoll T, Becker G, Spitzer RF, COMMITTEE C. Adolescent Pregnancy Guidelines. *J Obstet Gynaecol Can.* 2015;37(8):740–756.

73. Lozoff B, Georgieff MK. Iron deficiency and brain development. *Semin Pediatr Neurol.* 2006;13(3):158–165.

74. Nielsen JN, Gittelsohn J, Anliker J, O'Brien K. Interventions to improve diet and weight gain among pregnant adolescents and recommendations for future research. *J Am Diet Assoc.* 2006;106(11):1825–1840.

75. Story M. Promoting healthy eating and ensuring adequate weight gain in pregnant adolescents: issues and strategies. *Ann N Y Acad Sci.* 1997;817:321–333.

76. Substance Abuse and Mental Health Services Administration, Office of Applied Studies. *The NSDUH Report: Trends in Substance Use, Dependence or Abuse, and Treatment among Adolescents: 2002 to 2007.* Rockville, MD: SAMHSA; 2008.

77. Kann L, McManus T, Harris WA, et al. Youth Risk Behavior Surveillance - United States, 2015. *MMWR Surveill Summ.* 2016;65(6):1–174.

78. Center for Behavioral Health Statistics and Quality. Key substance use and mental health indicators in the United States: Results from the 2015 National Survey on Drug Use and Health. In. *HHS Publication No. SMA 16-4984, NSDUH Series H-51*2016.

79. Lowenberg ME, Development of food patterns in young children. In: Pipes PL, ed. *Nutrition Infancy and Childhood.* 4th ed. W.B. Saunders; 1989.

80. Committee on Injury, Violence, and Poison Prevention. Prevention of choking among children. *Pediatrics.* 2010;125(3):601–607.

81. Smith MM, Lifshitz F. Excess fruit juice consumption as a contributing factor in nonorganic failure to thrive. *Pediatrics.* 1994;93(3):438–443.

82. Nicklas T, O'Neill C, Fulgoni III V. Consumption of 100% fruit juice is associated with better nutrient intake and diet quality but not with weight status in children: NHANES 2007–2010. *Int J Child Health Nutr.* 2015;4:112–121.

83. United States. Department of Health and Human Services., United States. Department of Agriculture., United States. Dietary Guidelines Advisory Committee. *Dietary Guidelines for Americans, 2015–2020.* 8th ed. Washington, D.C.: U.S. Department of Health and Human Services and U.S. Department of Agriculture; 2015.

84. Auerbach BJ, Wolf FM, Hikida A, et al. Fruit juice and change in BMI: a meta-analysis. *Pediatrics.* 2017;139(4):e20162454.

85. Committee on Nutrition. American Academy of Pediatrics: The use and misuse of fruit juice in pediatrics. *Pediatrics.* 2001;107(5):1210–1213.

86. Fiorito LM, Marini M, Francis LA, Smiciklas-Wright H, Birch LL. Beverage intake of girls at age 5 y predicts adiposity and weight status in childhood and adolescence. *Am J Clin Nutr.* 2009;90(4):935–942.

87. Vikraman S, Fryar CD, Ogden CL. Caloric intake from fast food among children and adolescents in the United States, 2011–2012. *NCHS Data Brief.* 2015(213):1–8.

88. Alaimo K, Carlson JJ, Pfeiffer KA, et al. Project FIT: A school, community and social marketing intervention improves healthy eating among low-income elementary school children. *J Community Health.* 2015;40(4):815–826.

89. Blitstein JL, Cates SC, Hersey J, et al. Adding a social marketing campaign to a school-based nutrition education program improves children's dietary intake: a quasi-experimental study. *J Acad Nutr Diet.* 2016;116(8):1285–1294.

90. Story M, Neumark-Sztainer D, French S. Individual and environmental influences on adolescent eating behaviors. *J Am Diet Assoc.* 2002;102(suppl 3):S40–S51.

91. Caruso ML, Cullen KW. Quality and cost of student lunches brought from home. *JAMA Pediatr.* 2015;169(1):86–90.

92. Johnson DB, Podrabsky M, Rocha A, Otten JJ. Effect of the Healthy Hunger-Free Kids Act on the nutritional quality of meals selected by students and school lunch participation rates. *JAMA Pediatr.* 2016;170(1):e153918.

93. Welker E, Lott M, Story M. The School Food Environment and Obesity Prevention: progress over the last decade. *Curr Obes Rep.* 2016;5(2):145–155.

94. Briggs M, Mueller CG, Fleischhacker S, American Dietetic Association, School Nutrition Association, Society for Nutrition Education. Position of the American Dietetic Association, School Nutrition Association, and Society for Nutrition Education: comprehensive school nutrition services. *J Am Diet Assoc.* 2010;110(11):1738–1749.

95. U.S. Department of Health and Human Services, Office of Disease Prevention and Health Promotion. Healthy People 2020. Washington, DC: Available at: http://www.healthypeople.gov/2020/LHI/default.aspx. Accessed June 17, 2013.

96. Office of Disease Prevention & Health Promotion, U.S. Department of Health and Human Services. 2008 Physical Activity Guidelines for Americans Summary. 2008; Available at: http://www.health.gov/paguidelines/guidelines/summary.aspx. Accessed June 26, 2013.

97. Janssen I, Leblanc AG. Systematic review of the health benefits of physical activity and fitness in school-aged children and youth. *Int J Behav Nutr Phys Act*. 2010;7:40.

98. Subcommittee of the President's Council on Fitness, Sports, and Nutrition. *Physical Activity Guidelines for Americans Midcourse Report: Strategies to Increase Physical Activity Among Youth*. Washington, DC: U.S. Department of Health and Human Services; 2012.

99. Anderson SE, Economos CD, Must A. Active play and screen time in U.S. children aged 4 to 11 years in relation to sociodemographic and weight status characteristics: a nationally representative cross-sectional analysis. *BMC Public Health*. 2008;8:366.

100. Simeon DT, Grantham-McGregor S. Effects of missing breakfast on the cognitive functions of school children of differing nutritional status. *Am J Clin Nutr*. 1989;49(4):646–653.

101. Brown HE, Atkin AJ, Panter J, Wong G, Chinapaw MJ, van Sluijs EM. Family-based interventions to increase physical activity in children: a systematic review, meta-analysis and realist synthesis. *Obes Rev*. 2016;17(4):345–360.

102. LaBotz M, Griesemer BA, Council on Sports Medicine and Fitness. Use of performance-enhancing substances. *Pediatrics*. 2016;138(1).

103. Spear B. Sports nutrition for adolescents. *Building Block Life*. 2008;31(1):1–8.

104. Vos MB, Kaar JL, Welsh JA, et al. Added sugars and cardiovascular disease risk in children: a scientific statement from the American Heart Association. *Circulation*. 2017;135(19):e1017–e1034.

105. McGill CR, Fulgoni VL, Devareddy L. Ten-year trends in fiber and whole grain intakes and food sources for the United States population: National Health and Nutrition Examination Survey 2001–2010. *Nutrients*. 2015;7(2):1119–1130.

106. Adolphus K, Lawton CL, Champ CL, Dye L. The effects of breakfast and breakfast composition on cognition in children and adolescents: a systematic review. *Adv Nutr*. 2016;7(3):590S–612S.

107. Pollitt E, Cueto S, Jacoby ER. Fasting and cognition in well- and undernourished schoolchildren: a review of three experimental studies. *Am J Clin Nutr*. 1998;67(4):779S–784S.

108. Kleinman RE, Murphy JM, Little M, et al. Hunger in children in the United States: potential behavioral and emotional correlates. *Pediatrics*. 1998;101(1):E3.

109. Alaimo K, Olson CM, Frongillo EA. Food insufficiency and American school-aged children's cognitive, academic, and psychosocial development. *Pediatrics*. 2001;108(1):44–53.

110. Melina V, Craig W, Levin S. Position of the Academy of Nutrition and Dietetics: Vegetarian diets. *J Acad Nutr Diet*. 2016;116(12):1970–1980.

111. Vegetarian Resource Group. How many teens and other youth are vegetarian and vegan? Available at: http://www.vrg.org/blog/2014/05/30/how-many-teens-and-other-youth-are-vegetarian-and-vegan-the-vegetarian-resource-group-asks-in-a-2014-national-poll. Accessed November 21, 2017.

112. Robinson-O'Brien R, Perry CL, Wall MM, Story M, Neumark-Sztainer D. Adolescent and young adult vegetarianism: better dietary intake and weight outcomes but increased risk of disordered eating behaviors. *J Am Diet Assoc*. 2009;109(4):648–655.

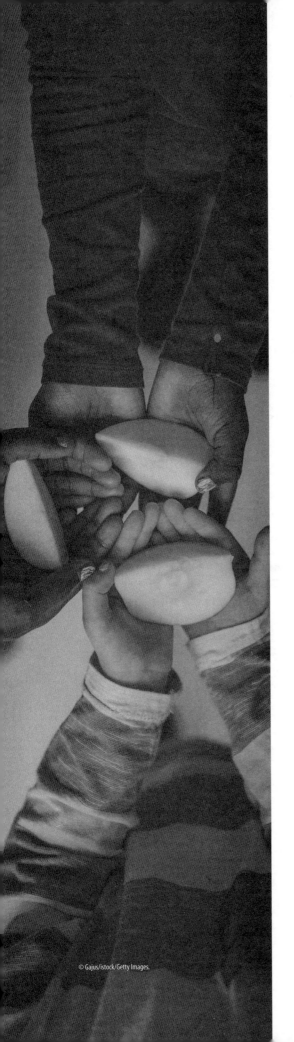

© Gajus/istock/Getty Images.

Nutrition Support

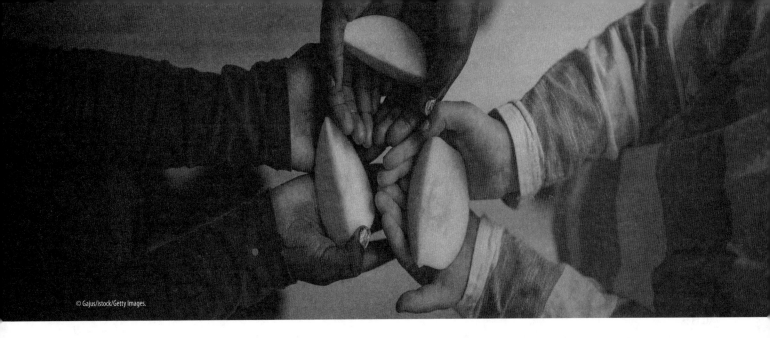

© Gajus/istock/Getty Images.

CHAPTER 10

Enteral Nutrition

Amy Coen and Alison Ruffin

LEARNING OBJECTIVES

- Selecting appropriate candidates for enteral nutrition, ranging in age from birth to 18 years.
- Selecting specific products.
- Administering and monitoring enteral feedings.
- Considering factors specific to the pediatric population.

▶ Introduction

Normal nutrition is received by voluntarily ingesting a variety of foods, both liquid and solid. Nutritional intake provides the required nutrients for the normal growth and development of infants and children. This process can be interrupted as a result of some acute or chronic conditions that affect an infant, child, or adolescent's ability to ingest, digest, or absorb nutrients. When these individuals are unable to obtain adequate nutrients from oral intake, supplemental feedings are warranted.

Enteral nutrition (EN) is the delivery of nutrition in the form of carbohydrate, protein, and/or fat directly into the **gastrointestinal tract** (GI) via a tube, catheter, or stoma. Indications for EN are a functioning GI tract of sufficient length and absorptive capacity. Infants and

children meeting these criteria who possess the inability to consume adequate nutrition via the oral cavity are candidates for EN.[1-3]

Enteral nutrition is preferred over parenteral nutrition because it is associated with fewer complications, is less expensive, and helps maintain the integrity of the GI mucosa.[2,3] Advances in commercial formulas and equipment for delivering EN have made enteral feeding safe and efficacious to administer to pediatric patients in either the hospital or home setting.

Condition Specific Nutrition Screening

The healthcare team should establish inpatient and outpatient criteria for the consideration of EN. Nutrition screening should identify patients who are at nutritional risk or malnourished and those who possess feeding disorders that affect their ability to ingest adequate nutrition. Factors to evaluate include:[4-6]

- Usual intake of less than 80% of calorie needs or less than 90% of fluid needs
- Weight loss or inadequate growth
- Weight-for-length or BMI z-score -1 or below
- Excessive feeding time
- Oral and/or texture aversion
- Mechanical problems with mastication, swallowing, or peristalsis

Pediatric patients with a variety of diseases who are at nutritional risk have been shown to benefit from EN (**FIGURE 10.1**).[3,5,7,8] Specific screens can be developed for a particular disease state or condition, as the need arises.

Patients with contraindications for receiving EN may be candidates for parenteral nutrition (**FIGURE 10.2**).[3,5,7,8] These patients should be continually re-evaluated for the ability to initiate or advance enteral or oral nutrition.

Functional:
- Inability to consume adequate intake
- Dysphagia
- Congenital malformations (i.e. cleft palate, Pierre Robin syndrome, tracheoesphageal fistula)
- Prematurity

Psychological:
- Anorexia
- Oral aversion

Injury:
- Trauma
- Burns
- Ingestion
- Sepsis

Obstruction:
- Intubation
- Head/neck cancer

Altered or Impaired absorption/digestion
- Cystic fibrosis
- Short bowel syndrome
- Food allergies
- Chronic liver disease
- Solid organ transplants

Additional Diseases and Disorders:
- Genetic/Metabolic Disorders
- Neurological disorders
- Congenital heart disease
- Chronic kidney disease
- Severe chronic lung disease

Data from Braegger C, Decsi T, Dias JA, et al. Practical approach to paediatric enteral nutrition: a comment by the ESPGHAN committee on nutrition. *J Pediatr Gastroenterol Nutr.* 2010;51(1):110–122.[3]
Axelrod D, Kazmerski K, Iyer K. Pediatric enteral nutrition. *J Parenter Enteral Nutr.*2006;30(1): S21–S26.[5]
Kleinman RE, Greer FR (eds). *Pediatric Nutrition Handbook.* 7th ed. Elk Grove Village, IL: American Academy of Pediatrics; 2014.[7]
Sonneville K, Duggan C (eds). *Manual of Pediatric Nutrition.* 5th ed. Shelton, CT: Peoples Medical Publishing House USA; 2014:158–433.[8]

FIGURE 10.1 Potential Indications for Enteral Nutrition in the Pediatric Patient[3,5,7,8]

- Gastrointestinal obstruction, ileus, or perforation
- Inflammatory bowel disease
- Intestinal atresia
- Intestinal dysmotility
- Limited or impaired absorptive surface
- Necrotizing enterocolitis
- Gastrointestinal bleed
- Side effects of cancer therapy

Data from Braegger C, Decsi T, Dias JA, et al. Practical approach to paediatric enteral nutrition: a comment by the ESPGHAN committee on nutrition. *J Pediatr Gastroenterol Nutr.* 2010;51(1):110–122.[3]
Axelrod D, Kazmerski K, Iyer K. Pediatric enteral nutrition. *J Parenter Enteral Nutr.* 2006;30(1):S21–S26.[5]
Kleinman RE, Greer FR (eds). *Pediatric Nutrition.* 7th ed. Elk Grove Village, IL: American Academy of Pediatrics; 2014.[7]
Hendricks KM. In: [8]Sonneville K, Duggan C (eds). *Manual of Pediatric Nutrition.* 5th ed. Shelton, CT; Peoples Medical Publishing House USA;2014:158–433.[8]

FIGURE 10.2 Potential Contraindications for Enteral Nutrition in the Pediatric Patient

Nutrition Assessment

Once an individual is flagged as a candidate for EN, an assessment can be completed by a **registered dietitian nutritionist** (RDN). Nutrition assessment is the first step in the Nutrition Care Process, described in full in Chapter 1 of this book. This section discusses relevant topics that should be considered when interpreting the data in order to implement appropriate EN interventions.

Nutrient Requirements

The DRIs (RDAs) are based on estimated needs for healthy individuals. When using DRIs as a standard for comparison, differences in the needs of nonambulatory, ill, or physically delayed children must be considered. In addition to using other predictive equations with activity factors, height has also been used to estimate calorie needs for individuals with various degrees of motor dysfunction. However, actual energy needs may still be lower or higher than potential therapeutic needs that are dictated by specific disease or deficiency states. Ideally, if equipment to perform an indirect calorimetry is available, **resting energy expenditure** (REE) should be measured for patients with suspected altered energy needs or for those who do not respond to nutrition support.[7,9]

In specific circumstances, both pediatric and adult formulas may require vitamin and/or mineral supplementation. Supplements may not be absorbed or utilized in the body as desired and should be evaluated frequently. Infant formulas generally provide adequate amounts of vitamins and minerals with a volume of 1000 mL; however, individuals with low calorie needs may require vitamin and mineral supplementation.

Adult enteral formulas are designed to provide the adult RDAs for vitamins and minerals when a volume of 1500–2000 mL/day is administered. When these adult enteral products are administered to children at lower volumes, some nutrients may not be adequate. A micro-nutrient analysis may be warranted.

Renal Solute Load and Fluid Balance

The **renal solute load** (RSL) of a formula consists primarily of electrolytes and metabolic end products of protein metabolism that the kidneys must excrete in the urine.[10] These solutes require water for urinary excretion and therefore have a major effect on water balance. Infants have an immature renal system with limited concentrating ability, and they require more free water to excrete solutes than do older children and adults. Therefore, infants are at particular risk for negative water balance and subsequent dehydration. **Potential renal solute load** (PRSL) does not need to be calculated routinely, but is important to determine with those patients who have medical problems or formula prescriptions that would influence renal metabolism. Equations for PRSL vary in the units of measurement for solute load. An example equation is:[7]

$$\text{PRSL (mOsm/L)} = \text{mEq sodium/L} + \text{mEq potassium/L} + \text{mEq chloride/L} + [4 \times \text{protein g/L}]$$

The renal solute load and fluid balance should be closely monitored when infants have a low fluid intake, are receiving calorically dense feedings, or have increased extrarenal fluid losses (i.e., fever, diarrhea, sweating) and/or impaired renal concentrating ability.[10] Neurologically impaired infants and children who are unable to indicate thirst may also be at risk for dehydration.

When determining fluid needs, it should be considered how much free water a patient's formula contains. Adult formulas are higher in protein and electrolytes, therefore they possess a higher RSL. In instances with a higher RSL, proper precautions should be taken; for example, additional water may be required and can usually be given while flushing the feeding tube.

Osmolality

Osmolality refers to the number of active particles in a kilogram of solution. The osmolality of a formula may affect tolerance. Feeding intolerances associated with delivering a hyperosmolar formula may include delayed gastric emptying, abdominal distention, vomiting, or diarrhea.

Carbohydrates, electrolytes, and amino acids are the major factors that determine the gastrointestinal osmotic load of a formula. Smaller particles, such as glucose and free amino acids, contribute more to a higher osmolality than do larger particles, such as polysaccharides or intact protein molecules. Thus, formulas that contain hydrolyzed protein and monosaccharides will tend to have a higher osmolality than will formulas with intact protein and glucose polymers.[8]

Osmolality of infant feeds typically range from 200 mOsm/kg to just over 400 mOsm/kg. Although there is little evidence regarding suggested upper limits for osmolality of EN feeds, current recommendations are that osmolality does not exceed 450 mOsm/kg (400 mOsm/L).[11]

Medications can also increase osmolality significantly and should be evaluated before selecting a formula.[12] The osmolality of Pregestimil, for example, concentrated to 27 kcal/oz is approximately 446 mOsm/kg, whereas a multivitamin with iron (Poly-Vi-Sol with Iron) at 10 mg/mL Fe is 10,683 mOsm/kg.[12]

Nutrition Diagnosis

Following completion of the nutrition assessment, one can identify an appropriate nutrition diagnosis. The nutrition diagnosis is something that can be improved (or resolved) through a nutrition intervention. **TABLE 10.1** includes examples of common nutrition diagnoses associated with EN.

Nutrition Intervention

Nutrition intervention should be focused on how to improve or resolve the nutrition problem. It is vital that the registered dietitian choose the most urgent nutrition diagnosis in order to choose the most appropriate enteral nutrition intervention. The nutrition interventions listed in this chapter will primarily focus on information/considerations related to food and nutrient delivery given that this is most closely associated with EN.

Product Selection

Enteral formulas are classified by the **US Food and Drug Administration** (FDA) under the heading of medical foods. Medical foods are described as "a food which is formulated to be consumed or administered enterally under the supervision of a physician."[13] **Medical foods** are not regulated as either conventional foods or drugs.[14] Infant formula must meet FDA assurance of nutrition quality, as well as labeling criteria, nutrient content, and manufacturers quality control procedures before marketing of the infant formula.

A wide variety of commercially prepared infant, pediatric, and adult enteral formulas can be utilized for pediatric patients requiring EN. The proper product selection is contingent on a number of factors related to the specific medical and nutritional status of the patient. Patient-specific factors include:[5,7]

- Age
- Medical history/current medical status
- Gastrointestinal function
- History of feeding tolerance
- Food allergies
- Nutrient requirements
- Feeding route

TABLE 10.1 Common Diagnoses Associated with Enteral Nutrition

Problem (P)	Etiology (E)	Signs/Symptoms (S)
Inadequate energy intake	Decreased oral intake, difficulty with feeding/prolonged feeding time, recent illness, respiratory distress/dyspnea	Weight loss Average intake of less than 50% of estimated calorie needs
Increased energy expenditure	Trauma, altered/impaired absorption, voluntary activity	Unintended weight loss of X% in Y months, inadequate weight gain, predicted need of approximately X calories per day, Indirect calorimetry result indicating need of X calories per day.
Inadequate oral intake	Inability to self-feed Lack of access to food	Reports of intake less than 50% of usual intake/estimated needs
Inadequate enteral nutrition infusion	Intolerance of feeds Increased energy needs	Emesis/diarrhea Results of indirect calorimetry
Swallowing difficulty	Oral motor dysfunction	Coughing and choking at meal times, aspiration during swallow study
Altered GI function	Gastroparesis, short bowel syndrome	Inability to tolerate 100% PO intake, inability to tolerate standard milk based formula, Emesis/diarrhea/constipation, inadequate weight gain/weight loss

Several formula-specific factors must also be considered before choosing an enteral formula; these include:[5,7]

- Osmolality
- Renal solute load
- Nutritional components
- Product availability
- Cost
- Caloric density

Infants Less than 1 Year of Age

Human milk and/or commercial infant formulas constitute the most appropriate feedings for infants who are less than 1 year of age. Human milk is the optimal choice when available. When human milk is not available, commercially prepared infant formulas are acceptable alternatives.

Breast Milk

Human milk provides the optimal food for infants and offers many immunologic and nutritional benefits. It is recommended that healthy, term infants receive breast milk exclusively for the first 6 months of life, with continuation of breastfeeding (in addition to introducing solid foods) through the first year of life. Contraindications for using breast milk include infants with classic galactosemia, an inborn error of metabolism that affects an individual's ability to metabolize the sugar galactose. In this case, a galactose and lactose free formula should be provided. The majority of other inborn errors of metabolism allow for at least a small amount of human milk to be provided in combination with a metabolic formula. Other contraindications for providing human milk include certain infections such as **human immunodeficiency virus (HIV)**, **T-cell lymphotrophic virus (HTLV)**, or untreated tuberculosis. For mothers requiring medications, there is a concern for the effects that certain drugs could have on the infant. Medications should be reviewed by appropriate health care professionals/resources in order to determine if it is safe for an infant to continue to receive mother's breast milk.[7,15]

Infants who are unable to nurse at the breast can receive pumped breast milk through a feeding tube; however, the delivery of breast milk by tube requires some unique considerations. First of all, the mother must be taught safe methods for collecting and storing her milk as well as proper care and sanitation of the delivery system.[7]

EN feedings of breast milk have been associated with appreciable fat losses, which result in a significant reduction of energy delivered to the infant. These losses occur because the fat in human milk separates and collects in the infusion system. A caloric loss of approximately 17–34% is typical depending on the method of delivery. Whenever possible, bolus feedings are preferred over continuous feeds due to increased fat loss using the continuous method of delivery.[16,17,18] It should be noted that when residual milk is flushed from the tubing, a large fat bolus may be delivered to the patient.[16–19] Patients with impaired gastrointestinal function may not tolerate a fat bolus.

Short-term refrigeration of human milk has been shown to increase the delivery of fat during continuous feedings.[20] Therefore, when delivering a continuous feeding of breast milk, the use of refrigerated milk may be advantageous. Unfortunately, significant fat losses still occur. Using a syringe pump helps to decrease the adherence of fat to the feeding pump bag and tubing. It is also advantageous to invert the syringe pump to encourage any separation of fat to be pushed through the pump first.[16]

Infant Formula Feedings

Iron-fortified infant formulas are an appropriate substitute for infants who are not able to receive breast milk. The most common breast milk substitutes are manufactured as dried powders, which then require reconstitution with water. Powdered formulas are usually the least expensive form of formula. Several manufacturing companies also offer a concentrated liquid formula that still requires reconstitution with water. Ready-to-feed infant formulas do not require mixing. They are provided by a small number of manufacturers and in a limited number of products. Typically ready-to-feed formulas are the most expensive form of formula. When available, the use of sterile liquid formula is preferred over powdered formulas. Powder formulas should be stored and prepared in a safe manner. Lids, scoops, and other mixing materials should be kept clean. It is best to use sterile water when reconstituting powdered formulas.[1,21–22]

A broad range of formulas are available with different characteristics. These products are suited for a variety of medical problems found in pediatrics, and are listed in **TABLE 10.2**. Most manufacturers' product guides have detailed information about the indicated use of formulas and absorption/utilization routes.[23–30] Infant formulas can be classified according to the protein source: cow's milk, soy, protein hydrolysate, or amino acid.

There is limited research available regarding the concentrated infant formula. It has been proposed that

an average density of 60–70 kcal/100 mL (18–21 kcal/oz) is appropriate for healthy term infants.[31] The standard dilution for infant formulas is typically 20 kcal/oz; however, there are some formulas that are now available in 19 kcal/oz. Infants who have increased metabolic needs and/or a decreased fluid tolerance may not be able to consume an adequate volume of standard formulas in order to promote growth. In this instance, a more concentrated formula may be needed. Infants and children with some conditions such as chronic lung disease, congenital heart disease, or chronic renal failure may require a formula with a caloric density greater than 20 kcal/oz. Concentrated infant formulas may also be useful for infants with malnutrition during periods of catch-up growth.

Infant formulas can be concentrated cautiously to a maximum of 30 kcal/oz by adding less water to a concentrated liquid or powdered formula base. If human milk is used instead of infant formulas, it can be "concentrated" with the addition of powdered infant formula. When this formula base (or human milk) is concentrated, the infant's water balance in relation to the RSL should be monitored. Patients receiving formula concentrated above 20 kcal/oz should be monitored frequently for signs of dehydration that include irregular output of urine, stool, emesis or high urine specific gravity or nutrient imbalances. Diluting formula to less than 20 kcal/oz should be done only with careful consideration and monitoring because of the risk of hyponatremia, diluted or insufficient nutrients, and/or excess fluid. A nutrient analysis should be completed for patients requiring formulas concentrated to 30 kcal/oz or diluted below 20 kcal/oz in order to determine if the patient is still receiving an appropriate distribution of macronutrients, vitamins, and minerals. Vitamin or mineral supplements may be needed for patients receiving diluted formulas in order to meet the DRI/RDA. The use of modulars are appropriate for patients requiring formula concentrated up to 30 kcal/oz in order to avoid excess macronutrients, vitamins, or minerals. It is important to ensure that caregivers clearly understand the instructions for mixing formulas correctly when counseling for either increased or decreased caloric density.

To ensure adequate hydration for the initial fluid prescription, maintenance fluid needs can be calculated by using the Holliday-Segar equation which includes 100 mL/kg for the first 10 kg of body weight. For weight between 10 and 20 kg, use 1000 mL plus 50 mL/kg for each kg over 10 kg; for weight over 20 kg, use 1500 mL plus 20 mL/kg for each kg over 20 kg.[32] Fluid should be adjusted frequently based on weight gain changes. Insensible water loss should be considered, as well as additional needs caused by any medical condition.

TABLE 10.2 Characteristics of Selected Enteral Formulas[23-30]

Formula Classification	Product Classification (may contain one or more of the following:)	Possible Indications for Use	Examples of Infant Formula up to 12 Months	Pediatric Formula 1 to 10 Years	Adult Formula 10 Years and Above
Standard milk-based (SMB)	Intact or partially hydrolyzed protein Contains lactose Long-chain triglycerides Low to moderate osmolality	Normal functioning GI tract Lactose tolerance	Similac Advance (Abbott Nutrition) Enfamil Infant/Newborn (Mead Johnson) Good Start Gentle (Gerber) Human milk		
Standard milk-based-altered	Intact or partially hydrolyzed protein Electrolyte manipulation (low iron, altered calcium, phosphorous) Low renal solute load Reduced lactose or lactose free Added starch Low protein Low residue Unique carbohydrate/fat blends	Renal disease, liver disease, endocrine conditions Lactose intolerant Mild reflux Metabolic stress	Similac PM 60/40 Similac Sensitive Similac Total Comfort (Abbott Nutrition) Enfamil AR Enfamil Gentlease Enfamil Reguline (Mead Johnson) Good Start Soothe (Gerber)	Pediasure (Abbott Nutrition) Boost Kid Essentials Compleat Pediatric Nutren Junior (Nestle Health Science) Renastart (Vitaflo/Nestle Health Science)	Carnation Breakfast Essentials Ensure Products Glucerna Products Jevity Nepro Carb Steady Osmolite Promote Suplena with Carb Steady TwoCal HN **(Abbott Nutrition)** Boost Impact Glytrol Novasource Renal Nutren Nutren Pulmonary Pulmocare RenalCal (Nestle Health Science)

Type	Characteristics	Indications			
Standard soy lactose free	Intact or partially hydrolyzed protein	Lactose intolerance Galactosemia	Similac Soy Isomil (Abbott Nutrition) Enfamil Prosobee (Mead Johnson) Good Start Soy (Gerber)	Bright Beginnings Soy Pediatric Drink (PBM Nutritionals)	
Added Fiber	Intact protein Lactose free 6–25 g fiber/1000 mL Low-moderate osmolality	Constipation Diarrhea Normal digestive/absorptive capacity	Similac Expect Care for Diarrhea (Abbott Nutrition)	Pediasure with fiber (Abbott Nutrition) Compleat Pediatric products Nutren Jr with fiber (Nestle Health Science) Nourish (Functional Formularies) Kate Farms products (Kate Farm)	Ensure with fiber Jevity Osmolite (Abbott Nutrition) Compleat Boost Nutren with fiber‡ (Nestle Health Science) Impact with fiber (Nestle Health Science) Liquid Hope (Functional Formularies) Kate Farms products (Kate Farm)
Modified fat	Intact protein 81%–87% of fat as MCT (depending on product used)	Chylothorax Intestinal lymphangiectasia severe steatorrhea Long chain fatty acid oxidation disorders	Monogen with DHA & ARA (Nutricia North America) Enfamil Enfaport (Mead Johnson)	Portagen (Mead Johnson) Lipistart (VitaFlo/Nestle Health Science)	Portagen (Mead Johnson) Lipistart (VitaFlo/Nestle Health Science)
Semi-elemental	Extensively hydrolyzed protein Lactose free Low-moderate osmolality Partial MCT content	Steatorrhea Intestinal resection Cystic fibrosis Chronic liver disease Inflammatory bowel disease Allergy to cow's milk and soy proteins	Similac Alimentum (Abbott Nutrition) Nutramigen Pregestimil (Mead Johnson)	Pediasure Peptide (Abbott Nutrition) Peptamen Junior (Nestle Health Science) Kate Farms Peptide Plus (Kate Farm)	Perative Vital Products (Abbott Nutrition) Vital Peptide - for ages 14+ (Abbott Nutrition) Peptamen (Nestle Health Science) Kate Farms Peptide Plus (Kate Farm)

(continues)

TABLE 10.2 Characteristics of Selected Enteral Formulas[23-30] *(continued)*

Formula Classification	Product Classification (may contain one or more of the following:)	Possible Indications for Use	Examples of Infant Formula up to 12 Months	Pediatric Formula 1 to 10 Years	Adult Formula 10 Years and Above
Elemental	Protein as free amino acids Lactose free High osmolality Partial MCT content	Multiple/severe food protein allergies Eosinophilic gastrointestinal disorders Reflux Inflammatory bowel disease Short bowel syndrome	Elecare (Abbott Nutrition) Puramino (Mead Johnson) Alfamino Infant (Nestle Health Science) Neocate Infant (Nutricia North America) Gerber Extensive HA (Gerber)	Elecare Junior (Abbott Nutrition) Alfamino Junior Vivonex Pediatric (Nestle Health Science) Neocate Junior Neocate Splash (Nutricia North America)	Vivonex Plus Vivonex RTF Vivonex TEN Tolerex (Nestle Health Science)
Real food formulas	Intact protein Include blend of real foods Nutritionally complete Lactose Free	Convenient alternative to home blenderized feeds		Compleat Pediatric Reduced Calorie (Nestle Health Science) Nourish (Functional Formularies) Kate Farms Komplete (Kate Farm)	Compleat (Nestle Health Science) Liquid Hope (Functional Formularies) Kate Farms Komplete (Kate Farm)

Calorically dense	Lactose free High renal solute load High osmolality 1.2–2.0 kcal/mL	Fluid restriction Increased metabolic needs	Boost Kid Essentials (Nestle Health Science) Liquid Hope (Functional Formularies)	Glucerna 1.2 Glucerna 1.5 Jevity 1.2 Jevity 1.5 Nepro Carb Steady Osmolite 1.2 Osmolite 1.5 Oxepa Perative 1.3 Pulmocare Suplena TwoCal HN Vital 1.2 Vital 1.5 (Abbott Nutrition) Boost High Protein Diabetisource AC Fibersource HN Impact 1.5 Isosource HN Isosource 1.5 Novasource Renal Nutrihep Nutren Replete Nutren 1.5 Nutren 2.0 Nutren Pulmonary Resource 2.0 (Nestle Health Science) Liquid Hope (Functional Formularies)

(continues)

TABLE 10.2 Characteristics of Selected Enteral Formulas[23–30] *(continued)*

Formula Classification	Product Classification (may contain one or more of the following:)	Possible Indications for Use	Examples of Infant Formula up to 12 Months	Pediatric Formula 1 to 10 Years	Adult Formula 10 Years and Above
Follow-up Toddler formulas	Over 1 year of age Iron fortified Balanced nutrition with vitamins and minerals	Over 1 year of age		Similac Go and Grow Toddler (Abbott Nutrition) Enfagrow Toddler Transitions Enfagrow Toddler Transitions Gentlease Enfagrow Toddler Transitions Soy Enfagrow Toddler Next Step Nutramigen Toddler Puramino Toddler (Mead Johnson) Stage 3 Gerber Good Start Grow Stage 3 Gerber Good Start Soy (Gerber)	
Transitional Premature Formulas	Post-discharge formula for pre-term infants Iron fortified Balanced nutrition Increased protein, vitamins, and minerals compared to standard infant formula		Similac Neosure (Abbott Nutrition) Enfamil Enfacare (Mead Johnson)		

Data from Abbott Nutrition. Available at: https://abbottnutrition.com. Accessed April 6, 2018.[23]
Gerber. Available at: https://www.gerber.com/products/formula. Accessed October 8, 2017.[24]
Mead Johnson. Available at: http://www.meadjohnson.com/pediatrics/us-en/product-information/products. Accessed October 8, 2017.[25]
Nestle NutritionHealth Science. Available at: https://www.nestlehealthscience.com. Accessed October 8, 2017.[26]
Nutricia North America. Available at: http://www.nutricia.com. Accessed October 8, 2017.[27]
Perrigo Nutritionals. Available at: http://www.perrigonutritionals.com/pediatric-nutritionals.aspx. Accessed October 8, 2017.[28]
Functional Formularies. Available at: http://www.functionalformularies.com/liquid-hope-information.html. Accessed October 8, 2017.[29]
Kate Farms. Available at: https://nutrition.katefarms.com/kate-farms-pro-portfolio/. Accessed October 8, 2017.[30]

Children Older than 1 Year

Feedings for children between 1 and 10 years of age include a choice of pediatric follow-up formulas, pediatric enteral formulas, and/or various homemade blenderized feedings. The caloric density of feedings utilized for children in this age group can range from 30 kcal/oz to 60 kcal/oz. A change to a more calorically dense formula may not always be appropriate. Therefore, the caloric density of an enteral formula may need to be increased by using a modular if the patient has increased metabolic needs and/or decreased fluid tolerance.

Enteral products for this age group are isotonic and lactose free, with a partial MCT content to facilitate absorption. These formulas can be concentrated to provide higher levels of nutrients, but also have a higher osmolality. Additional vitamin or mineral supplementation may also be needed, depending on the specific volume provided.

Adolescents

Standard milk-based, lactose-free, elemental, fiber-containing, and calorically dense formulas are commercially available for children between the ages of 10 and 18 years. For these children, many factors require consideration, such as physical ability or limitations, calorie requirements, and volume tolerance. Adolescent nutrient needs increase with the last growth phase. Their calorie and protein needs may be met in a pediatric formula but other nutrient needs, such as calcium, sodium, and iron, are not met. It is important to assess the adequacy of the micronutrients provided by the volume of formula, particularly when assessing the intake of a child who requires low volumes in order to promote growth. Micronutrient analysis is helpful in matching a formula or combination of pediatric and adult formulas to meet the unique needs of the teen.

A variety of computer nutrition assessment programs are available; when selecting one, pediatric parameters and pediatric formulas within the database should be considered in the selection criteria.

Blenderized Tube Feedings

Blenderized tube feedings consist of a mixture of various meats, fruits, vegetables, milk (or formula), carbohydrates, fats, water, vitamins, and minerals that have been blenderized, or pureed into liquid and strained. These blenderized feeds can be made for use in an institution or in the home setting. Interest from patients and families has been increasing in recent years which indicates a need for clinicians to become more knowledgeable about this as a potential tube feeding option.

There have been a number of concerns in the past regarding home blenderized feeds, including increased risk for bacterial contamination, cost, labor intensity, nutritional value, and the potential for obstruction of the feeding tube. Homemade blenderized feedings are moderate in residue and moderate to high in osmolality and viscosity. Because their high viscosity hinders flow through small feeding tubes, these feedings are most often administered as gastrostomy tube feedings.[33]

Because inappropriate homemade tube feedings can result in hypernatremic dehydration and a number of nutrient deficiencies, it is important to perform a periodic analysis of the recipe, including verifying how the family is making the formula at home, the adequacy of the nutrients, and the associated fluids. It is equally important to monitor the intake of protein and electrolytes because excess may lead to a negative water balance in the patient.[12,34,35] Despite the number of concerns from clinicians and limited research with the use of blenderized feeds, there have been benefits listed in the literature, including improved feeding tolerance. **FIGURE 10.3** indicates some of the benefits and risks of using blenderized tube feedings.[33,34,35]

There are a variety of commercial ready to use blenderized options now available for both pediatric and adult patients. These products are referenced in Table 10.2. Ready to use blenderized options are preferred (if covered through the patient's insurance) since they reduce many of the previous concerns associated with blenderized tube feedings. For example, they provide a consistent delivery of macronutrients, vitamins, and

Benefits:
- Decreased cost (if patient's previous commercial formula was not covered by insurance)
- Opportunity for more variety of EN feeds
- Increased emotional support for family
- Improved tolerance to feeding (i.e. decreased gagging/retching)

Risks:
- Increased cost (if patient's previous commercial formula was covered by insurance)
- Increased potential for bacterial contamination
- Increased potential for vitamin/mineral deficiencies
- Increased complications with delivery (i.e. clogging of tubing)
- More labor intensive

Data from Escuro AA. Blenderized tube feeding: suggested guidelines to clinicians. *Pract Gastroenterol.* 2014:58–66.[33]
Walia C, Hoorn MV, Edlbeck A, Feuling MB. The registered dietitian nutritionist's guide to homemade tube feeding. *J Acad Nutr Diet.* 2017;117(1):11–16.[34]
Adapted from Boullata JI, Carrera AL, Harvey L, et al. ASPEN safe practices for enteral nutrition therapy. *J Parenter Enteral Nutr.* 2017;41(1):15–103.[35]

FIGURE 10.3 Benefits and Risks of Homemade Blenderized Tube Feedings[33,34,35]

minerals, which decreases the risk for nutrient deficiencies. These products also eliminate the need for mixing which greatly reduces the risk for bacterial contamination.

In addition to the previously listed concerns, there are other considerations before transitioning a patient to a blenderized tube feeding. The patient should be slowly transitioned from a commercial formula, keeping in mind that many patients may have never been introduced to some of the foods included in the goal recipe. It is recommended that any new foods be introduced one at a time. The patient's family should keep a backup supply of commercial formula in case of travel or emergencies.[34]

Commercial Adult Formulas

A large variety of adult enteral products are commercially available primarily through Abbott Nutrition or Nestle Health Science.[23,26] These products contain macronutrients in various forms and amounts. As with adolescent formulas, they can also be divided into several general categories: standard milk-based, lactose-free, elemental, fiber-containing, and calorically dense. General characteristics of selected adult enteral products with possible indications for use are covered in Table 10.2. This list does not include all products that are commercially available, but is intended to provide examples of products that are available in each general category. Information regarding the complete nutrient composition of commercial adult formulas is readily available from the manufacturer.

It should be noted that adult enteral products are not designed for use in children and have not been extensively tested in the pediatric population. Specific concerns regarding using these products in children are addressed in the following discussions of RSL and nutrient requirements.

Formula Change and Acceptance

When a change in formula is indicated as part of the treatment of a gastrointestinal problem, there is concern about acceptance. As formulas become more elemental, the taste becomes less sweet and more bitter or sour. Partially hydrolyzed and elemental formulas often also have a less pleasant odor and an unpleasant aftertaste.[36] Amniotic fluid and breast milk are sweet and vary in flavor based on the mother's diet.[37] Clinicians have noted a difference between an infant who is initially offered a hydrolysate formula (and accepts it well) versus an older infant who is changed to the formula. The rejection does not occur until after 4 months of age. An interesting study by Mennella and associates looked at acceptance of a protein-hydrolysate formula after initially being given either a hydrolysate or a milk-based formula. Infants who were given a hydrolysate throughout infancy continued

to accept it at 7.5 months (and disliked the better tasting cow's milk–based formula) whereas an infant who is switched to a hydrolysate at 7.5 months rejects it.[36] Their research indicates that responses to olfactory components of flavor are influenced by the child's experience.[37] This is also shown in 4- to 5-year-old children who were fed hydrolysates as infants and had more positive responses to them years later.[38,39]

Adolescents with phenylketonuria who went off of their formula have been able to go back to the formula with some difficulty but with fewer problems than those who were not exposed as infants.[40] Infants will readily drink hydrolyzed formulas if introduced before 4 months of age. If required after this age, it should be mixed with a formula that is already accepted while gradually increasing the proportion of hydrolysate.[37] The parents are advised to work closely with a dietitian in order to make this transition acceptable to the child.

Product Availability and Cost

The cost of commercial enteral formulas may exceed the financial resources of some families. Therefore, whenever medically possible, the least specialized enteral product should be considered. The more specialized the feedings are (e.g., hydrolyzed protein and MCT oil), the higher the cost will be.

Formula costs do not necessarily constitute a socioeconomic barrier. Infants and children who range in age from birth to 5 years may be enrolled in the **Women, Infants, and Children** (WIC) nutrition program if their family income falls below a certain level. A variety of infant and pediatric formulas are available through this program. The Medicaid program and private insurance companies may cover enteral formulas and needed supplies, such as tubes, bags, or pumps. Coverage varies, and the healthcare team should work closely with home care companies and insurers in order to ensure that the patient obtains the best coverage possible. Letters of medical necessity are sometimes helpful in obtaining coverage for a specific enteral feeding product.

Selection of Specific Feeding Routes

When nutrition cannot be consumed orally, an **enteral access device** (AED) or feeding tube can be placed in order to provide EN into the stomach or intestines. Common routes for EN in pediatric patients include orogastric, nasogastric, nasoduodenal, nasojejunal, gastrostomy, and jejunostomy feeding tubes. **Orogastric** (OG) tubes are inserted through the mouth and have the tip in the stomach. **Nasogastric** (NG) tubes are inserted through the nose and end in the stomach. **Nasoduodenal**

(ND) and **nasojejunal** (NJ) tubes are inserted through the nose and end in the intestine, specifically in the duodenum or jejunum. **Gastrostomy** (G-tube) and **jejunostomy** (J-tube) tubes are placed during a procedure and result in a tube entering the stomach or jejunum from outside the abdomen. A GJ tube offers benefits of both a gastrostomy and a jejunostomy tube with the ability to provide some medications and nutrition into the stomach and the remainder into the jejunum, as specified by the medical team, or to vent the stomach while using mostly the jejunum for medications, nutrition, and hydration.

Nasoenteric tubes, tubes which are inserted into the nose and go into the stomach (NG) or intestine (ND or NJ), are the most common route of enteral access. Generally, nasoenteric or orogastric tubes are used when the anticipated need for a feeding tube is short-term, such as up to 4–6 weeks.[35] These tubes may fail secondary to tube occlusion or tube dislodgement, resulting in more frequent interruptions to EN and medication administration compared with semi-permanent enterostomy tubes (G-tubes and J-tubes).[41]

Bedside placement of nasoenteric feeding tubes is feasible, but correct placement must be confirmed. The most common type of nasoenteric tube confirmation is X-ray; nasogastric tube placement can also be confirmed by gastric pH testing and by aspirating, or removing, stomach contents via the tube.[35,41] Placement of some nasoenteric (NG and ND) feeding tubes can now be confirmed without X-ray by using an electromagnetic device, which shows real-time placement of the tip of the feeding tube on a screen as the tube is inserted into the patient.[42]

Semi-permanent enterostomy tubes (G-tubes and J-tubes) are generally considered for patients who expect to need feeding tubes for a period longer than 4–6 weeks.[35] Placement for semi-permanent tubes requires a more substantial procedure with sedation and can be placed endoscopically, radiologically, or surgically.[43]

Percutaneous endoscopic gastrostomies (PEG), which are placed endoscopically, are generally less invasive and require less time under anesthesia.[40,43] Low-profile gastrostomy devices are frequently used as replacement devices after the stoma tract is well healed (usually 6 to 8 weeks).[35,43] There are also low-profile devices that can be placed initially as a one-step procedure.[43]

The risk of aspiration becomes a major consideration when determining whether the tube should be placed in the stomach or the small intestine. The evaluation process for **gastroesophageal reflux** (GER) may include **upper gastrointestinal endoscopy** (UGI), modified barium swallow, pH probe, and occasionally, an esophageal motility or gastric emptying study. If the patient is determined to have a high risk of aspiration due to GER, placement of an ND or GJ tube is appropriate. Fundoplication, a surgical repair for severe gastroesophageal reflux, can sometimes be beneficial in reducing GER; however, postoperative complications may include retching, swallowing problems, dumping syndrome, impaired esophageal emptying, slow feeding, and abdominal distention.[44,45]

Gastric Feeding

Providing food or formula into the stomach is called a gastric feeding, which includes oral feedings and OG, NG, and G-tube feedings. A direct gastric feeding is preferable to an intestinal feeding because it allows for a more normal digestive process. This is generally true because the stomach serves as a reservoir and provides for a gradual release of nutrients into the small bowel. Gastric feedings are associated with tolerance of higher volume and osmolality, a more flexible feeding schedule, easier tube insertions, and a lower frequency of diarrhea and dumping syndrome. Additionally, gastric acid has a bactericidal effect that may be an important factor in decreasing the patient's susceptibility to various infections.[46] See **TABLE 10.3** for enteral feeding sites and routes.

Nasogastric (NG) feeding tubes are used for short-term periods of up to 4–6 weeks.[35] Patients requiring long-term EN are often evaluated after this time to determine the best enteral device to meet their needs, such as a gastrostomy or G-tube.

Nasogastric feeding is contraindicated in patients who have an obstruction between the nose and stomach and may be contraindicated or require special placement in patients with recent face, head, and/or neck trauma.[35] Additionally, nasogastric tubes may not be tolerated in neonates, who are obligate nose breathers.[41] To prevent airway occlusion in this instance, orogastric tubes are often used for premature infants before development of the gag reflex around 34 weeks gestational age.[41]

Transpyloric Feedings

Transpyloric feedings, also called post-pyloric feedings, refer to tube feedings that provide EN below the pylorus of the stomach. The pylorus is a flap-like opening from the stomach into the first part of the small intestine, the duodenum. Nasoduodenal, nasojejunal, jejunal, and gastrojejunal tubes provide transpyloric feedings, which are desirable for patients who are at high risk of aspiration or who are unable to tolerate feedings into the stomach. Typically, the at risk population includes patients who have a diminished gag reflex, delayed gastric emptying, frequent vomiting, or severe GER.

TABLE 10.3 Types of Feeding Tubes[35,41,43,47]

Location	Type of Tube	Advantages	Disadvantages	Indications	Contraindications
Gastric	Orogastric (OG)	Bedside placement possible; procedure not required Nasal passages are not obstructed Promotes normal digestion Offers feeding regimen flexibility Generally allows for tolerance of higher volumes and concentration	Prevents oral feeding Easily dislodged Uncomfortable for alert individuals	Anticipated use <4–6 weeks Neonate <34 weeks without gag reflex Patient without gag reflex (i.e. intubated without ability to place nasoenteric tube)	Neonate >34 weeks with gag reflex Patient with gag reflex Facial trauma or esophageal injury that prohibits safe placement
	Nasogastric (NG)	Simplest placement Bedside placement possible; procedure not required Promotes normal digestion Most cost effective Offers feeding regimen flexibility Generally allows for tolerance of higher volumes and concentration	Easily dislodged May cause nasal or esophageal irritation Difficult to conceal	Anticipated use <4–6 weeks Generally the preferred initial tube, when no contraindications exist	High risk of aspiration Severe GER Delayed gastric emptying Facial trauma or esophageal injury that prohibits safe placement
	Percutaneous Endoscopic Gastrostomy (PEG) or Gastrostomy (G-tube)	Promotes normal digestion Less visible Offers feeding regimen flexibility Generally allows for tolerance of higher volumes and formula concentration	Requires surgical, endoscopic, or radiologic procedure Skin breakdown or leaking are possible at the tube site	Anticipated use >4–6 weeks Congenital esophageal abnormalities Esophageal injury or obstruction	High risk of aspiration Severe GER Delayed gastric emptying

Post-Pyloric	Nasoduodenal (ND) or Nasojejunal (NJ)	Bedside placement possible Reduced risk of aspiration Improved tolerance of feedings for patients prone to vomiting	Prevents use of bolus feeds Easily dislodged Radiological confirmation required Difficult to conceal	Anticipated use <4–6 weeks High risk of aspiration Severe GER Delayed gastric emptying Intractable vomiting	Patient tolerates gastric feeds with low risk of aspiration
	Jejunostomy (J-tube)	Reduced risk of aspiration Improved tolerance of feedings for patients prone to vomiting Less visible	Requires surgical, endoscopic, or radiologic procedure Cannot access stomach Prevents use of bolus feeds Skin breakdown or leaking are possible at the tube site	Anticipated use >4–6 weeks High risk of aspiration Severe GER Delayed gastric emptying Intractable vomiting Congenital abnormalities of the upper GI tract Distal intestinal obstruction	Patient tolerates gastric feeds with low risk of aspiration Access to stomach is also desired
	Gastrostomy & Jejunostomy (GJ tube)	Reduced risk of aspiration Improved tolerance of feedings for patients prone to vomiting Less visible Allows access to stomach and jejunum for division of medication and nutrition delivery or to vent the stomach to reduce bloating	Requires surgical, endoscopic, or radiologic procedure Easily dislodged Prevents use of bolus feeds Skin breakdown or leaking are possible at the tube site	Anticipated use >4–6 weeks High risk of aspiration Severe GER Delayed gastric emptying Intractable vomiting Congenital abnormalities of the upper GI tract Distal intestinal obstruction	Patient tolerates gastric feeds with low risk of aspiration

Administration of Feeding

The method of delivery, formula type and concentration, additional fluid needs, and initiation and advancement of enteral feedings are other key factors that the practitioner must consider in providing EN for patients.

Methods of Delivery

The specific method utilized for feeding delivery is contingent on the clinical condition of the patient and the anatomic location of the tube (gastric or transpyloric). **Continuous and bolus** (or intermittent) **feeding** administration are the two methods most often used for delivering enteral feedings. Bolus feedings are generally delivered to the stomach by gravity over 15 to 30 minutes on a schedule of every 2–4 hours or via pump over a 1-hour period multiple times during a 24-hour period. Bolus feeding more closely mimics a normal oral feeding pattern and is often preferred for this reason. Bolus feeds are typically used during the day as opposed to overnight because there is an increased likelihood of GER with bolus feeds.[35,43] Bolus feedings may better facilitate transition to a home setting and eventually off enteral feeds.

In contrast, the continuous method provides an infusion of enteral nutrition at a constant rate over a period of hours up to 24-hours a day. Continuous feedings are beneficial for patients who cannot tolerate bolus feedings, for patients with altered gastrointestinal function, and in the critical care setting. Patients with transpyloric feeding tubes must receive continuous feeds. Bolus feedings are not tolerated when administered directly into the intestines, as with transpyloric tube feedings. Continuous feedings require using a feeding pump to deliver formula at a consistent rate over a period of time.

In practice, the individual patient's tolerance ultimately dictates the method and schedule of delivery. In many cases, patients receive a combination of bolus feeds during the day and a continuous feeding overnight. Each method of delivery provides a number of specific advantages and disadvantages (see **FIGURE 10.4**).

Pumps

Enteral feeding pumps are typically utilized to control the rate of delivery of continuous feedings and bolus feedings. A number of enteral feeding pumps are available

---

Continuous Feedings

Advantages

- Ability to increase the volume of formula more rapidly
- Greater caloric intake when volume tolerance may be a problem
- Associated with reduced incidence of vomiting in individuals with gastroesophageal reflux
- Improved absorption for people with intestinal disorders
- Increased tolerance during critical illness
- May be cycled over less than 24 hours to provide some time off feeds. Nocturnal cycled feeds may be used for ambulatory patients to provide extra calories

Disadvantages

- More expensive feeding method because a pump is required for delivery
- Patient is attached to the feeding pump for duration of the feeding
- Less physiologic
- Periods of NPO (nil per os or nothing by mouth/tube) are more likely to cause a barrier to adequate nutrition
- Continuous feedings are required for patients with post-pyloric feedings
- May prolong transition to oral feeding due to lack of hunger

Bolus Feedings

Advantages

- Preferred method for ambulatory patients, if tolerated
- More physiologic because a normal feeding schedule is mimicked
- Greater flexibility in feeding schedule
- Can be provided via syringe, gravity, or pump
- Gravity bolus feedings are less expensive because an enteral pump is not required
- Pump bolus feedings allow for longer boluses over 30–60 minutes to improve tolerance
- More time off feeds
- May promote sooner transition to oral feeding by promoting hunger between feeds

Disadvantages

- May increase risk of aspiration
- Poorly tolerated in cases of gastric reflux, gastroparesis, or large bore feeding tubes
- May cause nausea, vomiting, diarrhea, or abdominal distention for people with poor tolerance
- Reduced weight gain and nutrient absorption in individuals with malabsorption
- Larger-bore tube may be required for gravity administration
- More time required for administration than for pump-delivered feedings
- Not feasible for patients with post-pyloric feeds

FIGURE 10.4 Methods of Delivering Enteral Feedings[35,46,41]

for use in pediatric patients. Portable enteral pumps or backpack pumps allow for greater patient mobility while receiving their enteral feeding.[48]

Important features of enteral pumps for use in the pediatric population include the ability to provide low delivery rates (less than 5 mL/hour) and to advance in small increments (0.5–5 mL/hour).[43] Other desirable features of pediatric pumps include tamper-proof controls, an occlusion alarm, and a low-battery indicator.[43,48] The feeding pumps need to be calibrated periodically and formula delivery should be within five percent of the ordered daily volume.[43] These features all contribute to the safe and efficient delivery of continuous tube feedings for the pediatric population.

Delivery of human milk via enteral feeding requires a different system than that for infant, pediatric, or adult formulas. The loss of fat and fat-soluble vitamins due to the adherence of the fat to the enteral pump bag and tubing poses a unique complication. Because the required volumes of human milk are often low, particularly with continuous infusions, a syringe pump is typically used to deliver human milk via an enteral feeding system. Using a syringe pump helps reduce, but does not eliminate, fat loss compared with the use of an enteral pump bag.[19,20,49]

Bolus and Continuous Feedings

In cases where enteral feeding pumps are not used, enteral formula can be delivered as boluses by syringe push or open syringe to gravity. To provide continuous feedings via gravity without a pump, the feeding bag is suspended on a bedside pole where the rate is dependent only on the height of the feeding bag.[50] The delivery rate of gravity feedings is not precise and may predispose the patient to gastroesophageal reflux or aspiration.

Initiation and Advancement of Feedings

There are published recommendations for advancing EN in pediatric patients.[46,51,52] Many of these recommendations are based on institutional practices and modification of adult regimens. Generally, the rate of advancement of a feeding regimen (**FIGURE 10.5**) is

Type	Patient Age	Initial Infusion Rate	Advancement	Goal
Continuous	0–12 months	1–2 mL/kg/h	1–2 mL/kg every 8 hours	5–6 mL/kg/h
	1–3 years	1 mL/kg/h	1 mL/kg every 8 hours	4–5 mL/kg/h
	4–10 years	20–30 mL/h	20–30 mL every 8 hours	3–4 mL/kg/h
	11–18 years	30–60 mL/h	30 mL/h every 8 hours	100–150 mL/h
Bolus	0–12 months	30–60 mL every 2–3 hours	15–60 mL/feeding	150 mL every 4–5 hours
	1–3 years	30–90 mL every 2–3 hours	60 mL/feeding	180 mL every 4–5 hours
	4–10 years	75–90 mL every 3 hours	60 mL/feeding	210 mL every 4–5 hours
	11–18 years	90–120 mL every 3 hours	60 mL/feeding	240 mL every 4–5 hours
Cyclic	0–12 months	1–2 mL/kg/h	1–2 mL/kg/2 h	75 mL/h × 12–18 h per day
	1–3 years	1 mL/kg/h	1 mL/kg/2 h	90 mL/h × 8–16 h per day
	4–10 years	25 mL/h	25 mL every 2 hours	120 mL/h × 8–16 h per day
	11–18 years	30 mL/h	30 mL every 2 hours	150 mL/h × 12 h per day

Adapted from Singhal S, Baker SS, Bojczuk GA, Baker RD. Tube feeding in children. *Pediatr Rev.* 2017;38(1):23–32.[41]
Data from Baker SS, Baker RD, Davis AM. *Pediatric Nutrition Support.* Burlington, MA: Jones & Bartlett Learning;2007.[51]

FIGURE 10.5 Initiation and Advancement of Feedings[41,51]

contingent on the structure and function of the patient's gastrointestinal tract and should be guided by the patient's age, underlying disease, nutrition status, and nutritional requirements, enteral access device, and tolerance.[35,41,51] Figure 10.5 offers one example of guidelines for initiation, advancement, and goals for enteral tube feedings based on age. Some patients may be able to advance more quickly, may require more gradual advancement, or may require goals smaller or larger than those listed.

Enteral nutrition should be initiated at a low rate or volume and gradually advanced to goal. Patient tolerance should be the guide as to whether advancement is going too quickly or too slowly. Ideally, the goal should be achievable within 24–48 hours of initiation in order to minimize the period of inadequate nutrition.

To plan an enteral nutrition feeding regimen, the patient's estimated nutrition needs, desired formula, formula concentration, and additional fluid needs should be determined first. Once the total volume of formula and/or additional fluids are determined, Figure 10.5 may then be used as a guide for initiation and advancement.

Continuous feedings should be initiated at a low rate, approximately 25–30% of the goal rate, and gradually increased by a set amount every 2–8 hours until the goal is achieved. Many patients do well starting on continuous feeds and transitioning to bolus or cyclic feeds once tolerance has been established. For example, using Figure 10.5, a 5 kg infant could start at a rate of 5 mL/hr and increase by 5 mL/hr every 8 hours until a goal of 25 mL/hr was achieved.

Patients may also start EN with small bolus feeds that gradually increase in volume until the daily goal volume is achieved. For example, if a 10 year old patient's goal feeding plan provides 210 mL formula every 4 hours, a reasonable plan would be to initiate with a 90 mL bolus feeding and advance by 60 mL/feeding every 4 hours until a goal of 210 mL per feeding is achieved. The first feeding would be 90 mL, the second feeding would be 150 mL provided 4 hours after the first feeding, the third feeding would be 210 mL provided 4 hours after the second feeding, and all feedings afterwards would be 210 mL every 4 hours.

Cyclic feeds may be initiated as a first form of EN, or patients may transition to cyclic feeds by gradually increasing the rate and decreasing the number of hours infusing feeds daily. For an 18 year old patient starting cyclic feeds as a first form of EN, formula could be started at 30 mL/h and increased by 30 mL every 2 hours until a goal of 150 mL every 12 hours is achieved. Some patients may use feeding plans that provide bolus feedings during the day and nocturnal cyclic feeds. In the case of combined bolus and nocturnal feeding regimens, the desired daily volume of formula may be divided into daytime and nighttime portions. The daily boluses and cyclic nocturnal feeds should each be gradually advanced.

Once patients are established on an enteral nutrition regimen that is well tolerated, gradual initiation and advancement are not usually necessary. However, during acute illnesses or hospitalizations, patients on established EN plans may require gradual initiation and advancement if EN has not been well tolerated or gastrointestinal intolerance is anticipated.

Infants and children who are being weaned from parenteral nutrition and/or who are malnourished generally require a more conservative feeding progression than what is typically administered to children who have normal gastrointestinal function.

Prevention and Treatment of Complications

Enteral feedings, although safer than parenteral nutrition, are not without complications. Potential complications are generally classified into the following categories: gastrointestinal, mechanical (tube-related), fluid, electrolytes and nutrition, and psychologic. A summary of the most common complications and associated management suggestions is presented in **TABLE 10.4**.

▶ Special Considerations

Hang Time

Formulas that require reconstitution or manipulation (dilution or additives) present the greatest risk for bacterial contamination. In contrast, using sterile, undiluted, ready-to-feed products minimizes the risk of contamination (see **FIGURE 10.6**).[35,58,59]

Precautions to guard against the contamination of enteral feedings include frequently changing the feeding bag tubing, paying careful attention to clean technique during handling of the feedings, and limiting hang time of the formulas. Specific recommendations for preparing, administering, and monitoring enteral feedings in order to maximize bacteriologic safety have been published.[35,59] Of note, disposable enteral feeding bags should not be reused.

When nutritionally appropriate, sterile liquid formulas are recommended for all enteral feedings. Breast milk and all formulas either decanted with modular additives, reconstituted, or diluted should hang no longer than 4 hours. Recent research has indicated that using an enteral formula in a closed system is safe for a 24-hour hang time. Some pediatric and adult products are available in a closed system that can be hung for up to 48 hours as defined by the nursing policies of the hospital.[23,25,35,58,59]

Monitoring & Evaluation

After completing an initial nutrition assessment for a patient requiring enteral nutrition support, a plan for ongoing monitoring and evaluation should be

TABLE 10.4 Complications of Enteral Feeding

Complication	Possible Causes	Treatment/Prevention
Gastrointestinal		
Abdominal distention, bloating, gas	Rapid formula infusion Constipation Lactose intolerance Malabsorption Bacterial overgrowth Aerophagia (swallowing air) Air in tubing Gastrointestinal obstruction	Reduce or regulate infusion rate Treat constipation Use low lactose or lactose-free formula Use lower fat formula or formula with MCT oil Treat bacterial overgrowth Use a Farrell bag or manually vent the stomach Prime tubing with formula Stop enteral feeds and address obstruction
Aspiration, aspiration pneumonia	Dysphagia Gastrointestinal reflux Emesis Delayed gastric emptying Tube displaced or migrates out of position	Speech therapy feeding evaluation and/or modified barium swallow to evaluate safety of oral feedings Treat reflux Elevate head of bed by at least 30 degrees Address cause of emesis Transition from gastric to post-pyloric feeding tube Confirm correct tube placement before use
Constipation	Inadequate fluid provision Inadequate fiber provision Electrolyte abnormalities _mg? Na?_ Medication side-effect Physical inactivity Obstruction	Increase fluid provision Increase fiber provision Treat electrolyte abnormalities Modify or decrease medication causing constipation, if able Increase activity or physical/occupational therapy Rule out ileus Use laxative, stool softener, enema, and/or manual disimpaction

(continues)

TABLE 10.4 Complications of Enteral Feeding   *(continued)*

Complication	Possible Causes	Treatment/Prevention
Gastrointestinal		
Diarrhea	High osmotic load from formula/medications Rapid infusion rate Inadequate or excessive fiber provis on Malabsorption Food allergies or intolerances Infection Bacterial contamination of formula Medication side effect Aggressive bowel regimen	Consider changing formula to an isotonic formula Reduce infusion rate Increase or decrease fiber provision Consider changing to a MCT-containing, semi-elemental, or elemental formula Change formula to avoid allergen or offending substance Test for and treat infection, if present Ensure proper storage, handling, and administration of feeds Change feeding bag daily Limit prepared formula to a maximum of 4 hours Use undiluted ready-to-feed products to reduce risk Note medications which may cause diarrhea, avoid or reduce, if able Reduce frequency or dosage of laxatives and stool softeners Consider anti-diarrheal if appropriate and troubleshooting is ineffective
Nausea and vomiting	Formula intolerance Too rapid advancement of volume Too high of a concentration Gastroesophageal reflux Delayed gastric emptying Post-operative nausea and vomiting Incorrect tube position Gastrointestinal obstruction	Consider changing formula to an isotonic or semi-elemental product Advance volume more gradually Consider continuous infusion if using bolus or cycled feeds Reduce concentration of formula Elevate head of bed by at least 30 degrees Transition from gastric to post-pyloric feeding tube Use anti-emetics, hold feeds temporarily Replace or reposition feeding tube and confirm placement Hold feeds if obstruction is suspected or confirmed

Mechanical	Causes	Interventions
Clogged tube	Inadequate flushing of tube Residue from formula or medication Provision of crushed medications via tube Use of high fiber, highly concentrated, or real food formulas Use of cola, soda, or cranberry juice in an attempt to break down a clog may worsen the clog	Flush tube before and after administering formula or medication For continuous feedings, flush tube at least every 4–8 hours Use liquid medications, when possible If tablet medications are necessary, crush and dissolve in warm water before administering Do not mix formula and medication Flush tube with warm water to try to dislodge clog A combination of sodium bicarbonate and pancreatic enzymes may be used by trained professionals to try to dislodge a clog, when appropriate Replace feeding tube if clog cannot be dislodged
Tube displacement	Coughing Vomiting Accidental dislodgement Patient or parent removal	Reposition or replace feeding tube
Tube Site		
Skin breakdown	Pressure from nasoenteric tube resting on face Improper fit of semi-permanent tube Moisture at site Friction or use of abrasive product when cleaning the site of a semi-permanent tube	Alternate the site where nasoenteric tube is secured on the face Change to appropriate size tube Limit moisture at site by addressing leaking, drying the site after cleaning, and using moisture-wicking dressing at the site of semi-permanent tubes
Granulation tissue (semi-permanent tubes)	Moisture at the site Friction at the site Movement of the tube at the site Trauma at the site	To prevent, avoid moisture, friction, and movement at the site Clean twice daily with mild soap and water Ensure proper fit of semi-permanent tube Secure the tube to prevent movement Use appropriate moisture-wicking dressing and/or topical treatment Surgical excision may be necessary in severe cases

(continues)

TABLE 10.4 Complications of Enteral Feeding *(continued)*

Complication	Possible Causes	Treatment/Prevention
Leaking at site (semi-permanent tubes)	Tube is too narrow Balloon is inadequately filled	Change to appropriate size tube Check balloon volume and refill with correct amount
Tube cannot be rotated (semi-permanent tubes; skin dimples, possible irritation)	Tube is too tight	Change to appropriate size tube For tubes with balloons, check that volume is not too high
Buried bumper (semi-permanent tubes; becomes buried into the gastric wall)	Tube is too tight	Medical evaluation and treatment Change to appropriate size tube Ensure daily rotation of G-tubes
Tube hanging out of abdominal wall (semi-permanent tubes)	Tube is too long Internal balloon concerns (G-tubes)	Replace with appropriate size tube Check balloon structure and volume (if present)
Infection	Improper cleaning of the site Contamination of an open site Surgical complication	Clean with mild soap and water Prevent moisture, friction, and movement Ensure proper surgical procedure and care post-operatively
Fluid, Electrolytes, Nutrition		
Dehydration	Inadequate fluid intake Increased fluid losses Fluid restriction Medication side-effect Use of hyperosmolar formula within inadequate free water	Monitor intake and output for adequacy Ensure fluid provision matches maintenance needs or appropriate goal set by the team Modify fluid provision to match medication side-effect Assess renal solute load of formula Evaluate hydration status by looking at skin, mouth, and urine color Establish plan for regular nutrition assessment in inpatient, outpatient, and home care settings

Overhydration	Excessive fluid intake Fluid retention/inadequate urine output Medical status	Evaluate fluid intake from all sources including formula, food and beverage, intravenous fluids, and medications Reduce fluid provision Determine medical plan to diurese excess fluid, if needed Reevaluate fluid plan and increase, when appropriate, to avoid developing dehydration
Electrolyte imbalance	Inadequate or excessive electrolyte intake Fluid or formula composition Medical condition or diagnosis Increased electrolyte losses or inadequate electrolyte output Electrolyte supplementation Medication side effect	Evaluate electrolyte intake from all sources including formula, food and beverage, intravenous fluids, and supplements Note medications which may impact electrolytes Supplement for low electrolyte levels Select a modified nutrition plan when reduced electrolyte provision is needed to prevent excess provision
Weight loss or inadequate weight gain	Inadequate calorie intake Decrease in supplemental oral intake Estimated needs are less than actual needs Energy needs have increased due to increased activity or change in health Inadequate provision of EN Intolerance of EN Inability to afford formula	Evaluate adequacy of calorie intake and increase calorie provision, if appropriate Obtain indirect calorimetry, if possible Establish plan for regular nutrition assessment in inpatient, outpatient, and home care settings Verify home feeding plan and adequate support Identify cause of intolerance and alternate plan Help patient identify resources for financial support
Excessive weight gain	Excessive calorie intake Supplemental oral intake has improved Estimated needs are less than actual intake Energy needs have increased due to decrease in activity or change in health Excessive provision of EN	Evaluate calorie intake and decrease calorie provision, if appropriate Obtain indirect calorimetry, if possible Establish plan for regular nutrition assessment in inpatient, outpatient, and home care settings Re-educate patient and family/caregivers on appropriate nutrition plan if overfeeding is a concern

(continues)

TABLE 10.4 Complications of Enteral Feeding (continued)

Complication	Possible Causes	Treatment/Prevention
Fluid, Electrolytes, Nutrition		
Vitamin or Mineral Deficiency or Toxicity	Inadequate or excessive vitamin/mineral intake Fluid or formula composition Medical condition or diagnosis Increased vitamin/mineral needs or inadequate vitamin/mineral excretion Vitamin/mineral supplementation Medication side-effect	Evaluate vitamin/mineral intake from all sources including formula, food and beverage, intravenous fluids, and supplements Note medications which may impact vitamins/minerals Supplement for vitamin/mineral levels or intake Select a modified nutrition plan when reduced vitamin/mineral provision is necessary to prevent toxicity
Hypoglycemia or Hyperglycemia	Inadequate or excessive carbohydrate intake Overfeeding of total calories Diabetes may cause hypoglycemia or hyperglycemia Medication side-effect Hyperglycemia induced by stress response Hypoglycemia after period without carbohydrates (may be as short as a couple hours in infants) Abrupt disconnection from parenteral nutrition or intravenous fluids with high dextrose content may cause hypoglycemia Ketogenic diet may cause hypoglycemia	Reduce calories or carbohydrates, when appropriate, to reduce hyperglycemia Treat hyperglycemia with insulin or oral medication, when appropriate Discontinue or reduce medication causing hyperglycemia, when able Ensure adequate frequency and amount of carbohydrate provision Monitor glucose more frequently in patients at risk of hypoglycemia or hyperglycemia
Refeeding Syndrome	Renourishing a patient too rapidly in the setting of severe malnutrition or following a period of prolonged inadequate nutrition	Initiate and advance feedings slowly Allow a period of days (such as 5 days) to reach short-term nutritional goals Monitor potassium, phosphorus, magnesium, sodium fluid status, and glucose should be monitored frequently during advancement

Psychological		
Fear of tube placement	Psychologic trauma from a previous medical experience, such as previous feeding tube placement that caused pain, anxiety, or fear	Help the child use relaxation techniques Use medical play, allowing the child to play with a tube and engage in a positive pretend scenario first Offer comfort and praise after tube placement Sedation may be helpful before tube placement
Altered body image	Presence of a visible feeding tube such as a nasoenteric tube on the face or semi-permanent tube on the abdomen may have a negative impact on the person's self-image or cause others to notice the tube	Transition to nocturnal feedings with daily nasoenteric tube placement by the patient, when safe and with appropriate training Consider transition to low-profile G-tube, which is more discrete
Aversion to oral food and hydration	Inadequate exposure to normal oral feeding Traumatic experience consuming oral nutrition or hydration History of force feeding in a desperate attempt by family to meet nutrition needs	Initiate oral stimulation or oral feeding, as soon as medically able Promote positive oral feedings, such as offering a pacifier to infants during tube feedings Refer to speech language pathologist or interdisciplinary feeding team
Delayed feeding skills	Missed oral feedings during critical feeding skill development period around 6–7 months of age Late introduction of oral feedings or solid foods	Initiate oral stimulation or oral feeding, as soon as medically able Promote positive oral feedings, such as offering a pacifier to infants during tube feedings Refer to speech language pathologist or interdisciplinary feeding team

Data from Boullata JI, Carrera AL, Harvey L, et al. ASPEN safe practices for enteral nutrition therapy. *J of Parenter and Enteral Nutr.* 2017;41(1):15–103.[35]

Singhal S, Baker SS, Bojczuk GA, Baker RD. Tube feeding in children. *Pediatr Rev.* 2017; 38(1):23–32.[41]

Corkins MR, Balint J, Bobo E, Plogsted S, Yaworski JA, eds. The A.S.P.E.N. Pediatric Nutrition Support Core Curriculum. 2nd ed. American Society for Parenteral and Enteral Nutrition: 2015.[43]

Beer SS, Bunting KD, Canada N, et al. *Pediatric Nutrition Reference Guide.* 11th ed. Texas Children's Hospital: 2016.[47]

Blumenstein I, Shastri YM, Stein J. Gastroenteric tube feeding: techniques, problems and solutions. *World J Gastroenterol.* 2014;20(26):8505–8524.[53]

Children's Hospital of Philadelphia. Investigating and resolving feeding intolerance: definitions and recommendations. Available at: http://www.chop.edu/clinical-pathway/nutrition-picu-initiation-and-advancement-clinical-pathway-inpatient-intolerance. Accessed on October 30, 2017.[54]

Feeding Tube Awareness Foundation. Troubleshooting. Available at: http://www.feedingtubeawareness.org/troubleshooting/. Accessed on October 30, 2017.[55]

Tube feeding troubleshooting guide. The Oley Foundation. Tube feeding troubleshooting guide. Available at: http://cymcdn.com/sites/oley.org/resource/resmgr/Docs/TF_Troubleshooting_Guide_201.pdf. Accessed on October 30, 2017.[56]

Dandeles L, Lodolce AE. Efficacy of agents to prevent and treat enteral feeding tube clogs. *Ann Pharmacol.* 2011; 45:676–680.[57]

Product	Storage Time Room Temp	Storage Time in Refrigerator	Hang Time[1]	Bag Change	Tubing Change
EBM[2]	<4	24–72[3]	4	4	4
EBM with fortifiers[2]	2, <4[6]	24	2, <4[6]	4	4
Homemade blenderized formula	2	24	2	-	-
Concentrated liquids[4], nonsterile with additives, or powdered formula[5]	4	24	4	4	4
Infant, pediatric, and adult sterile, canned/bottled liquid products	8	48	4	8	Infant 8 Pediatric 8
Closed system formula	24	48	24	24	24

*See references for neonates and immune-compromised patients. Manufacturer's guidelines and/or hospital policy should be followed for any manipulation of enteral nutrition products. Equipment with ice packs may be used in overnight delivery, but temperatures must be checked routinely to ensure safety. All enteral nutrition products should be placed in food-grade containers.

1. Hang time includes all periods of time that the product is not refrigerated below 45°F (i.e., transport time; tubing or equipment setup).

2. For hospitalized infants.

3. Storage time for thawed EBM versus fresh EBM.

4. Sterile feeds include industrially produced, prepacked liquid formulas that are "commercially sterile."

5. Nonsterile feedings are those that may contain live bacteria and include hospital- or home-prepared formulas, reconstituted powdered feedings, and commercial liquid formulas to which nutrients and/or other supplements have been added in the hospital kitchen, pharmacy, unit, school, or home. Powdered formula is not recommended for neonates or immune-compromised patients, unless there is no alternative available.

6. One manufacturer recommends 2 hours and other companies recommend 4 hours.

Data from Abbott Nutrition. Available at: https://abbottnutrition.com. Accessed April 6, 2018.[23]

Mead Johnson Nutrition. Available at: http://www.meadjohnson.com/pediatrics/us en/product-information/products. Accessed October 8, 2017.[25]

Boullata JI, Carrera AL, Harvey L, et al. ASPEN safe practices for enteral nutrition therapy. *J Parenter Enteral Nutr.* 2017;41(1):15–103.[35]

Agostoni C, Axelsson I, Goutlet O, et al. Preparation and handling of powdered infant formula: a commentary by the ESPGHAN committee on nutrition. *J Pediatr Gastroenterol Nutr.* 2004;39(4):320–322.[58]

Robbins ST, Meyers R. *Infant Feedings: Guidelines for Preparation of Human Milk and Formula in Health Care Facilities.* 2nd ed. Chicago, IL: American Dietetic Association; 2011.[59]

FIGURE 10.6 Guidelines for Storage and Administration of Enteral Feedings (in hours)[23,25,35,58,59,*]

established. Follow-up may be completed in inpatient, outpatient, or home care settings. Nutrition monitoring and evaluation for patients receiving EN should include reviewing clinical data including intake and output, tolerance, updated anthropometric measurements, repeat nutrition-focused physical exam, pertinent laboratory values, nutrition-related medications, and ability to advance to or increase oral nutrition and hydration intake. The patient or family/caregiver should have an opportunity to express feelings or concerns about the current EN plan, available resources, and patient quality of life. Together with the patient and family/caregiver and interdisciplinary care team, the RDN should use the updated information to evaluate the current EN plan and recommend appropriate modifications, if needed, to best meet the patient's physical, nutritional, and psychosocial needs. The process of monitoring and evaluating should reoccur at set intervals throughout the entire duration of the patient's need for nutrition support and should offer the patient and family/caregiver the opportunity to

contact the care team between follow-ups should questions or concerns arise.

The following sections outline additional considerations for monitoring and evaluating patients who may be ready to start transitioning off EN including: weaning, feeding disorders, swallowing disorders, and planning for home nutrition support.

Transition to Oral Intake

Many factors must be considered before weaning the patient off a tube feeding. Typically, the transition is done slowly by introducing oral feedings and gradual reduction in tube feedings as oral intake increases. In the case of short term tube feeding in previously healthy individuals, the transition back to oral feedings may come naturally. For people who require tube feeding for longer periods, speech language pathologists often play a vital role in helping the individuals transition to safe oral feeding.

Weaning

When the patient's medical condition allows for normal oral feedings, weaning from tube feedings can be initiated. Managing the transition back to oral feedings is multifaceted and involves the interdisciplinary medical team, the patient, and the caregivers.[60–63] A complete weaning from EN should not be considered until the patient has achieved satisfactory nutritional status and oral-motor skills, because the patient may stop gaining weight for a time during the transition.

The weaning time may vary from a few days to several months or years, depending on the severity of oral feeding concerns. Children over 5 years of age may take longer to wean off tube feedings if they were not eating oral feeds during the critical period of feeding skill development in early childhood.[61] Careful records of the patient's oral intake should be kept during weaning because it is important to maintain an adequate intake from tube feedings and oral intake combined. Tube feedings should be continued until the patient can demonstrate that nutrient requirements can be met consistently by oral intake. Some patients use enteral tube feedings in combination with parenteral nutrition and oral intake, in which case, the parenteral nutrition would generally be weaned first as oral intake and/or EN increases and is tolerated.

A combination of enteral and oral feedings is difficult to project. Total daily requirements in fluid and calories are calculated, then enteral feedings are used to complete what the oral feedings lack. Ideally, the tube feeding schedule should mimic a normal meal and snack schedule from bolus feeds to allow for hunger between feedings.[35] To stimulate hunger, the enteral tube feeds may also need to be decreased. A conservative guideline is to begin with a 10–25% decrease in the caloric intake by tube, then start to offer oral feeds.[60,61,62] As part of a supervised interdisciplinary feeding therapy plan, feedings may be reduced up to 50% short-term in order to promote hunger in combination with medical, nutritional, behavioral, and feeding therapy interventions.[60,62] This transition will require frequent evaluation because of the risk of a decrease in growth with a lower caloric intake or if the child has trouble or if there is a delay in progressing. If the oral intake varies from day to day, a sliding scale for supplemental enteral feeds should be created.[35]

Feeding Disorders

Infant and toddler feeding disorders constitute a tube-feeding complication that is unique to the pediatric population. Many times, when a chronically ill infant or toddler is medically ready to begin oral feedings, the infant or toddler may display no interest in eating or may respond with manifested oral aversion when food, liquid, or utensils are near the face. In this situation, the child typically refuses, cries, gags, or vomits when offered feedings. This oral aversion can occur in children with or without mechanical eating problems.

Due to the emotional component of eating/feeding, a family may unintentionally worsen the trauma of eating by force feeding. Children who have been given EN often do not have normal hunger cycles, normal eating experiences at a table, or a mealtime routine. All of these points should be addressed when the transition to oral feeding occurs. Severe cases of oral aversion may require intervention and behavior modification from pediatric psychologists, as well as other health professionals such as speech language pathologists, dietitians, and occupational therapists.[60–62]

Illingsworth and Lister[63] suggest that resistant feeding behavior may be due to missing a "critical period" in the development of the child's feeding skills. They indicate that the critical period for the development of chewing skills is 6 to 7 months of age; if solids are not introduced during this time, the child typically will have difficulty accepting them later.

Other important oral experiences during the first year of life include developing the rooting and sucking reflexes, the oral exploration of objects, and the association of hunger with feeding. When a child is deprived of these normal oral feeding experiences during the first year of life, he or she may subsequently experience feeding difficulties that last throughout the toddler and preschool years. These children may also demonstrate significant delays in gross motor and personality development.[64] Daily oral therapy or "mouth play" can help to eliminate or reduce the problems that typically occur in the patient with non-oral nutrition support. Most feeding problems can be resolved or improved through medical, oral motor, and behavioral therapy.[60–62]

Initiating oral feedings as soon as medically possible can minimize feeding disorders. Concomitant speech or feeding therapy with EN can help to alleviate oral aversion.[35,43,61] Nonnutritive sucking during tube feedings in infancy can help to stimulate oral sucking and swallowing behavior. Pediatric speech pathologists or occupational therapists are the health professionals most qualified to assess an infant's feeding potential and to design an appropriate, ongoing oral motor stimulation program. Intervention should be considered during enteral feeding rather than at the termination of enteral feeding. Lastly, textured foods ideally should be offered, if medically feasible, when the infant is at a developmental age of 6 to 7 months. Positive caregiver–child mealtime interactions are critical for achieving feeding success.[35]

Swallowing Disorders

Eating/swallowing disorder therapy often includes recommendations to thicken liquids for therapy for managing an individual who has been diagnosed with dysphagia, or incorrect swallowing, by modified barium swallow studies using videofluoroscopy. This diagnosis means that, on regular fluid consistency, the patient is at risk for aspiration or actually aspirates the fluid into his or her lungs.

Swallowing dysfunction is compounded in infants or young children who have not learned the act of swallowing. Developmental progress, therapy, and nutrition all must be considered as the patient's plan is developed.[35]

Adding a thickening agent or food to the formula or liquid thickens the fluid so that the patient can swallow liquid with decreased risk of aspiration. Gel thickeners are preferred from a nutrition standpoint, as they are made from gum substances and contribute zero or minimal calories and carbohydrates compared with powdered thickeners and pulverized infant cereals. However, using gel-based thickeners in the premature and full-term infant populations should be avoided due to concern of increased risk of developing necrotizing enterocolitis.[65,66] Powdered thickeners and pulverized infant cereals have nutritional consequences. The more thickener that is required, the more the nutritional content of the intake is altered. Available powdered commercial thickening agents are carbohydrate based, with few or no other nutrients. Adding a powdered carbohydrate product will add calories, decrease the nutrient content per calorie, and increase free water needs in a medically unstable patient or one who is at risk for dehydration. The recipe for thickened consistency is included with the package label or provided by a speech language pathologist. The categories for thickening generally are nectar, honey, and pudding consistencies.

In all situations, there may be an increased need for fluid or free water with no method of delivery unless EN is considered as a means of alternative delivery. Because of these factors, judicious prescription and follow-up must be made. Time frames for trial therapy should be established. A well-developed behavioral and skill progression feeding plan is helpful and should include a multidisciplinary team familiar with pediatric dysphagia. Oral intake is important to encourage—as much as is medically safe. For a growing infant, 3 to 4 weeks on an altered regimen would be the maximum for a trial period; for a toddler or older child, 2 to 3 months would be the maximum. At the conclusion of the trial therapy, the patient should be evaluated for progress and/or the level of rehabilitation. If there has been no change in ability, a different modality for fluid delivery should be established, with swallowing therapy to work with oral skills.

In summary, the management plan for dysphagia should focus on reducing or eliminating factors that potentially contribute to airway compromise or aspiration, provide adequate nutrition and hydration, and facilitate a workable interaction between the caregiver and the child.[35]

Planning for Home Enteral Support

Whenever possible, EN should be provided in the home rather than in the hospital.

There are psychosocial benefits for the child and the family, and an economic benefit due to a reduced hospital stay. Often, third-party payers are making the decision of when to provide home enteral support because of the much-reduced cost of home management. A patient who is a candidate for home enteral feedings should be evaluated based on the following criteria:[35,67,68]

- The patient must be medically stable and have demonstrated a tolerance to the feeding regimen in the hospital.
- A safe home environment is required, with available running water, electricity, refrigeration, and adequate storage space.
- The family (or patient) must be educated and capable of preparing and administering the feedings at home, caring for the enteral access device, and cleaning and changing of equipment and supplies.
- A payment source is needed for the formula and tube-feeding equipment.
- A home care agency should be available to service the patient in his or her home locale. If an agency is not available, a hospital team that takes responsibility for home monitoring must be identified (pediatric nurse, dietitian, and pharmacist).
- A physician must be willing to assume responsibility for following the patient after discharge from the hospital.
- Supplies and equipment must be available.
- Patient/caregiver education must be arranged.
- A nutrition plan must be established.
- A social support system must be identified.
- Outpatient follow-up must be established.

Monitoring forms or electronic medical record templates should be used for these patients in order to document data collected between medical evaluations (see **FIGURE 10.7**). Lastly, arrangements should be made for outpatient follow-up including weight checks and nutrition analyses. The outpatient multi-disciplinary team should include at least a provider and a RDN; other key members of the team may include a nurse, speech language pathologist, social worker, case manager, pharmacist, and/or child life specialist.[35]

Successful EN can be delivered in the medical or home environment to provide for a patient's nutritional needs. The improvement in products and supplies and the reduction in complications of EN have enabled many ill children to improve nutrition and health outcomes in a more naturalized setting.

Date _____

Patient _____ DOB _____   Primary Care Physician _____
Caregiver _____   Hospital RD _____
Address _____   Monitoring Comments _____

Phone no. _____   Nutrition Support Contact Person _____

Age _____   Last measurements _____   Last nutrition Rx: Date _____
Wt _____   Wt _____   Formula _____
Ht _____   Ht _____   Total Volume _____
OFC _____   OFC _____   Delivery Schedule _____

Procurement   Enteral ☐   Parenteral ☐   Supporting Medical Equipment _____
Formula _____   Provider _____   Monitor   ☐   Provider _____
Equipment _____   Provider _____   Oxygen   ☐   Provider _____
Supplies _____   Provider _____   Other   ☐   Provider _____
Problems _____   Problems _____

Formula and Delivery   ☐ Same   ☐ Change to

Formula _____   Concentration _____
Vol/day _____   Substitute Formula _____
Planning for Home Enteral Support
Infusion and Schedule
☐ By mouth (PO)—attach diet history
☐ PO in combination with—attach diet history
☐ Bolus(es)   Infuse _____ mL over _____ minutes _____ times per day
☐ Continuous   Infuse _____ mL/hr for _____ hours from _____ to _____
☐ Parenteral   Infuse _____ mL/hr for _____ hours from _____ to _____
(See formula that follows)

Feeding Tube _____   Type _____   Size _____
☐ Nasogastric   ☐ PEG   ☐ Gastrostomy   ☐ Jejunostomy   ☐ Other

Water Flushes: Vol/day _____ mL   _____ mL water per flush _____ flushes/day

Medications and Methods of Delivery: _____

Monitoring Instructions (e.g., labs, anthropometrics, nutrition, specialists) _____

Referral Recommendations _____

Caregiver Issues _____

Home Nutrition Support Information Given to _____

Signature _____

Home Care Staff _____

Telephone _____

Comments _____
_____
_____

Problems: ☐ Vomiting   ☐ Reflux   ☐ Aspiration   ☐ Gagging   ☐ Diarrhea   ☐ Illness   ☐ Constipation
☐ Weight Loss   ☐ Behavioral   ☐ Sepsis   ☐ Equip. Malfunction   ☐ Other _____

FIGURE 10.7 Pediatric Home Care Monitoring Form

PLAN OF CARE

Signature_____

Parenteral Rx	Date _____
Dextrose	_____
Amino Acid	_____
NaCl	_____
KCl	_____
Kphos	_____
CaGlu	_____
Mg	_____
Na Acetate	_____
Other	_____
	_____
	_____
	_____
Calories Provided	_____
Amt. Protein	_____

FIGURE 10.7 *(continued)*

🔍 CASE STUDIES

Case Study #1: Nutrition Assessment of an Infant Transitioning from G-tube to GJ-tube

Nutrition Assessment

CR is a 10-month-old, full term infant male. He has daily seizures, dysphagia, and severe reflux. CR had a G-tube placed at 6 months of age after a modified barium swallow revealed aspiration with all consistencies. Despite treatment for reflux and trial of multiple formulas, he continues to vomit multiple times daily and was recently admitted a second time for aspiration pneumonia. He continues to grow, but his weight and weight-for-length percentiles have decreased. During this admission, he has been receiving continuous feedings equivalent to his home nutrition plan but has continued to vomit daily. Before discharge, the interdisciplinary care team would like to address CR's EN plan.

Home nutrition plan:

Formula: Standard milk-based 24 kcal/oz formula
Feedings: Four boluses of 150 mL administered over 1 hour each using a feeding pump at 0900, 1200, 1500, 1800 and nocturnal cycled feeds of 60 mL/hr x 8 hours from 2200–0600 via Gtube Provides (per 8 kg): 864 kcal (108 kcal/kg/d), 17.9 g protein (2.2 g/kg/d), 1080 mL (135 mL/kg/d)

Current inpatient nutrition plan:

Formula: Standard milk-based 24 kcal/oz formula
Feedings: 45 mL/hr via Gtube
Provides (per 8 kg): 864 kcal (108 kcal/kg/d), 17.9 g protein (2.2 g/kg/d), 1080 mL (135 mL/kg/d)

Anthropometrics measurements

Age	Weight	Length	Head Circumference	Weight-for-length
Birth	3.4 kg (54%, z = 0.11)	50 cm (51%, z = 0.03)	34.5 cm (51%, z = 0.03)	60% (z = 0.24)
3 months	6 kg (30%, z = −0.52)	61.5 cm (51%, z = 0.03)	40.5 cm (50%, z = −0.01)	22% (z = −0.78)
6 months	7.3 kg (22%, z = −0.76)	67.5 cm (48%, z = −0.06)	43 cm (39%, z = −0.27)	18% (z = −0.90)
8 months	7.8 kg (18%, z = −0.91)	70.5 cm (48%, z = −0.05)	44 cm (34%, z = −0.43)	13% (z = −1.11)
10 months	8 kg (11%, z = −1.24)	73 cm (45%, z = −0.12)	45 cm (37%, z = −0.32)	6% (z = −1.58)

Nutrition-focused physical exam:

CR appears slightly more pale than baseline. His mouth and lips are dry, likely from his fluid losses associated with vomiting. Otherwise, he appears small but well nourished.

Nutrition-related medication:

omeprazole

Nutrition-related labs:

Most recent BMP and CBC within normal limits
Estimated energy needs: ≥864 kcal per day using established nutrition history
Estimated protein needs: 9.6 grams per day using DRI of 1.2 gm/kg/day
Estimated fluid needs: 800 mL per day

Nutrition Diagnosis

Based on the nutrition assessment, a nutrition diagnosis or problem is identified.

Nutrition Intervention

Gastrojejunostomy (GJ-tube) placement is planned by the medical team. CR will receive medications via the G portion of the GJ-tube and formula and hydration via the J portion of the GJ-tube. His home nutrition regimen will need to be changed because bolus feedings cannot be provided by using a post-pyloric feeding method. Growth is a concern. The RDN recommends a conservative 5% calorie increase currently, with a plan to re-evaluate weight two weeks after discharge, as decreased vomiting may also help improve weight gain. CR's mother is concerned about having him hooked up 24/7, so a four hour break is incorporated into the plan to allow for bathing, tummy time, and easier cuddling.

New recommended nutrition plan:

Formula: Standard milk-based 24 kcal/oz formula
Initiation and advancement: Start at 10 mL/hr and increase by 10 mL/hr q 4 hours until goal of 57 mL/hr is achieved. Allow daily break from 3–7pm (time selected by family).
Goal feedings: 57 mL/hr x 20 hours daily (break 3–7pm) via J portion of GJ-tube
Provides (per 8 kg): 912 kcal (114 kcal/kg/d, 5.5% increase), 18.9 g protein (2.4 g/kg/d), 1140 mL (143 mL/kg/d)

Nutrition Education

Dietitian provides re-education on correct formula preparation and has family demonstrate understanding of how to prepare the correct amount and concentration of formula for CR's new home nutrition plan. The dietitian explains the new feeding schedule, why bolus feedings are no longer possible, addresses any family questions or concerns, and provides appropriate dietitian contact information for after discharge. The nurse and provider each provide education on caring for the GJ-tube, monitoring for any possible complications, and appropriate follow-up care.

Monitoring and Evaluation

CR should be seen as an outpatient by the provider or practice that placed the GJ-tube and by a dietitian for follow-up nutrition assessment. Home nutrition plan and formula preparation, feeding tolerance, intake and output, frequency of vomiting, risk of aspiration, updated anthropometrics, family questions or concerns, and patient quality of life should be reviewed in follow-up. The nutrition plan should be further modified, if needed, based on the follow-up nutrition and medical assessments, and additional plan for follow-up should be arranged.

Questions for the Reader

1) Write one PES statement for this case study.
   Altered gastrointestinal function as related to reflux and seizures as evidenced by daily vomiting. (Intervention by medical team is to place GJ tube; intervention by dietitian is to recommend modified home feeding regimen to eliminate bolus feedings)
   Inadequate calorie intake as related to daily vomiting as evidenced by decrease in weight-for-length from 18% to 6% in four months and average daily weight gain of only 3g/d in the last two months compared with expected 6–11 g/d for 8–12 month olds.[45]

2) At his follow-up appointment two weeks after discharge, CR's weight has increased to 8.2 kg. What was his average daily weight gain? Is his average daily weight gain sufficient, or should calories be increased again?
   Average daily weight gain was 14 g/d, which is slightly above expected for age of 6–11 g/d for 8–12 month olds and appropriate given recent history of inadequate weight gain.[45] Calories do not need to be increased again.

3) When would you recommend CR follow-up with a dietitian again?
   Two to four weeks to ensure continued adequate growth.

Case Study #2: Nutrition Assessment of 3 year old with Malnutrition

Nutriton Assessment

AK is a 3 year old female with history of developmental delay. She presents with malnutrition and was admitted for initiation of overnight NG feeds.

Parents report that AK is somewhat of a picky eater. Mother reports that meals are offered 3 times per day and last about 40 minutes to 1 hour. Family limits distractions during meal times. AK will typically only eat small portions of food and has difficulty with chewing meat. AK drinks 3 cans of Pediasure per day. Family has tried to increase Pediasure intake, but has been unsuccessful in doing so. Mother denies any coughing or gagging with feeding. AK does not take any additional supplements. They have been referred for feeding therapy, although therapy has not started yet.

Typical Intake

7 am: 4 ounces of Pediasure, 1–2 crackers
8:30 am: 4 ounces of Pediasure, 3 grapes
10 am: 4 ounces of Pediasure, couple bites of yogurt, 1–2 crackers
1 pm: 6 ounces of Pediasure
3 pm: 2 ounces of Pediasure, couple bites of mashed potatoes
6pm: 4 ounces of Pediasure, half of a banana

Weight History:

Age	Weight	Height	BMI
34 months	11.45 kg (z = −0.99)	89 cm (z = −0.96)	14.42 kg/m2 (z = −1.26)
35 months	11.5 kg (z = −1.63)	89.5 cm (z = −0.99)	14.4 kg/m2 (z = −1.26)
36 months	11.5 kg (z = −1.73)	90 cm (z = −1.44)	BMI 14.2 kg/m2 (z = −1.44)

IBW: 12.5 kg to achieve BMI at 50th percentile (z-score +0.06)
% IBW: 92%

Nutrition Focused Physical Exam:

This exam reveals no additional nutrition concerns other than a mid-upper arm circumference of 14.5 cm (z-score−1.62).

Nutrition-related Medication:

Miralax

Pertinent labs:

Most recent BMP and CBC within normal limits

Nutrition Diagnosis:

Based on the nutrition assessment, a nutrition diagnosis or problem is identified.

Nutrition Intervention:

Nocturnal feeds of Pediasure are to be provided using a volume of Pediasure to meet 50% of estimated calorie needs. Feeds are to run at 42 ml/hr for 12 hours overnight. AK has been seen by a speech therapist who has determined that it is safe for her to continue to take food and liquid by mouth.

Nutrition Education:

Family is to be educated on high calorie foods before discharge.
Limit oral feeds to 30 minutes
Family will need to be educated on NG feeding regimen prior to discharge.

Nutrition Monitoring/Evaluation

It is recommended that the patient follow up with a dietitian in the outpatient setting frequently so EN feeding regimen, oral intake, and weight gain can be reviewed in order to optimize growth. Once catch up growth has been achieved, the patient can follow up less frequently. The patient should receive feeding therapy in effort to optimize feeding experience and oral intake.

Questions for the Reader

1) Write one PES statement for this case study.
   Inadequate energy intake related to difficulty with feeding, prolonged feeding time, and inadequate oral intake as evidenced by average intake meeting only 70% of estimated calorie needs.
   Malnutrition (mild, chronic) related to energy expenditure exceeding energy intake as evidenced by family's report of decreased PO intake, BMI z-score of -1.73 and mid upper arm circumference z-score of −1.62.

2) What would you recommend as estimates for calorie, protein, and fluid needs for this patient?
   Estimated energy needs: 1025 kcal per day using DRI 82 kcal/kg/day and IBW
   Estimated protein needs: 13 grams per day using DRI of 1.05 gm/kg/day and IBW
   Estimated fluid needs: 1075 mL per day

3) What recommendations would you provide for advancing NG feeds for this patient?
   Feeds can be initiated at 10 ml/hr and can be advanced by 10 ml/hr every 8 hours to goal of 42 ml/hr.

▶ Conclusion

Nutrition screening should identify patients who have the inability to ingest adequate nutrition. If the gastrointestinal tract is functioning, EN is the preferred route for nutrition support. Each patient should receive an individualized EN regimen that meets estimated calorie, protein, and fluid needs in order to optimize growth and development. When indirect calorimetry is available, it is recommended for patients with suspected altered energy needs or for those who do not respond to nutrition support. Breast milk is the optimal choice for feeding in infants. There are a variety of infant formulas that can be provided if breast milk is not available or contraindicated. Cost and availability should be considered before selecting a formula for an individual of any age. A nutrient analysis should be completed for patients with altered energy needs or for those requiring diluted or concentrated formulas in order to ensure that the distribution of nutrients, vitamins, and minerals is still appropriate. Vitamin and mineral supplementation should be considered for patients receiving EN regimens that do not meet the RDA.

Selecting an appropriate feeding tube is an essential step in developing the EN plan. Nasoenteric tubes are available to feed through the stomach or intestine, are generally used for less than 4–6 weeks, and can be placed and removed without surgery. Semi-permanent tubes are also available to feed the stomach or intestine, are generally placed for anticipated need of greater than 4–6 weeks, and require surgical or endoscopic placement. Method of delivery of EN is also an important decision, since feedings can be provided as gravity boluses, as boluses using an enteral feeding pump, or as continuous or cycled feeds using an enteral feeding pump. Initiating and advancing enteral feeds should be gradual and individualized for the patient based on age, weight, tube type, method of delivery, nutrition goals,

and tolerance. While there are many benefits to providing EN, complications may also occur; prevention and prompt treatment of complications are important. The enteral nutrition plan should be continually monitored and re-evaluated in order to determine the need for any adjustments in the plan. A follow-up plan is essential for all patients receiving EN in inpatient, outpatient, or home care settings.

▶ Discussion Questions

1. What are important considerations for an infant with breastmilk available who requires tube feeding?

2. CJ is a 10 year old boy who weighs 30 kg and receives all of his nutrition and hydration via Gtube. He is growing well with 1200 calories per day. Using a standard pediatric 1 kcal/mL formula to meet his calorie needs, how much additional water does he need daily?

3. Patient MK needs 1680 mL of an adult ready-to-feed formula and an additional 500 mL water daily via Gtube. What would you recommend as a nutrition and hydration plan if the patient tolerates bolus feedings?

4. LB is a 10 month old infant with complex medical history including a trach and GJ-tube who is being discharged within the next 24 hours. He is on a hypoallergenic formula, and his concentration was increased this admission from 20 to 24 kcal/oz. He receives some formula through WIC and the rest through insurance. What steps would you take to make sure the family is ready for discharge?

5. What are potential benefits, risks, and options for families who desire blenderized real food options for their child's tube feeding?

Review Questions

1. List three indications and three contraindications to pediatric EN.

2. Create a nutrition diagnosis statement in PES format for a pediatric patient for whom you recommend initiating EN support.

3. Name three semi-elemental and three elemental formulas for infants and children.

4. List considerations involving product availability and cost when selecting formula for a patient.

5. What are appropriate indications for post-pyloric feeding tubes?

6. What are two nutrition-related and two tube-related complications that can occur with tube feeding? Choose from the following:

   - *Abdominal distention, bloating, gas*
   - *Aspiration pneumonia*
   - *Constipation*
   - *Diarrhea*
   - *Nausea and vomiting*
   - *Clogged tube*
   - *Tube displacement*
   - *Skin breakdown*
   - *Granulation tissue*
   - *Leaking at site*
   - *Infection*
   - *Dehydration*
   - *Overhydration*
   - *Electrolyte imbalance*
   - *Weight loss*
   - *Inadequate weight gain*
   - *Excessive weight gain*
   - *Vitamin or Mineral Deficiency or Toxicity*
   - *Hypoglycemia or Hyperglycemia*
   - *Refeeding Syndrome*
   - *Fear of tube placement*
   - *Altered body image*
   - *Aversion to oral food and hydration*
   - *Delayed feeding skills*

7. Which type of tube feeding delivery offers the most physiologic approach?

8. Describe three methods of bolus feeding delivery.

9. What is the maximum hang time for a prepared powdered infant formula?

10. Describe initiation, advancement, and goal rate of formula for continuous feeds via NG for a 5 kg infant on 20 kcal/oz formula that requires 540 calories daily?

References

1. ASPEN Board of Directors. Enteral nutrition practice recommendations. *J Parenter Enteral Nutr.* 2009;33(2):122–167.

2. Mehta NM, Skillman HE, Irving SY, et al. Guidelines for the provision and assessment of nutrition support therapy in the pediatric critically ill patient: Society of Critical Care Medicine and American Society for Parenteral and Enteral Nutrition. *J Parenter Enteral Nutr.* 2017;41: 706–742.

3. Braegger C, Decsi T, Dias JA, et al. Practical approach to paediatric enteral nutrition: a comment by the ESPGHAN committee on nutrition. *J Pediatr Gastroenterol Nutr.* 2010;51(1):110–122.

4. Becker P, Carney LN, Corkins MR, et al; Academy of Nutrition and Dietetics; American Society for Parenteral and Enteral Nutrition. Consensus Statement of the Academy of Nutrition and Dietetics / American Society for Parenteral and Enteral Nutrition: indicators recommended for the identification and documentation of pediatric malnutrition (undernutrition). *Nutr Clin Pract.* 2015; 30:147–161.

5. Axelrod D, Kazmerski K, Iyer K. Pediatric enteral nutrition. *J Parenter Enteral Nutr.* 2006;30(1): S21–S26.

6. DeVore J, Shotton A. *Academy of Nutrition and Dietetics Pocket Guide to Children with Special Health Care and Nutritional Needs.* Chicago, IL: Academy of Nutrition and Dietetics; 2012.

7. Kleinman RE, Greer FR (eds). *Pediatric Nutrition.* 7th ed. Elk Grove Village, IL: American Academy of Pediatrics; 2014.

8. Sonneville K, Duggan C (eds). *Manual of Pediatric Nutrition.* 5th ed. Shelton, CT: Peoples Medical Publishing House USA; 2013:158–433.

9. Psota T, Chen KY. Measuring energy expenditure in clinical populations: rewards and challenges. *Eur J Clin Nutr.* 2013;67(5):436–442.

10. Ziegler EE. Adverse effects of cow's milk in infants. Issues in complementary feeding In: Agostoni C, Brunser O,eds. *Nestlé Nutrition Workshop Series: Pediatric Program.* 2007;60:185–199.

11. Choi A, Fusch G, Rochow N, Fusch C. Target fortification of breast milk: predicting the final osmolality of the feeds. *Plos One.* 2016;11(2): doi:10.1371/journal.pone.0148941.

12. Jew RK, Owen D, Kaufman D, Balmer D. Osmolality of commonly used medications and formulas in the neonatal intensive care unit. *Nutr Clin Pract.* 1997;12:158–163.

13. U.S. Food and Drug Administration. Medical foods guidance documents and regulatory information. Available at: https://www.fda.gov/Food/GuidanceRegulation/GuidanceDocumentsRegulatoryInformation/Medical Foods/default.htm. Accessed October 6, 2017.

14. U.S. Food and Drug Administration. Frequently asked questions about medical foods; second edition. Available at: https://www.fda.gov/downloads/Food/GuidanceRegulation/GuidanceDocumentsRegulatoryInformation/UCM500094.pdf. Accessed October 6, 2017.

15. The American Academy of Pediatrics. Breastfeeding and the use of human milk. *Pediatrics*. 2012;129(3):e827–e841.

16. Greer FR, McCormick A, Loker J. Changes in fat concentration of human milk during delivery by intermittent bolus and continuous mechanical pump infusion. *J Pediatr*. 1984; 105:745–749.

17. Stocks RJ, Davies DP, Allen F, Sewell D. Loss of breast-milk nutrients during tube feeding. *Arch Dis Child*. 1985; 60:164–166.

18. Rogers SP, Hicks PD, Hamzo M, Veit LE, Abrams SA. Continuous feedings of fortified human milk lead to nutrient losses of fat, calcium and phosphorous. *Nutrients*. 2010;2(3):230–240.

19. Narayanan I, Singh B, Harvey D. Fat loss during feeding of human milk. *Arch Dis Child*. 1984;59(5):475–477.

20. Igawa M, Murase M, Mizuno K, Itabashi K. Is fat content of human milk decreased by infusion? *Pediatr Int*. 2014;56(2):230–233.

21. Food and Drug Administration. FDA takes final step on infant formula protection. Available at: https://www.fda.gov/ForConsumers/ConsumerUpdates/ucm048694.htm. Accessed October 15, 2017.

22. Centers for Disease Control and Prevention. Learn about cronobacter infection. Available at: https://www.cdc.gov/features/cronobacter/index.html. Accessed on October 15, 2017.

23. Abbott Nutrition. Available at: https://abbottnutrition.com/. Accessed April 6, 2018.

24. Gerber. Available at: https://www.gerber.com/products/formula. Accessed October 8, 2017.

25. Mead Johnson Nutrition. Available at: http://www.meadjohnson.com/pediatrics/us-en/product-information/products. Accessed October 8, 2017.

26. Nestle Health Science. Available at: https://www.nestlehealthscience.com/. Accessed October 8, 2017.

27. Nutricia North America. Available at: http://www.nutricia.com. Accessed October 8, 2017.

28. Perrigo Nutritionals. Available at: http://www.perrigonutritionals.com/pediatric-nutritionals.aspx. Accessed October 8, 2017.

29. Functional Formularies. Available at: http://www.functionalformularies.com. Accessed on October 8, 2017.

30. Kate Farms. Available at: https://nutrition.katefarms.com/kate-farms-pro-portfolio. Accessed on October 17, 2017.

31. Koletzko B, Baker S, Cleghorn G, et al. Global standard for the composition of infant formula: recommendations of an ESPGHAN Coordinated International Expert Group. *J Pediatr Gastroenterol Nutr*. 2005;41(5):584–599.

32. Holliday MA, Segar, WE. The maintenance need for water in parenteral fluid therapy. *Pediatrics*. 1957;19:823–832.

33. Escuro AA. Blenderized tube feeding: suggested guidelines to clinicians. *Pract Gastroenterol*. 2014:58–66.

34. Walia C, Hoorn MV, Edlbeck A, Feuling MB. The registered dietitian nutritionist's guide to homemade tube feeding *J Acad Nutr Diet*. 2017;117(1):11–16.

35. Boullata JI, Carrera AL, Harvey L, et al. ASPEN safe practices for enteral nutrition therapy. *J Parenter Enteral Nutr*. 2017;41(1):15–103.

36. Mennella JA, Griffin CE, Beauchamp GK. Flavor programming during infancy. *Pediatrics*. 2004; 113:840–845.

37. Mennella JA, Johnson A, Beauchamp GK. Garlic ingestion by pregnant women alters the odor of amniotic fluid. *Chem Senses*. 1995; 20:207–209.

38. Mennella JA, Beauchamp GK. Flavor experiences during formula feeding are related to preferences during childhood. *Early Human Dev*. 2002; 68:71–82.

39. Liem DG, Mennella JA. Sweet and sour preferences during childhood: role of early experiences. *Dev Psychobiol*. 2002; 41:388–395.

40. Owada M, Anki K, Kitagawa T. Taste preferences and feeding behavior in children with phenylketonuria on a semi-synthetic diet. *Eur J Pediatr*. 2000;159(11):846–850.

41. Singhal S, Baker SS, Bojczuk GA, Baker RD. Tube feeding in children. *Pediatr Rev*. 2017; 38(1):23–32.

42. Cortrack®2 enteral access system: Confident placement without X-ray™. Victus. Available at: = https://www.victus.com/?route=product/product&product_id=87Accessed =September 10, 2018.

43. Corkins MR, Balint J, Bobo E, Plogsted S, Yaworski JA. The A.S.P.E.N. Pediatric nutrition support core curriculum. 2nd ed. *American Society for Parenteral and Enteral Nutrition*; 2015; 567–573, 583–592.

44. Pascoe E, Falvey T, Jiwane A, Henry G, Krishnan U. Outcomes of fundoplication for paediatric gastroesophageal reflux disease. *Pediatr Surg Int*; 2016; 32:353–361.

45. Romano C, Wynckel M, Hulst J, et al. European Society for Paediatric Gastroenterology, Hepatology, and Nutrition guidelines for the evaluation and treatment of gastrointestinal and nutritional complications in children with neurological impairment. *J Pediatr Gastroenterol Nutr*. 2017;65:242–264.

46. Weissman TE, Wershil BK. Enteral feeding. *Pediatr Rev*. 2008; 29(3):105–106.

47. Beer SS, Bunting KD, Canada N, et al. *Pediatric Nutrition Reference Guide*, 11th ed. Texas Children's Hospital; 2016.

48. White H, King L. Enteral feeding pumps: efficacy, safety, and patient acceptability. *Med Devices*. 2014; 7:291–298.

49. Brooks C, Vickers AM, Aryal S. Comparison of lipid and calorie loss from donor human milk among 3 methods of simulated gavage feeding: one-hour, 2-hour, and intermittent gravity feedings. *Adv Neonatal Care*. 2013;13(2):131–138.

50. Feeding Tube Awareness Foundation. Bolus, gravity, and intermittent feeds. Available at: http://www.feedingtubeawareness.org/navigating-life/feeding-methods/bolus-gravity/. Accessed October 16, 2017.

51. Baker SS, Baker RD, Davis AM. *Pediatric Nutrition Support*. Burlington, MA: Jones & Bartlett Learning, 2007.

52. Chernoff R, Baker S, Baker R, Davis A. Guidelines for initiation and advancement of continuous and intermittent tube feedings. *Pediatric Enteral Nutrition in Clinical Nutrition*. New York, New York: Chapman & Hall, Inc;1994.

53. Blumenstein I, Shastri YM, Stein J. Gastroenteric tube feeding: Techniques, problems and solutions. *World J Gastroenterol*. 2014;20(26):8505–8524.

54. Children's Hospital of Philadelphia. Investigating and resolving feeding intolerance: definitions and recommendations. Available at: http://www.chop.edu/clinical-pathway/nutrition-picu-initiation-and-advancement-clinical-pathway-inpatient-intolerance. Accessed on October 30, 2017.

55. Feeding Tube Awareness Foundation. Troubleshooting. Available at: http://www.feedingtubeawareness.org/troubleshooting/. Accessed on October 30, 2017.

56. Agre A, Brown P, Stone K. The Oley Foundation. Tube feeding troubleshooting guide. Available at: http://c.ymcdn.com/sites/oley.org/resource/resmgr/Docs/TF_Troubleshooting_Guide_201.pdf. Accessed on October 30, 2017.

57. Dandeles L, Lodolce AE. Efficacy of agents to prevent and treat enteral feeding tube clogs. *Ann Pharmacol.* 2011;45:676–680.

58. Agostoni C, Axelsson I, Goutlet O, et al. Preparation and handling of powdered infant formula: a commentary by the ESPGHAN committee on nutrition. *J Pediatr Gastroenterol Nutr.* 2004;39(4):320–322.

59. Robbins ST, Meyers R. *Infant feedings: guidelines for preparation of human milk and formula in health care facilities.* 2nd ed. Chicago, IL: American Dietetic Association; 2011.

60. Krom H, Winter JP, Kindermann A. Development, prevention, and treatment of feeding tube dependency. *Eur J Pediatr.* 2017;176:683–688.

61. Wright CM, Smith KH, Morrison J. Withdrawing feeds from children on long term enteral feeding: factors associated with success and failure. *Arch Dis Child.* 2011;96:433–439.

62. Hartdorff CM, Kneepkens CMF, Stok-Akerboom AM, et al. Clinical tube weaning supported by hunger provocation in fully-tube-fed children. *J Pediatr Gastroenterol Nutr.* 2015; 60:538–543.

63. Illingsworth RS, Lister J. The critical or sensitive period, with special reference to certain feeding problems in infants and children. *J Pediatr.* 1964;65:839–848.

64. Rommel N, DeMeyer A, Feenstra L, Veereman-Wauters G. The complexity of feeding problems in 700 infants and young children presenting to a tertiary care institution. *J Pediatr Gastroenterol Nutr.* 2000;37:75–84.

65. Phagia-Gel Technologies. Simplythick easy mix. Available at: http://www.simplythick.com. Accessed September 30, 2017.

66. U.S. Food and Drug Administration. FDA expands caution about Simply Thick. Available at: https://www.fda.gov/ForConsumers/ConsumerUpdates/ucm256250.htm. Accessed October 30, 2017.

67. Vanderhoff JA, Young RJ. Overview of considerations for the pediatric patient receiving home parenteral and enteral nutrition. *Nutr Clin Pract.* 2003;18:221–226.

68. Sevilla WM, McElhanon B. Optimizing transiton to home enteral nutrition for pediatric patients. *J Parenter Enteral Nutr.* 2016;31(6):762–768.

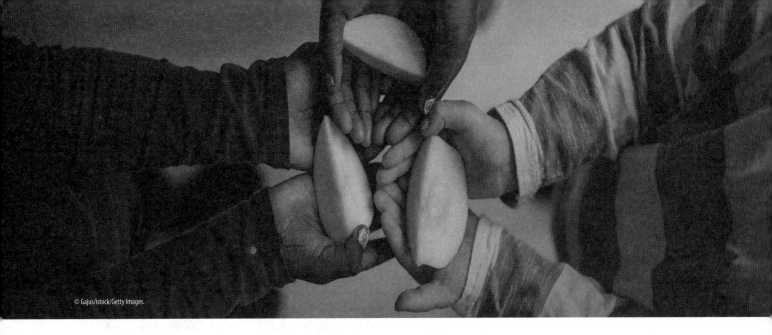
© Gajus/istock/Getty Images.

CHAPTER 11

Parenteral Nutrition

Kristy Paley

LEARNING OBJECTIVES

- Describe indications for providing parenteral nutrition.
- Identify the appropriate vascular access device that is dependent on clinical circumstances and duration of nutrition support.
- Explore and accurately prescribe the components of parenteral nutrition, including fluid and electrolytes, macronutrients, minerals, and trace elements.
- Recognize and manage the complications of parenteral nutrition.
- Define the monitoring parameters used to evaluate adequacy of parenteral nutrition.
- Identify the factors used to successfully transition to home parenteral nutrition support.

▶ Introduction

Parenteral nutrition (PN) is the intravenous delivery of nutrients, including carbohydrates, fat, protein, electrolytes, vitamins, minerals, trace elements, and water. The proportions of these nutrients are individualized, based on an assessment of the child's clinical and nutritional needs. The goal of PN is not to treat disease, but rather it is used as an adjunctive therapy to medical interventions in order to prevent malnutrition and provide nutrients necessary to support physiologic needs.[1] This chapter summarizes the complexities of pediatric PN as it is used both in the hospital and in the home setting.

▶ Clinical Indications

PN is needed when an infant or child is unable to meet ongoing nutrition needs with an oral diet and/or enteral feedings, the intestinal tract does not function properly, or the intestinal tract cannot be accessed.[2] The time frame to initiate PN can vary and depends on the age and nutritional status of the child, as these measures tend to correlate with somatic stores and energy requirements. PN should be initiated within 1–3 days in infants and within 3–5 days in children and adolescents who are anticipated to have an inability to achieve nutritional needs enterally.[1,3] In a well nourished child, initiating

PN is reasonable if inadequate enteral nutrition is anticipated longer than 5–7 days.[3] In the interim, intravenous fluids containing dextrose are typically provided in order to meet fluid needs and prevent hypoglycemia.

It is important to ensure that PN is used appropriately and that the infants and children who receive PN are managed effectively in order to support the best outcome at the lowest cost. PN policies and protocols, as well as nutrition support teams (physicians, dietitians, nurses, and pharmacists) have all been associated with fewer metabolic and mechanical complications and fewer days on PN.[1] Conditions that may require PN are listed in **TABLE 11.1**.

Vascular Access

PN may be delivered through a peripheral or central venous catheter, depending on the anticipated length of therapy, nutritional needs, and fluid allowance. Using a central versus peripheral venous access is an important factor to consider when providing PN to the patient.

Peripheral Venous Access

Peripheral PN is used when the anticipated length of therapy is less than 1 week, when central access is not possible, and when fluid volume is not limited.[1] Peripheral access may be more restrictive to normal activity than central access, depending on the site and stability. Because peripheral PN solutions are not as calorically dense as central PN solutions, greater fluid volumes up to 1.5 times maintainence are required in order to provide comparable nutrition.[1] Peripheral PN should not be considered in a child with moderate to severe nutrition deficits, since increased nutritional needs will unlikely be met given osmolality and dextrose limitations. The major complications associated with peripheral PN are soft tissue sloughs and phlebitis, which are more likely to occur if the infused solution has an osmolality greater than 900 mOsm/L. A final concentration of no more than 12.5% dextrose with a maximum solution osmolality less than 900 mOsm/L is recommended in the administration of peripheral PN.[4,5] Dextrose and amino acids are the main contributors to the osmolality of a PN solution. Computerized software for PN ordering and compounding can best determine the osmolality of a PN solution, since it considers all factors that may affect the osmolality not included in estimating equations. In the absence of computerized means, various equations exist to estimate the osmolarity of a PN solution; however, the ASPEN guidelines equation has been shown to correlate the best with measured osmolality.[6] Predictive equations for osmolarity should be used cautiously, since the actual measured osmolality may be 5–20% higher than estimated.[6] **FIGURE 11.1** provides information on the osmolarity of PN compoents.

TABLE 11.1 Conditions that May Require Parenteral Nutrition

GI Conditions		Other Circumstances
Bowel obstruction	Meconium ileus	Cancer cachexia
Diaphragmatic hernia	Necrotizing enterocolitis	Chylothorax
Gastroschisis	Neuromuscular intestinal disorders	Low-birth-weight neonate (< 1500 g)
High-output fistulas	Omphalocele	Single ventricle congenital heart disease
Intestinal atresia	Radiation enteritis	
Intractable diarrhea	Severe Hirschsprung's disease	
Intussusception	Short bowel syndrome	
Malrotation/volvulus	Graft versus host disease	
Small bowel mucosal disease	Prolonged ileus	
Impaired intestinal perfusion	Protein Losing Enteropathy	

> **Add the Osmolar Load of Each PN Component. Divide the Total Osmolar Load by the Total Volume of PN (in liters)**
>
> Total amino acid (g) × 10
> Total dextrose (g) × 5
> Total lipid (g) × 0.71*
> Total calcium gluconate (meq) × 1.4
> Total magnesium sulfate (meq) × 1
> Total potassium (meq) × 2**
> Total sodium (meq) × 2
>
> *20% intravenous lipid emulsion, product dependent
> **chloride, acetate, or phosphate salt
> PN: parenteral nutrition; g: grams; meq: milliequivalents
> Modified from Merritt R. *The A.S.P.E.N. Nutrition Support Practice Manual.* 2nd ed. Silver Spring, MD: A.S.P.E.N.; 2005.[7]

FIGURE 11.1 Equation to Estimate Osmolar Contribution of PN (mOsm/L)

Central Venous Access

Providing PN through a central vein is indicated when an infant or child requires long-term nutrition therapy or fluid restriction, or when an infant or child is a candidate for home PN. Central PN should be considered when the PN osmolarity needs to be greater than 900mOsm/L to meet nutritional needs, or when the duration of therapy is anticipated to be greater than 5 days.[1] The infusion of PN into a central vein allows the high blood flow to rapidly dilute the hypertonic solution. Hyperosmolar central PN solutions are best provided when the tip of the catheter is positioned in the distal third of the **superior vena cava** (SVC) near the junction with the right atrium.[1] Before PN administration, newly inserted **central venous catheters** (CVCs) should be confirmed either radiographically or fluoroscopically in order to ensure correct placement.[1] Intermittent re-verification of placement may be needed for long dwelling CVCs in children as they grow.[1] CVCs are also used to provide chemotherapy, prolonged antibiotic therapy, and blood components. The major complications associated with providing central PN are **central-line associated bloodstream infection** (CLABSI) and **deep vein thrombosis** (DVT).[1]

Central venous access can be temporary or permanent. In neonates, umbilical vessels may be used temporarily as a central route for PN. Due to the increased risk for thrombosis and infectious complications, umbilical lines are usually removed after 7 days.[8] In order to avoid complications associated with their use, many institutions restrict the use of umbilical catheters to lab and blood pressure monitoring, and PN is administered through a **peripherally inserted central catheter** (PICC) if central access is required.[8]

A PICC is a catheter inserted in a peripheral vein but with the distal tip located at the junction of the superior vena cava and right atrium.[9] A PICC line provides reliable central venous access and may be inserted at the bedside using strict sterile techniques.[10] Insertion-related complications inherent in the surgically placed CVC, such as pneumothorax and hemothorax, are virtually eliminated with the PICC line. PICC lines are commonly used in both neonates and older children because they provide central venous access less invasively, with lower risks and at lower cost than surgically placed CVCs or multiple insertions of peripheral lines.[11-14]

Permanent catheters are indicated when long-term access is needed. A tunneled catheter (i.e. Broviac, Hickman) is the most suitable CVC for pediatric patients who require long-term or home PN. The catheter is placed in the external jugular or the facial vein and threaded through the internal jugular vein and down into the SVC. Tip placement outside the pericardial sac avoids the risk of pericardial tamponade.[11] Location of the catheter tip should be verified every 6 to 12 months for children undergoing significant linear growth.[15] The distal end of the catheter is tunneled subcutaneously and exits mid-chest. The Dacron cuff affixed to the tunneled portion of the catheter helps secure the catheter because subcutaneous fibrous tissue adheres to the cuff. There is a decreased risk of dislodgement with the use of a tunneled catheter.[4]

Implanted catheters may be considered for intermittent PN and consist of a catheter connected to a chamber or port.[16] Implantable ports do not require routine site care when not in use and are ideal for intermittent intravenous therapies.[4] The advantages of the implantable port include reduced rate of infection and thrombis, and reduced disruption to body image.[4]

Although a single-lumen CVC is the venous access device most often used for the pediatric PN patient, two- and three-lumen CVCs also have been used for the pediatric population. Double- and triple-lumen catheters are particularly useful in patients who require frequent infusions of blood products and medications in addition to the nutrition solution. Designating one port exclusively for PN or for PN with compatible medications, and using the other ports for blood drawing, blood product delivery, and central venous pressure measurements may help decrease the risk for sepsis associated with multiple lumen catheters.[1,11] Lumens not in use must be heparinized and capped. Multiple-lumen catheters may be more suitable for the larger child rather than the neonate because of total catheter size. Strict aseptic technique is critical when a multiple-lumen CVC is in place.[17] **TABLE 11.2** describes the different types of access devices available for providing PN.

TABLE 11.2 Overview of Access Devices for Parenteral Nutrition

Access	Location	Duration of Use	Features
PIV	Peripheral; typical location forearm or hand; bedside insertion	72–96 hours	PPN osmolality <900mOsm/L; increased risk for phlebitis
Peripheral midline Catheter	Peripheral; proximal basilica or cephalic veins; ultrasound-guided placement	Up to 29 days	PPN osmolality <900mOsm/L; Unknown safety with PPN
Tunnelled CVC (Hickman, Broviac)	Central; surgical or fluoroscopic insertion	3 mon to years	Can be used for long-term TPN; no UE activity restrictions
Non-Tunnelled CVC	Central; subclavian, internal jugular veins primarily used; femoral vein optional (high infection risk); bedside insertion	5 days to a few weeks	Easily dislodged; not recommended for home TPN
PICC	Central; insertion into basilic, cephalic, or brachial veins however tip ends in superior vena cava; bedside insertion	Unknown maximum duration	Increased risk for DVT; antecubital exit site location limits activity/self care; central access device easy to remove; preferred CVC for neonates
Umbilical venous catheters	Central; surgical bedside insertion in critically ill neonates	14 days	Increased infection risk; short-term access
Totally implantable Venous-access port	Central; subclavian, internal jugular; surgical or fluoroscopic insertion	6 months to years	Requires surgical removal; intended for low-frequency, intermittent access; discretely covered under clothing

PICC: peripherally inserted central catheter, PIV: peripheral intravenous catheter, CVC: central venous catheter; DVT: deep vein thrombosis; PPN: peripheral parenteral nutrition; TPN: total (central) parenteral nutrition

Data from Worthington P, Balint J, Bechtold M, et al. When is parenteral nutrition appropriate? *JPEN.* 2017;41(3):324–377.[1]

Corkins MR, ed. *The A.S.P.E.N. Pediatric Nutrition Support Core Curriculum.* Silver Spring, MD: A.S.P.E.N.; 2010.[16]

Solution Administration

Due to the wide range in nutrient needs, fluid requirements, and clinical conditions of infants and children who require PN, individualized solutions are generally preferred over standard solutions.[11] Standard solutions may be used for short periods of time, particularly during the neonatal period, provided that electrolyte adjustment is possible and laboratory monitoring is consistent.[11,18] For individualized solutions, nutrient doses are calculated based on the infant's or child's weight (per kg) or daily need and ordered per day in a specified volume. When prescribing PN, standardized electronic PN order sets should be used to order PN for all pediatric patients.[19] Handwritten, verbal, and telephone orders should be avoided as these have a potential for error.[19] Recommendations are provided in **FIGURE 11.2**.

Parenteral nutrient solutions may be prepared as 2-in-1 solutions, or as 3-in-1 **total nutrient admixtures** (TNAs). In 2-in-1 solutions, dextrose and amino acids are combined with electrolytes, minerals, and trace elements. This solution is infused through one arm of a Y-connector, while lipids are infused in the other arm. Administering lipids separately allows for the

1. Use standardized PN order sets (electronic preferred).
2. Include patient identifiers (name, medical record number, date of birth).
3. Provide patient's current weight; provide dosing weight if different from current weight due to edema or obesity. Birth weight may be used in neonates in the first 1–2 weeks of life until the infant is back to birth weight (following post-natal weight loss).
4. Identify vascular access device and location (central, peripheral)
5. Include fluid prescription, accommodating other fluids needed for administration of flushes, medications, other intravenous fluids, and/or enteral feedings.
6. Specify total daily volume, hourly rate of delivery, and number of hours of delivery.
7. Each nutrient should be clearly identified, including chloride and acetate.
8. Order sets may include guidelines for nutrient requirements for various ages and/or acceptable ranges of nutrient concentration in admixture, including mineral content compatibility.
9. The list of nutrients in the prescription should be in the same order and units as in the guidelines and on the label. For example, do not use "mEq" for calcium in the prescription list but "mg" of calcium in the guidelines or "mL" of calcium gluconate on the label.
10. All PN ingredients should be ordered in amounts per kilogram per day or total per day for pediatric and neonatal patients. Avoid using percent concentration, amount per liter, or volume.
11. Specify type of formulation (2:1, 3:1).
12. If standard solutions are used, provide options for adjusting electrolytes; decreasing lipid, copper, and manganese; and other modifications that may be clinically indicated.
13. Establish standard guidelines for laboratory monitoring.

FIGURE 11.2 Recommendations for Writing Parenteral Nutrition Prescriptions

visualization of potential calcium phosphate precipitates in the dextrose/amino acid solution, but increases the risk for increased bacterial growth in the lipid emulsion, especially if the lipid is transferred from the original bottle into smaller syringes.[20] Vitamin stability may be greater if dosed in the lipid emulsion rather than the dextrose and amino acid solution.

A 3-in-1 or TNA combines the lipid emulsion, amino acid, and dextrose solutions in the same container. Although the TNA is more convenient to use, there has been concern about the stability and safety of these solutions. TNAs, unlike 2-in-1 solutions, are emulsions and therefore, are more significantly influenced by pH and temperature.[21,22] Optimum macronutrient dosing for TNA stability specify that final concentrations for amino acids total ≥4%, dextrose ≥10%, and lipid ≥2%.[5] As lipids are included in the admixture, there may also be a greater risk of incompatibility with medications, which may be especially problematic if access includes a single lumen.[5] Visual precipates, such as those resulting from calcium and phosphorus insolubilty, may also be more difficult to visually assess in a TNA given the opacity of the admixture, compared with a 2-in-1 solution. TNA are therefore not recommended for use in neonates and infants, since this population has the greatest calcium and phosphorus needs for bone mineral optimization. Trivalent cations also have a high risk of creating TNA instability, and therefore it is not recommended that iron dextran be provided in a TNA.[5] TNA require a larger pore size filter than a

2-in-1 solution, and does not eliminate as much particulate matter, including some bacteria, that a smaller filter would.[5]

Another concern is the potential peroxidation of lipid emulsions by ultraviolet lights.[23] Using aluminum foil to shield the bag and the tubing from ultraviolet lights can prevent this from happening. Opaque tubing is also available.[24] Infusion of a **multivitamin** (MVI) preparation along with shielding the tubing may fully protect the solution from peroxidation.[25]

Three main variables affect the overall stability of the final TNA[26–28]: (1) the final concentration of the macronutrients, (2) the amount of added cations (especially polyvalent cations such as iron, magnesium, calcium, and zinc), and (3) the compounding order. If parenteral medications are to be infused simultaneously via a Y-site, compatibility with the TNA solution should be verified.[29] Care must be taken to identify any precipitates or emulsion breakdown in the TNA before infusion occurs. The most commonly found precipitate is calcium phosphate. Emulsion breakdown or "creaming" (liberation of free oil) can result when higher amounts of cations are used in the mixture. The presence of yellow-brown oil droplets at or near the TNA surface is an indicator that the solution is unsafe for administration.[26] Various methods of in-process end-product testing are described in the **American Society for Parenteral and Enteral Nutrition** (ASPEN) guidelines to ensure and document the safety of the end TNAs.[26] Compounding PN solutions, either manually or using an automated compounding device, requires meticulous adherence to standards that ensure safety, sterility, accuracy, quality, and labeling. These standards are published and reviewed elsewhere.[2,5,19,30,31]

The solubility of calcium and phosphorus is a great concern with neonatal and pediatric PN solutions.[32] Many variables may affect calcium phosphorus solubility such as amino acids, volume, pH, temperature, PN mixing sequence, the presence or absence of lipid, and magnesium. Validated solubility curves and computerized PN ordering systems provide guidance on the maximum amount of calcium and phosphorus that can be added to PN.

For infants and children receiving home PN, the stability of the PN needs to be assured for longer periods of time. Using dual-chamber bags to separate the lipid from the rest of the solution and adding vitamins and trace minerals just before infusion helps improve the shelf-life of TNAs used in this setting.[27,33] Using a MCT/LCT-based TNA may also improve stability.[34,35] Caretakers administering PN in the home need to be trained on how to visually assess the stability of the emulsion.

Using filters with PN provides additional safety.[11,19,26] Filters can prevent the infusion of particulate matter, air, and microorganisms. Different types of filters are used for 2-in-1 and 3-in-1 solutions. 0.22-micron filters can be used with 2-in-1 solutions. These filters remove microorganisms and pyrogens (gram-negative endotoxins) and reduce the risk of air embolism. For TNAs, larger 1.2-micron filters are used to allow the administration of lipid droplets. These filter out particulate matter and larger organisms, such as *Candida albicans*, but are unable to filter out common smaller bacterial contaminants. Infusion sets for 2-in-1 solutions should be changed at least every 72 hours, or per manufacturer's instruction.[16] Infusion sets for TNAs or lipids administered separately should be changed within 24 hours of initiating the infusion.[2,11,26]

PN macronutrients, and occasionally fluid (in infants) are advanced gradually as the child's fluid and glucose tolerance permits. Infusion pumps are used to maintain a constant flow rate, thereby maintaining steady glucose delivery. If the PN infusion is interrupted or discontinued abruptly, IV fluids containing dextrose may be infused to maintain euglycemia until the PN solution can be replaced.

▶ Fluid and Electrolytes

Guidelines for administrating parenteral fluids to infants and children are based on normal maintenance estimates, with adjustments for increased or decreased losses due to disease or environmental conditions. Patients receiving PN who are at the greatest risk of dehydration include those with increased GI losses or those receiving inadequate PN volume.[36] Patients

receiving PN who are at greatest risk for fluid overload include those with cardiac, liver, and renal diseases or those receiving excessive volume via PN or other multiple intravenous sources (medications, IV fluids, electrolyte replacements).[36]

Frequent monitoring of fluid and electrolyte intake, serum and urine electrolyte levels, weight changes, and urine output may be needed to appropriately manage fluid and electrolyte balance during the neonatal period. During the first 12 to 36 hours of life, renal excretion of sodium, potassium, and fluid is minimal. Electrolytes may not be needed during the first 1–2 days, and fluid administration is conservative unless **insensible water loss** (IWL) is high. The onset of the diuretic phase usually occurs within the first 2 days and accounts for most of the weight, sodium, and potassium loss that occurs during the first week of life. The postdiuretic phase is characterized by improved homeostasis of fluid, sodium, and potassium.[37] The initial adjustment to extrauterine life usually results in up to 10% weight loss in term infants. Prematurely born infants may lose up to 20% of their body weight, due primarily to their greater percentage of total body water as extracellular water. Insensible water losses may be greater due to their greater body surface area to body mass ratio and their more permeable epidermis.[38] Low-birth-weight infants may require up to 200 mL/kg/day due to their renal immaturity and increased IWL. They may also be intolerant of excessive fluid intake. Weight loss greater than 15% to 20% of birth weight may represent some loss of lean tissue due to energy deficit.[39] Daily Maintenance fluid calculations are provided in **TABLE 11.3**.

Beyond the first week of life and throughout childhood, maintenance fluid and electrolyte requirements are directly related to metabolic rate.[41] Changes in metabolic rate, respiratory rate, insensible water loss, and water production from the oxidation of protein, carbohydrate, and fat also affect fluid needs. Older infants and children may initially require fluids and electrolytes in excess of maintenance requirements in order

TABLE 11.3 Daily Maintenance Fluid Requirements	
Body Weight	**Fluids Required per Day**
1–10 kg	100 mL/kg
11–20 kg	1000 mL + 50 mL/kg above 10 kg
Body weight above 20 kg	1500 mL + 20 mL/kg above 20 kg

Kg: kilogram, mL: milliliter
Data from Kleigman RM, Stanton BF, St Geme JN, Schor NF. *Nelson Textbook of Pediatrics.* 20th ed. Philadelphia, PA: Elsevier; 2016.[40]

to establish normal hydration if they have had prolonged or excessive vomiting, nasogastric suctioning, or diarrhea. In infants and children with unpredictable fluid loss requiring greater than maintainence fluid, it is common to provide PN near maintainence requirements and replace excessive fluid loss separately as they occur. This lessens the risk of reducing or discontinuing the PN should there be an abrupt change in the patients fluid loss.

Approximately 60% of water is lost in the urine, 5% in stool, and 35% via insensible losses (skin and lungs).[40] Fluid losses through urine and the gastrointestinal tract may be relatively easy to measure, although insensible water loss through the respiratory tract and skin is more elusive and may be affected by environmental conditions. Factors that may increase insensible water loss include radiant heat warmers, phototherapy, fever, excessive sweating, and tachypnea, while factors that may decrease insensible water loss include mechanical ventilation or the use of humidified air.[40]

Excessive sodium losses may occur in a variety of conditions. Inappropriate or excessive **antidiuretic hormone** (ADH) secretion, often associated with hypoxia, hemorrhage, central nervous system insult, hypotension, anesthesia, pneumothorax, or pain, requires fluid restriction and sodium supplementation in order to maintain normal extracellular fluid volumes and prevent hyponatremia.[42] Excessive gastric fluid output or stool output may also be a source of sodium loss, as the average sodium composition of gastric fluid and diarrhea is 60 meq/L and 55 meq/L, respectively.[40]

Potassium plays a significant role in the function of all cells in the body, and is especially important in cardiac function and smooth muscle contraction. Hyperkalemia may occur with impaired renal function, metabolic or respiratory acidosis, various medications, or excessive intravenous potassium provision.[36] Hypokalemia may be seen with intestinal malabsorption as a result of increased stool or urinary potassium loss, or when potassium is shifted intracellulary, as with refeeding syndrome or insulin administration.[36,40] Of note, magnesium deficiency increases renal potassium losses and disrupts the sodium-potassium adenosine triphosphatase pump.[36] Hypomagnesiumemia should be treated in order to effectively treat hypokalemia. Hypokalemia can be treated by increasing potassium in the PN solution; however, caution should be taken in order to avoid hyperkalemia, since the PN may need to be temporarily discontinued if hyperkalemia develops.

▶ Energy

Accurate assessment of energy requirements is crucial in order to avoid complications associated with over or underfeeding of parenteral substrates. This can be quite challenging given the variation in metabolic state of patients requiring PN and the lack of reliable, accessible methods to determine energy needs. Overfeeding may increase carbon dioxide production and respiratory burden, promote hyperglycemia and hypertriglyceridemia, worsen liver function, and increase obesity risk.[43] Underfeeding may result in growth failure, especially in infants considering their limited nutrient stores.

Energy needs during critical illness may be lower than normal due to the inability to achieve growth combined with a reduced metabolic rate while being mechanically ventilated and sedated. Anabolism is temporarily interrupted during critical illness, and providing calories above resting energy expenditure may increase the risk for overfeeding. It is important to maintain awareness of this risk during when the metabolic stress response is highest following the first few days of critical illness.[3] Measured energy expenditure by **indirect calorimetry** (IC) is recommended in order to determine energy requirements in this population.[44] Technical constraints and limited resources are the most often cited barriers to routine use of indirect calorimetry in the pediatric population. Numerous reports describe comparing established equations to indirect calorimetry for estimating individual energy needs.[10,43,45–48] When compared to IC, estimating equations are not accurate and can lead to unintended over or underfeeding. When IC is not feasible however, equations can be used to estimate the resting energy expenditure, without adding stress factors.[44,49] Caution should be taken in the pediatric critically ill obese patient, as predictive equations to estimate energy expenditure have been found to be inaccurate when compared with measured energy expenditure via indirect calorimetry.[50]

In the absence of critical illness, energy needs are more related to growth, activity, and the underlying illness.[11,51] When IC is not feasible, published predictive equations, such as the 2006 Dietary Reference Intakes or the 1989 **Recommended Dietary Allowance** (RDA), can be utilized as a method to estimate energy needs. These equations are published elsewhere.[52,53] **TABLE 11.4** provides the WHO equation for estimating resting energy. Of note, parenteral energy may be about 10% lower than estimated enteral needs for most infants and children due to reduced energy required for digestion and absorption.[53] Caution should be taken in providing calories for catch up growth via PN, since this may result in complications associated with PN-associated overfeeding, such as hyperglycemia, **parenteral nutrition-associated liver disease** (PNALD), increased infection risk, obesity, and difficulty weaning from the ventilator. Whichever method is used to estimate energy needs, frequent monitoring of anthropometric, clinical, and laboratory parameters allows adjusting energy delivery to meet individual

TABLE 11.4 World Health Organization Equation for Estimating Resting Energy Expenditure (kcal/day)

Age	Male	Female
0–3 years	60.9 × wt – 54	61 × wt – 51
3–10 years	22.7 × wt + 495	22.5 × wt + 499
10–18 years	17.5 × wt + 651	12.2 × wt + 746
≥ 18 years	15.3 × wt + 679	14.7 × wt + 496

Wt is in kilograms

Modified from World Health Association. Energy and protein requirements. Report of a Joint FAO/WHO/UNU expert consultation. Techanical report series 724. World Health Organization, Geneva; 1985.[54]

energy needs. Recommendations for other nutrients are listed in **TABLE 11.5**.

Carbohydrate

Dextrose (3.4 kcal/g) is the source of parenterally administered carbohydrate, and generally provides 50–60% of total calories. Dextrose is dosed in PN as **glucose infusion rate** (GIR). GIR describes the infusion of dextrose in mg/kg per minute of PN infusion time. Overall calorie requirement, macronutrient distribution, and glycemic need ultimately dictate GIR required GIR is typically advanced by 1–2 mg/kg/min daily until goal GIR achieved.[16] Baseline glucose utilization, GIR received from intravenous fluids, and glycemia should all be considered when dosing the GIR in the initial PN solution.

Baseline glucose utilization by infants is equal to a GIR of approximately 6–8 mg/kg/min, primarily due to brain metabolism. The brain requires glucose as the primary source of energy, and brain utilization of glucose may account for as much as 90% of basal glucose needs.[55,56] GIR above baseline utilization in infants is typically needed to support normal growth. Glucose infusions of less than 2 mg/kg/min may be insufficient to prevent ketosis caused by mobilization of fat stores as a source of energy. Maximum glucose tolerance varies with age, total energy expenditure, and clinical condition.[55–57] Parenteral provision of dextrose should not exceed the maximum glucose oxidation rate. In infants and young children (up to 2 years of age), exceeding a GIR of 12–14 mg/kg/min may increase the risk of hepatic steatosis.[57,58] Cautious advancement of GIR is recommended during critical illness. Hyperglycemia is more common during periods of stress and inflammation due to upregulated cytokines and counterregulatory hormones, thereby promoting decreased peripheral glucose uptake and increased hepatic glucose production.[36]

Generally, insulin is not added to parenteral nutrient admixtures because dose response varies widely, particularly in the low-birth-weight infant, as well as an increased risk for hypoglycemia. Symptoms of hypoglycemia in a neonate may include cyanotic spells, apnea, respiratory distress, or convulsions.[59] Providing insulin in PN solutions in order to prevent hyperglycemia is thereby not recommended in neonates within the first month of life.[59] Insulin can be considered when hyperglycemia persists despite both eliminating medications promoting hyperglycemia and reducing the GIR of the PN solution, or as needed in the presence of medical conditions promoting hyperglycemia, such as sepsis.[59] It is safest to utilize an insulin infusion, separate from the PN solution, so that the insulin dose can be easily adjusted based on clinical need. Insulin, when needed, should be initially dosed in the separate infusion starting at 0.05 U/kg/hour and increased or decreased as needed in order to maintain euglycemia.[16] Once the dose of insulin infusion and blood glucose have remained stable for at least 24 hours, one may consider adding the same insulin dose to the PN and discontinuing the separate insulin infusion.[16] This is however, also considering that the GIR will remain fairly constant. Early delivery of 2–3 g/kg/day of amino acids may also improve hyperglycemia in premature low birth weight infants, as it may stimulate endogenous insulin secretion.[57] Reduced glycogen stores in low-birth-weight infants and undernourished infants and children place them at a greater risk of developing hypoglycemia following abrupt cessation of parenteral glucose. Gradual weaning from parenteral glucose while advancing enteral feeding help prevent the development of hypoglycemia.

Protein

Crystalline amino acids (CAA) (4 kcal/g) are the source of parenterally administered protein, and generally provide 10–20% of total calories. Protein requirements during infancy and childhood are determined by taking into account the endogenous rate of protein turnover and what is required for overall growth.[60] This is typically the minimum intake required to ensure adequate growth in the presence of adequate energy intake. Protein requirements for healthy infants and children are expressed as the **Dietary Reference Intake**,(DRI), which is the amount to meet the needs of at least 97.5% of the population. Higher amounts of protein are indicated for infants born premature, as growth rates are highest during this time.[60] CAA are generally initiated between 1.5–3 g/kg/day in preterm and term infants, 1–2 g/kg/day in children 1–10 years of age, and 0.8–1.5 g/kg/day in adolescents, and further advanced by 1 g/kg/day until the goal is achieved.[16]

TABLE 11.5 Recommendations for Daily Parenteral Administration of Macronutrients, Electrolytes, and Minerals

	Dose Unit	Premature Infants	Term Infants	1–3 Years	4–6 Years	7–10 Years	11–18 Years
Dextrose[1]	mg/kg/min	8–12 (Max 14)	12 (Max 14)	8–10	8–10	8–10	5–6
Protein[2]	g/kg	3–4	2–3	1.5–3	1.5–3	1.5–3	0.8–2.5
Fat[3]	g/kg	3–3.5	3	2–3	2–3	2–3	1–2.5
Sodium	mEq/kg	2–5	2–5	2–5	2–5	2–5	1–2*
Potassium	mEq/kg	2–4	2–4	2–4	2–4	2–4	1–2*
Calcium[4]	mEq/kg	2–4	0.5–4	0.5–4	0.5–4	0.5–4	10–20 mEq/d*
Phosphorus[5]	mmol/kg	1–2	0.5–2	0.5–2	0.5–2	0.5–2	10–40 mEq/d*
Magnesium[6]	mEq/kg	0.3–0.5	0.3–0.5	0.3–0.5	0.3–0.5	0.3–0.5	10–30 mEq/d*
Chloride/Acetate	As needed to maintain acid base balance						
Zinc[7]	mcg/kg	400	50–250	50–125	50–125	50–125	2–5mg/d
Copper[7]	mcg/kg	20	20	5–20	5–20	5–20	200–500 mg/d
Chromium[7]	mcg/kg	0.05–0.2	0.2	0.14–0.2	0.14–0.2	0.14–0.2	5–15 mcg/d
Manganese[7]	mcg/kg	1	1	1	1	1	40–100 mcg/d
Selenium[7]	mcg/kg	1.5–2	2	1–2	1–2	1–2	40–60 mcg/d

[1] Peripheral venous access limits dextrose concentration to 12.5%.

[2] Protein needs may vary with diagnoses.

[3] Minimum fat dose to meet essential fatty acid requirements varies depending upon fat source and total energy needs. See text. Maximum lipid infusion: 0.17 mg/kg/hr preterm; 0.15 mg/kg/hr term.

[4] Calcium conversions: 1 mEq = 0.5 mmol = 20 mg elemental calcium; 1 mL calcium gluconate 10% contains 100 mg calcium gluconate = 9.3 mg elemental calcium = 0.47 mEq = 0.25 mmol calcium.

[5] Phosphorus conversions: 1 mmol = 31 mg elemental phosphorus; 1 mL sodium phosphate contains 3 mmol or 93 mg elemental phosphorus (and 4 mEq sodium); 1 mL potassium phosphate contains 3 mmol or 93 mg elemental phosphorus (and 4.4 mEq potassium).

[6] Magnesium conversions: 1 mEq = 0.5 mmol = 12.5 mg elemental magnesium; magnesium sulfate 50% contains 500 mg magnesium sulfate heptahydrate or 4.1 mEq (or 51.3 mg) elemental magnesium.

[7] Trace mineral additives are currently available individually and in various combinations/concentrations for various ages. Copper and manganese needs may be lower with cholestasis.

*adolescents and children >50 kg.

Data from Boullata JI, Gilbert K, Sacks G, et al. American Society for Parenteral and Enteral Nutrition. A.S.P.E.N. clinical guidelines: parenteral nutrition ordering, order review, compounding, labeling, and dispensing. *JPEN*. 2014;38(3):334–377.[5]

Corkins MR, ed. *The A.S.P.E.N. Pediatric Nutrition Support Core Curriculum*. Silver Spring, MD: A.S.P.E.N.; 2010.[16]

Nutrition therapy during critical illness should focus on providing optimal protein to offset the catabolic state, maximize nitrogen retention, and minimize cumulative nutritional deficits.

Increased endogenous protein catabolism coupled with reduced protein synthesis lead to a chronic state of protein deficiency and loss of lean body mass.[60] This may be further exacerbated if basal energy needs are not met. A minimum protein provision of 1.5 g/kg/day has been recommended in the presence of adequate energy in order to achieve positive nitrogen balance in critically ill infants and children,[61,62] although ASPEN guidelines for protein

TABLE 11.6 Protein Recommendations

Age	DRI (g/kg/day)	A.S.P.E.N Guidelines*
0–6 months	1.52	2-3
7–12 months	1.2	2-3
1–2 years	1.05	2-3
2–3 years	1.05	1.5-2
4–13 years	0.95	1.5-2
13–14 years	0.95	1.5
14–18 years	0.85	1.5

DRI: Dietary Reference Intake; ASPEN: American Society for Enteral and Parenteral Nutrition

*for critical illness

Data from Mehta NM, Compher C, A.S.P.E.N. Board of Directors. A.S.P.E.N. Clinical Guidelines: nutrition support of the critically ill child. *JPEN*. 2009;33(3):260–276.[45]

Otten JJ, Pitzi Hellwig J, Meyers LD, eds. *Dietary Reference Intakes: The Essential Guide to Nutrient Requirements.* Washington DC: The National Academies Press; 2006.[53]

provision may be higher, depending on age.[45] Obese, critically ill children may require at least 1.5 g/kg/day based on ideal body weight in order to mitigate negative protein balance.[44] General recommendations for parenteral protein administration for infants and children were presented in Table 11.5. ASPEN protein recommendations for critical illness, along with DRI reference for healthy infants and children, are listed in **TABLE 11.6**.

Parenteral amino acid solutions have been developed for infants reflecting the amino acid composition of human milk or plasma aminograms of healthy term infants fed mature human milk. Metabolic immaturity has also been considered, because cystine, taurine, tyrosine, and histidine may be essential amino acids for neonates and young children.[57,63] Methionine, phenylalanine, and glycine concentrations have been decreased in these solutions, while histidine, tyrosine, taurine, arginine, glutamic acid, and aspartic acid may be added or their concentrations increased.[63] These specialized amino acid solutions also have a lower pH allowing for increased provision of calcium and phosphorus.[16] Although the data are inconclusive, there may be a decreased incidence of cholestatic liver disease during specific pediatric CAA product administration.[64–66]

Although cystine may be a conditionally essential amino acid, it is not included in parenteral amino acids because it is unstable in solution for prolonged periods of time.[67] It is available as L-cystine hydrochloride and is added separately at the time of administration. The most commonly recommended dose for cystine is 30 to 40 mg/g of protein provided for pediatric CAA products, although cystine may not be needed for standard solutions due to higher methionine content.[68] Methionine, when provided in sufficient amounts, can produce cysteine via the trans-sulfuration pathway.[68] Adding L-cystine hydrochloride decreases the solution's pH, which increases calcium and phosphorus solubility, thus allowing for increased mineral delivery.[68]

Fat

Fat, known as **intravenous lipid** (IL), is included in PN regimens for infants and children as a source of **essential fatty acids** (EFA) and to provide optimal nutrition support. It is typically supplied as a 20% solution, provides a concentrated source of calories (2 calories per mL of 20% solution or 10 kcal/g regardless of solution), and contributes minimally to the osmolarity. IL bypasses the intestine, avoiding the need for hydrolysis by lipases and bile, and are not packaged into chylomicrons or require enterocyte absorption.[69] IL is thereby able to provide a concentrated energy source for patients with impaired enteral fat utilization, such as those with intestinal failure or chylous effusions. There are inconsistencies in the evidence to conclude superiority of one lipid emulsion over another regarding maintainence or gain in body weight, stature gain, or increase in head circumference in pediatric patients.[70]

Essential fatty acids include **alpha-linolenic acid** (ALA; n-3) and **linoleic acid** (LA; n-6), and are necessary for the integrity of cell membranes and for brain development during infancy. EFA deficiency can develop following inadequate IL and may include clinical manifestations such as dermatitis, poor growth, developmental delay, and increased infection risk.[69] Biochemical deficiency of EFA precedes these clinical manifestations and may be detected within a few days of lipid-free PN, especially in infants with reduced somatic stores.[57] Plasma levels of LA and **arachidonic acid** (AA) decline, and the ratio of plasma eicosatrienoic acid to AA (triene:tetraene) becomes elevated. A biochemical diagnosis of EFA deficiency is a triene:tetraene ratio of >0.2, however clinical manifestations may not be detected until a triene:tetraene ratio is >0.4.[69] Providing as little as 2% to 4% of the total daily caloric intake as LA (0.25 g/kg/day for infants and 0.1 g/kg/day in children) and 0.25% to 0.5% of the total daily caloric intake as LNA can prevent deficiency in most infants and children.[11,26,57,71] The fatty acid composition of parenteral lipid emulsions are listed elsewhere.[71] Total amount of lipid to prevent EFA deficiency will vary dependent upon the type of IL provided.

There are a variety of IL emulsions available in the United States. The most commonly used are soybean oil-based (i.e. Intralipid (Fresenius Kabi) or Liposyn III (Hospira)). These lipid emulsions have a higher concentration of EFAs than other lipid emulsions, making them ideal for use in children where IL dose may be reduced due to fluid restriction or hypertriglyceridemia. EFA deficiency can be prevented by providing a minimum of 0.5–1 g/kg/day of soybean oil-based IL.[16] These lipid emulsions also contain a high phytosterol concentration, low alpha-tocopherol content, both of which may be a contributing factor in the development of **parenteral nutrition associated liver disease** (PNALD).

SMOFlipid (Fresenius Kabi) is a 20% mixed lipid emulsion comprised of 30% soybean oil, 30% MCT oil, 25% olive oil, and 15% fish oil. It contains less phytosterols than soybean oil emulsions, and early clinical evidence in children and animal models suggests it may be helpful in preventing PNALD, although more data is needed.[69,72] When compared to soybean oil emulsions, greater amounts of SMOFlipid are required to meet EFA requirements.

Omegaven (Fresenius Kabi) is a commericially available lipid emulsion solely containing fish oil. It is a 10% solution providing 1.1 calories per mL. Although not currently FDA approved for routine use in the United States, it is permitted for treatment of PNALD in patients dependent on parenteral nutrition through a FDA compassionate-use allowance.[71] Unlike soybean oil-based IL, Omegaven contains negligible phytosterols and has reversed PNALD in PN-dependent pediatric patients when used as a replacement for soybean oil lipid emulsions.[69,73–75] The reduced n-6 content of Omegaven increases the risk for EFA deficiency; however, outcome reports of this treatment have not demonstrated clinical or biochemical evidence of EFA deficiency.[69]

Guidelines for parenteral macronutrient composition include 20–30% calories via lipid.[58] General recommendations for parenteral lipid administration in infants and children are given in Table 11.5. IL are generally initiated between 1–2 g/kg/day in infants and children up to 10 years of age, or initiated at 1 g/kg/day in adolescents.[16] IL are advanced by 1 g/kg/day until the goal is achieved.[16] The rate of administration may be just as significant a factor in lipid tolerance as the daily dose. Hypertriglyceridemia may occur if the lipid infusion rate exceeds the rate of triglyceride hydrolysis.[57] The research is inconclusive as to which lipid emulsion is preferred in order to reduce the risk of hypertriglyceridemia.[70] If triglycerides exceed 200 mg/dl, a reduction in lipid dose and/or intermittent provision of lipids (few days per week) may assist in lipid clearance.[16] Adverse effects of intravenous fat when given in boluses or in doses exceeding 0.15 g/kg/hour have been reported, including altered pulmonary function, impaired neutrophil function, and an increased risk of kernicterus in infants with elevated serum bilirubin level.[76–78] Preterm or malnourished infants and children may be at greater risk for impaired fat tolerance due to decreased adipose tissue mass, reduced lipoprotein lipase activity, hepatic immaturity, or carnitine deficiency. Recommendations for maximum lipid infusion include 0.17 g/kg/h in preterm infants and 0.15 g/kg/h in term infants.[16] Maximum lipid infusion for older children has been suggested at 0.08–0.13 g/kg/h.[57] Fat should not provide more than 60% of total calories in any patient, because ketotic acidosis may occur.[79]

Parenteral lipid emulsions contain egg phospholipid as an emulsifying agent. Because phospholipids interfere with enzymes that help metabolize and clear plasma lipids, 20% emulsions are recommended over 10% emulsions due to lower phospholipid-to-lipid ratio. Parenteral lipid emulsions also contain glycerol and are relatively isotonic and pH neutral, providing a favorable environment for the proliferation of several common pathogens. When infused separately, lipid emulsions are associated with an increased incidence of coagulase-negative staphylococcal bacteremia, particularly when hang times exceed 12 hours. Using administration sets up to 24 hours to accommodate a second lipid infusion has been suggested.[80] When administered as a component of a TNA, this association is no longer apparent, likely due to the hypertonic and relatively acidic environment provided by the presence of other nutrients.[78] Both of these factors may decrease the stability of the lipid emulsion, causing separation, particularly when higher amounts of amino acids and minerals are used, as for low-birth-weight infants. The opacity of TNAs may also mask the presence of incompatibilities and precipitates, resulting in adverse outcomes, although use of a 1.2-micron filter can remove larger organisms, particles, precipitates, and fat globules.[81]

Carnitine facilitates transport of long- and medium-chain fatty acids across mitochondrial membranes. Carnitine is normally synthesized in the liver and kidneys from methionine and lysine. It is found in human milk and infant formulas, however, it is typically void in pediatric PN solutions. Patients at highest risk for carnitine depletion include those who are less than 30 weeks' gestation, have a birth weight under 1500 g or a history of fetal malnutrition, or have hepatic or renal dysfunction, sepsis, trauma, or medium-chain acetyldehydrogenase deficiency.[58,82]

Carnitine deficiency may result in hypoglycemia, muscle weakness, and hypertriglyceridemia, although studies have found no significant changes in triglyceride values, weight gain, lipid utilization, or ketogensis with carnitine supplementation.[58] Carnitine may be considered in patients identified at high risk if parenteral nutrition is expected to be the single source of nutrition for longer than 2 weeks, or if hypertriglyceridemia, hypoglycemia, and low serum carnitine are present.[58,82] Dose recommendations for carnitine supplementation in pediatric PN vary from 10–20 mg/kg/day.[58,83]

Vitamins

Recommendations for term infants and children up to 11 years of age were established by the Nutrition Advisory Group of the American Medical Association in 1975.[84] They are based on the 1974 **recommended dietary allowances** (RDAs), which are guidelines for enteral nutrient intake. Recommendations for adolescents are based on guidelines for adults.

Parenteral vitamin preparations that are currently available are unlikely to meet the increased needs of vulnerable populations including premature infants, or infants and children with malabsorptive conditions or malnutrition.[16] Dosing recommendations for pediatric parenteral multivitamins include providing 2 ml/kg for infants weighing less than 2.5 kg, and providing 5ml per day for infants and children weighing greater than 2.5 kg.[16] Limited vitamin products available coupled with broad weight-based dosing categories result in inadequate micronutrient provision, especially in those vulnerable populations described above. Thiamin deficiency has been reported in infants and children during shortages of parenteral multivitamin products. A few days of inadequate thiamine intake can lead to severe lactic acidosis in children on PN.[57] Thiamin should be given as a separate intravenous additive during multivitamin shortages.[85] The vitamin content of commerically available intravenous pediatric multivitamin products are listed in **TABLE 11.7**.

Levels of several vitamins may decrease over time in parenteral nutrient admixtures due to light degradation, decomposition in the presence of bisulfite (an antioxidant additive) or varying pH, and adsorbance to plastic or glass. For these reasons, multivitamins should be added to TNA solutions immediately before administration, excessive light exposure (direct sunlight or phototherapy light) should be avoided, and administration of these admixtures completed within 24 hours. If lipids are given separately, adding both fat-soluble and water-soluble vitamins to the lipid emulsion may increase vitamin stability and delivery.[57]

Minerals

It is important to monitor key minerals such as magnesium, calcium, and phosphorus as well as trace minerals, and adjust the intake of these minerals accordingly while on PN.

Magnesium

Hypomagnesemia can occur in many conditions such as intestinal malabsorption, refeeding syndrome, hyperparathyroidism, or with increased renal magnesium losses with a variety of medications.[36] It may also occur in the setting of metabolic alkalosis, hypocalcemia, and/or hypokalemia.[36]

General magnesium dose recommendations for infants and children are 0.3 to 0.5 mEq/kg/day.[16] Further doses are listed in Table 11.5. Upper-range doses may be needed during rapid growth phases, diuretic therapy, or chronic malabsorption. Lower range doses may be indicated if renal function is impaired. Magnesium is added to parenteral admixtures as magnesium sulfate. Excessive doses may cause acute hypotonia, apena, hypotension, and refractory bradycardia.[86] Serum magnesium levels may be transiently elevated in preterm infants whose mothers received significant amounts of magnesium sulfate in order to prevent premature labor or treat preeclampsia. Magnesium may be withheld from PN solutions for these infants until serum levels are within normal limits.

Calcium

Calcium deficiency is not usually identified by low serum levels because serum calcium is usually maintained at the expense of bone stores.[87] Inadequate calcium provision increases the risk of impaired bone mineralization and fractures, especially among preterm infants. This population has the highest requirements of both calcium and phosphorus to promote optimum mineral accretion.[88] Hypocalcemia is most common during the neonatal period, particularly in infants born prematurely, due to their relatively low calcium stores and inappropriately low parathyroid hormone levels. Hypercalcemia can result from increased calcium intake or hypophosphatemia.[88] Hypercalciuria has been associated with furosemide therapy and inadequate phosphorus intake.[89,90] Older children receiving cyclic parenteral nutrition may have greater urinary losses of calcium due to higher rates of infusion.[91]

Recommendations for parenteral calcium administration are listed in Table 11.5. A calcium:phosphorus ratio of 1.7:1 (mg:mg) or 1.3:1 (mmol:mmol) has been recommended in short term PN (<6 weeks) in order to achieve optimum calcium and phosphorus retention in neonates.[5] Elemental calcium intake of 3.8 meq/kg/day (76 mg/kg/day) in neocates for short term PN has also been recommended to improve bone strength, especially when coupled with a PN phosphorus intake of 45 mg/kg/day (1.4 mmol/kg/day).[5] Calcium gluconate is the most common parenteral choice for calcium provision.

Phosphorus

Hypophosphatemia may occur with sepsis, respiratory or metabolic alkalosis, intestinal malabsorption, hyperparathyroidism, Vitamin D deficiency, or during refeeding syndrome.[36] Phosphorus depletion may be more pronounced when calcium is given without phosphorus,

TABLE 11.7 Commerically Available Intravenous Pediatric Multivitamin Products

	A (IU)	D (IU)	E (mg)	K (mcg)	C (mg)	Thiamin (mg)	Riboflavin (mg)	Niacin (mg)	Pyridoxine (mg)	B_{12} (mcg)	Folic acid (mcg)	Pantothenic Acid (mg)	Biotin (mcg)
MVI Pediatric (Hospira), per 5ml*	2310	400**	7	200	80	1.2	1.4	17	1	1	140	5	20
Infuvite Pediatric (Baxter), Per 5ml*	2300	400***	7	200	80	1.2	1.4	17	1	1	140	5	20

*Maximum dose not to exceed 5 ml per day

**ergocalciferol

***cholecalciferol

Modified from Gottschlich MM. *The A.S.P.E.N. Nutrition Support Core Curriculum: A Case-Based Approach-The Adult Patient.* Silver Spring, MD: A.S.P.E.N.; 2007.[4]

and is characterized by hypercalciuria, hypophosphatemia, and undetectable levels of urinary phosphorus excretion.[87,89,92,93] Hyperphosphatemia is typically seen with renal dysfunction, however, it may also be present when there is an extracellular shift of phosphorus, such as in tumor lysis syndrome or with metabolic acidosis.[36]

Recommendations for parenteral administration of phosphorus in infants and children are given in Table 11.5. As mentioned earlier, a calcium:phosphorus ratio of 1.7:1 (mg:mg) or 1.3:1 (mmol:mmol) has been recommended in short term PN (<6 weeks) in order to achieve optimum calcium and phosphorus retention in neonates.[5] Phosphorus is added to parenteral nutrient solutions as potassium phosphate or sodium phosphate salts. Potassium phosphate contains 93 mg (3 mmol) of phosphorus and 4.4 mEq of potassium per mL. Sodium phosphate contains 93 mg (3 mmol) of phosphorus and 4 mEq of sodium per mL. Phosphorus is also an inherent component of certain amino acids, as well as included in lipid emulsions via phospholipid.[36,94]

The greatest difficulty in providing adequate calcium and phosphorus parenterally is their relative insolubility in the same admixture. Calcium and phosphorus solubility is affected by many factors such as the final amino acid concentration, pH, temperature, compounding mixing sequence, presence or absence of lipid, and the total amount of calcium and phosphorus within the solution.[5,32] Providing calcium and phosphorus in concentrations above the saturation point in PN increase the risk for forming insoluble compounds known as precipitates. This is especially important to consider in pediatrics, specifically infants, where the calcium and phosphorus requirements are increased. TNA are generally not used in infants as visual identification of precipitates is difficult given the opacity of the admixture. 2:1 PN solutions are typically provided along with L-cystine hydrochloride, which decreases the solution's pH, increasing calcium and phosphorus solubility for increased provision of both minerals.[68] Solubility may be predicted by plotting the concentration of calcium and phosphorus in the compounded PN on a graph with a saturation curve specific to the concentration of amino acids, concentration of calcium and phosphorus, and temperature.[32]

Trace Minerals

Recommendations for daily parenteral doses of trace minerals are given in Table 11.5. Zinc, copper, chromium, manganese, selenium, and iodine are available singly or in combination for use in PN admixtures. Product information for available trace element products are given in **TABLE 11.8**. Neither clinical nor biochemical deficiency of molybdenum or iodine with parenteral nutrition has been reported in the literature, and they are generally not included in parenteral nutrition admixtures. Transdermal absorption of iodine from cleansing or disinfecting solutions or iodine received inadvertently as a contaminent of PN solutions may be an adequate source of iodine.[95] Fluorine is not added, because its role in human nutrition is limited primarily to dental health and may be of greater benefit when administered topically once teeth have erupted around 6 months of age.[96]

Very-low-birth-weight infants and infants and children with protein-calorie malnutrition, thermal injury, neoplasms, chronic diarrhea, enterocutaneous fistulas, malabsorptive disorders, or those receiving prolonged PN without trace elements are at greatest risk for developing trace element deficiencies.[98-100] Zinc should be included in the PN solution at the start of PN initiation for infants.[101] Zinc deficiency may promote increased infection risk, and may include symptoms such as impaired wound healing, skin lesions, and growth failure.[101] Serum zinc levels may not accurately reflect zinc status as serum levels are influenced by albumin levels, catabolism, and physiologic stress.[101] Alkaline phosphatase can be used in conjuction with serum zinc to assess zinc status, as alkaline phosphatase is a zinc metalloenyme, and may decrease in the presence of zinc deficiency.[101]

Copper doses are reduced or eliminated and manganese is often withheld for infants and children who develop cholestatic jaundice. These minerals are excreted primarily through bile and their accumulation is potentially hepatotoxic and, in the case of manganese, neurotoxic.[58,102] However, serum copper and manganese levels may not correlate with serum direct bilirubin levels, as copper deficiency has been reported when omitted from parenteral nutrition due to the presence of cholestasis.[98,103-107] Circulating copper levels may also be low in the first few months of life for a term infant due to low synthesis of ceruloplasmin.[98] Serum copper levels may be falsely increased due to the prescence of inflammation, thereby potentially masking a deficiency.[107] Clinical syptoms of copper deficiency include hypochromic, microcytic anemia, leukopenia, and various bone abnormalities.[98,107] Parenteral copper dose recommendations for infants and children is 20 mcg/kg/day, not to exceed 0.3 milligrams per day.[98,107] In the presence of liver disease one may consider reducing the copper content by half, with continued monitoring of copper status.[98] Serum manganese levels may become markedly elevated after several months of PN. Manganese is a contaminant of PN solutions, with non-manganese supplemented PN containing 5–38 micrograms of manganese per liter, strictly from contaminents.[102] Manganese may be included inherently within calcium gluconate, magnesium sulfate, potassium chloride, dextrose, and amino acid solutions.[36] Symptoms of manganese toxicity may resemble Parkinson's disease and include neurologic, psychiatric, and behavioral concerns with MRI demonstrating deposition in the basal ganglia of the brain.[36] The

TABLE 11.8 Available Trace Mineral Products

Products	mL	Zinc (mcg)	Copper (mcg)	Chromium (mcg)	Manganese (mcg)	Selenium[1] (mcg)
Multitrace-4 Neonatal[2]	1	1500	100	0.85	25	—
Multitrace-4 Pediatric	1	500 or 1000	100	1	25 or 30	—
Trace Elements-4 Pediatric	1	500	100	1	30	—
Multitrace-4 Pediatric	1	1000	100	1	25	—
Multitrace-4 (Adult)[3]	1	1000	400	4	100	—
Multitrace-4 Concentrate (Adult)[3]	1	5000	1000	10	500	—
Multitrace-5 (Adult)[3]	1	1000	400	4	100	20
Multitrace-5 Concentrate (Adult)[3]	1	5000	1000	10	500	60

[1]Neonatal, pediatric and select adult products do not contain selenium. These may be added separately when parenteral nutrition is required for longer than 4 weeks.

[2]Additional zinc is needed to meet recommendations for preterm neonates.

[3]Adult products are generally used for adolescents, or children over 10 years of age.

Data from Slicker J, Vermilyea S. Pediatric parenteral nutrition: putting the microscope on macronutrients and micronutrients. *Nutr Clin Pract*. 2009;24(4):481–486.[58]

Lexicomp. Trace elements (pediatric and neonatal lexi-drugs). Available at: http://online.lexi.com/lco/action/doc/retrieve/docid/pdh_f/130273. Accessed November 21, 2017.[97]

recommended dose of manganese is 1 mcg/kg/day with a maximum of 50 micrograms per day for children.[102] Manganese should be discontinued when bilirubin levels are greater than 2 mg/dl.[101] Whole blood manganese level is the most reliable marker of manganese status.[36]

Selenium deficiency can develop following 6 weeks of selenium-free PN, and may include symptoms such as cardiomyopathy, growth failure, pseudoalbinism, and skin disorders.[58] If the trace element preparation does not include selenium, it is recommended to supplement if exclusive PN is required for greater than 4 weeks.[58] Earlier supplementation may be required in patients with conditions promoting a high risk for selenium deficiency such as prematurity, short bowel syndrome, lymphangiomatosis, protein-losing enteropathy, or chylous leaks.[58,101] Dose recommendations for selenium include 2 micrograms per day for 0–6 years of age (term gestation), and 1–2 micrograms per day for children 7–10 years of age.[58] Selenium dose may need to be reduced or discontinued with renal insufficiency since the majority of selenium is excreted in the urine.[101] Whole blood and serum selenium concentrations are commonly used to assess selenium status.

Chromium functions to enhance the action of insulin and appears to be involved in glucose tolerance. It is a contaminent of PN, and contamination alone may be sufficient to exceed dosage recommendations. This may be especially concerning in a chronic home PN patient, where increased chromium concentrations have been found in the serum, urine, and autopsy tissues (heart, skeletal muscle, liver, and kidney) in pediatric patients receiving prescribed normal dosages of chromium in their PN.[108] Accumulation of chromium in the kidneys and prolonged excessive provision of parenteral chromium may contribute to ongoing renal damage.[108] It has been recommended that chromium supplementation be either reduced or discontinued in the setting of preexisting renal disease.[101,108]

Iron deficiency is a common cause of anemia in patients with prolonged PN dependency with limited enteral intake. Infants and children at risk for iron deficiency include those with prematurity, malabsorption, inadequate dietary iron as well as those who have significant unreplaced blood loss, or who receive unsupplemented parenteral nutrition for long periods of time.[36] It manifests as microcytic hypochromic anemia and is characterized by low serum hemoglobin and ferritin levels, low hematocrit, and low percent transferrin saturation.

There is some controversy over whether iron should be routinely included in parenteral nutrition therapy. Enteral iron supplementation is preferred and should be utilized as medically able. If provided parenterally, iron is given only for treating iron deficiency anemia, in infants and children dependent on PN, and when unable to provide enteral iron supplementation.[109] Iron provided in PN solutions is prone to disrupt lipid emulsions and form precipiates, especially when the cation load of the solution is already high.[109] Iron should thereby not be provided with PN containing lipid emulsion.[110] In many instutions lipid emulsions may be held on the day of the week that supplemental iron is given.

Iron dextran is available as the source of iron for parenteral use. It is typically provided a few times per month in order to avoid Fe overload. Iron toxicity may be difficult to ascertain because iron is quickly stored in hepatic tissue and serum iron levels may not reflect overload. Excess iron may also increase the risk of gram-negative septicemia and increase antioxidant requirements. These risks do not preclude using standard doses of parenteral iron, but higher doses must be used with caution beyond 4 weeks' duration.[87] The first dose of iron dextran should be ideally provided in the hospital setting to monitor for any adverse reaction, including hypersensitivity and anaphylactic-type reactions.[110] Infants and children may not need additional iron supplementation if they are receiving frequent blood transfusions.[16,111] Doses of 0.15 mg/kg/day up to 2 mg/day are recommended for infants and children.[110] Maximum daily doses are: infants <5 kg (25 mg), children 5–10 kg (50 mg), and children >10 kg (100 mg).[110] Additional guidelines for dosage and administration of iron dextran in treatment of iron deficiency are given in the manufacturer's package insert.

▶ Acid-Base Balance

Acid-base disorders should be recognized by clinicians ordering PN in order to adjust the acid-base balance of the solution accordingly. Acid-base homeostasis is maintained by the lungs, kidneys, and endogenous buffers.[112] Acid base disorders include acidosis or alkalosis of either metabolic or respiratory origin. Metabolic acidosis is characterized by an arterial pH <7.35 and/or a low serum bicarbonate.[112] Numerous causes exist for metabolic acidosis which may include renal failure, ketoacidosis, lactic acidosis, metabolism of parenteral amino acids, or medications.[112,113] Of note, gastrointestinal causes may include bicarbonate loss via diarrhea or pancreatic or small bowel fistula, or in the presence of excessive

chloride provision via PN.[112,113] Treating metabolic acidosis may include increasing the amount of acetate and reducing the amount of chloride in the PN solution. Metabolic alkalosis is characterized by an elevated pH on arterial blood gas coupled with an elevated bicarbonate. Metabolic alkalosis may occur due to the loss of gastric acid from vomiting or nasogastric suctioning, or loss of intravascular volume and chloride resulting from diuresis.[112] Excessive acetate in PN may also contribute to metabolic alkalosis, as acetate is converted endogenously to bicarbonate. Treating metabolic alkalosis may include increasing the amount of chloride and reducing the amount of acetate in the PN solution. A thorough discussion of both metabolic and respiratory acid base disorders, as well as further detail on etiology and compensatory mechanisms can be found elsewhere.[112]

▶ Special Considerations

PN provision is associated with various metabolic complications, both short- and long-term. Short-term complications may include fluid and electrolyte abnormalities, or hypo/hyperglycemia.[36] Long-term complications may include hepatobiliary disorders, metabolic bone disease, iron deficieny anemia, or trace element toxicities/deficiencies. Some of the more commonly seen complications with prolonged PN use are discussed in the next several sections.

Parenteral Nutrition-Associated Liver Disease

Parenteral nutrition-associated liver disease (PNALD) is characterized by serum direct bilirubin ≥2 mg/dL or liver histopathology showing a moderate –to-marked fibrosis in the setting of prolonged exposure (typically greater than 2 weeks) to PN.[43,58] PNALD includes hepatic steatosis, cholestasis, and cholelithiasis, however hepatic steatosis is most commonly seen in children.[58] There is a direct association between the development of PNALD and the duration of PN.[114]

Multiple factors that increase the risk of developing PNALD have been considered. Parenteral overfeeding in general, of any or all macronutrients, may promote hepatic fat deposition and lead to hepatic steatosis.[36] Providing GIR in excess of 12–14 mg/kg/min as well as providing parenteral calories in excess of needs may increase the risk for PNALD.[58] Research in premature infants has found that increased daily dextrose intake were associated with the development of PNALD.[112] Hepatocytes metabolize excess dextrose to either acetyl coenzyme A or store it as glycogen. When acetyl coenzyme A forms in excess, it may promote lipogenesis, increase liver triglyceride levels, and contribute to cholestasis.[115] As mentioned earlier, providing soybean oil based lipid emulsions may also increase the risk for PNALD. Uptake of parenteral phytosterols from intravenous lipids may precipitate cholestasis by accumulating in the circulation, liver, and bile, as has been suggested in animal models.[69] Other potential mechanisms exist, such as the generation of a proinflammatory state resulting from high levels of omega-6 fatty acids, and/or inadequate alpha-tocopherol provision.[58,72] Prolonged provision of >3 g/kg/day of amino acids, excluding in premature infants, may also play a role in PNALD development.[58]

There are numerous strategies one can utilize to both prevent and treat PNALD (see **TABLE 11.9**). Reducing the dose of soybean oil predominant lipid or using an alternate lipid emulsion containing n-3 may be beneficial. Caution must be taken when minimizing the dose of soybean oil predominant lipid to prevent PNALD in a child with early or no PNALD, since this may lead to growth failure, essential fatty acid deficiency, and/or negative impact on development.[72] A.S.P.E.N. clinical guideline recommendations in pediatric patients with intestinal failure include reducing soybean oil predominant lipids to less than or equal to 1 g/kg/day to treat PN associated cholestasis.[116] Avoiding the continuous infusion of dextrose via cycling PN may reduce the risk for PNALD by reducing insulin release, leading to reduced lipogenesis in the liver.[58,110] Cycling PN does typically lead to a subsequent increase in GIR if dextrose amount is maintained, however benefits are still maintained with this method. Providing any amount of enteral nutrition is encouraged, since this may stimulate enterohepatic circulation of bile acids and improve bile flow.[36] Balanced macronutrient composition also plays a role, with recommendations for caloric composition to include 50–60% carbohydrate, 10–20% protein, and 20–30% lipid.[58]

Metabolic Bone Disease

Patients receiving long-term PN therapy are at an increased risk for metabolic bone disease, or more specifically, osteopenia, osteoporosis, or osteomalacia. Numerous factors influence the development of metabolic bone disease, including nutrient composition of PN, medications, metabolic acidosis, aluminum contamination in PN, and nutrient deficiencies.[16] The inability to balance calcium and phosphorus, limited cysteine availability to increase solubility, and fluid restriction may all lead to inadequate parenteral calcium and phosphorus provision, which may contribute to poor bone mineralization. Inadequate parenteral copper provision leading to copper deficiency may also impair bone formation.[36] Clinical and laboratory parameters that may suggest metabolic bone disease include low to normal PTH, elevated alkaline phosphatase, altered Vitamin D levels,

TABLE 11.9 Approaches to Reduce the Occurance of PNALD
Provide a balanced macronutrient profile 50–60% calories from carbohydrate 10–20% calories from protein 20–30% calories from lipid
Avoid overfeeding of macronutrients and calories from parenteral nutrition.
Reduce soybean oil predominant lipid emulsion to ≤ 1 g/kg/day as appropriate
Consider alternate lipid emulsions containing n-3 fatty acids as appropriate.*
Cycle PN to <24 hours per day to allow time off from parenteral nutrition.
Initiate enteral nutrition as soon as medically appropriate (trophic feeds included).

PNALD, Parenteral Nutrition Associated Liver Disease

*Omegaven is not currently approved for routine use in the United States; permitted for treatment of PNALD through a FDA compassionate-use allowance

Data from Davila J, Konrad D. Metabolic complications of home parenteral nutrition. *Nutr Clin Pract.* 2017;32(6):753–768.[36]

Slicker J, Vermilyea S. Pediatric parenteral nutrition: putting the microscope on macronutrients and micronutrients. *Nutr Clin Pract.* 2009;24(4):481–486.[58]

Fell GL, Nandivada P, Gura KM, Puder M. Intravenous lipid emulsions in parenteral nutrition. *Adv Nutr.* 2015;6:600–610.[69]

Vanek V, Seidner DL, Allen P, et al. A.S.P.E.N. position paper: clinical role for alternative intravenous fat emulsion. *Nutr Clin Pract.* 2012;27(2):150–192.[71]

Diamond IR, Grant RC, Pencharz PB, et al. Preventing the progression of intestinal failure-associated liver disease in infants using a composite lipid emulsion: a pilot randomized controlled trial of SMOFlipid. *JPEN.* 2017 41(5):866–877.[72]

Norman JL, Crill CM. Optimizing the transition to home parenteral nutrition in pediatric patients. *Nutr Clin Pract.* 2011;26(3):273–285.[110]

Wales PW, Allen N, Worthington P, George D, Compher C, A.S.P.E.N., Teitelbaum D. A.S.P.E.N. clinical guidelines: support of pediatric patients with intestinal failure at risk of parenteral nutrition-associated liver disease. *JPEN.* 2014;38(5):538–557.[116]

changes in serum calcium, hypercalciuria, and the presence of fractures.[16] Preventing and treating metabolic bone disease includes providing adequate calcium, phosphorus, and Vitamin D in the PN solution, and avoiding both hypomagnesemia and metabolic acidosis.[36]

▶ Cycling

Administering PN in cycles provides for planned interruption of the nutrient infusion. Cycling more closely simulates normal patterns of food ingestion and fasting and may help prevent PN-associated hepatic complications.[110] Whether at home or in the hospital, cyclic PN allows a more normal daytime routine, enhancing mobility and activity patterns and also leaving a window of time for lipid clearance. It is reasonable to consider cycling PN once hemodynamic and electrolyte stability are achieved in all patients receiving long-term PN.

The nutrition needs of the child and the ability to tolerate oral/enteral feedings, in conjuction with age and nutrient reserves, should be taken into consideration when deciding on cyclic PN. Infants younger than 4 to 6 months of age who are receiving all of their nutrition parenterally may be able to tolerate breaks from PN up to 4 to 6 hours in duration.[1] Older infants and children may tolerate interruptions of up to 6 to 8 hours. Infants and children who are receiving enteral feedings or are eating in addition to their PN may receive adequate PN in shorter spans of time. Supplemental PN can usually be provided over 10–12 hours, dependent on fluid load and total required nutrition.

Glucose infusion rate should not exceed 18 mg/kg/min in order to prevent wide variations in serum glucose.[16] There is an increased risk for hypoglycemia in a child receiving cycled PN, especially in a younger child with reduced somatic stores. Gradually increasing the rate when starting the infusion and slowly weaning the rate at the end of the infusion may lessen the likelihood of hyper/hypoglycemia. The rate is adjusted over a period of 1 to 2 hours (i.e., run at half rate for the first hour and last hour) in order to maintain euglycemia. Infusion pumps that can be programmed to accomplish the gradual introduction and weaning of PN is available. A rate adjustment for cycling may not be necessary in children over 3 years of age.[1]

▶ Weaning

Minimal enteral feedings should be given whenever possible to prevent bowel atrophy and improve adaptation for tolerance of feeding advancement.[11] When increasing enteral feedings, making one change at a time in substrate, volume, or rate makes it easier to assess tolerance. Newborn infants are best weaned to mother's milk,

although fortification may be needed for preterm infants in order to adequately meet their nutrient needs. Older infants and children who recover gastrointestinal function quickly may be weaned to a diet that is age appropriate. When bowel function is expected to return gradually or remain somewhat compromised, mother's milk or hydrolyzed protein– or amino acid–based enteral products may be better tolerated.[11]

For the neonate whose feedings are limited or who is unable to take oral feedings, pleasant oral stimulation, nonnutritive sucking, and other sensory stimulation is needed to support normal oral development. When possible, the infant on PN should be offered some type of oral feeding, if only in very small amounts. If totally deprived of oral sustenance, the introduction of oral feedings may be met with gagging, vomiting, swallowing difficulties, or other signs of feeding aversion.

As an infant or child is able to make the transition to enteral/oral feedings, the volume of PN is gradually weaned by decreasing the hourly rate and/or decreasing the infusion time.[11] Total energy intake is adjusted as the percentage of enteral nutrition increases. Enteral energy needs are usually higher than PN needs because energy is required for digestion, and absorptive losses may be small or significant, depending on gastrointestinal function. When PN is cycled, providing PN at night offers supplemental nutrition with limited suppression of appetite during the day, which may better support a transition to oral feedings. Before PN discontinuation and removal of vascular access, a child should demonstrate appropriate weight gain velocity and adequate enteral nutrient intake.[2]

▶ Patient Monitoring

A comprehensive monitoring program for infants and children receiving PN includes evaluating growth parameters, laboratory measurements of metabolic and electrolyte status, fluid status, clinical status, tolerance to PN and enteral nutrition, medication changes that may affect nutrition prescription, and evaluation for PN complications. Metabolic complications that may occur during pediatric nutrition support are summarized in **TABLES 11.10** and **11.11.** Baseline and regularly scheduled laboratory measurements allow the timely identification of metabolic complications and assessment of nutritional adequacy. Laboratory monitoring protocols may vary from one setting to another, but should take into consideration smaller blood volumes in pediatric patients, using microtechniques whenever possible and avoiding unnecessary bloodwork. For patients on long-term PN, the need and frequency for some tests can be reevaluated once a stable regimen has been established. HPN patients may have laboratory values checked weekly for the first month, then spaced out to monthly if both the patient and HPN remains stable.[36] Increased monitoring may be necessary if there is a concern for fluid imbalance, changes to the patient's clinical condition, changes to medications, or for changes made to the HPN solution.[36] Tables 11.9 and 11.10 provide information on

growth parameters and suggested laboratory data that should be monitored in the pediatric patient receiving parenteral nutrition.

TABLE 11.12 provides information on metabolic complications that can occur in children on PN.

TABLE 11.10 Growth Parameters Monitored During Pediatric Parenteral Nutrition

Parameter	Frequency
Weight	Daily (neonates and infants) Daily to twice weekly (children, adolescents) Monthly (at a minimum) during provision of home PN (infants, children, adolescents)*
Length or height	Weekly (neonates) Monthly (infants, children, adolescents) Monthly during provision of home PN (infants, children, adolescents)
Head circumference	Weekly (neonates) Monthly (infants/children < 36 months of age) Monthly during provision of home PN (infants/children < 36 months of age)

*may need more frequent monitoring of weight for infants
Data from Worthington P, Balint J, Bechtold M, et al. When is parenteral nutrition appropriate? *JPEN*. 2017;41(3):324–377.[1]
Corkins MR, ed. *The A.S.P.E.N. Pediatric Nutrition Support Core Curriculum*. Silver Spring, MD: A.S.P.E.N.; 2010.[16]

TABLE 11.11 Suggested Laboratory Monitoring During Pediatric Parenteral Nutrition

Laboratory Index	Initial	Stable**	Home Monitoring**
Chemistry panel including BUN, creatinine, glucose, electrolytes, acid-base status, Ca, P, Mg	Daily	1-2x/week or as clinically indicated	Weekly until stable, then monthly
Total bilirubin, direct bilirubin, AP, ALT, AST, prealbumin, PT, INR	Baseline	Weekly	Monthly
Triglyceride	Daily	Weekly	Monthly
CBC with differential Platelets	Daily	1-2x/week	Weekly until stable, then monthly
Iron studies, zinc, selenium, manganese, copper, chromium	As clinically indicated*	As clinically indicated*	At 3 months, then every 3–6 months
Vitamin A, 25-OH Vitamin D, Vitamin E	As clinically indicated*	As clinically indicated*	At 3 months, then every 12 months
Vitamin B$_{12}$ and folate	As clinically indicated*	As clinically indicated*	At 3 months, then every 6–12 months

(continues)

TABLE 11.11 Suggested Laboratory Monitoring During Pediatric Parenteral Nutrition			*(continued)*
Laboratory Index	**Initial**	**Stable****	**Home Monitoring****
TSH	As clinically indicated	As clinically indicated	Every 12 months
Carnitine	As clinically indicated	As clinically indicated	At 3 months, then every 3–12 months

*As indicated by clinical condition or symptoms indicating deficiency, imbalance, or abnormality
**increased monitoring indicated if there are changes in clinical condition, fluid imbalance, medication changes that may affect PN or hydration, or changes made to PN solution
Abbreviations: BUN, blood urea nitrogen; Ca, calcium; P, phosphorus; Mg, magnesium; AP, alkaline phosphatase; ALT, alanine amino transferase; AST, aspartate amino transferase; PT, prothrombin time; INR, international normalized ratio; CBC, complete blood count; TSH, thyroid-stimulating hormone
Data from Worthington P, Balint J, Bechtold M, et al. When is parenteral nutrition appropriate? *JPEN.* 2017;41(3):324–377.[1]
Corkins MR, ed. *The A.S.P.E.N. Pediatric Nutrition Support Core Curriculum.* Silver Spring, MD:A.S.P.E.N.; 2010.[16]
Davila J, Konrad D. Metabolic complications of home parenteral nutrition. *Nutr Clin Pract.* 2017;32(6):753–768.[36]

TABLE 11.12 Metabolic Complications of Pediatric Parenteral Nutrition		
Complication	**Cause**	**Treatment**
Hyperglycemia, glycosuria, osmotic diuresis, hyperosmolar nonketotic dehydration, coma	Excessive dose or rate of glucose infusion	Decrease rate and concentration of glucose; use insulin with caution; results are often erratic in the very-low-birth-weight infant.
Hypoglycemia	Abrupt discontinuation of glucose infusion; excess insulin	Maintain constant glucose infusion; decrease glucose infusion rates slowly; decrease insulin.
Metabolic acidosis, hyperammonemia, prerenal azotemia	Excessive amino acid infusion	Decrease amino acids
Hyperchloremic metabolic acidosis	Excessive chloride administration causing cation gap	Provide equal amount of sodium and chloride in infusate; neutralize cation gap with acetate if respiratory status allows.
Hypokalemia	Inadequate potassium infusion relative to requirements	Increase potassium in infusate.
Hyperkalemia	Excessive potassium administration, especially in metabolic acidosis	Decrease potassium in infusate.
Volume overload, congestive heart failure	Excessive rate of fluid administration	Monitor weight daily; monitor intake and output daily to prevent volume overload; do not attempt to "catch up" by increasing rate of infusion; to treat, decrease rate of infusion.
Hypocalcemia	Inadequate calcium administration or phosphorus administration without simultaneous calcium infusion; hypomagnesemia or hypoalbuminemia	Increase calcium infusion, maintaining appropriate phosphorus and magnesium infusion.

Complication	Cause	Treatment
Hypophosphatemia	Inadequate phosphorus administration	Increase phosphorus infusion, maintaining appropriate calcium/phosphorus ratio.
Hypomagnesemia	Inadequate magnesium infusion relative to increased gastrointestinal losses in chronic diarrhea	Increase magnesium infusion.
Essential fatty acid deficiency	Inadequate linoleic and linolenic acid infusion	Provide at least 2–4% of total calories as linoleic acid, 0.25% to 0.5% of the total daily caloric intake as linolenic acid
Hypertriglyceridemia, hypercholesterolemia	Lipids infused at a rate greater than the capacity to metabolize	Decrease or interrupt lipid infusion
Anemia	Deficiency of iron, folic acid, vitamin B_{12}, or copper	Administer appropriate nutrient.

Data from Fusch C, Bauer K, Bohles HJ, et al. Working Group for Developing the Guidelines for Parenteral Nutrition of The German Society for Nutritional Medicine. Neonatology/Paediatrics – guidelines on parenteral nutrition, Chapter 13. *Ger Med Sci*. 2009;7:1–23.[57]
Hendricks KM, Walker WA. *Manual of Pediatric Nutrition*, 3rd ed. Philadelphia, PA: Decker, 2000:265–277.[118]

PN Shortages

PN product shortages are unfortunately becoming increasingly common, and the clinicians managing PN should be equipped to manage these shortages effectively. During shortages it is especially important to assess if PN is absolutely indicated, and to provide nutrition enterally as medically able. Depending on the exact product shortage (macro/micronutrient), consideration should be made to provide an enteral substitute as able. Intravenous products should be reserved for those receiving PN or those with a therapeutic medical need for such, in order to maintain the supply for those in need.[94] Institutional algorithms or protocols should be reconsidered to avoid the automatic provision of intravenous products that may be in shortage.[94] Clinicians should review other options of the product, since substitutes may be available in another form.[94] During prolonged shortages, the Food and Drug Administration may temporarily approve the alternative products imported from outside the United States.[94] Ultimately the product in shortage may need to be reduced, or in some cases, eliminated from the PN solution. Laboratory studies should be closely monitored for deficiencies, especially in the case of electrolyte, mineral, or lipid shortages. A.S.P.E.N. has developed parenteral nutrition shortage clinical recommendations to assist in effectively managing shortages while maintaining optimal patient care. These considerations, specific to the individual product in short supply, are published elsewhere.[94,117] For up-to-date product shortage information and recommendations, a list of available resources are provided in **TABLE 11.13**.

TABLE 11.13 PN Shortages: Up-to-Date Information	
Resource	**Website**
A.S.P.E.N. Product Shortage Latest News and Recommendations	www.nutritioncare.org/Guidelines_and_Clinical_Resources /Product_Shortages/Product_Shortage_Management/
US FDA Drug Shortages	www.accessdata.fda.gov/scripts/drugshortages/default.cfm
American Society of Health-System Pharmacists Drug Shortages Resource Center	www.ashp.org/shortages?WT.ac=hp_PopLinks_Drug_Shortages

Data from Plogsted S, Adams SC, Allen K, Breen HB, Petrea Cober M, Greaves J, Mogensen KM, Ralph A, Ward C, Ybarra J, Holcombe B, Clinical Practice Committee's Nutrition Product Shortage Subcommittee of A.S.P.E.N. Parenteral nutrition electrolyte and mineral product shortage considerations. *Nutr Clin Pract*. 2016;31(1):132–134.[94]
A.S.P.E.N. Clinical Practice Committee Shortage Subcommittee. A.S.P.E.N. parenteral nutrition trace element product shortage considerations. *Nutr Clin Pract*. 2014;29(2):249–251.[117]

Transition to Home Parenteral Nutrition Support

Home parenteral nutrition (HPN) is indicated in infants and children who require PN for an extended timeframe, coupled with impaired digestion and absorption, dysmotility, or unresponsiveness to enteral nutrition.[1] PN should always be initiated in the hospital setting first, allowing for placement of central access, macronutrient advancement, and close monitoring of glycemic tolerance to cycling, as indicated.[1] Candidates should be clinically stable, with stable fluid, electrolyte, and glucose requirements, before transitioning to HPN. Once the patient has been discharged from the hospital, micro- and macronutrients are typically adjusted on a weekly basis in order to ensure that needs are met and growth is adequate. Additional laboratory monitoring may include assessing vitamin and mineral deficiencies or toxicities, macro and microcytic anemia, PNALD, metabolic bone disease, and thyroid/endocrine disease.[110]

HPN requires collaboration between clinicians and the home care company. A primary and backup caregiver should receive appropriate training in order to provide HPN, and candidates should be followed by a qualified home infusion provider with pediatric experience.[110] The home referral process should initiate several weeks before discharge to ensure adequate training of caregivers and coordination with the home care company for processing of orders and necessary supplies.[110] A home glucose monitor should also be included in supplies for patients on cycled HPN.[110] Before hospital discharge, patients receiving HPN should receive a home safety evaluation, review of insurance coverage, and a comprehensive assessment including physical, psychological, and nutrition needs.[1] Patients and their families may also benefit from community and national support mechanisms that are available. The Oley Foundation (www.oley.org) is a non-profit organization that provides resources and psychosocial support for families and patients who receive HPN. Resources for children on home PN are described in **TABLE 11.14**.

TABLE 11.14 Resources that Support Successful Home Parenteral Nutrition	
Environment	Grounded electrical outlets.
	Backup electricity, either battery, generator, or power company priority for loss of power.
	Lack of physical barriers to maneuvering equipment or storing supplies.
	Refrigeration to store adequate supplies of solutions. Reliable telephone service.
	Convenient and safe water supply and hand-washing facilities.
Medical support	Convenient and reliable home healthcare agency for nursing care.
	Ongoing nutritional assessment, supplies, laboratory assessment.
	Local physician experienced and amenable to home parenteral nutrition.
	Responsive local community emergency care, both ambulance and local emergency room.
Family characteristics	At least two responsible adults who are competent to provide all care associated with home parenteral nutrition; extended family support.
	All children (both the patient and siblings, particularly small children) are protected from harm associated with home parenteral nutrition, such as needle sticks; damage to catheter, tubing, or other equipment; removal of catheter; etc.
Financial	Adequate medical insurance coverage with certified medical necessity for home parenteral nutrition.
Attitude	Family and patient must see home parenteral nutrition as having a positive influence on the life of the child.
	Respect for risks and safety issues associated with parenteral nutrition. Ability and willingness to comply with medical plan and techniques.

▶ Conclusion

In summary, the purpose of PN is: when an infant or child is unable to meet their ongoing nutrition needs with an oral diet and/or enteral feedings or the intestinal tract does not function properly, or the intestinal tract cannot be accessed, parenteral nutrition support should be provided.

So the old adage, if the gut works, use it, remains true.

The goal of this chapter is to provide resource information to the pediatric nutrition professional in providing parenteral nutrition safely and effectively. This complex therapy requires much care and skill. A team approach to the care of the child receiving parenteral nutrition support is recommended.

🔍 CASE STUDIES

Case Study
Patient History
Harrison is a 3 day old male, born at 40 1/7 weeks, presenting with an omphalacele, diagnosed shortly after birth. Enteral feeds have been withheld since birth, with plan to initiate central PN.

Nutrition Assessment
Anthropometric Measurements
Birth Anthropometrics:
Weight: 3.2 kg (38th percentile WHO growth standard, z score −0.3)
Length: 49.5 cm (42nd percentile WHO growth standard, z score −0.2)
Head Circumference: 35 cm (66th percentile WHO growth standard, z score 0.42)
Weight for Length: 46th percentile, z score −0.1
Weight at day of life three: 3.1 kg suggesting that the patient is 3% below birth weight

Laboratory results: chemistry within normal limits with the exception of hypophosphatemia (Phos 3.9 mg/dl) and hypomagnesemia (mg 1.8 mg/dl). Liver function tests and triglycerides within normal limits.

Total fluid order: 100 ml/kg/day however 25 ml/kg/day provided via medications and carrier fluids. Dextrose-containing intravenous fluids (10% dextrose) are infusing at 10ml/hour, providing a GIR of 5.2 mg/kg/min.

Energy needs are estimated at 90–100 kcal/kg/day, consistent with approximately 90% of the DRI for age (considering lack of thermogenesis of enteral substrates). Protein needs are estimated at 2–3 g/kg/day, consistent with A.S.P.E.N. guidelines for critical illness.

Nutrition Diagnosis
Altered GI function related to omphalacele as evidenced by provision of parenteral nutrition support.

Nutrition Intervention
Total volume available for PN is 10 ml/h (75 ml/kg/day). Dosing weight for PN is 3.2 kg, consistent with birth weight.

Day One PN order:
1g/kg/day 20% Intralipid = 3.2 g of lipid or 16 ml total lipid (infused at 0.67 ml/h)
    1 g × 3.2 kg = 3.2 grams lipid
    3.2 g ÷ 0.2 = 16 ml lipid
PN is provided as a 2:1 solution at 223 ml (9.3 ml/h) as follows:
    −2 g/kg amino acids
    −GIR 7.1 mg/kg/min (33 grams of dextrose)
    (33 g dextrose × 1000) ÷ 1440 minutes of infusion time ÷ 3.2 kg = 7.1 mg/kg/min
Total kcal:
Dextrose: 33 grams × 3.4 kcal per gram = 112.2 kcal
Amino acids: 6.4 grams × 4 kcal per gram = 25.6 kcal
Lipid: 16 ml lipid × 2 kcal per ml = 32 kcal
Total: 53 kcal/kg/day (169.8 kcal)

(continues)

🔍 CASE STUDIES   (continued)

Micronutrients ordered as follows:

2 meq/kg/day Na, 2 meq/kg/day K, 1 meq/kg/day Ca, 0.3 meq/kg/day Mg, 1 mmol/kg/day Phos, Cl:acetate in a 1:1 ratio, standard trace element and multivitamin preparations. Carnitine is provided at 10 mg/kg/day as PN duration is expected > 2 weeks.

Day Two PN order:

2 g/kg/day 20% Intralipid = 6.4 g of lipid or 32 ml total lipid (infused at 1.3 ml/h)

    2 g × 3.2 kg = 6.4 grams lipid

    6.4 g ÷ 0.2 = 32 ml lipid

PN is provided as a 2:1 solution at 208 ml (8.6 ml/h) as follows:

—3g/kg amino acids = 38.4 kcal

—GIR 9.1 mg/kg/min (42 grams of dextrose)

    (42 g dextrose × 1000) ÷ 1440 minutes of infusion time ÷ 3.2 kg = 9.1 mg/kg/min

Total kcal:

Dextrose: 42 grams × 3.4 kcal per gram = 142.8 kcal

Amino acids: 9.6 grams × 4 kcal per gram = 38.4 kcal

Lipid: 32 ml lipid × 2 kcal per ml = 64 kcal

Total: 76 kcal/kg/day (245.2 kcal)

Day Three PN order:

3 g/kg/day 20% Intralipid = 9.6 g of lipid or 48 ml total lipid (infused at 2 ml/h)

    3 g × 3.2 kg = 9.6 grams lipid

    9.6 g ÷ 0.2 = 48 ml lipid

PN is provided as a 2:1 solution at 192 ml (8 ml/h) as follows:

—3 g/kg amino acids

—GIR 11 mg/kg/min (51 grams of dextrose)

    (51 g dextrose × 1000) ÷ 1440 minutes of infusion time ÷ 3.2 kg = 11 mg/kg/min

Total kcal:

Dextrose: 51 grams × 3.4 kcal per gram = 173.4 kcal

Amino acids: 9.6 grams × 4 kcal per gram = 38.4 kcal

Lipid: 48 ml lipid × 2 kcal per ml = 96 kcal

Total: 96 kcal/kg/day (307.8 kcal)

Micronutrients adjusted daily based on serum levels. Calcium and phosphorus gradually increase in PN to achieve a calcium:phosphorus ratio of 1.7:1 (mg:mg) while maintaining normal serum levels.

Monitoring and Evaluation

Daily chemistry, weekly liver function tests, and triglycerides are obtained. Daily weights, weekly lengths, and weekly head circumferences are monitored. Once patient regains weight and exceeds birth weight, adjustment of PN dosing weight is considered.

Questions for the Reader

1. On day 7, PN fluid is restricted to half maintainence (50 ml/kg/day) due to concern for pulmonary edema. What macro/micronutrient adjustments would you make to the PN order? What concerns would you have regarding the PN solution?

2. Lab work on day 14 includes an elevated serum triglyceride level of 250 mg/dL. What adjustment would you recommend to the parenteral nutrition order?

3. Patient has remained on PN for 4 weeks. Serum direct bilirubin has demonstrated an upward trend, with current level of 2.2 mg/dL. What may this indicate? What adjustments to the PN should be considered?

References

1. Worthington P, Balint J, Bechtold M, et al. When is parenteral nutrition appropriate? *JPEN.* 2017;41(3):324–377.

2. Corkins MR, Griggs KC, Groh-Wargo S, et al; Task Force on Standards for Nutrition Support: Pediatric Hospitalized Patients, American Society for Parenteral and Enteral Nutrition Board of Directors. Standards for nutrition support: pediatric hospitalized patients. *Nutr Clin Pract.* 2013;28(2):263–276.

3. Jimenez L, Mehta NM, Duggan CP. Timing of the initiation of parenteral nutrition in critically ill children. *Curr Opin Clin Nutr Metab Care.* 2017;20:227–231.

4. Gottschlich MM. *The A.S.P.E.N. Nutrition Support Core Curriculum: A Case-Based Approach-The Adult Patient.* Silver Spring, MD: A.S.P.E.N.; 2007.

5. Boullata JI, Gilbert K, Sacks G, et al. American Society for Parenteral and Enteral Nutrition. A.S.P.E.N. clinical guidelines: parenteral nutrition ordering, order review, compounding, labeling, and dispensing. *JPEN.* 2014;38(3):334–377.

6. Valero Zanuy MA, Pablos Bravo S, Lazaro Cebas A, et al. Agreement between different equations to estimate osmolarity of parenteral nutrition solutions. *Nutr Hosp.* 2015;32(6):2757–2762.

7. Merritt R. *The A.S.P.E.N. Nutrition Support Practice Manual.* 2nd ed. Silver Spring, MD: A.S.P.E.N.; 2005.

8. Merenstein GB, Gardner SL. *Handbook of Neonatal Intensive Care.* 6th ed. St. Louis, MO: Mosby Elsevier; 2006.

9. Shin HS, Towbin AJ, Zhang B, Johnson ND, Goldstein SL. Venous thrombosis and stenosis after peripherally inserted central catheter placement in children. *Pediatr Radiol.* 2017;47(12):1670–1675.

10. Goodwin ML. The Seldinger method of PICC insertion. *J Intraven Nurs.* 1989;12:238–243.

11. Koletzko B, Goulet O, Hunt J, Krohn K, Shamir R for the Parenteral Nutrition Guidelines Working Group. Guidelines on paediatric parenteral nutrition of the European Society of Paediatric Gastroenterology, Hepatology and Nutrition (ESPGHAN) and the European Society for Clinical Nutrition and Metabolism (ESPEN), supported by the European Society of Paediatric Research (ESPR). *J Pediatr Gastroenterol Nutr.* 2005;41:S1–S87.

12. Dubois J, Garel L, Tapiero B, Dube J, Latramboise S, David M. Peripherally inserted central catheters in infants and children. *Radiology.* 1997;204(3):622–626.

13. Pettit J. Assessment of infants with peripherally inserted central catheters: part 1. Detecting the most frequently occurring complications. *Adv Neonatal Care.* 2002;2: 304–315.

14. Liossis G, Bardin C, Papageorgiou A. Comparison of risks from percutaneous central venous catheter and peripheral lines in infants of extremely low birth weight: a cohort controlled study of infants <1000 g. *J Matern Fetal Neonatal Med.* 2003;13(3):171–174.

15. Reed T, Phillips S. Management of central venous catheter occlusions and repairs. *J Intraven Nurs.* 1996;19: 289–294.

16. Corkins MR, ed. *The A.S.P.E.N. Pediatric Nutrition Support Core Curriculum.* Silver Spring, MD: A.S.P.E.N.; 2010.

17. Yeung C, May J, Hughes R. Infection rate for single lumen versus triple lumen subclavian catheters. *Inf Control Hosp Epidemiol.* 1988;9:154.

18. Valentine CJ, Puthoff TD. Enhancing parenteral nutrition therapy for the neonate. *Nutr Clin Pract.* 2007;22:183–193.

19. Ayers P, Adams S, Boullata J, et al. American Society for Parenteral and Enteral Nutrition. A.S.P.E.N. parenteral nutrition safety consensus recommendations *JPEN.* 2014;38(3):296–333.

20. Hardy G, Puzovic M. Formulation, stability, and administration of parenteral nutrition with new lipid emulsions. *Nutr Clin Pract.* 2009;24:616–625.

21. Mirtallo J. Should the use of total nutrient admixtures be limited? *Am J Hosp Pharm.* 1994;51:2831–2836.

22. Lee MD, Yoon JE, Kim, SI, Kim IC. Stability of total nutrient admixtures in reference to ambient temperatures. *Nutrition.* 2003;19(10):886–890.

23. Neuzil J, Darlow BA, Inder TE, Sluis KB, Winterbourn CC, Stocker R. Oxidation of parenteral lipid emulsion by ambient and phototherapy lights: potential toxicity of routine parenteral feeding. *J Pediatr.* 1995;126:785–790.

24. Laborie S, Lavoie JC. Protecting solutions of parenteral nutrition from peroxidation. *J Parenter Enteral Nutr.* 1999;23:104–108.

25. Silvers KM, Sluis KB. Limiting light-induced lipid peroxidation and vitamin loss in infant parenteral nutrition by adding multivitamin preparations to Intralipid. *Acta Paediatr.* 2001;90:242–249.

26. Mirtallo J, Canada T, Johnson D, et al. Task Force for the Revision of Safe Practices for Parenteral Nutrition. Safe practices for parenteral nutrition. *JPEN.* 2004;28(6):S39–S70.

27. Alwood M, Driscoll D, Sizer T, Ball P. Physicochemical assessment of total nutrient admixture stability and safety: quantifying the risk. *Nutrition.* 1998;14:166–167.

28. Skouroliakou M, Matthaiou C, Chiou A, et al. Physicochemical stability of parenteral nutrition supplied as all-in-one for neonates. *JPEN.* 2008;32:201–209.

29. Trissel LA, Gilbert DL. Compatibility of medications with 3-in-1 parenteral nutrition admixtures. *JPEN.* 1999;23: 67–74.

30. Pharmaceutical compounding—sterile preparations. In: *Revision Bulletin,* The United States Pharmacopeia. Rockville, MD: United States Pharmacopeial Convention; 2008:1–61.

31. Curtis C, Sacks GS. Compounding parenteral nutrition: reducing the risks. *Nutr Clin Pract.* 2009;24:441–446.

32. MacKay M, Jackson D, Eggert L, Fitzgerald K, Cash J. Practice-based validation of calcium and phosphorus solubility limits for pediatric parenteral nutrition solutions. *Nutr Clin Pract.* 2011;26(6):708–713.

33. Steger PJ, Muhlebach SF. Lipid peroxidation of intravenous lipid emulsions and all-in-one admixtures in total parenteral nutrition bags: the influence of trace elements. *JPEN.* 2000;24:37–41.

34. Driscoll DF, Bacon MN. Physicochemical stability of two types of intravenous lipid emulsion as total nutrient admixtures. *JPEN.* 2000;24:15–22.

35. Driscoll DF, Nehne J, Peterss H, Klutsch K, Bistrian BR, Niemann W. Physicochemical stability of intravenous lipid emulsions as all-in-one admixtures intended for the very young. *Clin Nutr.* 2003;22:489–495.

36. Davila J, Konrad D. Metabolic complications of home parenteral nutrition. *Nutr Clin Pract.* 2017;32(6):753–768.

37. O'Brien, F, Walker, IA. Fluid Homeostasis in the Neonate. *Pediatric Anesthesia.* 2014;24(1):49–59.

38. Lorenz JM, Kleinman LI, Ahmed G, Markarian K. Phases of fluid and electrolyte homeostasis in the extremely low birth weight infant. *Pediatrics.* 1995;96:484–489.

39. Heimler R, Doumas BT, Jendrzejcak BM, Nemeth PB, Hoffman RG, Nelin LD. Relationship between nutrition, weight change, and fluid compartments in preterm infants during the first week of life. *J Pediatr.* 1993;122:110–114.

40. Kleigman RM, Stanton BF, St Geme JW, Schor NF. *Nelson Textbook of Pediatrics.* 20th ed. Philadelphia, PA: Elsevier; 2016.

41. Rao M, Koenig E, Li S, et al. Estimation of insensible water loss in low birth weight infants by direct calorimetric measurement of metabolic heat release. *Pediatr Res.* 1989;25:295A.

42. Aperia A, Broberger O, Elinder G, Herin P, Zetterstrom R. Post-natal development of renal function in pre-term and full-term infants. *Acta Paediatr Scand.* 1981;70: 183–187.

43. Duro D, Mitchell PD, Mehta NM, et al. Variability of resting energy expenditure in infants and young children with intestinal failure-associated liver disease. *J Pediatr Gastroenterol Nutr.* 2014;58(5):637–641.

44. Mehta NM, Skillman HE, Irving SY, et al. Guidelines for the provision and assessment of nutrition support therapy in the pediatric critically ill patient: society of critical care medicine and american society for parenteral and enteral nutrition. *JPEN.* 2017;41(5):706–742.

45. Mehta NM, Compher C. A.S.P.E.N. clinical guidelines support of the critically ill child. *JPEN.* 2009;33:260–276.

46. Mehta NM, Bechard LJ, Leavitt K, Duggan C. Cumulative energy imbalance in the pediatric intensive care unit: role of targeted indirect calorimetry. *JPEN.* 2009;33:336–344.

47. Mellecker RR, McManus AM. Measurement of resting energy expenditure in healthy children. *JPEN.* 2009;33:640–645.

48. Soares FVM, Moreira MEL, Abranches AD, Ramos JR, Gomes Junior SC. Indirect calorimetry: a tool to adjust energy expenditure in very low birth weight infants. *J Pediatr (Rio J).* 2007;83:567–570.

49. Forchielli ML, Azzi N, Cadranel S, Paolucci G. Total parenteral nutrition in bone marrow transplant: what is the appropriate energy level? *Oncology.* 2003;64:7–13.

50. Martinez EE, Ariagno K, Arriola A, Lara K, Mehta NM. Challenges to nutrition therapy in the pediatric critically ill obese patient. *Nutr Clin Pract.* 2015;30(3):432–439.

51. Pierro A, Eaton S. Metabolism and nutrition in the surgical neonate. *Semin Pediatr Surg.* 2008;17:276–284.

52. Food and Nutrition Board, Committee on Dietary Allowances. *Recommended Dietary Allowances.* 10th ed. Washington DC: The National Academies Press; 1989.

53. Otten JJ, Pitzi Hellwig J, Meyers LD, eds. *Dietary Reference Intakes: The Essential Guide to Nutrient Requirements.* Washington DC: The National Academies Press; 2006.

54. World Health Association. Energy and protein requirements. Report of a Joint FAO/WHO/UNU expert consultation. Techanical report series 724. World Health Organization, Geneva; 1985.

55. Sunehag AL, Haymond MW. Glucose extremes in newborn infants. *Clin Perinatol.* 2002;29:245–260.

56. Kalhan SC, Kilic I. Carbohydrate as nutrient in the infant and child: range of acceptable intake. *Eur J Clin Nutr.* 1999;53:S94–S100.

57. Fusch C, Bauer K, Bohles HJ, et al. Working Group for developing the guidelines for parenteral nutrition of The German Society for Nutritional Medicine. Neonatology/ Paediatrics-guidelines on parenteral nutrition, Chapter 13. *Ger Med Sci.* 2009;7:1–23.

58. Slicker J, Vermilyea S. Pediatric parenteral nutrition: putting the microscope on macronutrients and micronutrients. *Nutr Clin Pract.* 2009;24(4):481–486.

59. Arsenault D, Brenn M, Kim S, Gura K, Compher C, Simpser E, American Society for Parenteral and Enteral Nutrition Board of Directors, Puder M. A.S.P.E.N. clinical guidelines: hyperglycemia and hypoglycemia in the neonate receiving parenteral nutrition. *JP E N.* 2012; 36(1):81–95.

60. Coss-Bu JA, Hamilton-Reeves J, Patel JJ, Morris CR, Hurt RT. Protein requirements of the critically ill pediatric patient. *Nutr Clin Pract.* 2017;32(s1):128s–141s.

61. Hurt RT, McClave SA, Martindale RG, et al. Summary points and consensus recommendations from the international protein summit. *Nutr Clin Pract.* 2017;32(s1):142s–151s.

62. Hauschild DB, Ventura JC, Mehta NM, Moreno YMF. Impact of the structure and dose of protein intake on clinical and metabolic outcomes in critically ill children: a systematic review. *Nutrition.* 2017;41:97–106.

63. Intravenous nutritional therapy. Crystalline amino acid infusions. *Drug Facts and Comparisons.* St. Louis, MO: Drug Facts & Comparisons; 2010;96–97.

64. Forchielli ML, Gura KM, Sandler R, Lo C. Aminosyn PF or Trophamine: which provides more protection from cholestasis associated with total parenteral nutrition? *J Pediatr Gastroenterol Nutr.* 1995;21:374–382.

65. Wright K, Ernst KD, Gaylord MS, Dawson JP, Burnette TM. Increased incidence of parenteral nutrition-associated cholestasis with Aminosyn PF compared to Trophamine. *J Perinatol.* 2003;23:444–450.

66. Adamkin DH. Total parenteral nutrition-associated cholestasis: prematurity or amino acids? *J Perinatol.* 2003;23:437–438.

67. Heird WC. Essentiality of cyst(e)ine for neonates. Clinical and biochemical effects of parenteral cysteine supplementation. In: Kinney JM, Borum PR, eds. *Perspectives in Clinical Nutrition.* Munich, Germany: Urban Schwarzenberg; 1989:275–282.

68. Plogsted S, Cober P, Gura K, Helms R, Robinson D. Parenteral nutrition L-cysteine product shortage considerations. *Nutr Clin Pract;* 2015;30(4):579–580.

69. Fell GL, Nandivada P, Gura KM, Puder M. Intravenous lipid emulsions in parenteral nutrition. *Adv Nutr.* 2015;6:600–610.

70. Edward R, Innes JK, Marino LV, Calder PC. Influence of different intravenous lipid emulsions on growth, development and laboratory and clinical outcomes in hospitalised paediatric patients: a systematic review. *Clin Nutr.* 2017; doi: 10.1016/j.clnu.2017.07.003.

71. Vanek VW, Seidner DL, Allen P, et al. Novel Nutrient Task Force, Intravenous Fat Emulsions Workgroup, American Society for Parenteral and Enteral Nutrition Board of Directors. A.S.P.E.N. postion paper: clinical role for alternative intravenous fat emulsions. *Nutr Clin Pract.* 2012;27(2):150–192.

72. Diamond IR, Grant RC, Pencharz PB, et al. Preventing the progression of intestinal failure-associated liver disease in infants using a composite lipid emulsion: a pilot randomized controlled trial of SMOFlipid. *JPEN.* 2017;41(5):866–877.

73. Sorrell M, Moreira A, Green K, et al. Favorable outcomes of preterm infants with parenteral nutrition-associated liver disease treated with intravenous fish oil-based lipid emulsion. *J Pediat Gastroenterol Nutr.* 2017;64:783–788.

74. deMeijer VE, Gura KM, Le HD, Meisel JA, Puder M. Fish oil–based lipid emulsions prevent and reverse parenteral nutrition-associated liver disease: the Boston experience. *JPEN.* 2009;33:541–547.

75. Gura KM, Lee S, Valim C, et al. Safety and efficacy of a fish-oil-based fat emulsion in the treatment of parenteral nutrition-associated liver disease. *Pediatrics.* 2008;121:e678–e686.

76. Mitton SG. Amino acids and lipid in the total parenteral nutrition for the newborn. *J Pediatr Gastroenterol Nutr.* 1994;18:25–31.

77. Pereira GR. Nutritional care of the extremely premature infant. *Clin Perinatol.* 1995;22:61–75.

78. American Academy of Pediatrics, Committee on Nutrition. Use of intravenous fat emulsions in pediatric patients. *Pediatrics.* 1981;68:738–743.

79. Sapsford A. Energy, carbohydrate, protein, and fat. In: Groh-Wargo S, Thompson M, Cox JH, eds. *Nutritional Care for High-Risk Newborns.* Chicago, Il: Precept Press; 1994:83.

80. Sacks GS, Driscoll DF. Does lipid hang time make a difference? Time is of the essence. *Nutr Clin Prac.* 2002;17:284–290.

81. Driscoll DF, Bacon MN, Bistrian BR. Effects of in-line filtration on lipid particle size distribution in total nutrient admixtures. *JPEN.* 1996;20:296–301.

82. McDonald CM, MacKay MW, Curtis J, et al. Carnitine and cholestasis: nutritional dilemmas for the parenterally nourished newborn. *Support Line.* 2003;25:10.

83. Crill CM, Wang B, Storm MC, et al. Carnitine: a conditionally essential nutrient in the neonatal population? *J Pediatr Pharmacol Ther.* 2001;6:225.

84. American Medical Association, Nutrition Advisory Group. Multivitamin preparations for parenteral use. *JPEN.* 1979;3:258–262.

85. Hahn JS, Berquist W, Alcorn DM, Chamberlain L, Bass D. Wernicke encephalopathy and beriberi during total parenteral nutrition attributable to multivitamin infusion shortage. *Pediatrics.* 1998;101:E10.

86. Ali A, Walentik C, Mantych GJ, Sadiq HF, Keenan WJ, Noguchi A. Iatrogenic actue hypermagnesemia after total parenteral nutrition infusion mimicking septic shock syndrome: two case reports. *Pediatrics*; 2003; 112:e70–e72.

87. Greene HL, Hambidge KM, Schanler R, Tsang RC. Guidelines for the use of vitamins, trace elements, calcium, magnesium, and phosphorus in infants and children receiving total parenteral nutrition: report of the Subcommittee on Pediatric Parenteral Nutrient Requirements from the Committee on Clinical Practice Issues of the American Society for Clinical Nutrition. *Am J Clin Nutr.* 1988;48(5):1324–1342.

88. Christmann V, de Grauw AM, Visser R, Matthijsse RP, van Goudoever JB, van Heijst AFJ. Early postnatal calcium and phosphorus metabolism in pretern infants. *J Ped GastroenterolNutr.* 2014;58(4):398–403.

89. Greer FR, Tsang RC. Calcium and vitamin D metabolism in term and low-birth-weight infants. *Perinatol Neonatol.* 1986:14.

90. Hufnagle KF, Khan SN, Penn D, Cacciarelli A, Williams P. Renal calcifications: a complication of long-term furosemide therapy in preterm infants. *Pediatrics.* 1982;70:360–363.

91. Wood RJ, Bengoa JM, Sitrin MD, Rosenberg IH. Calciuretic effect of cyclic versus continuous total parenteral nutrition. *Am J Clin Nutr.* 1985;41:614–619.

92. Aladjem M, Lotan D, Biochis H, Zohar Barzilay MD, Orda S. Changes in the electrolyte content of serum and urine during total parenteral nutrition. *J Pediatr.* 1980;97:437–439.

93. Giapros VI, Papdimitriou FK, Andronikou SK. Tubular disorders in low birth weight neonates after prolonged antibiotic treatment. *Neonatol.* 2007;91:140–144.

94. Plogsted S, Adams SC, Allen K, et al. Clinical Practice Committee's Nutrition Product Shortage Subcommittee of the American Society for Parenteral and Enteral Nutrition. Parenteral nutrition electrolyte and mineral product shortage considerations. *Nutr Clin Pract.* 2016;31(1):132–134.

95. Zimmermann, MB. Iodine: it's important in patients that require parenteral nutrition. *Gastroenterol.* 2009;137:S36–S46.

96. Kleinman RE. *Pediatric Nutrition Handbook.* 5th ed. American Academy of Pediatrics. 2004.

97. Lexicomp. Trace elements (pediatric and neonatal lexidrugs). Available at: http://online.lexi.com/lco/action/doc/retrieve/docid/pdh_f/130273. Accessed November 21, 2017.

98. Shike M. Copper in parenteral nutrition. *Gastroenterol.* 2009;137:s13–s17.

99. Shaw JC. Trace elements in the fetus and young infant II. Copper, manganese, selenium and chromium. *Am J Dis Child.* 1980;134:74–81.

100. Triplett WC. Clinical aspects of zinc, copper, manganese, chromium and selenium metabolism. *Nutr Int.* 1985;1:60.

101. Burjonrappa SC, Miller M. Role of trace elements in parenteral nutrition support of the surgical neonate. *J Ped Surg.* 2012;47:760–771.

102. Hardy G. Manganese in parenteral nutrition: who, when and why should we supplement? *Gastroenterol.* 2009;137:S29–S35.

103. McMillan NB, Mulroy C, MacKay MW, McDonald CM, Jackson WD. Correlation of cholestasis with serum copper and whole-blood manganese levels in pediatric patients. *Nutr Clin Pract.* 2008;23(2):161–165.

104. Hurwitz M, Garcia MG, Poole RL Kerner JA. Copper deficiency during parenteral nutrition: a report of four pediatric cases. *Nutr Clin Pract.* 2004;19(3):305–308.

105. Fuhrman MP, Herrmann V, Masidonski P, Eby C. Pancytopoenia after removal of copper from total parenteral nutrition. *JPEN.* 2000;24(6):361–366.

106. Zambrano E, El-Hennawy M, Ehrenkranz RA, Zelterman D, Reyes-Mugica M. Total parenteral nutrition induced liver pathology: an autopsy series of 24 newborn cases. *Pediatr Dev Pathol.* 2004;7:425–432.

107. MacKay M, Mulroy CW, Street J, et al. Assessing copper status in pediatric patients receiving parenteral nutrition. *Nutr Clin Pract.* 2015;30(1):117–121.

108. Moukarzel, A. Chromium in parenteral nutrition: too little or too much? *Gastroenterol.* 2009;137:s18–s28.

109. Forbes A. Iron and parenteral nutrition. *Gastroenterol.* 2009;137:s47–s54.

110. Norman JL, Crill CM. Optimizing the transition to home parenteral nutrition in pediatric patients. *Nutr Clin Pract.* 2011;26(3):273–285.

111. Ng PC, Lam CWK, Lee CH, et al. Hepatic iron storage in very low birthweight infants after multiple blood transfusions. *Arch Dis Child Fetal Neonatal Ed.* 2001;84:F101–F105.

112. Ayers P, Dixon C, Mays A. Acid-base disorders: learning the basics. *Nutr Clin Pract.* 2015;30(1):14–20.

113. Dounousi E, Zikou X, Koulouras V, Katopodis K. Metabolic acidosis during parenteral nutrition: pathophysiological mechanisms. *Indian J Crit Care Med.* 2015;19(5):270–274.

114. Lauriti G, Zani A, Aufieri R, et al. Incidence, prevention, and treatment of parenteral nutrition-associated cholestasis and intestinal failure-associated liver disease in infants and children: a systematic review. *JPEN.* 2014;38(1):70–85.

115. Gupta K, Wang H, Amin SB. Parenteral-nutrition-associated cholestasis in premature infants: role of macro-nutrients. *JPEN*. 2016;40(3):335–341.

116. Wales PW, Allen N, Worthington P, et al. American Society for Parenteral and Enteral Nutrition. A.S.P.E.N. clinical guidelines: support of pediatric patients with intestinal failure at risk of parenteral nutrition-associated liver disease. *JPEN*. 2014;38(5):538–557.

117. A.S.P.E.N. Clinical Practice Committee Shortage Subcommittee. A.S.P.E.N. parenteral nutrition trace element product shortage considerations. *Nutr Clin Pract*. 2014;29(2):249–251.

118. Hendricks KM, Walker WA. *Manual of Pediatric Nutrition*, 3rd ed. Philadelphia, PA: Decker, 2000:265–277.

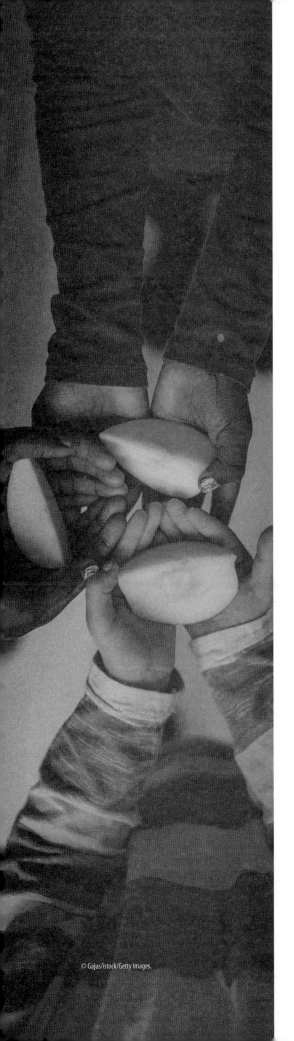

SECTION V

Pediatric Medical Nutrition Therapy

© Gajus/istock/Getty Images.

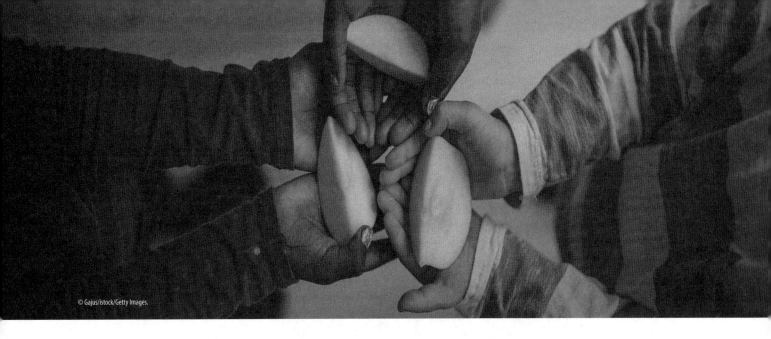

© Gajus/istock/Getty Images.

CHAPTER 12

Gastrointestinal Disorders

Jennifer Autodore, Julia Driggers, and Rebecca Wilhelm

LEARNING OBJECTIVES

- Explain how to assess, diagnose, and manage common pediatric gastrointestinal nutrition related topics such as celiac disease, lactose intolerance, inflammatory bowel disease, and pancreatitis
- Discuss normal digestion and absorption in the gastrointestinal tract
- Identify diagnosis related at-risk macro and micronutrients
- Interpret common diagnostic tests for pediatric gastrointestinal disorders

▶ Introduction

The gastrointestinal tract is an organ system that stretches from the mouth to the anus. It is a large muscular tube designed to ingest, digest, and absorb nutrients before expelling waste as feces. Functions of the gastrointestinal tract may be disrupted by disease, injury, chemotherapeutic agents, antibiotics, parasites, environmental toxins, and/or bacterial overgrowth, resulting in alterations in nutritional requirements. Many nutrients are absorbed throughout the intestinal tract, whereas others are absorbed only at specific sites. Absorption of the latter class of nutrients is particularly vulnerable to disease or surgical resection. **FIGURE 12.1** graphically portrays the principal sites of absorption of macro- and micronutrients, vitamins, and minerals.

Symptoms of gastrointestinal disease can arise from disorders located in a specific region of the bowel, the entire bowel, or distant sites (for example, vomiting can occur due to pyloric stenosis, gastroenteritis, or a brain tumor). Common pediatric disorders are listed in **TABLE 12.1** and common diagnostic tests are presented in **TABLE 12.2**. Many tests to evaluate gastrointestinal function as well as the presence or absence of disease are available.

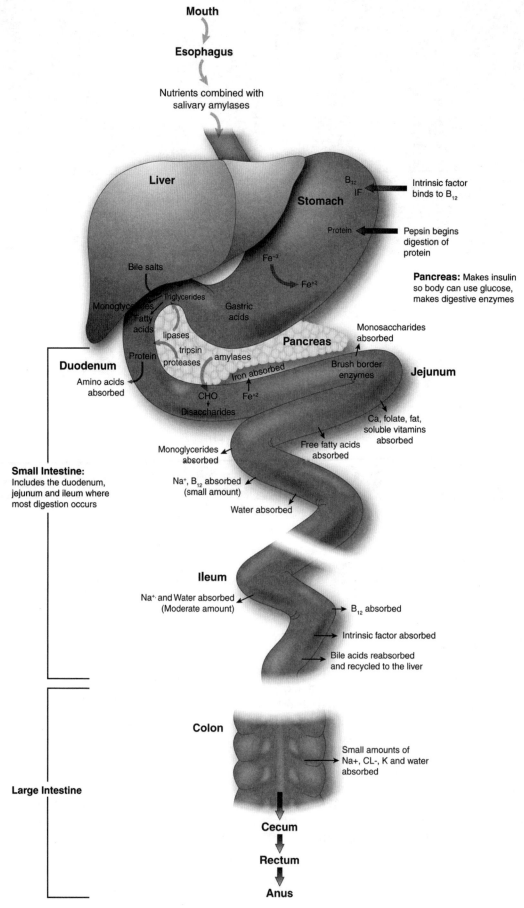

FIGURE 12.1 Normal Digestion and Absorption in the GI Tract.

TABLE 12.1 Common Pediatric Gastrointestinal Disorders

Presenting Symptom	Differential Diagnosis	Treatment
Stomach and Esophagus		
Vomiting/regurgitation	Congenital anomaly of the gastrointestinal tract	Surgery
	Gastroesophageal reflux	Infants: positioning, medications such as antacids, H2 blockers, and proton pump inhibitors (PPI). If preceding fails, consider surgical treatment.
		All ages: medications, antacids, H2 blockers, PPI, avoid caffeine-containing foods and other personal triggers
	Eosinophilic esophagitis	Elimination diet, swallowed steroids
	Eosinophilic gastritis	Steroids, immunosuppressive medication
	Peptic disease	Medications such as antacids, H2 blockers, and PPI; avoid caffeine-containing foods and other personal triggers
	H. pylori	Antibiotics, PPI
	Gastroparesis	Prokinetics, diet changes such as multiple small low-fat meals per day, or postpyloric feeds
Dysphagia (choking after eating), odynophagia (pain with swallowing)	Congenital anomalies, strictures, webs	Surgery
	Eosinophilic esophagitis	Elimination diet, swallowed steroids
	Esophageal spasms/dysmotility	Calcium channel blockers and nitrates; avoid extreme temperatures in foods
	Peptic strictures	Medications such as antacids, H2 blockers, and PPI; dilation
Liver and Pancreas		
Jaundice	Extrahepatic biliary tract obstruction, such as biliary atresia	Surgical correction; diet/formula with medium chain triglycerides (MCT), fat-soluble vitamin supplementation, choleretic agents such as ursodeoxycholate
	Autoimmune hepatitis	Steroids, evaluation for fat malabsorption, fat-soluble vitamin supplementation, protein restriction only if encephalopathic
Jaundice with recurrent abdominal pain	Gallstones	Surgery
	Choledochal cyst	Surgery
Nausea, vomiting, abdominal pain	Pancreatitis	NPO; if severe or prolonged course expected then postpyloric tube feeds or parenteral nutrition; pain control, H2 blockers; when clinically able, resume low-fat oral diet
	Pancreatic pseudocyst	Monitor cyst size; if cyst increases with enteral nutrition, may require parenteral nutrition

(continues)

TABLE 12.1 Common Pediatric Gastrointestinal Disorders   *(continued)*

Presenting Symptom	Differential Diagnosis	Treatment
Chronic diarrhea, failure to thrive	Pancreatic insufficiency, such as cystic fibrosis	Enzyme replacement therapy, fat-soluble vitamin supplementation, high calorie balanced diet
	Cholestatic disease	Diet/formula with MCT, fat-soluble vitamin supplementation
Small Bowel and Colon		
Anemia, gastrointestinal bleeding	Congenital malformations, such as Meckel's diverticulum, duplication cysts	Surgery
Vomiting	Food allergies	Hydrolysate formula, elimination diet
	Infectious enteropathies	Oral rehydration solutions, followed by lactose and/or sucrose restrictions
Diarrhea in neonatal period	Congenital disorders of carbohydrate absorption and transport	Restriction of the problematic carbohydrate, balanced nutrition, vitamin/mineral supplementation, enzyme replacement
Diarrhea, perioral and perianal rash	Zinc deficiency	Zinc supplementation
Diarrhea	Food allergies	Elemental formula and/or elimination diet
	Infectious enteropathies	Intravenous fluids, oral rehydration solutions, followed by lactose and/or sucrose restrictions if clinically indicated
	Crohn's disease	Enteral feeds for therapy and/or malnutrition, replete iron, fat-soluble vitamins, and zinc as necessary; monitor vitamin B_{12} if severe ileal disease or resection
	Ulcerative colitis	Enteral feeds for weight gain, replete iron as necessary, low-residue diet if strictures
	Celiac disease	Gluten-free diet
	Short bowel syndrome	Parenteral nutrition progressing to enteral nutrition to oral feeds; vitamin and mineral supplements specific to patient's condition
	Fructose intolerance	Dietary restrictions of fructose-containing foods
	Lactose intolerance	Dietary restrictions of lactose-containing foods
Diarrhea, normal growth pattern	Irritable bowel syndrome, chronic nonspecific diarrhea, toddler's diarrhea	Normal diet for age, increased soluble fiber intake, decreased intake of sorbitol-containing beverages (apple and pear juice) and other personal triggers

Presenting Symptom	Differential Diagnosis	Treatment
Abdominal distention/pain	Celiac disease	Gluten-free diet
	Short bowel syndrome	Total parenteral nutrition progressing to MCT-predominate hydrolysate formula; vitamin and mineral supplements
	Functional constipation	Complete bowel clean-out using saline enemas, mineral oil, Miralax; high-fiber diet and adequate fluids; bowel habit training
	Congenital disorders of carbohydrate absorption and transport	Restriction of the problematic carbohydrate, balanced nutrition, vitamin/mineral supplementation, enzyme replacement
	Fructose intolerance	Dietary restrictions of fructose-containing foods
	Lactose intolerance	Dietary restrictions of lactose-containing foods
Constipation	Hirschsprung's disease; post-NEC strictures	Surgery
	Functional constipation	Complete bowel clean-out using saline enemas, mineral oil, Miralax; high-fiber diet and adequate fluids; bowel habit training

TABLE 12.2 Common Diagnostic Tests for Pediatric Gastrointestinal Disorders

Test	Description	Useful to Help Diagnose
Barium enema	Barium sulfate administered by enema; colonic lumen and mucosa visualized by fluoroscopy.	<ul><li>Colonic strictures and obstructions</li><li>Hirschsprung's disease</li><li>Polyps</li></ul>
Barium swallow	Barium sulfate administered orally; upper gastrointestinal tract is visualized by fluoroscopy.	<ul><li>Aspiration</li><li>Dysmotility disorders</li><li>Hiatal hernias</li><li>Strictures</li><li>Varices</li></ul>
Breath hydrogen test	Oral administration of sugar and expiratory collection of hydrogen as an indirect measure of bacterial fermentation of unabsorbed carbohydrate.	<ul><li>Fructose malabsorption</li><li>Lactose malabsorption</li><li>Bacterial overgrowth</li></ul>
DXA (dual energy X-ray absorptiometry)	Measures bone density in the spine, hip, or forearm.	<ul><li>Osteomalacia</li><li>Osteopenia</li><li>Osteoporosis</li></ul>
Colonoscopy	Insertion of flexible fiber optic tube via anus into large bowel; visual examination of colonic lining, biopsies obtained.	<ul><li>Colitis</li><li>Polyps</li></ul>

(continues)

TABLE 12.2 Common Diagnostic Tests for Pediatric Gastrointestinal Disorders (*continued*)

Test	Description	Useful to Help Diagnose
CT (computed tomography scan) of abdomen	Multiple radiographs of abdomen with or without intraluminal and/or intravenous contrast; computer reconstructs multiple images to generate "slices" through the abdomen.	■ Areas of inflammation (e.g., abscess) ■ Blood vessel anatomy and obstructions ■ Organ size and consistency ■ Tumors
EGD (esophagogastroduodenoscopy)	Fiber optic tube is inserted into upper gastrointestinal tract allowing mucosal lining of upper GI tract to be visualized and biopsies to be taken.	■ Celiac disease ■ Duodenitis ■ Esophagitis, including eosinophilic esophagitis (EE) ■ Gastritis ■ Peptic ulcer disease
Fecal fat test	Concurrent 3-day diet record of fat intake and stool collection; comparison as percentage of total fat in 24 hours excreted in stool. Malabsorption indicated in children if greater than 7% of fat is excreted; for infants less than 6 months of age if greater than 15% of fat is excreted.	■ Fat malabsorption ■ Pancreatic insufficiency
pH probe	Tube with pH sensor is inserted into esophagus for 24 hours with feeding at regulated intervals.	■ Gold standard for gastroesophageal reflux
Scintigraphy ("milk scan")	Barium ingested with X-rays capturing movement through upper GI tract	■ Delayed gastric emptying ■ Pulmonary aspiration
Ultrasound	Can be of all abdominal organs or individual organs such as the stomach, intestines, gallbladder, liver, spleen, pancreas, kidney, and bladder	■ Anatomical abnormalities ■ Cysts ■ Obstructions ■ Stones ■ Tumors
Upper GI/upper GI with small bowel follow-through:	Barium ingested with X-ray monitoring of path in GI tract to duodenum or to ileum if small bowel follow through.	■ Anatomical abnormalities ■ Inflammation ■ Tumors
X-ray of abdomen		■ Bowel dilatation or obstruction ■ Calcified gall bladder stones ■ Gas patterns and free air ■ Presence of stool in GI tract ■ Pnuematosis ■ Toxic megacolon

Data from Corkins MR, Scolapino J. Diarrhea. In: Merritt R, ed. *The ASPEN Nutrition Support Practice Manual*, 2nd ed. Silver Spring, MD: ASPEN; 2005:207–210.[1]

Graham-Maar RC, French HM, Piccoli DA. Gastroenterology. In: Frank G, Shah SS, Catallozzi M, Zaoutis LB, eds. *The Philadelphia Guide: Inpatient Pediatrics*. Philadelphia, PA: Lippincott, Williams, and Wilkins; 2003:100–115.[2]

Leonberg BL. *ADA Pocket Guide to Pediatric Nutrition Assessment*. Chicago, Il: American Dietetic Association; 2008:106.[3]

Common gastrointestinal problems will be discussed in the first section of this chapter. These include acute diarrhea, chronic diarrhea, constipation, gastroesophageal reflux, and lactose intolerance. Discussions of celiac disease, inflammatory bowel disease, pancreatitis, cholestatic liver disease, liver transplant, short bowel syndrome, and intestinal transplant will be presented later.

▶ Diarrhea

Diarrheal illnesses in children follow a continuum from acute to chronic or persistent diarrhea. Acute diarrhea can be a common side effect of gastroenteritis, infectious diseases, foodborne illness, and chronic gastrointestinal diseases like Crohn's Disease and irritable bowel syndrome. Diarrhea has been defined by the World Health Organization as passage of three or more loose, watery stools per day or as 10 mL/kg liquid stool per day.[1,4] A child having diarrhea for 3–7 days is among the most common reasons for seeking the assistance of a pediatrician and is estimated to cost at least $1.5 billion yearly for evaluating and treating the population cared for.[5] Incidence of infectious diarrhea is estimated at approximately 99 million new cases each year in the United States.[6] Foodborne illness is a major cause of these cases.

Chronic or persistent diarrhea has been defined as "the passage of ≥3 watery stools per day for >2 weeks in a child who either fails to gain or loses weight."[7] Persistent diarrhea has many triggers, including acute diarrhea caused by an enteric infection, and more recently HIV infection and AIDS.[7] Chronic or persistent diarrhea (also called intractable diarrhea of infancy) has been thought of as a nutritional disorder, and certainly requires nutritional treatment for recovery. As with all diarrheal illnesses in infants, chronic diarrhea is dangerous if not treated promptly and appropriately, because it can result in dehydration and severe malnutrition.[8] Recent reports indicate that the incidence of chronic diarrhea has declined in the United States over the past two decades due to better treatment of acute diarrheal episodes.[9]

Anatomy, Physiology, Pathology & Diagnosis

Diarrhea is classified into five categories including: osmotic, secretory, dysmotility, malabsorption, and inflammatory. These classifications can be acute or chronic based on origin of causality.

Osmotic diarrhea occurs when active particles in the intestine pull water into the lumen in an attempt to normalize osmolality. As water passes through the lumen the bowel is unable to reabsorb fluid due to the presence of the nonabsorbable solutes. Stool volume is typically less than 1 liter per day.[10] Diarrhea stops when the dietary cause or solute particle is removed. Osmotic diarrhea can be caused by both dietary and pharmacological agents outlined below:

- Maldigestion of nutrients such as fat and carbohydrates
- Excessive sorbitol of >10 g/d (found in many liquid medications)[10]
- Medications including antihypertensives, cholinergics, glucose-lowering agents, anti-inflammatory drugs, laxatives, chemotherapy agents[10]
- Prokinetics (most common when receiving combination therapy of both erythromycin & metoclopramide)[10]
- Excessive fructose, lactose, or simple sugar
- Enteral formula feeding
- Overfeeding in infants and young children
- Food allergies
- "Starvation stools," defined as loose stool caused by a prolonged period of consuming only clear liquids[11]
- Laxatives

Secretory diarrhea results from excessive fluid and electrolyte secretions into the intestine. Increased fluid drawn into the intestinal lumen exceeds the absorption capacity of the bowel. Stool volume is typically greater than 1 liter per day.[10] The difference in the underlying disease is the factor causing the excessive secretions. Secretory diarrhea does not resolve when the patient is indicated as having nil per os, or nothing by mouth, status. Causes of secretory diarrhea are outlined below:

- Foodborne illnesses including *Escherichia coli*, clostridium difficile, and salmonella
- Medications, including antibiotic-associated diarrhea[10]
- Hormone-producing tumors
- Excessive prostaglandin production
- Excessive amounts of bile acids or unabsorbed fatty acids in the colon
- Rotavirus or *Clostridium difficile* ova and parasites
- Crohn's or celiac disease[12]
- Acquired immune deficiency syndrome[12]
- Pancreatic insufficiency or Cystic Fibrosis
- Zinc Deficiency

Diarrhea from dysmotility occurs when gastric, small bowel, or colonic motility alterations cause rapid transit time throughout the bowel. Diarrhea alternates with constipation and intermittent abdominal pain is present. Common causes include irritable bowel syndrome or gastrectomy. *Diarrhea from malabsorption* is caused by damage to the bowel or loss of bowel absorption causing maldigestion of nutrients. Symptoms include bloating, excessive gas, steatorrhea, and weight loss. Malabsorptive diarrhea can be caused from short bowel syndrome, bacterial overgrowth, pancreatic insufficiency, and **congenital-sucrose iso-maltase deficiency** (CSID).

Inflammatory diarrhea is due to intestinal inflammation that impairs the absorption of water and electrolytes. Characteristics include the presence of mucus, blood, and/or proteins in stool as well as an elevated white count. Intestinal lumen damage and small bowel disease are causes of inflammatory diarrhea.

An initial diagnosis of diarrhea is based on the degree of stool output and examination of stool cultures evaluating presence of blood, microorganisms, ova and parasites, leukocytes, and lactoferrin. Additional procedures to evaluate intestinal structure and function including upper endoscopy, flexible sigmoidoscopy or colonoscopy and bowel biopsy may be used to assist in diagnoses.

Nutrition Screening

Nutrition screening in pediatric patients with acute diarrhea should be consistent with clinical malnutrition (undernutrition) risk screening as defined by the **Academy of Nutrition and Dietetics** (AND) and the **American Society for Parenteral and Enteral Nutrition** (ASPEN).[13]

Nutrition Assessment

Patients with acute and chronic diarrhea presenting with signs of severe dehydration, poor oral intake, or malnutrition should be referred to a pediatric **registered dietitian/nutritionist** (RDN) with expertise in gastrointestinal disorders in order to receive individualized nutrition assessment. Nutrition assessment for patients with diarrhea consists of obtaining a thorough diet history with emphasis placed on fluid, fiber, and food intake or breastmilk/formula intake. If infection as a cause is excluded, other etiologies must be considered. Additional dietary history including food allergy, dietary protein intolerances, wheat intolerance, and lactose or other disaccharide intolerances should be gathered. In addition to nutritional intake, one should evaluate changes in appetite, as well as nausea and vomiting since these may coincide with underlying causes of diarrhea. Close attention should also be paid to anthropometric assessment, growth trends, electrolyte levels, and zinc deficiency with need for supplementation.

Nutrition Diagnostic Statements (PES)

- Altered GI function (NC-1.4) related to excessive intake of poorly absorbed carbohydrates as evidenced by cramping and loose stools.
- Food- and nutrition-related knowledge deficit (NB-1.1) related to frequent intake of apple juice and products containing sorbitol as evidenced by cramping and loose stools.
- Inadequate mineral intake: zinc (NI-5.10.1.8) related to environmental causes as evidence by altered GI function: diarrhea.

Management

The **American Academy of Pediatrics** (AAP) and the **Centers for Disease Control and Prevention** (CDC) have issued practice parameters and guidelines delineating treatment depending on the presence of dehydration.[5,14,15] "Gut rest," in which food is restricted, is an outdated concept and may result in malnutrition. General principles of diarrhea management are replacing fluid and electrolyte losses and nutritional therapy with early age-appropriate feeding.[4]

Replacing fluid and electrolyte losses is the primary medical management for acute diarrhea. Standard **oral rehydration solutions** (ORS) have been shown to replete electrolytes and fluid yet have not been shown to decrease fecal volume or duration of diarrhea. The investigative use of lower osmolality ORS have found some success in decreasing fecal volume and diarrhea duration.[16] Based on the severity of output, using an oral rehydration solution may be recommended. The composition of commonly used oral maintenance and rehydration solutions are presented in **TABLE 12.3**.

If commercial ORT are not available and rehydration is critical, home-made oral rehydration-like recipes may be tried. Homemade oral rehydration recipes do not contain the same electrolyte profile as commercial products. Examples of these types of solutions are presented in **TABLE 12.4**.

If oral rehydration fluids are unable to adequately rehydrate a patient, intravenous fluids may be required. Acute diarrhea often does not require **enteral nutrition** (EN) support for management. Chronic diarrhea, specifically malabsorptive and inflammatory, may require EN support when patients are malnourished, have inadequate oral intake or require slow continuous feeds to minimize osmotic load. In a patient with persistent diarrhea requiring long-term nutrition support, **parenteral nutrition** (PN) may be indicated if oral rehydration and enteral feedings are unable to provide adequate nutrition needs.[19]

In addition to rehydration, medical management focuses on treating the underlying gastrointestinal disorder associated with a diarrhea episode. If the diarrhea is infectious, antibiotics may be used as treatment. Anti-diarrheal agents are not recommended in those with infectious diarrhea. Patients without infection cause, specifically those with malabsorptive diarrhea, may benefit from intermittent use of anti-diarrheal agents.

Nutrition Intervention

Nutrition management varies with the degree of dehydration. The AAP has distinguished stages of dehydration using the following physical signs:

- *Mild:* Slightly dry mucous membranes, increased thirst

TABLE 12.3 Oral Rehydrating Solutions (ORS)

Solution	Glucose/CHO (g/L)	Sodium (mEq/L)	Potassium (mEq/L)	Osmolality (mmol/L)	CHO/Sodium
Pedialyte (Abbott, Columbus, Ohio)	25	45	20	250	3.1
Pediatric Electrolyte (PendoPharm, Montreal, Quebec)	25	45	30	250	3.1
Kaolectrolyte (Pfizer, New York, New York)	20	48	20	240	2.4
Rehydralyte (Abbott, Columbus, Ohio)	25	75	20	310	1.9
WHO, ORS, 2002 (reduced osmolarity)	75	75	30	224	1
WHO, ORS, 1975 (original formulation)	111	90	20	311	1.2
Cola*	126	2	0.1	750	1944
Apple juice*	125	3	32	730	1278
Gatorade* (Gatorade, Chicago, Illinois)	45	20	3	330	62.5
Whole cow's milk	12 (lactose)	40	1226	285	Not available

*Cola, juice, and Gatorade are shown for comparison only; they are not recommended for use.
Abbreviations: CHO, carbohydrate; WHO, World Health Organization.
Data from Oral therapy for acute diarrhea. In: Kleinman RE, ed. *Pediatric Nutrition Handbook*, 6th ed. Elk Grove Village, IL: American Academy of Pediatrics; 2009:651–659.[5]
Roberts J, Shilkofski N. *The Harriet Lane Handbook*, 17th ed. Elsevier Mosby; 2005:559, Table 20–14a.[17]

- *Moderate:* Sunken eyes, sunken fontanelle, loss of skin turgor, dry mucous membranes
- *Severe:* Signs of moderate dehydration plus one or more of the following: rapid thready (scarcely perceptible) pulse, cyanosis, rapid breathing, delayed capillary refill time, lethargy, coma[1]

Mild Diarrhea with No Dehydration

The AAP encourages continuing a normal diet throughout the acute illness, including breastfeeding or full strength infant formula and a regular diet, excluding beverages high in sugar (resulting in high osmolality) such as juices and sodas. Increased fluid intake is necessary to compensate for losses. Infants and children who are not dehydrated can be kept hydrated by using frequent breastfeeding, usual infant formula, and milk. The use of lactose-free formula is no longer recommended in managing acute diarrhea.[1] Infant formulas with added soy fiber have been reported to reduce liquid stools with no change in overall stool output in acute diarrhea and to reduce the length of antibiotic-associated diarrhea.[14,20,21] Using soy formula with added fiber is not a standard of care because continuation of breast feeding or usual

formula works to correct dehydration in most cases. Lactose-containing products, especially when given with complex carbohydrates, are no longer thought to increase diarrheal output or prolong the illness unless stool output clearly increases on a lactose-containing diet.[22]

Eating a regular diet during mild diarrhea does not change the volume of stool output. Parents should be educated to continue feeding their child a regular diet and offer adequate hydration.[5] Most infants and children demonstrate hunger and thirst during mild, acute diarrheal illness, and parents can respond to these cues. Historically, using the BRAT (bananas, rice, applesauce, and toast) diet guided the initial food choices for acute diarrhea; however, it is no longer recommended and should be avoided per the AAP nutrition guidelines.[23] However, foods that are high in carbohydrates, such as rice, wheat, peas, and potatoes, may slow diarrheal output.

Diarrhea with Mild to Moderate Dehydration

Increased fluid intake is necessary to compensate for losses and may require the use of ORS in addition

TABLE 12.4 Home-Made "Oral Rehydration-Like" Solutions Using Alternative Beverage Base

Recipe	Glucose/ CHO (g/L)	Sodium (mEq/L)	Potassium (mEq/L)	Calories per L	Osmolality (mmol/L)
Regular Gatorade® Drink ■ 1 ½ cup Gatorade® ■ 2 ½ cups water ■ ½ plus ¼ teaspoon salt	21	70	1.2	84	298
Powerade® ■ 1 ½ cups Powerade® ■ 2 ½ cups water ■ ¾ teaspoon salt	22	79	1.7	88	306
Grape or Cranberry Juice ■ ¾ cups juice ■ 3 ½ cups water ■ ¾ teaspoon salt	26/23	76/76	6.7/0.7	104/92	289/296
Chicken Broth ■ 4 cups water ■ 1 dry chicken broth cube ■ ¼ teaspoon slat ■ 2 tablespoons sugar	25	75	0.5	100	224
Vegetable Broth ■ 2 cubes vegetable bouillon ■ 4 cups water ■ 2 tablespoons sugar	25	77	1.3	100	228
Tomato Juice ■ 2 ½ cups tomato juice ■ 1 ½ cups water	20	74	27.5	122	259

Gatorade® is a registered trademark of PepsiCo
Powerade® is a registered trademark of Coca-Cola
Abbreviations: CHO, carbohydrate
Modified from Home-Made "Oral Rehydration-Like" Solutions Using Alternative Beverage Base In: Pocket Guide for Patients: Managing Short Bowel Syndrome 3rd Edition by Parrish RE, 2016.[18]

to the regular diet.[9] The use of ORS helps to replace fluid and electrolyte losses from diarrhea. Dehydration can be treated at home by giving an ORS solution by syringe at the rate of 1 teaspoon (5 mL) per minute over 4 hours for a child less than 15 kg or 2 teaspoons (5–10 mL) for children 15–20 kg. This method of fluid administration is adequate to replace the fluid deficit within a 4-hour period. After 1–2 hours of this treatment, the infant or child may begin voluntarily accepting the rehydration liquid. If the child or infant is unable to cooperate, a nasogastric (NG) tube may be used at home or in the hospital. After correction of dehydration, age-appropriate feeding should be initiated as described above.[9]

Diarrhea with Severe Dehydration

Severe dehydration in infants and children is a medical emergency and requires immediate hospitalization. Once rehydration is complete, age-appropriate feeding can be initiated.

Mild zinc deficiency may play a role in both acute and chronic diarrhea. Zinc supplementation in developing countries has been associated with a decrease in number of stools per day and decreased number of days with watery diarrhea in acute diarrhea and reduction of the duration of persistent diarrhea.[24] A randomized double-blind placebo-controlled trial of zinc supplementation in breastfed infants in the United States showed no significant difference in diarrhea frequency in the supplemented and not supplemented groups.[25] In a Cochrane review, zinc supplementation was not found statistically significant in reducing diarrhea. Zinc supplementation may be beneficial in patient populations susceptible to deficiency. The WHO recommends zinc supplementation in those susceptible at 20 mg per day for 7–14 days for children 6 months and older and 10 mg per day for children younger than 6 months.[16]

Prebiotics and Probiotics

Using probiotics and prebiotics in infant and enteral formulas and in foods has been proposed as beneficial for treating acute and chronic diarrhea of infancy and childhood. *Probiotics* are live microorganisms, historically available in fermented foods such as yogurt, that promote health by improving the balance of healthy organisms in the intestinal tract.[14] Additional proposed mechanisms are preventing adhesion of microbes to the gut mucosa, downregulation of inflammatory responses, and stimulation of immunoglobulin A production.[26,27] Technology has allowed beneficial bacteria to be freeze-dried, added to formula or foods, and be reactivated in the gut when consumed.[28] *Prebiotics* are complex carbohydrates, not microorganisms, that promote the growth of healthy microorganisms in the intestinal tract.[14] Human milk contains oligosaccharides (a type of prebiotic) that promote the growth of *lactobacilli* and *Bifidobacterium* in the colon of breastfed infants.[14,29] Higher intake of breast milk has been associated with a lowered incidence of acute diarrhea.[30]

Questions about consuming live probiotic bacteria and prebiotics include whether long-term consumption is safe and whether consumption has positive health effects. A randomized controlled trial has reported that healthy infants consuming a formula supplemented with prebiotic mixtures achieved normal growth and had stools more similar to breastfed infants when compared with infants fed an unsupplemented formula. The prebiotic mixtures included polydextrose and galacto-oligosaccharides in one group and polydextrose, galacto-oligosaccharides, and lactulose in the second group.[31] A double-blind randomized placebo-controlled trial evaluated the tolerance and safety of long-term consumption of different levels of cow's milk formula not supplemented and supplemented with different levels of *Bifidobacterium lactis* and *Streptococcus thermophilis* in infants 3–18 months of age. Healthy infants consuming the probiotic-supplemented formula reported a lower frequency of colic or irritability, and reduced severity of antibiotic-induced acute diarrhea.[32]

Manufacture of infant formulas with added prebiotics and probiotics have steadily increased in the past decade. Formula companies claim the benefits for inclusion, promoting digestive health, improving fussiness, and mimicking breast milk. Common prebiotic and probiotic additives in infant formulas include *Lactobacillus rhamnosus* GG and galactooligosaccharides. Pediatric enteral formula for children over 1 year of age with added pre- and probiotics are also on the rise. Examples include Boost Kids Essentials 1.0 and 1.5 (*L. reuteri* inserted in optional straw to use for drinking) by Nestlé,[33] Pediasure enteral formula with fiber (Nutra-Flora and scFOS) by Abbott;[34] Pediasure Peptide 1.0 and 1.5 (NutraFlora and scFOS), also from Abbott;[34] and Peptamen Jr with fiber (contains insoluble fiber and Prebio, a blend of FOS and inulin) and Peptamen Jr with Prebio (no insoluble fiber) by Nestlé.[33]

In pediatric patients with acute gastroenteritis using probiotics, specifically *Lactobacillus* GG (LGG) and *saccharomyces boulardii (s boulardii)*, may reduce the duration and intensity of symptoms in healthy children.[35] A meta-analysis showed that in children *LGG* reduced the duration of diarrhea, decreased mean stool frequency, and decreased the risk of diarrhea lasting 4 or more days.[35-36] Another meta-analysis study examining *s boulardii* showed similar results in healthy infants and children. Using *s boulardii* decreased duration of diarrhea by 1 day, decreased the risk of diarrhea lasting 4 or more days, and decreased the length of stay in hospitalized children.[37] In both meta-analysis high dose probiotics showed the most benefit in reducing diarrhea suggesting a dose of $\geq 10^{12}$ CFU per day LGG and 250–750 mg per day of *s boulardii* for a duration of 5–7 days.[35] Probiotics that show low efficacy for managing acute enteritis include *Lactobacillus reuteri Strain DSM 17938* and Heat Killed *L. acidophilus LB*.[38] In children, strong recommendations have been made to avoid the probiotic, *enterococcus faecium*, due to safety issues as a possible recipient of the vancomycin-resistant genes.[39]

There is still no consensus concerning the types and amounts of probiotics that are beneficial. More research is needed.

Diarrhea Associated with Enteral Nutrition Support

Diarrhea associated with enteral feeds have been seen in up to 95% of critically ill patients.[10] Causes for diarrhea on enteral feedings include an excessive rate or volume of feeding into the stomach or small intestine, the presence of unabsorbed carbohydrate in the large intestine, and diarrhea secondary to medications, especially those with sugar alcohols.[40] Gastric feedings versus post pyloric feedings have been shown to decrease diarrhea. Most patients are able to tolerate a polymeric formula; however, if diarrhea occurs, switching to a lower osmotic peptide based formula, specifically less than 300 mOsm, or high **medium-chain triglycerides** (MCT) may improve output.[40,41] Soluble liquid pectin at 1% to 3% mL per total formula volume and microlipids at 1–2 mL per 50 mL formula can be added to enteral formula in order to decrease and bulk stool output.[40] Using fiber containing formula in critically ill patients is discouraged due to the risk of splanchnic perfusion and mesenteric ischemia. ASPEN guidelines recommend 10–20 grams of fiber should be given in 24 hours if diarrhea is present.[42]

Monitoring and Evaluation

It is important to monitor patients closely to see if any adjustments are needed in nutrition intervention. These measurements can help monitor hydration status; intake/output records, stool consistency, laboratory values/electrolytes, and daily weights. As diarrhea improves and diet is advanced, it is important to monitor tolerance/intolerance to foods. Foods that exacerbate diarrhea can be eliminated from the diet temporarily.[19]

▶ Constipation

Constipation is a prevalent functional gastrointestinal disorder of childhood. The vast majority of constipation is termed *functional constipation*, which is idiopathic in nature and "characterized by the passing of infrequent, inconsistent, dry, hard, or painful stools"; whereas *anatomic constipation*, is experienced by individuals born with gastrointestinal and/or genitourinary tract anomalies.[43] Constipation presents with an estimated worldwide prevalence rate of 0.7 to 29.6 percent and it is reported that approximately 17 to 40 percent of children experience constipation within their first year of life. Additionally, constipation accounts for roughly 1 to 3 percent of all annual pediatric primary care visits and results in additional US healthcare costs estimated at $3.9 billion dollars or more precisely $3,362.00 per treated child.[43–47]

Risk factors for constipation have been identified and include intestinal causes such as Hirschsprung's disease, Celiac disease, or anatomic (anorectal) malformations; diseases or consequences of metabolic/endocrine origin (ex. vitamin D intoxication, diabetes mellitus, hypothyroidism), as well as medication/vitamin use (e.g. antidepressants, antihistamines, iron/calcium supplements, opioids). Additionally, those who have been diagnosed with anorexia nervosa, cystic fibrosis, or have experienced physical and psychological trauma, as well as emotional stress are also at an increased risk for constipation. Lastly, low consumption of dietary fiber, physical inactivity, genetic predisposition, and prematurity of birth also increase one's risk of experiencing constipation.[43,45] Whether or not infants and children diagnosed with a cow's milk protein allergy are at greater risk for constipation remains debatable since scientific evidence is inconclusive.[46]

Anatomy, Physiology, Pathology

The physiology and pathophysiology of pediatric constipation is multi-factorial. In some instances, constipation occurs secondary to innate defects in colonic function or a malfunction of the defecation process. Conversely, a fully functioning large intestine allows chyme (which enters the large intestine from the small intestine via the ileocecal sphincter) to move within the colon, promoting adequate absorption of fluid, electrolytes, and nutrients, all while converting digested food into waste (feces), which is then transported from the sigmoid colon to the rectum and then expelled. Any interruption experienced during this process can result in constipation. Lastly, the reabsorption of fluid and electrolytes that occurs during prolonged colonic transit time may result in constipation.[43,45]

When stooling is chronically difficult or painful, children may withhold stool, aggravating the existing problem. Encopresis may result due to the stretched rectal wall, allowing a softer stool to leak out involuntarily. A bowel program to treat encopresis, after a thorough clean-out, often includes a high-fiber diet, adequate fluid, and increased physical activity.[45]

Nutrition Screening

Nutrition screening in pediatric patients with constipation should be consistent with clinical malnutrition (undernutrition) risk screening as defined by the AND and ASPEN.[13]

Nutrition Assessment

Patients with constipation should be referred to a pediatric RDN with expertise in functional gastrointestinal disorders in order to receive individualized nutrition assessment. Nutrition assessment for patients with constipation consists of obtaining a thorough diet history with emphasis placed on food, fluid, and breastmilk/formula intake, as well as the amount of caffeine, psyllium, and dietary fiber detailed in the diet history. Inadequate fluid intake, excessive cow's milk intake, and suboptimal dietary fiber consumption contribute to constipation. Besides nutritional intake, one should also evaluate changes in feeding behaviors, food acceptance, appetite, nausea/vomiting/retching, as well signs/symptoms of **gastroesophageal reflux disease** GERD given the co-occurrence of GERD and constipation in the pediatric population.[43,45–46] Close attention should also be paid to anthropometric assessment, growth trends, and the need for multivitamin and mineral supplementation to help prevent and/or correct nutrient deficiency.[43,45]

Diagnosis

Presently, the diagnosis and classification of functional constipation is based on the Rome IV criteria (expert consensus criteria for diagnosing functional gastrointestinal disorders), history obtained, and physical examination.[43,46-47] Scientific evidence does not support the routine use of colonic transit studies, digital rectal examination, rectal ultrasound, or abdominal radiography to diagnose functional constipation in the pediatric population.[46]

Nutrition Diagnostic Statements (PES)

- Inadequate fiber intake (NI-5.8.5) related to limited oral consumption of fruits, vegetables, and whole grains as evidenced by a three-day diet history revealing an average fiber intake meeting less than the **Recommended Daily Allowance** (RDA) for age.
- Food and nutrition knowledge deficit (NB-1.1) related to patient and family presenting without prior knowledge of fiber-containing foods as evidenced by patient/family disclosure during clinic visit.

Management

Vital components for managing childhood constipation include medical education, nutrition intervention, treatment of fecal impaction to achieve disimpaction, maintenance therapy via osmotic or stimulant laxatives, and close follow-up.[45-46] Behavioral therapies aimed at decreasing defecation-related anxiety, discouraging the withholding of stools, and both improving and establishing toileting routines may serve as a beneficial non-invasive therapeutic intervention.[43,45] Lastly, surgical options may be considered in severe constipation cases when medical and nutrition therapy interventions have failed.[45]

To date, **polyethylene glycol** (PEG), an osmotic laxative not digested by colonic bacteria, is the primary laxative used for fecal disimpaction and maintenance treatment in the prevention of re-impaction.[45,48-49] PEG should not be used in children who are allergic, have a history of known or suspected bowel obstruction, and should be used prudently in children with swallowing difficulties secondary to an increased risk of aspiration occurrence.[48] The use of PEG has grown over recent years due to its efficacy, safety profile, and non-invasive administration route. Minor adverse reactions have been reported in the literature, which include bloating, increased flatulence, abdominal pain, nausea/vomiting, etc.[48] Recently, concerns have been raised regarding the lack of **Food and Drug Administration** (FDA)

approval for the use of PEG for functional constipation in the pediatric population as well as parental fears related to laxative addiction.[48-49] Neuropsychiatric events, such as tics, tremors, and obsessive compulsive behavior have been reported to the FDA; prompting an ongoing research study investigating the overall safety of PEG in children.[48-49]

Nutrition Intervention

The specific nutrition diagnosis established from the nutrition assessment helps determine the appropriate medical nutrition therapy intervention. Treatment in infants may include juices that contain natural sorbitol such as apple, pear, or prune (0.5 g/100 g, 2.1 g/100 g, and 12.7 g/100 g, respectively), increasing fluids, and verifying that infant formula is mixed correctly.[50-51] Rice cereal, a common first food for infants, as well as commercially available jarred baby foods, contain minimal amounts of fiber and may lead to constipation. Replacing rice cereal with oatmeal cereal and preparing homemade infant purees from fresh fruits and vegetables with the skin left on should be considered and may help resolve symptoms.[43] Higher fiber diets, alongside adequate fluid intake and physical activity is recommended as the first line of therapy in children with constipation.[43,45-46] Recommended fiber intake for individuals between the ages of 1 and 18 years is listed in **TABLE 12.5**. The fiber content of common foods is presented in **TABLE 12.6**. Fiber supplements may be considered when dietary intake is

TABLE 12.5 Adequate Intake of Fiber for Children

Age (in years)	Total Fiber Intake (g/day)
1–3	19
4–8	25
Boys	
9–13	31
14–18	38
Girls	
9–13	26
14–18	26

Data from National Academy of Sciences. Institute of Medicine. Food and Nutrition Board. Dietary Reference Intakes for Energy, Carbohydrate, Fiber, Fat, Fatty Acids, Cholesterol, Protein, and Amino Acids (Macronutrients) 2005. Available at: https://www .nap.edu/read/10490/chapter/32#1324. Accessed: October 18, 2017.[52]

TABLE 12.6 Good Sources of Dietary Fiber

	Grams of Fiber	Serving Size
Fruit		
Apple	2.2	1 med. w/skin
Apple	2	1 med. w/o skin
Apricot	7.8	dried, 3 oz
Blueberries	4.4	1 cup raw
Dates, dried	4.2	10
Kiwi	3.4	3 oz
Pear	4.1	1 med. raw
Prunes, dried	7.2	3 oz
Prunes, stewed	6.6	3 oz
Raisins	5.3	3 oz
Raspberries	5.8	1 cup
Strawberries, raw	2.8	1 cup
Vegetables and Legumes		
Avocado, California, raw	3	1 med.
Beans, black, boiled	7.2	1 cup
Beans, great northern, boiled	6	1 cup
Beans, kidney, boiled	6.4	1 cup
Beans, lima, boiled	6.2	1 cup
Beans, baby lima, boiled	7.8	1 cup
Beans, navy, boiled	6.6	1 cup
Beans, green, canned	6.8	½ cup
Broccoli, boiled	2.2	½ cup
Chickpeas (garbanzo beans)	5.7	1 cup
Cowpeas (black-eyed peas)	4.4	1 cup
Lentils, boiled	7.9	1 cup
Ready-to-Eat Cereal		
FiberOne (General Mills)	14	½ cup
All-Bran (Kellogg's)	10	½ cup
100% Bran (Post)	9	⅓ cup
Shredded Wheat and Bran (Post)	8	1¼ cup
Raisin Bran (Post)	8	1 cup
Grape-Nuts (Post)	7	½ cup
Multi Bran Chex (General Mills)	6	¾ cup
Cracklin' Oat Bran (Kellogg's)	6	¾ cup
Mini Wheats (Kellogg's)	6	1 cup (30 biscuits)
Frosted Mini Wheats with raisins (Kellogg's)	6	¾ cup (24 biscuits)
Shredded Wheat (Post)	6	1 cup
Mini Wheats with strawberries (Kellogg's)	5	¾ cup (24 biscuits)
Wheat Chex (General Mills)	5	¾ cup
Bran Flakes (Post)	5	¾ cup
Banana Nut Crunch (Post)	4	1 cup
Raisin Bran Pecan Date Crunch (Post)	4	½ cup
Cranberry Almond Crunch	3	¾ cup
Low Fat Granola (Kellogg's)	3	½ cup
Grape-Nut Flakes (Post)	3	¾ cup

Data from Data for sections on fruits and vegetables/legumes from: Pennington JAT. *Bowes and Church's Food Values of Portions Commonly Used*, 15th ed. Philadelphia: JB Lippincott; 1989[53]
U.S. Department of Agriculture. *USDA Provisional Table on the Dietary Fiber Content of Selected Foods*; 1988. HNIS/PT-106.[54]
Data for section on ready-to-eat cereals from a survey of manufacturer's Websites as of November 2009.

inadequate. Presently, insufficient evidence exists that supports the use of prebiotics and probiotics in the treatment of pediatric constipation.[43,46]

Monitoring and Evaluation

Ongoing monitoring and evaluation is essential for treating, maintaining, and preventing pediatric constipation. Following the initiation of treatment, 60 percent of children with functional constipation experience resolution of symptoms between 6 and 12 months, with the remaining 40 percent of children still reporting symptoms.[45–46] Additionally, approximately 30 percent of children continue to experience symptoms beyond puberty.[45] It is very important for parents to understand that the duration of maintenance therapy ranges from 6 to 24 months.[45] Therefore, individualized medical and nutrition follow up is paramount in order to allow for appropriate adjustments in the treatment plan and receive ongoing support to promote compliance. Focus should be placed on medical nutrition therapy components previously discussed, along with determining dietary compliance, goal achievement, and the current status of the patient's nutrition diagnosis (e.g. "resolved, improved, no change, worsened").[43] One should also assess the comprehension level of the patient and family, along with addressing individual questions/concerns and providing continued support in an effort to achieve improved quality of life.

▶ Gastroesophageal Reflux

Gastroesophageal reflux (GER) is the passage of gastric contents into the esophagus. GER is a normal physiologic process that occurs in healthy infants. GER may cause involuntary regurgitation or vomiting. GER is common in infants with more than 60% of infants regurgitating daily and over 25% regurgitating four or more times per day.[55] GER usually peaks at 4 months of age with tapering by 6 months and improvement of symptoms by 12–15 months when the child achieves a more upright posture.[55,56]

Anatomy, Physiology, Pathology

The primary physiologic cause of GER in infants is the transient relaxation of the lower esophageal sphincter allowing gastric contents to flow into the esophagus. Often, relaxation of the sphincter is spontaneous, however, increased abdominal pressure can cause reflux symptoms. Crawling, sitting, and coughing are common infant milestones that increase abdominal pressure and may worsen reflux.[57] When gastroesophageal reflux causes troublesome symptoms or complications of persistent GER such as recurrent regurgitation, weight loss, poor weight gain, dysphagia, or strider, it is classified as GERD.[58]

Nutrition Screening

Nutrition screening in pediatric patients with GERD should be consistent with clinical malnutrition (undernutrition) risk screening as defined by the AND and ASPEN.[13]

Nutrition Assessment

Patients with GER or GERD that present with growth related and intake related issues should be referred to a pediatric RDN with expertise in gastrointestinal disorders in order to receive an individualized nutrition assessment. A nutrition assessment for infants with GER/GERD consists of obtaining a thorough diet history with emphasis placed on breastmilk/formula intake, feeding position, frequency of feedings as well as using formula thickening agents. For children and adolescents, dietary recall, meal portion size, meal times, and frequency of meals should be assessed. Close attention should also be paid to anthropometric assessment and growth trends.[43]

Diagnosis

In most infants and children, a detailed history including feeding behavior, regurgitation occurrences, and a physical exam can diagnose uncomplicated GER.[46] To date, no set of symptoms or diagnostic test has been established to diagnosis GERD or identify what patients would respond to therapeutic interventions.[47] Diagnostic questionnaires related to reflux symptoms can be a useful tool in monitoring and detecting GERD in infants and children.[48] In certain cases a pH probe or impedance probe may be used to detect the number of reflux episodes and quantify GER, however, these test are unable to diagnosis GERD. An upper GI tract series or barium swallow test may be used in patients with troublesome GER/GERD symptoms in order to detect if there is a structural abnormality or motility disorder[58–61]; however, sensitivity and specificity of these test are low in the infant population.[62] In adolescent patients, there is a high reliability of diagnosing GER with the most common reported symptom being heartburn.[63]

Nutrition Diagnostic Statements (PES)

- Inadequate oral intake (NI-2.1) related to vomiting after feeding as evidenced by insufficient growth velocity
- Inadequate energy intake (NI-1.4) related to altered gastrointestinal function as evidence by weight for length z-score

Management

Thickening of feeds, formula modification, positioning changes, and changes in meal frequency are primary nonpharmacological management techniques for infants with GER. Pharmacological acid suppression medications like histamine2 (H_2) antagonists and proton pump inhibitors are used and have been shown to reduce gastric acidity and heal esophagitis in children.[64] Currently, there is minimal evidence of efficacy of using acid suppression in infants.[65,66] The **North American Society for Pediatric Gastroenterology, Hepatology, and Nutrition** (NASPGHAN) guidelines do not recommend using acid suppression therapy in healthy infants with regurgitation.[58] Shortterm use of acid-suppression therapy for infants with intractable or severe symptoms should only be considered after a hypoallergenic formula is trialed.[58] For patients with intractable GER, a surgical fundoplication in which the fundus of the stomach is wrapped around the lower end of the esophagus to prevent reflux, may be indicated.

Nutrition Intervention

In 2009, a joint committee of NASPGHAN and the **European Society for Pediatric Gastroenterology, Hepatology, and Nutrition** (ESPGHAN) revised clinical practice guidelines on pediatric GER and GERD.[58] The "happy spitter" is an infant who has frequent episodes of regurgitation but continues to grow well. Parental education concerning the expected improvement as the infant develops is all that is necessary. If the infant is not growing well or has increased irritability, changes in feeding are recommended. For recurrent regurgitation and poor weight gain, NASPGHAN guidelines suggest a 2 to 4-week trial of a hydrolyzed amino acid based formula in order to decrease reflux symptoms. If the infant is breastfed, eliminating cow's milk and/or soy from the mother's diet may be suggested. Discontinuing breastfeeding is rarely recommended. The exact mechanism for reducing reflux with a hypoallergenic formula is unknown. A common symptom of cow's milk protein allergy is reflux, however, milk protein allergy and GER are not mutually exclusive. No data exist to support the idea of an allergy to soy protein in infants that causes regurgitation and vomiting. Decreasing the volume of each feeding and offering more frequent feedings may also improve GER symptoms; however, total intake may decrease with this change.[58] Thickened formula may decrease the number of vomiting episodes and esophageal pain but does not reduce the number of reflux episodes.[58,67] Using infant rice or oatmeal cereal to thicken formula is the most common thickening technique in North America.[58] It is important to note that The Academy of Pediatrics does not recommend the introduction of infant cereal into a child's diet before 4 months of age and the early introduction through formula thickening has been linked to increase incidents of **necrotizing enterocolitis** (NEC) in preterm infants.[68,69] Recommendations on adding infant cereal per formula ounce varies with the minimum addition of 1 teaspoon

per ounce to a maximum addition of 1 tablespoon of infant cereal to 1 ounce of formula.[61] One tablespoon of infant cereal addition increases a 20 calorie per ounce formula to 34 calories per ounce. Formula with added infant cereal may require an enlarged nipple to allow flow, which may cause episodes of coughing.[58] Adding infant cereal can result in too rapid a weight gain and decrease the percentage of calories provided by protein and fat. Using antiregurgitant formulas such as Enfamil AR (Mead Johnson) may similarly reduce the number of vomiting episodes but not decrease the number of reflux episodes. If the infant is diagnosed with failure to thrive, increasing the caloric density of formula is recommended, especially if extensively hydrolyzed or amino acid formulas have improved symptoms. Although GER symptoms do improve in the flat, prone position, prone positioning is not recommended in infants because of its association with SIDS unless the infant is observed and awake, particularly in the postprandial phase.[70] The left-lateral feeding position has also been shown to decrease reflux symptoms and is considered safe.[71,72] The semi-supine position, such as in a car seat, does not offer any benefit and may worsen symptoms.[65]

Monitoring and Evaluation

Simple GER usually resolves around 18 months of age. GERD usually requires medical management including using acid suppression medications.[58] Using transpyloric feeds have been shown to decrease reflux episodes, but they may not completely eliminate the symptoms of GERD. When feeding modifications and use of medications do not improve GERD, surgical management such as a fundoplication, may be warranted. In older children and adolescents, there is no evidence that changes in diet improve symptoms, although in adults late night eating and obesity are associated with GER. Expert opinion suggests that children and adolescents eliminate caffeine, chocolate, and spicy foods. Alcohol use may also increase symptoms.[58] Elevating the head of the bed during sleeping in children and adolescents also may improve symptoms.

▶ Lactose Intolerance

Lactose intolerance is defined as the inability to metabolize and digest lactose, which is the sugar most commonly found in milk and milk products, due to lactase deficiency. It is a clinical syndrome characterized by abdominal cramping, bloating, flatulence, and diarrhea that occurs approximately 30 minutes to 12 hours following the ingestion of lactose containing food and beverage. Individual tolerance varies per individual and is based on one's degree of enzyme (lactase) deficiency, which directly influences how much lactose an individual can tolerate.[73,74] Throughout this section, four types of lactase deficiency will be discussed: primary lactase deficiency, secondary lactase deficiency, developmental lactase deficiency, and congenital lactase deficiency.

Anatomy, Physiology, and Pathology of Lactose Intolerance/Malabsorption

Lactose intolerance is caused by a shortage of the enzyme lactase, which is produced by the cells that line the small intestine. People who lack this enzyme are unable to metabolize and completely digest lactose (a disaccharide) into its simpler forms—glucose and galactose (monosaccharides)—following the ingestion of a lactose-containing food or beverage.[74–76] This results in digestive discomfort, such as abdominal cramping, bloating, flatulence, and diarrhea. The aforementioned symptoms result from bacterial fermentation of malabsorbed carbohydrate (undigested lactose) in the colon causing excess gas and increasing gut motility/osmotic load, which results in loose stools and/or diarrhea.[76]

Diagnosis

Lactose malabsorption is commonly diagnosed noninvasively via a breath hydrogen test. Following the ingestion of a lactose-containing beverage (typically 1–2 g lactose/kg body weight, up to a maximum of 25 grams lactose), the patient blows into a balloon-like bag at intervals for a specified amount of time (typically 2–3 hours).[74] Intermittent samples are taken and analyzed. Carbohydrate malabsorbed in the small intestine (undigested lactose) is fermented by colonic bacteria and released as hydrogen gas, allowing for the measurement of hydrogen in the breath. A raised hydrogen breath level greater than 20 ppm signifies the inability to digest lactose.[74–77] It is important to note that additional diagnostic tests are available such as the fecal pH test that measures the acidity of stool, small bowel biopsy that can determine lactase activity, and genotyping; however, the breath hydrogen test is considered the gold standard.[74]

Primary Lactase Deficiency

Primary lactase deficiency (PLD), also referred to as adult-type hypolactasia, lactase nonpersistence, and hereditary lactase deficiency occurs secondary to "relative or absolute absence" of the enzyme lactase.[74,77] PLD presents with a worldwide prevalence rate of 70 percent and is the most common enzyme deficiency known to cause lactose intolerance and/or malabsorption.[74,76,77] The prevalence and age of onset vary secondary to ethnicity and the overall use of dairy products in the diet.[74,76] Populations known to consume greater lactose containing diets present with lower prevalence rates (e.g. Europeans), whereas, populations with lower lactose

containing diets present with higher prevalence rates (e.g. Asia, Africa, American Indians, Ashkenazi Jewish people).[74–77] Individuals with PLD present with varying degrees of enzyme deficiency because **lactase-phlorizin hydrolase** (LPH), the enzyme responsible for digesting lactose, begins to decrease at 2 years of age, resulting in varying levels of lactose tolerance.[77] Nutrition management must be flexible and tailored to the individual (e.g. the complete removal of lactose from the diet vs. limited lactose dietary consumption).[74]

Secondary Lactase Deficiency

Secondary lactase deficiency may occur if the lining of the small intestine that houses lactase-containing epithelial cells is destroyed as a direct result of underlying disease (e.g. celiac disease), small intestinal resection, gastrectomy, chemotherapy treatments, viruses (e.g. rotavirus), bacteria, parasitic infections (e.g. giardiasis), or acute diarrheal disease.[74,75] Lactase deficient, underdeveloped epithelial cells replace those destroyed by disease, resulting in secondary lactase deficiency and lactose malabsorption.[74] According to the American Academy of Pediatrics Committee on Nutrition, eliminating lactose from the diet is generally not required for treating secondary lactase deficiency and lactose malabsorption.[74] Treating the underlying condition is key. Once the primary issue is resolved, lactose-containing products can be reintroduced according to individual tolerance.[74]

Developmental (Neonatal) Lactase Deficiency

Developmental or neonatal lactase deficiency occurs in premature infants as lactase is the last of the major intestinal disaccharidases to develop.[74,75] Therefore, the infant is born before the optimal development of the lactase enzyme.[75] Lactase activity is estimated at 30 percent (deficient) between 26 and 34 weeks of gestation and increases to an estimated 70 percent by gestation age range 35–38 weeks.[75] As a direct result, premature infants have lower levels of lactase activity and may be unable to digest and absorb lactose as well as their term counterparts.[75] Carlson and colleagues demonstrated that the "addition of lactase to preterm formula reduces the amount of lactose by 70% after a two hour incubation period at room temperature."[78] Therefore, using lactase to hydrolyze lactose in preterm formulas and maternal breast milk may aid in decreasing lactose malabsorption in preterm infants and further lead to enhanced weight gain and improved feeding tolerance.[74,79]

Congenital Lactase Deficiency

Congenital lactase deficiency is an extremely rare autosomal recessive disorder caused by coding mutations in the LPH gene, which results in the reduction or complete absence of LPH.[75,77,80] Primarily affecting those of Finnish decent, affected newborn infants present with severe diarrheal disease, metiorism (tympanites), and malnutrition immediately to a few days following the introduction of maternal breast milk or lactose-containing formula.[47,75,77,80] Treatment includes immediate and complete removal of lactose from the diet, followed by the replacement/consumption of a lactose-free formula during infancy and lactose-free milk products after infancy. If left untreated, congenital lactase deficiency can be life threatening as a result of dehydration and loss of electrolytes.[74,77,80]

Nutrition Screening

Nutrition screening in pediatric patients with lactose intolerance should be consistent with clinical malnutrition (undernutrition) risk screening as defined by the AND and ASPEN.[13]

Nutrition Assessment

Patients with lactose intolerance should be referred to a pediatric RDN in order to receive individualized nutrition assessment. Nutrition assessment consists of obtaining a thorough diet history with emphasis placed on both energy and nutrient intake, specifically calcium and vitamin D; two nutrients required for optimal bone health. Prolonged inadequate calcium and vitamin D intake are associated with reduced bone mass, osteoporosis, decreased bone mineral density, and osteomalacia. Close attention should also be paid to anthropometric assessment, growth trends, clinical data, and the need for multivitamin and mineral supplementation to help prevent and/or correct nutrient deficiency. The diet, clinical history, and additional data obtained by the pediatric dietitian may reveal a relationship between lactose ingestion and reported symptoms. Therefore, the nutrition assessment should also seek to identify potential hidden sources of lactose that may be continuing to cause reported discomfort, as well as assessing the patient/client and caregiver's readiness to make dietary changes and any barriers to learning or compliance.[73,74]

Nutrition Diagnostic Statements (PES)

Nutrition diagnosis is determined from information gathered during the nutrition assessment.

- Altered gastrointestinal function (NC-1.4) related to the inability to digest lactose as evidenced by hydrogen breath tests results greater than 20 ppm.
- Inadequate mineral intake (NI-5.10.1) related to eliminating calcium rich food and beverages from the diet as evidenced by 24-hour dietary recall of calcium rich foods meeting less than 50% RDA for age.

Nutrition Intervention

The specific nutrition diagnosis established from the nutrition assessment aids in determining the appropriate medical nutrition therapy intervention is nutrition education. The goal of nutrition education provided in the dietary management of lactose intolerance is to achieve resolution of symptoms and also prevent the onset and/or re-occurrence of symptoms. Clients and their caregiver(s) should receive nutrition education and resources related to reading food labels, identifying the lactose content of foods/beverages, meal preparation/planning, recipe modification, as well as how to gradually re-introduce lactose back into the diet & establish an individual threshold (when appropriate). Nutrition counseling should also focus on hidden sources of lactose, strategies for eating outside of the home, and identified age-related social situations that may require special attention in order to avoid feelings of depression, distress, or anxiety. Additionally, multivitamin with mineral supplementation may be recommended in addition to an increase in oral nutrient intake to aid in the prevention and/or correction of nutrient insufficiency vs. deficiency.[73,74,76] Lastly, one should always assess the comprehension level of the patient and caregiver, along with addressing individual questions/concerns. Please refer to the Pediatric Nutrition Care Manual for details on a Lactose Controlled Diet.[81]

Nutrition Monitoring and Evaluation

Ongoing monitoring and evaluation is essential to ensure that the nutrition intervention provided was effective and is sustainable. Feedback provided by the client and his/her caregiver(s) allows for appropriate adjustments in the dietary management plan to be made. Follow-up visits include the re-evaluation of diagnostic clinical markers, such as gastrointestinal symptoms/discomfort, growth trends, and review of food-symptom diary (if maintained) to reveal potential adverse relationships and to aid in establishing individual lactose tolerance/threshold. Nutrition-related vitamin/mineral lab results (ex. vitamin D) should also be monitored and addressed, with supplementation recommended and/or adjusted as appropriate. It is paramount that the caregiver and pediatric client receive continued support in an effort to achieve improved quality of life and for each to feel successful in their efforts.[73,74]

▶ Celiac Disease

Celiac disease (CD) is a multisystem, T-cell-mediated chronic autoimmune intestinal disorder that occurs in genetically predisposed individuals carrying human leukocyte antigen (HLA)-DQ2 and/or DQ8 haplotypes.

Both the incidence and prevalence of CD have risen in recent years due to increased awareness and it is now estimated to affect approximately 1% of the world's population with the exception of South East Asia, in which risk alleles of the populace are uncommon.[82–87] First degree relatives of individuals diagnosed with CD are at greatest risk with an estimated prevalence rate 10 times greater than that of the general population.[84] Additional at-risk populations include those previously diagnosed with type 1 diabetes mellitus, autoimmune thyroid disease, selective IgA deficiency, Trisomy 21, Turner Syndrome, and Williams Syndrome.[82,83,85,86]

Early Infant Feeding Practices and Celiac Disease

It was once believed that environmental factors, such as breastfeeding and the time in which gluten is introduced into an infant's diet were influential in the development and presentation of CD.[88,89] Over the last few years, research has revealed that the early introduction of gluten and breastfeeding have no effect on the risk of developing CD during childhood. However, whether or not delayed introduction of gluten into a genetically predisposed infant's diet increases versus decreases one's risk of developing CD during childhood remains highly debatable.[88–90] These new findings prompted ESPGHAN to update their 2008 recommendations and release a revised position paper in 2016. ESPGHAN recommends the safe introduction of gluten in all infants between the ages of 4 and 12 months and recommends avoiding consuming large amounts of gluten (quantity undefined) during the first few weeks that follow initial gluten introduction.[88,90] For a complete listing of position statements and recommendations, please refer to *Gluten Introduction and the Risk of Coeliac Disease: A Position Paper by the European Society for Pediatric Gastroenterology, Hepatology, and Nutrition.*[90]

Clinical Manifestations

The clinical presentation of CD is multi-systemic and ever changing. Classic gastrointestinal-related symptoms are most prominent in younger children and include diarrhea/steatorrhea, constipation, chronic abdominal pain, abdominal distention, and vomiting with associated malnutrition and growth failure.[83,91] A mild elevation of serum liver enzymes is also commonly seen within the pediatric population.[83] Non-gastrointestinal or extra-intestinal symptoms include short stature, inadequate weight gain, weight loss, delayed puberty, dental enamel defects, aphthous ulcers in the mouth, dermatitis herpetaformis, and reduced bone mineral density.[82,86,91] Although CD is traditionally associated with inadequate weight gain or weight loss, some children may initially present as overweight or obese.[82,83] Additionally, iron deficient anemia that is resistant to oral iron supplementation, fatigue, migraines, and

joint pain may also present as symptoms.[82,83,86,92] Lastly, anxiety, depression, hallucinations, panic attacks, and suicidal behavior have also been reported amongst adolescents.[83] Experts believe that CD remains underdiagnosed because of the great variability in clinical presentation, which often results in misdiagnoses of irritable bowel syndrome or lactose intolerance.[82,83]

Diagnosis

Those who present with symptoms suspicious of CD must first receive serology testing, which includes **immunoglobulin A** (IgA) antibody and **tissue transglutaminase** (TTG), along with **tissue transglutaminase immunoglobulin G** (TTG IgG) if IgA deficiency is present. For younger children than 2 years of age, research supports combining the tTG-IgA with a DGP-IgG to improve the accuracy of the result.[83] It is important that gluten remain in the diet to ensure reliable serology testing at a quantity of greater than 10 grams per day, which is the equivalent to 2 slices of bread, for no less than 8 weeks.[83] Formal diagnosis must be further confirmed via intestinal biopsy. In some cases, diagnosis may be uncertain. If this is the case, **human leukocyte antigen** (HLA) typing and repeat biopsy can be performed. A trial of a gluten-free diet may also be considered. After a trial of the gluten-free diet, repeat serology testing and intestinal biopsy are recommended. If once positive serology tests become negative after the trial of the gluten-free diet, this is tangible and supportive evidence for the diagnosis of CD.

While the diagnostic gold standard for CD is duodenal biopsy, ESPGHAN published evidence-based guidelines in 2012 that suggest that a formal diagnosis of CD may be made without performing a duodenal biopsy within pediatric patients who meet specified criteria. This specific subpopulation includes symptomatic individuals with a tTg-IgA greater than 10 times the upper normal limit for their age, present with a positive EMA-IgA antibody result, possess the HLA-DQ2 and/or HLA-DQ8 halpotypes, and experienced relief of symptoms following trial of a gluten-free diet.[82,94–96] However, discretion is advised even though a non-biopsy confirmed diagnosis of CD within the pediatric population is desirable with respect to avoiding sedation and endoscopy related risks, as well as decreasing overall diagnostic costs. Standardization of serological tests for CD in the United States does not exist and "variation in antibody levels between commercial assays when the same serum samples are tested" has been well documented; thus directly affecting the interpretation of results and leading to diagnostic inconsistencies.[83,94] Secondly, gastrointestinal disorders that may occur as comorbidities in those with CD, such as Eosinophilic Esophagitis, Helicobacter Pylori Gastritis, and Peptic Esophagitis, will remain undiagnosed in the absence of a biopsy.[83,97]

Nutrition Screening

Nutrition screening in pediatric patients with CD should be consistent with clinical malnutrition (undernutrition) risk screening as defined by the AND and ASPEN.[13]

Nutrition Assessment

All patients with CD should be referred to a RDN with expertise in celiac disease and the gluten free diet to receive individualized nutrition assessment. Nutrition assessment consists of obtaining a thorough diet history with emphasis placed on total energy intake, as well as both macronutrient and micronutrient intake. Close attention should also be paid to biochemical and clinical data results, anthropometric assessment, growth history/trends, and the need for multivitamin/mineral supplementation to aid in preventing and/or correcting nutrient deficiency. Lastly, the nutrition assessment should also seek to identify potential hidden sources of gluten that may be continuing to cause reported gastrointestinal discomfort, as well as assessing the patient/client and caregiver's readiness to make dietary changes and any barriers to learning or compliance, such as financial constraints.[82,88]

Nutrition Diagnostic Statements (PES)

Nutrition diagnosis is determined from information gathered during the nutrition assessment.

- Altered GI function (NC-1.4) related to damage to the intestinal villi as evidenced by elevated celiac antibody levels and positive duodenal biopsy.
- Food and nutrition related knowledge deficit (NB-1.1) related to lack of education in regard to the gluten free diet and its associated lifestyle as evidenced by new diagnosis of celiac disease.
- Limited adherence to nutrition related recommendations (NB-1.6) related to consumption of gluten-containing foods as evidenced by elevated celiac antibody tests, complaints of intermittent abdominal pain, and patient report of routinely eating gluten containing food items.

Nutrition Intervention

Immediately following diagnosis, affected individuals should be referred to a registered dietitian/nutritionist with expertise in CD in order to receive comprehensive nutrition education with emphasis placed on the importance of adhering to a gluten-free diet and the gluten-free lifestyle. When nutritive sources of gluten (e.g., wheat, rye, barley, and its derivatives) and nonnutritive sources of gluten (e.g., toothpaste) are completely eliminated from the diet, gastrointestinal and often extra-intestinal symptoms, serologic test results, histology, and growth

and development should normalize as celiac symptoms improve and move into a state of remission.[83,88,91]

Attendance of all primary caregivers should be encouraged during the initial nutrition consultation. Nutrition counseling should focus on nutritive and non-nutritive sources of gluten, gluten-free alternatives, hidden sources of gluten, various aspects of cross-contamination, where one can purchase gluten-free products; credible resources and support groups, eating outside of the home, and identified age-related social situations that may require special attention to avoid feelings of depression, distress, or anxiety. Close attention should also be paid to anthropometric assessment, growth trends, nutritional intake, and the need for multivitamin and mineral supplementation to aid in preventing and/or correcting nutrient deficiency.[88]

Inclusion of Oats in a Celiac Diet

Whether or not an individual with CD can safely consume oats remains controversial and is under scientific investigation. Oats may become contaminated by gluten during the harvesting and milling process, have been reported to cause gastrointestinal symptoms, induce an immunological response as confirmed via detection of serum anti-avenin antibodies, and cause small intestinal damage in some individuals with CD.[82,98,99] Clinical research supports the safe introduction and consumption of 20–25 grams per day (¼ cup gluten-free oats) in most children with CD following the resolution of symptoms and normalization of celiac antibody levels.[82] The patient should discuss including gluten-free oats with his or her gastroenterologist and/or registered dietitian/nutritionist before ingestion because individual tolerance varies and monitoring of antibody levels is required.[82]

Gluten Free Diet and Nutrient Deficiencies

Gluten is composed of two proteins, gliadin and glutenin. Gluten is the general name for storage proteins, referred to as prolamins that are found in wheat, rye, barley, and oats. Gliadin is the specific prolamin found in wheat, secalin is found in rye, and hordein is found in barley. When ingested, it is these specific prolamins that cause villous atrophy, which may further result in nutrient malabsorption and/or deficiency.[82,99]

Iron, calcium, and folate are key nutrients that are often affected in those with celiac disease, because these nutrients are absorbed in the proximal small bowel.[82,88,100] If the disease progresses further down the small intestinal tract, malabsorption of carbohydrates, fat, fat-soluble vitamins, and protein may also occur. The most common causes of anemia in those with celiac disease are iron, folate, or vitamin B_{12} deficiency. Calcium, phosphorus, and vitamin D deficiencies may also occur secondary to malabsorption or decreased intake of dairy products if lactose intolerance is present. Secondary lactose intolerance is commonly observed as the enterocytes at the tips of damaged villi are absent, and therefore unable to produce the enzyme lactase.[82,88,100]

Those diagnosed with celiac disease are at higher risk for developing metabolic bone disease secondary to "malabsorption, hypogonadism, and inflammation" and should receive dual energy x-ray absorpiometry (DXA scan), quantitative CT scan, or computerized bone age estimation; however, no guidelines exist regarding when or how often to assess bone mineral density via DXA in newly diagnosed pediatric patients.[101,102] Strict adherence to a gluten-free diet that contains sufficient nutrients required to achieve optimal bone health during childhood will result in improved bone mineral density in adulthood.[82,102]

Nutrition Monitoring and Evaluation

It is understood that individuals with CD have a permanent intolerance to gluten and must adhere to a gluten-free diet since this is the only known treatment. Ongoing monitoring and evaluation is essential in treating pediatric CD in order to achieve optimal health outcomes. Frequent medical and nutrition visits are recommended during the first one to two years following the initial diagnosis; however, no formal guideline exists.[83] Subsequent nutrition visits should encompass a complete review of new and pertinent data (e.g. repeat serology tests, DXA scan results), medical nutrition therapy components previously mentioned, along with determining dietary compliance, as well as addressing barriers to compliance (if applicable). One should also continue to assess the comprehension level of the patient and family, along with addressing individual questions/concerns and providing continued support in an effort to achieve improved quality of life.[82,83]

Special Considerations

The only known treatment for CD is strict adherence to a gluten-free diet. If left untreated, CD can result in nutritional deficiencies, decreased bone mineral density, and neurological disorders. Scientific research further suggests that if left untreated, affected individuals are at an increased risk for developing intestinal lymphoma, infertility, spontaneous abortion, and the delivery of low-birth-weight infants.[82,88,103,104] A gluten-free diet will allow for normal growth and development as well as relief from symptoms; however, some may continue to experience persistent symptoms despite adherence.[88] Alternative non-dietary therapeutic treatments, such as oral glutenase supplements (enzyme therapy), therapeutic vaccine, and zonulin inhibitors, for example, are currently in varying stages of development.[105,106] It is important to note that commercially available enzyme supplements are neither approved for use nor proven effective within the pediatric celiac population and therefore should not be recommended for use.[82]

▶ Inflammatory Bowel Disease

The two major types of **inflammatory bowel disease** (IBD) are **Crohn's disease** and **ulcerative colitis** (UC). Crohn's disease may occur in any portion of the gastrointestinal tract. Ulcerative colitis is by definition confined to the colon with minimal involvement of the terminal ileum.[107] Patients who develop nonspecific IBD-like symptoms are often temporarily termed as having indeterminate colitis. The two diseases have many features in common: diarrhea, gastrointestinal blood and protein loss, abdominal pain, weight loss, anemia, and growth failure. Children with IBD may experience growth failure because of inadequate intake, malabsorption, excessive nutrient losses, drug-nutrient interaction, and increased nutrient needs. Inadequate intake may be due to abdominal pain, gastritis, personal effort to decrease the incidence of diarrhea, and taste changes with zinc deficiency. The timing and referral to a gastroenterologist to endoscopically diagnose a patient with IBD is crucial as the symptoms can lead to growth impairment and malnutrition.

Condition Specific Nutrition Screening

Nutrition screening in pediatric patients with IBD should be consistent with clinical malnutrition (undernutrition) risk screening as defined by the AND and ASPEN.[13]

Nutrition Assessment

Nutrient deficits have been noted in 30–40% of adolescents and children with IBD.[108] At the time of diagnosis, about 85% of pediatric patients with Crohn's disease and 65% with UC present with weight loss.[109] A cohort study by Ricciuto et al, found that the median time of diagnosis is 4.5 months and that there is an independent association between delayed diagnosis and linear growth. Bone mass deficits in IBD children range between 10–40%.[110] Plateau linear growth may be the only presenting sign of IBD. Therefore, it is important to have early diagnosis in children in order to maximize growth potential.[111]

Malnutrition occurs in 32% of children at the time of diagnosis of IBD.[112] Patients who present in a flare, or active disease state, often have multiple macro- and micronutrient losses. Inflammation of the mucosa and bowel resections can lead to general malabsorption. Depending on the location and length of bowel resection, specific nutrients may no longer be absorbed and will need to be supplemented. Bacterial overgrowth due to altered motility or strictures can also lead to malabsorption. All these components can and do lead to malnutrition which is the key to identifying malnutrition and inflammation parameters in order to have improved patient outcomes.[113]

There has been a lack of consensus for estimated caloric needs in pediatric patients with IBD. In the Azcue, et al study, the authors looked at the **resting energy expenditure** (REE) and body composition of pediatric Crohn's patients. It was noted that Crohn's patients were similar to that of the control group per kilogram of lean body mass. The REE per kilogram of body mass was not regulated since it is in the starvation state.[114] A more recent study by Hill et al in 2011 compared four commonly used predicted equations for REE in children with IBD. The study concluded that the Schofield equation was more accurate at measuring and predicting REE for IBD patients.[115] In the adult population, it has been documented that total energy expenditure is not significantly elevated in active disease compared with remission or inactive disease.[116]

Protein requirements are likely elevated due to protein losses as well as increased needs for healing, especially in post-op patients. In patients with IBD who present with protein-losing enteropathy, the body cannot synthesize new proteins as fast as they are lost through the gastrointestinal tract.[117] The resulting hypoalbuminemia cannot be corrected by adding protein to the diet.

Bile malabsorption leads to decreased absorption of long-chain fatty acids but not medium chain fatty acids, because bile is not required for transporting medium-chain fatty acids through the mucosa. Fat malabsorption contributes to the malabsorption of fat-soluble vitamins.

All patients should be assessed for micronutrient deficiencies and repleted as necessary. Blood losses via the stool can lead to iron deficiency. Folate deficiency can result from drug-nutrient interactions as well as decreased intake of folate-rich food sources such as green leafy vegetables. The fat-soluble vitamins, A, D, E, and K as well as zinc, magnesium, and calcium are lost when steatorrhea is present. Zinc deficiency may be related to diarrheal, high-output fistula losses and inadequate dietary intake. Magnesium and potassium are also lost via diarrhea. Patients with resections of the stomach or ileum, or severe disease of the terminal ileum may not be able to absorb Vitamin B_{12}.[118,119] Patients should be on a daily multivitamin unless they are receiving enteral formula, which provides the equivalent of a multivitamin.[120] A study of 54 adults with Crohn's disease revealed that although those patients in clinical remission for longer than 3 months were able to meet macronutrient needs via food intake, micronutrient deficiencies remained. Low plasma levels of vitamin C, copper, niacin, and zinc were found in greater than 50% of the patients.[121]

Although bone disease in IBD is multifactorial, vitamin D and calcium are important nutrients to monitor. Pediatric patients with IBD are known to be at increased risk of osteopenia and osteoporosis.[122] Several factors along with medical treatment are thought to be the reason for impaired bone mineralization in children with IBD. Steroids are known to affect bone mineral density,[123] and new research shows that inflammatory cytokines lead to lower bone mineral density.[124] Even though calcium and vitamin D are not the sole answer in IBD-related low bone mineral density, blood levels should be kept within the normal range. Fat malabsorption can lead to low vitamin D levels, and vitamin D plays many roles beyond bone health in the body. A review article recommends 50,000 units of vitamin D_2 every week up to every day depending on the degree of fat malabsorption, or up to 10,000 units of vitamin D_3 every day for up to 5 months. This is followed by a maintenance dose of 50,000 units of vitamin D_2 every week. For children and adults without fat malabsorption, the recommendation ranges from 400 to 1000 units of vitamin D_3 every day.[125]

Nutrition Diagnostic Statements (PES)

Nutrition diagnosis is determined from information gathered during the nutrition assessment:

- Inadequate oral intake (NI-2.1) related to symptoms of IBD as evidenced by recording of about 50% or less of normal food intake per meals.
- Unintended weight loss (NC-3.2) related to increased needs resulting from active disease of IBD as evidenced by 10% weight loss.

Nutrition Intervention

Drug-nutrient interaction from the pharmacotherapy used in treating IBD may negatively affect nutrition. Sulfasalazine (azulfidine) interferes with folate absorption.[126] Methotrexate is a folic acid antagonist, and supplementation of folic acid helps reduce methotrexate's hepatic side effects.[127,128] Corticosteroid therapy interferes with absorption of calcium, phosphate and zinc.

Controlled studies have not supported using low-residue, high-fiber, or low-refined-sugar diet in order to maintain remission of Crohn's disease.[129,130] Dairy products need not be restricted in patients with IBD; however, lactose malabsorption is more common in patients with small bowel Crohn's disease than in patients with disease involving the colon or UC. Lactose intolerance is often temporary during times of active disease. Advice concerning the intake of dairy products should be individualized in order to avoid unnecessary dietary restrictions.[131]

Nutrition support has both primary and an adjunctive role in treating IBD.[108] Primary nutrition therapy appears to be more effective in treating Crohn's disease than ulcerative colitis.[107,132] In a pediatric study, patients with active Crohn's disease were treated with exclusive

EN therapy (multiple formulas) versus corticosteroids. The duration of clinical remission, degree of mucosal healing and improvement in mucosal inflammation, and improvements to linear growth were greater with any of the enteral formulas than with steroids.[113,133] These results are similar to another pediatric study that showed exclusive enteral feeds with intact proteins were just as effective as corticosteroids in inducing remission, and had a lower rate of relapse.[134] Borelli also looked at a polymeric diet versus corticosteroid therapy, and found that using polymeric formulas led to increased mucosal healing at the end of the 10-week study.[135] A randomized controlled trial of polymeric enteral formula and an elemental formula found similar results in inducing remission in children with Crohn's disease. Children given a polymeric diet, however, achieved better weight gain.[136]

Despite these positive studies in the pediatric population, a Cochrane review, including both pediatric and adult studies, reported that corticosteroids were more effective in inducing remission. The protein composition of the formulas did not reveal any difference in the effectiveness of the EN therapy,[137] however, for the maintenance of remission in Crohn's disease, enteral feeds were found to be beneficial in all age groups with no known side effects.[138] Due to lifestyle changes that accompany exclusive EN therapy, there is interest in the effectiveness of partial EN therapy. A pediatric study using elemental formula provided as either 50% or 100% of calorie needs showed higher remission rates and improved hemoglobin, albumin, and **erythrocyte sedimentation rate** (ESR) in those receiving 100% of their calorie needs from formula.[139] However, in a study of patients with steroid-dependent Crohn's disease in state of remission, adding enteral formula (either elemental or polymeric) taken orally along with a regular diet allowed 43% of patients to discontinue steroids and remain in remission at the 12-month follow-up.[140]

Bamba looked at elemental diets containing different amounts of **long-chain triglycerides** (LCT). The high LCT diet had a remission rate of 25% at 4 weeks, whereas the low LCT diet had a remission rate of 80%.[141] Other studies have found that formulas containing higher amounts of **medium-chain triglycerides** (MCT) have resulted in remission rates comparable to low-fat formulas or steroid therapy.[132-143] Per a Cochrane Review, there is inadequate evidence to support the use of omega-3 fatty acids for inducing or maintaining remission of ulcerative colitis[144,145] nor do they appear to be effective in maintaining remission in Crohn's disease.[146] Probiotics have not been shown to be effective for inducing and maintaining remission of Crohn's disease,[147,148] but when added to standard therapy for UC, they may lead to a reduction of disease activity.[149]

Enteral feeding has been shown to reduce inflammation and improve well-being, nutrition, and growth, but the exact mechanism is unknown. A study on the use of enteral feeding showed that inflammatory markers were significantly improved over the first 7 days of treatment; significant improvement in growth-related proteins and nutritional markers were not seen until day 14 or later.[150]

In patients not treated with EN therapy during periods of active disease and/or weight loss, oral nutritional beverages in addition to food can be useful. Because protein composition does not affect the rates of remission or disease improvement, formula choice should be based on palatability and patient tolerance. If voluntary intake is insufficient, nasogastric enteral supplementation may be considered. PN should be reserved for patients who have bowel obstructions or short bowel syndrome, or are unable to tolerate sufficient quantity of EN because of active disease. PN comes with greater risk as well as higher cost.

Most recently there has been more nutritional modifications done to the overall oral diet. Some of these new "diets" are gaining attention in treating symptoms of IBD. **Specific Carbohydrate diet** (SCD) and Cow's milk protein elimination diet have been used for inducing remission in pediatric IBD.[151] However, the available evidence is not strong enough to recommend this kind of nutrition intervention in the pediatric population.[151]

Nutrition Monitoring and Evaluation

Ongoing monitoring and evaluation is essential to ensure that the nutrition intervention provided was effective and is sustainable. Feedback provided by the client and his/her caregiver(s) will allow for appropriate adjustments in the dietary management plan. Follow-up visits include re-evaluating diagnostic clinical markers, such as gastrointestinal symptoms/discomfort, growth trends, and a review of the food-symptom diary. Nutrition related vitamin/mineral lab results should also be monitored and addressed, with supplementation recommended and/or adjusted as appropriate.

▶ Pancreatitis

Pancreatitis can be acute or chronic and divided into three groups: mild, moderate, and severe. Approximately 80% of all cases are mild and will often resolve within 5–7 days with bowel rest, fluid, and analgesic support.[152,153] The remaining cases are moderate to severe and require medical and nutritional therapy. Moderate and severe pancreatitis creates a state of hypermetabolism and catabolism with significant nitrogen losses, and results in an elevated systemic inflammatory response. It is often associated with infectious complications and in severe cases, multiple organ failure and pancreatic necrosis.[152-154]

Anatomy, Physiology, Pathology

Pancreatitis is the inflammation of the pancreas that occurs when pancreatic enzyme secretion accumulates in the pancreas, causing the organ to digest itself. In most cases, pancreatitis is an acute episode lasting a few days to a week, however, in rare circumstances, it can be a progressive chronic condition.

Acute pancreatitis occurs suddenly with rapid onset. Common causes of acute pancreatitis in pediatrics include physical injury, certain medications, gallstones, or problems in the anatomy of the ducts in the liver or pancreas. In 35% of children, acute pancreatitis is idiopathic.[155] Medications that are associated with pancreatitis include anti-seizure medications, chemotherapy agents, and certain antibiotics.

Chronic pancreatitis is a life-long condition with multiple episodes occurring over time. About 10% of children will have a recurrent episode of pancreatitis.[155] After the second episode of pancreatitis, additional genetic testing is required in order to evaluate the cause of recurrence. Children with genetic, metabolic, or anatomic abnormalities are at greatest risk of developing chronic pancreatitis.[156]

Pancreatitis can be categorized as mild, moderate, or severe. Based on laboratory markers, clinical findings, and CT-imaging severity of pancreatitis is classified.[157]

Nutrition Screening

Nutrition screening in pediatric patients with pancreatitis should be consistent with clinical malnutrition (undernutrition) risk screening as defined by the AND and ASPEN.[13]

Nutrition Assessment

Patients with pancreatitis should be referred to a pediatric RDN with expertise in gastrointestinal disorders in order to receive an individualized nutrition assessment. Nutrition assessment for patients with pancreatitis consists of obtaining a thorough diet history with emphasis placed on food and fluid intake both before and after onset of pancreatitis. Due to the acute nature of pancreatic episodes, decrease in oral intake may occur suddenly at the onset of abdominal discomfort. A thorough review of gastrointestinal systems including nausea, vomiting, and GERD should be evaluated. Close attention should also be paid to anthropometric assessment, growth trends, and feed tolerance. In patients with chronic pancreatitis, serum levels of fat soluble vitamins, vitamin B_{12}, calcium, folate, zinc, copper, and magnesium should be monitored and oral supplementation may be required.[156]

Diagnosis

The diagnosis of pancreatitis is based on multiple factors and includes clinical symptoms such as sudden abdominal or back pain, nausea, vomiting, loss of appetite, or sweating; abnormal blood tests, commonly elevated amylase and lipase levels; or radiographic images like ultrasound and CT scans showing inflammation in the pancreas. A diagnosis of acute pancreatitis can be made if two or more of these criteria are present.[155] Chronic pancreatitis is progressive and includes multiple episodes of pancreatitis throughout a lifetime. Diagnosis of chronic pancreatitis includes exocrine and/or endocrine insufficiency resulting in steatorrhea.[156]

Nutrition Diagnostic Statements (PES)

- Inadequate oral intake (NI-1.1) related to compromised pancreatic function as evidenced by need for enteral feedings to meet nutritional needs.
- Inadequate enteral intake (NI-2.3) related altered GI function as evidence by intolerance on enteral feeds.
- Impaired nutrient utilization (NC-2.1) related to compromised pancreatic function as evidenced by fat soluble vitamin deficiencies.

Management

Treating acute pancreatitis includes fluid resuscitation with intravenous hydration at up to 150% maintenance fluid requirement within the first 24 hours of hospitalization.[158] Antibiotics may also be used to manage inflammation as well as pain medication for discomfort.[154] Chronic pancreatitis may require daily enzyme supplementation and the possible need for surgery or islet cell transplant.[156]

Nutrition Intervention, Monitoring, and Evaluation for Mild Acute Pancreatitis

Traditionally in clinical practice, patients were often initially made NPO, and then advanced to a clear liquid diet as pain resolved. In a randomized controlled trial, patients with mild pancreatitis who resumed oral intake of liquids and solid foods before the resolution of pain were able to advance to a solid food diet sooner than those on bowel rest, thereby decreasing length of stay.[159] A study compared the initiation of a clear liquid diet versus soft solid food diet and found no significant difference between the two groups in cessation of feeds due to pain. Also, patients started on the soft solid diet took in significantly more calories and protein overall, with a decreased length of stay.[160] This research supports the initiation of oral feeds, both liquids and solids, during the first few days with the benefit of improved nutrient intake.

Nutrition Intervention, Monitoring, and Evaluation for Moderate to Severe Acute Pancreatitis

Early initiation of enteral feedings is highly recommended in patients with moderate to severe pancreatitis.[154] Studies have shown that by stimulating the gastrointestinal tract, early feeding has the potential to reverse organ failure with improvement in peristalsis and the return of gut function in those with ileus.[161] More so, jejunal feeds have been found most beneficial in resolution of ileus and gas stasis over PN and bowel rest.[162,163] EN provides adequate calories, protein, and vitamins to support organ recovery and decreases the risk of bacterial overgrowth and maintains gut integrity.[164] Traditionally, PN was used as first line therapy in patients with severe pancreatitis to minimize pancreatic stimulation and provide 'pancreatic rest.' Multiple studies now show that PN increases the proinflammatory response and contributes to gut atrophy, likely leading to bacterial translocation and increased infection rates.[165,166] A systematic review of 11 randomized controlled trials showed a statistically significant reduction in the risk of infectious complications and a statistically nonsignificant reduction in the risk of death with enteral feedings compared with PN.[167] The benefits of using EN over PN include a decrease in systemic inflammation markers[161] and a decrease in expense.[162,163] If PN must be used, it should not be initiated within the first 5 days of admission due to the higher inflammatory response that is present in the beginning of the disease process.[168]

Initiation of early enteral feeding should occur between 24 to 48 hours of admission to the hospital, especially in patients at risk for organ failure and pancreatic necrosis.[169] It is, however, recommended that patients are not fed within the first 24 hours of admission during the initial fluid resuscitation phase.[158] Feeding before fluid resuscitation can increase risk of an ileus and could result in feeding intolerance.[170] The route of enteral feeding is determined by the severity of disease. For patients with severe pancreatitis, a nasojejunal tube is recommended in an attempt to minimize or eliminate pancreatic secretion. A study of patients with severe pancreatitis found that patients on an elemental formula with a feeding tube 20 to 120 cm post the ligament of Treitz loss the stimulatory effect of the pancreas vs. a low-fat formula into the duodenum, which decreased secretory response but did not eliminate.[171] Additionally, patients with severe pancreatitis have a higher probability of gastroparesis due to decreased intake before hospitalization, increasing gastric feed intolerance.[154] Patients with peripancreatic collections also benefit from nasojejunal feeds as it offers a mechanism to splint the compressed stomach and duodenum.

This splint allows feeds to flow openly into the bowel without obstruction, unlike gastric feeds.[154,158] Patients with moderate pancreatitis have a greater probability of tolerating nasogastric feedings; however, in patients with gastric feeding intolerance a nasojejunal tube is preferred. The benefits of nasogastric feedings include ease of placement, quickness of initiation, and cost effectiveness.[158] Another review of 20 randomized controlled trials reported that using polymeric vs. semi-elemental formula showed no statistically significant difference in feeding tolerance, infectious complications, and mortality.[172]

As the patient improves clinically, low-fat oral feeds are initiated and slowly advanced, as enteral feeds are weaned to a normal diet.

Nutrition Intervention, Monitoring, and Evaluation for Chronic Pancreatitis

More than 80% of patients with chronic pancreatitis can follow a regular diet when macro and micro nutrients are met in addition to pancreatic enzyme supplementation.[156] Six to 8 small meals a day is recommended, especially in patients with early satiety. Patients with chronic pancreatitis have a 30–50% higher resting energy expenditure than healthy individuals and may require 35 kcal/kg/day to meet needs.[173] Adding a MCT like coconut oil and palm kernel oil to the diet will maximize fat absorption. In cases where oral nutrition cannot meet caloric demand, enteral feeding tubes are required. Less than 1% of patients with chronic pancreatitis will require long term PN.[174] Additionally, patients with chronic pancreatitis are at risk of nutritional deficiencies, most commonly vitamin K, vitamin D, vitamin E, and vitamin A, respectively.[175] Vitamin B_{12}, calcium, folate, zinc, copper, and magnesium are nutrients that may also be deficient in patients with chronic pancreatitis. These nutrients should be monitored with the addition of vitamin supplementation, if needed.[156]

Cholestatic Liver Disease

Introduction

Biliary atresia is one of the more common chronic cholestatic liver diseases that presents in infancy and requires surgical intervention. Alagille syndrome, Byler syndrome, primary biliary cirrhosis, and primary sclerosing cholangitis are cholestatic liver diseases seen in childhood through adulthood. Long-term use of PN can lead to cholestasis; a complete discussion of PN–induced cholestasis is found in Chapter 11. In cholestatic disease, a decrease in biliary bile acids results in fat and fat-soluble vitamin malabsorption. As the liver damage progresses, leading to cirrhosis, there is decreased synthesis of albumin and transport proteins, causing laboratory protein markers to become low. Nutritional concerns progress from fat malabsorption, protein-energy malnutrition, and excessive catabolism.[176]

Anatomy, Physiology, Pathology

Biliary atresia occurs only in infants. It is characterized by fibrotic obliteration or discontinuity of the extrahepatic biliary system, resulting in obstruction to bile flow. Bile ducts within the liver are initially patent during the first few weeks of life, but are progressively destroyed thereafter. This process occurs within the first 3 months of life.[177] If left untreated, biliary atresia progresses to cirrhosis and eventual death within 18 to 24 months of age.[178] The pathogenesis of biliary atresia is poorly understood.

Nutrition Screening

Nutrition screening in pediatric patients with cholestatic liver disease should be consistent with clinical malnutrition (undernutrition) risk screening as defined by the AND and ASPEN.[13]

Nutrition Assessment

Patients with cholestatic liver disease should be referred to a pediatric RDN with expertise in gastrointestinal disorders in order to receive individualized nutrition assessment. Nutrition assessment for patients with biliary atresia consists of obtaining a thorough diet history with emphasis placed on breastmilk/formula intake. Fat-soluble vitamins are malabsorbed in patients with biliary atresia and should be checked at the initial diagnosis and 1–3 months afterwards depending on the level. Patients with chronic cholestasis/cirrhosis can present with ascites and/or organomegaly, which will falsely elevate the patient's weight. Using this elevated weight would skew the results of a calculated BMI or the weight-for-length or weight/height assessment on a growth chart. These measurements can underestimate the degree of malnutrition. Using the mid-upper arm circumference and tricep skin folds to assess subcutaneous fat and skeletal muscle mass is the most accurate measurement of predicting malnutrition for patients with liver disease.[179] Mid-upper arm circumference z-scores can be used to assess the degree of malnutrition for infants greater than 3 months of age and children until age 5. For infants less than 3 months, serial MUAC measurements can be used to trend changes in nutrition status. For children over 5 years of age, MUAC percentile ranges can be used to predict BMI. Length/height-for-age and head circumference should be evaluated and monitored when appropriate. Infants with cholestatic liver disease are at risk for both stunting and microcephaly.[180]

Diagnosis

Infants with biliary atresia initially present to the doctor's office with jaundice, yellowing of the eyes, and acholic stools. Lab results are significant for elevated bilirubin and elevated **gamma-glutamyl transferase** (GGT).[181] Due to a range of cholestatic liver diseases, additional testing including ultrasound examination, X-rays, and liver biopsy are needed. Most commonly, a liver biopsy confirms diagnosis. Hallmark findings of biliary atresia found on biopsy include bile duct proliferation, portal tract expansion, and canalicular plugging.[182]

Nutrition Diagnostic Statements (PES)

- Malabsorption of fat related to altered gastrointestinal dysfunction as evidenced by need for modified diet high in medium chain triglycerides.
- Inadequate oral intake (NI-1.1) related to gastrointestinal dysfunction as evidenced by need for enteral nutrition to meet needs.

Management

According to the American Liver Foundation, there is no non-invasive treatment for biliary atresia. Patients identified to have biliary atresia will undergo a surgical procedure called a hepatoportoenterostomy, also known as a Kasai procedure, within days of diagnosis. This procedure reestablished bile flow in more than 80% of patients if performed within 60 days of birth. Endpoints include jaundice clearance, survival with native liver, and liver transplant. With a Kasai procedure, 35–50% of patients will survive with native liver at 3 years of age. This procedure improves outcomes and overall survival, however, about half of children will have a failed Kasai and require a liver transplant by 2 years of age.[178] Up to 85% of all patients with biliary atresia will require a liver transplant in their lifetime.

Nutrition Intervention

Chronic cholestasis in infancy and early childhood leads to increased calorie needs due to excessive catabolism. Calorie needs have been suggested to be 110–160% of the RDA for ideal body weight in children. Infants with biliary atresia require calories in the range of 120–200 kcal/kg/day.[183] Protein requirements should focus on providing equal to or greater than the RDA for protein in the nonencephalopathic patient. Recommendations for protein in infants have been made at 2–3 g/kg/day,[184] With encephalopathy, protein should be temporarily restricted below the RDA or a formula predominate in branch chain amino acids should be utilized until mental status returns to normal.[185]

Cholestatic liver disease leads to decreased biliary bile acids, resulting in malabsorption of LCT. Bile is not required for solubilization of MCT, which are absorbed unmodified into the portal circulation. Formulas containing a high percentage of MCT oil, in addition to emulsifiable MCT oil to formula, or supplementing foods with MCT oil is often recommended to provide fat and calories, while minimizing steatorrhea.[186] MCTs do not, however, provide essential fatty acids or help absorp fat-soluble vitamins;[187] thus, a source of linoleic acid is essential. In a study of infants on a formula containing 3% of calories from linoleic acid, they developed essential fatty acid deficiency. These results show that due to malabsorption with hepatobiliary disease, infants should receive well above 3% of calories from linoleic acid.[188] For infants with biliary atresia receiving formulas, those containing 40–60% of the fat from MCT are recommended. For premature infants, the formula Similac Special Care (Abbott) provides 50% of its fat source as MCT. For term infants, the formula Pregestimil (Mead Johnson) contains 55% of its fat source as MCT. For infants with milk protein allergy, Alfamino Infant (Nestle) a free amino acid based formula, contains 43% MCT. Liquigen (Nutricia) is an emulsifiable MCT oil that can be added to formula to increase caloric concentration and MCT content. Typically, 1 ml of Liquigen (0.5 gm fat, 4.5 calories) is added to 1 or 2 ounces of formula. Liquigen can be added to both oral and enteral formula regimens. For children over 1 year of age and older, Peptamen Junior (Nestlé) contains 60% of its fat as MCT. Additionally, oils naturally high in MCT like coconut oil and palm kernel oil can be added to soft foods. MCT oil given as an oral medication can be added in addition to formula in order to increase caloric intake of absorbable fats. Additional sources of MCT should be added gradually. Excessive intake of MCT oils and Liquigen can cause diarrhea.

To optimize nutrition after hepatoportoenterostomy or before liver transplant, using an enteral feeding tube may be warranted. A randomized study evaluating the use of a predominate MCT based formula showed a significant improvement in length and head circumference z-scores in patients who were enterally fed vs. PO ad libitum.[180] When initiating enteral feeds, continuous nocturnal feeds with PO ad libitum during the day is preferred to maintain oral skills. In cases of severe liver disease, continuous EN feeds may be required to maintain glucose levels by administering a constant **glucose infusion rate** (GIR).

Monitoring and Evaluation

In liver disease, the prevalence of fat-soluble vitamin deficiencies correlates with increasing bilirubin levels.[185] Infants with a total bilirubin greater than 2 mg/dL are at the highest risk for fat soluble vitamin malabsorption.[189] There is a wide array of supplemental and deficiency treatment doses throughout the literature. It is important to remember that the degree of fat malabsorption is unique to each patient's disease state and can change as treatments or medications are changed.

Prophylactically, a liquid water-soluble, fat-soluble multi-vitamin like aquADEKS can be started at the time of diagnosis for presumed fat-soluble malabsorption. Based on the child's age and weight, dosing can vary. When greater than 1 ml is given per day it is best to split the dose into two or three daily dose intervals in order to maximize absorption.

Vitamin A is stored in the liver and requires retinol-binding protein to circulate throughout the body. As liver disease progresses, there is impaired synthesis of retinol-binding protein, which leads to low vitamin A levels without a true deficiency. Clinical judgment needs to be used when reviewing both serum retinol and retinol-binding protein laboratory results. Of note, vitamin A is highly hepatotoxic and the risk benefit of under vs. oversupplementing should be considered before starting. Standard supplementation recommendations for Vitamin A range from 5000–15,000 International Units (IU)/day orally. For severe deficiency, intramuscular injections may be used.[176,186]

Vitamin E is stored in the liver and transported via lipoproteins. In patients with high triglycerides and cholesterol levels, the vitamin E level may be falsely elevated. It is best to check serum vitamin E levels in conjunction with total serum lipids to assess for deficiency. In children less than 12 years of age, a ratio of less than 0.6 mg/g and in children over 12 years of age, a ratio less than 0.8 mg/g is indicative of a deficiency. Supplementation recommendations in pediatrics range from 20–25 IU/kg/day of vitamin E or 10–200 IU/kg/day of alpha-tocopherol for intramuscular injections. Recommendations in adults range from 400–800 IU/day of alpha-tocopherol. The preferred source of vitamin E is D-alpha-tocopherol polyethylene glycol 1000 succinate TPGS vitamin E.[190,191] This suspension precludes the necessity of bile acid micellar solublization and is well absorbed in patients with severe cholestasis.[190]

In cholestatic and noncholestatic liver disease, metabolic bone disease has a multifactorial etiology that includes a decrease in insulin-like growth factor 1, hypogonadism, malnutrition, low BMI, loss of muscle mass, low calcium, and vitamin D deficiency. Vitamin D is hydroxylated in the liver, as one of the steps to forming its active state. Increased vitamin D levels lead to increased calcium and phosphorus absorption in the intestine. In cholestatic patients with fat malabsorption, less vitamin D is absorbed, which decreases calcium and phosphorus absorption. The nonabsorbed fatty acids bind to calcium in the intestine, further decreasing calcium absorption. Absorption of calcium is also reduced by corticosteroid therapy.[192,194] A 25-OH vitamin D level shows the pool of both dietary and endogenous vitamin D. One study recommends checking vitamin D levels every 1 to 2 months until it is within an appropriate range.[186] DEXA scans are the gold standard for assessing bone density, therefore all patients at risk should be screened.

Recommendations for supplementation of vitamin D differ significantly in light of the emerging research on vitamin D. In patients with biliary atresia, supplementation doses can range from 1200–8000 units per day for levels of Vitamin D less than 15 ng/mL.[189] In adults with primary biliary cirrhosis and primary sclerosing cholangitis, 400–800 IU/day of vitamin D in conjunction with TPGS vitamin E to enhance absorption has been recommended. In an adult-based review article, Holick, recommends 50,000 units of vitamin D_2 every week up to every day depending on the degree of fat malabsorption, or up to 10,000 units of vitamin D_3 every day for up to 5 months, then a maintenance dose of 50,000 units of vitamin D_2 every week.[105] Recent pediatric practice has shown wide use of 10,000–50,000 unit Vitamin D_2 per week in populations most susceptible to deficiency. The vast differences in these recommendations point to the importance of trending laboratory values and making dosage adjustments based on each patient's clinical response to supplementation.

Vitamin K deficiency is due to fat malabsorption and decreased absorption from gut flora alterations. This deficiency, as well as impaired hepatic synthesis of clotting factors, leads to prolonged **prothrombin time** (PT). If the abnormal PT is greater than 1.5, it is thought to be related to a vitamin K deficiency, the medical team can prescribe oral or intravenous supplementation. In a study of cholestatic children taking vitamin K supplementation with normal or near-normal PT, 54% were found to be vitamin K deficient per measure of a PIVKA-II level (protein induced by vitamin K absence).[194] Although following a PIVKA-II level is not widely done in clinical practice, it should be considered in order to assess for subclinical signs of vitamin K deficiency.

Liver Transplant

Introduction

The most common disease requiring liver transplantation in childhood is biliary atresia (over 50% of cases). Other less prominent causes are inherited metabolic disorders (e.g. alpha-1-antitrypsin deficiency, tyrosinemia, and urea cycle defects), intra-hepatic cholestasis syndromes (e.g. Alagille syndrome, Byler syndrome), chronic hepatitis with cirrhosis, and all forms of acute liver failure. Indications for transplantation include hepatic failure, complications of portal hypertension (e.g. variceal bleeding, ascites), specific metabolic disorders, and malignancy.

The patient with end-stage liver disease awaiting transplantation presents a formidable challenge to the medical and nutritional team. The particular liver disease involved, the magnitude of liver dysfunction, the presence of complications, and the transplantation procedure itself combine to present a complex treatment process including meeting nutritional needs for healing and growth.

Anatomy, Physiology, Pathology

Cirrhosis is a chronic disease of the liver marked by degeneration of cells, inflammation, and fibrous thickening of tissue. Cirrhosis may be caused by a degree of pediatric diseases discussed (See the discussion under "Cholestatic Liver Disease."). Without a liver transplant, cirrhosis left untreated results in death.

Nutrition Screening

Nutrition screening in pediatric patients requiring a liver transplant should be consistent with clinical malnutrition (undernutrition) risk screening as defined by the AND and ASPEN.[13]

Nutrition Assessment

Patients listed for liver transplant should be referred to a pediatric RDN who is a certified organ transplant provider in order to receive an individualized nutrition assessment. In most institutions, an RDN evaluation is required for a patient to be listed for liver transplant regardless of nutrition status. During the evaluation, the RDN determines if the patient is an appropriate candidate for organ transplant based on nutrition parameters. Nutrition assessment during liver transplant evaluation should consist of obtaining a thorough diet history with emphasis placed on food, fluid, and breastmilk/formula intake as well as the use of vitamin supplementation. Fat-soluble vitamins may need be checked at the initial diagnosis based on the pathophysiology of liver failure and in patients with cholestasis.[195]

Patients with chronic cholestasis/cirrhosis can present with ascites and/or organomegaly, which will falsely elevate the patient's weight as occurs in patients with cholestatic liver disease. (See the discussion under **Cholestatic Liver Disease**). In listing a patient for liver transplant, MUAC, length/height for age and head circumference are the preferred anthropometrics in evaluating nutrition status for determining PELD score.

Diagnosis

The need for a liver transplant is based on multiple factors. Institutions commonly have a liver transplant team composed of a transplant surgeon, hematologist, nurse practitioner, social work, psychiatrist, and dietitian that meet to discuss appropriate candidates for transplant based on the following criteria:

- Irreversible cirrhosis with at least two signs of liver insufficiency
- Fulminant hepatic failure: coma Grade 2
- Unresectable hepatic malignancy confined to the liver that is less than 5 cm in diameter
- Metabolic liver disease that would benefit from liver replacement

Factors that are listed below are often the precipitating reason for proceeding with liver transplantation:

- Severe fatigue
- Unacceptable quality of life
- Recurrent variceal bleeding
- Intractable ascites
- Recurrent or severe hepatic encephalopathy
- Spontaneous bacterial peritonitis
- Hepatorenal syndrome
- Development of small hepatocellular carcinoma on hepatic imaging

Nutrition Diagnostic Statements (PES)

- Inadequate oral intake related to cirrhosis as evidenced by EN to meet needs.
- Altered gastrointestinal function related to cirrhosis of the liver as evidence by fat-soluble vitamin supplementation.

Management

Once a patient is identified as a liver transplant candidate, they are listed on the national United Network for Organ Sharing (UNOS) roster.[196] Organ allocation for children is based on the Pediatric End-Stage Liver Disease (PELD) score.[196] The child in most urgent need of a transplant are placed highest on the status list and are given first priority.

As soon as a liver is available it is surgically placed into the recipient candidate. Post-liver transplant management requires a prolonged hospital stay with the use of multiple medications in order to decrease chances of rejection including using immunosuppressants and steroids.

Nutrition Intervention: Pre-transplant – End-stage liver disease creates a hypermetabolic state that elevates the REE.[197] In the hypermetabolic state, once the body's glucose stores are exhausted, lean body mass and proteins will be broken down for gluconeogenesis resulting in protein-energy malnutrition. In a study evaluating the use of predicted energy equations in the pediatric patient with liver disease, commonly used estimation methods, like Food and Agriculture Organization/World Health Organization/United Nations University (FAO/WHO/UNU) and Schofield were shown to underestimate calorie needs based on indirect calorimetry.[197] The study suggested that indirect calorimetry should be used when available in order to determine estimated needs in patients with liver disease who are malnourished.

Children with liver-disease have been found to have inadequate oral intake due to decreased appetite secondary to the anorexic effects of elevated serotonin levels[198] and increased serum leptin levels.[199] Long periods of suboptimal intake and fasting are not recommended in the pediatric population. For older children, small more frequent meals with a nighttime snack, specifically high in carbohydrates and branched-chain amino acids, can optimize nutrition intake and utilization.[200,201] Using oral nutrition supplements and/or enteral feedings may be required to provide adequate nutrition.[200] Protein should not be restricted in infants and children with end-stage liver disease and is often provided at levels above the RDA, unless encephalopathy is present.[183,185] **Branched-chain amino acid** requirements (BCAAs; leucine, isoleucine, valine) are increased in pediatrics patients with cholestatic liver disease at up to 142% of the recommended dietary allowance for the healthy child.[202] Additional supplementation with BCAA may be beneficial, however, dosing recommendations have not been established in children. Formulas with additional BCAA added has been shown to improve height, weight, and muscle mass in addition to decreased albumin infusions.[203]

If the end-stage liver disease is related to a cholestatic liver disease, then the decreased pool of bile acids will result in malabsorption of long-chain triglycerides. MCTs should be used to provide calories and minimize steatorrhea, but MCTs do not provide essential fatty acids or help absorp fat-soluble vitamins.[186] For more specific macro- and micronutrient information, please refer to the "Cholestatic Liver Disease" section of this chapter.

Multiple studies have shown that pre-operative malnutrition negatively affects the outcome of a liver transplant. Height z-score and head circumference is a good indicator of pre-transplant malnutrition. Severe growth retardation is linked to an increased length of stay and increased hospital costs after transplant.[204] In a study of infants with biliary atresia listed for liver transplant, researchers found the post-transplant mortality and graft failure risks include weight/height that is below two standard deviations at the time of listing.[205] Close nutrition monitoring in end-stage liver disease and optimizing nutritional intake will maximize growth potential and nutritional status going into transplant.

Monitoring and Evaluation: Post-Transplant – In many cases, the underlying disease is corrected by transplant; therefore, calorie and protein needs should be individualized to the patient's specific postoperative needs and nutritional status.

Immediately after transplant, early nutritional support should be implemented due to preoperative malnutrition, surgical stress, and postoperative catabolism.[206] Nutrition support should be initiated and slowly advanced to meet calorie and protein needs. The enteral formula should be chosen based on each patient's protein and fat composition needs. The continuation of a high MCT formula post-transplant is often not required. In a study evaluating tube feedings, nasointestinal tube feedings that were started post-transplant vs. maintenance intravenous fluids were maintained until an oral diet could be initiated and showed improved nitrogen balance by the fourth postoperative day and less overall infections.[207]

The nutritional goal is catch-up growth to achieve an age-appropriate weight and height. Post-transplant studies show that weight recovery is rapid and often normalizes within one year of transplant regardless of malnutrition status before transplant.[208] Long-term data evaluating height potential in patients from transplant to 15 years of age found that after transplant a growth spurt occurred with growth potential reaching its max by 10 years of age.[209,203] Deceleration of growth occurred by age 15 and was mostly related to graft dysfunction.[209] Catch-up growth potential was greatest in patients who had a transplant after 2 years of age and had the most growth retardation before transplant, although they remained significantly shorter and lighter at age 15 than age standards.[210] Overall, linear growth achievements should be analyzed by the underlying disease that necessitated transplant. Patients with biliary atresia and alpha-1-antitrypsin achieve better linear growth post-transplant than patients with fulminant liver failure, Alagille syndrome, or chronic hepatitis.[211]

Drug–nutrient interactions are key considerations post-transplant. Steroids are known to affect linear growth and bone health, and to contribute to hyperglycemia and diabetes mellitus.[212] Immunosuppressive medications also contribute to electrolyte and magnesium losses.

Concern regarding metabolic bone disease continues after liver transplant. Risk factors include continued corticosteroid use, malnutrition, muscle wasting, preexisting osteopenia/osteoporosis, and immunosuppressive agents. Bone loss is greatest in the first year after transplant.[168] Patients with cholestatic liver disease who undergo liver transplant improve their bone mineral density.[213] In a prospective pediatric study an increase in bone mineral density was noted at 3 months post-transplant along with improvements in 25-OH vitamin D levels.[214]

Using immune-suppressants after an organ transplant increases a patient's susceptibility to food-borne illness. Caregivers should be informed of safe food practices and receive information regarding cross-contamination and temperature danger-zones.

Short Bowel Syndrome
Introduction

Short bowel syndrome (SBS) is a condition in which the patient has an anatomic or functional loss of more than 50% of the intestine.[215] It has been defined as the reduction of functional gut mass below the minimal amount necessary for digestion and absorption adequate to satisfy the nutrient and fluid requirements for maintenance in adults or growth in children.[216,217] Typically, SBS results from NEC, volvulus, intestinal atresia, gastroschisis, ruptured omphalocele, or vascular infarct.[215,216,218,219] The result of the injury and/or resection is a decreased small intestinal surface area, which leads to malabsorption and large volume watery diarrhea.[220] Although most patients have had a significant bowel resection, some patients may have had a rather small amount of bowel removed, but have poor motility and absorption by the remaining intestine.[220,221] The degree of malabsorption is dependent upon the extent of missing or injured bowel; most affected individuals have difficulty sustaining appropriate growth and development without nutritional support. Growth is a major concern in this population, affected not only by adequate nutrient provision but also by absorption.

Intestinal adaptation is the process by which the remaining intestine grows, dilates, and changes via cellular hyperplasia and villous hypertrophy in order to compensate for its loss of surface area or function. Adaptation is the ultimate goal of treatment and it is dependent on small bowel length, intact **ileocecal valve** (ICV), intestinal continuity, and preservation of the colon.[222] Adaptation usually occurs within the first 3 years but it may take as long as 13.5 years.[222] A retrospective analysis of children with short bowel syndrome that required long-term PN by Quiros-Tejeira et al., found that patients with ICV even with USBS and patients with >15 cm of SBL without ICV have a chance of intestinal adaptation. The ability of the intestine to adapt is largely dependent on how much intestine remains, the health of the remaining intestine, the presence or absence of the ICV, and whether the colon is in continuity with the small bowel.[222]

Anatomy, Physiology, Pathology of Condition

Absorption of fluids and nutrients occurs throughout the small intestine and colon. Half of the mucosal surface is contained within the proximal one-fourth of the small intestine.[220] **TABLE 12.7** illustrates sites of nutrient absorption in the small intestine and colon, as well as the possible implications of intestinal resections of these areas.

The duodenum and jejunum are the primary sites of digestion and absorption of proteins, carbohydrates, lipids, and most vitamins and minerals. Resections in

TABLE 12.7 Intestinal Resection: Function Adaptation and Complications of Resection

Bowel Segment	Function	Adaptation	Complications of Resection
Duodenum	Absorption of CHO, FAT, Pro, Iron Calcium Phos, Mg, Folic Acid	Cannot adapt for the loss of other segments	Macronutrient malabsorption. Acidosis Anemia Osteopenia
Jejunum	Primary site of CHO & PRO absorption Water soluble vitamin absorption	Linger villi and large surface area can adapt for loss of the ileum and/or duodenum. Cannot absorb B_{12} or bile salts	Fluid/electrolyte losses Macronutrient and water soluble vitamin malabsorption
Ileum	Vitamin B_{12} & bile salt absorption Fat soluble vitamin absorption	Increased amount of water and CHO absorbed Does adapt for the Jejunum	Unable to absorb B_{12} Loss of fat soluble vitamins Increased risk of renal oxalate stones
Ileocecal Valve	Limits the reflux of colonic contents into the ileum Limits the rate of food passage into the cecum	Bowel cannot adapt for loss of the valve	Bacterial overgrowth causing inflammation and leading to further malabsorption Rapid transit time
Colon	Fluid absorption Na, Cl, K and fatty acid absorption	Can help in water absorption and enhance carbohydrate absorption (from short chain fatty acids)	Dehydration Electrolyte abnormalities Reduced ability to absorb bile salts Decrease in transit time

Beer S, Bunting KD, Canada N, Rich S, Spoede E, Turybury, K, eds. *Texas Children's Hospital Pediatric Nutrition Reference Guide.* Houston, Tx: Texas Children's Hospital; 2016:110.[223]

these areas result in a decreased surface area for absorption and cause increased osmotic diarrhea and loss of water-soluble vitamins.[224] Loss of calcium, iron, and magnesium can occur, as well as losses of trace minerals such as copper, chromium, and manganese. Decreased secretin, cholecystokinin, and pancreatic/biliary secretions result in decreased digestion and absorption of fats, proteins and fat-soluble vitamins. Decreased disaccharidase secretion allows increased substrate for bacterial overgrowth because carbohydrates are not fully metabolized when these enzymes are decreased.

Decreased surface area from ileal resection results in decreased vitamin B_{12} absorption. Decreased bile salt reabsorption in the ileum increases bile acid in the stool and decreases enterohepatic circulation.[224] This causes bile acid pools and decreased micelle formation. Decreased absorption of long chain fats results, as well as decreased absorption of fat-soluble vitamins. There is increased steatorrhea, and the potential for cholelithiasis and renal oxalate stones. Many gut hormones that affect GI motility are produced in the ileum, including entero-glucagon and peptide YY. Resection of the ileum can impair the nutrient-regulated gut motility.[216,225]

With jejunal resection, the ileum can assume the place of the jejunum in some ways to absorb less site-specific nutrients such as electrolytes and fluid, which the jejunum is responsible for when the bowel is intact.[226] However, due to some of the specific roles of the ileum, the jejunum cannot assume the role of the ileum. For example, loss of the terminal ileum requires B_{12} provision via intramuscular or nasal route for absorption because there are no other sites for B_{12} absorption in the proximal ileum, duodenum, or jejunum. With the loss of the jejunum there are no absolute requirements for supplementation, because absorption will vary depending on the individual child.

The ICV slows transit time and acts as a barrier to bacteria moving into the small bowel from the colon.[224] Resection of the ICV leads to vitamin B_{12} and possibly folate deficiency because the sites for absorption are often lost with adjacent ileum resections. Combined ICV and ileum resections lead to decreased transit time and large influx of nutrients into the large intestine, which can result in malabsorption. Bacterial overgrowth in the small bowel can be a major problem and lead to increased diarrhea and malabsorption.[215] Some centers routinely cycle patients on either a single antibiotic such as metronidazole for 1 to 2 weeks every month or a combination of two alternating antibiotics such as metronidazole and neomycin for overgrowth treatment. Length of treatment for overgrowth varies depending on the response to treatment; some children will continue treatment for only a few weeks whereas others can continue for several years.

The colon absorbs water, salvages malabsorbed carbohydrates and absorbs sodium. Colonic resection decreases water and sodium reabsorption and increases risk for dehydration.[224]

Nutrition Assessment

Growth is the ultimate measurement of nutritional adequacy. Caloric and protein needs are dependent on age and state of growth, as well as the degree of overall malabsorption. Caloric needs vary from child to child, and can be as low as normal for age or quite increased. No good studies or data exist for recommendations on specific calorie levels, and clinical judgment along with known intake levels and growth outcomes for the specific child should be used. Adequate carbohydrate, fat, micronutrients, and fluid provision are also dependent on age and state of growth; however, they are more influenced by resection site. Micronutrients should be monitored routinely depending upon the specific anatomy of the individual and should be replaced as needed in available forms (enteral, intramuscular, or parenteral.) The most common deficiencies are the fat-soluble vitamins, Vitamin B_{12}, zinc, and iron.

Nutritional management of the pediatric patient with short bowel syndrome can be divided into four phases. The first phase involves fluid, electrolyte, and hemodynamic stability, and PN initiation. The second phase is the initiation of EN. The third phase is weaning of PN and advancing oral nutrition and EN. The fourth phase is long-term nutrient provision and growth monitoring.

The first phase in treating a new patient with SBS is PN while the GI tract is recovering postoperatively. PN should be started as soon as possible via a central line.[221] Initial PN macronutrient needs vary depending on the infant and the clinical situation. Initiation of dextrose should be at 5–7 mg/kg/min and advancement by 1–3 mg/kg/min to endpoint goal of 12–14 mg/kg/min.[221] Various institutions are reporting anecdotal success with pushing the endpoint goal to as much as 16 mg/kg/min in order to use minimal lipids while providing adequate calories. Initiation of protein at 1–2 g/kg/day and advancement by 1–2 g/kg/day to endpoint of 3–3.5 g/kg/day is recommended.[221]

Initiation of lipid at 1 g/kg/day and advancing by 1 g/kg/day to an endpoint of no more than 3 g/kg/day is recommended.[221] Soy-based intravenous lipids have been associated with the development of liver disease.[216] Due to an increased risk of developing **intestinal failure-associated liver disease** (IFALD) many centers restrict lipids to 1 g/kg/day while adjusting other macronutrients within PN to meet calorie goals. Due to decrease/restriction of IV lipids, the clinician needs to be aware of essential fatty acid deficiency and monitor for those patients who are receiving less 1 g/kg/day.[216] Presently, there are newer lipid IV emulsions derived from fish oils that contain predominantly n-3 fatty acids, as opposed to the n-6 fatty acids that have been approved for adults.[216] These lipid emulsions are currently in clinical trials and long-term studies are needed to compare fat emulsions and examine the risk of hepatic cirrhosis in this patient population.[216]

Initial stool output, whether per rectum or ileostomy, typically increases the needs for sodium, magnesium, and zinc to compensate for losses.[221,227] Serum zinc is not always reflective of zinc status, but monitoring trends can be helpful. An infant not responding to adequate caloric and protein provision, but with high output stool volume may benefit from additional sodium and zinc supplementation despite normal serum values. PN should be monitored carefully to minimize complications associated with PN therapy. **Parenteral nutrition associated liver disease** (PNALD) is a major cause of death in patients with SBS.[228] See Chapter 11 on PN management details for maximizing calcium and phosphorus and for preventing associated complications with use of PN.

EN is the second phase of nutrition therapy and should be started as soon as the patient is stable and gastrointestinal motility has returned as a necessary component to promote intestinal adaptation.[219,229] A slow continuous infusion is thought to bathe the lumen and allow for better nutrient absorption.[219] In some conditions, if infants have a proximal high ostomy and a mucous fistula connected to a substantial portion of the bowel, refeeding the mucous fistula with the proximal bowel content can be done to prevent diffuse atrophy.[230]

If available from the mother or via donor, breast milk should be used in infants with SBS to initiate EN. The abundance of growth factor and nucleotides available in breast milk vs. formula makes it the ideal choice for these children.[219,221] If breast milk is unavailable, however, controversy exists as to the ideal formula for infants with SBS. Each infant is different, and a formula should be selected to start EN depending on his or her clinical situation.

Polymeric formulas have been shown to be better for mucosal adaptation in adults and in animal studies.[219,231,232] In pediatrics, hydrolyzed and even amino acid formulas are often preferred. In this population, mucosal breakdown, bowel dilation, and bacterial overgrowth all predispose the infants to higher rates of food allergies; thus, the provision of an amino acid formulation is a considerable advantage.[233] A 2001 prospective, randomized, crossover trial involving 10 children with SBS and lasting 60 days found no difference in energy and nitrogen balance when using a hydrolyzed protein formula versus an intact protein formula. This study is often cited in pediatric SBS guides.[234] It should be noted, however, that the study did not measure adaptation, diarrhea, or perceived tolerance to formulas. The study concluded that it is common practice that a semi-elemental diet is used to optimize absorption of the remaining bowel and that there was a difference in intestinal permeability, weight gain, and nitrogen balance in children with SBS whether they were receiving hydrolyzed or non-hydrolyzed protein formulas.[234] Also, some centers advocate amino acid formulations that were better tolerated and helpful in weaning from PN.[234]

If fat malabsorption exits from bile acid hypersecretion, PNALD, or pancreatic insufficiency, using a formula with a higher percentage of fat from MCTs is preferred.[233] Even though MCTs increase the osmotic load slightly and offer fewer calories per gram than LCTs, the lack of micelle needed for absorption makes them the ideal fats in this situation.[233] If bilirubin levels are elevated, using a very high MCT formula is recommended.[233,235] In rate studies, the use of LCTs have facilitated better adaptation of the remaining bowel than the use of MCTs.[233,235] Many have extrapolated this to indicate that LCTs are better than MCTs for infants with SBS and facilitate better intestinal adaption.[219,229,232] Interesting work has been done recently in adults with SBS indicating that the use of oleic acid (LCT) supplementation actually did not cause a delay in transit time (which is thought to stimulate adaption better) and actually decreased energy absorption by 14% vs. placebo overall.[236] The fact that this is an adult study with a small sample size (n=57) poses limitation for its use in pediatrics. However, it does make an argument in the setting of a human model with LCTs. Several institutions advocate using a blend of both MCTs and LCTs.[233,237] Most typically in practice, amino acid formulations with higher MCT content such as Elecare (33% MCT, Abbott Labs) and Neocate Infant DHA/ARA (33% MCT, Nutricia) are preferred formulas used for this patient population.

The third stage of nutritional management should be started while the infant is still hospitalized, if possible. PN should be weaned as EN and oral tolerance increases, stool output decreases, and growth is achieved. The ultimate goal is eliminating PN because cholestasis occurs in 30% to 60% of children with SBS; liver failure develops in 3% to 19% of children who acquired SBS in the neonatal period.[238-240] Gradual advances in EN/oral intake are dependent upon gastric tolerance, stool output (frequency and consistency), and rate of growth.[1] This stage can be quite lengthy, depending on setbacks and the rate of advancement. Stool should be monitored for frequency, acidosis, and reducing substances as EN and oral intake advances. PN should be cycled when 35–50% of EN goal has been achieved and if blood sugar levels are stable. Two to 6 hours off of PN each day allow for GI hormone release.[221,233] As PN is weaned, vitamin and mineral status should be closely monitored and supplemented as needed because the absorption route has changed and the potential for malabsorption has increased.

Oral feedings, even small amounts of volumes, should be started as soon as clinically stable and feasible, to prevent oral aversion.[1,219,229,233] Feeding aversions are common in this population for many reasons. First and foremost, prematurity and severe illness delay oral attempts and result in immature feeding skills.[224] Furthermore, frequent vomiting and diarrhea prevent pleasurable associations with food.[219] Oral feeds can be introduced as developmentally appropriate, and general precautions regarding monitoring for food allergies should be practiced. If the infant is unable to take any oral feedings, and oral motor stimulation program should be in place to help develop feeding skills. Feeding aversion in patients with SBS is notoriously difficult to treat, and the focus is on prevention of aversion as feasible.[1,232,241]

The fourth phase of management is long-term advancement of EN and maximizing oral intake. Once EN is at goal, it may be beneficial to start fiber therapy if the colon (or most of it) is present. The conversion of complex carbohydrate to **short-chain fatty acids** (SCFAs; acetate, propionate, and butyrate) in the colon can cause significant caloric reuptake by colonic cells.[1,232,240] Additionally, SCFAs also stimulate sodium and water reabsorption, which aids in fluid management. Adding a 1–3% pectin solution can decrease reducing substances and improve pH to allow for more fermentation of carbohydrates.[221] In orally fed patients, using guar gum fiber such as Nestlé's Resource Benefiber (hospital grade) at 0.5 g/kg/day may be used as a more palatable replacement for pectin.

As the intestine adapts, the goal is to normalize the EN schedule while promoting oral intake and growth. If possible, EN should be cycled overnight to maximize oral intake in the daytime hours. It is necessary that children find palatable beverages providing complete nutrition to help lessen EN dependence and increase oral intake. Higher calorie formulas typically have higher osmolarity and may interfere with desired weight gain. However, some nutritional products provide a high percentage of calories from fat, with lower osmolarity. Overly strict guidelines for oral intake should be discouraged. Each child needs to be carefully assessed because nutrient needs differ due to amount and location of the resections. General guidelines include:

- Limiting simple sugars (juice, candy) in order to minimize osmotic diarrhea.[1,219,221,232,233,235,242]
- Fat and protein should be adequate to support growth.
- Soluble fiber of at least 5–10 g/day as pectin/guar gum is beneficial to slow the gut transit time.[219,229,235] Those with a colon have an additional bonus of caloric reuptake from provision of soluble fiber in the diet.
- Lactose should be avoided only if symptoms are reported with ingestion.[1,235]
- Liberal salt intake at meals helps make the meal bolus isotonic in the gut.[235]

Much has been reported on the guidelines for adults with SBS, and many of these have been adapted to the child.[235] In adults with a colon, 50–60% of kcal from CHO and 20–30% of kcal from fat are recommended as a balance of LCT and MCT. Those without a colon are encouraged to consume 40–50% kcal from carbohydrates and 30–40% for kcal from fat with more LCTs than MCTs. Isotonic fluids are always encouraged, regardless of the presence or absence of a colon; however, hypoosmolar fluids that are higher sodium-containing fluids are encouraged for those without a colon. Sometimes oral rehydration solutions (ORS) are recommended for those without a colon (Table 12.3).

Increased renal oxalate stones occur with intestinal resections because of increased enteric absorption of oxalate (enteric hyperoxaluria).[243] Renal oxalate stones are well documented in the literature for adults with SBS, and up to 30% of this population develop stones.[1,235] However, the incidence is relatively rare in children.[243,244] A retrospective 5-year review at a tertiary pediatric medical center by Chang-Kit reported 72 causes of urolithiasis. Of note, seven patients had Crohn's disease, seven had cystic fibrosis, and four had SBS. It is not routine to restrict oxalates in patients with Crohn's disease or cystic fibrosis. Thus, empiric restrictions, especially in the setting of a history of food aversions, are not necessary. Allowing oxalated foods in diet or provision of extra calcium is recommended if 24-hour urinary oxalate levels are elevated.[235] Urinary oxalate levels should be monitored annually in this population.

Nutrition Diagnostic Statement (PES)

Nutrition diagnosis is determined from information gathered during the nutrition assessment.

- Altered GI function (NC 1.4) related to short bowel syndrome as evidenced by need for parenteral nutrition to support growth

- Inadequate oral intake (NC 2.1) related to oral aversion and oral diet modification as evidenced by need for enteral nutrition to maintain growth as advancing to oral autonomy

Nutrition Intervention

The overall nutrition goal is to achieve adaptation and autonomy and wean the patient off of PN. This includes careful consideration of managing the oral and enteral feeding regimen while weaning the patient off of PN and monitoring laboratory values and macro- and micronutrients.

Nutrition Monitoring and Evaluation

Ongoing monitoring and evaluation is essential to ensure that the nutrition intervention provided was effective and is sustainable. Feedback provided by the client and his/her caregiver(s) will allow for appropriate adjustments in the dietary management plan. Follow up visits include the re-evaluation of diagnostic clinical markers, such as gastrointestinal symptoms/discomfort, growth trends, and review of food-symptom diary. Nutrition-related vitamin/mineral lab results should also be monitored and addressed, with supplementation recommended and/or adjusted as appropriate.

Special Considerations

Although growth hormone and glutamine have been used in some adult studies,[242–246] more research is needed and there are no current recommendations for their use in pediatrics.[235,242–247] Alternative surgical procedures such as bowel lengthening, tapering enteroplasty, or intestinal transplant may be considered for those patients who are not making progress.[237,248–250]

Intestinal Transplantation
Introduction

An intestinal transplant is typically reserved for those pediatric patients who have developed PNALD and failed other nutrition modalities to wean off of PN or have had life-threatening line infections. Intestinal transplant is not limited to an isolated intestine, it can also be a modified multivisceral transplant, which includes the stomach and pancreas or a multivisceral transplant that includes stomach, pancreas, and liver.[251] Nutrition management both pre/post-transplant is varied from center to center. Managing children with intestinal failure has improved at centers that use a multidisciplinary team approach. Intestinal transplant is reserved for those who obtain life-threatening episodes of line sepsis, loss of venous access, and parenteral nutrition induced liver failure.[251] The overall postoperative management includes a complex treatment of immunosuppression and management of possible infectious complications as well as ongoing nutrition management that benefit from a multidisciplinary team approach. Grant et al reported that transplants since the year 2000 have a survival rate of 77% at year 1 and 55% at year 5. Sepsis remained the leading cause of graft loss.[252] The Intestinal Transplant Registry Report also noted that by 6 months after transplantation most recipients resume an oral diet and improved quality of life.[252]

Anatomy, Physiology, Pathology of Condition

Indications for intestinal transplant has not changed over time.[252] Intestinal transplant is not acceptable for all pediatric patients who have a diagnosis related to having intestinal failure. Transplantation should be considered when other modalities have not been successful. Recent advancements have been made in treating patients with intestinal failure such as restricting intralipids or even using other intravenous fat sources, rotating antibiotic therapy and medical advances to central line care as well as surgical procedures to help patients meet a more autonomy of enteral feeds and use less PN.[253] The primary indications for transplant of the intestine are not limited to: life-threatening episodes of line sepsis, loss of venous access, PNALD, or frequent life-threatening dehydration or electrolyte imbalances.[251] Intestinal transplant is not limited to an isolated intestine transplant, but may also be modified multivisceral and or a multivisceral transplant.[251] Overall intestinal transplant may include all of the following or selected organs with the intestine: stomach, liver, and pancreas.

Nutrition Assessment

Nutrition assessment is a complex assessment that entails growth history, feeding regimen, laboratory values, and nutrition-focus exam in developing and adjusting to meet the patient's nutritional requirements and aid in continued support of optimizing growth. These patients also typically have significant losses from output and need this volume and constituents replaced.

Nutrition Diagnostic Statement (PES)

Nutrition diagnosis is determined from information gathered during the nutrition assessment:

- Altered GI function (NC 1.4) related to short bowel syndrome as evidenced by the need for intestinal transplant due to PNALD.

Nutrition Intervention

Formalizing an individual nutrition regimen is based on findings from a patient's laboratory values, output losses, and growth. An early nutrition onset post-transplant complication seen is chylous ascites. Chylous ascites occur when lymphatic disruption is present in the abdominal cavity with resultant accumulation of chyle in the abdomen.[254] Post-transplant patients are started on a fat-free diet for the first 2–4 weeks after transplant and then the introduction of fat is adjusted after this time. Most patients receive gastrostomy or jejunostomy feedings to help achieve EN while weaning from PN.[255] The overall nutrition goal is to achieve autonomy and wean off of PN. Careful consideration of managing the oral and enteral feeding regimen while weaning PN is needed. Close monitoring of laboratory values and macro- and micronutrients is also required.

Nutrition Monitoring and Evaluation

Following a patient's individual growth, labs, and output is required as is adjusting these to continue to achieve appropriate growth. As immunosuppression is common, careful consideration in assessing vitamins and mineral levels and replenishment is needed. Since these patients are advanced on an EN regimen, feeds should be adjusted to prevent growth failure or the development of malnutrition.

Conclusion

The gastrointestinal tract is a complex organ system designed to ingest, digest, and absorb nutrients before waste expulsion. Its functions are essential to optimal health; however, if disrupted, alterations in nutritional requirements and status result. The clinical presentation of gastrointestinal disorders is multi-systemic and formal diagnoses are physician made and based on testing results. Nutrition screening in pediatric patients should be consistent with clinical malnutrition risk screening as defined by the AND and ASPEN. Additionally, pediatric patients benefit from receiving an individualized nutrition assessment from an experienced pediatric RDN, which often consists of obtaining a thorough diet history with emphasis placed on total energy intake, as well as both macronutrient and micronutrient intake, biochemical and clinical data results, anthropometric assessment, growth history/trends, and the need for multivitamin/mineral supplementation to aid in preventing and/or correcting nutrient deficiency. Information gathered during the nutrition assessment process allows for the determination of the nutrition diagnosis and appropriate intervention. Ongoing monitoring and evaluation is essential to achieve optimal health outcomes and improved quality of life within the pediatric gastrointestinal population.

🔍 CASE STUDY

LC is a 14-year 2 month-old female who was diagnosed with celiac disease one month ago. This is her first visit to the celiac clinic post diagnosis. Recent lab values reflect vitamin D of 28.1. DEXA revealed z-score of -0.8. LC has begun eliminating gluten from her diet. Weight at today's visit is 35.1 kg, height is 151.5 cm.

24 Hour Diet recall reveals:

Breakfast: 1 packet of Quaker oatmeal mixed with 1 cup skim milk, apple

Lunch: Dietz and Watson turkey and cheese on Udi's gluten-free bread, Snyder's gluten-free pretzels, carrots, water

Snack: Smartfood popcorn or Tostitos tortilla chips and salsa

Dinner: chicken, rice, green beans, apple juice

Snack: Schar gluten-free cookies

Please calculate the following:

Wt/age% tile: Ht/age %tile:
IBW (kg):   Stnd. Ht/age (cm):
% IBW: % Stnd Ht/age:
BMI:
BMI %tile:

Please classify LC's nutritional status:

☐ Normal   ☐ Wasted (mild/moderate/severe)   ☐ Stunted (mild/moderate/severe)

Please estimate needs:

Calories: per day   (REE x ___ used)
Protein (gm):   per kg
Fluid (ml):   per day

Calories: per day   (REE x ___ used)
Protein (gm):   per kg
Fluid (ml):   per day

Review Questions

1. Can you identify any sources of gluten that LC is currently receiving in her diet?
2. Comment on DEXA results and vitamin D level
3. Would you recommend vitamin/mineral supplementation? If so, please specify.
4. What are your MNT goals for LC?

Answer Key:

Wt/age %tile: <5th   Ht/age %tile: 5–10th
IBW (kg): 42   Stnd. Ht/age (cm): 161
% IBW: 83   % Stnd Ht/age: 94
BMI: 15.2 KG/M²
BMI %tile: <5th

Mild wasting
Mild stunting
1995 kcal/day (REE x 1.7) 1 gm protein/kg/day, 1802 ml/day (REE = 1174)

1. Quaker oats should be avoided due to cross contamination risk during milling and processing.
2. Introduction of certified gluten-free oats into diet (such as Bob's Red Mill brand) should be discussed with healthcare provider
3. DEXA normal and vitamin D insufficiency

4. Research reports that adherence to the gluten-free dietary pattern may result in a diet that is low in iron, folate, niacin, vitamin B$_{12}$, calcium, phosphorus and zinc. Therefore, a daily complete multivitamin is recommended. LC's dietary intake of calcium is also low. DRI for age indicates that LC should be taking in 1300 mg of calcium per day. In light of low vitamin D and suboptimal calcium intake, a calcium with vitamin D supplement is recommended. Ideally, a supplement that provides 1000 mg of calcium and 1000 IU of vitamin D.

Goals:

- Replete vitamin deficiencies and promote weight gain with diet and supplementation.
- Identify need for additional calorie boosting such as use of Ensure or Boost beverage.
- LC will verbalize good understanding of gluten-free diet.

▶ Websites

Websites that provide additional information on the various GI conditions are listed below.

General Gastrointestinal
https://www.gikids.org/http://www.naspghan.org

Celiac Disease
Foundations/Associations
Beyond Celiac
https://www.beyondceliac.org/
Celiac Disease Foundation
https://celiac.org/
National Celiac Association
https://www.nationalceliac.org/
Online resources for gluten-free food/recipes
https://simplygluten-free.com/
http://www.glutenfreemall.com
http://www.glutenfreeda.com
https://www.glutenfreeandmore.com/

Magazines for People with Celiac Disease & Other Food Allergies/Sensitivities
Gluten Free Living
http://www.glutenfreeliving.com
Simply Gluten Free
http://simplyglutenfreemag.com/

Crohn's and Colitis Foundation of America
http://www.ccfa.org

Review Questions

1. The gastrointestinal tract is a large muscular tube designed to ingest, digest, and absorb nutrients. Functions of the gastrointestinal tract may be disrupted by which of the following?
   A. Disease
   B. Antibiotics
   C. Environmental Toxins
   D. Bacterial Overgrowth
   E. All of the above

2. Approximately 95% of critically ill patients experience diarrhea associated with enteral feeds. Which feeding method has been shown to aid in decreasing diarrhea?
   A. Gastric feedings
   B. Post-pyloric feedings

3. The specific nutrition diagnosis established from the nutrition assessment aids in determining the appropriate medical nutrition therapy intervention. Which one of the following is NOT recommended as a first line of therapy in children with constipation?
   A. High Fiber Diet
   B. Use of Prebiotics and Probiotics
   C. Increased fluid intake
   D. Increased physical activity

4. The only known treatment for celiac disease is adherence to a gluten-free diet. Which of the following foods listed below **may** contain gluten?
   A. Baked Beans
   B. Hot chocolate mix
   C. French Fries
   D. Miso Soup
   E. All of the above

5. Crohn's disease may occur in any portion of the gastrointestinal tract; whereas, Ulcerative Colitis is confined to the colon with minimal involvement of the terminal ileum.
   A. True
   B. False

6. Early initiation of enteral feedings **is not** recommended in patients with moderate to severe pancreatitis.
   A. True
   B. False

7. Nutrition interventions in an infant/child with cholestatic liver disease includes all of the following **except**:
   A. Recommend infant formulas that contain 40–60% of the fat from medium chain triglycerides (MCT).
   B. Provide nutrition education regarding foods high in linoleic acid.
   C. Ensure that infants receive less than 3% of calories from linoleic acid.
   D. Ensure that additional sources of MCT are added gradually.

8. What nutrient deficiencies may be found in a child with Short Bowel Syndrome. Why?

9. Which of the following statements are true?
   A. Nutrition screening in pediatric patients should be consistent with clinical malnutrition risk screening as defined by the Academy of Nutrition and Dietetics and American Society for Parenteral and Enteral Nutrition.
   B. Information gathered during the nutrition assessment process allows for the determination of the nutrition diagnosis and appropriate intervention.
   C. Ongoing monitoring and evaluation is essential to achieve optimal health outcomes.
   D. All of the above

References

1. Corkins MR, Scolapino J. Diarrhea. In: Merritt R, ed. *The ASPEN Nutrition Support Practice Manual*, 2nd ed. Silver Spring, MD: ASPEN; 2005:207–210.

2. Graham-Maar RC, French HM, Piccoli DA. Gastroenterology. In: Frank G, Shah SS, Catallozzi M, Zaoutis LB, eds. *The Philadelphia Guide: Inpatient Pediatrics*. Philadelphia, PA: Lippincott, Williams, and Wilkins; 2003:100–115.

3. Leonberg BL. *ADA Pocket Guide to Pediatric Nutrition Assessment*. Chicago, Il: American Dietetic Association; 2008:106.

4. World Health Organization, Department of Child and Adolescent Health and Development. *The Treatment of Diarrhoea—A Manual for Physicians and Other Senior Health Care Workers*. 4th ed. Geneva, Switzerland: World Health Organization; 2005.

5. American Academy of Pediatrics. Oral therapy for acute diarrhea. In: Kleinman RE, ed. *Pediatric Nutrition Handbook*, 6th ed. Elk Grove Village, IL: American Academy of Pediatrics; 2009:651–659.

6. Nahikian-Nelms M, Sucher K, Long S. Diseases of the Lower Gastrointestinal Tract. In: *Nutrition Therapy and Pathophysiology*, 3ed. Belmont, CA: Wadsworth/Thomson Learning; 2015.

7. Bhutta ZA, Ghishan F, Lindley K, Memon IA, Mittal S, Rhoads JM. Persistent and chronic diarrhea and malabsorption: working group report of the Second World Congress of Pediatric Gastroenterology, Hepatology, and Nutrition. *J Pediatr Gastroenterol Nutr*. 2004;39:S711–S716.

8. Lo CW, Walker WA. Chronic protracted diarrhea of infancy: a nutritional disorder. *Pediatrics*. 1983;72:786.

9. American Academy of Pediatrics. Chronic diarrhea disease. In: Kleinman RE, ed. *Pediatric Nutrition Handbook*, 6th ed. Elk Grove Village, IL: American Academy of Pediatrics; 2009:637–649.

10. Brito-Ashurst I, Preiser JC. Diarrhea in critically ill patients: the role of enteral feeding. *JPEN*. 2016;40(7):913–923.

11. Fleisher G, Matson D. Patient education: acute diarrhea in children (beyond the basics). Available at: https://www.uptodate.com/contents/acute-diarrhea-in-children-beyond-the-basics. Accessed November 11, 2016.

12. Evans J. Protracted Diarrhea. In: Wyllie R, Hyams JS, Kay M. *Pediatric Gastrointestinal and Liver Disease*. 4th ed. Philadelphia, PA: Elsevier; 2011:350–359.

13. Becker P, Carney L, et al. Consensus statement of the Academy of Nutrition and Dietetics/American Society for Parenteral and Enteral Nutrition: Indicators recommended

for the identification and documentation of pediatric malnutrition (undernutrition). *J Acad Nutr Diet.* 2014;114(12): 1988–2000.

14. King CK, Glass R, Breese JS, Duggan C. Management of acute gastroenteritis among children: oral rehydration, maintenance and nutritional therapy. *MMWR.* 2003;52:1–16.

15. American Academy of Pediatrics, Provisional Committee on Quality Improvement, Subcommittee on Acute Gastroenteritis. Practice parameter: the management of acute gastroenteritis in young children. *Pediatrics.* 1996;97:424–435.

16. Sandhu B, Devadason D. Management of diarrhea. In: Wyllie R, Hyams JS, Kay M. *Pediatric Gastrointestinal and Liver Disease.* 4th ed. Philadelphia, PA: Elsevier; 2011:1002–1011.

17. Roberts J, Shilkofski N. *The Harriet Lane Handbook*, 17th ed. Elsevier Mosby; 2005:559, Table 20–14a.

18. Home-Made "Oral Rehydration-Like" Solutions Using Alternative Beverage Base In: Pocket Guide for Patients: Managing Short Bowel Syndrome 3rd Edition by Parrish RE, 2016.

19. Academy of Nutrition and Dietetics. Pediatric Nutrition Care Manual®. Diarrhea. Accessed November 7, 2017.

20. Brown KH, Perez F, Peerson J, et al. Effect of dietary fiber (soy polysaccharide) on the severity, duration, and nutritional outcome of acute, watery diarrhea in children. *Pediatrics.* 1993;92:241–247.

21. Burks AW, Vanderhoof JA, Mehra S, Ostrom KM, Baggs G. Randomized clinical trial of soy formula with and without added fiber in antibiotic-induced diarrhea. *J Pediatr.* 2001;139:578–582.

22. Brown KH, Peerson JM, Fontaine O. Use of non-human milks in the dietary management of young children with acute diarrhea: a meta-analysis of clinical trials. *Pediatrics.* 1994;93:17–27.

23. Samour P, King K. *Handbook of Pediatric Nutrition.* 4th ed. Sudbury, MA: Jones and Bartlett Publishers; 2012;279.

24. Sazawal S, Black RE, Bhan MK, Bhandari N, Sinha A, Jalla S. Zinc supplementation in young children with acute diarrhea in India. *N Engl J Med.* 1995;333:839–844.

25. Heinig MJ, Brown KH, Lonnerdal B, Dewey KG. Zinc supplementation does not affect growth, morbidity or motor development of U.S. term breastfed infants at 4–10 mo of age. *Am J Clin Nutr.* 2006;84:594–601.

26. Uauy R. Novel oligosaccharides in human milk: understanding mechanisms may lead to better prevention of enteric and other infections. *J Pediatr.* 2004:145(3):283–285.

27. Van Niel CW. Probiotics: not just for treatment anymore. *Pediatrics.* 2004;115(1):174–177.

28. Hattner JA. Digestive health: probiotics and prebiotics for children. *Nutr Focus.* 2009;24(3):1–2.

29. Dai D, Walker WA. Protective nutrients and bacterial colonization in the immature human gut. *Adv Pediatr.* 1999;46:353–382.

30. Morrow AL, Ruiz-Palacios GM, Altaye M, et al. Human milk oligosaccharides are associated with protection against diarrhea in breast-fed infants. *J Pediat.* 2004;145:297–303.

31. Ziegler E, Vanderhoof JA, Petschow B, Mitmesser SH et al. *J Pediatr Gastroenterol Nutr.* 2007;44;359–364.

32. Thibault H, Aubert-Jacquin C, Goulet O. Effects of long-term consumption of a fermented infant formula with (Bifidobacterium breve c50 and Streptococcus thermophilus 065) on acute diarrhea in healthy infants. *J Pediatr Gastroenterol Nutr.* 2004;39(2):147–152.

33. Nestle Health Science. 2016-2017 Product Guide. Available at: www.Nestlehealthscience.us. Accessed November 2017.

34. Abbott Laboratories. 2017-2018 Abbott Nutrition Product Reference.161624(1)/October 2017. Available at: https:// abbottnutrtion.com/product-handbook-landing.

35. Szajewska H, Guarino A, Hojsak I, Indrio F, et al. Use for probiotics for management of acute gastroenteritis: A position paper by ESPGHAN working group for probiotics and prebiotics. *JPGN.* 2014;58:531–539.

36. Allen SJ, Martinez EG, Gregorio GV, et al. Probiotics for treating acute infectious diarrhea. *Cochrane Database Syst Rev.* 2010;(11):CD003048.

37. Szajewska H, Skorka A, Ruszynski M, et al. Meta-analysis: Lactobacillus GG for treating acute gastroenteritis in children-updated analysis of randomized controlled trials. *Aliment Pharmacol Ther.* 2013;38:467–76.

38. Szajewska H, Skorka A. *Saccharomyce boulardii* for treating acute gastroenteritis in children: updated meta-analysis of randomized control trials. *Aliment Pharmacol Ther.* 2009;30:955–63.

39. Lund B, Edlund C. Probiotic *Enterococcus faecium* strain is a recipient of vanA gene cluster. *Clin Infect Dis.* 2001;32:1384–1385.

40. Cook R, Thane BA. Alleviation of retching and feeding intolerance after fundoplication. *Nutr Clin Pract.* 2014;29: 386–396.

41. Qiu C, Chen C, Zhang W, et al. Fat-modified enteral formula improves feeding tolerance in critically ill patients: a multicenter, single-blinded, randomized control trial *JPEN.* 2017;31(5):785–795.

42. McClave SA, Taylor BE, Martindale RG, et al. Guidelines for the provision and assessment of nutrition support therapy in the adult critically ill patient: Society of Critically Ill Medicine (SCCM) and American Society for Parenteral and Enteral Nutrition (A.S.P.E.N). *JPEN.* 2016;40(2):159–211.

43. Academy of Nutrition and Dietetics. Pediatric Nutrition Care Manual®. Constipation. Available at: https:// www.nutritioncaremanual.org/topic.cfm?ncm _category_id=13&lv1=144625&lv2=144769&ncm_toc _id=144769&ncm_heading=Nutrition%20Care. Accessed: September 19, 2017.

44. Mugie SM1, Benninga MA, Di Lorenzo C. Epidemiology of constipation in children and adults: a systematic review. *Best Pract Res Clin Gastroenterol.* 2011;25(1):3–18.

45. Rajindrajith S, Devanarayana NM. Constipation in children: novel insight into epidemiology, pathophysiology, and management. *J Neurogastroenterol Motil.* 2011;17(1): 35–47.

46. Tabbers MM, DiLorenzo C, et al. Evaluation and treatment of functional constipation in infants and children: evidence-based recommendations from ESPGHAN and NASPGHAN. *J Pediatr Gastroenterol Nutr.* 2014;58(2):258–274.

47. Vriesman MH, Velasco-Benitez CA, et al. Assessing children's report of stool consistency: agreement between the pediatric Rome III questionnaire and the Bristol stool scale. *J Pediatr.* 2017;190:69–73.

48. Koppen IJN, Broekaert IG, et al. Role of polyethylene glycol in the treatment of functional constipation in children. *J Pediatr Gastroenterol Nutr.* 2017;65(4):361–363.

49. Bekkali NLH, Hoekman DR, et al. Polyethylene glycol 3350 with electrolytes vs. polyethylene glycol 4000 for constipation: a randomized, controlled trial. *J Pediatr Gastroenterol Nutr.* 2017. PMID:28906317.

50. Heyman MB, Abrams S; Section of Gastroenterology, Hepatology, and Nutrition; Committee on Nutrition. Fruit juice in infants, children, and adolescents: current recommendations. *Pediatrics*. 2017;139(6):e20170967.

51. Baker SS, Liptak GS, et al. Constipation in infants and children: evaluation and treatment. A medical position statement of the North American Society of Pediatric Gastroenterology and Nutrition. *J Pediatr Gastroenterol Nutr*. 1999;29(5):612–626.

52. National Academy of Sciences. Institute of Medicine. Food and Nutrition Board. Dietary Reference Intakes for Energy, Carbohydrate, Fiber, Fat, Fatty Acids, Cholesterol, Protein, and Amino Acids (Macronutrients) 2005. Available at: https://www.nap.edu/read/10490/chapter/32#1324. Accessed: October 18, 2017.

53. Data for sections on fruits and vegetables/legumes from: Pennington JAT. *Bowes and Church's Food Values of Portions Commonly Used*, 15th ed. Philadelphia: JB Lippincott; 1989.

54. U.S. Department of Agriculture. *USDA Provisional Table on the Dietary Fiber Content of Selected Foods*; 1988. HNIS/PT-106.

55. Nelson SP, Chen EH, Syniar GM, Christoffel KK; Pediatric Practice Research Group. Prevalence of symptoms of gastroesophageal reflux during infancy: a pediatric practice-based survey. *Arch Pediatr Adolesc Med*. 1997;151(6):569–572.

56. Campanozzi A, Boccia G, Pensabene L, et al. Prevalence and natural history of gastroesophageal reflux. *Pediatrics*. 2009;123(3):779–783.

57. Rosen R. Gastroesophageal reflux in infants. More than just a phenomenon. *JAMA Pediatr*. 2014;168(1):83–89.

58. Vandenplas Y, Rudolph CD, Di Lorenzo C, et al. Pediatric gastroesophageal reflux clinical practice guidelines: joint recommendations of the North American Society for Pediatric Gastroenterology, Hepatology, and Nutrition and the European Society for Pediatric Gastroenterology, Hepatology, and Nutrition. *J Pediatr Gastroenterol Nutr*. 2009;49(4):498–547.

59. Lightdale J, Gremse D, Section on Gastroenterology, Hepatology, and Nutrition. Gastroesophageal reflux: Management guidance for the Pediatrician. *Pediatrics*. 2013;131: e1684.

60. Cameron AJ, Lagergren J, Henriksson C, Nyren O, Locke GR, III, Pedersen NL. Gastroesophageal reflux disease in monozygotic and dizygotic twins. *Gastroenterol*. 2002;122(1):55–59.

61. Kleinman L, Revicki DA, Flood E. Validation issues in questionnaires for diagnosis and monitoring of gastroesophageal reflux disease in children. *Curr Gastroenterol Rep*. 2006;8(3):230–236.

62. Aksglaede K, Pedersen JB, Lange A, Funch-Jensen P, Thommesen P. Gastro-esophageal reflux demonstrated by radiography in infants less than 1 year of age. *Acta Radiol*. 2003;44(2): 136–138.

63. Gold BD, Gunasekaran T, Tolia V, et al. Safety and symptom improvement with esomeprazole in adolescents with gastroesophageal reflux disease. *J Pediatr Gastroenterol Nutr*. 2007;45(5):520–529.

64. Tolia V, Youssef NN, Gilger MA, Traxler B, Illueca M. Esomeprazole for the treatment of erosive esophagitis in children: an international, multicenter, randomized, parallel-group, double-blind (for dose) study. *BMC Pediatr*. 2010;10:41.

65. Orenstein SR, Shalaby TM, Devandry SN, et al. Famotidine for infant gastro-oesophageal reflux: a multi-centre, randomized, placebo-controlled, withdrawal trial. *Aliment Pharmacol Ther*. 2003;17(9):1097–1107.

66. Jordan B, Heine RG, Meehan M, Catto-Smith AG, Lubitz L. Effect of antireflux medication, placebo and infant mental health intervention on persistent crying: a randomized clinical trial. *J Paediatr Child Health*. 2006;42(1-2):49–58.

67. Horvath A, Dziechciarz P, Szajewska H. The effect of thickened-feed interventions on gastroesophageal reflux in infants: systematic review and meta-analysis of randomized, controlled trials [review]. *Pediatrics*. 2008;122(6):e1268–e1277. Erratum in: *Pediatrics*. 2009; 123(4):1254.

68. Grummer-Strawn L, Kelley SS, Fein SB, Infant Feeding and Feeding Transitions during the First Year of Life. *Pediatrics*. 2008;122:S36–S42.

69. Clarke P, Robinson MJ. Thickening milk feeds may cause necrotising enterocolitis. *Arch Dis Child Fetal Neonatal Ed*. 2004;89(3):F280.

70. Jeske, HC. The influence of postural changes on gastroesophageal reflux and barrier pressure in nonfasting individuals. *Anesth Analg*. 2005;101:597–600.

71. Corvaglia L, Rotatori R, FerliniM, Aceti A, Ancora G, Faldella G. The effect of body positioning on gastroesophageal reflux in premature infants. *J Pediatr*. 2007;151(6):591–596.

72. Loots C, Smits M, Omari T, Bennink R, Benninga M, VanWijk M. Effect of lateral positioning on gastroesophageal reflux (GER) and underlying mechanisms in GER disease (GERD) patients and healthy controls. *Neurogastroenterol Motil*. 2013;25(3):222–229.

73. Lewis, Alexia. Professional Resources Development. Lactose intolerance: basics & beyond. Available at: https://www.pdresources.org/uploads/course/96b50.pdf. Accessed: October 26, 2017.

74. Heyman, MB, Committee on Nutrition. Lactose intolerance in infants, children, and adolescents. *Pediatrics*. 2006;118: 1279–1286.

75. Amiri M, Diekmann L, et al. The diverse forms of lactose intolerance and the putative linkage to several cancers. *Nutrients*. 2015;7(9):7209–7230.

76. Lember M. Hypolactasia: a common enzyme deficiency leading to lactose malabsorption and interolance. *Pol Arch Med Weiwn*. 2012:122; (suppl 1):60–64.

77. Berni C, Pezzella V, et al. Diagnosing and treating intolerance to carbohydrates in children. *Nutrients*. 2016;8(3):157.

78. Carlson SJ, Rogers RR, Lombard KA. Effect of a lactase preparation on lactose content and osmolality of preterm and term infant formulas. *J Parenteral Enteral Nutr*. 1991;15:564–566.

79. Erasmus H, Ludwig-Auser H, Paterson P, Sun Dongmei, Sankaran K. Enhanced weight gain in preterm infants receiving lactase-treated feeds: a randomized, double-blind, controlled trial. *J Pediatr*. 2002;141:532–537.

80. Diekmann L, Pfeiffer K, et al. Congenital lactose intolerance is triggered by severe mutations on both alleles of the lactose gene. *BMC Gastroenterol*. 2015;15:36.

81. Academy of Nutrition and Dietetics. Pediatric Nutrition Care Manual®. Lactose Controlled Nutrition Therapy. Available at: https://www.nutritioncaremanual.org/client_ed.cfm?ncm_client_ed_id=248. Accessed: October 26, 2017.

82. Case S. *Gluten Free: The Definitive Resource Guide*. Regina, Saskatchewan, Canada: Case Nutrition Consulting, Inc; 2016.

83. Hill ID, Fasano A, et al. NASPGHAN clinical report on the diagnosis and treatment of gluten-related disorders. *J Pediatr Gastroenterol Nutr*. 2016;63(1):156–165.

84. Galatola M, Cielo D, et al. Presymptomatic diagnosis of Celiac Disease in predisposed children: the role of gene expression profile. *J Pediatr Gastroenterol Nutr*. 2017; 65(3):314–320.

85. Lee GJ, Kao JY. Recent advances in pediatric celiac disease. *Exper Rev Gastroenterol Hepatol.* 2017;11(6):583–592.

86. Snyder J, Butzner D, et al. Evidence-informed expert recommendation for the management of Celiac Disease in children. *Pediatrics.* 2016;138(3):e20153147.

87. Szajewska H, Shamir R, et al. Gluten introduction and the risk of Coeliac Disease: a position paper by the European Society for Pediatric Gastroenterology, Hepatology, and Nutrition. *J Pediatr Gastroenterol Nutr.* 2016;62(3):507–513.

88. Academy of Nutrition and Dietetics. Pediatric Nutrition Care Manual®. Celiac Disease. Available at: https://www.nutritioncaremanual.org/topic.cfm?ncm_category_id=13&lv1=144625&lv2=144772&ncm_toc_id=144772&ncm_heading=Nutrition%20Care. Accessed: September 19, 2017.

89. Pinto-Sanchez M, Verdu E, et al. Gluten introduction to infant feeding and risk of celiac disease: Systematic review and meta-analysis. *J Pediatr.* 2016;168:132–143.e3.

90. Szajewska H, Shamir R, et al. Systematic review with meta-analysis: early infant feeding and coeliac disease-update 2015. *Aliment Pharmacol Ther.* 2015;41(11):1038–1054.

91. Fok C, Holland K, et al. The role of nurses and dietitians in managing paediatric coeliac disease. *Br J Nurs.* 2016;25(8):449–455.

92. Alehan F, Canan O, Cemil T, Erol I, Ozcay F. Increased risk for coeliac disease in paediatric patients with migraine. *Cephalalgia.* 2008;28:945–949.

93. Husby S, Koletzko S, et al. European Society of Gastroenterology, Hepatology and Nutrition for the diagnosis of coeliac disease. *J Pediatr Gastroenterol Nutr.* 2012;54(1):136–60.

94. Mills JR, Murray JA. Contemporary celiac disease diagnosis: is a biopsy avoidable? *Curr Opin Gastroenterol.* 2016;32(2):80–85.

95. Bozzola M, Meazza C, et al. Omitting duodenal biopsy in children with suspected celiac disease and extra-intestinal symptoms. *Ital J Pedatr.* 2017;43(1):59.

96. Tonutti E, Bizzaro N. Diagnosis and classification of celiac disease and gluten sensitivity. *Autoimmun Rev.* 2014;13(4-5):472–476.

97. Guandalini S, Newland C. Can we really skip the biopsy in diagnosing symptomatic children with celiac disease? *J Pediatr Gastroenterol Nutr.* 2013;57:e24.

98. Aaltonen K, Laurikka P, et al. The long-term consumption of oats in celiac disease patients is safe: a large cross-sectional study. *Nutrients.* 2017;9(6):e611.

99. Sjöberg V, Hollën E, et al. Noncontaminated dietary oats may hamper normalization of the intestinal immune status in childhood celiac disease. *Clin Transl Gastroenterol.* 2014;5:e58.

100. Vici G, Belli L, et al. Gluten free diet and nutrient deficiencies: A review. *Clin Nutr.* 2016;35(6):1236–1241.

101. Williams KM. Update on bone health in pediatric chronic disease. *Endocrinol Metab Clin North Am.* 2016;45(2):433–441.

102. Trovato, C, Albanese C, et al. Lack of clinical predictors for low mineral density in children with celiac disease. *J Pediatr Gastroenterol Nutr.* 2014;59(6):799–802.

103. Hill ID, Dirks MH, Liptak GS. Guidelines for the diagnosis and treatment of celiac disease in children: recommendations of the North American Society for Pediatric Gastroenterology, Hepatology and Nutrition. *J Ped Gastroenterol Nutr.* 2005;40(1):1–19.

104. Murray J, See J. Gluten-free diet: the medical and nutrition management of celiac disease. *Nutr Clin Prac.* 2006;21:1–15.

105. Mooney PD, Hadjivassiliou M, et al. Emerging drugs for coeliac disease. *Expert Opin Emerg Drugs.* 2014;19(4):533–544.

106. Plugis N, Khosla C. Therapeutic approaches for celiac disease. *Best Pract Res Clin Gastroenterol.* 2015;29(3):503–21.

107. Motil KJ, Grand RJ. Inflammatory bowel disease. In: Walker WA, Watkins JB, eds. *Nutrition in Pediatrics: Basic Science and Clinical Applications.* Hamilton, ON: Decker; 1997:516.

108. Motil KJ, Grand RJ. Nutritional management of inflammatory bowel disease. *Pediatr Clin North Am.* 1985;32:447.

109. Motil KJ, Grand RJ, Davis-Kraft L, Ferlic LL, Smith EO. Growth failure in children with inflammatory bowel disease: a prospective study. *United States Department of Agriculture/Agricultural Research Service Children's Nutrition Research Center, Houston, Texas Gastroenterology.* 1993;105(3):681–691.

110. DeFilippis EM, Sockolow R, Barfield E. Health care maintenance for pediatric patient with Inflammatory Bowel Disease. *Pediatrics.* 2016;3:1–11.

111. Ricciuto A, Fish J, Tomalty D, Carman N, Crowley E, Popalis C, Muise A, Walters TD, Griffiths AM, Church PC. Diagnostic delay in Canadian children with inflammatory bowel disease is more common in Crohn's disease and associated with decreased height. *Arch Dis Child.* 2018;103(4):319–326.

112. Wiech P, Binkowska-Bury M, Korczowski B. Body composition as an indication of nutritional status in children with newly diagnosed ulcerative colitis and Crohn's disease- Prospective study. *Gastroenterology Rev.* 2017;12(1):55–59.

113. Jansen I, Prager M, Valentini L, Buning C. Inflammation-driven malnutrition: a new screening tool predicts outcome in Crohn's disease. *Br J Nutr.* 2016;116:1061–1067.

114. Azcue M, Rashid M, Friffiths A, Pencharz PB. Energy expenditure and body composition in children with Crohn's disease: effect of enteral nutrition and treatment with prednisolone. *Gut.* 1997;41:203–208.

115. Hill RJ, Lewindon PJ, Withers GD, Connor FL, Ee LC, Cleghorn GJ, Davies PSW. Ability of commonly used prediction equations to predict resting energy expenditure in children with Inflammatory Bowel Disease. *Inflamm Bowel Dis.* 2011;17(7):1587–1593.

116. Stokes MA, Hill GL. Total energy expenditure in patients with Crohn's disease: measurement by the combined body scan technique. *J Parenter Enteral Nutr.* 1993;17:3–7.

117. Takeda H, Ishihama K, Fukui T, et al. Significance of rapid turnover proteins in protein-losing gastroenteropathy. *Hepatogastroenterol.* 2003;50(54):1963–1965.

118. Hartman C, Eliakim R, Shamir R. Nutritional status and nutritional therapy in inflammatory bowel diseases. *World J Gastroenterol.* 2009;15(21):2570–2578.

119. Frantz D, Munroe C, Parrish CR, Krenitsky J, Willcutts K, Fortune A. Gastrointestinal disease. In: Mueller CM, ed. *The ASPEN Nutrition Support Core Curriculum.* Silver Spring, MD: ASPEN; 2012:426–450.

120. Vagianos K, Bector S, McConnell J, Bernstein CN. Nutrition assessment of patients with inflammatory bowel disease. *J Parenter Enter Nutr.* 2007;31(4):311–319.

121. Filippi J, Al-Jaouni R, Wiroth JB, Hebuterne X, Schneider SM. Nutritional deficiencies in patients with Crohn's disease in remission. *Inflamm Bowel Dis.* 2006;12(3):185–191.

122. Kim S, Koh H. Nutritional aspect of pediatric inflammatory bowel disease: its clinical importance. *Korean J Pediatr.* 2015;58(10):363–368.

123. Semeao EJ, Jawad AF, Stouffer NO, Zemel BS, Piccoli DA, Stallings VA. Risk factors for low bone mineral density in

children and young adults with Crohn's disease. *J Pediatr.* 1999;135(5):593–600.

124. Paganelli M, Albanese C, Borrelli O, et al. Inflammation is the main determinant of low bone mineral density in pediatric inflammatory bowel disease. *Inflamm Bowel Dis.* 2007;13(4):416–423.

125. Holick MF. Vitamin D deficiency. *N Engl J Med.* 2007;357(3):266–280.

126. Davis AM, Baker SS, Baker RD Jr, et al. Pediatric gastrointestinal disorders. In: Meritt RM, ed. *The ASPEN Nutrition Support Practice Manual.* Silver Spring, MD: ASPEN;1998:27–30.

127. Prey S, Paul C. Effect of folic or folinic acid supplementation on methotrexate-associated safety and efficacy in inflammatory disease: a systematic review. *Br J Dermatol.* 2008;160(3):622–628.

128. Hyams JS. Crohn's disease. In: Hyams WS, Hyams JS, eds. *Pediatric Gastrointestinal Disease: Pathophysiology, Diagnosis, Management.* Philadelphia, PA: WB Saunders; 1993:750–764.

129. Levenstein S, Prantera C, Luzi C, et al. A low residue or normal diet in Crohn's disease: a prospective controlled trial of Italian patients. *Gut.* 1985;26:989.

130. Levi AJ. Diet in the management of Crohn's disease. *Gut.* 1985;26:985.

131. Mishkin S. Dairy sensitivity, lactose malabsorption, and elimination diets in inflammatory bowel disease. *Am J Clin Nutr.* 1997;65:564–567.

132. Siedman EG, Leliedo N, Ament M, et al. Nutritional issues in pediatric inflammatory bowel disease. *J Pediatr Gastroenterol Nutr.* 1991;12:424.

133. Berni Canani R, Terrin G, Borrelli O, et al. Short- and long-term therapeutic efficacy of nutritional therapy and corticosteroids in paediatric Crohn's disease. *Dig Liver Dis.* 2006;38(6):381–387.

134. Ruuska T, Savilahti E, Maki M, et al. Exclusive whole protein enteral diet versus prednisolone in the treatment of acute Crohn's disease in children. *J Pediatr Gastroenterol Nutr.* 1994;19(2):175–180.

135. Borrelli O, Cordischi L, Cirulli M, et al. Polymeric diet alone versus corticosteroids in the treatment of active pediatric Crohn's disease: a randomized controlled open-label trial. *Clin Gastroenterol Hepatol.* 2006;4(6):744–753.

136. Ludvigsson JF, Krantz M, Bodin L, et al. Elemental versus polymeric enteral nutrition in pediatric Crohn's disease: a multicentre randomized controlled trial. *Acta Paediatr.* 2004;93:327–335.

137. Zachos M, Tondeur M, Griffiths AM. Enteral nutritional therapy for induction of remission in Crohn's disease. *Cochrane Database Syst Rev.* 2007;1:CD000542.

138. Akobeng AK, Thomas AG. Enteral nutrition for maintenance of remission of Crohn's disease. *Cochrane Database Syst Rev.* 2007;3:CD005984.

139. Johnson T, Macdonald S, Hill SM, Thomas A, Murphy MS. Treatment of active Crohn's disease in children using partial enteral nutrition with liquid formula: a randomized controlled trial. *Gut.* 2006;55:356–361.

140. Verma S, Holdsworth CD, Giaffer GH. Does adjuvant nutritional support diminish steroid dependency in Crohn's disease? *Scand J Gastroenterol.* 2001;36:383–388.

141. Bamba T, Shimoyama T, Sadaki M, et al. Dietary fat attenuates the benefits of an elemental diet in active Crohn's disease: a randomized controlled trial. *Eur J Gastroenterol Hepatol.* 2003;15:151–157.

142. Gassull MA, Fernandez-Banares F, Cabre E, et al. Fat composition may be a clue to explain the primary therapeutic effect of enteral nutrition in Crohn's disease: results of a double blind randomized multicentre European trial. *Gut.* 2002;51(2):164–168.

143. Sakurai T, Matsui T, Yao T, et al. Short-term efficacy of enteral nutrition in the treatment of active Crohn's disease: a randomized, controlled trial comparing nutrient formulas. *JPEN.* 2002;26(2):98–103.

144. DeLey M, de Vos R, Hommes DW, Stokkers P. Fish oil for induction of remission of ulcerative colitis. *Cochrane DatabaseSyst Rev.* 2007;4:CD005573.

145. Turner D, Steinhart AH, Griffiths AM. Omega 3 fatty acids for maintenance of remission of ulcerative colitis. *Cochrane Database Syst Rev.* 2007;3:CD006443.

146. Turner D, Zlotkin SH, Shah PS, Griffiths AM. Omega 3 fatty acids for maintenance of remission of Crohn's disease. *Cochrane Database Syst Rev.* 2009;1:CD006320.

147. Butterworth AD, Thomas AG, Akobeng AK. Probiotics for induction of remission in Crohn's disease. *Cochrane Database Syst Rev.* 2008;3:CD006634.

148. Rolfe VE, Fortun PJ, Hawkey CJ, Bath-Hextall F. Probiotics for maintenance of remission in Crohn's disease. *Cochrane Database Syst Rev.* 2006;4:CD004826.

149. Mallon P, McKay D, Kirk S, Gardiner K. Probiotics for induction of remission in ulcerative colitis. *Cochrane Database Syst Rev.* 2007;4:CD005573.

150. Bannerjee K, Camacho-Hubner C, Babinska K, et al. Anti-inflammatory and growth-stimulating effects precede nutritional restitution during enteral feeding in Crohn disease. *JPEN.* 2004;38:270–275.

151. Penagini F, Dilillo D, Borsai B, et al.. Nutrition in Pediartic Inflammatory Bowel Disease: from etiology to treatment. a systematic review. *Nutrients.* 2016;8 (334):1–27.

152. Abou-Assi S, O'Keefe SJ. Nutrition support during acute pancreatitis. *Nutrition.* 2002;8(11–12):938–943.

153. Frossard JL, Steer ML, Pastor CM. Acute pancreatitis. *Lancet.* 2008;371(9607):143–152.

154. Seminerio J, O'Keefe SJ. Jejunal feeding in patients with pancreatitis. *Nutr Clin Pract.* 2014:29:283–286.

155. Lowe M, Greer J, Srinath A. Acute pancreatitis in children. Available at: https://pancreasfoundation.org/patient-information/childrenpediatric-pancreatitis/acute-pancreatitis-in-children/. Accessed November 6th 2017.

156. Afghani E, Sinha A, Singh V. An overview of the diagnosis and management of nutrition in chronic pancreatitis. *Nutr Clin Pract.* 2014;29:295–311.

157. Otsuki M, Takeda K, Matsuno S, Kihara Y, et al. Criteria for the diagnosis and severity stratification of acute pancreatitis. *World J Gastroenterol.* 2013;19(35):5798–5805.

158. Petrov MS. Gastric feeding and "Gut Rousing" in acute pancreatitis. *Nutr Clin Pract.* 2014; 29:287–290.

159. Eckerwall GE, Tingstedt BB, Bergenzaun PE, Andersson RG. Immediate oral feeding in patients with mild acute pancreatitis is safe and may accelerate recovery—a randomized clinical study. *Clin Nutr.* 2007;26(6):758–763.

160. Sathiaraj E, Murthy S, Mansard MJ, Rao GV, Mahukar S, Reddy DN. Clinical trial: oral feeding with a soft diet compared with clear liquid diet as initial meal in mild acute pancreatitis. *Aliment Pharmacol Ther.* 2008;28(6):777–781.

161. Duggan SN, Smyth MD, O'Sullivan M, et al. A transatlantic survey of nutrition practice in acute pancreatitis. *J Hum Nutr Diet*. 2012;25:388–397.

162. Abou-Assi S, Craig K, O'Keefe SJ. Hypocaloric jejunal feeding is better than total parenteral nutrition in acute pancreatitis: result of a randomized comparative study. *Am J Gastroenterol*. 2002;97:2255–2262.

163. Eatock FC, Chong P, Menezes N, et al. A randomized study of early nasogastric verses nasojejunal feeding in severe acute pancreatitis. *Am J Gastoenterol*. 2005;100:432–439.

164. Hegazi R, Raina A, Graham T, et al. Early jejunal feeding initiation and clinical outcomes in patients with severe acute pancreatitis. *JPEN*. 2011;35:91–96.

165. Marik PE, Zaloga GP. Meta-analysis of parenteral nutrition versus enteral nutrition in patients with acute pancreatitis. *BMJ*. 2004;328(7453):1407.

166. Marik PE. What is the best way to feed patients with pancreatitis? *Curr Opin Crit Care*. 2009;15(2):131–138.

167. Petrov MS, Pylypchuk RD, Emelyanov NV. Systematic review: nutritional support in acute pancreatitis. *Aliment Pharmacol Ther*. 2008;28(6):704–712.

168. McClave SA, Chang WK, Dhaliwal R, Heyland DK. Nutrition support in acute pancreatitis: a systematic review of the literature. *JPEN* 2006;30(2):143–156.

169. Sun JK, Mu XW, Li WQ, Tong ZH, Li J, Zheng SY. Effects of early enteral nutrition on immune function of severe acute pancreatitis. *World J Gastroenterol*. 2013;19:917–922.

170. Gatt M, MacFie J, Anderson AD et al. Changes in superior mesenteric artery blood flow after oral, enteral, and parenteral feeding in humans. *Crit Care Med*. 2009;37:171–176.

171. Kaushik N, Pietraszewski M, Holst JJ, O'Keefe SJ. Enteral feeding without pancreatic stimulation. *Pancreas*. 2005;31:353–359.

172. Petrov MS, Loveday BP, Pylypchuk RD, McIlroy K, Phillips AR, Windsor JA. Systematic review and meta-analysis of enteral nutrition formulations in acute pancreatitis. *Br J Surg*. 2009;96(11):1243–1252.

173. Dickerson RN, Vehe KL, Mullen JL, Feurer ID. Resting energy expenditure in patients with pancreatitis. *Crit Care Med*. 1991;19(4):484–490.

174. Gianotti L, Meier R, Lobo DN, et al. ESPEN guidelines on parenteral nutrition: pancreas. *Clin Nutr*. 2009;28(4):428–435.

175. Sikkens EC, Cahen DL, Koch AD et al. The prevalence of fat-soluble vitamin deficiencies and a decreased bone mass in patients with chronic pancreatitis. *Pancreatol*. 2013;13(3):238–242.

176. Alnounou M, Munoz SJ. Nutrition concerns of the patient with primary biliary cirrhosis or primary sclerosing cholangitis. *Pract Gastroenterol*. 2006;37:92–100.

177. Balistreri WE, Bezerra JA, Ryckman FC. Biliary atresia and other disorders of the extrahepatic bile ducts. In: Suchy FJ, Sokol RJ, Balistreri WF, eds. *Liver Disease in Children*. New York, NY: Cambridge University Press; 2007:248–61.

178. Sokol RJ, Shepherd RW, Superina R, et al. Screening and outcomes in biliary atresia: summery of a National Institutes of Health workshop. *Hepatol*. 2007;46:566–581.

179. Bakshi N, Singh K. Nutrition assessment in patients undergoing liver transplant. *Indian J. Crit. Care. Med*. 2014;18(10):672–681.

180. Macias-Rosales R, Larrosa-Haro A, Ortiz-Gabriel, Trujillo-Hernandez B. Effectivness of enteral verses oral nutrition with medium-chain triglycride formula to prevent

181. Tang K, Huang LT, Huang YH, Lai CY, et al. Gamma-glutamyl transferase in the diagnosis of biliary atresia. *Acta Paediatr Taiwan*. 2007;48(4):196–200.

182. Azar G, Beneck D, Lane B, Markowitz J, Daum F, Kahn E. Atypical Morphologic Presentation of Biliary Atresia and Value of Serial Liver Biopsies *JPGN*. 2002;34(2): 212–215.

183. Baker A, Amoroso P, Wilson S, et al. Increased resting energy expenditure: a cause of undernutrition in pediatric liver disease. *J Pediatr Gastroenterol Nutr*. 1991;13:318.

184. Sokol RJ, Stall C. Anthropometric evaluation of children with chronic liver disease. *Am J Clin Nutr*. 1990;52:203–208.

185. Delich PC, Siepler JK, Parker P. Liver disease. In: Gottschlich MM, ed. *The ASPEN Nutrition Support Core Curriculum*. Silver Spring, MD: ASPEN; 2007:540–557.

186. Ng VL, Balistreri WF. Treatment options for chronic cholestasis in infancy and childhood. *Curr Treat Options Gastroenterol*. 2005;8(5):419–430.

187. Kleiman R, Warman KY. Nutrition in liver disease. In: Baker SS, Baker RD Jr, Davis AM, eds. *Pediatric Enteral Nutrition*. New York, NY: Chapman and Hall; 1994:261.

188. Pettei MJ, Daftary S, Levine JJ. Essential fatty acid deficiency associated with the use of a medium-chain-triglyceride infant formula in pediatric hepatobiliary disease. *Am J Clin Nutr*. 1991;53:1217–1221.

189. Shneider BL, Magee JC, Bezera JA, Haber D, et al. Efficacy of fat-soluble vitamin supplementation in infants with biliary atresia. *Pediatrics*. 2012;130(3):607–614.

190. Sokol RJ, Butler-Simon N, Conner C, et al. Multicenter trial of d-alpha-tocopheryl poly-ethylene glycol 1000 succinate for treatment of vitamin E deficiency in children with chronic cholestasis. *Gastroenterol*. 1993:104(6):1727–1735.

191. Traber MG, Kayden HJ, Green JB, Green MH. Absorption of water-miscibile forms of vitamin E in a patient with cholestasis and in thoracic duct-cannulated rats. *Am J Clin Nutr*. 1986;44(6):914–923.

192. Sanchez AJ, Aranda-Michel J. Liver disease and osteoporosis. *Nutr Clin Pract*. 2006;21(3):273–278.

193. O'Brien A, Williams R. Nutrition in end-stage liver disease: principles and practice. *Gastroenterol*. 2008;134(6):1729–1740.

194. Mager DR, McGee PL, Furuya KN, Roberts EA. Prevalence of vitamin K deficiency in children with mild to moderate chronic liver disease. *J Pediatr Gastroenterol Nutr*. 2006;42(1): 71–76.

195. Mouzaki M, Ng V, Kamath BM, Selzner N, Pencharz P, Ling SC. Enteral energy and micronutrients in end-stage liver disease. *JPEN*. 2014;38(6):673–681.

196. Organ Procurement and Transplant Network. Liver and intestine. Available at: https://optn.transplant.hrsa.gov/resources/by-organ/liver-intestine/ Accessed November 11, 2017.

197. Carpenter A, Ng V, Chapman K, Ling SC, Mouzaki M. Predictive equations are inaccurate in the estimation of the resting energy expenditure of children with End-Stage Liver Disease. *JPEN*. 2017;41(3):507–511.

198. Laviano A, Cangiano C, Preziosa I, et al. Plasma tryptophan levels and anorexia in liver cirrhosis. *Int J Eat Disord*. 1997;21(2):181–186.

199. Testa R, Franceschini R, Giannini E, et al. Serum leptin levels in patients with viral chronic hepatitis or liver cirrhosis. *J Hepatol*. 2000;33(1):33–37.

malnutrition and growth impairment in infants with biliary atresia. *JPGN*. 2016;62:101–109.

200. Plauth M, Cabre E, Riggio O, et al. ESPEN guidelines on enteral nutrition: liver disease. *Clin Nutr*. 2006;25(2):285–294.

201. Yamanaka-Okumura H, Nakamura T, Takeuchi H, et al. Effect of late evening snack with rice ball on energy metabolism in liver cirrhosis. *Eur J Clin Nutr*. 2006;60(9):1067–1072.

202. Mager DR, Wykes LJ, Roberts EA, Ball RO, Pencharz PB. Branchedchain amino acid needs in children with mild-to-moderate chronic cholestatic liver disease. *J Nutr*. 2006;136(1):133–139.

203. Chin SE, Shepherd RW, Thomas BJ, et al. Nutritional support in children with end-stage liver disease: a randomized crossover trial of a branchedchain amino acid supplement. *Am J Clin Nutr*. 1992;56(1):158–163.

204. Barshes NR, Chang IF, Karpen SJ, Carter BA, Goss JA. Impact of pretransplant growth retardation in pediatric liver transplantation. *J Pediatr Gastroenterol Nutr*. 2006;43(1):89–94.

205. Utterson EC. Shepherd RW, Sokol RJ, et al. Biliary atresia: clinical profiles, risk factors, and outcomes of 755 patients listed for liver transplantation. *J Pediatr*. 2005;147(2):180–185.

206. Stickel F, Inderbitzin D, Candinas D. Role of nutrition in liver transplantation for end-stage chronic liver disease. *Nutr Rev*. 2008;66(1):47–54.

207. Hasse JM, Blue LS, Liepa GU, et al. Early enteral nutrition support in patients undergoing liver transplantation. *JPEN*. 1995;19(6):437–443.

208. Saito T, Mizuta K, Hishikawa S, Kawano Y, Sanada Y, Fujiwara T, et al. Growth curves of pediatric patients with biliary atresia following living donor liver transplantation: factors that influences posttransplantation growth. *Pediatr Transplant* 2007;11:764–770.

209. Moghazy W, Ogura Y, Harada K, Koizumi A, Uemoto S. Can children catch up in growth after living donor liver transplantation? *Liver Transpl*. 2010;16:453–460.

210. Ee LC, Beale K, Fawcett J, Cleghorn GJ. Long-term growth and anthropometry after childhood liver transplantation. *J Pediatr* 2013;163:537–542.

211. Van Mourik ID, Beath SV, Brook GA, et al. Long-term nutritional and neurodevelopmental outcome of liver transplantation in infants aged less than 12 months. *J Pediatr Gastroenterol Nutr*. 2000;30(3):269–275.

212. Viner RM, Forton JT, Cole TJ, Clark IH, Noble-Jamieson G, Barnes ND. Growth of long-term survivors of liver transplantation. *Arch Dis Child*. 1999;80(3):235–240.

213. Gasser RW. Cholestasis and metabolic bone disease—a clinical review. *Wein Med Wochenschr*. 2008;158(19–20):553–557.

214. Okajima H, Shigeno C, Inomata Y, et al. Long-term effects of liver transplantation on bone mineral density in children with end-stage liver disease: a 2-year prospective study. *Liver Transpl*. 2003;9(4):360–364.

215. Ziegler MM. Short bowel syndrome in infancy: Etiology and management. *Clin Perinatol*. 1986;13:167.

216. Duggan CP, Jaksic T. Pediatric Intestinal Failure. *N Engl J Med*. 2017;377:666–675.

217. Goulet O, Ruemmele F, Lacaille F, Colomb V. Irreversible intestinal failure. *J Pediatr Gastroenterol Nutr*. 2004;38:250–269.

218. Mazariegos GV, Squires RH, Sindhi RK. *Curr Gastroenterol Rep*. 2009;11(3):226–233.

219. King KL, Phillips SM. The ins and outs of pediatric short bowel. *Support Line*. 2009;31(3):18–26.

220. Taylor SF, Sokol RJ. Infants with short bowel syndrome. In: Hay WW, ed. *Neonatal Nutrition and Metabolism*. St. Louis, MO: Mosby Year Book; 1991;437.

221. Abad-Sinden A, Sutphen J. Nutritional management of pediatric short bowel syndrome. *Pract Gastro*. 2003;12:28–48.

222. Quiros-Tejeira RE, Ament ME, Reyen L, et al. Long-term parenteral nutrition support and intestinal adaptation in children with Short Bowel Syndrome: a 25- year experience. *J Pediatr*. 2004;145(2):157–163.

223. Beer S, Bunting KD, Canada N, Rich S, Spoede E, Turybury, K, eds. *Texas Children's Hospital Pediatric Nutrition Reference Guide*. Houston, Tx: Texas Children's Hospital; 2016:110.

224. Wessel JJ. Short bowel syndrome. In: Groh-Wargos S, Thompson M, Cox JH, eds. *Nutritional Care for High Risk Newborns*, 3rd ed. Chicago, IL: Precept Press; 2000:469–488.

225. Vanderhoof JA. Short bowel syndrome. In: Walker WA, Watkins JB, eds. *Nutrition in Pediatrics: Basic Science and Clinical Applications*. Hamilton, ON: Decker; 1997:610.

226. Klish WJ. The short gut. In: Walker WA, Watkins JB, eds. *Nutrition in Pediatrics*. Boston: Little, Brown; 1985:561.

227. Fleming CR, George L, Stoner GL, et al. The importance of urinary magnesium values in patients with gut failure. *Mao Clin Proc*. 1996;71:21–24.

228. Farrell MK. Physiologic effects of parenteral nutrition. In: Baker RD Jr, Baker SS, Davis AM, eds. *Pediatric Parenteral Nutrition*. New York, NY: Chapman and Hall;1997:36.

229. Abad-Jorge A, Roman B. Enteral nutrition management in pediatric patients with severe gastrointestinal impairment. *Support Line*. 2007;29(2):3–11.

230. Wong KY, Lan LC, Lin SC, et al. Mucous fistula refeeding in premature neonates with enterostomies. *J Pediatr Gastroenterol Nutr*. 2004;39:43–45.

231. Matarese LE, Costa G, Bond G, et al. Therapeutic efficacy of intestinal and multivisceral transplantation: survival and nutrition outcome. *Nutr Clin Pract*. 2007;22:474–481.

232. Parekh NR, Seidner DL. Advances in enteral feeding of the intestinal failure patient. *Support Line*. 2006;28(3):18–24.

233. Ching YA, Gura K, Modi B, Jaksic T. Pediatric intestinal failure: nutritional and pharmacological approaches. *Nutr Clin Pract*. 2007;22:653–663.

234. Ksiazyk J, Piena M, Kierkus J, Lyszkowska M. Hydrolyzed versus nonhydrolyzed protein diet in short bowel syndrome in children. *J Pediatr Gastroenterol Nutr*. 2002;35(5):615–618.

235. Matarese LE, O'Keefe SJ, Kandil HM, Bond G, Costa G, Abu-Elmagd K. Short bowel syndrome: clinical guidelines for nutrition management. *Nutr Clin Pract*. 2005;20:493–502.

236. Compher CW, Kinosian BP, Rubesin SE, Ratcliffe SJ, Metz DC. Energy absorption is reduced with oleic acid supplements in human short bowel syndrome. *JPEN*. 2009;33:102–108.

237. Vanderhoof JA, Grandjean CJ, Kaufman SS, Burkley KT, Antonson DL. Effect of high percentage medium-chain triglyceride diet on mucosal adaptation following massive bowel resection in rats. *JPEN*. 1984;(8):685–689.

238. Galea MH, Holliday H, Carachi R, et al. Short bowel syndrome: a collective review. *J Pediatr Surg*. 1992;27:592–596.

239. Cooper A, Floyd TF, Ross AJ. Morbidity and mortality of short bowel syndrome acquired in infancy: an update. *J Pediatr Surg*. 1984;19:711–717.

240. Linsheid TR, Tarnowski KJ, Rasnake LK, et al. Behavioral treatment of food refusal in a child with short gut syndrome. *J Pediatr Psych*. 1987;12:451.

241. Nordgaard I, Hansen BS, Mortensen PB. Importance of colonic support for energy absorption as small-bowel failure proceeds. *Am J Clin Nutr*. 1996;64:222–231.

242. Bryne TA, Morrissey TB, Nattakom TV, et al. Growth hormone, glutamine, and a modified diet enhance nutrient absorption in patients with severe short bowel syndrome. *JPEN*. 1995;19:296–302.

243. Rahman N, Hitchcock R. Case report of paediatric oxalate urolithiasis and a review of enteric hyperoxaluria. *J Pediatr Urol.* 2010:6(2):112–116.

244. Chang-Kit L, Filler G, Pike J, Leonard MP. Pediatric urolithiasis: experience at a tertiary care pediatric hospital. *Can Urol Assoc J.* 2008;2(4):381–386.

245. Szkudlarek J, Jeppesen PB, Mortensen PB. Effect of high dose growth hormone with glutamins and no change in diet on intestinal absorption in short bowel patients: a randomized, double blind, crossover, placebo controlled study. *Gut.* 2000;47:199–205.

246. Scolapio JS. Effect of growth hormone, glutamine, and diet on body composition in short bowel syndrome: a randomized, controlled study. *JPEN.* 1999;23:309–312.

247. Jeppesen PB, Hartmann B, Thulesen J, et al. Glucagon-like peptide 2 improves nutrient absorption and nutritional status in short-bowel patients with no colon. *Gastroenterol.* 2001;120:806–815.

248. Chaet MS, Warner BW, Farrell MF. Intensive nutritional support and remedial surgical intervention for extreme short bowel syndrome. *J Pediatr Gastroenterol Nutr.* 1994;19:295–298.

249. Thompson JS. Surgical management of short bowel syndrome. *Surgery.* 1993;113:4–7.

250. Warner BW, Chaet MS. Nontransplant surgical options for management of the short bowel syndrome. *J Pediatr Gastroenterol Nutr.* 1997;17:1–12.

251. Soltys KA, Bond G, Sindhi R, Rassmussen SK, Ganoza A, Khanna A, Mazariegos G. Pediatric Intestinal Transplantation. *Semin Pediatr Surg.* 2017;26:241–249.

252. Grant D, Abu-Elmagd K, Mazariegos G, et al. Intestinal Transplant Registry Report: global activity and trends. *Am J Transplantation.* 2015;15:210–219.

253. Hess RA, Welch KG, Brown PI, Teitelbaum DH. Survival outcomes of pediatric intestinal failure patients: analysis of factors contributing to improved survival over the past two decades. *J Surg Res.* 2011;170:27–31.

254. George D, Bobo K, Dorsey J. Gastrointestinal disease. In: Corkins MR, ed. *The ASPEN Pediatric Nutrition Support Core Curriculum.* Silver Spring, MD: ASPEN; 2015:387–409.

255. Squires RH, Iyer KR. Intestinal failure. In: Corkins MR, ed. *The ASPEN Pediatric Nutrition Support Core Curriculum.* Silver Spring, MD: ASPEN;427–440.

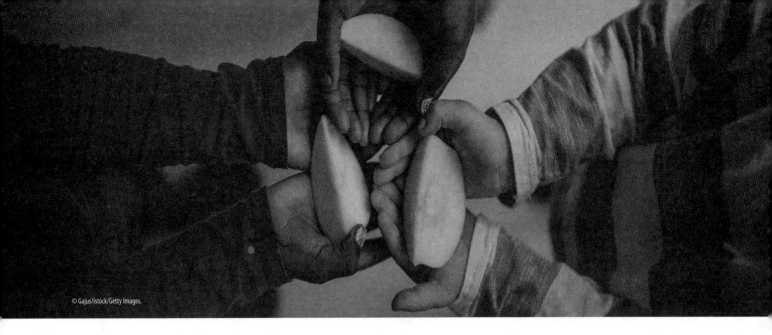

CHAPTER 13
Critical Care

Katelyn Ariagno, Nicolle Quinn and Lori J. Bechard

LEARNING OBJECTIVES

- Identify the key elements of the cascade of critical illness.
- Describe the relationships between critical illness and nutritional status.
- Assess the signs and symptoms of critical illness that impact nutrition interventions and delivery.
- Develop a nutrition care plan for the acute phase of pediatric critical illness.

▶ Introduction

Critically ill children have unique nutritional needs that are often unpredictable, especially by standard nutrition assessment methodologies. While the precise amount and preferred route of nutrition to optimize outcomes remains controversial, a hierarchical approach to planning nutrition prescriptions is widely accepted, and emphasizes the most physiological method that is tolerated in this highly medically complex setting. Despite concerted efforts, nutrition delivery rarely reaches the levels prescribed due to a variety of predictable events, including poor handling of volume, gastrointestinal intolerance, and interruptions for care and procedures. Several studies have described important associations between suboptimal nutrition (inadequate energy, inadequate protein, underweight) and clinical outcomes.[1–3]

Many questions remain unanswered regarding the amounts, route, and timing of specific nutrients. Guidelines have been developed and revised, but evidence to support these primarily consensus driven guidelines is scant. The heterogeneity of the typical population in the **pediatric intensive care unit** (PICU) complicates both the research questions and the clinical trial opportunities to answer these nutritional dilemmas. Novel approaches are needed to advance the science supporting best guidance for patient care.

▶ Anatomy, Physiology, Pathology of Condition

The metabolic response to an acute traumatic event or severe illness may vary by age, medical history, and stage of recovery as well as the type of insult (**FIGURE 13.1**).

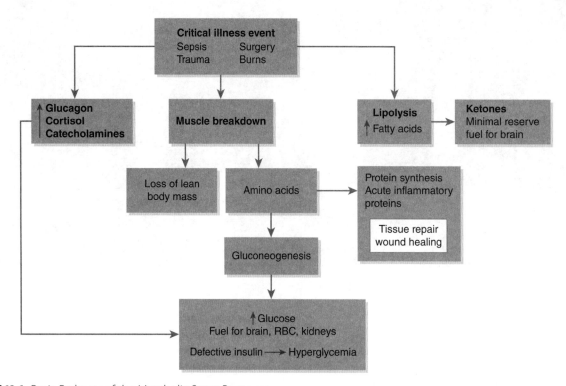

FIGURE 13.1 Basic Pathway of the Metabolic Stress Response

Modified from Sparks EA, Fisher JG, Khan FA, Mehta NM, Jaksic T. The Critically Ill Child. In: Duggan C, Watkins J, Koletzko B, Walker WA, eds. Nutrition in Pediatrics. 5th ed. Shelton, CT: People's Medical Publishing House - USA; 2016:958.[6]

The release of hormones, cytokines, and other proteins obligatory to the inflammatory process result in a net negative protein balance, despite the increased rates of protein turnover during critical illness.[4] The cytokine release related to acute injury also results in a counter-regulatory hormonal response, which includes increases in circulating catecholamines, glucagon, and cortisol. These hormones oppose the effect of insulin, leading to an insulin resistant state with hyperglycemia and accelerated protein catabolism with relatively stable protein rates of protein synthesis.[5] Provision of sufficient protein and energy to meet the increased demand related to the inflammatory response and healing is needed to preserve muscle mass and reduce morbidities associated with loss of lean body mass, though the optimal approach to achieving this goal remains unknown.

Condition Specific Nutrition Screening

Critically ill children are recognized to be at nutrition risk due to the severity of their illness and their likelihood of needing invasive nutrition support intervention. Specific risk screening tools have not been validated for critically ill children to date. In the adult critical care setting, the NUTRIC score (available at: https://www.criticalcarenutrition.com/resources/nutric-score), using a combination of variables including illness severity scores, comorbidities, length of stay, BMI, intake, weight loss and inflammatory markers has been validated against mortality.[7] Whether this score or an adapted variation of it might be valid or reliable in PICUs is as yet unknown.

▶ Nutrition Assessment

Malnutrition continues to be both under-reported and under-recognized, largely due to a lack of a unified definition within the pediatric population. Joosten et al. describe an increased prevalence of acute malnutrition upon admission to the hospital.[8] Awareness of a patient's underlying nutritional status upon admission to the PICU is crucial due to the known rapid nutritional deterioration that can occur following critical illness. Associations between malnutrition in the PICU setting and suboptimal patient-related outcomes, such as an increased infection morbidity, increased length of stay, increased ventilator days, as well as an increased risk of mortality has been described.[1] Nutritional status can be hard to define, however, especially in the absence of accurate weight and height measurements, which are notoriously difficult to obtain in the PICU setting. Over- and under-hydration may obfuscate true weight measurements. Reliance on biomarkers for nutritional assessment may also be futile. In critically ill children, no consistent relationships have been observed between commonly used nutrition-related biomarkers and clinical outcomes.[9]

A complete nutritional assessment is recommended within 48 hours of admission to the PICU.[10] Assessing the critically ill child begins with obtaining the nutritional history of the patient from the caregiver before the acute illness and compiling these data with anthropometric measurements in order to determine a baseline nutritional status. In 2006, the **Centers for Disease Control (CDC)** and the **American Academy of Pediatrics** (AAP) recommended using the **World Health Organization** (WHO) growth charts for children fewer than the age of 2 years and continued use of the CDC growth charts for children ages 2–19 years.[11]

Once a nutritional history is obtained from the caregivers and/or patient, a thorough physical exam of the patient should be completed. The Subjective Global Assessment[12,13] has been used for over 25 years, and was more recently validated in the pediatric population and termed the **subjective global nutrition assessment** (SGNA).[14] SGNA has been used in critically ill children[15] and is composed of two parts: the nutrition focused medical history and the nutrition focused physical exam. The nutritional status is rated; a numerical scoring system is not used. The rating form helps to give an overall sense of the child's nutritional status.[14] When completing the physical exam, it is also important to look at hair quality, nails, the presence of jaundice and overall skin integrity/turgor. The physical exam is a key piece to the nutrition assessment that completes the overall picture of a patient's nutritional status and may not be evident by evaluating the growth curve alone. Key elements of the nutritional assessment of critically ill children are listed in **TABLE 13.1**. Many children admitted to PICUs have chronic illnesses and may have significant medical and nutritional histories that accompany their acute condition.

A complete review of laboratory values is necessary to include in the nutritional assessment in order to evaluate protein stores, hydration status, recent or chronic changes in nutritional status, and a diagnosis of malnutrition (**TABLE 13.2**). A comprehensive understanding of blood chemistries provides information for developing a safe, customized nutrition support regimen.

Attention to medications used both before and during PICU admissions is also important for a thorough interpretation of the side effects and influence on past and present nutritional status (**TABLE 13.3**).

Anthropometry and Body Composition

Evaluating nutritional status by weight and height can be misleading. An assessment of body composition can reveal important information that could form a customized nutritional regimen for an individual patient.[17] However, many techniques used to measure body composition in the pediatric patient are not practical or reliable in the PICU setting. Weight, height, or length and head circumference measurements are necessary to help assess the risk of malnutrition, or the degree of malnutrition already present. Weight can be difficult to obtain if a patient is too unstable to be moved or if medical equipment or devices prohibit an accurate measurement. Alterations in hydration status also influence the accuracy and reliability of weight measurements. Heights or lengths may also be difficult to measure

TABLE 13.1 National Assessment for Critically Ill Children

A. Nutritional and Medical History

Admission anthropometrics (linear growth, weight relative to length/height)

Birth anthropometrics or recent growth history

Changes in body weight

Feeding history, adequacy of dietary intake

Review of usual intake/home nutrition support regimen

Review home medications

Review allergies

Physical activity level, limitations, functional impairment

Persistent gastrointestinal symptoms, changes in appetite

Metabolic stress

B. Nutrition Focused Physical Exam

Loss of subcutaneous fat	Examine the patient's face, arms, chest and buttocks looking for clear bony predominance and lack of fat stores in the face, between the fingers, biceps/triceps, depression between the ribs and flat buttocks.
Muscle wasting	Examine the patient's temple, clavicle, scapula, and extremities. Assess for hypotonia related to medical conditions
Edema	Test for edema by applying pressure near the foot or over the sacrum for 5 seconds and watching if the depression remains after lifting fingers.

in this setting. In patients who are contracted, a knee length can proxy for estimated height using standardized equations.[18] Serial tricep skinfold measurements are an inexpensive, portable way to track estimates of percent body fat, although inter-operator reliability may be low.

TABLE 13.2 Nutritional Monitoring and Associated Limitations During Critical Illness

Methodology	Clinical Indication/Use	Considerations During Critical Illness
Weight	Standard growth reference	Falsely affected by fluid shifts, edema. Difficult to obtain.
Height/Length	Standard growth reference	Difficult to obtain.
Serum Albumin	Visceral protein stores. Useful for long-term nutrition monitoring/assessments.	Falsely low due to immobility, capillary leak syndrome, renal or GI losses, or hepatic disease.
Serum Prealbumin	Visceral protein stores. Useful to detect acute changes in nutritional status	Falsely low during periods of inflammation. Influenced by liver and renal disease.
Hemoglobin	Iron status	Falsely low with phlebotomy, anemia of chronic disease.
Transferrin	Reflects protein depletion	Influenced by liver disease and inflammation.
Serum Retinol-Binding Protein	Vitamin A status. Often low with malnutrition	Falsely low during periods of inflammation. Influenced by liver and renal disease.
Urinary Nitrogen Excretion	Protein metabolism, specifically daily protein losses	Affected by diuretics, renal function, protein intake.

Joosten K, Hulst J. Nutrition Assessment of the Critically Ill Child. In: Goday PS, Mehta NM, eds. Pediatric Critical Care Nutrition: The McGraw-Hill Companies, Inc.; 2015:19-32.[16]

TABLE 13.3 Nutritional Consequences of Medications Used in Critical Illness

Medication	Nutritional Implications
Diuretics	Electrolyte wasting, long term use can affect bone density
Steroids	Hyperglycemia, long term use can affect bone density
Sedation	Can decrease GI motility
Paralytics	Can decrease GI motility
Antibiotics	Can cause diarrhea
Vasoactive Agents	At risk for decreased perfusion to the gut
Immunosuppressants	Hyperglycemia, electrolyte and mineral abnormalities
H_2 receptor antagonists	Hyperglycemia
Chemotherapy	Decreased appetite, nausea/vomiting, mucositis

These measurements may also be influenced by alterations in fluid status, depending on its distribution. **Mid upper arm circumference** (MUAC) is a quick, easy, and inexpensive indicator of malnutrition,[19] although it also can be affected by fluid status. **Bioelectrical impedance analysis** (BIA) is another quick, inexpensive tool to evaluate percent body fat. However, BIA assumes a balanced hydration status, which is often not the case in many critically ill patients. Other methods of body composition assessment not generally applicable in the PICU setting include dual-energy x-ray absorptiometry, stable isotopes, and air displacement plethysmography.[17]

Energy Expenditure and Critical Illness

The metabolic state following critical illness is often a dynamic process. Hypermetabolism may occur, depending on the level of stress or degree of inflammation; however, current treatment therapies including chemical paralysis, continuous sedation, and mechanical ventilator support may depress patients' energy demands and result in hypometabolism.

Accurate assessment of the metabolic state in the critically ill child remains challenging. Equations for estimating resting energy expenditure in critically ill children are known to be inaccurate.[19-22] Using stress factors is highly variable, resulting in both underfeeding and overfeeding.[20] Hardy et al. demonstrated that some of the more common predictive energy equations used in pediatric critical illness measured within 10% of the measured energy expenditure via **indirect calorimetry** (IC) only 45% of the time.[23] In a later study, Mehta et al. further demonstrated how inaccurate these equations were when compared with values obtained by IC.[24] In this single center study, greater than 50% of the PICU patients were hypometabolic compared with estimated energy expenditure by standard equations.[24] Average weekly cumulative energy balance was estimated to be greater than 2000 calories in excess of measured energy expenditure, if energy prescriptions were not altered following the IC measurement.[24] In a quality improvement initiative, Ladd et al conducted 35 ICs in 24 patients which led to adjustments in most of their energy prescriptions (47% were decreased and 22% were increased), underscoring the clinical value of indirect calorimetry in the PICU.[25] If IC is not available or contraindicated, then clinicians should use an appropriate predictive energy equation in order to estimate energy expenditure, with cautious consideration to the need for a stress factor to calculate an overall energy goal. Both underfeeding and overfeeding may be particularly deleterious to critically ill children (**TABLE 13.4**).

Indirect Calorimetry

IC remains the gold standard when striving to accurately determine a patient's energy expenditure.[10] IC should be utilized to measure **resting energy expenditure** (REE) in the PICU and inform energy goals of the nutrition regimen.

IC is a non-invasive procedure that can be performed on ventilated and non-ventilated PICU patients. Results provide valuable data to guide nutrition prescriptions throughout a patient's illness and recovery process.

The energy expenditure of a critically ill child does not remain constant; changes from hypometabolism to hypermetabolism may occur throughout a critical illness depending on the course of the individual patient.[27] The calorimeter can capture the REE at that moment by measuring **oxygen consumed** (VO_2) with **carbon dioxide exhaled** (VCO_2); results are entered into the Weir equation in order to determine the resting energy equation.

$$\text{Weir equation} = (3.94 \times VO_2) + (1.06 \times VCO_2) - (2.17 \times UUN)$$

The respiratory quotient is calculated as the ratio of the VCO_2 to VO_2, and can be used to confirm the clinical suspicion of overfeeding or underfeeding. A high RQ value (>1.0) is suggestive of overfeeding since it indicates a greater production of CO_2 than consumption of O_2. When long chain fat is oxidized, less CO_2 is utilized and the ratio is lower. The ideal RQ range indicating a mixed substrate is being used for energy is 0.7–1.0.[28] IC can be useful to capture measured REE at a critical time point that may fluctuate throughout a patient's PICU course. Serial IC measurements are beneficial in patients suspected to have ebbs and flows in their metabolic response, e.g. trauma patients, patients with large wounds or pressure ulcers, burn patients, and patients requiring multiple surgical interventions. IC measurements are typically contraindicated due to extreme inaccuracy in patients on **extracorporeal membrane oxygenation therapy** (ECMO), high frequency ventilation, patients who have a large ventilatory leak, the presence of a chest tube, or non-invasive oxygen support.

Resources to obtain IC measurements are often limited in PICUs due to the cost of equipment and labor intensity of the testing procedure. Therefore, it is useful to determine those patients in the PICU who are at the greatest risk for metabolic derangements and who might benefit the most from IC, as shown in **TABLE 13.5**.[20]

Protein Requirements

Energy intake is just one component of the nutrition intervention. Questions are now being raised about the association of protein intake, independent of energy intake, with patient-related outcomes in the critical care population. Inadequate protein intake remains widespread among PICUs worldwide, with patients receiving <50% of prescribed protein during the first 10 days of their PICU course.[2] While assessing the nitrogen balance may allow a clinician to more precisely estimate protein requirements, its feasibility for routine use at the bedside remains challenging. Loss of lean body mass related to protein breakdown can result in longer ventilation days and a higher risk of mortality.[29] In a multicenter, prospective cohort study of PICU patients, higher enteral protein adequacy was associated with lower 60-day mortality, with a significant dose-response independent of energy intake.[3] In a

TABLE 13.4 Consequences of Inaccurate Estimates of Energy Expenditure

Underfeeding	Overfeeding
Delayed wound healing	Hyperglycemia
Increased risk of infection	Hypertriglyceridemia
Delayed neurodevelopment	Hepatic steatosis
Increased mortality risk	Respiratory failure

Modified from Mehta NM, Duggan CP. Nutritional deficiencies during critical illness. *Pediatr Clin North Am.* 2009;56:1143–60.[26]

TABLE 13.5 Targeted Indirect Calorimetry During Pediatric Critical Illness

Underweight (body mass index [BMI] <5th percentile for age), at risk of overweight (BMI >85th percentile for age), or overweight (BMI >95th percentile for age)

Greater than 10% weight gain or loss during PICU stay

Failure to consistently meet prescribed caloric goals

Failure to wean or escalation in respiratory support

Need for muscle relaxants for >7 days

Neurologic trauma (traumatic, hypoxic, and/or ischemia) with evidence of dysautonomia

Oncologic diagnoses (including stem cell or bone marrow transplantation)

Need for mechanical ventilator support >7 days

Suspicion of severe hypermetabolism (status epilepticus, hyperthermia, systemic inflammatory response syndrome, dysautonomic storms) or hypometabolism (hypothermia, hypothyroidism, pentobarbital or midazolam coma)

Intensive care unit length of stay > 4 weeks

Mehta NM, Bechard LJ, Leavitt K, Duggan C. Cumulative energy imbalance in the pediatric intensive care unit: role of targeted indirect calorimetry. *J Parent Enteral Nutr.* 2009;33:336-44.[20]

systematic review of studies that included mechanically ventilated PICU patients, a minimum protein intake of 1.5 gm/kg/day and a minimum energy intake of 54 kcal/kg/day was associated with a positive nitrogen balance.[30] Certain pediatric patient populations and conditions may place patients at high risk for increased protein losses. Young infants and patients with burn injuries, increased losses with thoracic or peritoneal drains, severe wounds, or high stool or ostomy output should be evaluated in order to determine if protein intake goals exceeding 1.5 gm/kg/day could be warranted. In a randomized, controlled trial that included infants with viral bronchiolitis, anabolism was demonstrated with protein supplementation.[31] Based on these findings, dietitians should be cautious when using standard protein recommendations for healthy children, since providing these lower values might accelerate the negative nitrogen balance already likely to occur following critical illness.

During periods of critical illness, many challenges exist that limit the ability to deliver prescribed protein goals, despite the timely initiation of nutrition support. Organ dysfunction, such as acute kidney injury, and frequent interruptions to enteral feedings may result in inadequate protein delivery.[32] Additionally, pediatric enteral formulas may not meet recommended protein goals in the volumes needed for patients who are fluid restricted. In a single center, prospective cohort study, the feasibility of enteral protein supplementation was evaluated. In this study, using protein supplementation in patients receiving early enteral nutrition support led to a greater likelihood of meeting protein intake goals within 4 days. No changes in enteral tolerance were observed with the supplementation.[33]

The non-protein calorie to nitrogen ratio has been deliberated in the context of nutrition support in critical illness. This concept may be a way to ensure that protein intake is spared for lean body mass preservation and tissue recovery; however, an ideal ratio in children is unknown, and there is a concern that overfeeding may occur.[32] Future research is needed to help guide dietitians determine optimal protein amounts for the critically ill child.

Immunonutrition

Providing specific micronutrient blends has been investigated to determine if they might have any effect on the inflammatory response during critical illness. In the critically ill adult population, randomized, controlled trials have been conducted examining the effects of parenteral and enteral supplementation of antioxidant vitamins, trace elements, and varying combinations of macronutrients on patient-related outcomes. Specific nutrients under investigation have included glutamine, vitamins C and E, omega-3 fatty acids, selenium, and zinc.[34–36] These studies have had varying results, with some even suggesting increased harm, leaving clinicians with more questions than answers. It also remains unclear how to appropriately monitor the serum levels of these antioxidants during periods of critical illness or metabolic stress, since levels can be falsely impacted by undesired fluid distribution, unanticipated losses, altered protein binding, as well as inconsistent provision of nutrient intake, both before admission and during hospitalization. The heterogeneity of the PICU population also makes it challenging to identify a specific supplementation that can be targeted to meet the needs of an individual critically ill child.[37,38] Limited data is available on the use of micronutrient supplementation or specialized immune enhancing diets during pediatric critical illness.

▶ Nutrition Diagnosis

The PICU setting has a highly heterogeneous population of patients. As a result, nutrition diagnoses may vary widely from patient to patient depending on their

TABLE 13.6 Common Nutrition Diagnoses for the Critically Ill Child

Problem (P)		Etiology (E)		Signs/Symptoms (S)
Inadequate oral intake	*related to*	critical illness	*as evidenced by*	nothing by mouth (NPO) diet order, requiring mechanical ventilator support
Inadequate enteral nutrition infusion	*related to*	hemodynamic instability	*as evidenced by*	requiring ongoing fluid resuscitation and escalation of vasoactive agents
Enteral nutrition composition inconsistent with needs	*related to*	GI intolerance	*as evidenced by*	episodes of persistent vomiting and diarrhea
Inadequate parenteral nutrition infusion	*related to*	lack of IV access	*as evidenced by*	presence of only one peripheral IV that is prioritized for necessary medications
Parenteral nutrition composition inconsistent with needs	*related to*	fluid restriction	*as evidenced by*	prescribed parenteral solution only able to meet 50% of estimated energy and protein goals determined by the dietitian

underlying disease or condition as well as their nutritional status. The nutrition diagnosis may also change during a PICU course. For example, a patient initially admitted to the PICU who is acutely ill and hemodynamically unstable will have a different nutrition diagnosis than the same patient who is now extubated and being weaned off of increased support.

The nutrition diagnosis in a critically ill child should address the most acute nutrition problem targeted by the nutrition intervention while the patient is in the PICU. More commonly, the dietitian's immediate challenge is how to optimize energy and protein intake within the confines of fluid allotment and tolerance in this high-risk group of patients. Typically, nutrition support is provided through the enteral or parenteral route. See **TABLE 13.6.**

▶ Nutrition Intervention

Enteral nutrition (EN) and **parenteral nutrition** (PN) are the primary nutrition interventions used to deliver nutrients to a critically ill child. As discussed earlier, the metabolic stress response to critical illness places this vulnerable population at risk for loss of lean body mass. Hence, it is crucial for the dietitian to consider the optimal timing, appropriate route(s), as well as the appropriate amount of nutrition support to prescribe, in order to optimize energy and protein intake and attempt to attenuate negative nitrogen balance.

Enteral Nutrition

There are many benefits to EN compared with PN, often making it the preferred route when choosing a mode of nutrition support in the PICU setting. Considerations should be made for early EN, defined as 24–48 hours after admission to the PICU in eligible critically ill children.[10] Studies have investigated both the timing and route of nutrition support, in relation to patient-related outcomes.[9] In adults with critical illness, EN has been associated with lower infection morbidity and reduced length of stay;[39,40] however, despite the dietitian's best efforts in recommending and prescribing EN, many barriers exist that prevent adequate nutrient delivery via the enteral route. The nature of the PICU environment often leads to many delays in initiating EN. Furthermore, frequent interruptions of feedings commonly occur due to unplanned procedures or limitations in securing or maintaining enteral access. Also, the lack of a unified definition of feeding intolerance in the PICU patient has been shown to impede consistent nutrient delivery. In a prospective study examining bedside practices with EN, many of the identified barriers to full EN were avoidable.[41] Nutrition algorithms are a standardized method to improve nutrient delivery in the critical care setting by reducing or eliminating these avoidable barriers. Two single center studies; one retrospective[42] and one prospective,[43] followed nutrition support practices after instituting an EN algorithm. They reported substantial improvements in nutrient delivery by initiating EN early, while limiting the amount of avoidable barriers associated with intolerance as well as the general use of PN. Despite these findings, using nutrition algorithms in the PICU setting remain limited. In a review from an international multicenter cohort study in PICUs, only 9 out of 31 PICUs had established nutrition algorithms.[44]

Suboptimal EN delivery in the PICU has been associated with poor clinical outcomes, including a greater number of days on mechanical ventilation, an increased risk of infection, and mortality. Critically ill children who received at least 33–66% of prescribed energy goals during their PICU course had a reduced risk for mortality.[2,45,46]

Myths around avoiding enteral feeding in critically ill children on vasoactive support still exist. However, a recent study reported that neither severe enteral intolerance nor mortality increased when EN was received alongside vasoactive agents.[47] It is imperative for the PICU medical team and dietitian to consider each patient's hemodynamic status individually when deciding the route for nutrition support prescription.

Parenteral Nutrition

PN support should be considered in a critically ill child for whom EN is contraindicated or in patients who have failed to advance to adequate EN in order to meet appropriate energy and protein goals. A randomized controlled trial (PEPaNIC) was aimed at addressing the timing of supplemental PN in critically ill children. Patients were randomized to either "early" PN (PICU day 1) or "late" PN (PICU day 8). Results showed that patients in the late PN group had a lower number of new infections and a shorter PICU length of stay than those in the early PN group.[48] While a randomized controlled trial in the pediatric critical care population is exciting, this study had many limitations for which caution should be exercised regarding generalization to all critically ill children.[49] General guidelines suggest avoiding PN support within the first 24 hours of PICU admission. Critically ill children who are already assessed with malnutrition or who have a condition that places them at risk for rapid nutritional deterioration may incur harm from delaying PN support until PICU day 8.[10] Further studies are needed to be able to better guide dietitians in knowing the optimal timing for initiation of PN support, as well as the threshold of EN adequacy at which to provide PN as a supplement to EN.

▶ Nutrition Monitoring and Evaluation

Monitoring and evaluating the nutrition intervention in a critically ill child is a dynamic process. Many of the more common biomarkers and anthropometric data

dietitians rely on to assess if the nutrition intervention is effective are often unreliable during periods of critical illness. Edema, fluid shifts, lines, and tubes can affect the accuracy and ability to trend anthropometrics. Inflammation may affect the accuracy of biochemical data and it has been recommended that acute phase proteins be followed in combination with the monitoring of visceral proteins in order to appreciate when the acute-phase response following critical illness is subsiding and nutrient provision can be further optimized.[50]

Monitoring Enteral and Parenteral Intake

Nutritional intake adequacy is a fundamental component of nutrition care that the dietitian must carefully monitor in a critically ill child in the PICU. Adequacy of intake is based on what the patient actually received at the bedside compared with the prescribed values.

Adequacy of energy and protein intake should be assessed frequently during the acute period of critical illness in order to determine if significant cumulative deficits exist. This allows for prompt nutrition interventions to be adjusted by the dietitian and implemented in consultation with the PICU medical team. Indirect calorimetry studies, if locally available, should be conducted more than once during a critically ill child's PICU course. The metabolic stress response described earlier in this chapter is a dynamic process that supports the need for close monitoring of nutrition support and ongoing re-evaluation by the entire multidisciplinary PICU team.

Monitoring Anthropometric Measurements

Anthropometric measurements, if accurate, are considered to be the gold standard in determining if a child is receiving adequate energy and protein. These measurements include weights, lengths or heights, head circumferences (for children under 2 years of age), MUAC, and **triceps skinfold** (TSF).

As noted, many of the anthropometric measurements and biochemical data available may be falsely impacted by a patient's clinical condition or medical treatment, thus it is essential to consider each critically ill child individually. Younger children and infants, as well as patients assessed with malnutrition, may warrant daily monitoring of certain anthropometric measurements.

Monitoring Biochemical Data and Nutrition Focused Physical Findings

The dietitian and the PICU interdisciplinary team should monitor the tolerance to delivery of EN and PN. Daily intake totals compared with output totals is an easy yet effective way to follow along with weights for assessing overall hydration status. Fluid balance and biochemical data trends, along with anthropometric data, can help guide nutrition prescriptions. In patients receiving EN, vigilant monitoring for signs of enteral intolerance is important in the PICU. Patients with signs or symptoms of emesis or diarrhea, as well as increases in abdominal girths, may warrant a trial on a different formula, transition to post-pyloric feeds (from gastric), or a slower feeding advancement plan. In patients receiving PN, serum chemistries, including glucose, liver function tests, and triglycerides should be monitored regularly. Urinary output, losses from stool or ostomy(ies), chest tube losses, and any gastric output should also be monitored closely in patients receiving nutrition support. Frequency should be based on current individual clinical status as well as baseline nutritional status and goals.

▶ Conclusion

Nutrition intervention in the critically ill pediatric patient is recognized as a necessary and timely piece of their medical treatment. In this chapter, the nutritional assessment, nutrition intervention, and methods of evaluation are reviewed as well as the challenges that accompany each process. The risk of over and under feeding can be harmful and have impacts on the outcomes of a patient's stay in the PICU including potentially increasing the days of ventilation, a higher risk of infection and malnutrition, and ultimately increasing the risk of mortality. The authors have provided tools that best determine energy and protein needs, provide optimal nutrition support, and recommend methods to monitor nutritional status throughout a patient's critical illness. Two case studies are presented that incorporate key points addressed in the preceding pages.

🔍 CASE STUDIES

Critical Care Case #1

Four-year-old female with **acute lymphoblastic leukemia** (ALL), admitted to the PICU with concerns for septic shock following chemotherapy. She had been admitted to the Oncology floor 8 days prior for conditioning and treatment. Oral intake had significantly declined due to worsening mucositis, and more acutely developed episodes of vomiting and diarrhea. Upon transfer to the PICU, the patient was initiated on 2 vasoactive agents given her hemodynamic instability. She is febrile and hypotensive.

Diet Rx: NPO, receiving dextrose-containing intravenous fluids

Hospital Admission Anthropometrics

Weight:	14 kg	WAZ: -0.99
Height:	98 cm	HAZ: -0.64
Body Mass Index (BMI):	14.5 kg/m²	BMIZ: -0.65
PICU admission weight:	13.2 kg	
Estimated resting energy requirement:	55 kcal/kg/d (Schofield Weight-Height Equation)	
Recommended protein intake (RDA):	0.95 gm protein/kg/d	
Recommended protein intake (ASPEN):	1.5-2 gm protein/kg/d	
Fluid:	1200 ml/d	

Nutrition Diagnosis

Inadequate oral intake related to GI intolerance as evidenced by persistent vomiting and diarrhea.

Discussion

This patient could also be assessed with acute malnutrition given her weight loss; however, the higher priority nutrition problem is inadequate intake for 1 week, which is what the dietitian is prioritizing as her initial nutrition intervention. Also, this patient is receiving vasoactive agent therapy. As discussed earlier in this chapter, studies have supported the consideration of EN support while on vasoactive agents; however, when considering this patient's GI symptoms, the assessment would recommend against choosing EN over PN at this time.

Nutrition Intervention

Parenteral nutrition support to meet 100% of the initial energy and protein goals; 55 kcal/kg/d and 1.5 gm protein/kg/d. Enteral nutrition vs. oral intake should be considered when GI symptoms resolve. PN can be weaned off once oral/enteral nutrition tolerance is well established and meeting >50–75% of energy needs.

Nutrition Monitoring and Evaluation

Biochemical data while on PN support; specifically, daily chemistries during PN advancement in order to ensure stability and weekly gastrointestinal profile labs (liver function tests, total and direct bilirubin) to ensure overall tolerance to

PN support. Fluid balance and daily weights should also be monitored to ensure the patient is not fluid overloaded or potentially becoming dehydrated. Depending on the accuracy of weights, it could be beneficial to also trend MUAC and TSF in this patient. The nutrition focused physical exam, assessment of skin status, abdominal exam, and/or the presence of edema is crucial in this high-risk patient population.

Discussion Questions

1. Would you consider the use of a "stress factor" with the estimated resting energy expenditure obtained via predictive energy equation?
2. How would you manage advancement of PN support if the patient is at risk for refeeding syndrome and what monitoring aspects would you closely follow?
3. What micronutrients might this patient be deficient in given her clinical presentation?
4. Would the presence of inflammation make you consider waiting to assess these micronutrient levels?

Critical Care Case #2

Fourteen-year-old male with obesity, who presents to the PICU with respiratory failure secondary to **acute respiratory distress syndrome** (ARDS). Patient chemically paralyzed, sedated, and mechanically ventilated. Significant concerns for fluid overload; attempting diuresis. Patient with elevated inflammatory markers (C-reactive protein).

Current Diet Rx: NPO, receiving dextrose-containing intravenous fluids

Admitting PICU Anthropometrics

Weight:	77 kg	WAZ:	1.9
Height:	150 cm	HAZ:	-1.68
Body Mass Index (BMI):	34.2 kg/m^2	BMIZ:	2.41
Estimated resting energy expenditure:	1972 kcals/d (Schofield Weight-Height Equation)		
Recommended protein intake (RDA):	0.85 gm protein/kg/d		
Recommended protein intake (ASPEN):	1.5 gm protein/kg/d		
Fluid:	2640 ml/d		

Nutrition Diagnosis

Inadequate oral intake related to critical illness as evidenced by NPO status while mechanically ventilated.

Discussion

Standard energy estimation equations for children have been found to be highly inaccurate in the PICU setting. Indirect calorimetry, specifically in the pediatric obese population, is strongly recommended to measure energy expenditure. Indirect calorimetry would be beneficial in this scenario to more precisely target energy requirements with the current fluid restriction. Fluid restriction is common in the PICU, therefore avoiding overfeeding and prescribing energy based on IC results may facilitate achieving energy and protein goals with less volume, depending on the results. If indirect calorimetry is not available, use of additional stress factors with energy estimation equations should be cautioned against, given the risk of overfeeding.

Nutrition Intervention

Early enteral nutrition should be initiated and advanced to meet 100% of measured energy expenditure by IC. Consider protein supplementation if the patient is found to be hypometabolic and formula alone does not meet desired protein intake goals.

Nutrition Monitoring and Evaluation

Enteral tolerance with advancement of enteral feeds, along with urinary and stool output trends should be monitored daily. If the patient is fed gastric (vs. post-pyloric), trend abdominal girths during advancement of feeds since the patient is chemically paralyzed. Anthropometrics are more challenging to obtain in an obese patient; however, would aim to trend weights at least weekly. If feasible, regular indirect calorimetry measurements would be helpful to complete every 3–5 days to ensure adequacy of the nutrition support provided. During diuresis, chemistries should be monitored at least daily and it may also be helpful to trend inflammatory markers weekly.

Discussion Questions

1. What weight is recommended to use when determining energy and protein goals?
2. What micronutrient deficiencies might you be concerned about in the pediatric obese population?
3. Are there other alternative body composition measurements to consider obtaining in the critically ill pediatric obese patient?

Review Questions

1. Discuss some positive effects of initiating early enteral nutrition in critical care patients.

2. True or False? The hormones that are released during critical illness are called cytokines.

3. List three risk factors in underfeeding a critically ill pediatric patient.

4. For the critically ill patient, why is it important to monitor the following anthropometric measurements in children under 18 months?
   A. Weight
   B. Length/height
   C. Mid-upper arm circumference
   D. Head circumference

5. True or False? The risks associated with overfeeding include weight gain, carbon dioxide burden, and hepatic steatosis.

6. What is the gold standard for assessing energy expenditure in a critically ill pediatric patient?

References

1. Bechard LJ, Duggan C, Touger-Decker R, et al. Nutritional status based on Body Mass Index is associated with morbidity and mortality in mechanically ventilated critically ill children in the PICU. *Crit Care Med*. 2016;44:1530–1537.

2. Mehta NM, Bechard LJ, Cahill N, et al. Nutritional practices and their relationship to clinical outcomes in critically ill children—an international multicenter cohort study. *Crit Care Med* 2012;40:2204–2211.

3. Mehta NM, Bechard LJ, Zurakowski D, Duggan CP, Heyland DK. Adequate enteral protein intake is inversely associated with 60-d mortality in critically ill children: a multicenter, prospective, cohort study. *Am J Clin Nutr*. 2015;102:199–206.

4. Sparks EA, Fisher JG, Khan FA, Mehta NM, Jaksic T. The critically ill child. In: Duggan C, Watkins J, Koletzko B, Walker WA, eds. *Nutrition in Pediatrics*. 5th ed. Shelton, CT: People's Medical Publishing House - USA; 2016:958.

5. Chwals WJ. The acute metabolic response to injury. In: Goday PS, Mehta NM, eds. *Pediatric Critical Care Nutrition*. New York, NY: McGraw Hill Education Medical; 2015.

6. Sparks EA, Fisher JG, Khan FA, Mehta NM, Jaksic T. The Critically Ill Child. In: Duggan C, Watkins J, Koletzko B, Walker WA, eds. *Nutrition in Pediatrics*. 5th ed. Shelton, CT: People's Medical Publishing House - USA; 2016:958.

7. Heyland DK, Dhaliwal R, Jiang X, Day AG. Identifying critically ill patients who benefit the most from nutrition therapy: the development and initial validation of a novel risk assessment tool. *Crit Care*. 2011;15:R268.

8. Joosten KF, Hulst JM. Prevalence of malnutrition in pediatric hospital patients. Curr *Opin Pediatr*. 2008;20:590–596.

9. Ong C, Han WM, Wong JJ, Lee JH. Nutrition biomarkers and clinical outcomes in critically ill children: A critical appraisal of the literature. *Clin Nutr*. 2014;33:191–197.

10. Mehta NM, Skillman HE, Irving SY, et al. Guidelines for the provision and assessment of nutrition support therapy in the Pediatric Critically Ill Patient: Society of Critical Care Medicine and American Society for Parenteral and Enteral Nutrition. *Pediatr Crit Care Med*. 2017;18:675–715.

11. Grummer-Strawn LM, Reinold C, Krebs NF, Centers for Disease C, Prevention. Use of World Health Organization and CDC growth charts for children aged 0-59 months in the United States. *MMWR Recomm Rep*. 2010;59:1–15.

12. Baker JP, Detsky AS, Wesson DE, et al. Nutritional assessment: a comparison of clinical judgement and objective measurements. *N Engl J Med*. 1982;306:969–72.

13. Detsky AS, Smalley PS, Chang J. The rational clinical examination. Is this patient malnourished? *JAMA*. 1994;271:54–58.

14. Secker DJ, Jeejeebhoy KN. Subjective global nutritional assessment for children. *Am J Clin Nutr*. 2007;85:1083–1089.

15. Vermilyea S, Slicker J, El-Chammas K, et al. Subjective global nutritional assessment in critically ill children. *JPEN*. 2013;37:659–666.

16. Joosten K, Hulst J. Nutrition Assessment of the Critically Ill Child. In: Goday PS, Mehta NM, eds. Pediatric Critical Care Nutrition: The McGraw-Hill Companies, Inc.; 2015:19-32.

17. Ellis KJ. Body composition and growth. In: Duggan C, Watkins J, Koletzko B, Walker WA, eds. *Nutrition in Pediatrics*. 5th ed. Shelton, CT: People's Medical Publishing House - USA; 2016:37–54.

18. Stevenson RD. Use of segmental measures to estimate stature in children with cerebral palsy. *Arch Pediatr Adolesc Med*. 1995;149:658–662.

19. Rolland-Cachera MF, Brambilla P, Manzoni P, et al. Body composition assessed on the basis of arm circumference and triceps skinfold thickness: a new index validated in children by magnetic resonance imaging. *Am J Clin Nutr*. 1997;65:1709–1713.

20. Mehta NM, Bechard LJ, Leavitt K, Duggan C. Cumulative energy imbalance in the pediatric intensive care unit: role of targeted indirect calorimetry. *J Parent Enteral Nutr*. 2009;33:336–344.

21. Framson CM, LeLeiko NS, Dallal GE, Roubenoff R, Snelling LK, Dwyer JT. Energy expenditure in critically ill children. *Pediatr Critical Care Med*. 2007;8:264–267.

22. Jotterand Chaparro C, Taffe P, Moullet C, et al. Performance of predictive equations specifically developed to estimate resting energy expenditure in ventilated critically ill children. *J Pediatr*. 2017;184:220–226.e5.

23. Hardy CM, Dwyer J, Snelling LK, Dallal GE, Adelson JW. Pitfalls in predicting resting energy requirements in critically ill children: a comparison of predictive methods to indirect calorimetry. *Nutr Clin Pract.* 2002;17:182–189.

24. Mehta NM, Bechard LJ, Dolan M, Ariagno K, Jiang H, Duggan C. Energy imbalance and the risk of overfeeding in critically ill children. *Pediatr Critical Care Med.* 2011;12:398–405.

25. Ladd AK, Skillman HE, Haemer MA, Mourani PM. Preventing underfeeding and overfeeding: a clinician's guide to the acquisition and implementation of indirect calorimetry. *Nutr Clin Pract.* 2017:884533617710214.

26. Mehta NM, Duggan CP. Nutritional deficiencies during critical illness. *Pediatr Clin North Am.* 2009;56:1143–60.

27. Sion-Sarid R, Cohen J, Houri Z, Singer P. Indirect calorimetry: a guide for optimizing nutritional support in the critically ill child. *Nutrition.* 2013;29:1094–1099.

28. Ariagno K, Duggan C. Nutritional assessment in sick or hospitalized children. In: Sonneville K, Duggan C, eds. *Manual of Pediatric Nutrition.* 5th ed. Shelton, CT: People's Medical Publishing House- USA; 2014:146–157.

29. Cohen S, Nathan JA, Goldberg AL. Muscle wasting in disease: molecular mechanisms and promising therapies. *Nat Rev Drug Discov.* 2015;14:58–74.

30. Bechard LJ, Parrott JS, Mehta NM. Systematic review of the influence of energy and protein intake on protein balance in critically ill children. *J Pediatr.* 2012;161: 333–339 e1.

31. de Betue CT, van Waardenburg DA, Deutz NE, et al. Increased protein-energy intake promotes anabolism in critically ill infants with viral bronchiolitis: a double-blind randomised controlled trial. *Arch Dis Child.* 2011;96: 817–822.

32. Coss-Bu JA, Hamilton-Reeves J, Patel JJ, Morris CR, Hurt RT. Protein requirements of the critically ill pediatric patient. *Nutr Clin Pract.* 2017;32:128S–141S.

33. Moreno YMF, Hauschild DB, Martins MD, Bechard LJ, Mehta NM. Feasibility of enteral protein supplementation in critically ill children. *JPEN.* 2018;42:61–70.

34. Andrews PJ, Avenell A, Noble DW, et al. Randomised trial of glutamine, selenium, or both, to supplement parenteral nutrition for critically ill patients. *BMJ.* 2011;342:d1542.

35. Heyland D, Muscedere J, Wischmeyer PE, et al. A randomized trial of glutamine and antioxidants in critically ill patients. *N Engl J Med.* 2013;368:1489–1497.

36. van Zanten AR, Sztark F, Kaisers UX, et al. High-protein enteral nutrition enriched with immune-modulating nutrients vs standard high-protein enteral nutrition and nosocomial infections in the ICU: a randomized clinical trial. *JAMA.* 2014;312:514–524.

37. Koekkoek WA, van Zanten AR. Antioxidant vitamins and trace elements in critical illness. *Nutr Clin Pract.* 2016;31:457–474.

38. Carcillo JA, Dean JM, Holubkov R, et al. The randomized comparative pediatric critical illness stress-induced immune suppression (CRISIS) prevention trial. *Pediatr Crit Care Med.* 2012;13:165–173.

39. Gramlich L, Kichian K, Pinilla J, Rodych NJ, Dhaliwal R, Heyland DK. Does enteral nutrition compared to parenteral nutrition result in better outcomes in critically ill adult patients? A systematic review of the literature. *Nutrition.* 2004;20:843–848.

40. Simpson F, Doig GS. Parenteral vs. enteral nutrition in the critically ill patient: a meta-analysis of trials using the intention to treat principle. *Intensive Care Med.* 2005;31:12–23.

41. Mehta NM, McAleer D, Hamilton S, et al. Challenges to optimal enteral nutrition in a multidisciplinary pediatric intensive care unit. *JPEN.* 2010;34:38–45.

42. Petrillo-Albarano T, Pettignano R, Asfaw M, Easley K. Use of a feeding protocol to improve nutritional support through early, aggressive, enteral nutrition in the pediatric intensive care unit. *Pediatr Crit Care Med.* 2006;7:340–344.

43. Hamilton S, McAleer DM, Ariagno K, et al. A stepwise enteral nutrition algorithm for critically ill children helps achieve nutrient delivery goals. *Pediatr Crit Care Med.* 2014;15:583–589.

44. Martinez EE, Bechard LJ, Mehta NM. Nutrition algorithms and bedside nutrient delivery practices in pediatric intensive care units: an international multicenter cohort study. *Nutr Clin Pract.* 2014;29:360–367.

45. de Betue CT, van Steenselen WN, Hulst JM, et al. Achieving energy goals at day 4 after admission in critically ill children; predictive for outcome? *Clin Nutr.* 2015;34:115–122.

46. Mikhailov TA, Kuhn EM, Manzi J, et al. Early enteral nutrition is associated with lower mortality in critically ill children. *JPEN.* 2014;38:459–466.

47. Panchal AK, Manzi J, Connolly S, et al. Safety of enteral feedings in critically ill children Receiving vasoactive agents. *JPEN.* 2016;40:236–241.

48. Fivez T, Kerklaan D, Mesotten D, et al. Early versus late Parenteral Nutrition in critically ill children. *N Engl J Med.* 2016;374:1111–1122.

49. Koletzko B, Goulet O, Jochum F, Shamir R. Use of Parenteral Nutrition in the pediatric ICU: should we panic because of PEPaNIC? *Curr Opin Clin Nutr Metab Care.* 2017;20:201–203.

50. Chwals WJ. Metabolism and nutritional frontiers in pediatric surgical patients. *Surg Clin North Am.* 1992;72: 1237–1266.

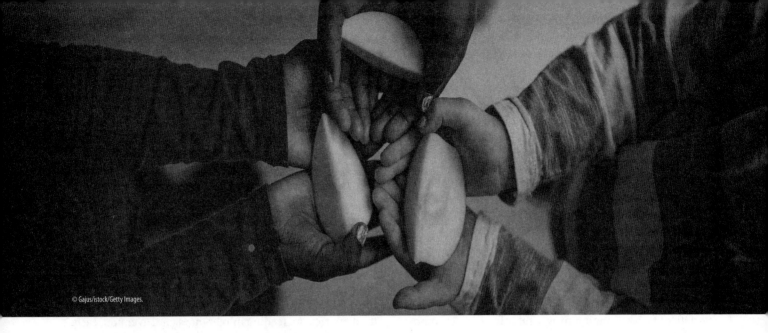

CHAPTER 14

Cardiology

Melanie Savoca and Megan Horsley

LEARNING OBJECTIVES

- Understand the anatomy of congenital heart disease and other cardiac diseases and associated nutrition problems contributing to malnutrition.
- Describe the nutritional interventions in the acute care of patients with congenital heart disease, including parenteral and enteral nutrition recommendations for patients before and after surgery.
- Describe the physiology and nutritional management of patients with particular types of cardiovascular disease, including patients on mechanical circulatory support, cardiomyopathy, pulmonary hypertension, lymphatic disorders, genetic syndromes, and hyperlipidemia.
- Review a case study and practice clinical decision making to gain a better understanding of the specific challenges related to growth assessment and nutrition provision of an infant with congenital heart disease.

▶ Introduction

Congenital heart disease (CHD) is one of the most common congenital defects in the United States (US) with an incidence of approximately 9 per 1000 live births.[1,2] In 2010, researchers estimated that approximately 1 million children and 1.4 million adults were living with CHD in the US.[2] Twenty-five percent of infants born with CHD are born with **critical congenital heart disease** (CCHD) and will require a corrective surgery or procedure within the first year of life. Life expectancy for children undergoing heart surgery has improved and mortality has decreased. However, there remains significant variability

in outcomes and resource utilization across hospitals.[3] Survival has been the greatest for those diagnosed before 1 day of age.[4] Although some types of CHD are not discovered until later in infancy, adolescence, or even adulthood, the majority of CCHD cases are diagnosed during routine prenatal care or shortly after birth.[5] In 2011, the US Secretary of Health and Human Services added pulse oximetry screening for CCHD to the Recommended Uniform Screening Panel, in order to help detect heart defects in newborns before they are discharged from the hospital.[6,7] Recommended and supported by the **American Academy of Pediatrics** (AAP), the **American College of Cardiology Foundation** (ACCF), and the

American Heart Association (AHA), many states have now implemented this cost-effective screening tool.[6,7]

CHD is a risk factor for growth failure. Malnutrition and growth impairment are common worldwide in infants and children with CHD.[8–21] Research has demonstrated that growth failure in cardiac patients is attributed to a variety of factors and is often multifactorial. Some of these factors include inadequate energy intake, poor feeding skills, increased metabolic demands, and disturbances in **gastrointestinal** (GI) function contributing to inefficient absorption and utilization. Associated genetic syndromes and chromosomal abnormalities may also influence growth patterns and nutritional intake.[22] In addition to CHD, the pediatric population may present at any age with acquired cardiac disease caused by a variety of factors ranging from viral infections, chromosomal abnormalities, abnormal rhythms, cardiac arrest, or as a secondary complication of other conditions. The combination of acute and chronic disease and malnutrition in pediatrics can have a detrimental effect on growth, development and disease-related morbidity and mortality.[23,24]

Nutritional support for infants and children with cardiac diseases covers a wide spectrum of disease severity and development, from critical care to chronic care and from infancy through adulthood. The magnitude of the effect of the cardiac defect on growth, development, and nutritional status depends on the particular lesion and its severity.[25] Additionally, children born with CHD are at an increased risk for developmental disabilities or developmental delay.[26] Ongoing surveillance, screening, evaluation, and reevaluation throughout the stages of growth may enhance early detection of deficits and allow for earlier intervention, ultimately improving nutritional and neurodevelopmental outcomes.

Corrective surgery for CHD has become increasingly possible in neonates and very young children, improving the nutritional status of infants with CHD during critical stages of development by eliminating cardiac factors that contribute to malnutrition.[27] Many studies from developed countries have documented normalization in growth when corrective surgeries are performed early. In developing countries, where resources are limited, corrective surgeries are generally performed later, leading to a higher incidence of heart failure, complications related to the effects of untreated cardiovascular disease on other organ systems, and infection.[28] Vaidyanathan and colleagues[28] studied this concept by evaluating the nutritional status of patients with CHD in a tertiary center in South India before and 2 years after corrective surgery. They demonstrated severe malnutrition in over half of the patients, which was not always reversed by intervention or surgery. Persistent malnutrition after intervention was predicted by nutritional status at presentation, birth weight ≤2.5 kg, and parental anthropometry. The results of the study highlight the importance of referring patients with CHD and **congestive heart failure** (CHF) for early corrective intervention before patients develop significant malnutrition.[28] If early cardiac surgery is not an option for an infant, then aggressive nutrition intervention and special nutritional considerations are warranted in order to prevent unsuccessful outcomes associated with malnutrition. However, if attempting aggressive calorie supplementation fails to improve growth, patients should be referred for corrective intervention.

Feeding difficulties and nutrition complications contributing to malnutrition often emerge shortly after surgery and persist throughout the first year or years of life despite advancements in surgical palliation. Impediments to optimal nutritional status after surgery include fluid restriction, feeding intolerances, oral aversion, early satiety, reflux, and developmental delay. Malnutrition in pediatric patients with CHD results in more frequent and lengthier hospital admissions, ultimately increasing the cost of their care.[29] Perhaps more alarming, a strong association has been reported between a decrease in weight-for-age following surgical correction of CHD and late mortality during the first year of life.[30]

Ongoing nutrition surveillance, screening, evaluation, and reevaluation throughout the stages of growth is crucial. It is important to continue to reevaluate caloric requirements of infants, children, and adolescents with CHD since they are not immune to the risk of becoming overweight and obese. Children with CHD may have more sedentary lifestyles secondary to limited physical activity due to developmental delays or restricted activity or exercise given a perceived strain on the heart. Families may also continue a high calorie diet that may have been previously encouraged during the period of time before surgery or resolution of heart failure.[31]

▶ Anatomy, Physiology, Pathology of Condition

Congenital heart diseases are classified as cyanotic or acyanotic (**TABLE 14.1**), depending on the patient's blood oxygen level and net of right-to-left vs. left-to-right shunt. The type of cardiac lesion, degree of hypoxemia, circulatory inefficiency, and associated respiratory considerations impact the patterns of pediatric growth failure. Cyanotic heart diseases are typically characterized by a large right-to-left intracardiac shunt and decreased effective pulmonary blood flow. Acyanotic heart diseases consist of lesions with varying degrees of compromised systemic output with or without a net left-to-right shunt. Lesions such as aortic stenosis, coarctation of the aorta, and interrupted aortic arch are characterized by systemic outflow obstruction and high left atrial pressure. Large left-to-right shunts, as are seen in lesions such as

TABLE 14.1 Congenital Heart Defects

Cyanotic	Acyanotic
Ebstein's Anomaly of the Tricuspid Valve	Atrial Septal Defect (ASD)
Hypoplastic Left Heart Syndrome (HLHS)	Atrioventricular Septal (AV Canal) Defect
Pulmonary Atresia with Intact Ventricular Septum (PA/IVS)	Patent Ductus Arteriosus (PDA)
Critical Pulmonary Stenosis (PS)	Truncus Arteriosus
Tetralogy of Fallot (TOF)	Ventricular Septal Defect (VSD)
Total Anomalous Pulmonary Venous Return (TAPVR)	Aortic Stenosis (AS)
Transposition of the Great Arteries (TGA)	Coarctation of the Aorta (CoA)
Tricuspid Atresia	Interrupted Aortic Arch (IAA)

Modified from The Cincinnati Children's Hospital Medical Center Heart Institute. Encyclopedia. Available at: https://www.cincinnatichildrens.org/patients/child/encyclopedia. Accessed April 6, 2018.[32]

VSD, PDA, truncus arteriosus and complete atrioventricular canal defects, resulting in excessive pulmonary blood flow, potentially at the expense of systemic cardiac output (so-called "pulmonary overcirculation"). In both cases, signs of CHF develop, including pulmonary edema, increased work of breathing, and impaired systemic perfusion. The impact of these cardiac lesions on development are complex, as are the nutritional requirements that must be met to achieve growth in the setting of increased cardiovascular and respiratory demand.

Condition Specific Nutrition Screening and Assessment

Pediatric patients with CHD or CHF have long been recognized to have an increased risk in the frequency and severity of acute and chronic malnutrition.[33–35] Most children with CHD have normal birth weights, but often develop malnutrition in the first few months of life leading to growth alterations on weight, stature, and head circumference. Chronic malnutrition and impaired growth have also been associated with worse neurodevelopmental outcomes and disabilities in infants and children with single ventricle physiology.[36] Risk factors associated with poor growth are multifactorial.[37] These patient populations require close nutrition monitoring from infancy through young adulthood. Nutrition screening in pediatric patients with CHD or CHF should be consistent with pediatric malnutrition risk screening and diagnostic criteria as defined by the consensus statement from the Academy of Nutrition and Dietetics and the **American Society for Parenteral and Enteral Nutrition** (ASPEN).[38]

Patients with cyanotic heart lesions usually exhibit reduced weight and linear growth.[10–12,20,39–41] The basal metabolic state of the heart in infants and children has been found to be significantly greater in the presence of cyanosis compared with acyanosis.[42] Cyanotic heart lesions when combined with pulmonary hypertension are also associated with a higher incidence of growth failure.[43] Acyanotic lesions with a large degree of left-to-right shunting typically affect weight while sparing height in the early stages before surgical repair.[10,39,44–46]

Inadequate energy intake has been frequently cited as the most important contributor of growth failure in infants and children with CHD.[27,34,39,47–54] Energy intake with aggressive nutritional support is also one of the most modifiable factors that may be associated with favorable growth.[55] Factors contributing to inadequate energy intake include oral feeding dysfunction, GI intolerance, limitations of fluid intake, and frequent interruptions in nutrient delivery during hospitalizations. A study by Hill and colleagues[56] indicated that adequate growth may be achieved for infants with CHD regardless of feeding modality with adequate provision of calories and close nutrition monitoring.

Hypermetabolism has also been well described in CHD and may contribute to malnutrition and growth failure.[51,57] **Total daily energy expenditure** (TDEE) was measured in infants with CHD by the doubly labeled water method. TDEE includes basal metabolism as well as the energy of activity, sweating, and the mechanical labor of the heart and lungs.[58] A significantly higher TDEE was found for infants with CHD (101 ± 3k cal/kg/day), compared with healthy infants (67 ± 14k cal/kg/day). The calculated increase in TDEE was 36% above that of healthy infants, except for one infant who had a very high TDEE.[58] On the contrary, one study by Irving and colleagues[59] found that **resting energy expenditure** (REE) at 3 months of age for infants following neonatal cardiac surgery did not differ between postsurgical infants with CHD and healthy infants. However, the infants with CHD were found to have lower growth z-scores and lower percent body fat.

Congestive heart failure is another factor that may impair growth. Heart failure is thought to increase metabolic rate, therefore increasing the energy required for growth. Some cardiac diseases that may cause CHF include atrioventricular canal defects, cardiomyopathy, or CHD with chronic hypoxemia. Additionally, patients with pulmonary hypertension in combination with CHD, particularly left-to-right shunts, have a higher risk for growth failure.[43] These children tend to weigh less than children with cyanotic heart lesions.[52,54] Obstructive malformations, such as pulmonary stenosis and coarctation of the aorta, typically result in impaired linear growth, with linear growth more affected than weight.[10,43,60]

Furthermore, there is evidence to support a neurohormonal relationship between heart failure and growth. Serum **brain type natriuretic peptide** (BNP) is a surrogate marker of heart failure. Elevated serum BNP concentrations have been associated with lower height z-scores.[36] Endocrine factors including **insulin-like growth factor** (IGF-1) and growth hormone are hormones essential for somatic growth. Many authors have detected reduced IGF-1 levels in children with CHD and pulmonary hypertension.[10,43,60–63] Another study found higher BNP and lower systemic flow in children with Fontan physiology to be associated with lower IGF-1 z-scores.[64]

Anthropometrics measurements, including weight, length/height, head circumference (<2 years of age) should be measured frequently, both inpatient and outpatient, to closely monitor growth velocity. **Mid-upper arm circumference** (MUAC) may also be trended for patients who have fluid shifts or ascites where weight-for-length or BMI-for-age may be unreliable measurements. **Nutrition focused physical exams** (NFPE) are imperative for understanding nutritional status. Assessing muscle mass, subcutaneous fat stores, edema, skin, hair, and nails can identify and uncover nutrient deficiencies, toxicities, and signs of malnutrition. NFPE should be part of each assessment. A registered dietitian is a vital member of the interdisciplinary team to assess nutrition intake and anthropometrics, diagnose malnutrition, and provide appropriate medical nutrition interventions as needed.

Nutrition Diagnostic Statements

- Increased energy expenditure (NI-1.1) related to congestive heart failure as evidenced by suboptimal weight gain velocity with age-appropriate energy intake.
- Inadequate oral intake (NI-2.1) related to difficulty feeding and decreased ability to consume sufficient energy as evidenced by insufficient growth velocity.
- Inadequate enteral nutrition (NI-2.3) related to altered gastrointestinal function as evidenced by intolerance of enteral feeds and need for parenteral nutrition.
- Suboptimal growth rate (NS-3.5) related to decreased ability to consume sufficient energy as evidenced by anthropometric measurements consistent with mild to severe malnutrition.

- Swallowing difficulty (NC-1.1) related to vocal cord dysfunction as evidenced by abnormal swallow study or signs/symptoms of aspiration with oral feeds.

Nutrition Intervention, Monitoring and Evaluation

In the next few sections, the different phases of care from acute to chronic care that cardiac patients often experience will be discussed. Specific cardiac conditions will also be reviewed in detail. The nutritional interventions often times overlap but all require appropriate levels of monitoring. Due to varying degrees of critical cardiac anomalies, heart failure, and stages of palliation, it is imperative for frequent monitoring and evaluation of nutritional plans. Monitoring and evaluating for adequate nutrient intake, tolerance, adherence, anthropometrics, and neurodevelopmental outcomes may improve quality of life and decrease incidence of malnutrition for these complex patients.

Acute Care

Critically ill neonates are at high risk for malnutrition due to metabolic stress, limited reserves and inadequate supply of nutrients.[65–67] The metabolic state is very heterogeneous during critical illness and one's response to injury, surgery, stress or inflammation is unpredictable. Therefore, overfeeding and underfeeding in the intensive care setting is prevalent. Protein-energy malnutrition in hospitalized children is associated with increased physiological instability and increased resource utilization potentially affecting outcomes.[68,69] The goal of nutrition support is to mitigate the stress response, preserve muscle mass, promote recovery after surgery, and minimize long term harmful consequences.

Preoperative nutrition support: For neonates diagnosed with CHD, the primary nutrition goal after birth is to minimize neonatal weight loss during the preoperative period. Research has shown that preoperative malnutrition is associated with a longer intensive care unit length of stay.[70] Benefits and safety of early enteral feeding has been widely recognized in preterm and term neonates. Hesitance with early feeding practices in critical cardiac neonates is the result of concerns of increased risk of **necrotizing enterocolitis** (NEC) from cyanosis, **prostaglandin E$_1$** (PGE) administration, or the presence of **umbilical arterial catheters** (UAC) before surgery. Infants with ductal-dependent pulmonary or systemic circulation are believed to be at most risk for intestinal hypoperfusion, increasing their risk for NEC. A study by Becker and colleagues[71] examined the incidence of NEC in a large cohort of infants with CHD between 1997 and 2010 receiving PGE. The results of the study demonstrated a low incidence of NEC at 0.3%, supporting the practice of enteral feeding in infants requiring PGE. ASPEN clinical guidelines recommend initiating minimal **enteral nutrition** (EN) within two days of life for those at risk for NEC along with the preferential use of human milk over formula.[72] Feeding of infants with cyanosis has not been shown to date to be associated with an elevated incidence of NEC, and in hemodynamically stable infants, PGE administration has not been shown to be a risk factor for adverse events associated with enteral feeding.[73] Although the presence of UAC has been a theoretical risk factor for gut hypoperfusion, in one large series, there was no significant increase in NEC in infants fed with UAC in place,[74] irrespective of placement: high vs. low lying.[75]

A survey by Howley and colleagues[76] demonstrates notable variation in preoperative feeding practices around the world and consensus on timing and method is lacking. Slicker and colleagues[77] echoed Howley's survey results looking at perioperative feeding approaches specifically in single ventricle centers. Two-thirds of centers permit feeding infants with single ventricle physiology before surgical palliation, although there is large variation in the methods of feeding across centers. In some infants, this period of EN deprivation is inevitable. However, literature has shown that a cautious introduction of early postnatal EN may be largely beneficial. Additional

suspected benefits for preoperative feeding include oromotor skill and neurodevelopment, maternal bonding, improved hemodynamics of the infant, and protective health benefits to the GI tract.

Postoperative nutrition support: The best surgical outcomes are achieved in patients with good nutritional status and positive nitrogen balance. For this reason, protocols for initiating and advancing enteral feeding postoperatively are advantageous. Assessing energy needs is challenging during the critical postoperative illness. **Indirect calorimetry** (IC) is the gold standard for determining energy needs in the critically ill.[68] This is due to the moving metabolic targets and inaccuracies of predictive equations. There are specific criteria for implementing IC, which at many times limits the use of IC in small infants. If IC is unavailable, literature recommends initially aiming for basal energy expenditure using the **World Health Organization** (WHO) tables during the first 3–5 days, then multiplying basal energy expenditure by stress or injury factors after postoperative days 5–7.[78] Alternate predictive equations to consider are the Dietary Reference Intakes from 2002 and resting energy expenditure tables by Page and colleagues.[79,80] **TABLE 14.2** is a brief reference summarizing postoperative nutrition guidelines:

TABLE 14.2 Nutrition Guidelines for Neonates Undergoing Surgery for CHD

	Postoperative Guidelines	Acute Care Guidelines
Energy	Determined by indirect calorimetry* 55–65 kcal/kg for first 3–5 days	Advance to 120–150+ kcal/kg**
Protein	Preterm: 3–4.5 g/kg Term: 3–4 g/kg Protein needs lower with acute kidney injury (AKI) or higher with CRRT/Peritoneal dialysis	2.2–3.5 g/kg
Carbohydrate	40–60% of total calories Initiate GIR 4–8 mg/kg/min Advance to max GIR 12–14 mg/kg/min	
Lipid	1.5–3 g/kg***	
Fluid	Fluid restriction 50–85%mIVF mIVF fluid: 100 mL/kg	Advance to 100–150 mL/kg Increased 10–15% with insensible losses due to fever, tachypnea, tachycardia, diarrhea

* If available, results may be affected by ventilation, sedation, medications.
** Estimated needs from EN.
*** Limited with cholestasis or hypertriglyceridemia.
Abbreviations: GIR (glucose infusion rate); mIVF (maintenance intravenous fluids)
Data from Nydegger A, Bines JE. Energy metabolism in infants with congenital heart disease. *Nutr.* 2006;22: 697–704.[22]
Owens JL, Musa N. Nutrition support after neonatal cardiac surgery. *Nutr Clin Pract.* 2009;24:242–249.[81]
Pronsky ZM. *Food-Medication Interactions.* rev ed. Birchrunville, PA: Food-Medication Interactions; 2004.[82]

During the immediate postoperative period, nutrition support should be initiated as early as 24–48 hours in order to promote wound healing, minimize the loss of lean body mass, and support vital organ function. Barriers may preclude the delivery of adequate calories for growth at this time. These barriers include hemodynamic instability, hypotension, hyperglycemia, electrolyte derangements, fluid restrictions, impaired renal function, and mechanical ventilation.[81] Although infants have a fundamental need to grow, growth is not a critical priority during the immediate postoperative period. Growth cannot occur until the infant begins to recover from the postoperative stress response and positive nitrogen balance is achieved.[65] Additionally, overfeeding is associated with increased carbon dioxide (CO_2) production, difficulties weaning from ventilator support, and impaired immune and organ function.[81] Nutrition support in the acutely ill infant typically involves the use of **parenteral nutrition** (PN) and **intravenous** (IV) fluids. The infant may be fluid restricted to 50–80% maintenance in the first 24 hours. There may be multiple lines requiring 0.5–1mL/hr each for patency. Medications and infusions may use a significant amount of fluid or be incompatible with PN. Fluid allotment should be liberalized as the patient becomes more stable.

Laboratory values may be abnormal. The use of diuretics may deplete total body sodium and potassium; calcium, phosphorus, and magnesium levels may also be abnormal.[82] The renal lab values may reflect some degree of dehydration due to the need for fluid restriction, with elevated sodium and blood urea nitrogen. Acid–base status may also be altered, complicating electrolyte management. Metabolic alkalosis is common with excessive use of loop and thiazide diuretics due to hypochloremia and hypokalemia.

Furthermore, other end organ dysfunction is often common. **Acute kidney injury** (AKI) is the most common complication following pediatric heart surgery.[83] It is postulated that the use of **cardiopulmonary bypass** (CPB), the time on CPB, aortic cross clamp time, and high levels of vasopressors increase the patient's risk for AKI.[83] In addition to these characteristics, low body weight, stunting, and mechanical ventilation are risk factors for developing AKI postoperatively. Some infants may temporarily need dialysis via peritoneal dialysis catheter or continuous renal replacement therapy, further complicating nutrition support. For infants and children unable to be weaned from cardiopulmonary bypass after surgery, **extracorporeal life support** (ECLS) may be used.[84–86]

EN should be introduced as determined appropriate by the multidisciplinary medical team. PN and EN should be used simultaneously in the gradual transition to full enteral feedings. Once full EN is achieved, nutrition support should provide adequate calories and protein for optimal growth. Anthropometric measurements and growth trends should be regularly monitored. Developing feeding skills may also be an integral component of care as EN is advanced. A feeding therapist should be consulted if difficulties or concerns are noted with oral feeding.

Parenteral Nutrition Support

PN should be initiated for patients when enteral feeding is contraindicated, including times of hemodynamic instability, acute decompensated heart failure, escalating pressor support, or concern for NEC. The postoperative period for neonates who have undergone cardiac surgery is often associated with undernutrition. Providing adequate nutrition is an integral component of postoperative management.

To plan the nutrition support for an acutely ill infant or child, the multidisciplinary team should review all fluids objectively. The volume of PN is driven by the total fluid limit of each patient. Laboratory tests, including basic metabolic and renal panels, glucose, ionized calcium, phosphorus, and magnesium should be monitored daily until stable. Hepatic function should be checked weekly or as indicated. Nursing should obtain daily weights to evaluate fluid status. The pharmacist or front line clinician can determine whether the medication infusions are concentrated appropriately to maximize fluid allotted for PN. Any dextrose used in fluid administration should be counted toward the overall **glucose infusion rate** (GIR) and carbohydrate and calorie intake. Sodium used in medication infusions or fluids should be calculated since it can provide a significant and unexpected amount. Line patency fluids should be counted toward the total fluid limit. PN volume should be written last, accounting for the content of the other fluids. Since there can be significant medication incompatibility and varying intravenous access, PN and fat emulsion should run separately and PN admixtures should not be used.

Energy requirements in the immediate postoperative period of the stressed infant may be decreased because of growth inhibition resulting from a catabolic stress mechanism, decreased insensible losses, and inactivity. Giving patients high calories during this acute period can lead to overfeeding, resulting in increased CO_2 production since they cannot utilize the nutrients. The period of metabolic stress after surgery can be relatively short, often less than 48 hours, although it may be slightly prolonged with additional injuries, infection, or complications. Once cytokines released during stress have dissipated and the metabolic response shifts from a catabolic to anabolic state, calories should be adjusted in order to provide adequate calories for growth and healing.[87] Li and colleagues[88] measured energy expenditure in neonates for the first 3 days following the Norwood procedure and found energy expenditure on days 0, 1, 2, and 3 was 43, 39, 39, and 41 kcal/kg/day, respectively. Another study found average inadequate energy intake of <63 kcal/kg/day in infants after open heart surgery was associated with adverse outcomes in the **intensive care unit** (ICU), including increased duration of ventilation days, delayed chest closure, and length of ICU and hospital stay.[90] PN may be used to improve nutrition delivery to high risk neonates until clinical status improves and initiation of EN is appropriate.

PN is usually very concentrated in the cardiac infant due to fluid restrictions. Central lines are generally used because peripheral PN lines are at increased risk of IV infiltration and should not contain more than 12.5% dextrose. With increasing dextrose concentrations, the osmolarity of solutions increases dramatically. Typically, the maximum dextrose concentration used in central lines is 25%. Higher dextrose percentages increase the risk of thrombosis. The tip of venous lines should be verified by radiology film before initiation of PN in order to determine the maximum dextrose concentration that can be safely infused. The risks and benefits of providing higher calories through a higher percentage of glucose should be considered carefully. Hyperglycemia is common early after infant cardiac surgery. Insulin is not often used in infants after cardiac surgery because glucose usually normalizes within 24–48 hours. Tight glycemic control using insulin to maintain target glucose level between 80–110mg/dL has not been shown to impact neurodevelopmental outcomes at 1 year of age compared with standard care.[90,91] However, moderate to severe hypoglycemia is associated with poor neurodevelopmental outcomes at 1 year of age.[90] PN can be initiated postoperatively with a GIR of 4–8mg/kg/min, and may be advanced as tolerated. Postoperative infants may tolerate a GIR of only 10–12mg/kg/min.

Intravenous lipids are a concentrated source of calories and a source of essential fatty acids. The most commonly used 20% fat emulsions are Intralipids® and Smoflipids®. Triglyceride levels should be monitored to assess tolerance to this therapy. For patients on ECLS, fat emulsion should be infused through a separate intravenous site other than the ECLS circuit secondary to layering, agglutination, and adhesion of the fat emulsion to the circuit forming clots, which may result in disruption of blood flow.[92,93]

Protein needs are important to consider in this stressed population. Chaloupecky and colleagues[94] found that providing a small amount of intravenous protein, 0.8 g/kg/day, blunted the muscle proteolysis hypercatabolic response in infants after cardiac surgery, in contrast to an isocaloric maintenance dextrose solution. Teixeira-Cintra and colleagues[95] demonstrated that children undergoing surgery for CHD were able to achieve anabolism during postoperative days 3 to 10 with energy and protein intakes >55 kcal/kg/day and >1 g/kg/day of protein, respectively. Starting PN with protein immediately postoperatively would seem to be warranted, even if only half of maintenance fluids can be used for this endeavor, due to electrolyte fluctuations. Careful attention to providing dextrose, protein, and electrolytes should be made if urine output is temporarily reduced after cardiopulmonary bypass, or with increased electrolyte losses that may occur with diuretic administration.

Additionally, it may not be possible for mineral needs for bone development to be met in the short term, due to the use of PN, intravenous shortages affecting PN prescription, and fluid limitations. Diuretic use may alter calcium status through increased urinary excretion of calcium. Premature and term infant calcium and phosphorus requirements for bone mineralization often cannot be optimized from PN alone. Signs of cholestasis and bone demineralization should be monitored closely for patients requiring long term PN.[96]

Enteral Nutrition Support

EN is the preferred mode of nutrient delivery when the gut is functional. Infants and children requiring EN via enteral tube feeding are unable to meet optimal calories from oral feeding alone for reasons such as heart failure, **gastroesophageal reflux** (GER), swallowing dysfunction, dysphagia, oral aversion, and other endocrine and genetic factors. Given the vast consensus of growth concerns and the increased need for nutrition support in this population, establishing best nutritional practices may mitigate growth failure. The National Pediatric Cardiology Quality Improvement Collaborative has developed best practice recommendations to target optimizing nutritional intake in order to mitigate poor growth in children with CHD.[97] Due to the acknowledgement of the high incidence of feeding difficulties and growth failure in this population, there is wide interest in developing nutrition pathways or protocols in an attempt to standardize management and decrease variability in provider recommendations in order to improve outcomes in neonates undergoing surgery for CHD.[97] Using enteral feeding protocols has been shown to be a safe and effective method of initiating and advancing enteral nutrition and achieving adequate nutrient delivery.[98-100]

Early trophic EN should be initiated as soon as the patient is hemodynamically stable. A trophic rate of 10–20mL/kg/day is recommended. PN should be weaned down as EN is advanced while ensuring combined adequate caloric intake. Human milk is recommended, although standard infant formula may be an appropriate alternative. The enteral formulas used for infants and children with CHD are often the same as for other children. Infants with compromised systemic cardiac output, high prevalence of feeding difficulties or concerns for malabsorption may require semi-elemental or elemental formulas for improved enteral tolerance and absorption. EN may be trialed in the stomach, although patients may temporarily require post-pyloric feeding if on high non-invasive respiratory support, or if there are concerns for gastroparesis or reflux.

Since infants with CHD need additional calories, it may be necessary to titrate the caloric density of breast milk or formulas greater than 20 kcal/oz, ranging frequently from 22 to 30 kcal/oz. Once full volume of enteral feeds is achieved, caloric density can be increased gradually. The multidisciplinary team should determine the volume of enteral fluid tolerated by each patient; however, the amount of fluid available is often related to the amount of diuretic therapy. Diuretics may be used to lessen the effects of high-volume feedings, although side effects of potassium wasting, acid–base problems, and potential for altered calcium and magnesium excretion exist.[101] The literature indicates that infants tolerate feeds if the calorie increase is done slowly, increasing by approximately 2kcal/oz at a time.[102]

To increase the caloric density, formulas can be made using less water with formula powder or liquid concentrate while keeping the original proportion of carbohydrate, protein, and fat the same. However, the amount of electrolytes and minerals is also increased when the caloric density of formulas is increased and should be taken into consideration. If patients have signs of osmotic diarrhea or are exceeding micronutrient and mineral intake, modulars may be added to increase caloric density without significant increase in osmolality or micronutrients. Enteral medications should also be considered when enteral intolerance is present as they may contribute significant osmotic load to a much greater extent than formula alone. In practice, some clinicians use an intravenous preparation of a medicine, such as intravenous potassium chloride instead of the oral form, which has a greater osmolality due to the syrup suspension of the medication.[102]

Calorie needs of infants and children with CHD are most often greater than those without cardiac problems. Studies using nutrition intervention in either the inpatient or outpatient setting have shown that normal growth can be achieved using higher calorie intakes. One study using 24-hour continuous enteral infusion showed a growth improvement of 198% with infants age 1 week to 9 months who had previously displayed poor growth. The calorie range used was 120–150kcal/kg with a 24–30 kcal/oz range in caloric densities of the formulas.[103] Infants with mild CHD were given higher calorie formula recipes to increase calorie intake by 20% in oral feedings. Favorable growth was seen in 60% of the group with the higher calorie intake.[104] Higher calorie formulas were used in a study with oral feedings and infants with CHD. Calories were increased by 32%, and weight gain improved significantly. The authors' recommendation is to begin supplementation from the time of diagnosis to optimize growth.[105]

The precise energy needs of infants with CHD are difficult to estimate, but many infants will need 120–150 kcal/kg or even greater if additional calories are required for catch-up growth.[27] Toddlers and children may need 20–33% more than normal estimated needs. After cardiac repair, the calorie needs will usually decrease but may stay 10–15 kcal/kg above the average for some infants or children, especially if additional calories are needed to achieve catch-up growth due to presence of malnutrition before surgery.[21] Calorie needs may be estimated using IC while in the hospital; however, many institutions do not have the equipment to accurately assess infants under 5 kg or infants who are mechanically ventilated. The best method is to set an estimated goal, assess growth parameters, and make adjustments as needed until appropriate growth velocity is achieved.

Special Considerations
Gastrointestinal Function

Gastrointestinal disturbances and feeding dysfunction are frequently seen complications of hospitalized infants and children with cardiac disorders and may have a significant negative impact on outcomes and burden of illness. Inadequate enteral intake, GI morbidity, and feeding problems can affect growth and recovery and can influence short and long term outcomes.[43] The challenges of supporting nutrition in children with CHD are discussed in the sections highlighting specific conditions and points in the course of treatment. A number of GI concerns, including fat and/or protein malabsorption, are common in many of infants with CHD.[27,106] In addition to causing early satiety and vomiting, decreased cardiac output may also cause decreased nutrient absorption.[54] Furthermore, some children with CHD have GI malformations that will affect their ability to be nourished. These may include pyloric stenosis, duodenal atresia, malrotation, and severe defects such as gastroschisis, all requiring surgical repair. Reduced gut perfusion is another factor recognized as a complication often present in infants with cardiac insufficiency. NEC prevention from the aforementioned ASPEN clinical guidelines should be considered when concerns for reduced gut perfusion are present.[72]

Inadequate energy intake and impaired utilization is felt to be the predominant cause of growth failure in infants with CHD. Achieving adequate calories through oral feedings is difficult and often challenging. Oral feeding, even if the patient's condition allows, requires a great deal of energy expenditure and may result in symptoms like tachypnea, sweating, discoordination, and fatigue during feeding. For this reason, it is difficult to achieve adequate oral intake to support nutritional needs and modifications to nutrition support are often required. Other factors contributing to inadequate intake include early satiety, decreased gastric capacity related to hepatomegaly, and delayed gastric emptying as a result of low cardiac output or medication side effect.

One study compared the impact of acyanotic and cyanotic CHD in neonates on enteral feeding milestones.[107] Those children with cyanotic CHD had significant delays in time to initiate and achieve maximal gavage feeds and maximal nipple feeds, and prolonged lengths of hospital stay. Even so, a high percentage of infants in both groups eventually were able to achieve adequate nipple feedings upon discharge. This study also found that prolonged respiratory support had a negative effect on maximal nippling skills and delaying achievement of maximal tube feeds. It was noted in another study of infants with cyanotic and acyanotic heart lesions that feeding practices, rather than the type of heart defects, predicted weight gain postoperatively.[108] Feeding guidelines and protocols can improve nutrient delivery and decrease time to goal feeds, ultimately leading to shorter length of stay and improved weight gain. Using necessary feeding modalities will support optimal growth velocity.

In planning for transition to enteral feeding, it is important to remember the impact of the cardiorespiratory system on the achievement of EN support.[107] Infants with a history of cardiopulmonary bypass and prolonged respiratory support showed abnormalities in oromotor feeding skills. For pediatric patients intubated for more than 7 days, the risk of dysphagia increases, as does the inability to feed orally by hospital discharge.[109,110] Jadcherla and colleagues[107] noted that other covariates, including narcotic use, vasopressor support, and cardiopulmonary bypass, may also negatively impact oral feeding ability. Tachypnea may cause an uncoordinated suck, swallow, and breathe pattern necessary for successful oral feeding. When prolonged stridor is present, concern for vocal cord dysfunction should be considered. Aspiration and dysphagia may be present in patients with vocal cord paralysis. Fatigue is common in these infants and respiratory and heart rates should be closely monitored with oral trials. Infants with CHD often cannot feed long enough to support their nutritional needs.

Sluggish reflexes, decreased sensory input, hypoxemia, neurological insults, or bowel ischemia may impair the GI system. In the event of gut hypoperfusion, waiting for bowel recovery may cause delayed initiation of EN. GER is common in up to 65% of healthy infants[111,112] but may play a more significant role in infants with CHD. Using a nasogastric tube may result in increased reflux symptoms. Aggressive management to reduce the symptoms of reflux, delayed gastric emptying, or slow gut motility when tube feedings is required and intolerance is present are common in this population.

Neurologic maturation is another key factor that should be considered in the ability of an infant to reach optimal oral intake.[113] Although the majority of infants with CHD are full term at birth, evidence suggests they may be neurologically immature and suffer early neurological insults that may have profound effects on impaired feeding ability.[114] Infants with CHD have a higher risk for neurologic sequelae, including bleeds or strokes. Children with CHD are often found to have neurologic disabilities.[115] Depending on the severity of deficits, infants with these complications are most often supported by long term tube feedings.

Another surgical complication includes injury to the recurrent laryngeal nerve. Injury to this nerve can be caused by a variety of operative events, such as arch augmentation, and results in vocal cord paresis or paralysis and often GER.[116] It has been reported that laryngopharyngeal dysfunction presents after the Norwood procedure in about 48% of patients, with resultant dysphagia, aspiration, and left recurrent laryngeal nerve injury.[117] For these reasons, vocal cord dysfunction will often result in the need for gavage feedings to support nutrition. These factors that affect GI function require consideration to EN regimens.

Mechanical Circulatory Support

Mechanical circulatory support (MCS) has become an indispensable tool when caring for patients with cardiac and respiratory failure. Advances in MCS have revolutionized in the last several years leading to more utilization of both temporary and long term support devices (**TABLE 14.3**).[118] **Temporary circulatory support** (TCS) strategies can now be effectively utilized as a bridge to decision, to recovery, to long term support devices and/or heart transplantation.[119] **Extracorporeal membrane oxygenation** (ECMO) has long served as the standard of care for short term support but statistics demonstrate that approximately one half of children fail to survive to hospital discharge.[120,121] There has also been a dramatic rise in the use of TCS over the last 10 years and a longer supportive duration over ECMO.[120]

A **ventricular assist device** (VAD) is a medical device that can be implanted or sit external to the patient. VADs are used to partially or completely replace the circulatory function of the heart and are often intended as a bridge to transplantation or destination therapy. There are **left ventricular assist devices** (LVAD), **right ventricular assist devices** (RVAD) or **bi-ventricular assist devices** (BiVAD) available depending on the extent of failure. Montgomery and colleagues[122] describe these more in detail, but all have been shown to improve morbidity and mortality, increase the quality of life, and improve the functional capacity of patients with heart failure. Timely insertion of long term support devices is vital to minimizing morbidity and mortality.[119] Table 14.3 is an overview of available temporary and long term support devices.

TABLE 14.3 Mechanical Circulatory Support Devices

Temporary Circulatory Support Devices	Long Term Circulatory Support Devices
ECMO Heart and lung machine	**Berlin Heart EXCOR** Pumping chamber that rests outside the body and assists the heart to get blood flow to all vital organs while awaiting a transplant.
RotaFlow Centrifugal Pump A Pump that assists the heart but not the lungs	**HeartMate II** Internally housed (inside the body) continuous flow pump that can support an older child/adult until transplantation. This device can be used to support a patient for the duration of their lifetime.
Centrimag/Pedimag Pump that assists the heart but not the lungs	**SynCardia Total Artificial Heart and the Freedom Driver** Internally housed pump that replaces the whole heart until transplantation. Patients can go home with this device by transitioning to the Freedom driver.
CardioHelp Device for patients who need short-term respiratory and/or circulatory support	**HeartWare Ventricular Assist Device System** Internally housed continuous flow pump that can support a patient until transplantation.

Data from The Cincinnati Children's Hospital Medical Center. Ventricular Assist Device (VAD) Program. Available at: [electronic resource]. 2018; https://www.cincinnatichildrens.org/service/v/ventricular-assist-device/devices. Accessed 30 April 30, 2018.[123]

Kozick, Deborah J and Mark D Plunkett. Mechanical circulatory support. *Organogenesis* 7(1):50–63.[124]

Additional information can be found at the following websites:

https://pulmccm.org/review-articles/mechanical-circulatory-support-devices/

https://www.berlinheart.com/

http://www.thoratec.com/

https://syncardia.com/

http://www.heartware.com/

https://www.uptodate.com/contents/intermediate-and-long-term-mechanical-circulatory-support

Nutritional studies and assessment guidelines for patients with VADs is lacking, although there is much paucity regarding their nutritional complications such as wound healing and feeding intolerance. A considerable number of VAD patients have minimal nutritional reserves and ongoing nutritional challenges before VAD placement. Due to limited nutritional guidelines, management is often similar to that of critically ill patients. A detailed nutrition assessment before VAD placement is extremely important to provide optimal care. Similarly, the nutrition goals for patients on all forms of MCS are to provide adequate calories and protein to minimize catabolism and promote wound healing. ASPEN guidelines of neonates on ECMO recommends initiating nutrition support expeditiously given their limited reserves and high protein catabolic rates. Although critically ill patients on MCS are severely stressed, catabolic, and have an increased metabolic burden of wound healing, caloric requirements may be initially decreased as neonates redirect energy, normally used for growth, to fuel the stress response.[125] Research has estimated calorie needs for infants on MCS, specifically ECLS, also called ECMO, to initially range between 70–80kcal/kg/day. For older children, estimated energy needs may be 70–90% of the REE.[125–127] However, calorie needs may need to be increased the longer patients require ECMO support or as support is weaned.

Nevertheless, providing adequate caloric intake is paramount in this patient population. Fluid restriction, difficulties with glucose control, end organ dysfunction, anticoagulation management, GI complications, early satiety, and nutritional deficiencies pose challenges of meeting calorie, protein and micronutrient needs. The key to nutritional management of the patient on MCS is to provide optimal nutrition within the limits of restricted fluid intake. Total PN and EN are initiated as early as possible with maximized caloric density. The use of post-pyloric feeding may be beneficial in decreasing the risk of aspiration and GER along with improved time to reach goal feeding.[122]

Due to renal dysfunction, fluid resuscitation, and endocrine problems, electrolyte derangements are frequent occurrences among patients on MCS. Careful attention to electrolyte supplementation, particularly optimization of potassium, calcium, and magnesium, is of prime importance in order to avoid dysrhythmias. In addition to electrolyte abnormalities, specific vitamin deficiencies have been identified in patients with heart failure and those requiring MCS. Vitamin B deficiencies have also been closely studied in patients with heart failure.[122] For this reason, particular attention to thiamine (B$_1$), riboflavin (B$_2$) and pyridoxine (B$_6$) may be warranted and supplementation may be necessary.[122] Another vitamin of particular interest in heart failure and cardiomyopathy is vitamin D. Emerging evidence suggests that vitamin D has additional roles in the musculoskeletal system and extraskeletal functions like immune cell proliferation, anti-inflammatory effect, and malignancies.[122,128,129] Available research suggests a strong prevalence of vitamin D deficiency in patients with cardiac failure and those who have undergone transplantation. Graham and colleagues[129] suggest that vitamin D deficiency may play a role in myocardial injury in neonates undergoing cardiopulmonary bypass. Given the challenges with wound healing in those on MCS, zinc deficiency should also be considered. More studies are needed on wound healing supplementation due to lacking evidence, but nonetheless, supplementation is reasonable if clinical signs of poor wound healing are present.

Multiple complications can arise after initiating MCS support. Capillary leak syndrome is caused by increased vascular permeability due to prolonged hypoxia and hypotension, and can cause severe edema, particularly in neonates, with as much as a 50–75% weight increase. A systemic inflammatory response syndrome most often occurs related to blood exposure to foreign material, but is self-limited to 24–72 hours after initiating MCS or after a circuit change. Hemorrhagic or bleeding complications can also occur and are related to systemic heparinization, which makes the blood twice as thin as normal. Cholestasis may be seen, but often resolves without long term hepatic complications.[130] Delayed gastric emptying, GER, and reduced gut motility are also seen in critically ill patients.[131]

In the past, EN has been restricted in patients on ECMO and may be delayed extensively with other forms of MCS. This practice has been based on concerns of compromised splanchnic perfusion secondary to periods of hypoxia and vasopressor therapy in patients on ECMO. These factors may result in an increased risk of NEC, bacterial translocation, and sepsis.[132] However, recent data show that EN in ECMO patients is not only safe,[133] but also maintains gut mucosal integrity, improves GI immunologic function, and minimizes the risk of sepsis.[134] Feeding on MCS remains varied across centers. Research has determined that pediatric patients on ECMO have adequate gut hormone profiles. Initiation

of EN may be safely administered and is highly recommended since it has been shown to promote gut mucosal integrity and blood flow, secrete GI hormones that enhance cell growth and development, improve glucose tolerance, stimulate motor activity, improve GI mucosal immune function, and reduce morbidity in critically ill patients.[135–138] Trophic feeds may also help reduce gallbladder sludge or cholelithiasis as fasting decreases gallbladder movement, which causes bile to become over concentrated. Despite which form of MCS, the patients on EN should be monitored very closely for early signs of feeding intolerance.

Pediatric Cardiomyopathy

Pediatric cardiomyopathy is a serious disorder of the heart muscle that is responsible for significant morbidity and mortality among affected children. The estimated incidence is between 1.1 and 1.5 cases per 100,000 children 18 years of age and younger, with the highest incidence among children less than 1 year of age.[139,140] Children with cardiomyopathy have some of the worst clinical outcomes compared with other heart diseases in children. Within 2 years of diagnosis, 40 percent of children die or undergo transplantation.[140] Cardiomyopathy is the second most common indication for transplantation for infants less than 1 year of age (40%); whereas, cardiomyopathy predominates as the most common indication for heart transplantation in older children (63%).[141] Heart transplantation remains the standard of care for children who fail medical therapy.

Cardiomyopathy can be classified into different categories:[142–144]

1. Dilated cardiomyopathy is characterized by pathologic stretching of the myocardial fibers, causing dilatation of the ventricles, decreased contractility, and predominant systolic dysfunction.

2. Hypertrophic cardiomyopathy is an abnormal growth or arrangement of myocardial fibers that leads to a thickening of the ventricular walls and reduction in size of the pumping chamber; it is often associated with obstruction of the left ventricular outflow tract.

3. Restrictive cardiomyopathy is stiffening of the walls of the ventricles and loss of ventricular compliance, resulting in decreased cardiac filling and predominant diastolic dysfunction.

4. Arrythmogenic right ventricular cardiomyopathy is characterized by the replacement of myocytes in the right ventricle with fatty, fibrous tissue.

5. Left ventricular non-compaction cardiomyopathy is characterized by arrhythmias, myocardial trabeculations, systemic thrombotic embolism and heart failure.

6. Myocarditis, mostly viral induced, has been considered among secondary cardiomyopathies as the pathogenesis of myocardial damage may evolve toward dilated cardiomyopathy.

Malnutrition is a significant clinical problem in children with cardiomyopathy due to an imbalance between nutritional intake and requirement. Nearly one-third of this high risk population will have some degree of malnutrition over the duration of their disease.[145] The disease is associated with increased caloric demands of the failing heart, increased work of breathing, and a general catabolic state of chronic illness. The most common reported causes include increased energy expenditure secondary to chronic disease, malabsorption, decreased appetite and chronically suboptimal oral intake, and psychosocial problems. Although it is apparent these patients are at increased nutritional risk, it is important to consider that poor nutrition may further lead to complications that may directly or indirectly impact heart function and overall clinical status.[145] Malnutrition has been shown to negatively affect mortality in infants awaiting heart transplant.[146] Infants, children, and adolescents with cardiomyopathy may also have need for a VAD as a bridge to transplantation.

One study evaluating cardiac outcomes in chronically ill children revealed that nutritional status was a strong and independent predictor of mortality and cardiac function.[147] Adequate nutrition forms an integral part of managing heart failure associated with cardiomyopathy. Nutritional rehabilitation should be instituted early and aggressively to compensate for heart failure and prevent a vicious downward cycle of growth failure and worsened clinical outcome. Optimal nutrition is usually estimated to be approximately 110–125% normal estimated energy requirements and is critical in providing affected children the means to withstand the detrimental metabolic effects of the disease, participate in rehabilitation, and recover from their illness.[145] The goal of therapy remains adequate EN; however, the hospitalized acutely ill patient with decompensated heart failure may not tolerate oral or enteral feeds. In such cases, PN should be initiated until transition to enteral feeds is tolerated.

Pulmonary Hypertension

New guidelines from the American Heart Association and American Thoracic Society were recently published in *Circulation* addressing diagnosis, evaluation, and treatment of pediatric pulmonary hypertension. Pulmonary hypertension is defined as a resting mean pulmonary artery pressure >25mm Hg beyond the first few months of life.[148] Varan and colleagues[43] investigated the prevalence of malnutrition and growth in 89 patients with CHD aged 1–45 months. Results showed 41.5%

were found to be below the 5th percentile for both weight-for-age and height-for-age. Nutritional complications have been underappreciated and guidelines are lacking, but it is well known that pulmonary hypertension can cause significant morbidity and mortality. Many patients with pulmonary hypertension or related pulmonary vascular disease have poor growth, impressive physical exam findings indicative of malnutrition, and feeding difficulties. Attention to nutritional needs and deficiencies is warranted. More research is needed to further develop nutritional guidelines for patients with pulmonary hypertension.

Lymphatic Disorders

The lymphatic system is a complex network of channels that transports lymphatic fluid produced in the tissues or organs. The lymphatic system plays a key role in immunity, active absorption and transport of cells, dietary fatty acids, proteins, macromolecules, and is vital to the circulatory system where it returns excess interstitial fluid from the tissues to the venous system.[149-151] The lymphatic system can be divided into three distinct sections: soft tissue lymphatics, intestinal lymphatics, and liver lymphatics.[150] Liver and intestinal lymphatics produce the majority of lymphatic fluid in the body. Fluid composition sampled from different areas of the lymphatic system can vary. The intestinal lymphatics transport chylomicrons and some proteins, whereas the liver is the largest producer of lymph and carriers a significant amount of proteins, particularly albumin.

There have been multiple lymphatic disorders described in the literature. One frequently seen complication or disorder in patients with CHD is chylothorax. Chylothorax is the presence of lymphatic fluid in the pleural space caused by damage to the thoracic duct or lympho-venous connections or secondary to lymphatic abnormalities. It is often a result of iatrogenic complications of cardiothoracic surgery, commonly caused by trauma to the thoracic duct or other surrounding lymphatic tributaries.[152-154] It has also been described in children with genetic syndromes associated with CHD, including trisomy 21, Noonan's and Turner's syndromes, and cardio-facio-cutaneous syndrome.[155-161] Furthermore, chylothorax can result from high central venous pressure within the **superior vena cava** (SVC), thereby affecting the pressure in the lymphatic system and inability of the lymphatic system to adequately drain into the bloodstream.[152,162] This is seen mainly in operations that cause increased SVC pressure, such as the hemi-Fontan or bidirectional Glenn, Fontan, and Senning procedures, and can also be seen in patients with thrombus occluding the SVC or subclavian vessels.[162]

Chyle is a white, milky-appearing substance composed of chylomicrons and lymph. Lymph fluid from the intestines, as well as the lower extremities and liver are transported by lymphatic channels that converge into the thoracic duct at the level of the cisterna chyli. The majority of terminal drainage of lymphatic fluid into the venous system is through the thoracic duct and main connection at the junction of the left subclavian and internal jugular veins.[150] The primary purpose of chyle is the absorption and transportation of **long-chain triglycerides** (LCT) in the intestines. Chyle is formed in the lacteals of the intestines during digestion in response to the presence of intraluminal fat. The chyle binds with LCT to form chylomicrons, which are then absorbed and transported by the intestinal lymphatics to the bloodstream. Chyle is also rich in proteins and is responsible for absorbing fat-soluble vitamins; therefore, high losses are of great nutritional concern.[153] When a person is fasting, the fluid can appear less white, and more yellowish or clear. Diagnosis of chyle can be made if there are elevated lymphocytes >80% absolute cell count, triglycerides >110mg/dL, white blood cell count >1000/μL, and high total protein content of 2–6g/dL in a sample of the pleural fluid.[153,162–165] Treating chylothorax can be multifactorial, but the primary goal remains conservative therapies directed to reduce intestinal lymphatic flow through dietary modifications and/or medications. The main therapies used in reducing chylous effusions include pleural drainage, initiating a restricted fat diet that contains minimal LCT and enriched with **medium-chain triglycerides** (MCT).[166] MCT are absorbed directly from the intestinal lumen into the portal system, as are carbohydrates and amino acids, and thus do not stimulate an increase in lymphatic flow. Nutritional management usually starts with trialing a low LCT and MCT-enriched formula or diet, observing for a reduction in chylous output, and if ineffective, providing gut rest with PN.[153,167] Formulas containing high amounts of MCT may not meet patients' minimum **essential fatty acid** (EFA) needs.

Essential fatty acid deficiency results when there is insufficient dietary intake of **linoleic acid** (LA) and **alpha-linolenic acid** (ALA). Deficiency is further exaggerated by increased metabolic demands required for growth and hypermetabolism after stress, injury, surgery, or sepsis. Therefore, it may be necessary in patients that are fed long term with specialty formulas restricting LCT to supplement with EFA in order to provide 1–4% and 0.2–1% of the total daily caloric intake from dietary LA and ALA, respectively, in order to prevent EFA.[153,167–169] Adequate intakes for LA and ALA are also defined by age group in the Dietary Reference Intake macronutrient guidelines.[170]

Clinical symptoms of a long term EFA deficiency may include growth retardation, impaired cell membrane and skin integrity, eczematous dermatitis, impaired cholesterol metabolism, poor neurocognitive development, poor wound healing and alopecia.[171] The biochemical changes in the presence of EFA deficiency can result in a reduced LA, reduced ALA, elevated mead acid or an elevated triene:tetraene ratio, which is calculated from the ratio of mead acid to arachidonic acid.[171,172] Periodic laboratory monitoring of EFA biochemical profiles should be monitored for patients on a restricted fat diet. Abnormal triene:tetraene (T:T) ratios have been classified as follows: mild deficiency (≥0.05), moderate deficiency (≥0.2), and severe deficiency (≥0.4).[173] Although a T:T ratio >0.2 is considered a biochemical EFA deficiency, clinical signs and symptoms of EFA deficiency may be more clinically detected at ratios ≥0.4.[171] Good concentrated sources of EFA that include both LA and ALA are walnut oil and flaxseed oil.[174,175] It is imperative that dietitians and clinicians promptly identify and treat subclinical EFA deficiency.

Formulas commonly used for managing chylothorax and other lymphatic disorders are listed in **TABLE 14.4** for comparison purposes. The literature has also demonstrated safety and efficacy in the medical nutrition treatment of chylothorax in infants with skimmed breast milk, with the fat removed via centrifugation.[176–178] Young infants with chylothorax may benefit from using skimmed breast milk given the immunological properties and improved GI tolerance.[175] Several published protocols for treating chylothorax have recommended continuing a low-fat, MCT-enriched diet for four to six weeks after resolution of chylous drainage, then resuming a regular diet, breast milk or standard formula.[179–184]

Medical management of chylous effusions may include using somatostatin and its analogue octreotide. It is known to reduce intestinal secretions and inhibit lymph excretion.[185] Caution must be used when enterally feeding patients receiving somatostatin or octreotide because splanchnic circulation may be diminished; GI side effects should be closely monitored.[185]

Protein losing enteropathy (PLE) is a devastating disease characterized by the severe loss of enteric proteins, predominantly albumin, through the intestinal tract. Clinical symptoms of PLE include diarrhea, ascites and abdominal distention, malabsorption, and soft tissue swelling. Itkin and colleagues[186] have demonstrated through liver lymphangiography that PLE in patients with CHD and elevated central venous pressures is caused by lymphatic leakage into the intestines. Patients with CHF were studied and imaging showed increased liver lymph production. The increase in flow of lymphatic fluid in the liver results in dilation of the hepatoduodenal lymphatic vessels and lacteals in the duodenum, which subsequently causes leakage of lymph fluid rich in proteins into the intestine. MUAC measurements should be part of the anthropometric assessment for patients with PLE as weight may be falsely affected by ascites, steroids, or shifts in fluid status.

TABLE 14.4 Formulas with Low LCT and/or High MCT Content for Lymphatic Disorders

Formula	Type	MCT:LCT Ratio	Percent Calories from LCT Fat	LCT Fat g per 100 Calories	Protein g per 100 Calories
Enfaport™* (Mead Johnson)	Liq Concentrate 30 cal/ounce	83:17	7.8	0.9	3.5
Lipistart™* (Néstle)	Powder	80:20	7.6	0.82	3
Monogen®* (Nutricia)	Powder	83:17	4.5	0.5	2.9
Portagen®*a (Mead Johnson)	Powder	87:13	5.5	0.6	3.5
Tolerex®*** (Néstle)	Powder	0:100	2	0.2	2.1
Vivonex Pediatric®*** (Néstle)	Powder	70:30	7.5	0.87	3
Vivonex TEN®*** (Néstle)	Powder	0:100	3	0.3	3.8

*Contains milk proteins.

**Elemental, 100% free amino acids.

aLong Term Usage: Portagen powder is not nutritionally complete. If used long term, supplementation of essential fatty acids and ultra-trace minerals should be considered [manufacturer's notation].

Abbreviations: MCT, medium chain triglycerides; LCT, long chain triglycerides; g, grams.

Data from manufacturers' product labels as of 11/2017. Please note product composition may be changed by the discretion of manufacturers. Information may be obtained at the following websits:

https://www.meadjohnson.com/pediatrics/us-en/
https://www.nestlehealthscience.us/
https://www.nutricia-na.com/

Furthermore, fat-soluble vitamins and B-vitamin levels should be screened and monitored for patients with persistent high output chylous effusions or prolonged malabsorption in patients with PLE as they are at high risk for deficiencies.[153,164,167] Large volume output from chylothorax can cause high protein losses, resulting in low albumin levels, and losses of fat, electrolytes, immunoglobulins, and other minerals that may be protein-bound, such as zinc, copper, and selenium. Chylous losses may also lead to hypovolemia, which can lead to hemodynamic instability.[153] Sodium and calcium levels may be decreased, and metabolic acidosis may be seen in patients with high output. One study measured fat-soluble vitamins and plasma and erythrocyte membrane fatty acid levels in patients with CHD who developed chylothorax after cardiac surgery. Laboratory values were taken at baseline and after 28 days on a MCT-rich diet. Results showed that administration of a MCT-rich diet for 28 days (range 27–31 days) was an effective treatment in the resolution of chylothorax. Data also showed a reduction in vitamin E status and linoleic acid levels from baseline, but without any symptoms of deficiency. Maintaining a restricted fat diet longer than 4 weeks may put individuals at increased risk for deficiencies.

Genetic Syndromes and Chromosome Anomalies

Many genetic syndromes and chromosome anomalies are associated with CHD, including Down syndrome (Trisomy 21), Trisomy 13 and 18, Turner's syndrome, William's syndrome, DiGeorge and/or velo-cardio-facial syndrome, Marfan syndrome, Ellis-van Crevald syndrome, Noonan's syndrome, VACTERL syndrome (tracheal and esophageal malformations associated with vertebral, anorectal, cardiac, renal, radial, and limb abnormalities), and CHARGE syndrome, which includes coloboma, heart defect, atresia choanae, retardation of growth and development, genital hypoplasia, ear anomalies and deafness.

Within the spectrum of genetic syndromes, many of these infants and children are likely to have feeding difficulties and may be genetically prone to growth disturbances. For infants with Down syndrome, low muscle tone may contribute to poor oromotor skills, as well as constipation and other digestive problems.[187,188] DiGeorge syndrome is a genetic disorder with varying conditions present in each infant with the syndrome. An estimated 90% of patients with DiGeorge syndrome have a chromosomal 22q11 deletion, which is associated with a wide range of CHD.[189,190] Other conditions common to this syndrome include hypocalcemia, immunodeficiency, dysmorphic facial appearance, palate anomalies, speech and feeding disorders, lack of or underdeveloped thymus and parathyroid glands, and neurocognitive and behavioral disorders.[191,192]

Infants and children with CHARGE syndrome should be monitored closely for feeding difficulties, growth, and adequacy of nutrition intake.[193] At birth, children with CHARGE syndrome usually have normal weights and lengths; however, growth and developmental retardation may become more apparent as the child matures.[194] CHARGE syndrome characteristics also include cranial nerve dysfunction in 86–100% of patients, which causes abnormal suck-swallow coordination, gastrointestinal peristalsis, GER, esophageal dyskinesia, and abdominal constipation.[195] Aspiration is also a frequent problem due to swallowing abnormalities, but can also be secondary to severe GER disease. Approximately 90% of children with CHARGE syndrome require gastrostomy, jejunostomy, and/or nasogastric tubes.[194]

Feeding in children with genetic and chromosomal anomalies can be a significant challenge for families and medical professionals. These children may require aggressive medical nutrition management, often requiring long term enteral access via gastrostomy and jejunostomy feeding tubes. Gastroesophageal fundoplication may be indicated for GER that does not respond to conventional medical therapy.

Chronic Care

Feeding methodology often becomes a concern in the follow up care of infants and children with cardiac anomalies. In infancy, when caloric needs are very high, an infant may eat eagerly for a short time and then tire quickly. Parents and caregivers may assume the infant is full, but it may be that the infant lacks the energy needed to adequately feed. Other infants and children may refuse to eat or feed very poorly. Thommessen and associates[196] found 65% of parents of infants and children with CHD document feeding problems. The reported feeding problems were a good predictor of low voluntary food intake and suboptimal growth outcome.

As previously noted, higher calorie formulas or supplements may be used to decrease the volume needed for optimal caloric intake. For infants who may orally feed, oral feedings should typically not exceed 20–30 minutes so that energy expenditure does not exceed caloric intake. If an infant is unable to take a desired volume within that time, an indwelling nasogastric tube may be used to give the remainder of the feed. If an infant is close to goal, he or she may be able to feed by mouth during the day and receive overnight tube feedings to make up the daytime deficit. Frequent follow up care with an outpatient dietitian should be recommended to ensure that projected goal volumes and the rate of growth are appropriate for age. For some infants, 24-hour continuous enteral infusions may be needed. Attempts can be made to compress feedings into a shorter infusion time, giving a few hours off for social and developmental purposes. For infants and children not able to take oral feeds, an oral stimulation program should be initiated. Oral motor therapies can be instituted by an experienced occupational therapist or speech-language pathologist.

For infants and children who are thought to need tube feeding assistance for more than 3 months, a **gastric tube** (G-tube) is a positive step toward simplifying the care. G-tubes can be inserted surgically or endoscopically (percutaneous endoscopic gastrostomy). G-tubes and tube feedings should be viewed as tools to improve the quality of life. Without the pressure of forced or unpleasant mealtimes or around-the-clock marathons, feeding can be pleasurable, with the best possible behavioral and developmental outcome. Oral feedings should be a pleasant time for both the caregiver and the infant or child.

Monitoring growth velocity is vital in infants and children with CHD. It is important to screen those at risk for malnutrition during follow up care. Preventive measures and early nutritional interventions are the best approach to correcting growth problems in childhood. Multidisciplinary teamwork is again important; growth or appetite problems can be caused by a change in clinical course or by a change in medication. It is necessary to consider all possibilities for malnutrition when cardiac status is stable and calorie intake appears sufficient for age-appropriate growth. Reevaluation of all parameters on an ongoing basis provides the best outcome.

Special considerations and support should be given to parents and caregivers of infants with complex CHD, especially those requiring tube feeding at home. Parents of infants with complex CHD have been shown to have higher parenteral stress and anxiety than parents of healthy infants and children.[197,198] Focus group sessions of mothers of infants with CHD requiring home tube feeds has shown that growth and feeding contributes to ongoing family stress. Mothers have expressed particular concerns with meeting infant weight gain goals, the demands around feeding times, the energy and time involved administering tube feeds, and cleaning and replacing the tube should it become dislodged. Stress was also increased with frequent vomiting, confused hunger cues, nighttime tube feedings with lack of sleep, and long term worrying about the effects of tube feedings on their infants' ability to have normal feeding in the future.[33] Early family interventions and considerations to EN regimen schedules for ease at home may promote parental compliance and ease anxiety.

Pediatric Obesity and Hyperlipidemia

Childhood overnight and obesity rates have increased at alarming rates and may lead to comorbidities such as diabetes mellitus, coronary artery disease, hypertension, pulmonary disease, and peripheral vascular disease. Children with congenital and acquired heart disease are not immune to the growing obesity epidemic and may suffer the complications of obesity more so than children without heart disease.[31] In a multicenter cohort study, obesity was associated with increased risk of adverse perioperative outcomes in children, adolescents and young adults between the ages of 10–35 years undergoing a cardiothoracic operation with or without CPB.[199] Obesity was significantly correlated with an increased incidence of wound infection or dehiscence, hospital length of stay, and operative mortality. Furthermore, obese patients who have been converted to the Fontan circulation may suffer the consequences of having an increased afterload and ventricular mass.[200]

Several theoretical possibilities explain why this population may be at higher risk for obesity. Parents are often misinformed regarding physical activity restrictions.[201] Patients with heart disease infrequently require strict limitations on activity, but may be perceived as more fragile and thus still avoid participation in activities that may put additional stress on the heart. Patients with heart disease who were advised to restrict their activity and lead a more sedentary lifestyle have been found to be more likely to become either overweight or obese.[202] Furthermore, children with a history of heart failure who had previous difficulties gaining weight during infancy and early childhood and fed high calorie formulas or diets may also continue a high calorie diet even after surgical repair or resolution of heart failure, when high energy requirements are no longer needed.

Pediatric cardiologists who have traditionally focused on assessing the adequacy of surgical repairs and progression of heart disease are now faced with managing the consequences of a preventable condition. Cardiologists should discuss diet and nutrition, weight, and activity with their patients and ensure that they are receiving preventative counseling on the basis of age, degree of excessive weight, and the presence of comorbidities. Nutrition counseling should be recommended when needed. A well-defined exercise program should be created for each individual patient based on the severity of the cardiac disease.[31] Children with mild forms of disease should be allowed to participate in most sports. Participation in intermediate sports should be based on an individual assessment for children with moderate disease, with

consideration of exercise testing. For children with severe heart disease, specific programs delineating the type of sport and limitations should be developed on an individual basis. If patients are advised against physical exertion, they should subsequently be counseled on appropriate dietary habits.[202] As rates of survival to adulthood for patients with CHD have markedly improved and are estimated to be as much as 85%,[203] the importance of preventative counseling and understanding the consequences of obesity with consequent atherosclerosis and hyperlipidemia increases.

Hyperlipidemia is an elevation of lipids in the bloodstream. These lipids include cholesterol, cholesterol esters, phospholipids, and triglycerides. They are transported in the blood as part of lipoproteins. The aim of nutrition management in pediatric hyperlipidemia is to provide nutrition for normal growth and development, as well as to normalize lipid levels as much as possible to decrease the risk of cardiovascular disease.[204] The Centers for Disease Control and Prevention[205] analyzed results from the **National Health and Nutrition Examination Survey** (NHANES) for 2011–2014 on the prevalence of elevated total cholesterol, low **high density lipoprotein** (HDL) cholesterol, and high non-HDL cholesterol among children and adolescents ages 6–19 years. Results showed that one in five youths had high total cholesterol, low HDL or high non-HDL cholesterol. Prevalence of abnormal cholesterol among children and adolescents with obesity was almost 3–5 times higher than for those youths of normal weight. The **National Cholesterol Education Program** (NCEP) and the AHA advocate dietary changes for all healthy children over 2 years of age and for adolescents.[206,207] The **Therapeutic Lifestyle Changes** (TLC) diet macronutrients recommendations are 50–60% of total calories from carbohydrates, 15% of total calories from protein, and limiting total fat to 25–35% of total calories.[206] Saturated fat should be limited to less than 7% of total calories. Therapeutic options for lowering LDL cholesterol include consuming 2g/day of plant stanols/sterols and increased viscous (soluble) fiber.[206] Before the age of 2 years, restriction of fat intake may result in altered growth.[208] The **American Academy of Pediatrics** (AAP) recommends that total fat intake should not fall below 20% of total calories for children and adolescents.[208]

The 2015–2020 Dietary Guidelines for Americans emphasize the importance of a diet low in saturated and trans fat, and rich in fruits, vegetables, whole grains, fat-free and low-fat dairy products, and lean meat, fish, and poultry.[209] For children at higher risk, the NCEP TLC guidelines offer dietary therapy for subgroups of people with specific medical conditions and risk factors, which include high LDL cholesterol, dyslipidemia, coronary heart disease or other cardiovascular disease, diabetes mellitus, insulin resistance, or metabolic syndrome. Refer to the NCEP guidelines for medical and dietary management of lipid serum levels.[206] If serum levels are not improved with dietary intervention alone, medication may be considered for children over 10 years of age.[208] Strong evidence from both prospective and randomized controlled trials has shown that *dietary patterns* that reduce intake of dietary cholesterol are associated with decreased risk of cardiovascular disease, and moderate evidence suggests a further association with reduced obesity risk.[209]

Increasing fiber intake is advocated for all children over 2 years of age. The Academy of Nutrition and Dietetics recommends children consume a number of grams of fiber each day that equals their age plus 5 additional grams.[210] This rule should be applied throughout adolescence until the age of 20, at which time adult guidelines should be followed. Fiber may be helpful in reducing serum cholesterol. Studies on the lipid-lowering effect of fiber in children have been inconclusive.[211] However, one study found water-soluble fibers, such as psyllium, enhanced the hypocholesterolemia effect of NCEP dietary changes by lowering LDL cholesterol an additional 5–10%.[212] A dietary intervention program designed for preschoolers, Healthy Start has been shown to reduce serum cholesterol when measured over the course of the school year. This program in a largely minority Head Start preschool population reduced the total and saturated fat content of snacks and meals.[213]

A few studies indicate that nutrition education and dietary intervention can improve weight loss in obese children, reduce obesity-related health risks, and improve dyslipidemias.[213-217] In a study by Reinehr and Andler,[218] weight loss and a reduction in body mass index were shown to improve the atherogenic profile and insulin resistance in children 4–15 years of age. Activity is important in reducing the likelihood of childhood obesity, and it is also an important facet of promoting cardiovascular health.[219] Playing outdoors and high-activity playing have been shown to have positive effects on cardiovascular health in children ages 4–7 years.[220] The activity level of the family influences the activity of the children. A family commitment to a healthy lifestyle, including diet and physical activity, is essential.

▶ Conclusion

In summary, congenital cardiac defects remain one of the most common defects in the US with approximately one fourth of defects labeled as critical, requiring surgery within the first year of life. Advances in early detection of cardiac anomalies is ongoing and can impact outcomes. Often these patients undergo an array of medical and surgical management to correct or palliate one's cardiac lesion. Because of this variation, cardiac patients often demonstrate some form of growth failure and remain at increased risk for malnutrition. Research has identified that growth failure in cardiac patients is attributed to a variety of factors. Some of these factors include inadequate energy intake, poor feeding skills, increased metabolic demands, and disturbances in GI function contributing to inefficient absorption and utilization.

Aggressive nutritional intervention is often warranted to attenuate complications. This may include: supplemental EN and/or PN while critically ill; or high calorie concentration of enteral feeds if fluid is restricted; protocolized feeding and oral strategies if concern for intolerance or poor oral skills; and unique diet modification or supplementation. Preventive strategies like the use of human milk or algorithms in nutrition management for chylothorax are potential therapies believed to contribute to reducing poor nutritional outcomes. Appropriate monitoring and follow up is ongoing and imperative throughout each phase of care in order to improve the nutritional status for each cardiac patient. Adherence and tolerance to nutritional interventions should be assessed heterogeneously. With concrete understanding of one's cardiac anatomy and through optimal interventions, monitoring and evaluation, normal growth and neurodevelopment outcomes can be achieved in complex cardiac patients.

🔍 CASE STUDY

Nutrition Assessment

Client History

JL is a male delivered at an outside hospital with suspected coarctation of the aorta by cesarean delivery at 38 weeks 5 days gestation to a 39 year old mother and birth weight of 3430 grams (42nd percentile, z-score -0.18). Complications of pregnancy included insufficient prenatal care, poorly controlled type 1 diabetes mellitus and breech presentation. He had persistent respiratory distress requiring escalation to **Continuous Positive Airway Pressure** (CPAP) after birth. Initial glucose at the outside hospital was 30mg/dL, requiring a dextrose bolus. He was placed on 12.5% dextrose fluids at 80mL/kg upon arrival. His echocardiogram confirmed a diagnosis of coarctation and **ventricular septal defect** (VSD). Preoperative course was complicated by hypoglycemia and respiratory status. He was managed on PGE and **high flow nasal cannula** (HFNC) until he underwent repair of coarctation and VSD closure, **patent ductus arteriosus** (PDA) ligation on **day of life** (DOL) 8. He was extubated on postoperative day (POD) 3 with notable stridor.

(continues)

🔍 CASE STUDY (continued)

Food/Nutrition-Related History

No enteral feeds were started in the preoperative period due to high respiratory support. PN was started on DOL2 and continued until surgery. Preoperatively, he was prescribed to receive 109 mL/kg/day and 3.5 g/kg of protein, 2 g/kg of **intralipids** (IL) and **glucose infusion rate** (GIR) of 15.4 mg/kg/min for a total calorie of 109 kcal/kg/day. Postoperatively, due to fluid restriction, nutrition was delayed until POD4 and **nasoduodenal** (ND) feeds on a standard enteral formula were then initiated. He reached goal feed rate of 21 mL/hr × 24 hours within 26 hours of starting and began fortification to 22 kcal/oz on POD6/DOL14. Concentrating caloric density further was delayed secondary to frequent interruptions to enteral feeds. During his feed advancement, he was also noted to have persistent hypocalcemia (low ionized calcium) requiring multiple calcium boluses. Genetics labs (FISH testing) were sent. Otolaryngology was also consulted due to stridor and poor vocal quality, with identification of bilateral vocal cord immobility. Feeds were therefore kept nasoduodenal at this time. Enteral feeds were interrupted again on POD8 due to escalation in respiratory support and need for reintubation. His feeds were restarted at full rate shortly after intubation. On POD10, JL was extubated for a second time to HFNC. During POD6–10, he received 50% of his prescribed enteral nutrition goal due to interruptions to feeding and slow advancement. PN was not initiated postoperatively due to fluid restriction and aggressive diuresis. On POD13, feeds were fortified to 24 kcal/oz to provide 119 kcal/kg and 2.7 g/kg of protein.

On POD14, a **videos swallow study** (VSS) was completed per routine swallowing protocol following coarctation and found deep penetration with ultra-preemie nipple. He was subsequently only allowed to eat by mouth with speech therapy. After his VSS, JL continued to require non-invasive respiratory support and intermittent interruptions to EN. He was increased to 26 kcal/oz on POD17 to promote weight gain as anthropometrics showed he had lost 11% body weight since birth. At this time, a wound **vacuum-assisted closure** (VAC) was placed for mediastinal dehiscence and poor healing. Scheduled wound healing vitamins were initiated as well as calcium supplementation for persistent hypocalcemia.

On POD25, JL required reintubation again due to hypercarbia/hypoxia event. At this time, JL remained ND fed and was on full nutrition receiving 132 kcal/kg, 3 g protein/kg. He is now being assessed for tracheostomy placement. Sternal wound is showing slow improvement now with more consistent nutrition intake.

Anthropometric Measurements

Birth	Weight: 3.43 kg z-score −0.18	Length: 49 cm z-score −0.37	Wt/length: 50th–75th percentile z-score 0.77
DOL14	Weight: 3.04 kg z-score −1.98	Length: 49 cm z-score −1.89	Wt/length:15th–50th percentile z-score −0.33
DOL28	Weight: 3.42 kg z-score −1.65	Length: 49 cm z-score −1.89	Wt/length: 25th–50th percentile z-score −0.33
DOL35	Weight: 3.7 kg z-score −1.6	Length: 49.5 cm z-score −2.97	Wt/length: 93% z-score 1.5

Estimated Nutrition Needs

Calories: Dietary Reference Intake (DRI) + catch-up growth to equal 115–135 kcal/kg/day
Protein: >2.4–4 g/kg/day
Fluid: <150 mL/kg/day for enteral nutrition given diuresis
Biochemical Data, Medical Tests, and Procedures
Labs on DOL35: ↓ below normal; ↑ above normal)

Na: 140	Cl: 96 ↓	BUN: 23	Gluc: 97	Mg: 2.3	Ionized Ca: 1.33
K: 3.3 ↓	CO_2: 37 ↑	Creat: 0.24	Ca: 9.7	Phos: 4.9	Alb: 2.7

Vitamin 25(OH)D: 40.4 (normal)
FISH: no genetic deletion per report

Current Medications

Zinc sulfate, ranitidine, vitamin C, folic acid, furosemide, lansoprazole, calcitriol, calcium carbonate, poly-vi-sol 1 mL/day, propranolol.

Assessment on DOL35

JL is currently receiving standard infant formula fortified to 26 kcal/oz at 23 mL/hr × 24 hr via ND tube. Current weight is 3.7 kg. He remains intubated. Continues to show improvement in sternal wound healing.

 Weight gain velocity is suboptimal for age, and linear growth z-score is declining. He may benefit from increasing total caloric and protein intake in order to achieve optimal growth. JL is on a proton pump inhibitor for reflux precautions given complicated respiratory course. Labs reflect low creatinine and, chloride, and elevated CO_2 levels. His ionized calcium and vitamin D levels represent adequate intake of these nutrients with current supplementation and feeds.

Nutrition Diagnosis

Based on the information detailed above, a nutritional problem or diagnosis is made.

Nutrition Interventions

Because JL's weight gain has been suboptimal, recommend additional protein supplementation to provide 3.5 g/kg/day and weight-adjust volume to provide 150 mL/kg (24 mL/hr) at current body weight of 3.7 kg.

Questions for the Reader

1. How would you classify JL's nutritional status on DOL14?
2. What was the nutrition prescription on POD6? Fluid (mL/kg/day)? Calories (kcal/kg/day)? Protein (g/kg/day) based on birth weight? (Standard formula providing 2.2 grams (g) protein per 100 calories)
3. On average, how many grams per day per World Health Organization (WHO) growth velocity guidelines[221] should JL gain given his current age? How many grams per day did JL gain over the past 7 days (between DOL28 and DOL35)?
4. Write one Nutrition Diagnosis (PES) statement that describes one nutrition problem, etiology and signs/symptoms identified at DOL35.
5. How many calories and protein per kg are provided in his feeding regimen on DOL35? (assuming protein intake is 2.2 grams per 100 calories)
6. What nutritional parameters would you want to continue to monitor?
7. How would you diagnose JL's pediatric malnutrition on DOL35?
8. Describe some nutritional interventions that may have improved his nutrient delivery throughout the course of his admission and overall nutritional outcome.
9. Discuss your goals for nutrition before discharge?

Review Questions

1. Describe common risk factors associated with malnutrition and growth failure in CHD patients.

2. Name the two classifications of CHD and provide an example defect in each. Describe the characteristics of each classification.

3. What hormones are believed to play a role in heart failure and growth?

4. At what day of life (DOL) does ASPEN clinical guidelines recommend initiating enteral nutrition for those at high risk for NEC?

5. What barriers may preclude the cardiac patient from receiving optimal nutrition during the critical phase of care, specifically postoperatively?

6. Name the most common complication following pediatric heart surgery. Can you provide two additional post-operative surgical complications?

7. What calorie per kg do cardiac infants typically require for catch-up growth?

8. Please list the specific vitamin deficiencies one may be concerned with in patients with heart failure or on MCS?

9. What are the classifications of cardiomyopathy? Please describe.

10. What diet modification is used in the treatment of chylothorax? What type of nutritional deficiency may result from this modification? How would you monitor for this deficiency?

References

1. Kay JD, Colan SD, Graham TP. Congestive heart failure in pediatric patients. *Am Heart J.* 2001;142(5):923–928.

2. Gilboa SM, Devine OJ, Kucik JE, et al. Congenital heart defects in the United States: estimating the magnitude of the affected population in 2010. *Circulation.* 2016;134(2):101–109.

3. Pasquali SK., Sun JL, d'Almada P, et al. Center variation in cost and outcomes for congenital heart surgery. *Circ Cardiovasc Qual Outcomes.* 2011;4(3):306–312.

4. Oster ME, Lee KA, Honein MA, et al. Temporal trends in survival among infants with critical congenital heart defects. *Pediatrics.* 2013;131(5):e1502–e1508.

5. Levey A, Glickstein JS, Kleinman CS, et al. The impact of prenatal diagnosis of complex congenital heart disease on neonatal outcomes. *Pediatr Cardiol.* 2010;31(5):587–597.

6. Grosse SD, Riehle-Colarusso T, Gaffney M, et al. CDC Grand Rounds: Newborn screening for hearing loss and critical congenital heart disease. *MMWR Morb Mortal Wkly Rep.* 2017;66(33):888–890.

7. Engle, MS, Kochilas, LK. Pulse Oximetry screening: a review of diagnosing critical congenital heart disease in newborns. *Med Devices:Evidence Res.* 2016;9:199–203.

8. Floh AA, Slicker J, Schwartz SM. Nutrition and mesenteric issues in pediatric cardiac critical care. *Pediatr Crit Care Med.* 2016;17(8):S243–S249.

9. Davis D., Davis S, Cotman K, et al. Feeding difficulties and growth delay in children with hypoplastic left heart syndrome versus d-transportation of the great arteries. *Pediatr Cardiol.* 2008;29(2):328–33.

10. Mehrizi A, Drash A. Growth disturbance in congenital heart disease. *J Pediatr.* 1962;61:418–429.

11. Glassman MS, Woolf PK, Schwarz SM. Nutritional considerations in children with congenital heart disease. In: Baker SB, Baker RD Jr, Davis A, eds. *Pediatric Enteral Nutrition.* New York, NY: Chapman & Hall; 1994:340.

12. Venogopalan P, Akinbami FO, Al-Minai KM, et al. Malnutrition in children with congenital heart disease. *J Saudi Med J.* 2001;22:1964–1967.

13. Cameron JW, Rosenthal A, Olson AD. Malnutrition in hospitalized children with congenital heart disease. *Arch Pediatr Adolesc Med.* 1995;149:1098–1102.

14. Villasis-Keever MA, Aquiles Pineda-Cruz R, Halley-Castillo E, et al. Frequency and risk factors associated with malnutrition in children with congenital cardiopathy. *Saluda Publica Mex.* 2001;43:313–323.

15. Thompson Chagoyan OC, Reyes Tsubaki N, Rubiela Barrios OL, et al. The nutritional status of the child with congenital cardiopathy. *Arch Inst Cardiol Mex.* 1998;68:119–123.

16. Dimiti AI, Anabwani GM. Anthropometric measurements in children with congenital heart disease at Kenyatta National Hospital (1985–1986). *East Afr Med J.* 1991;68:757–764.

17. Leite HP, de Camargo Carvalho AC, Fisberg M. Nutritional status of children with congenital heart disease and left-to-right shunt. The importance of the presence of pulmonary hypertension. *Arq Bras Cardiol.* 1995;65:403–407.

18. Miyague NI, Cardoso SM, Meyer F, et al. Epidemiological study of congenital heart defects in children and adolescents. Analysis of 4,538 cases. *Arq Bras Cardiol.* 2003;80:269–278.

19. Jacobs EG, Leung ML, Karlberg JP. Postnatal growth in southern Chinese children with symptomatic congenital heart disease. *J Pediatr Endocrinol Metab.* 2000;3:387–401.

20. Tambic-Bukovac L, Malcic I. Growth and development in children with congenital heart disease. *Lijec Vjesh.* 1993;115:79–84.

21. Mitchell IM, Logan RW, Pollock JCS, et al. Nutritional status of children with congenital heart disease. *Br Heart J.* 1995;73(3): 277–283.

22. Nydegger A, Bines JE. Energy metabolism in infants with congenital heart disease. *Nutr.* 2006;22:697–704.

23. Steltzer M, Rudd N, Pick B. Nutrition care for newborns with congenital heart disease. *Clin Perinatol.* 2005;32:1017–1030.

24. Anderson JB, Iyer SB, Schidlow DN, et al. Variation in growth of infants with a single ventricle. *J Pediatr.* 2012;161(1):16–21.

25. Carlson SJ, Ryan JM. Congenital heart disease. In: Groh-Wargo S, Thompson M, Cox J, eds. *Nutritional Care for High Risk Newborns*, rev ed. Chicago, IL: Precept Press, Inc.; 2000:397–408.

26. Marino BS, Lipkin PH, Newburger JW, et al. Neurodevelopmental outcomes in children with congenital heart disease: evaluation and management: a scientific statement from the American Heart Association. *Cir.* 2012;126(9):1143–1172.

27. Leitch CA. Growth, nutrition and energy expenditure in pediatric heart failure. *Prog Pediatr Cardiol.* 2000;11:195–202.

28. Vaidyanathan B, Radhakrishnan R, Sarala DA, et al. What determines nutritional recovery in malnourished children after correction of congenital heart defects? *Pediatr.* 2009;124(2):e294–e299.

29. Silberback M, Shumaker D, Menshe V, Cobanoglu A, Morris C. Predicting hospital discharge and length of stay for congenital heart surgery. *Am J Cardiol.* 1993;72:958–963.

30. Eskedal LT, Hagemo PS, Seem E, et al. Impaired weight gain predicts risk of late death after surgery for congenital heart defects. *Arch Dis Child.* 2008;93(6):495–501.

31. Shustak RJ, McGuire SB, October TW, Phoon CK, Chun AJ. Prevalence of obesity among patients with congenital and acquired heart disease. *Pediatr Cardiol.* 2012;33(1):8–14.

32. The Cincinnati Children's Hospital Medical Center. Heart Institute Encyclopedia. Available at: https://www.cincinnatichildrens.org/patients/child/encyclopedia. Accessed April 16, 2018.

33. Medoff-Cooper B, Naim M, Torowicz D, et al. Feeding, growth, and nutrition in children with congenitally malformed hearts. *Cardiol Young.* 2010;20(Suppl 3):149–153.

34. Blasquez A, Clouzeau H, Fayon M, et al. Evaluation of nutritional status and support in children with congenital heart disease. *Eur J Clin Nutr.* 2016;70:528–531.

35. Toole BJ, Toole LE, Kyle UG, et al. Perioperative nutritional support and malnutrition in infants and children with congenital heart disease. *Congenit Heart Dis.* 2014;9(1):15–25.

36. Ravishankar C, Zak V, Williams IA, et al. Association of impaired linear growth and worse neurodevelopmental outcome in infants with single ventricle physiology: a report from the pediatric heart network infant single ventricle trial. *J Pediatr.* 2013;162(2):250–256.

37. Daymont C, Neal A, Prosnitz A, Cohen M. Growth in children with congenital heart disease. *Pediatr.* 2012;131(1):236–242.

38. Becker PJ, Nieman-Carney L, Corkins MR. Consensus Statement of the Academy of Nutrition and Dietetics/American Society for Parenteral and Enteral Nutrition: indicators recommended for the identification and documentation of pediatric malnutrition (undernutrition). *J Acad Nutr Diet.* 2014;114:1988–2000.

39. Forchielli ML, McColl R, Walker WA, et al. Children with congenital heart disease: a nutrition challenge. *Nutr Rev.* 1994;52:348–353.

40. Cheung MMH, Davis AM, Wilkinson JL, Weintraub RG. Long term somatic growth after repair of tetralogy of Fallot: evidence for restoration of genetic growth potential. *Heart.* 2003;89:1340–1343.

41. Vogt KN, Manlhiot C, Van Arsdell G, et al. Somatic growth in children with single ventricle physiology impact of physiologic state. *J Am Coll Cardiol.* 2007;50(19):1876–1883.

42. Modi P, Suleiman MS, Reeves BC, et al. Basal metabolic state of hearts of patients with congenital heart disease: the effects of cyanosis, age, and pathology. *Ann Thorac Surg.* 2004;78(5):1710–1716.

43. Varan B, Tokel K, Yilmaz G. Malnutrition and growth failure in cyanotic and acyanotic congenital heart disease with and without pulmonary hypertension. *Arch Dis Child.* 1999;81(1):49–52.

44. Umansky R, Hauck AJ. Factors in the growth of children with patent ductus arteriosis. *Pediatrics.* 1992;146:1078–1084.

45. Okoromah C, Ekure E, Lesi F. Prevalence, profile and predictors of malnutrition in children with congenital heart defects: a case-control observational study. *Arch Dis Child.* 2011;96:354–360.

46. Hsu D, Pearson G. Heart failure in children: Part 1: history, etiology, and pathophysiology. *Circ Heart Fail.* 2009;2:63–70.

47. Krieger I. Growth failure and congenital heart disease. Energy and nitrogen balance in infants. *Am J Dis Child.* 1970;120:497–502.

48. Huse DM, Feldt RH, Nelson RA, et al. Infants with congenital heart disease. *Am J Dis Child.* 1975;129:65–69.

49. Yahav J, Avigad S, Frand M, et al. Assessment of intestinal and cardiorespiratory function in children with congenital heart disease on high calorie formulas. *J Pediatr Gastroenterol Nutr.* 1985;4:778–785.

50. Hansen SR, Dorup I. Energy and nutrient intakes in congenital heart disease. *Acta Paediatr.* 1993;82:166–172.

51. Barton JS, Hindmarsh PC, Scrimgeour CM, et al. Energy expenditure in congenital heart disease. *Arch Dis Child.* 1994;70:5–9.

52. Van Der Kuip M, Hoos MB, Forget PP, Westerterp KR, Gemke RJ, De Meer K. Energy expenditure in infants with congenital heart disease, including a meta-analysis. *Acta Paediatr.* 2003;92:921–927.

53. Davis D, Davis S, Cotman K, et al. Feeding difficulties and growth delay in children with hypoplastic left heart syndrome versus d-transposition of the great arteries. *Pediatr Cardiol.* 2008;29(2):328–333.

54. Kelleher D, Lauseen P, Teixeira-Pinto M, Duggan C. Growth and correlates of nutrition status among infants with hypoplastic left heart syndrome (HLHS) after stage 1 Norwood procedure. *Nutrition.* 2006;22:237–244.

55. Williams RV, Zak V, Ravishankar C, et al. Factors affecting growth in infants with single ventricle physiology: a report from the Pediatric Heart Network Infant Single Ventricle Trial. *J Pediatr.* 2011;159(6):1017–1022.

56. Hill GD, Hehir DA, Bartz PJ, et al. Effect of feeding modality on interstage growth after stage I palliation: a report from the National Pediatric Cardiology Quality Improvement Collaborative. *J Thorac Cardiovasc Surg.* 2014;148(4):1534–1539.

57. Leitch CA, Karn CA, Peppard RJ, et al. Increased energy expenditure in infants with cyanotic congenital heart disease. *J Pediatr.* 1998;133:755–760.

58. Broekhoff C, Houwen RHJ, de Meer K. Energy expenditure in congenital heart disease [commentary]. *J Pediatr Gastroenterol Nutr.* 1995;21:322–323.

59. Irving SY, Medoff-Cooper B, Stouffer NO, et al. Resting energy expenditure at 3 months of age following neonatal surgery for congenital heart disease. *Congenit Heart Dis.* 2013;8(4):343–351.

60. Stranway A, Fowler R, Cunningkam K, et al. Diet and growth in congenital heart disease. *Pediatrics.* 1976;57:75–86.

61. Dinleyici EC, Kilic Z, Buyukkaragoz B, et al. Serum IGF-1, IGFBP-3 and growth hormone levels in children with congenital heart disease: relationship with nutritional status, cyanosis and left ventricular functions. *Neuro Endocrinol Lett.* 2007;28(3):279–283.

62. Surmeli-Onay O, Cindik N, Kinik ST, et al. The effect of corrective surgery on serum IGF-1, IGFBP-3 levels and growth in children with congenital heart disease. *J Pediatr Endocrinol Metab.* 2011;24(7–8):483–487.

63. Barton JS, Hindmarsh PC, Preece MA. Serum insulin-like growth factor1 in congenital heart disease. *Arch Dis Child.* 1996;75:162–163.

64. Avitabile CM, Leonard MB, Brodsky JL, et al. Usefulness of insulin like growth factor 1 as a marker of heart failure in children and young adults after the Fontan palliation procedure. *Am J Cardiol.* 2015;115(6):816–820.

65. Agus MS, Jaksic T. Nutritional support of the critically ill child. *Curr Opin Pediatr.* 2002;14:470–481.

66. Wang KS, Ford HR, Upperman JS. Metabolic response to stress in the neonate who has surgery. *Neoreviews.* 2006;7:410–418.

67. Madhok AB, Ojamaa K, Haridas V, Parnell VA, Pahwa S, Chowdhury D. Cytokine response to children undergoing surgery for congenital heart disease. *Pediatr Cardiol.* 2006;27:408–413.

68. Mehta NM, Compher C. ASPEN Clinical Guidelines: Nutrition Support of the Critically Ill Child. *JPEN.* 2009;33(3):260–276.

69. Pollack NM, Ruttinmann UE, Wiley JS. Nutritional depletions in critically ill children: associations with physiologic instability and increased quantity of care. *JPEN.* 1985;9(3):309–313.

70. Gillespie M, Kuijpers M, Van Rossem M, et al. Determinants of intensive care unit length of stay for infants undergoing cardiac surgery. *Congenit Heart Dis.* 2006;1:152–160.

71. Becker KC, Hornik CP, et al. Necrotizing enterocolitis in infants with ductal-dependent congenital heart disease. *Am J Perinatol.* 2015;32(7):633–638.

72. Fallon EM, et al. ASPEN Clinical Guidelines: nutrition support of neonatal patients at risk for Necrotizing Enterocolitis. *JPEN.* 2012;36(5):506–523.

73. Bellander M, Ley D, Polberger S, Hellström-Westas L. Tolerance to early human milk feeding is not compromised by indomethacin in preterm infants with persistent ductus arteriosus. *Acta Paediatrica*. 2003;92(9):1074–1078.

74. Davey AM, Wagner CL, Cox C, Kendig JW. Feeding premature infants while low umbilical artery catheters are in place: a prospective, randomized trial. *J Pediatr*. 1994;124:795–799.

75. Barrington KJ. Umbilical artery catheters in the newborn: effects of position of the catheter tip. *Cochrane Database Syst Rev*. 1999;1:CD000505.

76. Howley LW, Kaufman J, et al. Enteral feeding in neonates with prostaglandin-dependent congenital cardiac disease: international survey on current trends and variations in practice. *Cardiol Young*. 2012;222(2):121–127.

77. Slicker J. et al. Perioperative Feeding Approaches in Single Ventricle Infants: A Survey of 46 Centers. *Congenit Heart Dis*. 2016;11(6):707–715.

78. Abad-Jorge A. Nutrition management of the critically ill pediatric patient: minimizing barriers to optimal nutrition support. *ICAN*. 2103;5:221.

79. Trumbo P, Schlicker S, Yates AA, Poos M; Food and Nutrition Board of the Institute of Medicine, The National Academies. Dietary reference intakes for energy, carbohydrate, fiber, fat, fatty acids, cholesterol, protein and amino acids. *J Am Diet Assoc*. 2002;102(11):1621–1630.

80. Page CP, Hardin TC, Melnik G. *Nutritional Assessment and Support*. 2nd ed. Baltimore, MD: Williams & Wilkins, 1994.

81. Owens JL, Musa N. Nutrition support after neonatal cardiac surgery. *Nutr Clin Pract*. 2009;24:242–249.

82. Pronsky ZM. *Food-Medication Interactions*, rev ed. Birchrunville, PA: Food-Medication Interactions; 2004.

83. Lee SH, Kim SJ, Kim HJ, et al. Acute kidney injury following cardiopulmonary bypass in children: risk factors and outcomes. *Circ J*. 2017;81(10):1522–1527.

84. Walters HL III, Hakimi M, Rice MD, et al. Pediatric cardiac surgical ECMO: multivariate analysis of risk factors for hospital death. *Am Thorac Surg*. 1995;60:329–336.

85. Ishino K, Wong Y, Alexi-Meskishvili V, et al. Extracorporeal membrane oxygenation as a bridge to cardiac transplantation. *Artif Organs*. 1996;30:728–732.

86. Keckler SJ, Laituri CA, Ostlie DJ, Peter SD. A review of venovenus and venoarterial extracorporeal membrane oxygenation in neonates and children. *Eur J Pediatr Surg*. 2010;20(1):1–4.

87. Chwals WJ. The metabolic response to surgery in neonates. *Curr Opin Pediatr*. 1994;6(3):334–340.

88. Li J, Zhang G, Herridge J, et al. Energy expenditure and caloric and protein intake in infants following the Norwood procedure. *Pediatr Crit Care Med*. 2008;9:55–61.

89. Larsen BMK, Goonewardene LA, Field CJ, et al. Low energy intakes are associated with adverse outcomes in infants after open heart surgery. *JPEN*. 2013;37:254–260.

90. Sadhwani A, Asaro LA, Goldberg C, et al. Impact of tight glycemic control on neurodevelopmental outcomes at 1 year of age for children with congenital heart disease: a randomized controlled trial. *J Pediatr*. 2016;174:193–198.

91. Ballweg JA, Ittenbach RF, Bernbaum J, et al. Hyperglycaemia after stage I palliation does not adversely affect neurodevelopmental outcome at 1 year of age in patients with single-ventricle physiology. *Eur J Cardiothorac Surg*. 2009;36(4):688–693.

92. Buck ML, Ksenich RA, Wooldridge P. Effect of infusing fat emulsion into extracorporeal membrane oxygenation circuits. *Pharmacother*. 1997;17(6):1292–1295.

93. Buck ML, Wooldridge P, Ksenich RA. Comparison of methods for intravenous infusion of fat emulsion during extracorporeal membrane oxygenation. *Pharmacother*. 2005;25(11):1536–1540.

94. Chaloupecky V, Hucin B, Tlaskal T, et al. Nitrogen balance, 3-methylhistidine excretion, and plasma amino acid profile in infants after cardiac operations for congenital heart defects: the effect of early nutritional support. *J Thorac Cardiovasc Surg*. 1997;14:1053.

95. Teixeira-Cintra MA, Monteiro JP, Tremeschin M, et al. Monitoring of protein catabolism in neonates and young infants post-cardiac surgery. *Acta Paediatr*. 2011;100(7):977–982.

96. Hartl WH, Jauch KW, Parhofer K, Rittler P. Working group for developing the guidelines for parenteral nutrition of the German Association for Nutritional Medicine. Complications and Monitoring—Guidelines on Parenteral Nutrition, Chapter 11. *GMS Ger Med Sci*. 2009;7.

97. Slicker J, Hehir DA, Horsley M, et al. Nutrition algorithms for infants with hypoplastic left heart syndrome; birth through the first interstage period. *Congenit Heart Dis*. 2013;8(2):89–102.

98. Braudis NJ, Curley MA, Beaupre K, et al. Enteral feeding algorithm for infants with hypoplastic left heart syndrome poststage I palliation. *Pediatr Crit Care Med*. 2009;10(4):460–466.

99. Hamilton S, McAleer DM, Ariagno K, et al. A stepwise enteral nutrition algorithm for critically ill children helps achieve nutrient delivery goals. *Pediatr Crit Care Med*. 2014;15(7):583–589.

100. Kaufman J, Vichayavilas P, Rannie M, et al. Improved nutrition delivery and nutrition status in critically ill children with heart disease. *Pediatr*. 2015;135(3):717–725.

101. Cavell B. Gastric emptying in infants with congenital heart disease. *Acta Paediatr Scand*. 1981;70:517–520.

102. Sapsford A. Enteral nutrition products. In: Groh-Wargo S, Thompson M, Cox J, eds. *Nutritional Care for High Risk Newborns*, rev ed. Chicago, IL: Precept Press; 1994:176.

103. Vanderhoof JA, Hofshire PJ, Baluff MA, et al. Continuous enteral feedings: an important adjunct in the management of complex congenital heart disease. *Am J Dis Child*. 1982;136:825–827.

104. Khajuria R, Grover A, Bidwai PS. Effect of nutritional supplementation on growth of infants with congenital heart diseases. *Indian Pediatr*. 1989;26:76–79.

105. Jackson M, Poskitt EM. The effects of high energy feeding on energy balance and growth in infants with congenital heart disease and failure to thrive. *Br J Nutr*. 1991;65:131–143.

106. Vaisman N, Leigh T, Voet H, et al. Malabsorption in infants with congenital heart disease with diuretic treatment. *Pediatr Res*. 1994;36:545–549.

107. Jadcherla SR, Vijayapal AS, Leuthner S. Feeding abilities in neonates with congenital heart disease: a retrospective study. *J Perinatol*. 2009;29:112–118.

108. Boctor DL, Pillo-Blocka F, McCrindle BW. Nutrition after cardiac surgery for infants with congenital heart disease. *Nutr Clin Pract*. 1999;14(3):111–115.

109. Einerson KD, Arthur HM. Predictors of oral feeding difficulty in cardiac surgical infants. *Pediatr Nurs*. 2003;29:315–319.

110. Kohr L, Dargan M, Hauge A, et al. The incidence of dysphagia in pediatric patients after open heart procedures with transesophageal echocardiography. *Ann Thorac Surg.* 2003;76:1450–1456.

111. Krebs N. Gastrointestinal problems and disorders. In: Kessler D, Dawson P, eds. *Failure to Thrive and Pediatric Undernutrition: A Transdisciplinary Approach.* Baltimore, MD: Paul H. Brookes; 1999:215–226.

112. Jung AD. Gastroesophageal reflux in infants and children. *Am Fam Physician.* 2001;64(11):1853–1860.

113. Medoff-Cooper B, Irving SY. Innovative strategies for feeding and nutrition in infants with congenitally malformed hearts. *Cardiol Young.* 2009;19(Suppl 2):90–99.

114. Licht DJ, Shera DM, Clancy RR, et al. Brain maturation is delayed in infants with complex congenital heart defects. *J Thorac Cardiovasc Surg.* 2009;137:529–536.

115. Maher KO, Giddings SS, Baffa JM, Pizzaro C, Norwood WI Jr. New developments in the treatment of hypoplastic left heart syndrome. *Minerva Pediatr.* 2004;56(1):41–49.

116. Daya H, Hosni A, Bejar-Solar J, Evans M. Pediatric vocal fold paralysis: a long term retrospective study. *Arch Otolaryngol Head Neck Surg.* 2000;126:21–25.

117. Skinner ML, Halstead LA, Rubinstein CS, Atz AM, Andrews D, Bradley SM. Laryngopharyngeal dysfunction after Norwood procedure. *J Thoracic Cardiovasc Surg.* 2005;130:1293–1301.

118. Van Dorn CS, Aganga DO, Johnson JN. Extracorporeal membrane oxygenation, Berlin, and ventricular assist devices: a primer for the cardiologist. *Curr Opin Cardiol.* 2018; 33(1):87-94.

119. Shekar, K, Gregory SD, Fraser JF. Mechanical circulatory support in the new era: an overview. *Critical Care.* 2016;20:66.

120. Yarlagadda VV, Maeda K, Zhang Y, Chen S, et al. Temporary circulatory support in U.S. Children awaiting heart transplantation. *J Am Coll Cardiol.* 2017;70(18):2250–2260.

121. Paden ML, Rycus PT, Thiagarajan RR, ELSO Registry. Update and outcomes in extracorporeal life support. *Semin Perinatol.* 2014;38(2):65–70.

122. Montgomery TD, Cohen AE, Garnick J, et al. Nutrition assessment, care, and considerations of ventricular assist device patients. *Nutr Clin Pract.* 2012;27(3):352–362.

123. The Cincinnati Children's Hospital Medical Center. Ventricular Assist Device (VAD) Program. Available at: https://www.cincinnatichildrens.org/service/v/ventricular-assist-device/devices. Accessed April 30, 2018.

124. Kozick, Plunkett, MD. Mechanical circulatory support. *Organogenesis 7(1):50–63.*

125. Jaksic T, Shew SB, Keshen TH, Dzakovic A, Jahoor F. Do critically ill surgical neonates have increased energy expenditure? *J Pediatr Surg.* 2001;36(1):63–67.

126. Brown RL, Wessel J, Warner BW. Nutrition considerations in the neonatal extracorporeal life support patient. *Nutr Clin Pract.* 1994;9(1):22–27.

127. Keshen TH, Miller RG, Jahoor F, Jaksic T. Stable isotopic quantitation of protein metabolism and energy expenditure in neonates on and post-extracorporeal life support. *J Pediatr Surg.* 1997;32(7):958–962.

128. Holick MF. Vitamin D Deficiency. *N Engl J Med.* 2007;357(3):266–281.

129. Graham EM, Taylor SN, Zyblewski SC, et al. Vitamin D status in neonates undergoing cardiac operations: relationship to cardiopulmonary bypass and association with outcomes. *J Pediatr.* 2013;162(4):823–826.

130. Abbasi S, Stewart DL, Radmacher P, Adamkin D. Natural course of cholestasis in neonates on extracorporeal membrane oxygenation (ECMO): 10-year experience at a single institution. *Am Soc Artif Org J.* 2008;54(4):436–438.

131. Ukleja A. Altered GI motility in critically ill patients: current understanding of pathophysiology, clinical impact, and diagnostic approach. *Nutr Clin Pract.* 2010;25:16–25.

132. Crissinger KD. Regulation of hemodynamics and oxygenation in developing intestine: insight into the pathogenesis of necrotizing enterocolitis. *Acta Paediatr Suppl.* 1994;396:8–10.

133. Pettignano R, Heard M, Davis R, Labuz M, Hart M. Total enteral nutrition versus total parenteral nutrition during pediatric extracorporeal membrane oxygenation. *Crit Care Med.* 1998;26(2):358–363.

134. Hanekamp MN, Spoel M, Sharman-Koendjbiharie I, Peters JW, Albers MJ, Tibboel D. Routine enteral nutrition in neonates on extracorporeal membrane oxygenation. *Pediatr Crit Care Med.* 2005;6(3):275–279.

135. Tyson JE, Kennedy KA. Trophic feedings for parenterally fed infants. *Cochrane Database Syst Rev.* 2005;3: CD000504.

136. Okada Y, Klein N, van Saene HK, et al. Small volumes of enteral feedings normalise immune function in infants receiving parenteral nutrition. *J Pediatr Surg.* 1998; 33:16–19.

137. Hadfield RJ, Sinclair DG, Houldsworth PE, Evans TW. Effects of enteral and parenteral nutrition on gut mucosal permeability in the critically ill. *Am J Respir Crit Care Med.* 1995;152:1545–1548.

138. Hanekamp MN, Spoel M, Sharman-Koendjbiharie M, et al. Gut hormone profiles in critically ill neonates on extracorporeal membrane oxygenation. *Pediatr Gastroenterol Nutr.* 2005;40(2):175–179.

139. Lipchultz SE, Sleeper LA, Towbin JA, et al. The incidence of pediatric cardiomyopathy in two regions of the United States. *N Engl J Med.* 2003;348(17):1647–1655.

140. Lee TM, Hsu DT, Kantor P, et al. Pediatric Cardiomyopathies. *Circ Res.* 2017;121(7):855–873.

141. Kirk R, Dipchand AI, Edwards LB, et al. The Registry of the International Society for Heart and Lung Transplantation: fifteenth pediatric heart transplantation report—2012. *J Heart Lung Transplant.* 2012;31(10):1065–1072.

142. Grenier MA, Osganian SK, Cox GF, et al. Design and implementation of the North American Pediatric Cardiomyopathy Registry. *Am Heart J.* 2000;129:S86–S95.

143. McKenna WJ, Maron BJ, Thiene G. Classification, epidemiology, and global burden of Cardiomyopathies. *Circ Res.* 2017;121(7):722–730.

144. Haland TF, Saberniak J, Leren IS, et al. Echocardiographic comparison between left ventricular non-compaction and hypertrophic cardiomyopathy. *Int J Cardiol.* 2017;228:900–905.

145. Miller TL, Neri D, Extein J, Somarriba G, Strickman-Stein N. Nutrition in pediatric cardiomyopathy. *Prog Pediatr Cardiol.* 2007;24(1):59–71.

146. Berger S, Slicker J. Abnormal nutrition impacts waitlist mortality in infants awaiting heart transplantation. *J Heart Lung Transplant.* 2014;33(3):229–30.

147. Al-Attar I, Orav EJ, Exil V, Vlach SA, Lipshultz SE. Predictors of cardiac morbidity and related mortality in children with acquired immunodeficiency syndrome. *J Am Coll Cardiol.* 2003;41(9):1598–1605.

148. Abman S, Hansmann G, Archer SL, et al. Pediatric Pulmonary Hypertension: Guidelines From the American Heart Association and American Thoracic Society. *Circ.* 2015;132(21):2037–2099.

149. Dori Y. Novel lymphatic imaging techniques. *Tech Vasc Interv Radiol.* 2016;19(4):255–261.

150. Hsu MC, Itkin M. Lymphatic anatomy. *Tech Vasc Interv Radiol.* 2016;19(4):247–254.

151. Loukas M, Bellary SS, Kuklinski M, et al. The lymphatic system: a historical perspective. *Clin Anat.* 2011;24(7):807–816.

152. Beghetti M, La Scala G, Belli D, et al. Etiology and management of pediatric chylothorax. *J Pediatr.* 2000;136:653–658.

153. Spain DA, McClave SA. Chylothorax and chylous ascites. In: Gottschlich MM, ed. *The ASPEN Nutrition Support Core Curriculum: A Case Based Approach—The Adult Patient.* Silver Spring, MD: ASPEN; 2007:477–486.

154. Savla JJ, Itkin M, Rossano JW, Dori Y. Post-operative chylothorax in patients with congenital heart disease. *J Am Coll Cardiol.* 2017;69(19):2410–2422.

155. Prasad R, Singh K, Singh R. Bilateral congenital chylothorax with Nona syndrome. *Indian Pediatr.* 2002;39:975–976.

156. Lanning P, Simia S, Saramo I, et al. Lymphatic abnormalities in Noonan's syndrome. *Pediatr Radiol.* 1978;7:106–109.

157. Munoz Conde J, Gomez de Terroros I, Sanchez Ruiz F. Chylothorax associated with Turner's syndrome in a child. *An Esp Pediatr.* 1975;8:449–454.

158. Goens MB, Campbell D, Willins JW. Spontaneous chylothorax in Noonan syndrome. *Am J Dis Child.* 1992;146:1453–1456.

159. Hamada H, Fujita K, Kubo T, et al. Congenital chylothorax in a trisomy 21 newborn. *Arch Gynecol Obstet.* 1992;252:55–58.

160. Chan PC, Chiu HC, Hwu WL. Spontaneous chylothorax in a case of cardio-facio-cutaneous syndrome. *Clin Dysmorph.* 2002;11:297–298.

161. Bellini C, Mazzella M, Arioni C, et al. Hennekam syndrome presenting as non immune hydrops fetalis, congenital chylothorax, and congenital lymphangiectasis. *Am J Med Genetics.* 2003;120A:92–96.

162. Suddaby E and Schiller S. Management of chylothorax in children. *Pediatr Nurs.* 2004;30(4):290–295.

163. Büttiker V, Fanconi S, Burger R. Chylothorax in children: guidelines for diagnosis and management. *Chest.* 1999;116:662–687.

164. Winkler MF. Nutrition management of the patient with chylous fistula. *Support Line.* 2003;25:8–13.

165. Soto-Martinez M, Massie J. Chylothorax: diagnosis and management in children. *Ped Resp Rev.* 2009;10:199–207.

166. Chan EH, Russell JL, Williams WG, Van Arsdell GS, Coles JG, McCrindle BW. Postoperative chylothorax after cardiothoracic surgery in children. *Ann Thorac Surg.* 2005;80:1864–1871.

167. Parrish C, McCray SR. When chyle leaks: nutrition management options. *Pract Gastroenterol.* 2004;26(5):60–76.

168. Sardesai VM. The essential fatty acids. *Nutr Clin Pract.* 1992;7(4): 179–186.

169. Innis SM. Essential fatty acids in growth and development. *Prog Lipid Res.* 1991;30:39–103.

170. Dietary Reference Intake macronutrient guidelines: Available at: http://nationalacademies.org/hmd/~/media/Files/Activity%20Files/Nutrition/DRI-Tables/8_Macronutrient%20Summary.pdf?la=en. Accessed April 16, 2018.

171. Anez-Bustillos L, Dao DT, Fell GL, et al. Redefining essential fatty acids in the era of novel intravenous lipid emulsions. *Clin Nutr.* 2018;37(3):784–789.

172. Holman RT. The ratio of trienoic: tetraenoic acids in tissue lipids as a measure of essential fatty acid requirement. *J Nutr.* 1960;70:405–410.

173. Anez-Bustillos L, Dao DT, Fell GL, et al. Redefining essential fatty acids in the era of novel intravenous lipid emulsions. *Clin Nutr.* 2018;37(3):784–789.

174. Lagerstedt SA, Hinrichs DR, Batt SM, et al. Quantitative determination of plasma c8-c26 total fatty acids for the biochemical diagnosis of nutritional and metabolic disorders. *Mol Genet Metab.* 2001;73(1):38–45.

175. United States Department of Agriculture, Agricultural Research Service. USDA Food Composition Databases. Available at: https://ndb.nal.usda.gov/ndb/search/list. Accessed November 1, /2017.

176. Lessen R. Use of skim breast milk for an infant with chylothorax. *Infant Child Adolesc Nutr.* 2009;1(6):303–310.

177. Chan GM, Lechtenberg E. The use of fat-free human milk in infants with chylous pleural effusion. *J Perinatol.* 2007;27:434–436.

178. Fogg KL, DellaValle DM, Buckley JR, et al. Feasibility and efficacy of defatted human milk in the treatment for chylothorax after cardiac surgery in infants. *Pediatr Cardiol.* 2016;37(6):1072–1077.

179. Kocel SL, Russell J, O'Connor DL. Fat-modified breast milk resolves chylous pleural effusion in infants with postsurgical chylothorax but is associated with slow growth. *JPEN.* 2016;40(4):543–551.

180. Wu JM, Yao CT, Kan CD, et al. Postoperative chylothorax: differences between patients who received median sternotomy or lateral thoracotomy for congenital heart disease. *J Card Surg.* 2006;21(3):249–253.

181. Densupsoontorn N, Jirapinyo P, Tirapongporn H, et al. Fat-soluble vitamins and plasma and erythrocyte membrane fatty acids in chylothorax pediatric patients receiving a medium-chain triglyceride-rich diet. *J Clin Biochem Nutr.* 2014;55(3):174–177.

182. Panthongviriyakul C, Bines JE. Post-operative chylothorax in children: an evidence-based management algorithm. *J Paediatr Child Health.* 2008;44(12):716–721.

183. Cormack BE, Wilson NJ, Finucane K, West TM. Use of Monogen for pediatric postoperative chylothorax. *Ann Thorac Surg.* 2004;77(1):301–305.

184. Cabrera AG, Prodhan P, Bhutta AT. Nutritional challenges and outcomes after surgery for congenital heart disease. *Curr Opin Cardiol.* 2010;25(2):88–94.

185. Beghetti M, La Scala G, Belli D, et al. Etiology and management of pediatric chylothorax. *J Pediatr.* 2000;136(5):653–658.

186. Roehr CC, Jung A, Proquitté H, et al. Somatostatin or octreotide as treatment options for chylothorax in young children: a systematic review. *Intensive Care Med.* 2006;32:650–657.

187. Itkin M, Piccoli DA, Nadolski G, et al. Protein-losing enteropathy in patients with congenital heart disease. *J Am Coll Cardiol.* 2017;69(24):2929–2937.

188. Hawli Y, Nasrallah M, El-Hajj Fuleihan G. Endocrine and musculoskeletal abnormalities in patients with Down syndrome. *Nat Rev Endocrinol.* 2009;5(6):327–334.

189. Mizuno K, Ueda A. Development of sucking behavior in infants with Down's syndrome. *Acta Paediatr.* 2001;90(12):1384–1388.

190. Thomas JA, Graham JM Jr. Chromosomes 22q11 deletion syndrome: an update and review for the primary. *Clin Pediatr (Phila)*. 1997;36(5):253–266.

191. Khositseth A, Tocharoentanaphol C, Khowsathit P, Ruangdaraganon N. Chromosome 22q11 deletions in patients with conotruncal heart defects. *Pediatr Cardiol*. 2005;26(5):570–573.

192. Goldmuntz E. DiGeorge syndrome: new insights. *Clin Perinatol*. 2005;32(4):963–978.

193. Eicher PS, McDonald-McGinn DM, Fox CA, Driscoll DA, Emanuel BS, Zackai EH. Dysphagia in children with a 22q11.2 deletion: unusual pattern found on modified barium swallow. *J Pediatr*. 2000;137(2):158–164.

194. Blake KD, Prasad C. CHARGE syndrome. *Orphanet J Rare Dis*. 2006;1:34.

195. Dobbelsteyn C, Peacocke SD, Blake K, Crist W, Rashid M. Feeding difficulties in children with CHARGE syndrome: prevalence, risk factors, and prognosis. *Dysphagia*. 2008;23(2):127–135.

196. Blake KD, Hudson AS. Gastrointestinal and feeding difficulties in CHARGE syndrome: A review from head-to-toe. *Am J Med Genet*. 2017;175(4):496–506.

197. Thommessen M, Heiberg A, Kase BF. Feeding problems with children with congenital heart disease: the impact on energy intake and growth outcomes. *Eur J Clin Nutr*. 1992;46:457–464.

198. Golfenshtein N, Hanlon AL, Deatrick JA, Medoff-Cooper B. Parenting stress in parents of infants with congenital heart disease and parents of healthy infants: the first year of life. *Compr Child Adolesc Nurs*. 2017;17:1–21.

199. Lisanti AJ, Allen LR, Kelly L, Medoff-Cooper B. Maternal stress and anxiety in the pediatric cardiac intensive care unit. *Am J Crit Care*. 2017;26(2):118–125.

200. O'Byrne ML, Kim S, Hornik CP, et al. Effect of obesity and underweight status on perioperative outcomes of congenital heart operations in children, adolescents, and young adults: an analysis of data from the Society of Thoracic Surgeons Database. *Circulation*. 2017;136(8):704–718.

201. Pinto NM, Marino BS, Wernovsky G, et al. Obesity is a common comorbidity in children with congenital and acquired heart disease. *Pediatr*. 2007;120:e1157–e1164.

202. Cheuk DK, Wong SM, Choi YP, et al. Parents' understanding of their child's congenital heart disease. *Heart*. 2004;90(4):435–439.

203. Stefan MA, Hopman WM, Smythe JF. Effects of activity restriction owing to heart disease on obesity. *Arch Pediatr Adolesc Med*. 2005;159:477–481.

204. Greutmann M, Tobler D. Changing epidemiology and mortality in adult congenital heart disease: looking into the future. *Future Cardiol*. 2012;8(2):171–177.

205. American Academy of Pediatrics Committee on Nutrition. Statement on cholesterol. *Pediatr*. 1992;90:469–473.

206. Nguyen D, Kit B, Carroll M. Abnormal Cholesterol Among Children and Adolescents in the United States, 2011–2014. *NCHS Data Brief*. 2015;(228):1–8.

207. National Cholesterol Education Program Expert Panel Detection, Evaluation, and Treatment of High Blood Cholesterol in Adults (Adult Treatment Panel III). Third report of the National Cholesterol Education Program (NCEP) Expert Panel on Detection, Evaluation, and Treatment of High Blood Cholesterol in Adults (Adult Treatment Panel III): final report. *Circulation*. 2002;106:3143–3421.

208. Krauss RM, Eckel RH, Howard B, et al. AHA dietary guidelines: revision 2000: a statement for healthcare professionals from the Nutrition Committee of the American Heart Association. *Circ*. 2000;102(18):2284–2299.

209. NCEP Expert Panel on Blood Cholesterol Levels in Children and Adolescents. National Cholesterol Education Program (NCEP). Highlights of the report of the Expert Panel on Blood Cholesterol Levels in Children and Adolescents. *Pediatrics*. 1992;89:525–527.

210. U.S. Department of Health and Human Services and U.S. Department of Agriculture. *2015–2020 Dietary Guidelines for Americans*. 8th ed. Available at: Health.gov/DietaryGuidelines/2015/guidelines. 2016.

211. Marcason W. What is the "age15" rule for fiber? *J Am Diet Assoc*. 2005;105(2):301–302.

212. Kwiterovitch PO. The role of fiber in the treatment of hypercholesterolemia in children and adolescents. *J Pediatr*. 1995;96:1005–1009.

213. Kwiterovich PO Jr. Recognition and management of dyslipidemia in children and adolescents. *J Clin Endocrinol Metab*. 2008;93(11):4200–4209.

214. Williams CL, Stobino BA, Bollella M, et al. Cardiovascular risk reduction in preschool children: the "Healthy Start" project. *J Am Coll Nutr*. 2004;23:117–123.

215. Wabitsch M, Hauner H, Heinze E, et al. Body fat distribution and changes in atherogenic risk factor profile in obese adolescent girls during weight loss. *Am J Clin Nutr*. 1994;60:54–60.

216. Sothern MS. Obesity prevention in children: physical activity and nutrition. *Nutrition*. 2004;20(7–8):704–708.

217. Cotts TB, Goldberg CS, Palma Davis LM, et al. A school-based health education program can improve cholesterol values for middle school students. *Pediatr Cardiol*. 2008;29(5):940–945.

218. Bond M, Wyatt K, Lloyd J, Taylor R. Systematic review of the effectiveness of weight management schemes for the under fives. *Obes Rev*. 2010;12(4):242–253.

219. Reinehr T, Andler W. Changes in the atherogenic risk factor profile according to degree of weight loss. *Arch Dis Child*. 2004;89:419–422.

220. Nutrition management of hyperlipidemia. In: William CP, ed. *Pediatric Manual of Clinical Dietetics*. Chicago, IL: American Dietetic Association; 1998:265–283.

221. Saakslahti A, Numminen P, Varstala V, et al. Physical activity as a preventive measure for coronary heart disease risk factors in early childhood. *Scand J Med Sci Sports*. 2004;14:143–149.

222. World Health Organization (WHO). The WHO Child Growth Standards. Available at: http://www.who.int/childgrowth/standards/en/. Assessed April 16, 2018.

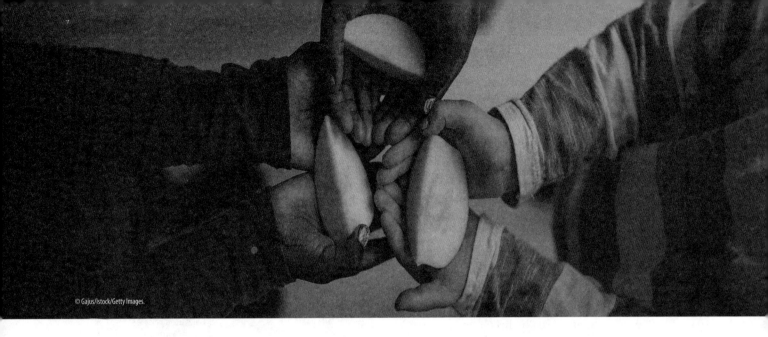

© Gajus/istock/Getty Images.

CHAPTER 15

Pulmonary Diseases

Laura Grande Padula, Emily Bingham and Andrea Nepa

LEARNING OBJECTIVES

- Understand the role of nutrition in pediatric pulmonary diseases including cystic fibrosis, bronchopulmonary dysplasia, and asthma.
- Discuss nutrition and how it is related to the complications of cystic fibrosis, including pancreatic insufficiency, micronutrient deficiencies, and CF-related diabetes.
- Identify potential barriers for meeting increased nutrient needs in the BPD population.
- Identify the role nutrition plays in the risk of developing asthma.

▶ Introduction

Promoting optimal growth and development is important for any child, but it is especially important for the child with chronic pulmonary disease. In this chapter, the nutritional management of **cystic fibrosis** (CF), **bronchopulmonary dysplasia** (BPD), and asthma will be discussed. Adequate nutrition in the care of the child with CF or BPD plays an important prognostic role in the outcome of these diseases. A discussion on asthma is included because it is one of the most common chronic diseases of childhood, and nutrition may play an important role in its management. In each of these three pulmonary-related disease states, nutrition plays an integral role and a nutrition assessment, diagnosis, and care plan are essential for appropriate nutritional care.

▶ Cystic Fibrosis

CF is a life-threatening disorder and is the most common genetic disease amongst Caucasians affecting approximately 30,000 people in the United States.[1] The disease is characterized by an abnormality in the **CF transmembrane conductance regulator** (CFTR) protein, causing increased sodium reabsorption and a decreased chloride secretion. This results in the production of abnormally thick and viscous mucus, which affects various organs of the body. In the lungs, the thick mucus clogs the airways causing obstruction, subsequent bacterial infections, and progressive lung disease. In the pancreas, the thick mucus prevents the release of pancreatic enzymes into the small intestine for the digestion of foods. Blockage of ducts eventually causes pancreatic

351

fibrosis and cyst formation. About 90% of CF patients have **pancreatic insufficiency** (PI),[2] exhibited by such gastrointestinal symptoms as frequent, foul-smelling stools, increased flatus, and abdominal cramping. In a small percentage of patients, the ducts and tubules of the liver are obstructed by mucus, resulting in liver disease that may progress to cirrhosis. Common complications in the CF population include **CF-related diabetes** (CFRD) and bone disease. A unique characteristic of CF is an increased loss of sodium and chloride in the sweat. Sterility due to the bilateral absence of the vas deferens in males and decreased fertility in females is also seen.

The life expectancy of CF patients has greatly improved since the disease was first described as a distinct clinical entity by Andersen in 1938.[3] During the 1930s to 1950s, CF patients usually died at an early age, secondary to malabsorption and malnutrition. Pancreatic enzyme therapy, antibiotic therapy, nutrition therapy, CFTR modulator drugs, and early diagnosis due to newborn screening have been major contributing factors to the improvement in the prognosis for patients with CF. The CF Foundation currently reports the median age of survival to be 43 years for people with CF born between 2012 and 2016, an increase from 31 years for people born between 1992 and 1996.[1]

Genetics/Incidence

CF is transmitted as an autosomal recessive trait. Both parents are carriers of the defective gene but exhibit no symptoms of the disease themselves. Each offspring of two carriers of the defective gene has a 25% chance of having the disease, a 50% chance of being a carrier of the defective gene, and a 25% chance of neither having the disease nor being a carrier.

The CF gene was discovered in 1989 on the long arm of chromosome 7.[4] The CF gene product is a protein called the CFTR, which is a cyclic adenosine monophosphate (cAMP)-regulated chloride channel and regulator of secondary chloride and sodium channels normally present in epithelial cells.[5–10] The most common mutation is called F508del, and it accounts for the majority of CF alleles among the Caucasian population worldwide.[11] However, over 2000 mutations of the CFTR gene have been identified,[12] which accounts for the variability of disease symptoms and severity that is seen among patients with CF. It is hoped that these genetic discoveries will continue to lead to improved treatment, including CFTR modulator therapy and ultimately a cure for the disease.

Manifestations/Diagnosis

Manifestations of the disease are numerous and vary greatly from patient to patient, due in part to the large numbers of mutations of the defective gene. A summary

TABLE 15.1 Manifestations of Cystic Fibrosis

Pulmonary	Gastrointestinal
Chronic cough	Malnutrition
Repeated bronchial infections	Steatorrhea
Increased work of breathing	Hypoalbuminemia
Digital clubbing	Rectal prolapse
Bronchospasm	Frequent, greasy, foul-smelling stools
Cyanosis	Abdominal cramping
Chronic pneumonia	Poor weight gain despite a good appetite
Nasal polyps	Anemia
Chronic sinusitis	Intussusception of the small and large bowel
Salty tasting skin	Fat soluble vitamin deficiences

of common pulmonary and gastrointestinal manifestations of CF is depicted in **TABLE 15.1**. Any child or adult who repeatedly exhibits any of these symptoms should be tested for CF.

According to the consensus statement on the diagnosis of CF published by the CF Foundation,[12] CF is diagnosed when a person clinically presents with signs of the disease and evidence of CFTR dysfunction is confirmed. CFTR dysfunction is typically confirmed with an elevated sweat test; however, all patients with CF should have CFTR genetic analysis performed. Most patients are referred for a sweat test as a result of an elevated newborn screening and may often be asymptomatic of the disease at that time.

Sweat chloride is measured by a quantitative pilocarpine iontophoresis sweat test. A sweat chloride concentration greater than 60 mmol/L is indicative of the diagnosis of CF. Patients with an intermediate sweat chloride concentration (30–59 mmol/L) should undergo CFTR mutation analysis in order to confirm or rule out the diagnosis of CF. The diagnosis can also be made with the identification of CF mutations on both alleles of the CFTR gene, which is sometimes even seen in patients who have a normal sweat test (<30 mmol/L).[12]

The CF Foundation recommends that all states routinely conduct newborn screening for CF. Research has revealed that earlier diagnosis of CF is linked with improved growth and lung function, reduced hospital stays, and increased life expectancy. This is due largely to more prompt medical treatment and nutrition intervention. A positive CF newborn screen does not always mean that the patient has CF, so further medical testing such as a sweat test must be done to confirm the diagnosis.

Management

Rigorous daily management is required to control the symptoms of the disease. Daily chest percussion therapy and postural drainage, along with aerosolized medications, help to clear the airways of mucus, improve existing lung compromise, and delay future deterioration. Aerosolized, oral, or intravenous antibiotics are used to control pulmonary infections. Pancreatic enzyme replacement therapy is a crucial part of managing GI symptoms in patients who exhibit PI. These patients are required to take pancreatic enzymes before each meal and a snack containing fat, protein, and/or complex carbohydrates. The dosage of pancreatic enzymes is individualized, depending on factors such as the extent of pancreatic involvement, dietary intake, and the weight and age of the patient. Vitamin, mineral, and salt supplementation are also recommended and are discussed in detail in the nutrition management section of this chapter. Providing adequate nutrition for normal growth and development is one of the primary goals of disease management in CF, and the CF Foundation recommends that every patient with CF be assessed by a registered dietitian at least once a year. The complex and multifaceted nature of the disease requires an interdisciplinary team approach with patient and family involvement in decision making in order to optimize disease management and improve health outcomes.

Effects of CF on Nutritional Status

CF is a disease with many nutrition implications. The following section will further explain the nutritional manifestations of this disease and how and why it is important to monitor the nutritional status of patients with CF.

Chronic Energy Deficit

Many aspects of CF stress the nutritional status of the patient directly or indirectly by affecting the patient's appetite and subsequent intake. Aspects of pulmonary and GI involvement affecting nutritional status are summarized in **TABLE 15.2**. CFRD and liver disease also impact nutritional status. Bile salts and bile acid losses contribute to fat malabsorption. Gastrointestinal losses

TABLE 15.2 Aspects of Cystic Fibrosis that Affect Nutritional Status

Pulmonary	Gastrointestinal
Increased work of breathing	Malabsorption of fat
Chronic cough	Loss of fat-soluble vitamins
Cough-emesis cycle	Loss of essential fatty acids
Chronic antibiotic therapy	Malabsorption of protein
Fatigue, anxiety	Anorexia
Decreased tolerance for exercise	Gastroesophageal reflux/esophagitis
Repeated pulmonary infections	Bile salts and bile acid loss
Distal intestinal obstructive syndrome (DIOS)

occur in spite of optimized dosing of pancreatic enzyme replacement therapy. Also, the catch-up growth that is often needed after diagnosis requires additional calories. The energy metabolism of CF patients has been studied and generally an increase in resting energy expenditure has been found, when compared with controls and/or predicted resting energy expenditure.[13–17] It is estimated that energy requirements for patients with CF range from 110–200% of the calories recommended for healthy individuals of the same age, gender, and size.[18,19] All of these factors can contribute to a chronic energy deficit which, if left untreated, can lead to a marasmic type of malnutrition. The primary goal of nutritional therapy is to overcome this energy deficit and to promote normal growth and development for CF patients in an effort to optimize lung function and increase longevity.

Appetite

Many references have been made to the voracious appetites of CF patients. This may be true of undiagnosed and untreated patients, particularly infants. In practice, however, dietetics professionals often treat patients with CF who have very poor appetites and early satiety. As previously mentioned, Table 15.2 delineates some aspects of CF that can contribute to poor appetite and malnutrition. Psychosocial issues that the patient may be dealing with may cause depression, anxiety, fatigue, and anorexia that will also impact appetite and nutritional status. Behavioral issues related to eating and ineffective parenting strategies may play a role in a child's poor appetite and intake as well. Studies of the use of medications for appetite stimulation, such as megestrol acetate and cyproheptadine hydrochloride, as part of therapy for CF have been conducted with positive short-term results.[20-23]

Weight Gain, Growth, and Nutrition as a Prognostic Indicator

The expectation of the CF Foundation is that children with cystic fibrosis should grow and develop like their peers without CF. Additionally, adults are expected to maintain a nutrition status similar to healthy individuals of the same age. The CF Foundation has established the following updated age-specific goals for patients with CF:[18]

- *Infants and children 2 years or younger:* Achieve weight for length ≥50th percentile by 2 years
- *Children and adolescents 2 years old to 20 years old:* Achieve ≥50th percentile body mass index (BMI) for age
- *Females 20 years or older:* Achieve or exceed a BMI of 22 kg/m^2
- *Males 20 years or older:* Achieve or exceed a BMI of 23 kg/m^2

Studies have begun to show that better nutritional status early in life is associated with improved pulmonary outcomes and survival.[24,25] Beker and colleagues[26] found height to be an important prognostic indicator of survival for both male and female patients with CF. Yen et al prospectively studied patients with CF and found that weight-for-age percentile >50% at age 4 years was positively correlated with improved height percentile

and lung function in addition to improved survival at age 18 years.[24] Lai et al also found that children who achieve catch-up weight gain and recover back to their birth weight z-score by age 2 years had better outcomes and improved lung function at age 6 years.[25] Close attention to weight gain and nutritional status in the early years is imperative and close follow-up is recommended if patients are not meeting their nutritional goals.

FIGURE 15.1 demonstrates the relationship between FEV$_1$ and BMI percentiles. It is clear that there is an association between growth parameters and lung function. Due to the fact that progressive lung disease is usually what causes the morbidity and mortality of CF, the CF Foundation recognizes the importance of nutrition intervention to optimize growth and help improve lung function.

Nutritional Screening and Assessment

Because nutrition plays such an important role in the treatment of CF, routine nutritional screenings and thorough assessments are very important. The CF Foundation recommends that every patient with CF should be assessed by a registered dietitian annually. Some patients who are at increased nutrition risk may benefit from meeting with a registered dietitian more frequently. In this section, anthropometric, biochemical, clinical, dietary, and drug–nutrient interaction evaluations will be discussed. The CF Foundation has published a consensus report on pediatric nutrition for patients with CF, which includes nutrition management information.[27] Refer to **FIGURE 15.2** for the CF Foundation's recommendations for nutritional status assessment.

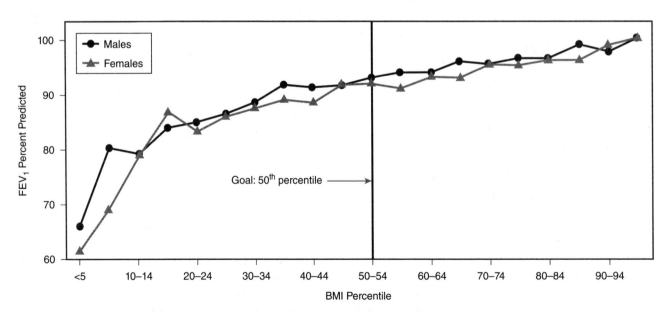

FIGURE 15.1 FEV$_1$ Percent Predicted vs. BMI Percentiles in Patients 6 to 19 Years

Anthropometrics

Monitoring growth parameters is an important component of the screening, assessment, and follow-up of CF patients. As with any child, CF patients should be weighed and measured routinely by trained individuals using appropriate techniques and equipment, such as those described by Fomon[28] and the CF Foundation.[27]

For children less than 24 months of age, weight-for-age, recumbent length-for-age, weight-for-height, and head circumference-for-age should be accurately measured and plotted on the appropriate growth curves at each clinic visit or hospitalization. For children 2 years of age or older who are measured standing, weight-for-age, height-for-age, and BMI-for-age should be measured,

	At Diagnosis	Every 3 Months Birth to 24 Months	Every 3 Months	Annually
Head circumference	X[a]	X		
Weight (to 0.1 kg)	X	X	X	
Length (to 0.1 cm)	X	X		
Height (to 0.1 cm)	X		X	
Mid-arm circumference (MAC) (to 0.1 cm)	X			X
Triceps skinfold (TSF) (to 1.0 mm)	X[b]			X
Mid-arm muscle area, mm² (calculated from MAC and TSF)	X[b]			X
Mid-arm fat area, mm² (calculated from MAC and TSF)	X[b]			X
Biological parents' heights[c]	X			
Pubertal status, female				X[d]
Pubertal status, male				X[e]
24-hour diet recall				X
Nutritional supplement intake[f]				X
Anticipatory dietary and feeding behavior guidance		X	X[g]	X

[a] If younger than 24 months of age at diagnosis.
[b] Only in patients older than 1 year of age.
[c] Record in cm and gender-specific height percentile; note patient's target height percentile on all growth charts.
[d] Starting at age 9 years, annual pubertal self-assessment form (patient or parent and patient) or physician examination for breast and pubic hair Tanner-stage determination; annual question as to menarchal status. Record month and year of menarche on all growth charts.
[e] Starting at age 12 years, annual pubertal self-assessment form (patient or parent and patient) or physician examination for genital development and pubic hair Tanner-stage determination.
[f] A review of enzymes, vitamins, minerals, oral and enteral formulas, herbal, botanical, and other CAM products.
[g] Routine surveillance may be done informally by other team members, but the annual assessment and every 3 month visits in the first 2 years of life and quarterly visits for patients at nutritional risk should be done by the center's registered dietitian.
Reproduced with Borowitz D, Baker R, Stallings V. Consensus report on nutrition for pediatric patients with cystic fibrosis. *J Pediatr Gastroenterol Nutr.* 2002;35(3):246–259.[27]

FIGURE 15.2 Nutritional Assessment in Routine CF Center Care

plotted, and calculated. (See Appendix B for growth charts and Chapter 3 for additional information.)

It is important to note that the **Cystic Fibrosis Foundation** (CFF) recommendation for weight-for-length to be ≥50th percentile is based on using the CDC growth charts. Since it is standard practice in pediatrics to plot children <2 years on the WHO growth chart, the weight-for-length goals must be adjusted if these growth charts are being used. The CFF has released a statement recommending a weight-for-length goal of ≥75th percentile for children aged 12–24 months on the WHO growth chart which correlates with the 50th percentile goal on the CDC chart. Alternatively, younger children may be plotted on the CDC growth chart instead of the WHO chart and the 50th percentile goal can still be used.[29] Further research is needed in this area to ensure adequate nutritional goals for young children with CF.

According to the CF Foundation, anthropometric measurements, including mid-arm circumference and triceps skinfold thickness, should be obtained according to standard procedures by a registered dietitian at least once a year on all patients greater than 1 year of age.[27] From these measurements, mid-arm muscle circumference, mid-arm muscle area (mm^2) and mid-arm fat area (mm^2) should be calculated and compared with gender- and age-specific normative data.[30] (See Appendix D.) Measurements provide information about fat and somatic protein stores and are particularly beneficial when monitoring the effects of nutrition intervention over time. They are also useful in monitoring the nutrition status of CF patients with liver disease and ascites, in which case weight may not be a good indicator of nutrition status.

It is important to determine whether patients with CF are achieving their full genetic potential in terms of height growth. One method used is to determine mid-parental height, plot this height on the growth chart at age 20, and use this percentile as the target for the individual patient. The CF Foundation suggests calculating target height as follows: Add 13 centimeters to the mother's height if the patient is a boy, or subtract 13 centimeters from the father's height if the patient is a girl. Obtain the average of the two parents' adjusted heights. To calculate the patient's target height range, adjust +/− 10 cm for a boy and +/− 9 cm for a girl.[27]

Biochemical

Laboratory monitoring of nutritional status as recommended by the CF Foundation at diagnosis and annually is outlined in **FIGURE 15.3**.

Protein Status Undiagnosed infants, particularly those who are breastfed, often present with hypoalbuminemia and subsequent edema. The malabsorption that occurs in undiagnosed CF causes inadequate absorption of protein. Upon diagnosis of CF and the initiation of pancreatic enzyme therapy, hypoalbuminemia is usually corrected because the infant is no longer malabsorbing protein. Any time an inadequate protein intake is suspected, it may be beneficial to assess the albumin or prealbumin level. However, it is important to remember that other potential causes of an abnormal albumin value include infection and other physiologic stress, fluid overload, congestive heart failure, and severe hepatic insufficiency.[31] CF patients, who chronically have inadequate calorie intakes, usually have a marasmic type of malnutrition. Their visceral protein levels are usually in the normal range, whereas somatic protein stores are low.[31]

Iron Status Hemoglobin and hematocrit are checked annually. If there is evidence of anemia, further iron studies should be obtained, including serum iron, iron-binding capacity, ferritin, transferrin, and reticulocyte count.[27] A trial of iron therapy will help determine if the anemia is caused by iron deficiency or anemia of chronic disease.

Fat-Soluble Vitamins Even patients who are adequately treated with pancreatic enzymes may continue to malabsorb fat and consequently fat-soluble vitamins, so it is important that fat-soluble vitamin levels are checked annually. Vitamin A levels should not be drawn during an acute illness because vitamin A is a negative acute phase reactant and will be decreased with acute illness and inflammation.[27] Vitamin E deficiency is less common with various formulations of CF-specific multivitamins now readily available. Serum levels are ideally measured in the fasting state.[32] Vitamin E is dependent on serum lipid levels and can be reported as a ratio to total cholesterol[33] or total lipids[34] to confirm vitamin E deficiency. Supplementation of vitamin E can be provided if deficiency occurs. All patients should have a serum 25-hydroxyvitamin D level measured. Many CF patients, especially those in northern latitudes, among certain cultures, or with limited sun exposure, may not be exposed to enough sunlight in order to meet vitamin D needs. This in conjunction with fat malabsorption seen in CF, which makes vitamin D deficiency common in this CF population. All patients should have a serum 25-hydroxyvitamin D level measured annually and the level should be maintained at 30 ng/mL or above.[35]

The long-term antibiotic therapy commonly used in the treatment of CF alters the gut flora. Because an important source of vitamin K is microbiologic synthesis in the gut, vitamin K status is often negatively affected. For this reason, it is important to monitor serum vitamin K status. It is preferable to monitor proteins induced by vitamin K absence or antagonism (PIVKA-II), but this measurement is not always available in the clinical setting. **Prothrombin time** (PT) is an indirect measurement of vitamin K status and is more widely utilized. PT may also be a useful measure of hepatic synthetic function in patients with nutritional failure or biliary cirrhosis.[27]

	How Often to Monitor			
	At Diagnosis	**Anually**	**Other**	**Tests**
Beta Carotene			At physician's discretion	Serum levels
Vitamin A	x[1]	x		Vitamin A (retinol)
Vitamin D	x[1]	x		25-OH-D
Vitamin E	x[1]	x		α-tocopherol
Vitamin K	x[1]		If patient has hemoptysis or hematemesis; in patients with liver disease	PIVKA-II (preferably) or prothrombin time
Essential Fatty Acids			Consider checking in infants or those with FTT	Triene; tetraene
Calcium/Bone Status			> age 8 years if risk factors are present	Calcium, phosphorus, ionized PTH, DEXA scan
Iron	x	x	Consider in-depth evaluation for patients with poor appetite	Hemoglobin, hematocrit
Zinc			Consider 6-month supplementation trial and follow growth	No acceptable measurement
Sodium			Consider checking if exposed to heat stress and becomes dehydrated	Serum sodium; spot urine sodium if total body sodium depletion suspected
Protein Stores	x	x	Check in patients with nutritional failure or those at risk	Albumin

[1]Patients diagnosed by neonatal screening do not need these measured.

Abbreviations: FTT, failure to thrive; PTH, parathyroid hormone; DEXA, dual energy x-ray absorptiometry; PIVKA, protein induced by vitamin K antagonistism or absence.

Reproduced with Borowitz D, Baker R, Stallings V. Consensus report on nutrition for pediatric patients with cystic fibrosis. *J Pediatr Gastroenterol Nutr.* 2002;35(3):252.[27]

FIGURE 15.3 Laboratory Monitoring of Nutritional Status

Essential Fatty Acids Patients with CF are also at risk of **essential fatty acid** (EFA) deficiency. The etiology of EFA deficiency can be multifactorial, including fat malabsorption and abnormal fatty acid oxidation. It also has been associated with certain CF genotypes and pancreatic status. Some of the clinical manifestations of EFA deficiency include scaly rash, poor growth, and alopecia. EFA deficiency is also correlated with an increased inflammatory response in patients with CF. Checking a triene to tetraene ratio has often been the common way to assess for EFA deficiency in patients exhibiting poor growth; however, more recent studies have shown serum linoleic acid status to be associated with improved growth and pulmonary status.[32] The goal of nutrition care is to prevent EFA deficiency. A minimum of 3–5% of total calories should come from EFAs.[36] Some sources of EFAs include soybean oil, canola oil, walnuts, fatty fish, and flaxseed.

CF-Related Diabetes (CFRD) Screening

With the increased life expectancy of CF patients, the frequency of glucose intolerance in this population has increased.[37] CFRD is most commonly diagnosed after the age of 10 years, but it has been observed in younger children. In patients with CF above 30 years old, up to 50% prevalence has been reported. Changes in screening practices have increased the number of reported patients with CFRD.[37] CFRD is a distinct clinical entity because it has features of both type 1 and type 2 diabetes.[38] Clinical symptoms of CFRD include polydipsia, polyuria, fatigue, unintentional weight loss, and decreased lung function. **TABLE 15.3** outlines how CFRD is diagnosed.

Pancreatic Function/Malabsorption

PI is often inferred based on a patient presenting with symptoms of malabsorption. Stool fecal elastase-I1is

considered a highly sensitive and specific way to measure pancreatic function and is generally tested at the time of diagnosis. Patients who are initially pancreatic sufficient can become pancreatic insufficient over time. This is especially true of those who have an identified mutation that is associated with PI. These patients should have their pancreatic function evaluated annually by checking a stool fecal elastase-I.[27]

When a patient is pancreatic insufficient and on pancreatic enzyme therapy, it is important to evaluate the appropriateness of their enzyme regimen at regular intervals. In some rare instances, a 72-hour fecal fat test is used to assess fat absorption. Although 72-hour fecal

TABLE 15.3 Diagnosis of Cystic Fibrosis Related Diabetes

Test	Time	Blood Glucose Level	Diagnosis	Action
Fasting blood glucose	Done first thing in the morning after an 8-hour fast	< 100 mg/dL (< 5.6 mmol/L)	Normal	Starting at age 10, or earlier if symptoms occur, do OGTT annually.
		100–125 mg/dL (5.6–6.9 mmol/L)	*Impaired fasting glucose (IFG)*	You are more likely to develop diabetes; you will be closely monitored by your CF team. Repeat OGTT annually or earlier if symptoms occur.
		≥126 mg/dL (≥7.0 mmol/L)	CFRD	You will be followed by your CF and endocrinology team and treated with insulin.
Casual (random) blood glucose	Done at any time regardless of time of last meal or snack	<200 mg/dL (11.2 mmol/L)	*Non-diagnostic*	Starting at age 10, or earlier if symptoms occur, do OGTT annually.
		≥200 mg/dL (≥11.1 mmol/L)	High risk of CFRD	If symptoms are present, do a fasting blood glucose test, otherwise OGTT.
OGTT	Done in the morning after an 8-hour fast	2-hour glucose ≥200 mg/dL (≥11.1 mmol/L)	CFRD	You will be followed by your CF and endocrinology team and treated with insulin.
		2-hour glucose 140–199 mg/dL (7.8–11.0 mmol/L)	*Impaired glucose tolerance (IGT)*	You are at higher risk for developing diabetes; you will be closely monitored by your CF team. Repeat OGTT annually or earlier if symptoms occur.
		Mid-OGTT glucose ≥200 mg/dL (≥11.1 mmol/L), OGTT otherwise normal	*Indeterminate glycemia (INDET)*	You are at higher risk for developing diabetes; you will be closely monitored by your CF team. Repeat OGTT annually or earlier if symptoms occur.
		2-hour glucose	Normal	Repeat OGTT annually

Abbreviations: CFRD, cystic fibrosis related diabetes; OGTT, oral glucose tolerance test.
Courtesy of Brunzell C, Hardin D, Kogler A, Schindler T, Moran A. Managing Cystic Fibrosis Related Diabetes (CFRD): *An Instruction Guide for Patients and Families*, 6th ed. Bethesda, MD: Cystic Fibrosis Foundation; 2015.[38]

fat tests are an accurate way of assessing fat absorption, the steps that must be completed are cumbersome for patients and families. Additionally, older patients are uncomfortable or embarrassed collecting their stools. For these reasons, it can be difficult to complete a 72-hour fecal fat test, and adjustments are often made to pancreatic enzyme dosages based on reported symptoms of malabsorption or poor weight gain in the setting of adequate caloric intake.

Clinical

Assessing the patient's overall health status should be obtained. Questions about activity and energy levels should be asked. Any missed school or work days should be noted. A general review of systems should be performed by the physician and a description of the patient's Tanner stage should be noted.[27] (See Appendix E, Progression of Sexual Development.) Co-morbid medical conditions such as active pulmonary or sinus disease, **gastroesophageal reflux disease** (GERD), CFRD, hepatobiliary disease, or history of gut resection should be noted.[27] These conditions will also have a direct impact on the patient's nutritional status by affecting appetite, intake, and disease state. Questions about the patient's use of alternative/complementary medicine therapies should be asked in addition to questions about using routine medications.

Stool Pattern Information about the patient's stool pattern should be monitored carefully at each clinic visit because this is a good indication of the adequacy of the enzyme therapy. Questions to be asked during a nutrition screening and assessment should include:

- Number of stools per day
- Consistency of stools
- Presence of oily discharge
- Rectal prolapse
- Foul-smelling, floating stools and/or flatus
- Abdominal cramping
- Protruding abdomen

Increased frequency or volume of stool output, notable oil in stools or in toilet water, extremely malodorous stools, increased gassiness and abdominal distention, and/or stools that float instead of sinking to the bottom of the toilet are all signs that a patient may be experiencing malabsorption. Some patients with persistent malabsorptive symptoms should also be evaluated for nonpancreatic causes of malabsorption such as lactose intolerance, bacterial overgrowth of the small intestine, giardia or other parasites, celiac disease, or inflammatory bowel disease.[27] It is also important to ask about constipation. Constipation can be a symptom of distal intestinal obstructive syndrome (DIOS), which is also a complication of PI.

Enzyme Therapy Important aspects of enzyme replacement therapy that need to be checked during every clinic visit and hospitalization are:

- Type of enzymes
- Brand
- Amount taken
- When taken
- Method of administration
- Timing with meals
- Calculation of units of lipase/kg body weight/meal and total units of lipase/kg body weight/day
- Adherence
- Where enzymes are being stored

Enzymes should be stored at room temperature because they may be deactivated by extreme heat or cold. The expiration date should be monitored closely because enzymes become less potent when expired. Generic enzymes should never be used.

Other Medications It is important to keep track of other medications the patient may be taking at each clinic visit, including antibiotics (oral and inhaled), bronchodilators, H_2 blockers, proton pump inhibitors, prokinetic agents, steroids, diuretics, cardiac medications, appetite stimulants, probiotics, vitamins, minerals, and CFTR modulators.

Pulmonary Status The pulmonary status of the patient will directly influence the patient's nutritional status. The dietetics professional should note the presence of an acute pulmonary exacerbation and chronic disease. CF patients older than about 6 years of age will be able to perform pulmonary function tests to assess the extent of their pulmonary involvement.

Bone Health Indices Patients with CF are at risk for developing osteopenia and osteoporosis. The origin of bone disease in CF appears to be multifactorial (**FIGURE 15.4**). Important contributing factors include malabsorption of vitamins D and K, malnutrition, delayed puberty, physical inactivity, and the use of corticosteroid medications. The prevalence of bone disease appears to increase with severity of lung disease and malnutrition.[39] Several studies have demonstrated a positive correlation between **bone mineral density** (BMD) z-scores, FEV_1, and BMI.[40–43] Patients with severe pulmonary disease ($FEV_1 < 30\%$) often have severe bone disease with a high rate of kyphosis and fractures of long bones, vertebrae, and ribs.[41,44]

According to the CFF bone health consensus statement, patients older than 8 years of age should have a dual energy x-ray absorptiometry (DXA) as a measure of bone mineral density if <90% ideal body weight, FEV_1 <50% predicted, glucocorticoids ≥5 mg/day

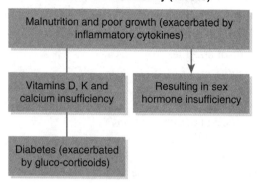

FIGURE 15.4 Pathogenesis of Bone Disease in CF

Courtesy of Aris RM, Merkel PA, Bachrach LK, et al. Consensus statement: guide to bone health and disease in cystic fibrosis. *J Clin Endocrinol Metab*. 2005;90:1888–1896

for ≥90 days/yr, delayed puberty, or history of fractures.[39] In addition to the DXA, children at risk for poor bone health should be assessed for appropriate vitamin D, vitamin K, and calcium status.[45] Normative data for DXA are not available for children younger than 3 years of age. All patients should have DXA scans by age 18 years if the scans have not been previously obtained for other reasons.[39]

Dietary

As part of the nutritional assessment, dietary analysis provides important information about what, where, and how much the CF patient is eating. Several methods of gathering the data can be utilized, including a 24-hour dietary recall, a 3–5 day food record, and a food frequency questionnaire. The dietetics professional should analyze the diet's adequacy in terms of energy, protein, and other key nutrients, such as calcium and iron, by looking for a variety of foods in adequate amounts. During this interview, information about the patient's appetite, eating patterns, consumption of sweetened beverages, and behavioral issues related to feeding should be noted.[27] The Behavioral Pediatrics Feeding Assessment Scale, which is a self-reported measure of meal-time problems, may be administered to identify and evaluate behavioral issues related to eating.[27,46]

Drug–Nutrient Interactions

It is important to consider drug–nutrient interactions when assessing any patient, and CF patients are often on a long list of medications. A dietitian or other healthcare provider should take into account how these medications may impact the patient's appetite, if there are dietary restrictions related to any of the patient's medications, and/or what biochemical data may need to be evaluated with the use of certain medications. For example, prolonged antibiotic therapy can alter the gut flora and subsequently influence vitamin K status. Additionally, some of the intravenous antibiotics can cause nausea in a number of patients. CF patients with an asthma component of their disease may be on steroids periodically. As the CF patient's pulmonary disease progresses, issues with fluid status may develop. If diuretics are prescribed, fluid and electrolyte status need to be carefully monitored.

Nutritional Management

The overall goal of nutrition management is to promote normal growth and development for the patient with CF. The main components of nutrition management in CF are providing adequate energy, protein, and nutrients, pancreatic enzyme therapy, and vitamin and mineral supplementation.

Adequate Diet for Normal Growth and Development

In the past, the GI symptoms of the disease, such as the increased number of bulky, foul-smelling stools, increased flatus, and abdominal cramping were treated with a low-fat diet. Today, with the advent of better enzyme replacement therapy, fat restriction is no longer routinely imposed on all patients. Health professionals now appreciate the tremendous energy demands of the disease, and there is good evidence to support that higher energy intake results in improved weight gain.[18] Estimated energy recommendations to support age-appropriate growth in children with CF over the age of 2 years range from 110%–200% of energy needs for the healthy population of similar age, gender, and size.[18] This can be accomplished by increasing both the amount and caloric density of foods consumed. To achieve this energy goal, patients with CF often require a greater amount of dietary fat, 35–40% of total energy.[27] It is appropriate to encourage the use of polyunsaturated fats that are good sources of the EFAs, linoleic acid and alpha-linolenic acid, rather than saturated fats. Vegetable oils such as flax, canola, and soy and cold-water marine fish are high in calories and a good source of these fats.[27] Limited information is available describing specific dietary protein recommendations for children with CF[32]; however, protein intake is correlated with overall calorie intake and, in general, patients with CF who consume adequate calories also consume adequate protein.[47,48] Defining energy needs in patients with CF can be a challenge due to many individual variables. It is suggested that formulas be used as a starting point, but gain in weight and height, velocity of weight and height gain, and fat stores may provide a more objective measure of energy balance.[32]

1. Infant
   - Breast milk or standard iron-fortified infant formula should be recommended. Protein hydrolysate formulas containing medium-chain triglycerides, can be recommended for infants in special situations, such as bowel resection or those with milk protein allergy.
   - Pancreatic enzymes should be given before feedings.
   - CF-specific multivitamin should be given.
   - Introducing solid foods and advancing the diet should proceed as recommended by the **American Academy of Pediatrics** (AAP). The RD should guide parents toward foods that will enhance weight gain. Meat, a good source of iron and zinc, may be recommended as a first food for infants consuming human milk and fats may be added to solid foods in order to increase the caloric density of fruits and vegetables.
   - Salt should be added to breast milk or infant formula. When solid foods are added to the infant's diet, salt should be added to these foods.
   - Referrals should be made to community programs such as the WIC program.

2. Toddler
   - Toddlers' diets should be based on a normal healthy diet for age with a variety of foods.
   - Regular meal and snack times should be encouraged.
   - Constant snacking or "grazing" should be discouraged.
   - Drinking of sweetened beverages should be discouraged.
   - Pancreatic enzymes are continued.
   - CF vitamin therapy is continued.
   - Continue communication with community programs such as the WIC program.

3. Preschool and school age
   - A normal healthy diet with a variety of foods should continue to form the basis of the diet.
   - Limit sweetened beverages.
   - Parents lose control of what the child eats away from home at preschool, child care, and school.
   - Arrangements need to be made for the child to take enzymes during the school day.
   - CF vitamin therapy is continued.
   - Diet prescriptions for a high-calorie, high-protein, high-salt diet can be sent to the school.

4. Adolescent
   - Patients are exercising more independence in food choices.
   - Parents can provide an appropriate food environment at home.
   - Patients can be taught to include quick-to-prepare high-calorie foods in their daily diet.
   - Snack and fast foods can add a significant amount of calories to the diet and should not be discouraged.
   - Limit sweetened beverages.
   - Health professionals should emphasize the importance of high-calorie intake and enzyme and vitamin therapy directly to the patient and not via the parents.
   - Nutrition needs increase before and during an adolescent growth spurt.

FIGURE 15.5 Nutritional Management of CF Patients

Age-specific considerations in the nutritional management of CF are summarized in **FIGURE 15.5**. Infants with CF may be successfully breastfed, as long as pancreatic enzymes are administered before each feeding. Standard iron-fortified infant formulas are alternatives to breast milk but also require administering pancreatic enzymes before each feeding. A study of newly diagnosed infants with CF compared nutrition and growth parameters of those infants fed standard infant formula with those fed a protein hydrolysate formula.[49] There was no significant difference in growth parameters between the two groups of infants. Therefore, standard infant formulas should be used for the routine care of newly diagnosed infants with CF rather than expensive hydrolyzed formulas.[49]

To close the gap between energy needs and the amount of calories the patient is able to consume, energy-dense foods can be added to the patient's diet. Since fat is the most calorie dense macronutrient, it is often used to add to foods to increase the caloric density. Heart healthy fats are encouraged although a wide variety of energy boosters can be used. **FIGURE 15.6** depicts various methods to boost calories.

Pregnancy

With the increased life expectancy of patients with CF, more women with the disease are becoming pregnant. In addition to the usual nutrient recommendations of CF, the increased energy needs of pregnancy must be

Calorie-Protein Boosters

—Some ways to hide extra calories and protein—

Powdered milk (33cal/tbsp, 3g pro/tbsp)

Add 2–4 tbsp to 1 cup milk. Mix into puddings, potatoes, soups, ground meats, vegetables, and cooked cereal.

Eggs (80cal/egg, 7g pro/tbsp)

Add to casseroles, meat loaf, mashed potatoes, cooked cereal, and macaroni & cheese. Add extra to pancake batter and french toast. (Do not use raw eggs in uncooked items.)

Butter or margarine (45cal/tsp)

Add to puddings, casseroles, sandwiches, vegetables, and cooked cereal.

Cheeses (100cal/oz, 7 gpro/oz)

Give as snacks or in sandwiches. Add melted to casseroles, potatoes, vegetables, and soup.

Wheat germ (25cal/tbsp)

Add a tablespoon or two to cereal. Mix into meat dishes, cookie batter, casseroles, etc.

Mayonnaise or salad dressings (45cal/tsp)

Use liberally on sandwiches, on salads, as a dip for raw vegetables, or as a sauce on cooked vegetables.

Evaporated milk (25cal/tbsp, 1g pro/tbsp)

Use in place of whole milk, in desserts, baked goods, meat dishes, and cooked cereals.

Sour cream (26cal/tbsp)

Add to potatoes, casseroles, dips; use in sauces, baked goods, etc.

Sweetened condensed milk (60cal/tbsp, 1g pro/tbsp)

Add to pies, puddings, milkshakes. Mix 1–2 tbsp with peanut butter and spread on toast.

Peanut butter (95cal/tbsp, 4g pro/tbsp)

Serve on toast, crackers, bananas, apples, and celery.

Carnation Instant Breakfast (130cal/pckt, 7g pro/pckt)

Add to milk and milkshakes.

Gravies (40cal/tbsp)

Use liberally on mashed potatoes and meats.

High Protein Foods

MEATS—Beef, Chicken, Fish, Turkey, Lamb

MILK & CHEESE—Yogurt, Cottage Cheese, Cream Cheese

EGGS

PEANUT BUTTER (with Bread or Crackers)

DRIED BEANS & PEAS (with Bread, Cornbread, Rice)

Courtesy of Pediatric Pulmonary Center, ©1990. University of Alabama at Birmingham, Birmingham, Alabama.[50]

FIGURE 15.6 Instructional Handout on Increasing Calories

taken into consideration. Emphasis needs to be put on proper weight gain. The woman's weight before and during pregnancy has a tremendous impact on the outcome for both mother and infant. Oral supplements and/or enteral feeds should be considered to promote adequate weight gain during the period of pregnancy.[51] Special attention should be made to serum retinol levels because excessive vitamin A intake during pregnancy could be teratogenic to the fetus. Levels should be monitored closely and supplementation adjusted as necessary. There are no specific recommendations for folic acid or minerals for pregnant women with CF so standard advice should be given.[52]

CF-Related Diabetes (CFRD)

As with any patient with CF, the treatment goal for CFRD is to provide a diet that promotes optimal growth and development in children and adolescents, achieves and maintains normal weight in adults, as well as optimal nutritional status.[37,53] Other treatment goals include controlling hyperglycemia to reduce diabetes complications, avoiding severe hypoglycemia, and assisting the patient in adapting to another chronic illness from a psychological standpoint.[37] The primary goal remains meeting the patient's energy needs. Foods with carbohydrates have the greatest impact on blood sugar. Simple sugars can be included in the diet plan, but regular sodas and other sweetened beverages should be discouraged. The patient needs to learn how to recognize the carbohydrate content of foods, such as with the carbohydrate counting method, which is used when taking rapid acting insulin to cover meals.[41] For those on a fixed insulin regimen, blood sugars can be better managed by eating a consistent amount of carbohydrate at each of the three meals and three snacks in addition to eating at the same time each day.[41] Eating protein and fat-containing foods along with simple sugars slows the absorption of the simple sugars from the intestinal tract. Calories should not be restricted.

Patient/Family Education

Patient and family education on nutrition management and its importance in the patient's overall health care is an integral component of the individual patient's care plan. A qualified, registered dietitian should be available to the patient and family in order to assist them in meeting the nutritional needs of the patient in the least invasive way possible. Information about the nutrient content of foods and suggestions for increasing the patient's caloric intake should be available.

For children with CF ages 1–12 years with or at risk of growth deficits, the CF Foundation recommends that intensive treatment with behavioral intervention in conjunction with nutrition counseling be used to promote weight gain.[18] Some strategies include complimenting children for appropriate feeding behaviors (e.g., trying a new food, taking consecutive bites), paying minimal attention to behaviors not compatible with eating (e.g., refusing food), and limiting mealtimes to 15 minutes specifically for toddlers.[54]

Supplemental Nutrition

Oral supplements, milkshakes, and other high-calorie drinks may be used to supplement oral intake. Commercially made oral supplements can also be used to boost calories, but they often require additional expense if they are not covered by the patient's insurance. A recent Cochran review also showed that oral supplements did not improve the nutritional status of patients with CF and they should not be considered an essential piece of nutritional care.[55]

Oftentimes, in spite of vigorous efforts by the patient, the family, and the CF team, it is very difficult to meet the patient's energy needs by the oral route alone. The CFF consensus committee for enteral tube feeding recommends that using supplemental tube feedings be considered when optimizing feeding behaviors and oral calories have not achieved adequate weight gain or growth parameters.[56] The patient and family need to be given the facts about available adjunct therapies in a positive way and be involved in the decision making.[27] CF centers have reported using various forms of tube feedings, including nasogastric, gastrostomy, and jejunostomy feedings; however, gastrostomy tubes are the most commonly placed. Tube feedings are most often administered on a continuous basis while the patient is asleep in order to cause the least disruption to their daily life. There are a variety of formulas available, some with a fairly high concentrations of MCT oil, which can be helpful with fat absorption issues. However, the CFF does not recommend using any specific formula and polymeric formulas may be used successfully especially if cost is a concern.[56] Pancreatic enzyme administration with overnight tube feeds will be discussed briefly in the "Pancreatic Enzyme Replacement Therapy" section of this chapter. The CFF does not recommend for or against any specific method for providing pancreatic enzymes for tube feedings.[56]

Vitamin and Mineral Supplementation

Vitamins CFF recommendations for pediatric nutrition for patients with CF regarding vitamin supplementation can be found in **FIGURE 15.7**.[27] CF-specific multivitamin preparations are available on the market that contain high amounts of the fat-soluble vitamins A, D, E, and K in a water-miscible form to meet the needs of patients with CF. **TABLE 15.4** compares the amounts of fat-soluble vitamins in different CF-specific vitamins to a standard multivitamin. Using CF-specific multivitamins simplifies a patient's vitamin regimen and helps to improve patient compliance. Not all of the commercially available products contain the recommended level of vitamin K, so vitamin K status needs to be monitored carefully.

In addition to a standard, age-appropriate dose of nonfat-soluble multivitamins, the following should be given:

Individual Vitamin Daily Supplementation				
	Vitamin A (IU)	Vitamin E (IU)	Vitamin D (IU)	Vitamin K (mg)
0–12 months	1500	40–50	400	0.3–0.5*
1–3 years	5000	80–150	400–800	0.3–0.5*
4–8 years	5000–10,000	100–200	400–800	0.3–0.5*
> 8 years	10,000	200–400	400–800	0.3–0.5*

*Currently, commercially available products do not have ideal doses for supplementation. In a recent review, no adverse effects have been reported at any dosage level of vitamin K. Clinicians should try to follow these recommendations as closely as possible until better dosage forms are available. Prothrombin time or, ideally, PIVKA-II levels should be checked in patients with liver disease, and vitamin K dose titrated as indicated.

Reproduced with Borowitz D, Baker R, Stallings V. Consensus report on nutrition for pediatric patients with cystic fibrosis. *J. Pediatric Gastroenterology & Nutrition.* 2002;35(3):251.[27]

FIGURE 15.7 Recommendations for Vitamin Supplementation

TABLE 15.4 Examples of Pancreatic Enzymes

Enzyme	Form*	Lipase USP Units	Protease USP Units	Amylase USP Units
Creon 3,000[1]	Delayed release capsules	3,000	9,500	15,000
Creon 6,000[1]	Delayed release capsules	6,000	19,000	30,000
Creon 12,000[1]	Delayed release capsules	12,000	38,000	60,000
Creon 24,000[1]	Delayed release capsules	24,000	76,000	120,000
Creon 36,000[1]	Delayed release capsules	36,000	114,000	180,000
Pancreaze MT2[2]	Delayed release capsules	2,600	6,200	10,850
Pancreaze MT4[2]	Delayed release capsules	4,200	14,200	24,600
Pancreaze MT10[2]	Delayed release capsules	10,500	35,500	61,500
Pancreaze MT16[2]	Delayed release capsules	16,800	56,800	98,400
Pancreaze MT20[2]	Delayed release capsules	21,000	54,700	83,900
Zenpep 3,000[3]	Delayed release capsules	3,000	10,000	14,000
5,000[3]	Delayed release capsules	5,000	17,000	24,000
ZENPEP 10,000[3]	Delayed release capsules	10,000	32,000	42,000
ZENPEP 15,000[3]	Delayed release capsules	15,000	47,000	63,000
ZENPEP 20,000[3]	Delayed release capsules	20,000	63,000	84,000
Zenpep 25,000[3]	Delayed release capsules	25,000	79,000	105,000
Zenpep 40,000[3]	Delayed release capsules	40,000	126,000	168,000
Pertzye 4,000[4]	Delayed release capsules	4,000	14,375	15,125
Pertzye 8,000[4]	Delayed release capsules	8,000	28,750	30,250
Pertzye 16,000[4]	Delayed release capsules	16,000	57,500	60,500
Pertzye 24,000[4]	Delayed release capsules	24,000	86,250	90,750
Viokace 10,440[3]	Tablets	10,440	39,150	39,150
Viokace 20,880[3]	Tablets	20,880	78,300	78,300

*Form as described by respective company
[1] Abbvie, Inc: http://www.creon-us.com/default.htm
[2] Janssen Pharmaceuticals, Inc: http://www.pancreaze.net
[3] Allergan, Inc: http://www.zenpep.com
[4] Digestive Care, Inc: https://www.pertzyecf.com/

The CFF has published specific consensus guidelines on screening, diagnosing, and treating vitamin D deficiency in CF. All patients should be treated with cholecalciferol (vitamin D_3) to treat deficiency which is defined as a 25-hydroxy vitamin D level <30 ng/mL. Cholecalciferol (vitamin D_3) is recommended as the form of vitamin D for repletion in CF. Refer to the vitamin D consensus statement for detailed guidelines on how to treat vitamin D deficiency in CF in all age groups. If vitamin D levels remain low after following the recommended treatment algorithm, and the levels are still less than 30 ng/mL after treatment with additional cholecalciferol per the guidelines, a referral to endocrinology should be considered for alternative options of repleting vitamin D.[35]

Minerals Minerals such as zinc, iron, and selenium have been studied in the CF population. Additional study is needed before specific supplementation recommendations can be made. A trial of zinc supplementation for 6 months may be initiated for patients with CF who have poor growth.[54] All patients with CF should be encouraged to consume at least the DRIs for calcium for their age group.[57] CF patients who are on steroids, who have decreased dietary intake of calcium, and/or who are found to have decreased bone density may benefit from calcium supplementation. These minerals as well as other macro- and micronutrients are important to the overall nutritional status of the patient with CF. Therefore, eating a variety of foods should be encouraged.

Additional salt should be added to the diet during times of increased sweating, such as:

- During hot weather
- With fevers
- During strenuous physical activity
- With profuse diarrhea

The additional salt compensates for the increased losses of sodium and chloride through perspiration. In most instances, the liberal use of the salt shaker and the inclusion of high-salt foods in the diet will supply the needed sodium and chloride. Salt supplements may be used in instances of very heavy sweating. Both breastfed and formula-fed infants need supplementation with sodium chloride, particularly during hot weather.[27] Infants without CF require 2–4 mEq/kg/day of sodium; infants with CF are likely to require the upper end of this normal range, even when not exposed to heat stress.[27] In practice, 1/8 teaspoon per day of table salt is recommended for infants less than 6 months of age, and 1/4 teaspoon per day is recommended for infants greater than 6 months of age. The table salt is typically added to the infant's formula throughout the day.[54]

Pancreatic Enzyme Replacement Therapy

Types of Available Enzymes In an effort to confirm safety and efficacy of pancreatic enzymes, a new rule was issued in 2004 requiring makers of pancreatic enzyme products to obtain approval by the **US Food and Drug Administration** (FDA) by April 28, 2010. There are currently five brands which are FDA approved (**TABLE 15.5**), and they contain varying amounts of lipase, which breaks down fat; protease, which breaks down protein; and amylase, which breaks down carbohydrate.

The nonproprietary name of these products is pancrelipase. The products are available in capsule form

TABLE 15.5 BPD Drug–Nutrient Interactions

Medication	Nutrients Affected (lowers all)	Other Effects
Diuretics (e.g., furosemide)	Na, K, Cl, Mg, Ca, Zn	Volume depletion Metabolic alkalosis Anorexia Diarrhea Hyperuricemia Gastrointestinal irritant
Bronchodilators (e.g., theophylline)		Gastrointestinal distress Nausea Vomiting Diarrhea
Steroids (e.g., dexamethasone)	Ca, P	Growth suppression

and most feature an enteric coating that protects the enzymes from inactivation in the acid environment of the stomach. The enzymes become activated in the alkaline pH of the duodenum.

Dosage/Administration There is a CF consensus statement on the use of pancreatic enzyme supplements.[58] Extremely high doses of pancreatic enzymes have been associated with fibrosing colonopathy or strictures in the colon in CF patients.[59,60] A recommended starting dose for infants is 2000 to 5000 units of lipase per 4 oz feeding, though this may be less in newborns who take less volume at each feeding.[54] Another proposed weight-based enzyme dosing schedule starts with 1000 units of lipase/kg body weight/meal for children younger than 4 years of age and 500 units of lipase/kilogram body weight/meal for those over age 4.[58] The usual enzyme dose for snacks is one-half of the mealtime dose. It is recommended not to exceed 2500 units of lipase/kg body weight/meal, with a maximum daily dose of 10,000 units lipase/kg body weight. Calculating units of lipase/kilogram body weight/meal has become an integral component of routine care. For example, a 10-year-old child weighing 35.7 kg who takes a mealtime dose of three capsules of a pancreatic enzyme preparation containing 20,000 units of lipase per capsule will receive 1681 units of lipase/kg body weight/meal (60,000 units of lipase divided by 35.7 kg equals 1681 units of lipase/kg body weight/meal). Careful monitoring of the patient's growth, stool pattern, and the absence or presence of gastrointestinal symptoms is necessary in order to determine the adequacy of therapy. Monitoring and adjusting the dosage as needed should be continued throughout the patient's treatment. If the patient with CF is still exhibiting symptoms of malabsorption after reaching a maximum enzyme dose, it may be because the stomach contents are too acidic when reaching the small intestine and are inactivating the enzymes. In these cases, addingbicarbonate or other drugs that inhibit gastric acidity may be helpful.[58] Nonpancreatic reasons for malabsorption should also be considered.

Enzymes should be taken immediately before meals and snacks that contain fat, protein, and/or complex carbohydrate. The enterically coated enzymes should not be chewed or crushed. For infants and small children who are unable to swallow a capsule, the capsule can be opened and the contents mixed with a soft, acidic food such as applesauce. Enzymes mixed with food should be used within 30 minutes of mixing. When the enterically coated enzymes are mixed with a higher pH food such as pudding or milk, the enzymes may become activated and begin breaking down the food. Older patients swallow their enzymes whole before eating a meal or snack.

There is currently no consensus on enzyme dosing for gastrostomy tube feedings and often it can be difficult to dose enzymes appropriately. The previously most common method was for patients to take their usual meal dose of pancreatic enzymes by mouth before initiating the feeding.[27] If receiving continuous overnight tube feeds, some patients may need to take additional enzymes during the middle of the night or at the end of their feeding.[27] Some other CF centers suggest crushing Viokace™ which is a non-enteric coated version of pancrealipase. The Viokace™ tablets can be crushed into powder form and added to the enteral formula to pre-digest the fat in the formula prior to the patient receiving it.[61] If non-enteric coated enzymes are unavailable, another option described is to mix enteric-coated beads or microspheres in nectar thick juice or a bicarbonate solution and infuse directly into the feeding tube.[62,63] When used like this, pancreatic enzymes are often dosed by units lipase per gram of fat with the range being 500–4000 units lipase per gram of fat.[61] The options described above should be used with caution, however, because they are an off-label use of pancrealipase and may cause problems by clogging the feeding tube. Alternatively, Pertzye® 4,000 was recently FDA approved to go through a feeding tube of French size 14 or larger. Contents of no more than 2 capsules may be administered at one time and the microscpheres must be given in applesauce and then plunged directly into the feeding tube.[64]

Recently, the first FDA-approved method of giving pancreatic enzymes with tube feeds was made available. Relizorb® (immobilized lipase) is a digestive enzyme cartridge placed in-line with the enteral feeding system. The cartridge is filled with lipase beads and as the formula flows through the cartridge it is able to hydrolyze the fat before reaching the patient.[65] The cartridge is approved as a device and the dosing is one cartridge per 500 mL formula with the maximum dose of two cartridges used in a 24-hour period. Currently, Relizorb® is only approved for patients age 5 years and up and is limited to overnight feedings given at a rate of 24–120 mL/hr. It is not compatible with formulas that contain fiber. A randomized, double-blind, placebo-controlled trial showed that patients receiving Relizorb® with their overnight feeds had an increase in their plasma concentration of EHA and DHA which suggests an overall improvement in fat absorption.[66] Patients also described a decrease in the frequency and severity of their malabsorption symptoms when using Relizorb® over other traditional enzyme methods.[66] Decisions regarding the best method of giving pancreatic enzymes with enteral feeds should be a joint decision between the patient, their family, and the CF team. A patient's tolerance to their tube feeds, as well as if the patient will be able to comply with the enzyme regimen at home need to be assessed. It is important to tailor the enzyme regimen to the individual needs of each patient.

Patient Compliance Administering enzymes to an extremely young infant can be a frustrating endeavor for the parent or caretaker, primarily because of the young infant's natural extrusion reflex. After a few months of age, taking enzymes becomes part of a patient's daily routine. Parents of toddlers should be warned against allowing the child to "graze" throughout the day because this makes enzyme dosing difficult. In the preadolescent and adolescent age groups, patient adherence with enzyme administration can become a big issue. Some schools require the child to come to the school office for medications, and this may be a source of embarrassment and alienation from peers for the child with CF. The lack of compliance needs to be discussed with the child and a solution must be found that is agreeable to the child, the parents, and the school authorities.

Pancreatic enzyme therapy is very expensive and contributes significantly to the overall cost of disease management. Enzymes are often covered by third-party payers and some state programs for children with special healthcare needs.

Referral to Food/Nutrition and Other Resources

Referral to food and nutrition resources such as the USDA's **Special Supplemental Nutrition Program for Women, Infants, and Children** (WIC) program and the **Supplemental Nutrition Assistance Program** (SNAP) should be made based on the individual's needs and eligibility. In some states, referrals can be made to the state program for children with special healthcare needs to help obtain supplemental feedings, enzymes, and vitamins. Children who participate in the Child Nutrition Program at their school will need diet prescriptions for high-calorie, high-protein diets sent to their schools.

CF has a tremendous impact on patients and their families emotionally, physically, and financially. CF centers provide an interdisciplinary team approach to the care of these children and their families to better help them meet their many needs.

Alternative/Complementary Medicine

As with other chronic diseases, the use of alternative/complementary medicine in CF care has sparked the interest of patients with CF, their families, and health professionals. To date, little published science-based research exists in the area of alternative and complementary medicine in CF care. More and more CF centers are surveying their patients to ascertain the extent of alternative medicine practices. Currently, patients with CF are obtaining a lot of their information from the Internet, with many CF Internet sites having links to alternative

medicine sites. CF centers need to study alternative medicine practices further so that CF caregivers can advise patients and their families as to the safety and efficacy of various therapies.

It is important that CF caregivers ask questions about alternative/complementary medicine practices when interviewing patients with CF and their family members, especially in regard to ingested substances. This is especially important information to obtain from patients who may be participating in studies with experimental drugs because the possibility exists that substances such as unregulated botanical products may confound the study results.

▶ Lung Transplant

Lung transplantation is now becoming more common as a treatment of end-stage CF.[67] Patients become eligible for lung transplant when their lung function is significantly below normal and their health is declining despite aggressive pulmonary and nutrition interventions. Feeding tubes are often placed before transplant to improve nutritional status in preparation for major surgery. After the transplant is complete and lung function begins to improve, nutritional status usually also improves as energy expenditure from increased work of breathing and chronic infection is less.[68]

CF is a complicated disease, affecting many organs of the body, and the disease process is highly variable. Proper nutritional care is an integral part of its therapy. Therefore, every patient and family deserves individualized treatment and support from an interdisciplinary team of health professionals, including a qualified dietetics professional who is trained in the care of patients with CF.

▶ Bronchopulmonary Dysplasia

Bronchopulmonary dysplasia (BPD) was first described by Northway and colleagues[69] in 1967 as a form of chronic lung disease seen in infants with severe hyaline membrane disease who required mechanical ventilation and high concentrations of oxygen for prolonged periods of time. Since that time, improvements in neonatal intensive care and the changing epidemiology of prematurity have resulted in changes in both the definitions of BPD and the pathology of the lung disease. Most recently, clinical practice has advanced, resulting in a decrease in lung injury in larger (greater than 1200 gram birth weight) and more mature infants. At the same time, more and more premature infants are surviving at earlier gestational ages and lower birth weights. The National Institute of Child Health and Human Development/National Heart, Lung and Blood

Institute refined the definition of BPD to reflect differing criteria for infants born at less than or greater than 32 weeks gestation.[70] The expanded definition includes different diagnostic criteria for mild, moderate, and severe forms of the disease.[70] For example, the definition of severe BPD for an infant with a gestational age of less than 32 weeks is the need for 30% oxygen or more and/or positive pressure at 36 weeks postmenstrual age or discharge, whichever comes first.[70]

Today's definition of BPD includes infants who have had an acute lung injury with minimal clinical and radiographic findings, as well as those with major radiographic abnormalities. BPD represents a continuum of lung disease. The pathogenesis of BPD is multifactorial. Premature infants are born with few tiny air sacs of the lung, called alveoli. The alveoli that are present are often not mature enough to function normally, and as a result, the infant requires respiratory support with oxygen and/or mechanical ventilation. Severe, diffuse, acute lung injury and an early inflammatory response exacerbate the abnormal lung development due to primary injury and inadequate immature repair mechanisms. The lungs may be damaged by the barotrauma from using intermittent positive pressure ventilation (IPPV) and by oxygen toxicity from the high concentrations of oxygen required by these infants early in life.[71,72] The damage affects existing alveoli and those that develop after birth. This often leads to the need for prolonged periods of support on a ventilator and/or oxygen. Infection may play a role in the pathogenesis of BPD.[71] Other factors that may contribute to the development of the disease include increased fluids contributing to pulmonary edema[73] and inadequate early nutrition impeding lung reparative processes.[74,75]

Today, younger and smaller preterm infants are surviving with the aid of mechanical ventilation. Consequently, BPD has become one of the most common sequelae of newborn intensive care unit stays. BPD has become rare in premature infants weighing 1500 grams or more with uncomplicated respiratory distress syndrome. This is due to the use of antenatal steroids, surfactant replacement therapy, gentler ventilation that reduces barotrauma, better nutrition, and careful use of supplemental oxygen.[76] However, the incidence of BPD is about 30% of infants with birth weight under 1000 grams and is higher in lower birth weight infants. Between 2000 and 2009 the rates of **chronic lung disease** (CLD) reported by the Vermont Oxford Network in Infants born 501–1500 grams ranged from 26.2% to 30.4% with only a slight gradual decline during this period.[77]

Signs of respiratory distress, such as chest retractions, tachypnea, crackles, and wheezing, characterize BPD. Supplemental oxygen therapy may be required,

and there may be changes on the patient's chest radiograph. Pulmonary complications of BPD may include recurrent atelectasis, pulmonary infections, and respiratory failure requiring mechanical ventilation. The passage of blood through the lungs can also be difficult due to damage to surrounding blood vessels. This can subsequently lead to pulmonary hypertension and strain of the heart which may cause heart failure. Decreased lung reserves can often cause infants to breathe harder and faster than other infants. This is thought to affect growth due to potentially increased energy needs and decreased oral intake. Other complications of BPD include an increased need for hospital readmissions, persistent respiratory symptoms, decreased lung function, and neurodevelopmental delays.[78] As BPD patients are followed over time, chronic lung disease remains a major clinical problem for many of these patients into late childhood and even adulthood.

Prematurity and low birth weight are predictors of BPD. Infants born with intrauterine growth restriction and those born small for gestational age are also at an increased risk for developing BPD.[79]

The primary goal of BPD management is to provide the patient with the necessary pulmonary support during the acute and chronic phases of the disease to minimize lung damage and to maintain optimal oxygen saturation. Of equal importance is providing adequate nutrition, not only for growth and development, but also to compensate for the demands of the disease. Growth of new lung tissue can occur in humans until about 8 years of age. Theoretically, a BPD patient can "outgrow" the disease if adequate pulmonary and nutritional support can be provided.

▶ Nutritional Implications and Factors Affecting Growth

Adequate nutrition is important for patients with BPD but can often be a challenge for parents and health providers. The following section will further explore the nutrition implications of BPD.

Effects of Prematurity

Most babies who develop BPD are premature infants, so it is easy to see that these infants have little fat, glycogen, or other nutrients in reserve, particularly iron, zinc, calcium, and phosphorus. Faced with the demands of prematurity and the stress of BPD, the infant can quickly develop a state of negative nutrient balance. Small premature infants have frequent respiratory decompensation events that may cause interruptions in feedings that can result in greater deficits.

Effects of Bronchopulmonary Dysplasia

It has been reported that energy expenditures are higher with BPD. Several factors can increase the energy and nutrient requirements of BPD patients, including:

- Increased basal metabolic rate
- Increased work of breathing
- Chronic hypoxia
- Chronic illness/infections
- Respiratory distress/metabolic complications
- Tissue repair/catch-up growth
- Drug–nutrient interactions

Weinstein and Oh[80] reported that resting oxygen consumption was approximately 25% higher in eight infants with BPD, when compared with controls. Kurzner and colleagues[81] found that infants with BPD and growth failure had increased resting oxygen consumption, compared with control infants and infants with BPD and normal growth. Other investigators have also found an increase in resting energy expenditure in infants with BPD compared with controls, ranging from 125–150%.[82–84]

Treating the BPD patient usually includes a wide array of medications, including diuretics, steroids, and bronchodilators. Large variations in the use of these medications among institutions have been reported.[85,86] Using some diuretics may cause hyponatremia, hypochloremia, and/or hypokalemia requiring electrolyte supplementation. Using sodium chloride and potassium chloride is common. Potassium chloride has a high osmolarity and can cause gastrointestinal symptoms including nausea, vomiting, gas, or diarrhea. Diuretics could also cause increased urinary zinc losses. This places preterm infants at a higher risk for zinc deficiency due to low body stores of zinc due to the reduced time for placental transfer. Steroids are used to help facilitate extubation and improve lung function. Long-term steroid courses were common in the 1990s, but their use has decreased due to reports of an increased risk for negative neurodevelopmental outcomes. Steroids are associated with negative effects on growth and altered composition of weight gain by increasing fat deposition.[87] The impact of these drugs on the patient's nutritional status is further summarized in **TABLE 15.6**.

Decreased Nutrient Consumption

Infants with BPD are fluid sensitive because of the acute lung disease and the possible complication of cor pulmonale, or right-sided heart failure. When fluid restrictions are imposed, this potentially places a limitation on the provision of energy and nutrients. Thus, infants with BPD often require higher caloric concentrations in order to meet their energy needs for adequate growth.

TABLE 15.6 BPD Drug–Nutrient Interactions

Medication	Nutrients Affected (lowers all)	Other Effects
Diuretics (e.g., furosemide)	Na, K, Cl, Mg, Ca, Zn	Volume depletion Metabolic alkalosis Anorexia Diarrhea Hyperuricemia Gastrointestinal irritant
Bronchodilators (e.g., theophylline)		Gastrointestinal distress Nausea Vomiting Diarrhea
Steroids (e.g., dexamethasone)	Ca, P	Growth suppression

Frequent intubations and mechanical ventilation interfere with the normal feeding sequence and feeding-skill development. Therefore, these infants may be poor oral feeders and develop aversive oral behavior.[88] Also, these patients may experience fatigue or decreased oxygen saturation during feeding because of their underlying pulmonary disease.[89,90] Infants with BPD also may have associated gastroesophageal reflux, causing an impediment to feeding.[91]

▶ Growth of Infants with BPD

Growth failure is a reported complication of BPD. Suggested explanations for poor growth in this population include increased caloric needs related to both prematurity and the demands of the disease including increased work of breathing and higher metabolic rates. Premature infants are also more prone to acute life-threatening events, such as respiratory failure and necrotizing enterocolitis, which would cause periods of instability and subsequent interruptions to nutrient delivery. Older studies that documented poor growth patterns may be reflective of older management strategies for infants with BPD such as a higher incidence of early steroids and less aggressive nutrition intervention. Early nutrition intervention for critically ill, very low birth weight infants, including parenteral and enteral nutrition, has become standard practice and is associated with improved growth without an increased risk of negative clinical outcomes.[92]

In a recent study, Gianni and colleagues reported that increasing energy intakes of preterm infants with BPD improved their weight gain velocity. Enteral calorie intake was higher in the intervention group, which received individually tailored fortified breast milk and/or preterm formula in order to reach 120–150 kcal/kg/day. In the historical control group, breast milk was fortified as indicated by the instructions of the manufacturer of the fortifier, or preterm formula was used. Enteral protein intake was the same. Improvements in weight gain did not correlate with an improvement in linear growth. This raises concerns about the quality of growth as the infants could have increased fat deposition. Body composition was not assessed.[93]

Huysman and colleagues studied 29 preterm infants with BPD and compared their growth and body composition to healthy term infants during the first year of life. The preterm infants with BPD had lower total body fat and fat free mass by 6 weeks post term. These markers continued to remain low throughout the first year of life. Infants with BPD had lower mean length z-scores at 6 weeks post term. The length scores did improve between 6 weeks and 12 months; however, in girls with BPD the mean length scores were still significantly lower than term infants at 12 months post term. There was no correlation between energy and protein intake and the differences. Since the study compared preterm infants with BPD to health term infants, it is not known whether the effects on body composition are due to BPD or prematurity.[94]

Sanchez-Solis et al studied 71 preterm infants with BPD and measured lung function at 6 months corrected age and 1 year later. Infants with BPD had lower lung function at both time points. There was a significant correlation between an increase in lung function with an increase in linear growth velocity, but not with an increase in weight.[95] Many studies only report weight gain, but this reinforces the need for adequate linear growth which can be a better indicator of long-term growth and lean body mass accretion.

Nutritional Screening and Assessment

It is important to monitor the nutritional status of patients with BPD in order to ensure they are receiving adequate nutrition for growth and development and to compensate for the demands of the disease. Nutrition assessment in infants with BPD includes the same components evaluated in other populations with the addition of classification of gestational age and size for gestational age. These classifications can also help guide clinical care needs. Infants born with intrauterine growth restriction are at a higher risk for BPD.

Anthropometric

Weight, length, and head circumference measurements are used to monitor post-natal growth and nutritional status. Serial measurements are plotted on growth curves and compared to established reference data. Intrauterine growth curves are used for premature infants. Once corrected to term age, the **Centers for Disease Control and Prevention** (CDC) recommends using the **World Health Organization** (WHO) growth charts published in 2006, which establish the growth of breastfed infants as the norm, to monitor growth for infants and children age 0–2 years. The CDC growth charts are recommended to monitor growth for children age 2 years and older. Measurements are usually corrected for gestational age until 24 months.

Obtaining daily weights in a BPD patient is essential during early hospitalizations and critical stages of the disease. Weight data can help to identify fluid overload as well as monitor growth. For premature infants the goal weight gain is between 15–20 grams/kg/day after regaining birth weight. For term infants, and preterm infants who correct to term, the goal weight gain is about 25–35 grams/day. In 2006 the WHO published weight gain velocity charts that reflect the growth of term infants in conditions researchers felt were ideal.[96] Weight gain velocities are higher right after birth and in earlier infancy, and then continue to decrease throughout the first year of life.

Length should be measured on an infant length board. Weekly length measurements have advantages over weight measurements. Length more accurately reflects lean body tissue mass and is not influenced by fluid status or edema. Linear growth is a better marker for long-term growth. Goal incremental gain in length for low birth weight infants is about 0.9 cm per week.[97] The goal is less for full term infants and the goal for linear growth velocity also gradually decreases over time.

Head circumference should also be measured weekly. Situations such as edema and the use of certain devices can affect the accuracy of the measurements. Other situations, such as hydrocephalus, may require more frequent measurements.

Weight-for-length reflects body weight in proportion to attained growth in length; it is useful in assessing the symmetry of growth. Infants with low weight-for-length may be malnourished. Using z-scores for this measure can identify the severity of malnutrition.[98] The more negative the z-score is indicative of how many standards deviations it is away from the mean. Infants with high weight-for-length z-scores may be over-nourished and at risk of becoming overweight or obese.

Additional measurements such as mid-arm circumference and triceps skinfold can help determine whether weight gain is secondary to growth or edema. See also Chapter 4 "Malnutrition Related to Undernutrition."

Biochemical

Biochemical monitoring of the BPD patient is individualized based on the patient's clinical status, the type and amount of diuretic therapy, and the protocol of the individual institution. During diuretic therapy, electrolytes need to be monitored, especially sodium, chloride, and potassium. Mineral status should be monitored including calcium, phosphorus, and magnesium. Other helpful measurements may include prealbumin or albumin as a measure of visceral protein stores, a complete blood count, alkaline phosphatase, parathyroid hormone, and 25-hydroxyvitamin D.

Clinical

The patient's pulmonary status will have an impact on nutritional needs and intake. If a patient with BPD is ventilator dependent, this is an indication of respiratory failure and severe lung disease. Ventilator-dependent BPD patients require close follow-up because it may be difficult initially to determine their nutritional needs. Many chronic ventilator-dependent patients with BPD have very low energy needs and yet their other nutrient needs are the same as other infants with BPD. For these patients, feedings must be adjusted to meet nutrient needs without providing too many calories. This may require protein and vitamin and/or mineral supplementation. A patient who has a low arterial partial pressure of oxygen is not properly oxygenating tissue, which may contribute to growth failure. These patients may require supplemental oxygen for tissue oxygenation and growth. Noting a patient's oximetry reading is important. An increase in pulmonary symptoms such as the presence of tachypnea, rales, rhonchi, and bronchiolitis/pneumonia is indicative of active pulmonary disease. The presence of chronic pulmonary disease and acute pulmonary exacerbations in BPD patients increases energy needs and at the same time may increase their sensitivity to fluids.

Other medical conditions, such as cor pulmonale, gastroesophageal reflux with or without aspiration, esophagitis, repeated emesis, and the patient's medication regimen, should also be noted. Table 15.6 lists drug–nutrient interactions of medications commonly prescribed for BPD patients. It is important to note a patient's input and output to complete the clinical assessment.

Dietary Intake

The BPD patient's dietary intake needs to be evaluated for calories, protein, fluid, electrolytes, and other key components including calcium, phosphorus, vitamin D, iron, and zinc. The type of feeding (enteral versus parenteral) should be noted, as well as the route of administration and additional vitamin, mineral, and/or electrolyte supplementation. This can then be compared with the patient's estimated nutrient and fluid requirements.

Of particular importance in the nutrition assessment of BPD patients is careful monitoring of the patient's ability to suck and swallow and the patient's feeding skill development. The sucking reflex does not develop until between 32–34 weeks gestational age. Alternate methods of feeding are required until this reflex develops. Neurologic impairment may prevent the patient from being able to coordinate sucking and swallowing. Noxious stimuli to the patient's mouth, such as frequent intubations and suctioning, may seriously affect normal feeding skill development. Maintaining adequate oxygenation during feedings is essential.[89,90] It is important to note whether the patient tires during feedings and whether he or she turns blue around the mouth or fingertips, indicating a drop in oxygen saturation. It is imperative that these problems are identified early and appropriate intervention instituted.

Nutrition Management

After the nutritional assessment of a patient with BPD is complete, it is important to provide appropriate nutrition interventions that will support the infant's specific nutritional requirements. There are many factors that need to be taken into consideration when establishing these interventions. The next section will explore in more detail the nutrition management of patients with BPD.

Nutrients of Concern

It is important to assess and monitor intake of macronutrients as well as several key micronutrients in the BPD patient.

Energy The caloric requirement for infants with BPD can initially be higher than normal and could range from 120–150 kcal/kg/day.[91,99] Higher ranges would be more common with rapidly growing low birth weight infants. As these infants approach term age and weight, calorie needs may be closer to what is appropriate at term. Meeting these high levels of intake can be a challenge, especially when other problems exist such as fluid restrictions, gastrointestinal immaturity, and renal immaturity.

Protein Protein needs for preterm infants are high and range from 3.8–4.4 grams/kg/day for extremely low birth weight infants and 3.4–4.2 grams/kg/day for very low birth weight infants.[100] Providing adequate protein for corrected gestational age is essential to promote linear growth. Protein needs will continue to be high during catabolic states. Steroid use can impact body composition and linear growth and so aiming toward the higher range for protein provision may be beneficial.

Vitamins A and E Many older studies have examined the role of vitamin A (retinol) in animals and premature infants who develop chronic lung disease.[101] Vitamin A is essential in the respiratory tract for maintaining the integrity and differentiation of epithelial cells. Deficiency of vitamin A results in loss of cilia and other changes in the airways, which resemble the changes seen in BPD. Vitamin A adequacy may decrease the incidence of BPD in infants with very low birth weight.[102] Administering 5000 IU vitamin A intramuscularly three times a week to infants at risk for developing BPD may be advantageous.[103,104] Some newborn intensive care units administer vitamin A in an attempt to protect against BPD.[105]

Adequate vitamin E status is particularly important in premature infants with BPD who are on oxygen therapy because vitamin E is a major antioxidant. Vitamin E acts as an oxygen free radical scavenger and membrane stabilizer, protecting lipid-containing cell membranes from oxidation. Infants are most likely to receive adequate vitamin E when fed human milk or commercial formulas. Large doses of vitamin E appear to offer no additional protection against BPD.[106]

Zinc Zinc is an essential micronutrient that plays an important role in growth and the production of enzymes. It is also a structural component of certain proteins and hormones.[107] Most fetal accretion of zinc occurs in the third trimester. Premature infants are at high risk for zinc deficiency due to decreased body stores related to less time for placental transfer. The risk of zinc deficiency is also increased with other conditions such as intestinal failure which may be associated with increased stool losses. Zinc levels can also be decreased with diuretic therapy. Zinc deficiency is associated with stunted growth, decreased immune function, and poor wound healing.[108] Plasma zinc concentration is a biomarker of zinc status, but it has limitations.[108] Alkaline phosphatase is a zinc-dependent metalloenzyme that is thought to be lower with zinc deficiency[108] but some studies do not show a correlation.[109]

Zinc supplementation has been shown to have a positive effect on linear growth in premature infants.[107] In a recent study, researchers evaluated the effect of enteral zinc supplementation on weight gain and linear growth in extremely low birth weight infants with BPD. Most of the infants received fortified human milk which may vary in zinc concentration and is lower in zinc compared with formula. Both rates of weight gain and linear growth increased after zinc supplementation. The limitations of the study include its small sample size and retrospective nature.[109] Larger, prospective studies are needed to further evaluate the relationship between zinc supplementation and growth in preterm infants with BPD.

Enteral requirements for zinc for growing extremely low birth weight and very low birth weight infants are between 1000–3000 mcg/kg/day.[100] Adequate intakes for infants 0–6 months old and 7–12 months old are 2 mg/day and 3 mg/day, respectively.[100] Zinc supplementation above estimated requirements could potentially inhibit copper and iron absorption. An older study did not show that zinc supplementation affected copper or iron status,[110] however, it may be beneficial to monitor copper and iron status during long periods of supplementation.

Iron The recommended iron intake is 2–4 mg of elemental iron/kg/day,[111] and the supplementation should begin no later than 2 months of age. Iron can be provided through a supplement or through the use of iron-fortified formulas.

Calcium and Phosphorus Metabolic bone disease (MBD), or osteopenia of prematurity, due to inadequate calcium and phosphorus is common. Infants born prematurely are born without the benefit of the calcium and phosphorus accretion of the third trimester of pregnancy. Additionally, the calcium and phosphorus status of premature infants with BPD can be further compromised by diuretic therapy, steroid therapy, and feeding delays. Complications of severe prematurity could require long-term use of parenteral nutrition. Severe respiratory decompensation may lead to feeding intolerance and infants with BPD could also require intermittent use of parenteral nutrition. The solubility of calcium and phosphorus in parenteral nutrition limits their intake during its use. MBD is diagnosed by decreased bone density on X-rays and is correlated with elevated alkaline phosphatase levels. Often serum calcium levels are normal while serum phosphorus levels are low. Enteral calcium requirements for ELBW and VLBW infants are 100–220 mg/kg/day.[100] Enteral phosphorus requirements for ELBW and VLBW infants are 60–140 mg/kg/day.[100] Adequate vitamin D (400 IU/d) intake is also important.[111]

Electrolytes Electrolyte imbalance may result, especially when the infant is receiving diuretic therapy. Potassium, chloride, and/or sodium may need to be supplemented depending on the diuretic therapy.[72,73] Electrolye levels should be closely monitored when sodium chloride and/or potassium chloride are being added to the infant's feedings.

Barriers to Meeting Increased Needs

Many barriers must be overcome in order to meet the increased nutrient needs of the infant with BPD. These barriers include:

- Fluid restriction for infants with cor pulmonale or right-sided heart failure and those who are fluid sensitive
- Gastrointestinal limitations such as an immature gut
- Immature renal function, making renal solute load of feedings a potential issue
- Chronic hypoxia, especially during feedings and sleep

- Feeding difficulties, including lack of sucking reflex and feeding aversions
- Significant gastroesophageal reflux resulting in vomiting or discomfort with feeding

Meeting Nutritional Needs

Translating these energy, protein, and other nutrient needs into a feeding order can be challenging.

Parenteral Nutrition (PN)

PN is used for preterm infants in order to prevent negative energy and protein balance and support growth until enteral feeds can be initiated and advanced. During an acute phase of BPD, parenteral nutrition is often employed when it is anticipated that adequate enteral nutrition will not be tolerated. See chapter 11 for specific guidelines for PN in the early postnatal period for premature infants.

Enteral Nutrition

Enteral feedings must be begun at a slow rate in order to allow the immature intestine of the premature infant to adapt to the feedings. During this transitional phase, PN is continued, but decreased as the volume of enteral feeds is gradually increased, in order to meet the increased energy needs of the patient. It is important to maintain the delivery of adequate energy and protein while tolerance to enteral feedings is being established. PN is usually continued until volumes of enteral nutrition reach 100–120 ml/kg/day.

Breast milk (maternal or donor) is preferred initially for the premature gastrointestinal tract because it is easily tolerated and associated with a decreased incidence of necrotizing enterocolitis.[112,113] As described, enteral nutrient requirements are higher in preterm infants than in term infants because of decreased nutrient stores and more rapid rates of weight gain. The higher need for calories, protein, calcium, phosphorus, vitamins, and minerals can usually be met if a human milk fortifier (HMF) is added to the breast milk, or if a premature formula is used. One commercial fortifier is made from concentrated and fortified donor breast milk. Other HMF products are made from bovine milk. Breast milk is typically fortified with HMF to 24 kcal/oz and the typical concentration for preterm formula is 24 kcal/oz. At enteral feeding volumes of 150–160 ml/kg/day, a 24 kcal/oz formula will provide 120–130 kcal/kg/day. In some cases it may be necessary to use a higher caloric concentration; for example if energy needs for adequate growth are higher or if fluid is restricted. Modular fat can be added to further increase the breast milk to 26 or 28 kcal/oz as needed. Formula can be concentrated to 27 or 30 kcal/oz. Concentrating formula in this manner keeps the nutrient distribution in balance, but careful monitoring of electrolytes and fluid status are warranted.

The infant should continue on breast milk fortified with a HMF or with a premature formula until they correct to post-term, reach a weight of at least 3000 grams, or as the clinical situation indicates. At this point, the infant can likely be transitioned to a premature discharge formula or to breast milk fortified with a premature discharge formula.

A recent review on the effects of premature discharge formula compared with term formula indicated that when energy intakes are sufficient, increased protein intake resulted in at least short term increased growth and lean mass accretion.[114] The additional protein and selected minerals in premature discharge formulas may be especially beneficial to support linear growth in the BPD population.

Premature infants display a nutritional suck between 32–34 weeks gestation, but their swallowing function could still be immature. Oral feeding before this time is not indicated as it may cause apnea or aspiration due to uncoordinated airway protective mechanisms. Infants with BPD are often not candidates for oral feeding even at higher gestational ages due to respiratory compromise requiring the need for supplemental oxygen and other support. Most premature infants with or without BPD begin enteral feeding by tube feeding. Nasogastric and orogastric tubes are the most common. Feeds can be given via an intermittent bolus. If there is emesis, reflux or concern for malabsorption, continuous feeds can be tried. For infants with severe reflux and aspiration risk, post-pyloric feeds can be used. Nasoduodenal or nasojejunal feeds must always be given continuously due to the osmotic load being given past the stomach if bolus feeds are used. Long term gastrostomy tubes can be placed when the need for tube feeding is greater than 2–3 months. Sometimes infants are able to consume small amounts of formula by mouth and then the rest can be given via the feeding tube in order to achieve adequate intake.

Addressing Feeding Difficulties

The patient's ability to suck and swallow must be assessed. Abnormalities in the developmental patterns of suck-and-swallow rhythms during feeding in preterm infants with BPD have been reported.[115] Feeding behavior should be assessed for age appropriateness based on corrected age.

Patients with BPD are susceptible to developing feeding difficulties because of their usual prematurity and because of the nature of the life-sustaining respiratory therapy that they receive. Intubations and suctioning are noxious stimuli to the oral area and can interfere with normal feeding development.

Speech language pathologists identify feeding problems and design treatment plans. Nonnutritive sucking can be instituted during a tube feeding so that the infant can begin to associate feelings of satiety with sucking. Overlooking problems in the development of feeding skills can result in serious aversions to eating or decreased and inadequate intake. A comprehensive behavioral feeding program may be necessary to help initiate and advance oral feeds in growing premature infants.

Singer and associates[116] found that mothers of infants with BPD spent more time prompting the infants to feed, but these infants took in less formula and spent less time sucking than the two control groups of premature infants without BPD and term infants. In another study, parents often expressed concern about getting their infant with BPD to take enough food and reported long feeding times.[117] Problematic feeding interactions between the caregiver and the infant may develop. It is important that the healthcare professional be aware of this potential problem and provide the family with anticipatory guidance in this area. If the patient's oral intake is not adequate to meet nutritional needs, then tube feedings are necessary. A plan for balancing tube feedings with oral feedings must be designed to establish hunger and appetite for feedings by mouth but providing the balance of nutrition via the tube feeding.

Family/Caretaker Education

The home care of the patient with BPD can be quite complex and may include supplemental oxygen and multiple medications and therapies as well as nutrition management. Family and caretaker education by a registered dietitian is an important component of the nutrition care plan, and adequate time must be devoted to education during the discharge-planning process. Written instructions for mixing formulas in common household measures for volumes that will be used in 24 hours or less should be given to families. It is important to have the family member or caretaker demonstrate the proper mixing of formulas, especially formula that is being concentrated or contains additives. Reinforcing these instructions needs to take place on an ongoing basis in outpatient follow-up. It is important to consistently ask the family how they are mixing the formula at home to ensure that they are following the correct recipe and the infant is getting the calories that he or she needs to demonstrate adequate growth.

Referral to Food/Nutrition Resources

Caring for a patient with BPD can be very draining for the patient's family from emotional, physical, and financial standpoints. It is important to assess the patient's and family's needs with regard to food and nutrition resources. Appropriate referrals must be made. Often,

this can be done in cooperation with the nurse and/or social worker.

Medical and Nutrition Follow-up

After discharge from the hospital, the infant with BPD will require regular medical and nutrition follow-up. Feedings will need to be adjusted as the patient grows and develops. Many patients benefit from being enrolled in early intervention programs that can provide nutrition, occupational therapy, physical therapy, and speech therapy as needed by the individual patient.

Identification of Areas Needing Further Research

The effects of early onset of respiratory failure and vigorous ventilator support on nutrient and energy requirements for patients with BPD should be assessed at various stages of the disease, particularly regarding energy, protein, calcium, phosphorus and zinc. General growth studies that measure linear growth and symmetry of growth using weight-for-length z-scores for patients with BPD would provide guidance for healthcare practitioners. Nutritional requirements of BPD patients at various stages of the disease and appropriate methods and timing of nutrition intervention in BPD treatment require further study. The long-term sequelae of BPD and its current treatment modalities require ongoing investigation.

▶ Asthma

Asthma is a common chronic disease of childhood, affecting 9.5% of children from birth until 17 years of age.[118] Overall asthma occurs more often among females than in males.[118] Disparities exist among racial/ethnic populations, with the highest prevalence seen in whites and the lowest among Asians. Black, American Indian and Alaskan natives have a higher incidence of asthma compared with whites, and people of Puerto Rican descent have the highest rate of all groups.[118]

Asthma is defined by the National Heart, Lung and Blood Institute[119] as a chronic inflammatory disorder of the airways. Symptoms of this inflammation include recurrent episodes of wheezing, breathlessness, chest tightness, and cough, particularly at night and early in the morning and during or after exercise.[120] These asthma episodes are associated with widespread but variable obstruction of airflow. Inflammation of the airways also causes an associated increase in airway responsiveness to a variety of stimuli.[120] Inflammation causes airway narrowing and increased airway secretions. Chronic inflammation can lead to airway remodeling, which can cause progressive loss of pulmonary function.[120]

A major goal of asthma treatment is reducing inflammation. The first step toward this is for the patient to recognize and avoid the triggers of asthma. Triggers may include indoor allergens such as dust mites, cockroaches, and animal dander, and outdoor allergens such as trees, grasses, weeds, pollens, and mold.[120] Environmental tobacco smoke, air pollutants, exercise, weather/humidity changes, and some medications (particularly aspirin, beta blockers, and non steroidal anti-inflammatory drugs) can also precipitate asthma symptoms in children.[120] Viral respiratory infections can also influence the development and severity of asthma.[120] Other factors contributing to asthma severity include rhinitis, sinusitis, gastroesophageal reflux, obstructive sleep apnea, and obesity.[120] Food allergies may also cause asthma symptoms.[121]

In addition to reducing factors that increase the patient's asthma symptoms, pharmacologic therapy is an important component of asthma management. The choice of specific medicines is based on asthma severity and the classification of asthma. The goal is to optimize pharmacotherapy while minimizing side effects. Long-term control medicines are taken daily in order to achieve and maintain control of persistent asthma by reducing inflammation. Long-term control medicines include inhaled corticosteroids, long-acting beta$_2$ agonists, cromolyn sodium or nedocromil (inhaled), omalizumab, leukotriene modifiers, and rarely, methylxanthine.[120] Quick relief medications, including inhaled short-acting beta$_2$ agonists, anticholinergics, and short-course systemic corticosteroids are used to treat acute symptoms and exacerbations.[120]

Food Allergies and Asthma

The rates of food allergies and asthma are rising, and it appears that there may be more of a correlation between the two than was once thought. Infants diagnosed with an allergy in early infancy have been shown to have an increased risk of asthma.[121,122] There appears to be an even stronger association between the diagnosis of food allergies and asthma in children who have multiple or more severe food allergies.[123]

The role of food allergies in the exacerbation of asthma symptoms is controversial. In a study by Adler and associates,[124] 14.5% of children with asthma were reported by their parents to have food-provoked asthma symptoms. Several studies have been reported in the scientific literature investigating the true incidence of asthma symptoms caused by food allergies using double-blind, placebo-controlled food challenges.[125–127] The results of these investigations thus far include findings that IgE-mediated reactions to food can cause respiratory symptoms, including wheezing, but that this is uncommon, even in children with histories of other adverse reactions to food. According to Ozol and Mete, only 6–8% of children with asthma have respiratory symptoms triggered by foods.[121] Although rare, it should be noted that patients with asthma are more likely to have a life-threatening reaction if they are exposed to foods they are allergic to because of the potential for respiratory system involvement.[122] It is important that patients receive a thorough education on how to safely avoid foods they have been diagnosed as allergic to while still maintaining a balanced diet.

Milk and Mucus

It is a common misconception among lay people that drinking milk causes an increased production of mucus and may be a trigger for asthma. However, there is no scientific evidence to support this claim. This belief may persist because milk, particularly whole milk, coats the tongue and mouth and some people may have the sensation that they have an increase in mucus production or that their mucus is thicker after milk consumption. In an Australian study, believers and nonbelievers of the milk–mucus connection were studied.[128] Clearing their throats was the most common symptom described by both the believers and nonbelievers after drinking milk. Words commonly used to describe the sensation associated with drinking milk were "thick," "blocked," and "clogged."[128] These same researchers administered chocolate cow's milk or chocolate soy milk in a randomized trial.[129] They found that the same type of sensory perceptions of milk were described by believers and nonbelievers of the milk–mucus connection theory for both types of milk. These researchers concluded that these same perceptions extended to milk substitute beverages as well as milk. Further studies found the ingestion of a cow milk solution powder dissolved in a strawberry-flavored beverage to have no effect versus placebo on the pulmonary function in a group of adult mild asthmatics in a double-blind placebo-controlled study.[128] Individuals may have bona fide milk allergy, but these numbers are relatively low. Indiscriminate elimination of a whole food group such as dairy products from the diet of a child with asthma may be totally unnecessary and may deprive the child of an important source of nutrients such as calcium.

Role of Breastfeeding in the Prevention of Asthma

The relationship of breastfeeding to asthma prevention has been studied using data from the **National Health and Nutrition Examination Survey** (NHANES III) with conflicting interpretations. One group of investigators found that breastfed children compared with never breastfed children "may" have a delay in the onset of asthma or recurrent wheeze or they "may" actually be actively protected against asthma.[130] However, Rust and colleagues[131] found that breastfeeding "did not appear" to have an impact on asthma prevention or a reduction in its severity. According to the NHANES III data, the relationship between breastfeeding and asthma prevention is not strong. Wright and associates[132] found that longer durations of exclusive breastfeeding increased the risk of reported asthma among children with asthmatic mothers, whereas a meta-analysis showed evidence that longer duration of breast feeding in infancy is associated with lower risk of asthma later on in children ages 5–18 years of age.[133] Other studies have demonstrated conflicting results in exclusive breastfeeding impact upon later development of asthma.[134,135] One study demonstrated that breast feeding for the first twelve months may be protective against asthma, but this decreased after eighteen months and actually increased the risk for children who were breast fed for over twenty four months.[136] Additionally, there is no evidence to justify delaying the introduction of solid foods in infants older than 4 to 6 months of age in order to prevent asthma.[137]

Relationship Between Asthma and Obesity

Both asthma and obesity have been increasing at alarming rates in the United States. This epidemiological observation prompted studies conducted during the 1980s, which generated the hypothesis of an association between asthma and obesity.[138] This association has been studied in adults and children.

Studies in adults have found that obesity does affect pulmonary function. The prospective Nurses' Health Study II found that BMI was a strong, independent, positive risk factor for the onset of asthma.[139]Other investigators in Finland have shown improvements in lung function, symptoms, morbidity, and health status with weight reduction in obese patients with asthma.[140] Possible explanations for the association between asthma and obesity include the possibilities that gastroesophageal reflux due to obesity exacerbates asthma, that physical inactivity may promote both diseases, and that the high-fat diets of obese patients may promote airway inflammation and asthma.[138]

The relationship between asthma and obesity also has been studied in the pediatric population. Many of these studies have been conducted with inner city, minority populations because these populations have the highest prevalence of asthma and are at greatest risk of experiencing the morbidity and mortality of this chronic disease.

Luder and associates[141] compared a group of inner city children with asthma to a group of their peers. The prevalence of overweight was significantly higher in children with moderate to severe asthma than in their peers. In the asthma group, a higher BMI was associated with significantly more severe asthma symptoms, such as lower pulmonary function measurements, more school absenteeism, and a greater number of prescribed asthma medications.[141] These investigators recommend studying the effect of weight reduction in asthma patients with a high BMI on asthma symptoms. Gennuso and colleagues[142] studied urban minority children and adolescents who had asthma and non-asthma controls. These investigators found an increase in obesity among children with asthma for both sexes and across ages compared with controls. The severity of asthma was not related to obesity. These investigators concluded that asthma is a risk factor for obesity in children. As part of the National Cooperative Inner City Asthma Study, Belamarich and colleagues[143] found that 19% of the asthma patients ages 4 to 9 years had BMIs over the 95th percentile, as compared with 11% of all children in the NHANES III survey. The investigators also found that obese children with asthma required more asthma medication, reported more days of wheezing, and visited the emergency department more than nonobese children with asthma.

The Tucson Children's Respiratory Study found that female subjects who were overweight or obese between 6 and 11 years of age were seven times more likely to develop new asthma symptoms at age 11 and 13 years.[144] These investigators hypothesized that being overweight may influence female sex hormones, which in turn increase asthma risk. Gilliland and associates[145] studied almost 4000 school-age children in the longitudinal Children's Health Study in southern California. These investigators found that overweight was associated with increased risk of new onset asthma in boys and in non-allergic children. Tantisira and colleagues[146] studied children with mild to moderate asthma who were enrolled in the Childhood Asthma Management Program (CAMP). They found that although an increasing BMI was associated with an increase in forced expiratory volume in 1 second (FEV_1) and forced vital capacity (FVC), the ratio of FEV_1 to FVC was reduced. There was a positive association between BMI and cough/wheeze with exercise. This study did not support the hypothesis that an increase in BMI increases asthma severity, but the increase in exercise-induced bronchospasm with increasing BMI suggests a relationship between increased airway responsiveness and BMI. Conversely, one large study found that although school aged children who are persistently overweight or who become overweight during childhood are at increased risk of asthma, persistently underweight children have an increased risk of allergic asthma as well.[147] The conclusions that can be drawn regarding the association of overweight and asthma from these studies in pediatrics include:

- There is a higher prevalence of overweight in children with asthma.
- Overweight children with asthma have increased asthma symptoms.
- Overweight may influence asthma risk.

Effects of Nutrients on Asthma

Because asthma affects the lives of so many adults and children, much research has been done in the area of asthma treatment and preventing asthma exacerbations, including the impact of nutrition on asthma patients. Many studies have been performed investigating the role of various nutrients in protecting against asthma, as well as their effects on improving asthma symptoms. Nutrients that have been studied include vitamin C, fish oils, selenium, and electrolytes, including sodium and magnesium.

Vitamin C

Antioxidants protect cell membranes from damage caused by free radicals and chemical oxidants. Of the antioxidant vitamins, vitamin C has received the most attention, with most of the studies involving adult subjects. According to NHANES I, lower dietary vitamin C intakes were associated with lower FEV_1. However, the difference in this pulmonary function test between the highest and lowest levels of dietary vitamin C was not great and the clinical significance of this finding was questioned.[148] In one pediatric study, children ages 8 to 11 years who never ate fresh fruit had 4.3% lower pulmonary function and had a 25.3% higher incidence of wheezing than did children who ate fruit more than once a day.[149] However, vitamin C intake was not specifically analyzed in this study. Other studies have suggested possible short-term protective effects of vitamin C on airway responsiveness.[150] This area warrants further investigation before routine supplementation can be recommended for asthma patients. However, encouraging children with asthma to include a daily source of vitamin C in their diets is sound advice.

Fish Oils

The ingestion of fish oils, which contain omega-3 fatty acids, causes **arachidonic acid** (AA) to be replaced by **eicosapentaenoic acid** (EPA) and **docosahexaenoic acid** (DHA) in cell membranes. This replacement leads to a decrease in the production of the inflammatory metabolites of AA, including leukotrienes. It is thought that this change in metabolites could have potential effects on airway inflammation, which is why fish oil ingestion and its relationship to asthma has been studied.[151,152]

As with the antioxidants, most of the studies have been with adult asthma patients.[121] A positive relationship between dietary fish intake and higher pulmonary function was found when the data from NHANES I were examined.[152] A study of Australian schoolchildren found an association between oily fish intake and a reduction in prevalence of increased airway responsiveness and in the incidence of asthma.[153] Another group of investigators compared the clinical effects of fish oil supplementation and a diet that increases omega-3 polyunsaturated fatty acids with a diet enriched in omega-6 fatty acids in a double-blind, randomized trial of 39 children with asthma. No significant changes in clinical severity of asthma were found.[154] Other investigators found decreased asthma symptoms when fish oil capsules were given to 29 children with asthma who participated in a randomized controlled trial in a controlled environment in terms of inhalant allergens and diet.[155] The majority of the studies do not show significant clinical improvement in asthma patients with the use of fish oils, with the exception of an inverse relationship between fish intake in pregnant mothers and infant fish intake with the development of asthma.[156] Another question that remains is whether dietary fatty acids play a role in the development of asthma. The data are inconclusive at this point and do not support using fish oil to treat asthma.[156] Further investigation is warranted, but recommending the inclusion of fatty fish in the diets of children with asthma is simply consistent with current healthy diet recommendations.

Selenium

The relationship of selenium to asthma has been studied because of selenium's role as an antioxidant. No current data demonstrate a beneficial effect of selenium supplementation on pulmonary function tests in asthma patients. Although some studies have indicated a possible correlation between low serum levels of selenium and asthma symptoms, there is insufficient evidence to advocate using selenium supplementation to treat asthma.[157]

The role that specific nutrients may play in asthma has sparked much interest in the scientific community. More research in this area is needed before specific recommendations can be made. Interest in this area will probably continue to grow, especially as the practice of alternative/complementary medicine receives more attention. The data gathered to date reinforce the importance to asthma patients of a diet containing a variety of food sources.

Electrolytes

The relationship of increased sodium intake and asthma has been investigated by several groups of researchers.[158] These studies have been performed because it was hypothesized that diets high in salt may increase bronchial reactivity. Although the data have shown some benefit in improving lunch function after exercise in exercise-induced asthma, no significant effects on the clinical symptoms of asthma have been found.[158] Also, the data from many of the studies are confounded by other variables, such as other dietary constituents. Currently, there are little scientific data to support using low-salt diets to treat asthma.[158-160] Magnesium administered intravenously may play a role in treating acute asthma exacerbations in children.[161] Several studies concluded that IV magnesium decreases the need for hospital admission in children with moderate to severe asthma flare-ups; however, all of these studies are very small.[161] One study in England[162] evaluated the relationship between magnesium intake assessed from food frequency questionnaires, and pulmonary function FEV_1, airway reactivity to methacholine, and self-reported wheezing. A magnesium intake of 100mg per day or higher was associated with a 27.7 mL higher FEV_1, a reduction in relative odds of airway hyper-responsiveness of 0.82 and a reduction in wheeze symptoms.[162] One study showed no evidence of intracellular magnesium deficiency in children with chronic bronchial asthma.[163] Another small study showed a negative correlation between magnesium level and degree of asthma severity among adults in India, with almost 60% of the asthma patients showing hypomagnesemia compared with only 5% of the control group.[164] These studies indicate that although intravenous magnesium supplementation may have a minimal role in treating acute asthma, further study is needed of the role of magnesium supplementation in the treatment of chronic asthma.

Effects of Asthma Treatment on Nutritional Status

Most of the effects of asthma treatment on the nutritional status of patients are related to the use of oral steroids and high-dose inhaled steroids. According to the NHLBI guidelines, medium- to high-dose inhaled corticosteroids may be needed daily for long-term control in patients whose disease is classified as moderate persistent.[119] For patients whose disease is in the severe persistent classification, long-term control may require high-dose inhaled corticosteroids as well as a long-acting bronchodilator plus oral corticosteroids.[119] The primary goal is to treat the asthma with the smallest doses of medicines that will control the symptoms in order to minimize side effects.

Linear Growth

According to the NHLBI guidelines, poorly controlled asthma may delay growth in children.[119] Generally, children with asthma tend to have longer periods of reduced growth rates before puberty, however, this delay in puberty does not appear to affect final adult height.[165] This delay in puberty also is not associated with the use of inhaled corticosteroids.[166] The potential for adverse effects on linear growth from inhaled corticosteroids appears to be dose dependent.[166–169] High doses of inhaled corticosteroids have greater potential for growth suppression than lower doses. When inhaled corticosteroids are used as recommended, the majority of studies report no change in expected growth velocity.[167,168] In contrast,

a few studies have demonstrated a small growth delay in children on inhaled corticosteroids, but the delay in growth velocity is not sustained, is not progressive, and may be reversible.[170,171] A meta-analysis of the effect of inhaled steroids found decreased growth velocity with inhaled steroids, but the effect on final adult height was unknown.[169] A study by Agertoft and Pedersen[170] in Denmark showed that expected adult height was attained for asthma patients on inhaled steroids. This is an area of asthma management that warrants further study, especially in young, preschool-age children. Using high doses of inhaled corticosteroids with children having severe persistent asthma has less potential for decreasing linear growth than does using oral systemic corticosteroids.[172] Using oral corticosteroids on a prolonged basis does stunt linear growth.[172]

Bone Density

Chronic corticosteroid use does induce osteoporosis.[173] Corticosteroids decrease calcium absorption from the gastrointestinal tract and decrease renal calcium reabsorption, which leads to a decrease in plasma calcium. At the same time, there is an increase in parathyroid hormone secretion and an increase in bone resorption, all of which lead to osteoporosis. That is why it is important that the smallest possible dose be used to control asthma symptoms. Many studies—again mainly in adults—have been performed on the effect of inhaled corticosteroids on bone density, with varying results reported. Short-term effects on markers of bone turnover, such as osteocalcin, have been reported, but the long-term risk of osteoporosis is not clear.[174, 175] Collagen turnover was found to be reduced in children receiving long-term (over 12 months) inhaled steroid treatment.[176] Martinati and colleagues[177] found no adverse effect on bone mass in prepubertal children with mild to moderate asthma when treated with beclomethasone dipropionate, compared with children treated with cromolyn sodium, a nonsteroidal anti-inflammatory drug. Most long-term studies indicate that inhaled corticosteroids have a negligible effect, if any, on bone mineral density. However, more research is needed before there is agreement as to the effect of the dose and duration of inhaled corticosteroids on bone density in patients, especially children with asthma.

Investigators conclude that attention should be given to maintaining adequate calcium and vitamin D intake in patients on chronic steroid therapy.[178] Calcium supplementation may be necessary in some patients, especially if dietary intake of calcium is low.[161] Other factors that may benefit the patient are weight-bearing exercise and avoiding other inhibitors of osteoblast production, such as alcohol excess.[178] In a study of adult asthmatic patients, Gagnon and associates[179] did find a significant positive correlation between bone density and calcium intake in asthmatic patients. This is another compelling reason why indiscriminate elimination of dairy products from the diet of a child with asthma may be harmful.

Excessive Weight Gain

Common, well-known side effects of oral corticosteroid therapy include appetite stimulation, central distribution of fat, sodium and fluid retention, and steroid-induced glucose intolerance. For the asthma patient whose disease is in the persistent severe classification and who may require chronic oral steroid therapy to control asthma symptoms, anticipatory dietary guidance as to how to combat some of these side effects, such as limiting salt intake or limiting concentrated sweets and high fat foods, will be beneficial.

Nutritional Management

The growth of children with asthma should be monitored on a regular basis. Any deviation in growth parameters should be investigated. BMI (2–20 years of age) or weight for length (up to 24 months of age)[36] should be calculated and the age-appropriate growth charts used to monitor overweight asthma patients and those at risk for overweight. Nutrition counseling and lifestyle changes need to be emphasized by the healthcare practitioner at the first sign that an asthma patient may be at risk for overweight.

Based on the available data, a diet that provides a variety of foods, including fruits, vegetables, and dairy products, should be encouraged. Educational tools such as the USDA Choose My Plate[180] can be utilized. Patients and family members should be warned against eliminating whole food groups from the diet indiscriminately. Preadolescent and adolescent patients should receive information about healthy weight control practices, including regular exercise. Chronically ill adolescents, including asthma patients, were found to have increased body dissatisfaction and to be at increased risk of engaging in unhealthy weight-loss practices.[181]

Some patients with asthma who have a true food allergy will require an allergen elimination diet. (See Chapter 25 – "Food Allergy").

Combating Steroid Side Effects

For those asthma patients who must take oral corticosteroids on a regular basis, additional factors should be closely monitored. An adequate calcium intake is essential. These patients should be receiving at least the DRIs[57] for calcium and in some instances may require calcium supplementation. Adequate vitamin D intake is also important. The patient may need to modify kilocalorie intake to maintain weight control. The registered dietitian can assist the patient in identifying ways to accomplish a healthy diet, especially if the patient develops steroid-induced hyperglycemia. Moderate exercise should be encouraged because this will help maintain bone density and will assist with weight control. Individuals with risk factors for developing diabetes (such as obesity or family history) should be monitored for hyperglycemia, even on inhaled steroids.[172]

Alternative/Complementary Medicine

Many asthma patients and their families have turned to alternative/complementary medicine therapies. Relaxation techniques, such as biofeedback training and yoga, are commonly practiced. Acupuncture has also been tried and although there is a very low risk associated with acupuncture in pediatrics, controlled studies of acupuncture for asthma in children are limited.[169] It is important to ask about the use of specific herbal products when obtaining a diet history. Several recent studies reported that traditional Chinese medicine (TCM) herbal formulas are safe and had a positive effect on symptoms and/or lung function in children when used as monotherapy or complementary therapy.[182] Investigation of TCM herbal therapy for children with asthma is an active area of research and may have potential as a complementary and alternative medicine therapy for asthma.[182]

Identification of Areas for Further Research

The areas needing further research have been indicated throughout this section. Additional scientific study of the role of specific nutrients in asthma must be done before precise recommendations for supplementation can be made. The effects of chronic steroid therapy and chronic inhaled steroid therapy on growth in children, especially in infants and young children, and on bone density require continued study. The relationship between being overweight and asthma requires further investigation. It is exciting to realize that nutrition may play a major role in treating this significant public health problem.

▶ Conclusion

CF is the most common genetic disease among Caucasians and its manifestation of symptoms require significant nutritional interventions. Most patients with CF are pancreatic insufficient, which results in malabsorption of fat in addition to putting patients at risk of fat soluble vitamin deficiencies, decreased bone density, and CF-related diabetes. BPD is common in infants born prematurely and it requires aggressive nutrition intervention to promote normal growth and support the patient through the high pulmonary demands of the disease. Asthma is the most common chronic disease of childhood and is more common among overweight children. Long-term use of steroids in asthma treatment can contribute to excessive weight gain as well as delayed growth, hyperglycemia, and reduced bone density. Nutrition intervention is of utmost importance in managing these pediatric pulmonary diseases to foster normal weight, growth, and development of the children who have them.

🔍 CASE STUDY

Nutrition Assessment

Client History
GB is an 11.5-year-old male with cystic fibrosis, mild lung disease, and PI. He presents to the outpatient nutrition clinic for annual nutrition evaluation.

Food/Nutrition-Related History
Patient reports that he generally has a good appetite. He always eats three meals per day and two to three snacks. Dietary intake from yesterday reported as:

Breakfast: 1 slice of toast with peanut butter, 8 oz whole milk with chocolate syrup, ½ banana
Snack: 1 cup pretzels, water
Lunch: ½ hamburger, 1 cup French fries, ½ cup peaches, 8 oz apple juice
Dinner: 1 cup spaghetti with beef marinara sauce, ½ cup cooked carrots, 8 oz whole milk
Snack: apple with peanut butter

Patient and mom both agree that above intake is consistent with a typical day of eating for GB. Caloric intake is estimated approximately 1900kcal/day. He appears to be eating a variety of foods and choosing some higher fat options for additional calories.

GB is currently swimming three to four times a week outdoors on his local swim team. He also plays basketball and baseball with his friends for fun. Mom reports that he is usually pretty active and likes to be outside with his friends.

Current nutrition-related medications include 1 MVW Complete Formulation soft gel daily, ZENPEP 20,000 (3 with meals, 1 with snacks), and Prevacid. GB reports compliance with these meds as they are ordered every day. Mom confirms his compliance and states, "He always takes his enzymes before eating. I don't even have to remind him." He has been taking all of these medications at their current dosage for at least a year.

Nutrition-Related Physical Findings
He complains of increased gassiness and abdominal pain after some of his meals over the past 3–4 months. He is stooling 2–3/day. He reports that his stools float about half of the time and recently he's noticed that there is an oil ring in the toilet. He denies weight loss.

Biochemical Data, Medical Tests, and Procedures
Chem 10 WNL, CRP WNL, vitamin A slightly low, vitamin E slightly low, vitamin D (WNL), PT WNL

Anthropometric Measurements
35 kg, 144 cm

Comparative Standards
REE: (Schofield) 1289 kcal/day (37 kcal/kg) × 1.5–1.75 1950–2190 kcal/day
Estimated protein needs: (RDA) 1 g protein/kg/day

Nutrition Diagnosis
Increased energy expenditure related to high pulmonary and gastrointestinal demands of CF and PI as evidenced by need for a high calorie diet to promote adequate weight gain and growth.

Nutrition Intervention

Nutrition prescription
High-calorie, high-protein diet, compliance with enzymes, and CF-specific vitamin

Monitoring and Evaluation

1. Growth pattern indices/percentile rankings
2. Biochemical data (vitamins A and E)
3. Total energy intake
4. Intestinal (signs and symptoms of malabsorption)

Questions for the Reader

1. How many units of lipase/kg/meal is GB's current enzyme regimen providing? What is the maximum recommended unit of lipase/kg/meal?
2. His serum vitamin A and E are slightly low. Is he on the recommended dose of his CF-specific MVI (MVW Complete Formulation softgel) for his age?
3. Calculate GB's BMI and plot on the correct NCHS growth chart in order to determine his BMI percentile for age. What is the CF Foundation's goal BMI percentile for his age? Is he currently meeting this goal?
4. Using this data and taking into account the information presented above, please develop at least one appropriate Nutrition Diagnosis.
5. Using NCP terminology, identify an appropriate nutrition intervention based on the etiology of your PES statement(s). Define an ideal goal of your intervention based on the signs and symptoms mentioned in your PES statement.

Review Questions

1. What is the relationship between nutrition status and lung function in cystic fibrosis?

2. What are some reasons why children with cystic fibrosis require higher caloric needs?

3. What are some common nutritional concerns in children with cystic fibrosis and pancreatic insufficiency?

4. How does cystic fibrosis diabetes differ from type 1 and type 2 diabetes?

5. What are some factors that can be used to identify infants at an increased risk for developing BPD?

6. What are common medications used in the treatment of infants with BPD?

7. Why should future research studies related to growth in the BPD population describe changes in linear growth?

8. Why is obesity associated with asthma?

9. What are some nutritional consequences of long term oral steroid use in treating asthma?

10. Are there any micronutrient supplements that would benefit children with asthma?

11. Does breastfeeding in infancy play a role in the risk of developing asthma?

12. Are there any diet restrictions indicated for asthma?

References

1. Cystic Fibrosis Foundation. Cystic fibrosis foundation patient registry. [2016 Annual Data Report to the Center Directors]. 2017.
2. Borowitz D, Durie PR, Clarke LL, et al. Gastrointestinal outcomes and confounders in cystic fibrosis. *J Pediatr Gastroenterol Nutr.* 2005;41:273–285.
3. Andersen DH. Cystic fibrosis of the pancreas and its relation to celiac disease: a clinical and pathologic study. *Am J Dis Child.* 1938;56:344–399.
4. Riordan JR, Rommens JM, Kerem B, et al. Identification of the cystic fibrosis gene: cloning and characterization of complementary DNA. *Science.* 1989;245:1066–1073.
5. Anderson MP, Gregory RJ, Thompson S, et al. Demonstration that CFTR is a chloride channel by alteration of its anion selectivity. *Science.* 1991;253:202–205.
6. Bear CE, Li CH, Kartner N, et al. Purification and functional reconstitution of the cystic fibrosis transmembrane conductance regulator (CFTR). *Cell.* 1992;68:809–818.
7. Cheng SH, Rich DP, Marshall J, et al. Phosphorylation of the R domain by cAMP-dependent protein kinase regulates the CFTR chloride channel. *Cell.* 1991;66:1027–1036.
8. Schwiebert EM, Egan ME, Hwang TH, et al. CFTR regulates outwardly rectifying chloride channels through an autocrine mechanism involving ATP. *Cell.* 1995;81:1063–1073.
9. Stutts MJ, Canessa CM, Olsen JC, et al. CFTR as a cAMP-dependent regulator of sodium channels. *Science.* 1995;269:847–850.
10. Welsh MJ, Smith AE. Molecular mechanisms of CFTR chloride channel dysfunction in cystic fibrosis. *Cell.* 1993;73:1251–1254.

11. Cystic Fibrosis Genetic Analysis Consortium. Population variation of common cystic fibrosis mutations. *Hum Mutat*. 1994;4:167–177.

12. Farrell PM, White TB, Ren CM, et al. Diagnosis of Cystic Fibrosis: Consensus Guidelines from the Cystic Fibrosis Foundation. *J Pediatr*. 2017;181S:S4–S15.

13. Tomezsko JL, Stallings VA, Kawchak DA, et al. Energy expenditure and genotype of children with cystic fibrosis. *Pediatr Res*. 1994;35:451–460.

14. O'Rawe A, McIntosh I, Dodge JA, et al. Increased energy expenditure in cystic fibrosis is associated with specific mutations. *Clin Sci*. 1992;82:71–76.

15. Murphy M, Ireton-Jones CS, Hilman BC, et al. Resting energy expenditures measured by indirect calorimetry are higher in preadolescent children with cystic fibrosis than expenditures calculated from prediction equations. *J Am Diet Assoc*. 1995;95:30–33.

16. Shepherd RW, Vasques-Velasquez L, Prentice A, et al. Increased energy expenditure in young children with cystic fibrosis. *Lancet*. 1988;135:1300–1303.

17. Vaisman N, Pencharz PB, Corey M, et al. Energy expenditure of patients with cystic fibrosis. *J Pediatr*. 1987;111:137–141.

18. Stallings VA, Stark LJ, Robinson KA, et al. Evidence-based practice recommendations for nutrition-related management of children and adults with cystic fibrosis and pancreatic insufficiency: results of a systematic review. *J Am Diet Assoc*. 2008;108:832–839.

19. Food and Nutrition Board. *Recommended Dietary Allowances*, 10th ed. Washington, DC:National Academies Press;1989.

20. Marchand V, Baker SS, Stark TJ, Baker RD. Randomized, double-blind, placebo-controlled pilot trial of megestrol acetate in malnourished children with cystic fibrosis. *J Pediatr Gastroenterol Nutr*. 2000;31(3):264–269.

21. Homnick DN, Homnick BD, Reeves AJ, et al. Cyproheptadine is an effective appetite stimulant in cystic fibrosis. *Pediatr Pulmonol*. 2004;l38:129–134.

22. Homnick DN, Marks JH, Hare KL, et al. Long-term trial of cyrpoheptadine as an appetite stimulant in cystic fibrosis. *Pediatr Pulmonol*. 2005;40:251–256.

23. Eubanks V, Koppersmith N, Wooldridge N, et al. Effects of megestrol acetate on weight gain, body composition, and pulmonary function in patients with cystic fibrosis. *J Pediatr*. 2002;140:393–395.

24. Yen EH, Quinton H, Borowitz D. Better nutritional status in early childhood is associated with improved clinical outcomes and survival in patients with cystic fibrosis. *J Pediatr*. 2013;162:530–535.

25. Lai HJ, Shoff SM, Farrell PM, et al. Recovery of birth weight z score within 2 years of diagnosis is positively associated with pulmonary status at 6 years of age in children with cystic fibrosis. *J Pediatr*. 2009;123:714–722.

26. Beker LT, Russek-Cohen E, Fink RJ. Stature as a prognostic factor in cystic fibrosis survival. *J Am Diet Assoc*. 2001;101:438–442.

27. Borowitz D, Baker RD, Stallings V. Consensus report on nutrition for pediatric patients with cystic fibrosis. *J Pediatr Gastroenterol Nutr*. 2002;35:246–259.

28. Fomon SJ. *Nutrition of Normal Infants*. Philadelphia, PA:Mosby;1993.

29. Usatin D, Yen EH, McDonald C, et al. Differences between WHO and CDC early growth measurements in the

30. Frisancho AR. New norms of upper limb fat and muscle areas for assessment of nutritional status. *Am J Clin Nutr*. 1981;34:2540–2545.

assessment of cystic fibrosis clinical outcomes. *J Cyst Fibros*. 2017;16:503–509.

31. Heimburger DC, Ard J. *Handbook of Clinical Nutrition*, 4th ed. St. Louis, MO: Mosby; 2006.

32. Michel SH, Maqbool A, Hanna MD, et al. Nutrition management of pediatric patients who have cystic fibrosis. *Pediatr Clin N Am*. 2009;56:1123–1141.

33. Huang SH, Schall JI, Zemel BS, et al. Vitamin E status in children with cystic fibrosis and pancreatic insufficiency. *J Pediatr*. 2006;148(4):556–559.

34. Sokol RJ. Selection bias and vitamin E status in cystic fibrosis. *J Pediatr*. 2007;150(5):e85.

35. Tangpricha V, Stephenson A, et al. An update on the screening, diagnosis, management, and treatment of vitamin D deficiency in individuals with cystic fibrosis: evidence-based recommendations from the Cystic Fibrosis Foundation. *J Clin Endocrinol Metab*. 2012;97:1082–1093.

36. Sonneville K, Duggan C. *Manual of Pediatric Nutrition*, 5th ed. Shelton, CT: People's Medical Publishing House; 2014.

37. Moheet A, Moran A. CF-related diabetes: Containing the metabolic miscreant of cystic fibrosis. *Pediatr Pulmonol*. 2017;52(S48):S37–S43.

38. Brunzell C, Hardin D, Kogler A, Moran A, Schindler, T. Managing cystic fibrosis related diabetes (CFRD). In: *An Instruction Guide for Patients and Families*, 6th ed. Bethesda, MD: Cystic Fibrosis Foundation; 2015.

39. Aris RM, Merkel PA, Bachrach LK, et al. Consensus statement: guide to bone health and disease in cystic fibrosis. *J Clin Endocrinol Metab*. 2005;90:1888–1896.

40. Elkin SL, Fairney A, et al. Vertebral deformities and low bone mineral density in adults with cystic fibrosis: a cross sectional study. *Osteoporos Int*. 2001:12;366–372.

41. Aris R, Renner JB, Winders AD, Buell HE, et al. Increased rate of fractures and severe kyphosis: sequelae of living to adulthood with cystic fibrosis. *Ann Intern Med*. 1998;128:186–193.

42. Henderson R, Madsen C. Bone mineral content and body composition in children and young adults with cystic fibrosis. *Pediatr Pulmonol*. 1999;27:80–84.

43. Haworth C, Selby PL, Webb AK, Dodd ME, Musson H, et al. Low bone mineral density in adults with cystic fibrosis. *Thorax*. 1999;54:961–967.

44. Shane E, Silverberg S, Silverberg SJ, Donovan D, Papadopoulos A, et al. Osteoporosis in lung transplantation candidates with end stage pulmonary disease. *Am J Med*. 1996;101:262–269.

45. Marquette M and Haworth CS. Bone health and disease in cystic fibrosis. *Paediatr Respir Rev*. 2016;20:2–5.

46. Crist W, McDonnell P, Beck M, et al. Behavior at mealtimes in the young child with cystic fibrosis. *J Devel Behav Pediatr*. 1994;15:157–161.

47. Kawchak D, Zhoa H, Scanlin TF, Tomezsko JL, et al. Longitudinal, prospective analysis of dietary intake in children with cystic fibrosis. *J Pediatr*. 1996;129:119–129.

48. White H, Morton A, Peckham DG, Conway SP, et al. Dietary intakes in adult patients with cystic fibrosis—do they achieve guidelines? *J Cystic Fibrosis*. 2003;3:1–7.

49. Ellis L, Kalnins D, Corey M, et al. Do infants with cystic fibrosis need a protein hydrolysate formula? A

prospective, randomized, comparative study. *J Pediatr.* 1998;132:270–276.

50. Pediatric Pulmonary Center, ©1990. University of Alabama at Birmingham, Birmingham, Alabama.

51. Edenborough FP, Borgo G, Knoop C, et al. Guidelines for the management of pregnancy in women with cystic fibrosis. *J Cyst Fibros.* 2008;7:S2–S32.

52. Michel SH and Mueller DH. Nutrition for pregnant women who have cystic fibrosis. *J Acad Nutr Diet.* 2012;112:1943–1948.

53. Moran A et al. Clinical care guidelines for cystic fibrosis-related diabetes: a position statement of the American Diabetes Association and a clinical practice guideline of the Cystic Fibrosis Foundation, endorsed by the Pediatric Endocrine Society. *Diabetes Care.* 2010;33(12):2697–2708.

54. Borowitz D, Robinson KA, Rosenfield M, et al. Cystic Fibrosis Foundation evidence-based guidelines for management of infants with cystic fibrosis. *J Pediatr.* 2009;155:S73–S93.

55. Smyth RL and Rayner O. Oral calorie supplements for cystic fibrosis (review). *Cochrane Database Syst Rev.* 2017;5.

56. Schwarzenberg SJ, Hempstead SE, McDonald CM, et al. Enteral tube feeding for individuals with cystic fibrosis: Cystic Fibrosis Foundation evidence-informed guidelines. *J Cyst Fibros.* 2016;16:724–735.

57. Institute of Medicine. *Dietary Reference Intakes for Calcium and Vitamin D.* Washington, DC: National Academies Press;2010.

58. Borowitz DS, Grand RJ, Durie PR, Consensus Committee. Use of pancreatic enzyme supplements for patients with cystic fibrosis in the context of fibrosing colonopathy. *J Pediatr.* 1995;127:681–684.

59. FitzSimmons SC, Burkhart GA, Borowitz D, et al. High-dose pancreatic enzyme supplements and fibrosing colonopathy in children with cystic fibrosis. *N Eng J Med.* 1997;336:1283–1289.

60. Schwarzenberg SJ, Wielinski CL, Shamieh I, et al. Cystic fibrosis-associated colitis and fibrosing colonopathy. *J Pediatr.* 1995;127:565–570.

61. Berry AJ. Pancreatic enzyme replacement therapy during pancreatic insufficiency. *Nutr Clin Pract.* 204;29:312–321.

62. Ferrie S, Graham C, Hoyle M. Pancreatic enzyme supplementation for patients receiving enteral feeds. *Nutr Clin Pract.* 2011;26:349–351.

63. Nicolo M, Stratton KW, Rooney W, et al. Pancreatic enzyme replacement therapy for enterally fed patients with cystic fibrosis. *Nutr Clin Pract.* 2013;28:485–489.

64. Pertzye [package insert]. Bethlehem, PA. Digestive Care, Inc; 2017.

65. Freedman S. Options for addressing exocrine pancreatic insufficiency in patients receiving enteral nutrition supplementation. *Am J Manag Care.* 2017;23:S220–S228.

66. Freedman S, Orenstein D, Black P, et al. Increased fat absorption from enteral formula through an in-line digestive cartridge in patients with cystic fibrosis. *JPGN.* 2017;65:97–101.

67. Thiou TG, Cahill BC. Pediatric lung transplantation for cystic fibrosis. *Transplantation.* 2008;86:636–637.

68. Hadiljiadis D. Special considerations for patients with cystic fibrosis undergoing lung transplantation. *Chest.* 2007;131:1224–1231.

69. Northway WH, Rosan RCC, Porter DY. Pulmonary disease following respiratory therapy of hyaline membrane disease. *N Engl J Med.* 1967;276:357–368.

70. Jobe AH, Bancalari E. Bronchopulmonary dysplasia. *Am J Respir Crit Care Med.* 2001;163:1723–1729.

71. Abman SH, Groothius JR. Pathophysiology and treatment of bronchopulmonary dysplasia. Current issues. *Pediatr Clinics.* 1994;41:277–315.

72. Cox JH. Bronchopulmonary dysplasia. In: Groh-Wargo S, Thompson M, Cox J, eds. *Nutritional Care for High-Risk Newborns*, 3rd ed. Chicago, IL: Precept Press; 2000:369–390.

73. Tammela OKT, Lanning FP, Koivisto ME. The relationship of fluid restriction during the 1st month of life to the occurrence and severity of bronchopulmonary dysplasia in low birth weight infants: a 1-year radiological follow up. *Eur J Pediatr.* 1992;151:367–371.

74. Wilson DC, McClure G, Halliday HL, et al. Nutrition and bronchopulmonary dysplasia. *Arch Dis Child.* 1991;66:37–38.

75. Frank L, Sosenko IR. Undernutrition as a major contributing factor in the pathogenesis of bronchopulmonary dysplasia. *Am Rev Respir Dis.* 1988;138:725–729.

76. Northway WH. Bronchopulmonary dysplasia: thirty-three years later. *Pediatr Pulmonol.* 2001; Suppl 23:5–7.

77. Horbar JD, Carpenter JH, Badger GJ, et al. Mortality and Neonatal Morbidity Among Infants 501 to 1500 Grams From 2000 to 2009. *Pediatr.* 2012;129:1019–1026.

78. Jensen EA, Schmidt B. Epidemiology of Bronchopulmonary Dysplasia. *Wiley Periodicals.* 2014;100:145–157.

79. Bose, C, Van Marter LJ, Laughon, M, et al. Fetal growth restriction and risk of chronic lung disease among infants born before the 28th week of gestation. *Pediatr.* 2009 September;124(3)e450–e458.

80. Weinstein MR, Oh W. Oxygen consumption in infants with bronchopulmonary dysplasia. *J Pediatr.* 1981;99:958–960.

81. Kurzner WI, Garg M, Bautista DB, et al. Growth failure in infants with bronchopulmonary dysplasia: nutrition and elevated resting metabolic expenditure. *Pediatrics.* 1988;81:379–384.

82. Yunis KA, Oh W. Effects of intravenous glucose loading on oxygen consumption, carbon dioxide production, and resting energy expenditure in infants with bronchopulmonary dysplasia. *J Pediatr.* 1989;115:127–132.

83. Yeh TF, McClenan DA, Ajayi OA, Pildes RS. Metabolic rate and energy balance in infants with bronchopulmonary dysplasia. *J Pediatr.* 1989;114:448–451.

84. deGamarra E. Energy expenditure in premature newborns with bronchopulmonary dysplasia. *Biol Neonate.* 1992;61:337–344.

85. Cuevas Guaman M, Gien J, Baker CD, et al. Point Prevalence, Clinical Characteristics, and Treatment Variation for Infants with Severe Bronchopulmonary Dysplasia. *Am J Perinatol.* 2015;32:960–967.

86. Slaughter JL, Stenger MR, Reagan PB, Jadcherla SR. Inhaled Bronchodilator Use For Infants with Bronchopulmonary Dysplasia. *J Perinatol.* 2015 January;35(1):61–66.

87. Leitch CA, Ahlrichs J, Karn C, Denne SC. Energy expenditure and energy intake during dexamethasone therapy from chronic lung disease. *Pediatr Res.* 1999 Jul;46(1):109–113.

88. Farrell PA, Fiascone JM. Bronchopulmonary dysplasia in the 1990s: a review for the pediatrician. *Curr Probl Pediatr.* 1997;27:129–163.

89. Singer L, Martin RJ, Hawkins SW, et al. Oxygen desaturation complicates feeding in infants with bronchopulmonary dysplasia after discharge. *Pediatr.* 1992;90:380–384.

90. Garg M, Kurzner SI, Bautista DB, Keens TG. Clinically unsuspected hypoxia during sleep and feeding in infants with bronchopulmonary dysplasia. *Pediatr.* 1988;81:635–642.

91. Biniwale MA, Ehrenkranz RA. The role of nutrition in the prevention and management of bronchopulmonary dysplasia. *Semin Perinatol.* 2006;30:200–208.

92. Ehrenkranz RA, Das A, Wrage LA, et al. Early Nutrition Mediates the Influence of Severity of Illness on Extremely LBW Infants. *Pediatr Res.* 2011;69(6):522–529.

93. Gianni ML, Roggero P, Colnaghi MR, et al. The role of nutrition in promoting growth in pre-term infants with bronchopulmonary dysplasia: a prospective non-randomised interventional cohort study. *BMC Pediatr.* 2014;14:235.

94. Huysman WA, de Ridder M, de Bruin NC, et al. Growth and body composition in preterm infants with bronchopulmonary dysplasia. *Arch Dis Child Fetal Neonatal Ed.* 2003;88:F46–F51.

95. Sanchez-Solis M, Perez-Fernandez V, Bosch-Gimenez V, et al. Lung function Gain in Preterm Infants With and Without Bronchopulmonary Dysplasia. *Pediatr Pulmonol.* 2016;51:936–942.

96. WHO Multicentre Growth Reference Study Group. *WHO Child Growth Standards: Growth Velocity Based on Weight, Length and Head Circumference: Methods and Development.* Geneva, Switzerland: World Health Organization;2009 (242 pages).

97. Anderson DM. Nutritional assessment and therapeutic interventions for the preterm infant. *Clin Perinatol.* 2002:29:313–326.

98. Becker PJ, Nieman Carney L, Corkins MR, et al. Consensus Statement of the Academy of Nutrition and Dietetics/American Society for Parenteral and Enteral Nutrition: indicators recommended for the identification and documentation of Pediatric Malnutrition (Undernutrition). *J Acad Nutr Diet.* 2014;114:1988–2000.

99. Oh W. Nutritional management of infants with bronchopulmonary dysplasia. In: Farrell PM, Taussig LM, eds. *Bronchopulmonary Dysplasia and Related Chronic Respiratory Disorders.* Columbus, OH: Ross Laboratories;1986:96–101.

100. Groh-Wargo S, Thompson M, Hovasi Cox J, editors. *ADA Pocket Guide to Neonatal Nutrition.* Chicago, IL. American Dietetic Association. 2009.

101. Zachman RD. Role of vitamin A in lung development. *J Nutr.* 1995;125:1634S–1638S.

102. Robbins ST, Fletcher AB. Early vs. delayed vitamin A supplementation in very-low-birth-weight infants. *J Parenter Enteral Nutr.* 1993;17:220–225.

103. Kennedy KA, Stoll BJ, Ehrenkranz RA, et al. Vitamin A to prevent bronchopulmonary dysplasia in very-low-birth-weight infants: has the dose been too low? *Early Human Dev.* 1997;49:19–31.

104. Tyson JE, Wright LL, Oh W, et al. Vitamin A supplementation for extremely-low-birth-weight infants. *New Eng J Med.* 1999;340:1962–1968.

105. Shenai JP. Vitamin A supplementation in very low birth weight neonates: rationale and evidence. *Pediatr.* 1999;104:1369–1374.

106. Atkinson SA. Special nutritional needs of infants for prevention of and recovery from bronchopulmonary dysplasia. *J Nutr.* 2001;131:942S–946S.

107. Diaz-Gomez NM, Domenech E, Barroso F, et al. The Effect of Zinc Supplementation on Linear Growth, Body Composition, and Growth Factors in Preterm Infants. *Pediatr.* 2003;111(5):1002–1009.

108. Lowe NM, Fekete K, Decsi T. Methods of assessment of zinc status in humans: a systematic review. *Am J Clin Nutr.* 2009;89(suppl):2040S–2051S.

109. Shaikhkhalil AK, Curtiss J, Puthoff TD, Valentine CJ. Enteral Zinc Supplementation and Growth in Extremely-Low-Birth-Weight Infants With Chronic Lung Disease. *J Pediatr Gastroenterol Nutr.* 2014;58(2): 183–187.

110. Walravens PA and Hambridge KM. Growth of infants fed a zinc supplemented formula. *Am J Clin Nutr.* 1976;29:1114–1121.

111. American Academy of Pediatrics, Committee on Nutrition. Kleinman RE, ed., *Pediatric Nutrition Handbook,* 5th ed. Elk Grove Village, IL: American Academy of Pediatrics; 2004.

112. Lucas A, Cole TJ. Breast milk and neonatal necrotizing enterocolitis. *Lancet.* 1990;336(8730):1519–1523.

113. Sisk PM, Loevlady CA, Gruber KJ, et al. Early human milk feeding is associated with a lower risk of necrotizing enterocolitis in very low birth weight infants. *J Perinatol.* 2007;27(7):428–433.

114. Teller IC, Embleton ND, Griffin IJ, van Elburg RM. Post-discharge formula feeding in preterm infants: A systematic review mapping evidence about the role of macronutrient enrichment. *Clin Nutr.* 2016;35:791–801.

115. Gewolb IH, Bosma JF, Taciak VL, Vice FL. Abnormal developmental patterns of suck and swallow rhythms during feeding in preterm infants with bronchopulmonary dysplasia. *Dev Med Child Neur.* 2001;43:454–459.

116. Singer LT, Davillier M, Preuss L, et al. Feeding interactions in infants with very low birth weight and bronchopulmonary dysplasia. *J Dev Behav Pediatr.* 1996;17:69–76.

117. Johnson DB, Cheney C, Monsen ER. Nutrition and feeding in infants with bronchopulmonary dysplasia after initial hospital discharge: risk factors for growth failure. *J Am Diet Assoc.* 1998;98:649–656.

118. Akinbami L, Moorman J, Bailey C et al. *Trends in Asthma Prevalence, Health Care Use, and Mortality in the United States, 2001–2010.* NCHS Data Brief. May 2012;94:1–8.

119. National Heart, Lung and Blood Institute. Expert panel report 3: guidelines for the diagnosis and management of asthma. August 2007. Available at: http://www.nhlbi.nih.gov/guidelines/asthma/asthgdln.htm. Accessed January 27, 2010.

120. Silbert-Flagg, J, Sloand Elizabeth D. *Pediatric Nurse Practitioner Certification Review Guide,* 6th edition. Burlington, MA:Jones & Bartlett Learning;2017; 143–145.

121. Ozol D, Mete E. Asthma and food allergy. *Curr Opin Pulm Med.* 2008;14(1):9.

122. Beausoleil J, Fiedler J, Spergel J. Food intolerance and childhood asthma: what is the link? *Paediatr Drugs.* 2007;9(3):157–163.

123. Schroeder A, Kumar R. Food allergy is associated with an increased risk of asthma. *Clin Exp Allergy.* 2009;39(2):261–270.

124. Adler BR, Assadullahi T, Warner JA, Warner JO. Evaluation of a multiple food specific IgE antibody test compared to parental perception, allergy skin tests and RAST. *Clin Exp Allergy*. 1991;21:683–688.

125. Bock SA. Respiratory reactions induced by food challenges in children with pulmonary disease. *Pediatr Allergy Immunol*. 1992;3:188–194.

126. James JM, Berhisel-Broadbent J, Sampson HA. Respiratory reactions provoked by doubleblind food challenges in children. *Am J Respir Crit Care Med*. 1994;149:59–64.

127. Onorato J, Merland N, Terral C, et al. Placebo-controlled double-blind food challenge in asthma. *J Allergy Clin Immunol*. 1986;78:1139–1146.

128. Pinnock CB, Arney WK. The milk-mucus belief: sensory analysis comparing cow's milk and a soy placebo. *Appetite*. 1993;20:61–70.

129. Nguyen MT. Effect of cow milk on pulmonary function in atopic asthmatic patients. *Ann Allergy Asthma Immunol*. 1997;79:62–64.

130. Chulada PC, Arbes SJ, Dunson D, Zeldin DC. Breastfeeding and the prevalence of asthma and wheeze in children: analyses from the Third National Health and Nutrition Examination Survey. *J Allergy Clin Immunol*. 2003;112:328–336.

131. Rust GS, Thompson CJ, Minor P, et al. Does breastfeeding protect children from asthma? Analysis of NHANES III survey data. *J Nat Med Assoc*. 2001;93:139–148.

132. Wright AL, Holberg CJ, Taussig LM, Martinez F. Maternal asthma status alters relation of infant feeding to asthma in childhood. *Advances Exp Med Biol*. 2000;478:131–137.

133. Lodge CJ, Tan DJ, MX L et al. Breastfeeding and asthma and allergies: a systemic review and meta-analysis. *Acta Paediatr*. 2015;104(467):38–53.

134. Jelding-Dannemand E, Schoos M, Bisgaard H. Breastfeeding does not protect against allergic sensitization in early childhood and allergy-associated disease at age 7 years. *J Allergy Clin Immunol*. 2015;136(5):1302–1308.

135. Silvers KM, Frampton CM, Wickens K et al. Breastfeeding protects against current asthma up to 6 years of age. *J Pediatr*. 2012;160(6):991–996.

136. Arif AA, Racine EF. Does longer duration of breastfeeding prevent childhood asthma in low-income families? *J Asthma*. 2017;54(6):600–605.

137. Zutavern A, Brockow I, Schaaf B et al. Timing of Solid Food Introduction in Relation to Eczema, Asthma, Allergic Rhinitis, and Food and Inhalant Sensitization at the Age of 6 Years: Results From the Prospective Birth Cohort Study LISA. *Pediatrics*. 2017;121(1):e44–e52.

138. Chinn S. Obesity and asthma: evidence for and against a causal relation. *J Asthma*. 2003;40:1–16.

139. Camargo CA, Weiss ST, Zhang S, Willett WC, Speizer FE. Prospective study of body mass index, weight change, and risk of adult-onset asthma in women. *Arch Intern Med*. 1999;159:2582–2588.

140. Stenius-Aarniala B, Poussa T, Kvarnstrom J, et al. Immediate and long term effects of weight reduction in obese people with asthma: randomized controlled study. *BMJ*. 2000;320:827–832.

141. Luder E, Melnik TA, DiMaio M. Association of being overweight with greater asthma symptoms in inner city black and Hispanic children. *J Pediatr*. 1998;132:699–703.

142. Gennuso J, Epstein LH, Paluch RA, Cerny F. The relationship between asthma and obesity in urban minority children and adolescents. *Arch Pediatr Adolesc Med*. 1998;152:1197–1200.

143. Belamarich PF, Luder E, Kattan M, et al. Do obese inner-city children with asthma have more symptoms than non-obese children with asthma? *Pediatr*. 2000;106:1436–1441.

144. Castro-Rodriguez JA, Holbert CJ, Morgan WJ, Wright AL, Martinez FD. Increased incidence of asthma like symptoms in girls who become overweight or obese during the school years. *Am J Respir Crit Care Med*. 2001;163:1344–1349.

145. Gilliland FD, Berhane K, Islam T, et al. Obesity and the risk of newly diagnosed asthma in school-age children. *Am J Epi*. 2003;158:406–415.

146. Tantisira KG, Litonjua AA, Weiss ST, Fuhlbrigge AL, for the Childhood Asthma Management Program Research Group. Association of body mass with pulmonary function in the Childhood Asthma Management Program (CAMP). *Thorax*. 2003;58(12):1036–1041.

147. Chastang J, Baiz N. Parnet L et al. Changes in body mass index during childhood and risk of various phenotypes: a retrospective analysis. *Pediatr Allergy Immunol* 2017; 28(3): 273–279.

148. Shwartz J, Weiss ST. Relationship between dietary vitamin C intake and pulmonary function in the first National Health and Nutrition Examination Survey (NHANES I). *Amer J Clin Nutr*. 1994;59:110–114.

149. Cook DG, Carey IM, Whincup PH, et al. Effect of fresh fruit consumption on lung function and wheeze in children. *Thorax*. 1997;52:628–633.

150. Baker J, Ayres J. Diet and Asthma. *Respir Med*. 2000;94:925–934.

151. Spector SL, Surette ME. Diet and asthma: has the role of dietary lipids been overlooked in the management of asthma? *Ann Allergy Asthma Immunol*. 2003;90:371–377.

152. Schwartz J, Weiss ST. The relationship of dietary fish intake to level of pulmonary function in the first National Health and Nutrition Examination Survey (NHANES I). *Eur Respir J*. 1994;7:1821–1824.

153. Peat JK, Salome CM, Woolcock AJ. Factors associated with bronchial hyperresponsiveness in Australian adults and children. *Eur Respir J*. 1992;5:921–929.

154. Hodge L, Salome CM, Hughes JM, et al. Effect of dietary intake of omega-3 and omega-6 fatty acids on severity of asthma in children. *Eur Respir J*. 1998;11:361–365.

155. Nagakura T, Matsuda S, Shichijyo K, et al. Dietary supplementation with fish oil rich in omega-3 polyunsaturated fatty acids in children with bronchial asthma. *Eur Respir J*. 2000;16:861–865.

156. Hardy M, Kekic A, Graybill N, Lancaster Z. A systematic review of the association between fish oil supplementation and the development of asthma exacerbations. *Sage Open Medicine*. 2016; volume 4:1–6.

157. Norton R, Hoffmann P. Selenium and asthma. *Mol Aspects Med*. 2012; 33(1):98–106.

158. Pogson Z, McKeever T. Dietary sodium manipulation and asthma. *Cochrane Database Syst Rev*. 2011 March 16;(3):CD000436.

159. Demissie K, Ernst P, Gray D, Joseph L. Usual dietary salt intake and asthma in children: a case-controlled study. *Thorax*. 1996 Jan;51(1):59–63.

160. Pogson ZE, Antoniak MD, Pacey SJ, Lewis SA, Britton JR, Fogarty AW. Does a low sodium diet improve asthma

control? A randomized controlled study. *Am J Respir Crit Care Med.* 2008 Jul 15;178(2):132–138.

161. Griffiths B, Kew KM. Intravenous magnesium sulfate for treating children with acute asthma in the emergency department. *Cochrane Database Syst Rev.* 2016;29(4):CD011050.

162. Britton J, Pavord I, Wisniewski A, et al. Dietary magnesium, lung function, wheezing, and airway hyperreactivity in a random adult population. *Lancet.* 1994;344:357–363.

163. Sein HH, Lian W, Loong J et al. Relationship between Intracellular Magnesium Level, Lung Function, and Level of Asthma Control in Children with Chronic Bronchial Asthma. *Malays J Med Sci.* 2014;21(5):30–36.

164. Shaikh, M, Malapati B, Gokani R, et al. Serum magnesium and vitamin D levels as indicators of asthma severity. *Pulm Med.* 2016;1643717.

165. Price JF. Asthma, growth and inhaled corticosteroids. *Resp Med.* 1993;87:23–26.

166. Merkus PJFM, van Essen-Zandvliet EEM, Duiverman EJ, et al. Long-term effect of inhaled corticosteroids on growth rate in adolescents with asthma. *Pediatr.* 1993;91:1121–1126.

167. Agertoft L, Pedersen S. Effects of long-term treatment with an inhaled corticosteroid on growth and pulmonary function in asthmatic children. *Resp Med.* 1994;88:373–381.

168. Allen DB, Bronshky EA, LaForce CF, et al. Growth in asthmatic children treated with fluticasone propionate. *J Pediatr.* 1998;132:472–477.

169. Sharek PJ, Bergman DA. The effect of inhaled steroids on the linear growth of children with asthma: a meta-analysis. *Pediatr.* 2000;106. Available at: http://www.pediatrics.org/cgi/content/full/106/1/e8. Accessed February 1, 2002.

170. Agertoft L, Pedersen S. Effect of long-term treatment with inhaled budesonide on adult height in children with asthma. *N Eng J Med.* 2000;343:1064–1069.

171. Allen DB. Inhaled corticosteroid therapy for asthma in preschool children: growth issues. *Pediatr.* 2002;109:373–380.

172. Kapadia C, Nebesio T, Myers S et al. Endocrine effects of inhaled corticosteroids in children. *JAMA Pediatr.* 2016;170(2):163–170.

173. Hosking DJ. Effects of corticosteroids on bone turnover. *Resp Med.* 1993;87:15–21.

174. Barnes NC. Safety of high-dose inhaled corticosteroids. *Resp Med.* 1993;87:27–31.

175. Boner AL, Piacentini GL. Inhaled corticosteroids in children. Is there a "safe" dosage? *Drug Safety.* 1993;9:9–20.

176. Crowley S, Trivedi P, Risteli L, et al. Collagen metabolism and growth in prepubertal children with asthma treated with inhaled steroids. *J Pediatr.* 1998;132:409–413.

177. Martinati LC, Bertoldo F, Gasperi E, et al. Effect on cortical and trabecular bone mass of different anti-inflammatory treatments in preadolescent children with chronic asthma. *Am J Respir Crit Care Med.* 1996;153:232–236.

178. Picado C, Luengo M. Corticosteroid-induced bone loss. *Drug Safety.* 1996;15:347–359.

179. Gagnon L, Boulet LP, Brown J, Desrosiers T. Influence of inhaled corticosteroids and dietary intake on bone density and metabolism in patients with moderate to severe asthma. *J Amer Diet Assoc.* 1997;97:1401–1406.

180. U.S. Department of Agriculture. Choose My Plate.gov. Available at: https://www.choosemyplate.gov. Accessed May 7, 2018.

181. Neumark-Sztainer D, Story M, Resnick MD, et al. Body dissatisfaction and unhealthy weight-control practices among adolescents with and without chronic illness: a populationbased study. *Arch Pediatr Adolesc Med.* 1995;149:1330–1335.

182. Xiu-Min L. Complementary and alternative medicine in pediatric allergic disorders. *Curr Opin Allergy Clin Immunol.* 2009;9:161–167.

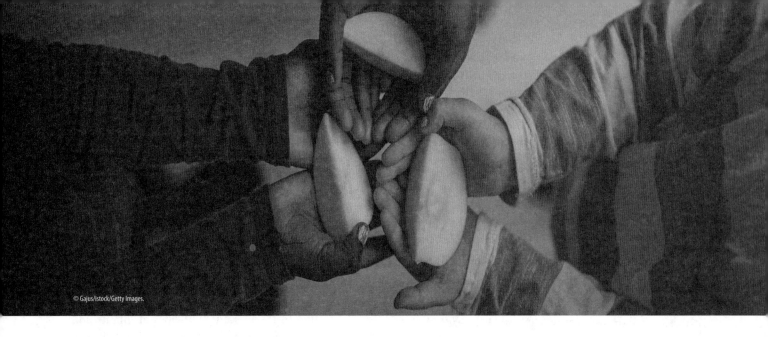

© Gajus/istock/Getty Images.

CHAPTER 16

Oncology and Hematology*

Kathryn Hunt and Paula Charuhas Macris

LEARNING OBJECTIVES

- Identify nutrition assessment and monitoring parameters for pediatric oncology patients.
- Review appropriate nutrition support practices related to pediatric oncology.
- Discuss nutrition management of children with cancer undergoing oncologic therapy.
- Describe long-term nutritional sequelae associated with pediatric malignancies.

▶ Introduction

Despite recent advances in research and treatment, cancer is still the leading cause of death by disease for all children past infancy in the United States. As recent as 2014, researchers estimated 10,450 new cancer cases and 1350 cancer deaths among children from birth to 14 years, and an additional 5330 new cases and 610 deaths were expected in adolescents between 15–19 years old.[1]

Progress in survival rates is nevertheless being made nationwide. An estimated 379,112 survivors of childhood cancer were in remission in the United States as of January 1, 2010,[1] The five-year relative survival rate for all children diagnosed with cancer under age 20 years increased from 58% in the late 1970s (1975–1979) to over 83% between 2007–2013.[2] This dramatic increase in childhood cancer survival is due to multiple factors, including success in identifying effective treatments for certain cancers such as **acute lymphoblastic leukemia** (ALL) and improved treatment protocols for Wilms tumor, **non-Hodgkin lymphoma** (NHL), Hodgkin lymphoma and germ cell tumors.[3] The opportunity for children and adolescents to participate in sophisticated clinical trials, such as those from Children's Oncology Group

---

*Parts of this chapter have been reprinted with permission from *Nutrition Focus* 2017;30(2)1–17.

and the increasing acceptance of interdisciplinary supportive care teams that specialize in treating and caring for children undergoing treatment, have also contributed.[4]

More recently, researchers and treating providers have developed, and are now administering, new therapeutic options for specific pediatric malignancies. These "novel" treatments, include biologic and immune-based therapies, harvesting the patient's own T-Cells, genetically modifying them and reintroducing the cells into the body. This complex process is intended to boost the immune system in order to eradicate malignant tissues and lessen side effects caused by some cancer treatments.[5] A recently published phase 1 trial of 45 children and young adults with relapsed or refractory CD 19* B-lineage ALL with a dismal prognosis were treated with CD19 CAR-T cells. The trial outcome showed that patients can achieve remission of disease, without the need for prolonged chemotherapy or allogeneic **hematopoietic cell transplantation** (HCT).[5]

As further progress is made towards curing childhood malignancies, researchers will continue to focus on improving outcomes for all pediatric cancers by incorporating more precision treatment strategies based on specific tumor targets and approaches to new therapies. The challenge for oncology dietitians will be to continue to define and address the nutritional status of this patient population, to focus on reliable standards of care to prevent malnutrition, and to support the child though their treatment process.

▶ Anatomy, Physiology, Pathology of Condition

Common Childhood Cancers

The prevalence of childhood cancer types varies by age of the child. **TABLE 16.1** shows the incidence of the most common childhood cancers by age group and their comparative prevalence.[2] Infants are at the greatest risk of being diagnosed with neuroblastoma, which they acquire at the rate of over 49 per 1 million infants.[2] The vast majority of infants with neuroblastoma acquire a low-risk subtype that can be cured by observation or surgical resection and do not require chemotherapy.[6] Intermediate high risk neuroblastoma is more prevalent in children in the 1–4-year-old age category and presents with the most nutrition support complications. Neuroblastoma is rarely diagnosed in children over ten years of age.[1]

Children between ages 1–4 years are at greatest risk of acquiring ALL, and are diagnosed at a frequency of

more than two times the rate of any other age group. Children in the age groups 5–9 years, 10–14 years, and 15–19 years are also most at risk of developing ALL, but they acquire it at less than one-half the rate of children ages 1–4 years.[1,2] Finally, children ages 10–19 years have an elevated incidence of serious bone tumors, including osteosarcoma, Ewings sarcoma and other soft tissue sarcomas when compared with the younger age groups.[1,2]

Malnutrition in Childhood Cancer

Unintended weight loss (NC-3.2) related to inadequate oral intake during therapy as evidenced by 10% weight loss in the past two weeks.

According to the literature, 10–50% of infants and children (hereafter, unless otherwise noted, infants are included in the term "children") experience malnutrition either at diagnosis or during cancer treatment.[7,8] Children may present malnourished at diagnosis due to tumor histology, stage of disease, and location of the tumor.[4] Malnutrition at diagnosis is more commonly seen in children with solid tumors such as sarcomas, hepatoblastoma, neuroblastoma, and Wilms tumor.[4]

Once treatment is initiated, there may be increased metabolic demands from the disease, or from treatment-related factors from chemotherapy, radiation, surgery, or HCT. A child's compromised nutritional status may influence prognosis by contributing to decreased immune function, an increased risk of infection, delayed wound healing, and altered drug metabolism.[8] Tolerance to treatment, response to therapy, quality of life, and other clinical outcomes all improve if malnutrition is prevented during treatment.

Infants and toddlers (children 1–4 years) are in various stages of oral feeding development during this time and eating is frequently interrupted due to cancer treatment and related side-effects. Children commonly suffer pain, nausea, vomiting, and mucositis, and therefore are often unable to accept breast milk, formula, or solid foods at sufficient energy and protein levels to sustain appropriate growth and weight gain.

Adolescent cancer patients are equally vulnerable to therapy-induced malnutrition. Adolescence is the second period in the human lifecycle where significant gains in growth and development must occur. This age group presents special challenges for the health care team due to their increased nutrient needs and to achieve and maintain appropriate growth and weight gain. These needs, coupled with aggressive cancer treatment protocols, often cause rapid weight loss from nausea, vomiting, and mucositis. Pediatric oncology dietitians play an important role in helping the child and adolescent navigate the complexities of how to receive adequate calories, protein, and nutrients when eating is no

TABLE 16.1 Incidence of Cancer Types by Age Group (Per 1,000,000 Children)

Cancer Types – Leukemias	Total	Infants	1–4	5–9	10–14	15–19
■ Acute Lymphoblastic Leukemia (ALL)	175.1	20.1(11.5%)	78.6 (44.9%)	36.6 (20.9%)	22.4 (12.8%)	17.4 (9.9%)
■ Acute Myeloid Leukemia	53.6	19.2 (35.8%)	11.6 (21.6%)	4.8 (9.0%)	7.8 (14.6%)	10.2 (19.0%)
Cancer Types – Brain and Central Nervous System Tumors (SNC)						
■ Astrocytoma	71.2	13.9 (19.5%)	19.9 (27.9)	18.0 (25.3%)	16.2 (22.8%)	13.2 (18.5%)
■ Ependymomas and Choroid Plexus Tumor	23.3	8.6 (36.9%)	6.8 (29.2%)	2.5 (10.7%)	2.5 (10.7%)	2.9 (12.4%)
■ Embryonal Tumors, Including Medulloblastoma	35.3	11.6 (32.9%)	10.3 (29.2%)	7.2 (20.4%)	3.8 (10.8%)	2.4 (6.8%)
Cancer Types – Lymphomas						
■ Non-Hodgkin Lymphoma	38.8	0	5.4 (13.9%)	8.0 (20.6%)	10.7 (27.6%)	14.7 (37.9%)
■ Burkitt Lymphoma	9.8	0	1.3 (13.3%)	3.5 (35.7%)	2.5 (25.5%)	2.5 (25.5%)
■ Cancer Types – Neuroblastoma	77.7	49.6 (63.8%)	21.8 (28.1%)	4.0 (5.1%)	1.4 (1.8%)	0.9 (1.5%)
Cancer Types – Renal Tumors						
■ Wilms Tumor (Most Common)	38.9	13.9 (35.7%)	19.0 (48.8%)	5.3 (13.6%)	0.7 (1.8%)	0
Cancer Types – Bone Tumors						
■ Osteosarcoma	20.2	0	0	3.4 (16.8%)	8.5 (42.1%)	8.3 (42.1%)
■ Ewings Tumor and Related Sarcomas	11.4	0	1.1 (9.6%)	2.3 (20.2%)	4.3 (37.7%)	3.7 (32.5%)
Cancer Types – Soft Tissue Sarcomas						
■ Rhabdomyosarcoma	24.8	5.6 (22.6%)	7.4 (29.8%)	4.4 (17.7%)	3.8 (15.3)	3.6 (14.5%)

Data from National Cancer Institute, Surveillance, Epidemiology, and End Results Program. Available at: https://seer.cancer.gov/archive/csr/1975_2013/browse_csr.php?sectionSEL=29&pageSEL=sect_29_table.01.html. Accessed November 1, 2017.[2]

longer about enjoyment of food. The primary objective of nutritional intervention then is to increase toleration of the cancer treatment by maintaining body stores as close to the ideal weight as possible and minimizing muscle wasting.[8]

Malnutrition is not the only risk factor for morbidity during cancer treatment. Childhood obesity also presents various risks. Orgel and colleagues studied the impact of obesity during treatment of high-risk ALL.[9] The study found that children with sustained underweight or obese status during intensive phases of treatment were at significantly greater risk of relapse, or death, and that they developed treatment-related toxicities more frequently than normal weight patients.[9] Increased toxicities from chemotherapy are of particular concern for obese children with acute leukemia. The cause of increased morbidity in obese patients is likely multifactorial, including altered drug clearance due to increased body fat and a higher rate of developing liver and pancreatic toxicities due to accumulation of adiposity. Studies have also shown that improved survival outcomes for childhood ALL were associated with normalization of weight as the child, whether underweight or overweight, progressed through treatment.[9,10]

Common childhood cancers associated with high risk of developing malnutrition during treatment are presented in **TABLE 16.2**.

Nutritional Effects of Cancer Therapy

Children with cancer are often treated with multimodal therapies, depending on the type and stage of the malignancy. Cancer therapies may produce only mild, transient nutrition issues or may lead to severe, permanent problems, which impact nutritional status. Historically, the four main treatments were chemotherapy, surgery, radiation therapy, and HCT. In the past decade, however, there has been an emergence of cutting edge cancer therapies, including targeted therapies, immunotherapy, and biotherapy.

Chemotherapy

Chemotherapeutic agents work by inhibiting DNA synthesis of both normal tissues and malignant cells. Most of the adverse effects associated with chemotherapy are caused by damage to rapidly proliferating cells including the epithelial cells of the gastrointestinal (GI) tract. The degree of the GI alterations depends upon the specific medication, dosage, duration, rate of metabolism, and the child's susceptibility to the agents.

Nutritional complications of chemotherapy are described in **TABLE 16.3**. Nausea and vomiting, which are associated with chemotherapy, are the most common problems interfering with adequate oral intake. These symptoms occur as a result of a direct central nervous system effect, as well as the emetogenicity of the drug administered. Complications of chemotherapy-induced emesis include weight loss, dehydration, fluid and electrolyte imbalances, and metabolic alkalosis. Managing chemotherapy-induced nausea and vomiting includes the judicious use of antiemetics. Single agent or combination antiemetics are frequently used and can decrease the child's discomfort.

Immunotherapy and Biotherapy

Decades of cancer research and advances in molecular biology have led to the development of new cancer treatments that are now helping to cure cancer. Immunotherapies and biotherapeutic agents, known as targeted therapies, are combined with traditional cancer treatment to enhance the immune system response to eradicate disease and lessen treatment side-effects. Some treatments target extracellular receptors on cell surfaces while others target intracellular processes. These complex therapies, when combined with conventional chemotherapy, have increasingly improved patient response and treatment outcome.[5,17,20]

Radiation Therapy

Pediatric brain tumors are the most common solid tumor malignancies. They are often treated with surgery, chemotherapy, and radiation. While traditional radiation therapy with X-ray beams has improved treatment outcomes, it has also produced documented long-term side effects in some children, such as a decrease in bone and soft tissue growth in the treated area, hormonal deficiencies, intellectual impairment, including neuro-cognitive deficits, and secondary cancers later in life.[14]

A newer radiotherapy technique called **proton beam radiation therapy** (PBRT) has the ability to precisely target tumors, with less scatter of radiation to surrounding healthy brain tissue.[22,23] The use of PBRT provides accurate treatment of tumors near or within sensitive organs while limiting radiation exposure to healthy tissues. This is vital in children whose bodies are still growing and developing and reduces both immediate and long-term side effects during treatment. Studies show that PBRT can result in fewer effects later in life from treatment, a major concern among physicians and families when a young child (3 years of age or younger) is undergoing radiation treatment. This includes potentially less toxicity related to brain development and cognitive function for children who have been treated for brain tumors.[14]

Nutritional implications of radiation depend upon many factors such as the region of the body radiated; dosage, fractionation, duration of treatment, field size of the radiation administered, concurrent use of other antitumor therapy (surgery or chemotherapy), and the child's baseline nutritional status. Nutritional sequelae associated with radiation therapy are detailed in **TABLE 16.4**.

Surgery

Pediatric solid tumors often require surgical resection as first line treatment. This is the case for certain brain tumors such as medulloblastoma, and for kidney tumors such as Wilms tumor. Surgery is an important component of treating hepatoblastoma and various risk stratifications for neuroblastoma. A recent Children's Oncology Group study of low risk neuroblastoma showed 5-year overall survival was achieved with

TABLE 16.2 Common Childhood Cancers Associated with High Nutrition Risk

ANC: absolute neutrophil count
ARMS: alveolar rhabdomyosarcoma
AVN: avascular necrosis
CNS: central nervous system
ERMS: embryonal rhabdomyosarcoma
HCT: hematopoietic cell transplantation
MRD: minimal residual disease
NG: nasogastric
NPO: non per os (nothing by mouth)
PN: parenteral nutrition
SIADH: syndrome of inappropriate anti-diuretic hormone
TBI: total body irradiation

Childhood Cancer	High Risk Clinical Factors Affecting Prognosis	Treatments	Factors Affecting Nutritional Status

Leukemias
Acute Lymphoblastic Leukemia (ALL)
	▪ White blood cell count ≥50,000 mm³ in B-cell precursor ALL
	▪ ≥ 10 years of age at diagnosis
	▪ Infants < 12 months especially those with mixed lineage leukemia
	▪ Relapsed or refractory disease
	▪ MRD after initial 1–3 months of therapy
		▪ Corticosteroids
		▪ Chemotherapy
		▪ HCT
		▪ Cranial radiation therapy in special cases:
		  • CNS 3 disease, especially in T-cell ALL
		  • CNS relapse
		  • HCT regimens that require TBI
			Side-effects of corticosteroids may include:
			▪ Diabetes requiring insulin management
			▪ Muscle wasting
			▪ Alterations in bone health (osteopenia, AVN)
			Chemotherapy related treatment toxicities may include:
			▪ Risk for tumor lysis syndrome: high white count at diagnosis may result in increased serum potassium and phosphorus levels as cells break apart; may result in need for short term kidney dialysis to remove potassium and phosphorus
			▪ Vincristine related constipation and SIADH
			▪ Asparaginase-induced pancreatitis
			▪ Mucositis
			▪ Pneumatosis/typhlitis
			Other:
			▪ Frequent NPO status for procedures and intrathecal chemotherapy contributes to weight loss

(continues)

TABLE 16.2 Common Childhood Cancers Associated with High Nutrition Risk *(continued)*

Childhood Cancer	High Risk Clinical Factors Affecting Prognosis	Treatments	Factors Affecting Nutritional Status
Acute Myeloid Leukemia (AML)	■ High white blood cell counts at diagnosis (arbitrary definition: WBC ≥ 100 x 10⁹/L ■ Unfavorable cytogenetics such as monosomy 7, certain 11.23 translocations ■ Molecular features including FLT3-ITD ■ Relapsed disease ■ MRD at the end of induction	■ Chemotherapy ■ HCT (is used as post-remission consolidation therapy; both autologous and allogeneic HCT have been studied)	Chemotherapy side-effects: ■ Nausea ■ Anorexia ■ Mucositis ■ Prolonged immune-suppression: time to count recovery, defined as ANC ≥ 200 mm³ may take up to 6 weeks Prolonged immunosuppression may lead to development of: ■ Bacterial infections ■ Invasive fungal infections ■ Poor oral intake from lack of food variety while hospitalized
Brain and CNS Tumors ■ Astrocytomas ■ Ependymomas and Choroid Plexus Tumor ■ Intracranial and intraspinal embryonal tumors which includes medulloblastoma	■ Metastatic disease at diagnosis ■ Young age at diagnosis: birth to 4 years ■ Tumors in this age group (birth to 4 years of age): ■ Are more biologically aggressive ■ Recur more frequently ■ Cause higher rates of neuropsychologic dysfunction ■ Cause other long term side-effects	■ Surgery: to resect/remove the tumor ■ Intensive chemotherapy regimens used first in infancy to 4 years to delay or replace radiation therapy, with or without autologous stem cell rescue ■ Radiation therapy plus cisplatin-based chemotherapy in age group 5–19 years; note: radiation therapy may still be necessary in some patients < 5 years of age	Chemotherapy side-effects: ■ Nausea, vomiting ■ Electrolyte disturbances ■ SIADH Radiation: ■ If indicated, treatment course is typically 6 weeks ■ Sedation is often necessary in younger children (NPO for up to 8 hours per day which interferes with oral and enteral feeding) ■ Dysphagia ■ Fatigue ■ Anorexia ■ Dysgeusia
Non-Hodgkin Lymphomas Most common subtypes: ■ Burkitt ■ Diffuse large B-cell ■ Lymphoblastic ■ Anaplastic large-cell		■ Chemotherapy	■ Risk for tumor lysis syndrome: high white count at diagnosis may result in increased serum potassium and phosphorus levels as cells break apart; may result in need for short term kidney dialysis to remove potassium and phosphorus ■ Mucositis ■ Anorexia ■ Early satiety ■ Weight loss ■ Frequent NPO status for procedures and intrathecal chemotherapy

Neuroblastoma	• High risk, stage III/IV and presence of metastatic disease • MYCN* oncogene amplification • Older age at diagnosis (> 5 years of age) • Relapsed disease	• High dose chemotherapy (6 cycles) • Surgical resection of tumor • Autologous HCT • Post-transplant radiation therapy • Immunotherapy with anti-GD2 antibodies • Isotretinoin therapy (cis-retinoic acid)	Chemotherapy side-effects: ■ Nausea and vomiting ■ Mucositis ■ Interruption in breastfeeding, oral feeding ■ Need for enteral tube feeding given young age and treatment side-effects Post-surgery: ■ Possible need for PN for post-operative recovery HCT: ■ Need for PN with transition to enteral/oral feeding Post-transplant radiation therapy: ■ Continued need for enteral nutrition via NG tube ■ Mucositis ■ Radiation induced diarrhea Immunotherapy plus isotretinoin: ■ Continued need for enteral nutrition via NG tube ■ Avoid vitamin A containing supplements while on cis-retinoic acid ■ Intensive feeding therapy upon completion of therapy often required to relearn oral feeding skills due to prolongec need for nutrition support during treatment
Renal Tumors Wilms Tumor (most common)	• High risk: stage III/IV and anaplastic • Unfavorable histology • Relapsed disease • Young age at diagnosis (usually occurs in children < than 5 years of age)	• Surgery • Chemotherapy • Radiation therapy (in some cases)	Surgery: ■ Resection of tumor at diagnosis ■ Post-operative resection may require nutrition support Chemotherapy side-effects: ■ Constipation ■ Loss of appetite ■ Early satiety ■ High need for enteral nutrition support during treatment

(continues)

(continued)

TABLE 16.2 Common Childhood Cancers Associated with High Nutrition Risk

Childhood Cancer	High Risk Clinical Factors Affecting Prognosis	Treatments	Factors Affecting Nutritional Status
Bone Tumors ■ Osteosarcoma (most common) ■ Ewing sarcoma	■ Period of adolescence (increased growth requirements) ■ Metastatic disease	■ Chemotherapy (cycles every 2–3 weeks) ■ Surgery (osteosarcoma): limb-sparing or amputation	Chemotherapy side-effects: ■ Nausea, vomiting ■ Weight loss ■ Anorexia ■ Magnesium, potassium, and phosphorus wasting due to kidney damage Other: ■ Compressed chemotherapy cycles contribute to shortened time intervals between treatments to regain lost weight ■ Increased energy and protein needs due to demands of growth in this age group ■ Poor wound healing post limb sparing surgery or amputations
Soft Tissue Sarcomas Rhabdomyosarcoma (most common) 2 major histologic subtypes: ■ ERMS (most common in children < 10 years) ■ ARMS (most common in children ≥ 10 years)	■ Presence of metastatic disease at diagnosis ■ Alveolar subtype	■ Chemotherapy ■ Surgery or radiation for local tumor control	Chemotherapy side-effects: ■ Mucositis ■ Diarrhea ■ Nausea and vomiting ■ Early satiety ■ Alterations in taste and smell of food Radiation: ■ Depends upon tumor location

*MYCN is an oncogene present on chromosome 2. The MYCN gene is amplified (has more than ten copies instead of two copies) in a subset of neuroblastoma tumors and the amplification of the MYCN gene is associated with poor outcome.

Data from Ward E, DeSantis C, Robbins A, et al. Childhood and adolescent cancer statistics, 2014. *CA Cancer J Clin*. 2014;64:83–103.[1]

Creutzig U, van den Heuvel-Elbrink MM, Gibson B, et al. Diagnosis and management of acute myeloid leukemia in children and adolescents: recommendations from an international expert panel. *Blood*. 2012;120:3187–3205.[11]

Gorlick R, Janeway K, Lessnick S. Review. Children's Oncology Group's 2013 blueprint for research: bone tumors. *Pediatr Blood Cancer*. 2013;60:1009–1015.[12]

Malempati S, Hawkins D. Rhabdomyosarcoma: Review of the Children's Oncology Group (COG) Soft-Tissue Sarcoma Committee experience and rationale for current COG Studies. *Pediatr Blood Cancer*. 2012;59:5–10.[13]

Cohen BH, Geyer JR, Miller CD, et al. Pilot study of intensive chemotherapy with peripheral hematopoietic cell support for children less than 3 years of age with malignant brain tumors, the CCG-99703 phase I/II study. A report from the Children's Oncology Group. *Pediatr Neuro*. 2015;53:31–46.[14]

Pui CH, Robison LL, Look AT. Acute lymphoblastic leukemia. *Lancet*. 2008;371:1030–1043.[15]

Patrick K, Vora A. Update on biology and treatment of T-cell acute lymphoblastic leukemia. *Curr Opin Pediatr*. 2015;27:44–49.[16]

Pinto NR, Applebaum MA, Volchenboum SL et al. Advances in risk classification and treatment strategies for neuroblastoma. *J Clin Oncol*. 2015;33:3008–3017.[17]

TABLE 16.3 Chemotherapeutic and Biotherapy Agents with Nutritional Implications

Drug	Common Pediatric Uses	Nausea & Vomiting	Anorexia	Mucositis	Diarrhea (D) or Constipation (C)	Electrolyte Imbalance	Hepatic Effects	Other
Alkylating Agents								
Bendamustine	Hodgkin lymphoma	++	+	+	C	+		Constipation, xerostomia, hypokalemia, weight loss
Busulfan *(intravenous and oral)*	HCT conditioning	++	+	+	D	+	+	SOS with HCT doses, hyperglycemia, hypokalemia, hypomagnesemia
Carboplatin	CNS tumors, germ cell tumors, HCT conditioning	+++	+		D	+	+	Prolonged electrolyte wasting, abdominal pain
Cisplatin	Germ cell tumors, osteosarcoma, neuroblastoma, CNS tumors	+++	+		D	++		Severe acute or delayed nausea and vomiting, up to 6 days after administration, SIADH, electrolyte wasting due to renal tubular necrosis, hypomagnesemia, metallic taste
Cyclophosphamide	ALL, lymphomas, sarcomas, CNS tumors, neuroblastoma, HCT conditioning & lymphodepletion for CAR-T cells	+++ (DD)	+		D	+	+	SIADH, abdominal discomfort, loss of appetite, hydration +/− to prevent cystitis
Ifosfamide	Sarcoma	++	+	+	D	+	+	Abdominal pain, hyponatremia, hypokalemia, hydration/mesna required to prevent cystitis, anorexia, SIADH

(continues)

TABLE 16.3 Chemotherapeutic and Biotherapy Agents with Nutritional Implications *(continued)*

Drug	Common Pediatric Uses	Nausea & Vomiting	Anorexia	Mucositis	Diarrhea (D) or Constipation (C)	Electrolyte Imbalance	Hepatic Effects	Other
Lomustine (CCNU)	CNS tumors	++	+	+			+	Renal toxicity, anorexia, related to cumulative dose
Melphalan	HCT conditioning	++ (DD)		+	D	+		Hypokalemia, hypophosphatemia
Procarbazine	Hodgkin lymphoma	+++	+		D			Dysphagia, xerostomia. Avoid foods high in tyramine, such as aged cheeses, cured meats, fava or broad beans, beer, wine, vermouth, sauerkraut, soy sauce, other soybean foods as procarbazine inhibits MAOI
Temozolomide *(Oral)*	CNS tumors	++	+		C		+	Fatigue, nausea & vomiting (best to take on an empty stomach to reduce nausea and vomiting), transaminitis
Thiotepa	CNS tumors, HCT conditioning	+++ (DD)	+	++	D	+	+	SOS, dose dependent nausea and vomiting
Antimetabolites								
Azacitidine	MDS, relapsed AML	++	+		D and C	+	+	Elevated serum creatinine, hypokalemia, hypophosphatemia, diarrhea and constipation
Cladribine	Langerhans cell histiocytosis		+		D			Nephrotoxicity, fatigue, mild nausea

Drug	Indication							Comments
Clofarabine	Relapsed or refractory leukemia	++	+	+	D	+	+	Pancreatitis, abdominal pain, gum bleeding, loss of appetite
Cytarabine	AML, ALL, lymphoblastic lymphoma	++ (DD)	+	+	D	+	+	Abdominal pain, esophageal ulceration, metallic taste, dysphagia, severe GI ulceration
Fludarabine	AML, HCT conditioning, Lymphodepletion for CAR-T cells	+	+		D			Mild abdominal pain
Fluorouracil (5-FU)	Colorectal carcinoma hepatoblastoma	+	+	++	D		+	Taste alterations, avoid pyridoxine supplementation, ascites
Mercaptopurine (6-MP)	ALL, lymphoblastic lymphoma		+	+	D	+	+	Biliary stasis, cholestatic jaundice, increased serum ALT, abdominal pain.***
Methotrexate	NHL, ALL, osteosarcoma	+++ (DD)	+	++	D	+	+	GI ulceration, enteritis, taste alterations, osteoporosis, decreased absorption of vitamin B$_{12}$. Avoid administration in patients with pleural or pericardial effusions, or ascites
Nelarabine	T-cell ALL, T-cell lymphoblastic lymphoma	+			D and C			Diarrhea, constipation, fatigue
Thioguanine (6-TG)	ALL		+	+	D	+	+	SOS, mild mucositis, diarrhea

(continues)

TABLE 16.3 Chemotherapeutic and Biotherapy Agents with Nutritional Implications *(continued)*

Drug	Common Pediatric Uses	Nausea & Vomiting	Anorexia	Mucositis	Diarrhea (D) or Constipation (C)	Electrolyte Imbalance	Hepatic Effects	Other
Antitumor Antibiotics								
Bleomycin	Hodgkin lymphoma, Germ cell tumors		++	+	D		+	
Dactinomycin	Wilms tumor	+++	+	+				Weight loss, xerostomia, taste alterations
Daunorubicin	ALL, lymphoblastic lymphoma, AML	++	+	+	D			Xerostomia, taste alterations, occasional diarrhea
Doxorubicin	ALL, lymphomas, neuroblastoma, Wilms tumor, sarcomas	++	+	+	D		+	Xerostomia, taste alterations
Idarubicin	AML	++		+	D			
Mitoxantrone	AML	+		+				
Plant Alkaloids								
Etoposide	AML, relapsed ALL, lymphomas, sarcomas, neuroblastoma, CNS tumors, HCT conditioning, HLH	++	+		D			High dose: mucositis, diarrhea (mild)
Irinotecan	Sarcoma, CNS tumors, relapsed solid tumors	++	+	+	D+	+	+	Abdominal pain, early and/or late diarrhea. Early diarrhea is a cholinergic driven process requiring atropine treatment. Late diarrhea often-requires loperamide to decrease stooling

Drug	Indication						C and D	Side effects
Topotecan	Neuroblastoma	+	+	+			C and D	Abdominal pain, constipation or diarrhea, fatigue
Vinblastine	Langerhans cell histiocytosis, Hodgkins lymphoma, CNS tumors			+		+	C	Paralytic ileus, SIADH, abdominal pain
Vincristine	ALL, lymphoma, Wilms tumor, sarcomas, CNS tumors, neuroblastoma			+	+	+	C+	Abdominal pain, SIADH, paralytic ileus, jaw pain
Retinoids								
Isotretinoin	Neuroblastoma					+		Hypertriglyceridemia, hypercholesterolemia, xerostomia, taste alterations. Give medication with MCT oil or foods high in fat for best absorption. Avoid supplements containing vitamin A
All trans retinoic acid	APL	+	+				C and D	Hypertriglyceridemia, hypercholesterolemia, xerostomia, taste alterations. Give medication with MCT oil or foods high in fat for best absorption. Avoid supplements containing vitamin A

(continues)

TABLE 16.3 Chemotherapeutic and Biotherapy Agents with Nutritional Implications *(continued)*

Drug	Common Pediatric Uses	Nausea & Vomiting	Anorexia	Mucositis	Diarrhea (D) or Constipation (C)	Electrolyte Imbalance	Hepatic Effects	Other
Adrenocorticosteroids								
Prednisone and Dexamethasone	Leukemia, lymphoma, CNS tumors, HCT immunosuppression							Hyperphagia, sodium and fluid retention, gastric ulceration, glucose intolerance, hyperlipidemia, osteoporosis, muscle wasting
Enzyme								
Erwinia Asparaginase and Pegasparaginase	ALL						+	Hypoalbuminemia, hyperglycemia/diabetes, pancreatitis, weight loss
Monoclonal Antibodies								
Brentuximab	Hodgkin lymphoma	+	+		D+			
Protein-Targeted Therapies: Small Molecule Inhibitors Tyrosine Kinase Inhibitors (TKI's)								
Imatinib Mesylate	CML, Ph+ ALL,	++	+		D	+	+	Weight gain, edema, GI reflux, hypokalemia, hypophosphatemia and pancreatitis. Avoid grapefruit juice

Dasatinib	CML and Ph+ ALL	+	+		D	+	+	Severe fluid retention, hypocalcemia, hypophosphatemia, abdominal pain
Nilotinib	CML	+	+	+	C	+	+	Hyperglycemia, hyperkalemia, hypokalemia, hyponatremia, hypophosphatemia, abdominal pain
Sorafenib	FLT-3 ITD AML	+	+		C and D	+	+	Increased lipase and amylase
mTOR Inhibitors								
Temsirolimus	Relapsed solid tumors			+	C and D	+		Fatigue, hyperlipidemia, hypercholesterolemia
Proteasome Inhibitor								
Bortezomib	Relapsed/refractory malignancy in combination with standard chemotherapy	+			D		+	Fatigue, avoid grapefruit juice and other drinks containing bergamottin

(continues)

TABLE 16.3 Chemotherapeutic and Biotherapy Agents with Nutritional Implications *(continued)*

Drug	Common Pediatric Uses	Nausea & Vomiting	Anorexia	Mucositis	Diarrhea (D) or Constipation (C)	Electrolyte Imbalance	Hepatic Effects	Other
Angiogenesis Inhibitors								
Bevacizumab	High grade gliomas, relapsed CNS tumors		+	+	D	+		Hyponatremia, weight loss, abdominal pain, taste alterations, GI perforation

Key: Nausea and vomiting:

+++: high level of emetic risk (>90% frequency of emesis in absence of prophylaxis)

++: moderate level of emetic risk (30–90% frequency of emesis in absence of prophylaxis)

+: low level of emetic risk (10–<30% frequency of emesis in absence of prophylaxis)

no +: minimal emetic risk (<10% frequency of emesis in absence of prophylaxis)

DD: level of emetic risk is also <u>Dose Dependent</u>

*** commonly practiced restrictions to avoid food and dairy 2 hours before taking 6-MP may no longer be warranted with this medication (source: Landier – see below).

Abbreviations:

ALL: acute lymphoblastic leukemia;
AML: acute myeloid leukemia
APL: acute promyelocytic leukemia
CML: chronic myeloid leukemia
CNS: central nervous system
GI: gastrointestinal
HCT: hematopoietic cell transplantation
HLH: hemolytic lymphocytic histiocytosis
MAOI: monoamine oxidase inhibitor
MCT: medium chain triglyceride
MDS: myelodysplastic syndrome
NHL: non-Hodgkin lymphoma
SIADH: syndrome of inappropriate anti-diuretic hormone
SOS: sinusoidal obstructive syndrome

Data from The Children's Oncology Group, Guideline for the Prevention of Nausea and Vomiting due to Antineoplastic Medication in Pediatric Cancer Patients. Available at: https://childrensoncologygroup.org/downloads/COG_SC_CINV_Guideline_Document.pdf. Accessed November 17, 2017.[18]

Macris PC (ed). *Nutrition Care Criteria.* 3rd ed. Seattle, WA: Seattle Cancer Care Alliance; 2012.[19]

Polovich M, Whitford JM, Olsen M (eds). *Chemotherapy and Biotherapy Guidelines and Recommendations for Practice.* Pittsburgh, PA: Oncology Nursing Society;2014:27–91.[20]

Landier W, Hageman L, Chen Y, et al. Mercaptopurine ingestion habits, red cell thioguanine nucleotide levels, and relapse risk in children with acute lymphoblastic leukemia: A report from the Children's Oncology Group Study AALL03N1. *J Clin Oncol.* 2017;35:1730–1736.[21]

TABLE 16.4 Nutritional Implications of Radiation Therapy

Central Nervous System
- Anorexia
- Nausea and vomiting
- Growth disturbances

Head and Neck
- Xerostomia (oral dryness)
- Nausea
- Mucositis and esophagitis
- Dysgeusia (impaired taste) and dysosmia (impaired smell)
- Tooth decay
- Altered salivation (saliva becomes thick and viscous)
- Dysphagia

GI Tract
- Nausea and vomiting
- Diarrhea
- Steatorrhea and malabsorption
- Fluid and electrolyte imbalances

Total Body
- Nausea, vomiting, diarrhea
- Mucositis and esophagitis
- Altered taste acuity and salivation
- Anorexia
- Delayed growth and development

Data from Macris PC (ed). *Nutrition Care Criteria*. 3rd ed. Seattle, WA: Seattle Cancer Care Alliance; 2012.[19]

Macris PC, Hunt K. Hematology and oncology. In: Queen PS, King K, (eds). *Pediatric Nutrition*. 4th ed. Sudbury, MA: Jones and Bartlett Publishers, Inc; 2012:363–383.[24]

surgery alone for patients with asymptomatic stage 2a or 2b neuroblastoma.[17] Surgery is also a planned part of treatment to resect residual or necrotic tumor after four or five cycles of chemotherapy in high-risk neuroblastoma patients. Surgical removal of a tumor may lead to insufficient nutritional intake over several days during a time of increased requirements of energy and protein. Depending on the surgical site, nutrient intake via the oral route may be impaired due to unsafe swallowing issues (dysphagia) following surgical resection of brain tumors. If the tumor is located in the abdominal region, **parenteral nutrition** (PN) support may be required to treat post operative ileus in the area of resection. Surgery in these areas may result in profound nutritional implications including chewing and swallowing issues, diarrhea, malabsorption of vitamins and minerals, and fluid and electrolyte imbalances.

Hematopoietic Cell Transplantation (HCT)

Treatment with HCT is an established therapeutic modality for select hematologic malignancies and solid tumors. It is also a treatment for hematologic disorders, immunodeficiency diseases, and pediatric non-neoplastic conditions. **TABLE 16.5** outlines pediatric diseases and conditions treated by HCT.[25]

Children receiving a traditional myeloablative regimen are prepared with high doses of chemotherapy and possibly TBI and local irradiation; lower dose chemotherapy and radiation are delivered to children receiving a nonmyeloablative conditioning regimen.[26] Children with relapsed malignancy following myeloablative HCT or those with nonmalignant disorders may be candidates for the nonmyeloablative regimens.

TABLE 16.5 Conditions for Application of Pediatric Hematopoietic Cell Transplantation

Hematologic malignancies
- Acute leukemia
- Chronic leukemia
- Myelodysplastic syndrome

Malignant solid tumors
- Advanced-stage neuroblastoma
- Refractory Ewing's sarcoma
- Recurrent lymphomas

Immunodeficiency disorders
- Severe combined immunodeficiency disease
- Wiskott-Aldrich syndrome
- Hyper IgM syndrome
- Other cellular immunodeficiencies

Nonneoplastic disorders
- Severe aplastic anemia
- Thalassemia major
- Fanconi anemia
- Diamond-Blackfan syndrome
- Sickle cell disease
- Paroxysmal nocturnal hemoglobinuria
- Shwachman Diamond syndrome
- Lysosomal storage diseases (e.g., Gaucher's disease, metachromatic leukodystrophy, Niemann-Pick disease)
- Mucopolysaccharidoses (e.g., Hunter's disease, Hurler's disease)
- Infantile osteopetrosis
- Hemophagocytic lymphohistiocytosis
- Refractory autoimmune disorders
- Tay-Sachs Disease

Data from Locatelli F, Giorgiani G, Di-Cesare-Merlone A, et al. The changing role of stem cell transplantation in childhood. *Bone Marrow Transplant*. 2008;41:S3–S7.[25]

The intense conditioning regimen is designed to eliminate active and residual malignant cells or a defective hematopoietic system in order to restore normal hematopoiesis and immunologic function.[26] An intravenous infusion of autologous (child's own), syngeneic (identical twin), or allogeneic (from a histocompatible related or unrelated donor) stem cells follows the conditioning regimen. The source of the stem cells may be bone marrow, peripheral blood, or umbilical cord blood.[19]

Posttransplant course: Severe pancytopenia (low blood counts) lasts from two to six weeks posttransplant. Children are at the greatest risk for bacterial and fungal infections until the stem cells engraft. During this period, supportive care including frequent red blood cell and platelet transfusions, systemic antibiotic therapy, and PN support are instituted.

Nutrition effects of HCT are due to the conditioning therapy, infections, graft-versus-host disease (GVHD), and medications, including anti-infectious and immunosuppressive agents.[27] Complications interfering with nutrient intake include mucositis; esophagitis; dysgeusia (impaired taste); xerostomia (oral dryness); thick, viscous saliva; nausea; vomiting; anorexia; diarrhea; steatorrhea; and multiple-organ dysfunction.[28] The duration and intensity of symptoms, as well as the stress of treatment, preclude oral intake for a minimum of three to four weeks post-transplant and necessitate using PN support. Oral intake is encouraged as soon as tolerated. Energy, protein, and fluid goals should be defined for each child.

At hospital discharge, some children are still unable to eat an adequate amount of nutrients, and partial PN and/or enteral tube feeding may be prescribed, especially for children with chronic food aversions and long-term anorexia. Supplemental intravenous hydration may also be necessary. Follow-up nutrition counseling and assessment are imperative throughout the child's post-transplant course in order to ensure provision of adequate nutrition support.

Graft-Versus-Host disease: Children who receive allogeneic transplants are at risk for the development of GVHD, an immunologic reaction in which the newly engrafted stem cells react against the host's tissue antigens following engraftment. The ensuing immunologic response can cause multiple-organ damage.[27] The GVHD may occur as an acute reaction early posttransplant or progress to a chronic condition. Because of its potentially devastating effects, efforts are directed at prevention of GVHD. Medications and therapy used for prophylaxis and treatment of GVHD are shown in **TABLE 16.6**.

TABLE 16.6 Therapies Used for Prophylaxis and Treatment of GVHD

Therapy	Nutritional Effects
Antithymocyte globulin	Nausea and vomiting, diarrhea, stomatitis
Beclomethasone dipropionate	Xerostomia, dysgeusia, nausea
Budesonide	Nausea, diarrhea
Corticosteroids	Sodium and fluid retention resulting in weight gain or hypertension, hyperphagia, weight gain, hypokalemia, skeletal muscle catabolism and atrophy, gastric irritation and peptic ulceration, osteoporosis, growth retardation in children, decreased insulin sensitivity and impaired glucose tolerance, hyperglycemia or steroid-induced diabetes, hypertriglyceridemia
Cyclosporine	Nausea and vomiting, renal insufficiency, magnesium wasting, potassium wasting
Extracorporeal photopheresis	Intravenous fluid may be necessary to maintain adequate hydration status; monitor calcium status if citrate anticoagulant is used because it may bind calcium and induce hypocalcemia
Methotrexate	Nausea and vomiting (mild to moderate); anorexia; mucositis and esophagitis; diarrhea; renal and hepatic changes; decreased absorption of vitamin B_{12}, fat, and D-xylose; hepatic fibrosis; change in taste acuity
Methoxsalen (in conjunction with Psoralen 1 ultraviolet A light)	Nausea, hepatotoxicity

Therapy	Nutritional Effects
Monoclonal antibodies	Nausea and vomiting
Mycophenolate mofetil	Nausea and vomiting, diarrhea
Sirolimus	Hypertriglyceridemia
Tacrolimus	Nephrotoxicity, hyperglycemia, hyperkalemia, hypomagnesemia
Ursodeoxycholic acid	Nausea and vomiting, diarrhea, dyspepsia

Data from Macris PC (ed). *Nutrition Care Criteria*. 3rd ed. Seattle, WA: Seattle Cancer Care Alliance; 2012.[19]

Acute GVHD can affect the skin, liver, or GI tract. Clinical symptoms include a maculopapular rash, cholestatic liver dysfunction, or anorexia, nausea, vomiting, and diarrhea. Intestinal GVHD can involve either the upper or lower GI tract.[28] Upper intestinal GVHD symptoms include early satiety, anorexia, nausea, and vomiting. In lower intestinal GVHD, diarrhea may be severe and, at its worst, associated with crampy abdominal pain and bleeding. Children with severe disease often require a period of bowel rest with PN support. Refeeding guidelines include slow diet progression and feeding one new food at a time, as presented in **TABLE 16.7**. Children who develop steatorrhea or pancreatic insufficiency often benefit from pancreatic enzyme replacement therapy.[27,28]

TABLE 16.7 Gastrointestinal GVHD Diet Progression

Phase	Clinical Symptoms	Diet	Nutrition Support
1. Bowel rest	GI cramping Large volume watery diarrhea or active GI bleeding Depressed serum albumin Severely reduced transit time Small-bowel obstruction or diminished bowel sounds Nausea and vomiting	Oral: NPO	PN with supplemental zinc and possibly copper
2. Introduction of oral feeding	Minimal GI cramping Diarrhea less than 500 mL/day Guaiac-negative stools Improved transit time (minimum 1.5 hours) Infrequent nausea and vomiting	Oral: Isosmotic, low-residue, low-lactose beverages, initially 60 mL every 2 to 3 hours, for several days	PN Trophic enteral feeds of semi-elemental formula if patient unable to eat
3. Introduction of solids	Minimal or no GI cramping Formed stool	Oral: Allow introduction of solid food, once every 3 to 4 hours: minimal lactose, low fiber, low fat (20–40 g/day), low total acidity, no gastric irritants	Begin to cycle and decrease PN Advance feeds slowly (small boluses or continuous infusion) if patient unable to eat

(continues)

TABLE 16.7 Gastrointestinal GVHD Diet Progression *(continued)*

Phase	Clinical Symptoms	Diet	Nutrition Support
4. Expansion of diet	Minimal or no GI cramping Formed stool	Oral: Minimal lactose, low fiber, low total acidity, no gastric irritants; if stools indicate fat malabsorption, low fat	Nighttime supplemental PN if oral intake less than needs or patient unable to maintain weight owing to malabsorption Enteral feed schedule and formula dependent on any residual GI symptoms
5. Resumption of regular diet	No GI cramping Normal stool Normal transit time Normal albumin	Oral: Progress to regular diet by introducing one restricted food per day; acid foods with meals, fiber-containing foods, lactose-containing foods; order of addition will vary depending on individual tolerances and preferences; patients no longer exhibiting steatorrhea should have the fat restriction liberalized slowly	Discontinue PN Supplemental enteral feeds if patient unable to consume adequate nutrients

Abbreviations: GI, gastrointestinal; GVHD, graft-versus-host disease; NPO, nil per os (nothing by mouth); PN, parenteral nutrition.
Data from Gauvreau JM, Lenssen P, Cheney CL, et al. Nutritional management of patients with intestinal graft-versus-host disease. *J Am Diet Assoc.* 1981;79:673–677.[29]

▶ Condition Specific Nutrition Screening, Nutrition Assessment, and Nutrition Diagnosis

Nutrition assessment should begin at diagnosis and continue throughout treatment. A comprehensive baseline assessment identifies high risk patients. Serial measurements throughout the child's treatment course allows for rapid response to sudden changes in clinic status. Techniques for the newly diagnosed child do not differ from normal nutrition assessment recommendations as presented in Chapter 1. The pediatric oncology dietitian, however, should have a clear understanding of the specific type and stage of cancer, treatment protocol, and effects of therapy to better formulate an appropriate nutrition care plan for the child undergoing therapy.

Nutrition History

Altered GI function (NC-1.4) related to cancer therapy as evidenced by need for nutrition support (EN or PN) to maintain nutritional status.

The nutrition history includes a comprehensive assessment of current oral and GI symptoms (i.e., chewing or swallowing difficulties, mucositis and esophagitis, taste alterations, xerostomia, heartburn, nausea and vomiting, early satiety, changes in appetite, and altered bowel habits). Current dietary modifications including using special diets; presence of food allergies; food aversions or intolerances; using vitamin, mineral, and herbal supplements; and integrative medicine therapies should be included in the initial evaluation. Current or past need for nutrition support interventions (enteral nutrition [EN] and PN or intravenous fluid [IVF]) support should also be assessed.

For infants and young children, stage of eating development (self-feeding skills; puree versus table food; cup versus bottle) and use of infant formulas or breast-feeding should be evaluated. For children undergoing HCT who are breastfed, the mother's cytomegalovirus serology must be negative to prevent transmission of the virus to the infant (Institutional reference: Seattle Cancer Care Alliance, HCT Standard Practice Guideline: "Breast Feeding of Hematopoietic Cell Transplant Recipients," 2014).

Physical Assessment

A nutrition-focused physical examination is valuable to detect the presence of obesity, emaciation, dehydration, or edema. The physical assessment should also include a careful examination of hair, eyes, mouth, skin, and nails to look for signs of micronutrient deficiency.[30]

Biochemistry

Finding reliable measures to detect malnutrition in the pediatric cancer patient can be challenging. Both the disease itself and the treatment can affect laboratory data used for nutrition assessment. Hematologic parameters, such as hemoglobin and hematocrit, often reflect the disease state and treatment with blood transfusions, rather than nutritional status. Many chemotherapy agents will suppress bone marrow production and cause some degree of myelosuppression, which is the decrease in number of neutrophils, megakaryocytes and erythrocytes within the bone marrow; therefore, the complete blood count must be interpreted cautiously once therapy begins. Biochemical indices on renal and hepatic function as well as serum lipids, glucose, and electrolytes should always be reviewed for detection of nutritional deficiencies.

Serum albumin, a marker of internal protein status, is no longer considered a meaningful biomarker for diagnosing malnutrition, because infection, excessive GI or renal losses, impaired liver function, certain chemotherapy agents, and overhydration can each depress serum albumin levels.[30] Prealbumin, an acute-phase protein-like albumin, is less influenced by changes in body fluids than serum albumin, making it a more reliable test with which to evaluate nutritional status. However, both biomarkers are affected by inflammation, and lack the sensitivity and specificity required to stand alone as indicators of malnutrition.[30,31] Identifying malnutrition that is otherwise undetectable by anthropometric data such as weight loss, **body mass index** (BMI), or hypoalbuminemia, serial **mid-upper arm circumference** (MUAC) measurements can be used to monitor changes in body composition using the child as his or her own control.[31]

The **C-reactive protein** (CRP) test is another laboratory value that measures general levels of body inflammation. High CRP levels are caused by infections and many chronic diseases such as cancer. Inflammation can impact appetite and alter nutrient utilization.[30]

It is paramount to closely monitor fluid and electrolyte parameters as some chemotherapeutic agents induce the **syndrome of inappropriate antidiuretic hormone** (SIADH), a disorder of water intoxication. The release of anti-diuretic hormone causes the kidneys to resorb water, leading to hyponatremia. Chemotherapy agents that can contribute to SIADH include cyclophosphamide, vincristine, cisplatin, docetaxel, melphalan, and ifosfamide.[19,20] Managing presenting symptoms may include fluid restriction and diuresis.

Anthropometry

Obtaining accurate initial measurements of height or recumbent length, weight, and occipital frontal circumference, in children less than two years of age, provides baseline data for serial measurements. Any measurement below the 10th percentile should be investigated as a sign of growth impairment possibly due to inadequate nutrition. Children undergoing HCT who present at <95% ideal weight, have a significantly poor prognosis; those <85% ideal weight have an even poorer prognosis.[32] Conversely, overweight children have a higher risk of poorer survival following HCT.[33]

A landmark paper by Mehta and colleagues highlighted a paradigm toward etiology-related definitions of malnutrition.[34] Using anthropometric z-scores to help identify and describe malnutrition is now a common practice in the pediatric oncology population. Using z-scores to determine mild (z-score: –1 to –1.99), moderate (z-score: –2 to –2.99), and severe (z-score: ≥ –3) malnutrition has provided a uniform way for clinicians to understand and communicate the degree of wellness or undernutrition in pediatric diseases such as cancer.[34]

From the baseline anthropometry information, the child's body surface area and ideal weight, which are often used to calculate medication dosages, can be determined.

For pre-pubertal children (females less than 12 years old; males less than 14 years old), ideal weight is determined by matching the weight at the 50th percentile for height on the age- and gender-specific **Centers for Disease Control** (CDC) Growth Charts: United States.[35] For post-pubertal children, an estimation of the ideal weight is determined using the **body mass index** (BMI) CDC growth charts for age. If the child's BMI is between the 25th to 75th percentiles, this may be considered an ideal weight. An adjusted weight is calculated for children greater than 120% ideal weight:

Adjusted weight = [actual weight (kg) − ideal weight (kg)] × 0.25 + ideal weight (kg).[36]

It is important to assess both growth history and current height (or length) for age, weight for age, and weight for length or BMI.

Arm anthropometry, including baseline measurements of MUAC and triceps skinfold, is a tool that can assess the child's somatic muscle protein and adipose reserves. MUAC and triceps skinfold measurements are more reliable to interpret nutritional status since they are unaffected by fluid shifts and tumor mass.[10] Specific to the HCT population, arm anthropometry should be assessed during the initial nutrition evaluation in order to provide baseline data for subsequent measurements. In a retrospective review of over 700 pediatric HCT recipients, children who presented with low baseline somatic muscle reserves had poorer outcomes.[37]

Other Assessment Tools

The child's medical history, including past surgeries and endocrine or cardiac complications, current medications (for drug-nutrient interactions), physical strength, activity level, organ function, and level of pain and pain control, which may interfere with oral intake, should be evaluated.

Nutrient Requirements

Increased nutrient needs (NI-5.1) related to oncologic therapy as evidenced by elevated energy and protein requirements.

Nutrient requirements during childhood cancer are described in **TABLE 16.8**. The goals are to:

- Provide adequate nutrition to preserve lean body mass and promote growth and development
- Identify and prevent or correct protein-energy malnutrition
- Prevent or correct metabolic abnormalities
- Prevent or correct micronutrient deficiencies
- Maximize quality of life

Energy and Protein Requirements

It is critical to evaluate and monitor the ongoing energy needs of each child undergoing cancer treatment in order to ensure expected growth is occurring. Energy needs can be measured by indirect calorimetry or estimated through the use of standard equations.[39] All methods determine energy needs at least in part by measuring the child's age, weight, gender, therapy, and growth requirements.

TABLE 16.8 Nutrient Requirements During Childhood Cancer

Nutrient Requirements	Recommendations
Calories	- Infants: Birth to 12 months: Use RDA for age for appropriate weight infants. Use catch-up growth calculation if underweight: (Kcal/kg/day = Kcal/kg/day for weight age × ideal weight age (kg) + actual weight in kg) - Older children (> than 1 year): Use BMR table multiplied by additional factors: - Appropriate weight for height: BMR × 1.6 - Obese: BMR × 1.3 - Sedentary with 5% weight loss: BMR × 1.4–1.6 - 10% weight loss from usual weight or weight is 90% or less of usual or ideal weight: BMR × 1.8–2.0 - Use adjusted weight calculation for obese children; BMI weight at the 75th percentile may also be used to calculate energy needs in obese children - HCT: BEE/BMR × 1.6 (or 1.8 for children <2 years old) during immediate posttransplant course; BEE/BMR × 1.4 following engraftment and medically stable (use BEE for patients >16 years old >75 kg)
Protein	- Infants birth to 6 months: 3 g/kg/day - Infants 6 to 12 months: 2.5–3 g/kg/day - Children: 2–2.5 g/kg/day (in most cases) - Adolescents with increased lean body mass: 1.5–1.8 g/kg/day
Fat	- 10–30% total calories
Fluid	- 1–10 kg: 100 mL/kg/day - 11–20 kg: 1000 mL plus 50 ml for every kg > 10 per day - 21–40 kg: 1500 mL plus 20 mL for every kg > 20 per day - > 40 kg: 1500 mL/m2 body surface area

Nutrient Requirements	Recommendations
Vitamins	<ul><li>Use ASPEN parenteral vitamin guidelines for age</li><li>After PN discontinued, oral multiple vitamin/mineral without iron, during antineoplastic therapy</li><li>Provide additional vitamin C during HCT:<ul><li>< 31 kg, additional 250 mg vitamin C per day</li><li>> 31 kg, additional 500 mg vitamin C per day</li></ul></li></ul>
Minerals and electrolytes	<ul><li>Iron supplementation contraindicated during oncologic therapy and HCT</li><li>Eliminate copper and manganese from PN in presence of hepatic dysfunction (i.e., serum bilirubin > 10.0 mg/dL)</li><li>Closely monitor serum electrolytes during therapy</li><li>Calcium (milligrams) and /vitamin D (units) recommendations during steroid therapy:<ul><li>Birth to 1 year: 500 milligrams/400 units</li><li>1–3 years: 1,000 milligrams/800 units</li><li>4–8 years: 1,200 milligrams/800 units</li><li>9–18 years: 1,500 milligrams/1,000 units</li></ul></li></ul>

Abbreviations: ASPEN, American Society for Parenteral and Enteral Nutrition; BEE, basal energy expenditure; BMI, body mass index; BMR, basal metabolic rate; HCT, hematopoietic cell transplantation; PN, parenteral nutrition; RDA, recommended dietary allowance.

Data from Macris PC, McMillen K. Nutrition support of the hematopoietic cell transplant recipient. In: Forman SJ, Negrin RS, Antin JH, Appelbaum FR, (eds). Thomas' *Hematopoietic Cell Transplantation*. 5th ed. Hoboken, NJ: Wiley Blackwell; 2016:1216–1224.[27]

Task Force for the Revision of Sale Practices for Parenteral Nutrition. Mirtallo J, Canada T, Johnson D, et al. Safe practices for parenteral nutrition. *JPEN J Parenter Enteral Nutr 2004*; 28:S39–S70.[38]

The 2005 **Dietary Reference Intakes** (DRIs) set forth specific equations for calculating energy and protein, categorized by age and gender, however, this method of measurement may underestimate energy needs in the pediatric oncology population, since equations were determined solely from children with normal growth and activity, especially in children younger than 5 years old.[40]

The 1989 **Recommended Dietary Allowance** (RDA) calculations for infants and children and the WHO equation, which uses the basal metabolic rate with additions for growth, infection, stress, and inactivity, are commonly used to estimate energy needs.[41] Multiplying the basal metabolic rate by a stress factor of 1.6 to 1.8 for very young or malnourished children will allow for growth, stress, and light activity.[42] The Harris-Benedict formula and other equations have been used to estimate calorie needs in adults and may be appropriate for children who have completed their growth.[43] Protein needs are also increased during oncologic treatment in order to counteract the catabolic demands associated with multimodal therapies.

Vitamin, Mineral and Electrolyte Requirements

Vitamin and mineral requirements have not been determined for children with cancer. Recommendations are based on the DRI (https://www.ncbi.nlm.nih.gov/books/NBK56068/table/summarytables.t2/?report=objectonly).

Extensive radiation or surgical damage to the GI tract and treatment with long-term antibiotic therapy for chronic infections may also increase the child's need for vitamins and minerals. Specific nutrient deficiencies may occur from therapy-related treatments; however, they are difficult to identify without laboratory assay. Most children receiving cancer treatment benefit from taking an age-specific multivitamin/mineral supplement without iron, to prevent iron overload, which may develop due to red cell transfusions during therapy.

Children diagnosed with ALL, non-Hodgkin's lymphoma, or those who develop GVHD following HCT are especially at risk for developing osteopenia and fractures due to the use of corticosteroids during treatment.[44,45] As corticosteroids disrupt calcium absorption, the natural intake of calcium and vitamin D from the child's own diet is often insufficient to meet increased needs. Therefore, calcium and vitamin D supplementation, in addition to the multivitamin/mineral supplement, is often necessary to maintain bone health. Calcium and vitamin D recommendations for children maintained on corticosteroid therapy are outlined Table 16.8[27,38] Bisphosphonate therapy, in addition to calcium and vitamin D supplementation has also shown to be effective in reversing bone loss in children undergoing HCT.[45]

Pediatric HCT patients require additional vitamin C to promote tissue recovery via collagen biosynthesis after cytoreductive therapy.[19] Some chemotherapies, as well as medications used to treat fungal and viral infections (e.g., ambisone, foscarnet) are nephrotoxic and may cause increased losses of certain minerals. For example, cisplatin commonly causes magnesium, phosphorus, potassium, and zinc wasting.[19,20] Children undergoing cancer treatment with nephrotoxic chemotherapy agents may require long-term supplementation of these nutrients.

Vitamin D plays an essential role in maintaining bone health through regulating calcium concentrations in the body.[46] Historically, the majority of research has centered on the link between vitamin D deficiency and rickets in children and exacerbation of osteoporosis in children and adults. Currently, there are ongoing prospective studies evaluating the relationship between vitamin D deficiency and risk for developing cancer and other chronic diseases.[47] Although determining a clear relationship between vitamin D deficiency and the development of certain diseases is in the early stages of research, practitioners who care for children with cancer should routinely measure the serum 25-OH vitamin D level to evaluate for deficiency.[47]

Specific to the HCT population, prevalence of vitamin D deficiency occurs more commonly than in the healthy pediatric population.[48] Low serum 25-OH vitamin D[49] and vitamin A levels[50] have also been associated with increased incidence of GVHD in children. Close monitoring of serum levels is necessary with supplementation as indicated.

Omega-3 Fatty Acids

Certain medications, including cyclosporine, corticosteroids, and all-trans retinoic acid, are known to cause a fluctuation and possible increase in serum triglyceride levels.[19] Because clinical trials have shown that fish oil (omega-3 fatty acids including docosahexaenoic and eicosapentaenoic acid) supplementation can improve hypertriglyceridemia (≥ 500mg/dL) in adults,[51] it is an accepted practice among pediatric practitioners to use this **Food and Drug Administration** (FDA) approved therapy for children with cancer; it is generally provided when the child is tolerating oral medications.

Nutrition Intervention

The practice of nutrition support widely ranges in the timing, duration, and method of intervention in children with cancer. However, despite the well-documented connection between adequate nutrition and positive long-term outcomes, the practice still lacks standardized assessment criteria, or aligned strategies to prevent or treat nutrition failure in this population.[8] The literature continues to support early detection of pre-existing malnutrition in children at diagnosis and nutrition therapy during treatment to sustain and promote normal growth and development for the most positive outcomes possible.

Oral Diet

As described earlier, pediatric oncology patients experience multiple oral and GI issues that interfere with nutrient intake and nutritional status. Dietary guidelines for managing these common nutrition issues are detailed in **TABLE 16.9**.

While an oral diet is always indicated for a child with a functional GI tract, feeding a child during intense

TABLE 16.9 Guidelines for Increasing Nutrient Density	
Butter, margarine, and oils ■ Add to soup, mashed and baked potatoes, hot cereal, grits, rice, noodles, and cooked vegetables.	■ Stir into sauces and gravies.
Cream ■ Use on desserts, gelatin, pudding, fruit, pancakes, waffles, and mashed potatoes. ■ Use in soups, sauces, egg dishes, batters, puddings, and custards; put on cereals.	■ Mix with pasta, mashed potatoes, and rice. ■ Substitute for milk in recipes. ■ Make cocoa with cream and add marshmallows.
Sour cream ■ Add to soups, baked potatoes, vegetables, sauces, salad dressings, gelatin desserts, bread, and muffin batter.	■ Use as dip for raw fruits and vegetables.
Mayonnaise ■ Add to salad dressing. ■ Spread on sandwiches and crackers.	■ Use in sauces and gelatin desserts.

Honey (use in children over 1 year of age) • Add to cereal, milk drinks, fruit desserts, smoothies, or yogurt.	• Use as a glaze for meats such as chicken.
Granola • Use in cookie, muffin, and bread batters. • Sprinkle on vegetables, yogurt, ice cream, pudding, custard, and fruit.	• Mix with dried fruits and nuts for a snack. • Substitute for bread or rice in pudding recipes.
Dried fruits and nuts • Cook and serve dried fruits for breakfast or as dessert. • Add to muffins, cookies, breads, cakes, rice and grain dishes, cereals, puddings, and stuffing.	• Bake in pies and turnovers. • Combine with cooked vegetables such as carrots, sweet potatoes, or acorn and butternut squash.
Milk and cheese • Mix one cup dry milk powder in four cups of liquid milk; use this milk for cooking and baking. • Add milk powder directly to hot or cold cereals, scrambled eggs, soups, gravies, casserole dishes, and desserts.	• Add grated cheese or chunks of cheese to sauces, vegetables, soups, salads, and casseroles. • Spread cream cheese on hot buttered bread.
Eggs • Add eggs to soups and casseroles.	• Slice boiled eggs in sauces and serve over rice, cooked noodles, buttered toast, or hot biscuits.
Peanut butter • Add peanut butter to sauces; use on crackers, waffles, or celery sticks.	• Spread peanut butter on hot buttered bread.

Reproduced from Seattle Cancer Care Alliance. Medical Nutrition Therapy Services. Seattle, Washington.[52]

therapy may be a slow process since appetite and tolerance for food fluctuate widely. Individualizing the child's diet by offering small and frequent servings of nutrient dense foods and fluids he/she enjoys and encouraging parental involvement may enhance oral intake. Suggestions for boosting the nutrient density of foods consumed are shown in **TABLE 16.10**. Young children with preexisting delays in feeding development should have intervention from a feeding team.

Diet for the pediatric oncology patient: Because food may serve as a potential infection source, "low microbial" or "neutropenic" diets have often been used with the pediatric oncology population. While the protective benefits of a neutropenic diet have not been established, most cancer centers utilize some type of low microbial diet.[53–55] In a survey of 198 member institutions of the Children's Oncology Group, 84% recommended a neutropenic diet for HCT patients.[54] Immununosuppressed diet guidelines for children undergoing oncologic therapy are presented in **TABLE 16.11**.

Food safety: Providing education on food safety may be more important in reducing foodborne illness than extensive diet restrictions.[55] Education should emphasize handwashing; high-risk foods; proper temperatures for storage, defrosting, and cooking; cross-contamination issues; correct cooling and reheating procedures; and sanitation.

Probiotics during cancer therapy: The intestinal microbiota helps to maintain the physical, functional, and immunologic barriers within the GI tract. There is growing evidence that decreased intestinal microbiota diversity may result in aberrant systemic immune responses, such as GVHD. Prebiotics and probiotics have the potential to change the gut flora to support the development and sustainability of a healthier microbiota.[56] The concern, however, is sepsis as a result of bacterial translocation or viral infection in immunosuppressed children. A small, pilot human study showed no increase in infection in pediatric transplant recipients supplemented with *Lactobacillus plantarum*.[57] For now, pasteurized food sources of probiotics, such as yogurt, kefir, etc., are recommended during the immediate post-transplant course. More human studies are needed in the pediatric oncology population before specific recommendations can be made.

TABLE 16.10 Dietary Guidelines for Managing Common Nutrition Problems of Children with Cancer

Oral and esophageal mucositis (inflammation of the oral and esophageal mucosa)
- Try soft or pureed foods or a blenderized liquid diet.
- Offer soft, nonirritating, cold foods (popsicles, ice cream, frozen yogurt, slushes) and smooth, bland, moist foods (custard, cream soups, mashed potatoes).
- Encourage frequent mouth rinsing to remove food and bacteria and promote healing.

Xerostomia (oral dryness)
- Offer moist foods (stews, casseroles, canned fruit) and liquids.
- Add sauce, gravy, margarine, butter, or broth to dry foods.
- Drink liquids with meals.
- Offer sugar-free lemon-flavored candy to help stimulate saliva.
- Encourage good oral hygiene.

Thick, viscous saliva and mucous
- Try club soda, hot tea with lemon, or a beverage with citric acid.
- Encourage adequate fluid intake.
- Encourage good oral hygiene.

Dysgeusia (impaired taste)
- Enhance food taste with herbs, spices, flavor extracts, and marinades.
- Offer cold foods.
- Offer fruit-flavored beverages.
- Try tart foods like oranges or lemonade, which may have more taste.
- Encourage good oral hygiene.
- Offer fluids with meals to help take away a bad taste in the mouth.

Nausea and vomiting
- Try high carbohydrate foods and fluids (crackers, toast, gelatin) and nonacidic juices.
- Try small, frequent feedings.
- Offer cold, clear liquids and solids.
- Avoid overly sweet or high fat foods.
- Avoid feeding in a stuffy, too-warm room or one filled with cooking odors or other odors that might be disagreeable.
- Encourage drinking or sipping liquids frequently throughout the day; using a straw may help.
- Encourage rest periods after meals.
- Avoid offering favorite foods when nauseated; it may cause a permanent dislike of the food.

Diarrhea
- Try a low-fat, low-fiber, low-lactose diet.
- Avoid caffeine.
- Eat warm or room temperature foods because hot foods may increase bowel motility
- Encourage adequate fluids to prevent dehydration.

Constipation
- Encourage fluids.
- Drink hot liquids to increase bowel activity.
- Offer high-fiber foods.

Other helpful hints
- Take the child's sports bottle filled with a favorite beverage when going shopping or to a clinic appointment.
- If lack of appetite is a problem at mealtimes, limit snacks and fluids for 1 to 2 hours before the meal.
- Serve food "family style" to allow the child to dish out his or her own food portions.
- Serve very small servings on a large dinner plate so that portions will not look as overwhelming.
- Arrange foods creatively on plates.
- Serve brightly colored foods and different food shapes together.
- Offer new foods along with favorite foods.
- Allow the child to help prepare the food.

Reproduced from Seattle Cancer Care Alliance. Medical Nutrition Therapy Services. Seattle, Washington.[52]

TABLE 16.11 Diet Guidelines for Immunosuppressed Patients

These guidelines are intended to minimize the introduction of pathogenic organisms into the GI tract by food while maximizing healthy food options for immunosuppressed children. These guidelines should be coupled with food safety education to assume proper food preparation and storage in the home and hospital kitchen. High-risk foods, identified as potential sources of organisms known to cause infection in immunosuppressed children, are restricted.

Generally, these guidelines should be followed by children who have an absolute neutrophil count of below 1×10^3 Children receiving an autologous transplant should follow the diet for the first 3 months after HCT; children receiving an allogeneic transplant should follow the diet until off all immunosuppressive therapy (i.e., cyclosporine, tacrolimus, prednisone).

Food Restrictions

Contraindicated:

- Raw and undercooked meat (including game), fish, shellfish, poultry, eggs, sausage, and bacon
- Raw tofu, unless pasteurized or aseptically packaged
- Luncheon meats (including salami, bologna, hot dogs, ham, and others) unless heated until steaming
- Refrigerated smoked seafood typically labeled as lox, kippered, nova-style, or smoked or fish jerky (unless contained in a cooked dish); pickled fish
- Nonpasteurized milk and raw milk products, nonpasteurized cheese, and nonpasteurized yogurt
- Blue-veined cheeses, including blue, Gorgonzola, Roquefort, and Stilton
- Uncooked soft cheeses including brie, camembert, feta, and farmer's
- Mexican-style soft cheese, including queso blanco and queso fresco unless made with pasteurized milk
- Cheese containing chili peppers or other uncooked vegetables
- Fresh salad dressings (stored in the grocer's refrigerated case) containing raw eggs or contraindicated cheeses
- Unwashed raw and frozen fruits and vegetables and those with visible mold; all raw vegetable sprouts (alfalfa, mung bean, all others)
- Raw or unpasteurized honey
- Unpasteurized commercial fruit and vegetable juices

Reproduced from Seattle Cancer Care Alliance. Medical Nutrition Therapy Services. Seattle, Washington.[52]

Hospital food service and patient satisfaction: The goals of a hospital food service are to provide patients with nutritious meals that promote healing, restore any loss of weight, and improve recovery from illness.[58] This is especially important for pediatric oncology patients who are frequently admitted to the hospital for extended periods, and rely on hospital food to meet their nutrition needs. Also, important for this patient population is that the food service be flexible and accommodating to both the child and family around food choice and timing of meals. Cancer therapies often cause side-effects that make it difficult for the nutrition team to determine what food(s) the child desires or tolerates. Traditional hospital food services with set menus, tray line service, rigid meal hours, and 24-hour advance menu selection often do not meet the needs of many pediatric oncology and transplant patients.

Although very few data are available on pediatric hospital food satisfaction, many cancer centers have implemented hotel-style room service with extended hours (up to 24 hours/day), telephone ordering systems, short delivery times, and elimination of wasted trays.[58]

Allowing the child or parent to order food by telephone when they are ready to eat ensures a higher probability that the child will eat the meal when it arrives to the room, as it is aligned with their schedule and on their terms. At one facility, children's caloric intake improved significantly (>28% + change in intake) and protein intake increased by 18% after the introduction of room service. Satisfaction with hospital food also improved, with excellent ratings increasing by 35%.[58]

Feeding dynamics in young children undergoing cancer treatment: An often overlooked and unintended consequence of pediatric cancer therapy is the disruption to the relationship between parents and their children in the area of food and nutrition. Because side-effects of cancer therapy often cause nausea, vomiting, loss of appetite, and taste alterations, children lose the pleasure of eating. By nature, children look to their parents for their daily food intake, and parents instinctively assume and guard their nurturing role as the primary food provider. Frequently, neither children nor parents are prepared for the intervening influence and directives of the pediatric oncology dietitian, whose responsibilities include counseling parents and age-appropriate children in new eating habits, patterns, and food choices critical to cancer treatment. Parents can quickly sense a loss of control in their role as providers, and children can suffer from the loss of their comfort foods and mealtime rituals and routines.

The potential disruption to eating patterns and habits can be a source of stress and anxiety for the child and can lead to a family that becomes overly-focused on food. Therefore, it is essential that the pediatric oncology dietitian understand and appreciate the parent-child-food relationship and support both the parent's role and the child's need for his or her parent to continue as the food provider. While educating the parents and age-appropriate children on their essential diet and nutritional needs and the side-effects of therapy, the pediatric oncology dietitian must reinforce and support, both the parents' needs to make appropriate dietary decisions for their children, and the children's needs for security, familiarity, and routine. Respecting the feeding dynamics between parents and children is an essential component of pediatric cancer treatment.

Enteral Nutrition Support

Inadequate oral intake (NI-2.1) and limited food acceptance (NI-2.9) related to oncologic therapy as evidenced by need for EN support.

EN is now recognized as the accepted nutrition support strategy for children and adolescents undergoing cancer treatment. Benefits of EN support in the pediatric oncology population include:

- Maintenance of mucosal integrity/normal gut barrier function
- Stimulation of mucosal repair
- Decreased incidence of hyperglycemia
- Decreased incidence of infection
- Decreased cost

Children unable to meet their nutritional needs solely by oral intake will require nutrition intervention. The literature supports using EN over PN when clinically necessary.

Current practice at Seattle Children's Hospital is for nasogastric (NG) tube placement in all patients from birth to young adulthood, whose weight meets criteria for placing a feeding tube (see below), or if the child is unable to meet calorie, protein, or fluid goals for any reasons, including dysphagia, anorexia, or treatment-related side-effects.

Pediatric oncology patients who meet the following criteria may be candidates for enteral tube feedings:

- Interval or total weight loss of >5% (10% for children 9 years or older) of pre-illness body weight (usual weight)

- Weight for height reaches ≤ 90% of ideal weight for height, adjusted for height and age
- BMI falls to or below the 10th percentile
- Repeated attempts to meet nutrient needs orally have failed
- Functional GI tract
- Unintentional weight loss before diagnosis should be taken into account, as this may predispose patients to malnutrition

The guidelines above also apply to patients obese at diagnosis.

Lowest weight threshold or NG tube cut-off weight: an agreed upon weight, determined by healthcare providers and parents, below which it is unsafe for the patient to proceed with therapy without EN support.

The NG tube cut-off weight is primarily based on the following criteria:

- Birth – 6 months: no allowance for weight loss; recommend NG tube placement if no weight gain for 2 consecutive measurements
- 7–12 months: if > 100% of ideal weight/length, cut-off assessed at 5% loss from baseline/dry weight
- 1–5 years: allow for 5% loss of baseline weight (if usual weight is > ideal for height age)
- 6–8 years: allow for 8% loss of baseline weight (if usual weight > ideal for height age)
- 9 years–adulthood: allow for 10% loss from baseline weight in patients who present at diagnosis >ideal weight

Historically, cancer patients have been treated with chemotherapy, IVF, medications, and the administration of blood products through a central line. However, the central line began to serve a double purpose, since it was also used by oncologists and dietitians to administer PN to patients who could not maintain their weight through oral intake.

As EN support maintains the function and integrity of the GI tract, it has additional benefits, including reducing the risk of infection, helping reduce anxiety in patients, parents, and providers from failures to meet calorie, protein, and mineral goals via oral feeding, and providing a more cost-effective therapy than PN. For children having difficulty taking oral medications, a feeding tube provides a safe route for administration. A feeding tube may also be used for supplemental fluid administration when needs are high and the child cannot consume adequate amounts. Therefore, EN support has become the preferred method of providing the patient with safe, beneficial, and physiologic nutrition support.

Nasogastric feeding tubes are most commonly used since they can be easily placed at the child's bedside and used immediately. Successfully overcoming patient and parent resistance to NG tube placement requires a team approach with skilled and dedicated oncology dietitians, nurses, and health care providers. Child life specialists are invaluable in helping children and parents better understand and cope with the fear and discomfort of the tube placement. Thus, the health care team should present the necessity for NG tube placement to the child and family in a positive manner, explaining its effectiveness to restore a malnourished child back to normal weight and health, and/or to protect at-risk patients from nutrition deficits.

The use of EN support for the HCT population has increased in the past decade and may have a protective benefit against the development of acute GVHD and survival.[59] Children undergoing HCT may be candidates for EN support during the following conditions:[27]

- Intact and functional GI tract
- Non-myeloablative or reduced intensity conditioning regimens
- Low risk transplant (autologous or matched sibling) with long-term eating problems
- Chronic oral/esophageal GVHD with need for long-term nutrition support
- Ongoing weight loss
- Ventilation

For safe tube placement during HCT, the absolute neutrophil count should be >1,000 mm^2 and the platelet count >50,000 mm^2. A variety of nasoenteric and enterostomy feeding tubes and enteral formulas (pediatric/adult specific; semi-elemental; renal; concentrated) have been used with pediatric HCT recipients.[27] Children receiving EN support during HCT should be closely monitored since reports of tube dislodgment, delayed gastric emptying, suboptimal electrolyte and mineral intake, and inadequate energy intake, resulting in weight loss and decreased body cell mass have been reported.[27]

Parenteral Nutrition Support

Altered GI function (NI-1.4) related to high volume diarrhea due to intestinal GVHD as evidenced by need for PN support.

During cancer therapy, the child's GI tract may not be usable for oral diet or EN due to complications associated with surgery, nausea and vomiting, diarrhea, colitis, typhilitis, pneumatosis, pancreatitis, intestinal GVHD, ileus, or radiation enteritis. In these situations, PN is indicated. The decision to use PN is often based upon the child's nutritional status, type of therapy, and expected oral and GI complications associated with the chosen treatment. As multiple lumen central venous catheters are often placed at the start of treatment for delivery of medications and blood products, an access device is often available for PN and hydration fluids. Children maintained on PN support during cancer therapy must be closely monitored to ensure that nutrient

and fluid requirements are met (see Table 16.8) and that any serum electrolyte alterations or changes in glucose or lipid tolerance, especially as a result of medications, be promptly corrected.

Special Considerations
CAM and Integrative Medicine

The National Center for Complementary and Integrative Health, a center within the National Institute of Health, defines **complementary and alternative medicine** (CAM) as a group of diverse medical and health care systems, practices, and products that are not generally considered part of conventional medicine.[60] Integrated medicine is defined as relationship-centered care that focuses on the whole person, is informed by evidence, and makes use of all appropriate therapeutic approaches, healthcare professionals, and disciplines in order to achieve optimal health and healing.[60] Complementary or integrative therapies by the pediatric oncology population is reported to be increasing; however, the literature shows a wide range of use between 12%–85%.[61] Recent surveys and studies show that children use CAM treatments more readily if their parents have also used them.[62,63] Parents seek out these therapies for their children undergoing conventional cancer treatments in order to address many medical issues, including managing the symptoms and side effects caused by chemotherapy over extended periods of treatment[62] relief of pain, and enhancement of immune defenses. Parents also request CAM treatments to help their children cope with emotional effects, to improve quality of life, and to feel more hopeful.[62] Parents also frequently choose mind-body interventions, such as meditation or prayer, art or music therapy, or nonconventional therapies such as herbs, high-dose antioxidants, homeopathy, and botanicals that they believe may help soothe and comfort their children. Parents of children with relapsed cancer will more frequently use alternative therapies than those with an initial diagnosis.[64] Acupuncture and massage are the integrative therapies most frequently used and reported to help alleviate treatment side-effects, including nausea, vomiting, pain, and anxiety.[64]

While some CAM therapies may help promote healing during treatment, others may have potential harmful effects or interfere with conventional treatment. Using herbal, botanical, and megavitamin therapy to treat childhood cancer raises several concerns, including:

- Unexpected or undesirable interactions with preparations and prescribed medications, which may affect the action of drugs routinely used during the course of chemotherapy and HCT
- Potential for side effects associated with using some herbal supplements which include: nausea,

vomiting, skin irritation, sleep disturbances, diarrhea, and unpleasant taste

- Potential contamination of preparations derived from plants, which may pose the risk of bacterial, fungal, or parasitic infections; a few specific preparations have been associated with serious toxic side effects or infections
- The possibility that the alternative nutrition therapy may be chosen by a parent as the sole source of treatment

There is ongoing debate regarding the potential interaction of concurrently used dietary antioxidants with chemotherapeutic agents.[64] Those who support using antioxidants believe there is evidence that they protect healthy cells from the toxic effects of chemotherapy drugs while at the same time leaving the cancer cells exposed to the drugs. Those who argue against using antioxidants during chemotherapy are concerned that these nutrients will interfere with or reduce the efficacy of chemotherapeutic agents that use reactive oxygen species as a mechanism for cytotoxicity.[64]

Herbal and botanical preparations are derived directly from plants and may be sold as tablets, capsules, liquids, extracts, teas, powders, or topical preparations; however, the dose is dependent on the potency of the preparation.

Some herbals are contraindicated in children with cancer, as described in **TABLE 16.12**, because of their association with serious side effects; herbal preparations should be discontinued during HCT.[19] The pediatric oncology dietitian must be sensitive to the family's views and biases and educate the healthcare team appropriately.

Long-term Complications and Management

As advances in technology and supportive care measures have improved, the number of childhood cancer survivors continues to increase. Concomitant with increased survival comes the possibility of more long-term nutrition related complications. These late effects are often associated with poor health and functional status.

Chronic complications associated with cancer therapy may impact a child's nutrition status and require intervention for several years. Growth and development issues, endocrine complications (gonadal dysfunction; hypothyroidism), metabolic syndrome, neuropsychological implications, cardiac complications, bone density changes, avascular necrosis, iron overload, and dental abnormalities have been reported.[65,66]

Specific to the HCT population is the issue of chronic GVHD, which develops beyond day 80–100 post-transplant. Chronic GVHD is associated with multiple nutritional implications including weight gain

TABLE 16.12 Contraindicated Herbal Supplements During Cancer Therapy
- Alfalfa
- Botanicals containing pyrrolizidine alkaloids (borage, coltsfoot, comfrey, groundsel, valerian, mate' tea)
- Botanicals that react with drugs utilizing the cytochrome P450 enzyme system (echinacea, garlic, ginkgo, ginseng, grape seed, kava)
- Chaparral
- Chinese/oriental herbs
- DHEA
- Dieter's tea
- Ephedra
- Laetrile
- Licorice root
- Lobelia
- L-Tryptophan
- Pau D'arco
- Pennyroyal
- Sassafras
- St. John's wort
- Yohimbe
- Yohimbine

Modified from Maurs PC (ed). *Nutrition Care Criteria.* 3rd ed. Seattle, WA: Seattle Cancer Care Alliance; 2012.[19]

(due to corticosteroid therapy), weight loss, oral sensitivity to spicy or acidic foods, xerostomia, reflux symptoms, and diarrhea.

Metabolic syndrome, characterized by hyperlipidemia, insulin resistance, obesity, and hypertension, has been reported in the pediatric HCT population. Pediatric HCT survivors are more likely to develop diabetes as well as hypertension compared to the general population and should be monitored through adulthood.[67]

Adolescents and young adults: The experience of cancer among adolescents and young adults has its' own unique challenges. Because of the formative transitions that occur during these ages, (14–25 years), such as establishing independence, social circles, sexual identity, and sense of self working to understand the psychosocial benefits and burdens of this age group as they go through cancer treatment is vital to help with coping to life adaptation, both during and after cancer treatment.[68,69]

Sickle Cell Disease

Sickle cell disease (SCD) is a genetic disorder characterized by the production of abnormal hemoglobin, which causes red blood cells to become sickle shaped. Sickle-shaped red blood cells trigger inflammation, coagulation, and platelet aggregation resulting in inadequate tissue blood flow and chronic anemia. Manifestations of SCD include severe painful crises, acute chest syndrome, splenic sequestration, clinical stroke, chronic pulmonary and renal dysfunction, delayed growth, neuropsychological deficits, and premature death.[70] According to the National Institute of Health, it is estimated that between 70,000–100,000 individuals in the United States are effected by SCD, primarily African Americans.[71]

Paramount in supportive care for SCD is the prevention of pain crises. Chronic blood transfusions, pain management, antibiotics to prevent infections, and immunizations are also necessary. With this type of care, most children survive into adulthood; however, these treatments do not cure the disease. The only curative treatment for SCD is HCT.[72]

Nutrition assessment, nutrient requirements, and nutrition support practices for children with SCD do not differ from pediatric patients with other oncologic or hematologic disorders; however, children with SCD may be at risk for specific nutrient deficiencies.[73] Altered zinc, vitamin C, and vitamin E levels have been described and emphasize the need for regular monitoring and supplementation as indicated.[74] As folate deficiency has been reported in observational studies, most children with SCD require folic acid supplementation.[75] Vitamin D deficiency and suboptimal dietary calcium intake are also common and may contribute to delayed skeletal maturation with altered bone development, so supplementation may be necessary.[76,77] One study also showed that vitamin D supplementation in children with SCD was associated with decreased chronic pain.[78] Hepatic iron overload is another serious complication of SCD due to chronic transfusion therapy.[79] Treating iron overload includes chelation therapy, which may cause depletion of divalent cations such as calcium and magnesium. Delayed growth has generally been observed in children with SCD[80], however, one multi-center trial showed improved linear growth following HCT.[81] Finally, researchers are examining the promising role of glutamine as an adjunctive treatment for SCD.

Two recent double-blind studies showed decreased frequency of sickle cell crises in patients maintained on glutamine supplementation.[82,83] More research, however, is necessary before specific recommendations can be made regarding glutamine supplementation for the SCD population.

As oral intake may be compromised during acute pain crises in children with SCD, a diet emphasizing nutrient-dense foods with provision of adequate calories and protein should be emphasized. Long-term suboptimal nutrition support may impact growth and development. Maintaining an adequate hydration status is also necessary because dehydration may cause sickling of red blood cells. An iron-free multivitamin/mineral supplement is recommended for all children with SCD.

▶ Conclusion

As novel immunotherapies emerge to treat relapsed or refractory ALL and neuroblastoma, there is hope that the same T-cell immunotherapy trials open for children with these cancers will expand to treat other malignancies. However, the acute and long-term burdens of cancer therapy remain high for some children in remission and many challenges remain for those uncured when frontline treatments fail. These patients often experience malnutrition and deconditioned states from the disease progression and treatment side effects. Children with cancer experience multiple adverse oral and GI nutritional implications so dietary modifications are frequently necessary to promote an adequate intake of energy and nutrients. Specialized nutrition support may be required to ensure that nutrient needs are met for both adequate growth and development, and survival of the disease. As advances in technology and support care measures improve, the number of long-term pediatric survivors will continue to increase and with this comes the need for close nutrition monitoring as they reach adulthood. The pediatric oncology dietitian plays a vital role in providing optimum nutrition management of this highly complex population.

🔍 CASE STUDY

Patient History

Marie was a previously healthy 7-year-old female presented to her primary care physician for a well-child visit. During the appointment, it was observed that the child was pale. Parents gave a history of easy bruising, which had persisted for the past 2 months. A complete blood count with differential showed anemia, thrombocytopenia, and a white blood cell count of 65,000 thou/rcL (normal: 4500–13,500 thou/rcL). A diagnosis of acute myeloid leukemia (AML)-M4 (select

(continues)

marker) was confirmed by bone marrow biopsy. Other markers notable for central nervous system: negative disease with FLT 3 marker (poor prognostic indicator).

Marie's caregiver denied oral or gastrointestinal symptoms before her diagnosis. Her diet history included the following typical day's intake: breakfast: pancakes or cereal with 2% milk or yogurt and cheese; lunch: sandwich (ham or turkey with cheese and butter) or Caesar salad with ranch dressing or macaroni and cheese; dinner: chicken or pasta with butter (no sauce) or steak or pizza, vegetables; snacks: carrots, broccoli, bananas, apples, melon, grapes, or strawberries. She had no known food allergies. Marie was taking a pediatric multivitamin supplement.

Assessment

Age: 7 years

Gender: Female

Weight: 24.2 kg (64th%ile)

Weight for age z-score: 0.37

Height: 128.1 cm (88th%ile)

Height for age z-score: 1.16

Ideal weight for height: 26 kg (50th percentile CDC height)

BMI: 14.8 kg/m2, 31st%ile, −0.50 z-score

Estimated daily nutrient needs: 1565 calories (BMR = 979 × 1.6), 58 g protein (2.4 g/kg) and 1580 ml fluids.

During the first round of induction chemotherapy, Marie's weight decreased to a nadir of 22.2 kg, 6 days into treatment (85% of ideal weight for height). She also had symptoms of nausea, vomiting, and increased stooling.

A nasogastric (NG) enteral tube was placed for initiation of a 1 kcal/mL pediatric elemental formula; however, due to mucositis and bloody stools, she did not tolerate NG feeds well.

A computed tomography (CT) scan, confirmed typhlitis and pancolitis. Marie was placed NPO and maintained on full parenteral nutrition support (PN).

Diagnosis

Inadequate energy intake (NI-1.2) related to altered gastrointestinal (GI) function and increased energy needs as evidenced by bloody diarrhea and weight loss of > 8% of usual body weight in one week.

Intervention

1. Marie placed NPO with institution of PN support until resolution of typhlitis and pancolitis.
2. Educate Marie/caregivers on need to remain NPO, to allow gut rest for healing of current GI symptoms.

Monitoring and Evaluation

Marie to remain NPO with PN support until resolution of typhlitis and pancolitis. When symptoms have resolved, reinstitute NG feeds as tolerated and educate patient/caregivers on appropriate food/fluid choices. Work regularly with medical team (e.g., primary provider, team nurse) following her.

After placing Marie NPO for 12 days, a low-lactose, low-fiber, low-acid diet, with three to four foods per tray, was instituted. NG feeds were reinitiated, with a 1 kcal/mL pediatric elemental formula, at an infusion rate of 10 mL/hour. Feeds were slowly advanced over 1 week until a goal of 65 mL/hour × 24 hrs was achieved, at which point PN was discontinued.

Review Questions

1. Describe how immune-based therapies work to achieve remission in patients with B-cell leukemia.

2. True or False: Neuroblastoma is the most common childhood cancer diagnosed in children over 10 years of age?

3. What are two morbidities, if present during cancer treatment, pose relative risk for disease relapse or contribute to negative survival outcomes?

4. True or False: Radiation therapy is the preferred treatment in children 1–2 years of age with brain tumors?

5. What are the main associated risks to patients less than 3 years of age who require radiation therapy to the brain?

6. List 3 assessment methods, other than height and weight, that identify or define malnutrition.

7. Identify cancer populations at risk of developing diminished bone health during treatment. What are the best interventions to maintain optimal bone health?

8. What diet modifications may be necessary if a child develops gut GVHD?

9. What nutritional implications are associated with corticoid therapy for gut GVHD?

10. List components of a comprehensive nutrition assessment for a child undergoing HCT.

11. What are the long-term complications associated with HCT?

12. What are some of the micronutrient deficiencies reported in children with sickle cell disease?

References

1. Ward E, DeSantis C, Robbins A, et al. Childhood and adolescent cancer statistics, 2014. *CA Cancer J Clin.* 2014;64(2):83–103.

2. National Cancer Institute, Surveillance, Epidemiology, and End Results Program. Available at: https://seer.cancer.gov/archive/csr/1975_2013/browse_csr.php?sectionSEL=29&pageSEL=sect_29_table.01.html. Accessed November 1, 2017.

3. Smith MA, Altekruse SF, Adamson PC, et al. Declining childhood and adolescent cancer mortality. *Cancer.* 2014;120:2497–2506.

4. Ladas E, Sacks N, Meacham L, et al. A multidisciplinary review of nutrition considerations in the pediatric oncology population: a perspective from Children's Oncology Group. *Nutr Clin Pract.* 2005;20:377–393.

5. Lee DW, Gardner R, Porter, DL, et al. Current concepts in the diagnosis and management of cytokine release syndrome. *Blood.* 2014;124:188–195.

6. Maris JM. Recent advances in neuroblastoma. *N Engl J Med.* 2010;362:2202–2211.

7. Steele C, Salazar A, Rypkema L. Utilization of a nutrition support algorithm reduces unnecessary parenteral nutrition use in pediatric oncology inpatients. *J Acad Nutr Diet.* 2016;116:1235–1238.

8. Bauer J, Jurgens, H, Fruhwald MC. Important aspects of nutrition in children with cancer. *Adv Nutr.* 2011;2:67–77.

9. Orgel E, Spasto R, Malvar J, et al. Impact on survival and toxicity by duration of weight extremes during treatment for pediatric acute lymphoblastic leukemia: a report from the Children's Oncology Group. *J Clin Oncol.* 2014;32:1331–1337.

10. Rogers PCJ. Nutritional status as a prognostic indicator for pediatric malignancies. *J Clin Oncol.* 2014;32:1293–1294.

11. Creutzig U, van den Heuvel-Elbrink MM, Gibson B, et al. Diagnosis and management of acute myeloid leukemia in children and adolescents: recommendations from an international expert panel. *Blood.* 2012;120:3187–3205.

12. Gorlick R, Janeway K, Lessnick S. Review. Children's Oncology Group's 2013 blueprint for research: bone tumors. *Pediatr Blood Cancer.* 2013;60:1009–1015.

13. Malempati S, Hawkins D. Rhabdomyosarcoma: Review of the Children's Oncology Group (COG) Soft-Tissue Sarcoma Committee experience and rationale for current COG Studies. *Pediatr Blood Cancer.* 2012;59:5–10.

14. Cohen BH, Geyer JR, Miller CD, et al. Pilot study of intensive chemotherapy with peripheral hematopoietic cell support for children less than 3 years of age with malignant brain tumors, the CCG-99703 phase I/II study. A report from the Children's Oncology Group. *Pediatr Neuro.* 2015;53:31–46.

15. Pui CH, Robison LL, Look AT. Acute lymphoblastic leukemia. *Lancet.* 2008; 371:1030–1043.

16. Patrick K, Vora A. Update on biology and treatment of T-cell acute lymphoblastic leukemia. *Curr Opin Pediatr.* 2015;27:44–49.

17. Pinto NR, Applebaum MA, Volchenboum SL et al. Advances in risk classification and treatment strategies for neuroblastoma. *J Clin Oncol.* 2015;33:3008–3017.

18. The Children's Oncology Group. Guideline for the Prevention of Nausea and Vomiting due to Antineoplastic Medication in Pediatric Cancer Patients. Available at: https://childrensoncologygroup.org/downloads/COG_SC_CINV_Guideline_Document.pdf. Accessed November 17, 2017.

19. Macris PC (ed). *Nutrition Care Criteria.* 3rd ed. Seattle, WA: Seattle Cancer Care Alliance; 2012.

20. Polovich M, Whitford JM, Olsen M (eds). *Chemotherapy and Biotherapy Guidelines and Recommendations for Practice.* Pittsburgh, PA: Oncology Nursing Society;2014:27–91.

21. Landier W, Hageman L, Chen Y, et al. Mercaptopurine ingestion habits, red cell thioguanine nucleotide levels, and relapse risk in children with acute lymphoblastic leukemia: A report from the Children's Oncology Group Study AALL03N1. *J Clin Oncol.* 2017;35:1730–1736.

22. Sands S. Proton beam radiation therapy: The future may prove brighter for pediatric patients with brain tumors. *J Clin Oncol.* 2016;34:1024–1026.

23. Mizumoto M, Oshiro Y, Yamamoto T, et al. Proton beam therapy for pediatric brain tumor. *Neurologia Med.* 2017;57:1–13.

24. Macris PC, Hunt K. Hematology and oncology. In: Queen PS, King K, (eds). *Pediatric Nutrition.* 4th ed. Sudbury, MA: Jones and Bartlett Publishers, Inc; 2012:363–383.

25. Locatelli F, Giorgiani G, Di-Cesare-Merlone A, et al. The changing role of stem cell transplantation in childhood. *Bone Marrow Transplant.* 2008;41:S3–S7.

26. Gyurkocza B, Sandmeier BM. Conditioning regimens for hematopoietic cell transplantation: one size does not fit all. *Blood.* 2014;17:344–353.

27. Macris PC, McMillen K. Nutrition support of the hematopoietic cell transplant recipient. In: Forman SJ, Negrin RS, Antin JH, Appelbaum FR, (eds). Thomas' *Hematopoietic Cell Transplantation*. 5th ed. Hoboken, NJ: Wiley Blackwell; 2016:1216–1224.

28. McDonald GB. How I treat acute graft-versus-host disease of the gastrointestinal tract and the liver. *Blood.* 2016;128:1449–1457.

29. Gauvreau JM, Lenssen P, Cheney CL, et al. Nutritional management of patients with intestinal graft-versus-host disease. *J Am Diet Assoc.*1981;79:673–677.

30. Bouma S. Diagnosing pediatric malnutrition: Paradigm shifts of etiology-related definitions and appraisal of the indicators. *Nutr Clin Pract.* 2017;32:52–67.

31. Becker BJ, Carney LN, Corkins MR, et al. Concensus statement of the Academy of Nutrition and Dietetics/American Society for Parenteral and Enteral Nutrition: indicators recommended for the identification and documentation of pediatric malnutrition (undernutrition). *Nutr Clin Pract.* 2015;30:147–161.

32. Deeg HJ, Seidel K, Bruemmer B, et al. Impact of weight on non-relapse mortality after marrow transplantation. *Bone Marrow Transplant.* 1995;15:461–468.

33. White M, Murphy AJ, Hallahan A, et al. Survival in overweight and underweight children undergoing hematopoietic stem cell transplant. *Eur J Clin Nutr.* 2012;66:1120–1123.

34. Mehta NM, Corkins MR, Lyman B, et al. Defining pediatric malnutrition: A paradigm shift towards etiology-related definitions. *JPEN.* 2013;37:460–481.

35. Kuczmarski RJ, Ogden CL, Guo SS, et al. 2000 CDC growth charts for the United States: methods and development. *Vital Health Stat.* 2002;246:1–190.

36. Wiggins KL (ed). *Guidelines for Nutrition of Renal Patients.* 3rd ed. Renal Dietitians Dietetic Practice Group. Chicago IL:American Dietetic Association;2002:113.

37. Hoffmeister PA, Storer BE, Macris PC, et al. Body mass index and arm anthropometry predict outcomes after pediatric allogeneic hematopoietic cell transplantation for hematologic malignancies. *Biol Blood Marrow Transplant.* 2013;19:1081–1086.

38. Task Force for the Revision of Sale Practices for Parenteral Nutrition. Mirtallo J, Canada T, Johnson D, et al. Safe practices for parenteral nutrition. *JPEN.* 2004;28: S39–S70.

39. Carney LN, Blair J. Assessment of nutritional status and determining nutrient needs. In Corkins MR (ed). *The A.S.P.E.N. Pediatric Nutrition Support Core Curriculum.* Silver Springs, MD: American Society for Parenteral and Enteral Nutrition; 2010;409–432.

40. Institute of Medicine, Food and Nutrition Board. *Dietary Reference Intakes for Energy, Carbohydrate, Fiber, Fat, Fatty Acids, Cholesterol, Protein and Amino Acids.* Washington, DC:National Academies Press;2005.

41. National Research Council. *Recommended Dietary Allowances.* 10th ed. Washington, DC: National Academies Press;1989.

42. Hunt KL, Nowak-Cooperman K, Verbovski M, et al. Nutrition for health and disease infancy and childhood. In: Bernstein M, McMahon K (eds). *Nutrition Across Life Stages.* Burlington, MA:Jones & Bartlett Learning, LLC;2016:226–227.

43. Bechard LJ, Adiv OE, Jaksic T, et al. Nutritional supportive care. In: Pizzo PA, Poplac D, eds. *Principles and Practice of Pediatric Oncology,* 5th ed. Philadelphia, PA:Lippincott Williams & Wilkins;2006:1330–1335.

44. Wilson CL, Ness KK. Bone mineral density deficits and fractures in survivors of childhood cancer. *Curr Osteoporos Rep.* 2013;11:329–337.

45. Carpenter PA, Hoffmeister P, Chesnut CH, et al. Bisphosphonate therapy for reduced bone mineral density in children with chronic graft-versus-host disease. *Biol Blood Marrow Transplant.* 2007;13:683–690.

46. Lee JY, So, TY, Thackray J. A review on vitamin D deficiency treatment in pediatric patients. *J Pediatr Pharmacol Ther.* 2013;18:227–291.

47. Misra M, Pacaud D, Petryk A, et al.Vitamin D deficiency in children and its management: review of current knowledge and recommendations. *Pediatrics.* 2008; 122:398–417.

48. Simmons J, Sheedy C, Lee H, et al. Prevalence of 25-hydroxyvitamin D deficiency in child and adolescent patients undergoing hematopoietic cell transplantation compared to a healthy population. *Pedatr Blood Cancer.* 2013;60:2025–2030.

49. von Bahr L, Blennow O, Alm J, et al. Increased incidence of chronic GVHD and CMV disease in patients with vitamin D deficiency before allogeneic stem cell transplantation. *Bone Marrow Transplant.* 2015;50:1217–1223.

50. Lounder DT, Khandelwal P, Dandoy CE, et al. Lower levels of vitamin A are associated with increased gastrointestinal graft-versus-host disease in children. *Blood.* 2017;129:2801–2807.

51. Bays II. Clinical overview of omacor: a concentrated formulation of omega-3 polyunsaturated fatty acids. *Am J Cardiol.*2006;98:71i–76i.

52. Seattle Cancer Care Alliance. Medical Nutrition Therapy Services. Seattle, Washington.

53. Trifilio S, Helenowski I, Giel M, et al. Questioning the role of a neutropenic diet following hematopoetic stem cell transplantation. *Biol Blood Marrow Transplant.* 2012;18:1385–1390.

54. Braun LE, Chen H, Frangoul H. Significant inconsistency among pediatric oncologists in the use of the neutropenic diet. *Pediatr Blood Cancer.* 2014;61:1806–1810.

55. Fox N, Freifeld AG. The neutropenic diet reviewed: moving toward a safe food handling approach. *Oncology.* 2012;26:572–575.

56. Andermann TM, Rezvani A, Bhatt AS. Microbiota manipulation with prebiotics and probiotics in patients undergoing stem cell transplantation. *Curr Hematol Malig Rep.* 2016;11:19–28.

57. Ladas EJ, Bhatia M, Chen L, et al. The safety and feasibility of probiotics in children and adolescents undergoing hematopoietic cell transplantation. *Bone Marrow Transplant.* 2016;51:262–266.

58. Dall-Oglio I, Nicolo R, Di Ciommo V, et al. A systematic review of hospital foodservice patient satisfaction studies. *J Acad Nutr Diet.* 2015;115:567–584.

59. Seguy D, Duhamel A, Rejeb MB, et al. Better outcome of patients undergoing enteral tube feeding after myeloablative conditioning for allogeneic stem cell transplantation. *Transplantation.* 2012;94:287–294.

60. Vohra S, Surette S, Mittra D, et al. Pediatric integrative medicine: pediatrics' newest subspecialty? *BMD Pediatrics.* 2012;12:1–8.

61. Clerici CA, Veneroni L, Giancon B. Complementary and alternative medical therapies used by children with cancer treated at an Italian pediatric oncology unit. *Pediatr Blood Cancer.* 2009;44:599–604.

62. Post-White J, Fitzgerald M, Hageness S, et al. Complementary and alternative medicine use in children with cancer and general and specialty pediatrics. *J Pediatr Oncol Nursing.* 2009;26:7–15.

63. Nathanson I, Sandler E, Ramirez-Garnica G, et al. Factors influencing complementary and alternative medicine use in a multisite pediatric oncology practice. *J Pediatr Hematol Oncol.* 2007;29:705–708.

64. Langler A, Mansky PJ, Seifert G (eds). *Integrative Pediatric Oncology.* Springer: Heidelberg New York Dordrecht London;2012;5–17.

65. Chow EJ, Simmons JH, Roth CL, et al. Increased cardiometabolic traits in pediatric survivors of acute lymphoblastic leukemia treated with total body irradiation. *Biol Blood Marrow Transplant.* 2010;16:1674–1681.

66. Baker KS, Ness KK, Weisdorf D, et al. Late effects in survivors of acute leukemia treated with hematopoietic cell transplantation: a report from the Bone Marrow Transplant Survivor Study. *Leukemia.* 2010;24:2039–2047.

67. Baker KS, Ness KK, Steinberger J, et al. Diabetes, hypertension, and cardiovascular events in survivors of hematopoietic cell transplantation: a report from the bone marrow transplantation survivor study. *Blood.* 2007;109:1765–1772.

68. Eshelman D, Landier L, Sweeney T, et al. Facilitating care for childhood cancer survivors: integrating children's oncology group long-term follow-up guidelines and health links in clinical practice. *J Pediatr Oncol Nurs.* 2004;21:271–280.

69. Straehla JP, Barton KS, Yi-Frazier JP, et al. The benefits and burdens of cancer: a prospective longitudinal cohort study of adolescents and young adults. *J Palliative Med.* 2017;20:494–501.

70. National Heart, Lung, and Blood Institute. What is Sickle Cell Disease? Available at: https://www.nhlbi.nih.gov/health/health-topics/topics/sca. Accessed November 17, 2017.

71. National Heart, Lung, and Blood Institute. Expert Panel Report. Evidence Based Management of Sickle Cell Disease. Available at: https://www.nhlbi.nih.gov/guidelines. Accessed November 17, 2017.

72. Nickel RS, Kamiani NR. Ethical challenges in hematopoietic cell transplantation for sickle cell disease. *Biol Blood Marrow Transplant.* 2017; Sep 1. pii: S1083–8791(17)30689-4. doi: 10.1016/j.bbmt.2017.08.034. [Epub ahead of print].

73. Ohemeng A, Boadu I. The role of nutrition in the pathophysiology and management of sickle cell disease among children: A review of literature. *Crit Rev Food Sci Nutr.* 2017;7:1–7.

74. Wasnik RR, Akarte NR. Evaluation of serum zinc and antioxidant vitamins in adolescent homozygous sickle cell patients in Wardha, district of central India. *J Clin Diagn Res.* 2017;11:BC01–BC03.

75. Kennedy TS, Fung EB, Kawchak DA, et al. Red blood cell folate and serum vitamin B_{12} status in children with sickle cell disase. *J Pediatr Hematol Oncol.* 2001;23:165–169.

76. Buison AM, Kawchak DA, Schall J, et al. Low vitamin D status in children with sickle cell disease. *J Pediatr.* 2004;145:622–627.

77. Buison AM, Kawchak DA, Schall JI, et al. Bone area and bone mineral content deficits in children with sickle cell disease. *Pediatrics.* 2005;116:943–949.

78. Osunkwo I, Ziegler TR, Alvarez J. High dose vitamin D therapy for chronic pain in children and adolescents with sickle cell disease: results of a randomized double blind pilot study. *Br J Haematol.* 2012;159:211–215.

79. Brown K, Subramony C, May W, et al. Hepatic iron overload in children with sickle cell anemia on chronic transfusion therapy. *J Pediatr Hematol Oncol.* 2009;31:309–312.

80. Lukusa Kazadi A, Ngiyulu RM, Gini-Ehungu JL, et al. Factors associated with growth retardation in children suffering from sickle cell anemia: first report from Central Africa. *Anemia.* 2017;7916348.

81. Eggleston B, Patience M, Edwards S, et al. Effect of myeloablative bone marrow transplantation on the growth in children with sickle cell anaemia: results of the multicenter study of haematopoietic cell transplantation for sickle cell anaemia. *Br J Haematol.* 2007;136:673–676.

82. Niihara Y, Macan H, Eckman JR, et. Al. L-glutamine therapy reduces hospitalization for sickle cell anemia and sickle B-thalassemia patients at six month-a phase II randomized trial. *Clin Pharmacol Biopham.* 2014;3:1–5.

83. Emmaus Medical. *Oral L-Glutamine Powder for the Treatment of Sickle Cell Disease.* Torrance, CA: Emmaus Medical: 2017. Sponsors briefing document NDA 208587.

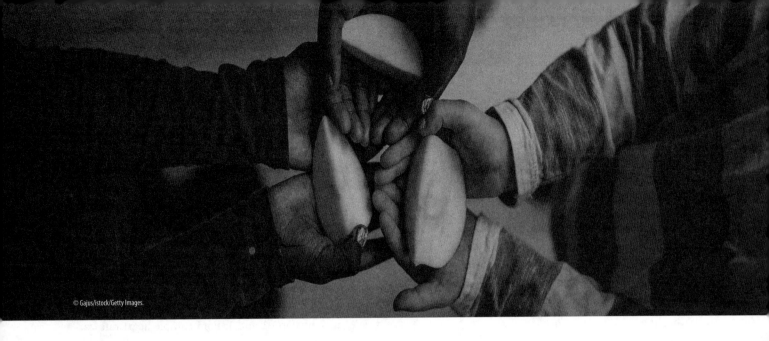

© Gajus/istock/Getty Images.

CHAPTER 17

Pediatric Surgical Nutrition: Principles and Techniques

Robin C. Cook and Thane Blinman

LEARNING OBJECTIVES

- Understand the role of nutrition in infants and children with congenital surgical anomalies.
- Discuss the calorie and protein needs of the pediatric surgical patient.
- Recognize potential causes of retching in the pediatric patient following fundoplication.
- Identify nutritional additives that may benefit a pediatric surgical patient.

▶ Introduction

Often relegated to afterthought, nutritional support nevertheless speeds healing and supports recovery after surgery. It is not too strong a statement to say that, after meticulous operative technique, no intervention does more for a good surgical outcome than providing the right form, amount, and composition of "substrate delivery" to the patient recovering from surgical intervention. Success here is enhanced whenever the clinician grasps the peculiar structural alterations of common pediatric surgical problems (and their surgical remedies), and the physiological constraints imposed by those mechanical changes. These limits are further delimited by the non-linearities of physiological scaling.

These and other factors must inform successful nutritional support of the pediatric surgical patient. However, in typical medical training, scant attention is paid to scaling, protein composition, osmolarity, and mechanical limits from altered anatomy, fat metabolism, etc. As a result, practitioners often fall back on imitative (but uninformed) heuristics ("I guess tube feeds should equal maintenance fluids"), or avoid the problem altogether ("He might eat in a day or two," "I'm going off service tomorrow and don't want to rock the boat," and so on). The first response can

423

transform a good surgical intervention into a bad result, and the second produces starvation and diminished surgical results.

But it doesn't have to be this way. This chapter briefly outlines principles for nutritional support of the pediatric surgical patient. Good principles drive out bad heuristics, and handy tricks yield definitive action steps. Underlying all discussion are limits imposed by scaling, motility, absorptive surface, gut perfusion, and other mechanical constraints. The end result is intended to be a collection of nutritional "whats," each paired with a surgical or physiological "why." As with oxygen delivery, substrate delivery for the surgical child need not be a guessing game but can consist of a series of targeted interventions designed to support healthy growth and faster healing.

▶ An Introduction to Physiological Scaling

Pediatric patients range in body mass from 100s of grams to over 100 kilograms, a range of nearly 3 orders of magnitude. Over this range, there are huge, usually nonlinear differences in physiological parameters such as energy expenditure, heart rate, respiratory rate, lung volume, gastric volume, cardiac output, CO_2 production, intestinal surface area, etc. Most practitioners have a fuzzy conception of how physiology changes as body size changes, but there is a single equation that captures most of this variability:

$$Y(m) \cong (A \cdot m^b) \cdot \varepsilon$$

This equation says that any physiological function $Y(m)$ that varies by mass m can be approximated by a scaling factor A multiplied by mass raised to a scaling exponent b, all multiplied by an error term ε. The general name for this type of equation is a power law, and physiological scaling is sometimes referred to as power-law scaling. Let's see how it works.

For now, ignore the scaling factor A. First consider the mathematically trivial case for the scaling equation and its exponent, the case in which $b = 0$. In this case, there is no variation in the physiological parameter. Examples include erythrocyte size, skeletal muscle cross sectional tension, and (curiously), time required to empty the bladder. Baby red blood cells are the same size as adult red blood cells; baby enterocytes have similar microvilli length as adults, and so on. A graph of this equation would just be a horizontal line when plotted against body mass.

Next, consider the case where $b = 1$. In this case, the physiological function $Y(m)$ scales linearly as body mass increases. Some examples of this include total blood volume

(around 85 ml/kg), gastric capacity (around 22 ml/kg), and pulmonary tidal volume (around 7.8 ml/kg/breath for mammals). The error term E captures unusual circumstances of clinical context. For example, pregnant women have a blood volume expanded by around 20% (or an E value of about 1.2), even considering the added mass of pregnancy. Essentially, one can imagine E shifting the curve up or down on the vertical axis, based on local context. For example, energy expenditure can be shifted upward with fever according to predictable amounts. Implicitly, most people imagine all physiology scales in a linear way, but instead these examples are exceptions.

Most physiological functions scale non-linearly with body mass. In this case, b will be some positive or negative value between −1 and 1. For example heart rate varies according to:

$$HR(m) \cong 160 \cdot m^{-1/4}$$

This gives a curve as seen in **FIGURE 17.1**. This type of curve is sometimes called an inverse power law. Physiologically, it means that in humans, heart rate rises disproportionately with body mass. A similar effect can be seen with energy expenditure (**FIGURE 17.2**). This shows that as humans get larger they require more energy overall, but this energy demand is decelerating as mass increases. This relationship between mass and energy expenditure is seen more prominently when energy expenditure is plotted on a per kg basis, which gives us the inverse power law again (**FIGURE 17.3**).

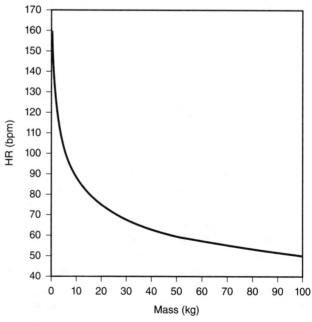

FIGURE 17.1 Physiological Scaling of Heartrate

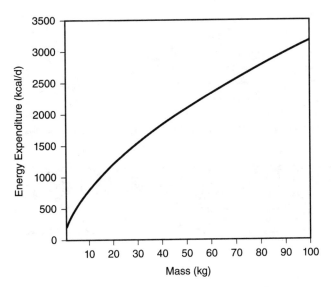

FIGURE 17.2 Physiological Scaling Energy Expenditure (Kcal/day)

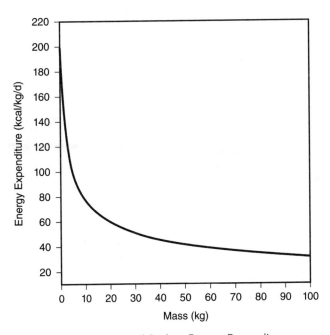

FIGURE 17.3 Physiological Scaling Energy Expenditure (Kcal/kg)

This shows that small children are "little furnaces of metabolic fire," at least on a per-kg basis. The implications of this nonlinearity are enormous for nutritional management. For example, the combination of linear scaling of the stomach and nonlinear scaling of energy expenditure explains why human infants need to eat 8 times/day. If this was scaled (incorrectly!) to the adult circumstance, the milk intake of an infant would be like an adult having to drink 3–4 gallons of whole milk every day! Many constraints on feeding small children (especially those who have their energy requirements scaled upward by heart disease, increased work of breathing, or other stressors) are explained by these scaling relationships.

In pediatric practice, nothing makes sense physiologically without considering these relationships based on *mass* (not age, height, or other variables). Traditionally, allopathic medicine has tried to handle scaling relationships with regression equations (e.g. energy equations), body surface area (e.g. some pharmacological dosing), or look-up tables based on age ranges (like the descriptions of vital signs seen in most texts). But all of these methods have been shown to be imprecise, based on faulty models of physiology, or both.

► Estimating Nutrition Needs

Calories

Providing adequate calories is the first step in providing adequate nutrition support. In children, energy is partitioned between resting metabolism, thermoregulation, muscular activity, and growth. Though surgery has been shown to increase energy expenditure in adults, this same effect has not been evidenced in children, suggesting that energy normally utilized for growth may be initially diverted to tissue repair.[1,2]

Resting Energy Expenditure (REE) can be estimated by using predictive equations, including World Health Organization and Schofield though multiple studies have demonstrated the inaccuracy of predictive equations to estimate energy needs in pediatric surgical patients, especially those who are critically ill, which can lead to unintentional overfeeding and underfeeding.[3–6] While indirect calorimetry remains the gold standard, it is often unavailable or not feasible in many institutions. Moreover, indirect calorimetry as typically used doesn't return energy expenditure, but REE, a metabolic rate artificially suppressed by fasting and sedation. This value is not particularly useful at real bedsides.

Generally, we follow a strategy of weight based calorie estimation using the allometric energy estimate (AE)[7] plus repeated measures of weight and laboratory values in an iterated "calculate-intervene-measure" strategy (see **FIGURE 17.4**). That is, we start with a calculated energy estimate using the power-law based equation below, and then adjust interventions based on serial measures of outcome parameters (especially rate of weight gain). The AE allows for a quick bedside estimate of calorie needs based on body weight alone, and generally produces a surprisingly accurate "first guess":

Allometric Energy Estimate (AE) — $AE = 200 \times M^{-0.4}$

where M is body mass in kilograms (kg) and AE is allometric energy (kcals/kg/day). Though this equation does not account for extremes of age (prematurity, elderly), body habitus (obesity, malnutrition), or clinical condition (fevers, sedations, paralytics), it acts as a good first approximation and can be adjusted based on the clinical context of the patient. For example, patients with congenital anomalies leading to pulmonary hypoplasia, including congenital diaphragmatic hernia (CDH) and giant omphalocele (GO) generally require 110–120% of calculated AE while those surgical patients requiring ventilator support and sedation may require 80–90% of the calculated AE. **TABLE 17.1** can be used as a guide for applying stress factors for various surgical scenarios utilizing both the AE and REE.

TABLE 17.1 Stress Factors for Various Surgical Scenarios Utilizing Both the AE and REE

Description	Stress Factors	
Intubated/Sedated/Use of Paralytic	REE × <1.0	AE × 0.8
Intubated/Sedated Trauma Intubated/Sedated ARDS ECMO Chronic Respiratory Failure with Tracheostomy/Ventilator	REE × 1.1−1.3	AE × 0.9
Gastroschisis Hirschsprung Disease TEF/EA Intubated/Sedated Trauma with Pulmonary Injury Extensive Wounds Sepsis	REE × 1.3−1.5	AE × 1.0
Trauma Open Abdomen Malnutrition CDH GO SBS	REE × 1.5−1.7+	AE × 1.1−1.2+

REE = Resting Energy Expenditure, AE = Allometric Equation, ARDS = Acute Respiratory Distress Syndrome, ECMO = Extracorporeal Membrane Oxygenation, TEF = Tracheoesophageal Fistula, EA = Esophageal Atresia, CDH = Congenital Diaphragmatic Hernia, GO = Giant Omphalocele, SBS = Short Bowel Syndrome

FIGURE 17.4 Allometric Energy Estimate (AE) – a Method of Calculating Energy Requirements

Protein

Humans have stores of fat and carbohydrate, but not of protein; there is no protein reserve. Instead, amino acids required for protein synthesis must be supplied by diet, generated de novo (except essential amino acids), or recruited from existing, functioning proteins. Proteins undergo a constant state of degradation and resynthesis known as protein turnover. Protein turnover is higher in newborns (6 g/kg/day) compared with adults (3.5 g/kg/day)[8] with this high rate serving to increase the pool of amino acids available for energy and other functions. In order to allow for the synthesis of acutely needed enzymes, serum proteins, and glucose, protein turnover produces a net redistribution of amino acids away from skeletal muscle to the wound, acute phase reactants, and the liver. This protein flux is even higher following trauma (remember that surgery itself is considered trauma), which likely translates to maximal adaptability.

In patients suffering from **traumatic brain injury** (TBI), protein catabolism appears to peak 8–14 days after injury[9] while children undergoing thoracic surgery with a mean surgical time of 3.7 hours demonstrated a higher rate of protein breakdown than protein synthesis post-operatively resulting in a net negative protein balance.[10] Providing adequate protein aims to shorten recovery time but it remains difficult, especially in the critically ill patient, in order to achieve adequate delivery.

A study of 519 pediatric surgical patients by Velazco et al[11] found that protein and energy delivery by EN alone and by EN supplemented by PN were all significantly less in the surgical cohort compared with the medical cohort with only 15% of the surgical cohort receiving 60% of their protein goal by day seven compared with 60% of the medical cohort.

In the 2017 publication, *Guidelines for the Provision and Assessment of Nutrition Support Therapy in the Pediatric Critically Ill Patient*, the authors recommend providing a minimum of 1.5 g/kg/day of protein.[12] Note that this value meets or exceeds the Dietary Reference Intake for all age groups. Research in pediatric surgical patients has demonstrated that 15–20% of total calories from protein, or 2–3 g/kg/d for infants less than 2 years of age, 1.5–2 g/kg/d for children ages 2–13 years, and 1.5 g/kg/d for adolescents, supports resistance to infection, replenish preexisting or injury-driven depletion, and maintain muscle mass.[13,14]

Though it is well known that the same intervention within medical and surgical *adult* patients tends to yield vastly different results, there is not yet a differentiation between interventions for medical and surgical pediatric patients within the *Guidelines for the Provision and Assessment of Nutrition Support Therapy in the Pediatric Critically Ill Patient* due to the paucity of research in critically ill children. In the *Guidelines for the Provision and Assessment of Nutrition Therapy in the Adult Critically Ill Patient*, protein recommendations are 1.2–2 g/kg/day in the traumatically injured and post-operative patients with needs likely at the higher end of the provision range and 1.5–2.5 g/kg/day in the patient with traumatic brain injury.[15] There are certain clinical situations where protein needs will exceed the recommendations above. For instance, patients with an open abdomen will require an additional 15–30 g protein per liter of exudate.[15]

Fluid

Traditional estimates of fluid relied on the Holliday Segar method (e.g. 100 mL/kg for 1–10 kg + 50 mL/kg for 11–20 kg + 20 mL/kg for >20 kg).[16] Clinicians intuitively know that in patients ≤10 kg, the Holliday Segar method dramatically underestimates fluid requirements. This is evidenced by **total fluid limits (TFL)** that are regularly set to 120–150 mL/kg/day in the **Neonatal Intensive Care Unit** (NICU). Few remember that Holliday and Segar based their fluid estimate on the premise that ml/day equaled kcal/day. That is, the fluid estimator was really an energy estimator. They also recognized that energy (and in their reckoning, fluid) needs varied nonlinearly by mass. Rather than give a single equation that modeled this nonlinear relationship, they approximated it with three integrated linear relations, producing the 4-2-1 rule used heuristically today.

Holliday and Segar's rule misses the mark however in very small patients, less than 10 kg. Instead, much like energy, fluid can also be calculated using an allometric estimate:

$$F = 300 \times M^{-0.5}$$

where M is mass in kg and F is fluid in mL/kg/day. This equation closely matches the well-known Holliday-Segar rule, but corrects the underestimate in small patients. Note that the two allometric equations (for energy and for fluid needs) shown in this chapter have not been validated for babies less than 2 kg in body mass.

▶ Useful Tips and Methods

Know Your Protein Source

It is well known that human milk has a faster gastric emptying time than formula, but the composition of the formula, including protein source and osmolarity, contributes to gastric emptying. Numerous studies have found more rapid gastric emptying in formulas containing whey compared with casein.[17-20] Upon reaching the acidic environment of the stomach, whey remains in a liquid state while casein curdles. This coagulation slows the digestion of amino acids and the subsequent gastric emptying of casein. When human milk is unavailable or requires fortification to greater than 20 kcals/oz, we recommend using whey-based formulas.

These differences in protein handling by the human become important in a number of surgical conditions. For example, **gastroesophageal reflux disease** (GERD) is a common problem in infants and children with a number of congenital surgical anomalies.[21,22] For example, in tracheoesophageal fistula/esophageal atresia (TEF/EA), around 85% of patients suffer from esophageal dysmotility at one year of age, and GERD is widespread.[23] **Giant omphalocele** (GO) is a midline defect of the ventral abdominal wall wherein the abdominal organs herniate outside the abdominal wall while remaining encased in a membranous sac. By nature of the defect, all patients with GO have malrotation, which can delay gastric emptying and slow bowel transit. Worse, because of increased intra-abdominal pressure, increased work of breathing, and elevated calorie needs, GERD is common in these patients.[22] GERD also plagues gastroschisis (which carries elevated probabilities of both dysmotility and hiatal hernia), congenital diaphragmatic hernia (which carries risk of poor gastric emptying, increased kcal needs, and disrupted lower esophageal sphincter integrity), and other pediatric surgical conditions. For all these conditions, utilizing a protein source which improves gastric emptying may reduce manifestations of GERD, improve tolerance, and aid growth. Moreover, careful feeding strategies that aim to improve (or at least not impede) gastric emptying may even forestall other invasive interventions such as fundoplication or distal feeding tubes, both of which carry a panoply of added risks. In contrast, a clumsy feeding strategy can lead to a spiral of interventions and complications from malnutrition to gas bloat to blood sugar instability. Protein source is important, but not the only factor the clinician can manipulate.

Control the Osmolarity

Few practitioners attend to osmolar effects of formula, but reducing the osmolarity of the formula is one of the surest ways to promote a successful feeding regimen. Hyperosmolar solutions not only delay gastric emptying but also increase gastric irritation.[24,25] Through both intrinsic autonomic nerves and the enteric neurons, chemoreceptors in the duodenum trigger inhibition of gastric emptying through a direct effect on the stomach.[21,25] The delayed emptying causes discomfort, distension, retching, reflux, and emesis, all of which are usually lumped under the fuzzy moniker of "feeding intolerance."

Generally, elemental formulas tend to have higher osmolarity than those with an intact protein source. Remember that a change in the standard concentration of a product will affect the overall osmolarity although the net change will differ based on the formula's composition. For example, when Good Start® Soothe (a 100% partially hydrolyzed whey protein infant formula with 70% maltodextrin and 30% lactose by Nestlé, Vevey Switzerland) is concentrated from 20 kcal/oz to 24 kcal/oz, the osmolarity changes from 195 mOsm/L to ~234 mOsm/L while the same increase in concentration of Alfamino® Infant (an amino acid based infant formula by Nestlé, Vevey Switzerland) will increase the osmolarity from 330 mOsm/L to 396 mOsm/L. Compare these values to the osmolarity of breast milk or serum at around 290 mOsm/L (**FIGURE 17.5**). Keeping osmolarity in check is not only the goal for children with congenital anomalies which increase the prevalence of GERD but is essential in those who have undergone fundoplication, or surgical treatment of GERD. In a retrospective review, we found that the most frequent cause of retching after fundoplication was high osmolarity of feeds.[21] By the same mechanism discussed

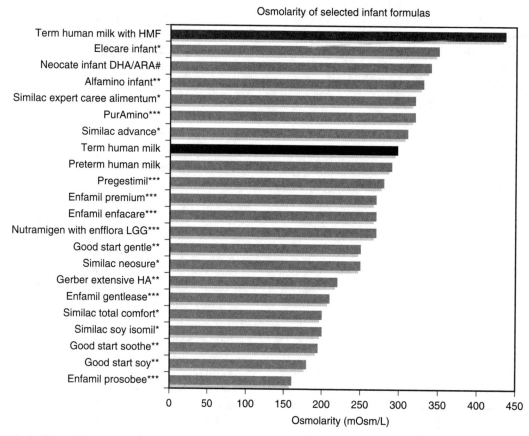

FIGURE 17.5 Osmolarity of Selected Infant Formulas

Data from *Abbott Nutrition, referenced on January 28, 2018 https://abbottnutrition.com;
**Gerber, referenced on January 28, 2018 https://www.gerber.com/products/formula;
**Nestle Nutrition Health Science, referenced on January 28, 2018, https://www.nestlehealthscience.com/;
***Mead Johnson, referenced on January 28, 2018, http://www.meadjohnson.com/pediatrics/us-en/product-information/products;
#Nutricia North America, referenced on January 28, 2018, http://www.nutricia.com;
Kreissl A, Zwiauer V, Repa A, et al. Effect of fortifiers and additional protein on the osmolarity of human milk: is it still safe for the premature infant? *J Pediatr Gastroenterol Nutr.* 2013;57(4):432–437.[26]

above, osmolarity of medications can also negatively influence gastric emptying and accounted for 14% of retching at initial presentation. As a result, one helpful strategy is to "divide-decrease-dilute-discontinue" medications whenever possible.

Helpful Additives

Sodium

Enteral sodium is another often overlooked topic, but in surgical patients with ostomies, attention to enteral sodium intake divides good growth from static growth. This effect seems to be conveyed via two mechanisms. First, repletion of enteral chloride losses appears to be essential to growth. Although the physiological reason is not clear, infants and small children simply will not grow without chloride repletion, regardless of the calories delivered. At the same time, a threshold of enteral sodium content is needed to allow function of sodium-glucose cotransporters in the gut to drive efficient glucose absorption by the small bowel mucosa.

In the pediatric surgical population, ostomies may be found in a variety of patients, including those with surgical NEC, imperforate anus, following traumatic injury to the bowel (such as gunshot wound), and in **Hirschsprung's Disease** (HD). Total body sodium depletion can lead to poor growth in infants and children with ostomies.[27-29] A study by O'Neil et al documented four cases of total body sodium depletion (as determined by urine sodium <10 mmol/L), which led to unintentional weight loss despite adequate caloric provision.[27] Weight gain resumed and urine sodium levels rose above 10 mmol/L with sodium supplementation of 5–10 mEq/kg/day. Sodium requirements are multifactorial but may be particularly dependent on the volume of ostomy output and the location of the stoma (that is, how proximal it is). Because sodium absorption occurs predominantly in the colon, children with small bowel ostomies and proximal colostomies are at the greatest risk.

The recommendation above aligns closely to those of both Bower et al and Sacher et al. Bower et al found that sodium intakes of 4–8 mEq/kg/day were associated with resumption of normal weight gain in seven infants who had an ileostomy as a result of necrotizing enterocolitis or meconium ileus[28] while Sacher et al determined that sodium requirements in infants with an ileostomy may be as high as 6–10 mEq/kg/day.[29] In both studies, it was noted that volume of ostomy output was directly related to the amount of sodium supplementation required.

Occasionally, practitioners fear adding sodium to feeds, believing it will contribute to edematous states, fluid retention, or hypernatremia. This fear is generally unfounded. The amount of supplementation is actually quite low and monitoring urine sodium (to keep levels just over 30 mmol/L) and utilizing a sodium chloride solution prepared by a pharmacy rather than addition of table salt can easily avoid oversupply of sodium.

Long Chain Triglycerides (LCT)

Enteral supplementation of LCTs may confer numerous advantages to the pediatric surgical patient, especially those with osmotic sensitivity (e.g. post-fundoplication), reduced mucosal surface area (e.g. after intestinal resection), or volume restrictions (e.g. some cardiac patients). LCT supplementation has not only been shown to activate the "ileal brake" to slow motility in the small bowel but also increases calories without increasing osmolarity. The ileal brake works to slow small bowel transit through the activation of a distal to proximal intestino-intestinal feedback loop activated by the presence of nutrients in the distal small bowel.[30] In a study by Malcolm et al,[31] ten infants with temporary enterostomies were supplemented with 1mL of a commercially prepared LCT solution to every 50 mL of formula. A 32% decrease in ostomy output was observed despite an increase in the volume of enteral nutrition delivery. The result was predominantly attributed to the ileal brake.

Another potential benefit of LCT supplementation is an increase in calories without increasing respiratory quotient. High CO_2 levels have been shown to increase pulmonary hypertension, exacerbate acidosis, and increase work of breathing thereby decreasing ability to wean the ventilator.

LCT supplementation offers benefits to patients after fundoplication as well. Following ingestion of a meal, the proximal stomach possesses the ability to distend with little change in intragastric pressure which enables the ingestion of a meal without post-prandial discomfort.[21] Fundoplication causes a decrease in gastric accommodation. Barbera et al[32] found that infusion of LCT induced a rapid and sustained relaxation of the stomach through the stimulation of **cholecystokinin** (CCK). Supplementation of LCT following fundoplasty may improve gastric accommodation and as a result of the ileal brake phenomena may improve symptoms of early dumping syndrome.

Pectin

Soluble fiber supplements, such as pectin, have a number of beneficial effects including prolongation of gastrointestinal transit time, improving fluid absorption, and enhancing energy assimilation through the production of **short chain fatty acids** (SCFA) in the colon. Chief among these SCFAs is butyrate, which may contribute 5–15% of total energy absorbed in normal individuals and substantially more in those with short bowel syndrome (SBS).[33] Butyrate upregulates one of the sodium-hydrogen exchangers enhancing water and sodium absorption in the colon.[34] Importantly, concentrations greater than 3% (that is, adding more than 3 mL of liquid pectin to each 100 mL of formula) can worsen diarrhea as the osmotic load outweighs the water absorptive effect across the sodium hydrogen exchangers. Because the increase in sodium-hydrogen exchangers occurs on a molecular level, it may take 58–72 hours to see the improvement in fluid absorption.[35] Pectin is very good for the colon but more is not better.

Immunonutrition

Immunonutrition can be defined as using specific nutritional elements in an attempt to modulate the immune system in a way that benefits a certain injury or disease state. It is well studied in the *adult* surgical and trauma population with the most recent guidelines recommending the routine usage of immune-enhancing formulas containing arginine and ω-3 fatty acids in patients with severe trauma, traumatic brain injury and during the post-operative period in the surgical intensive care unit.[15] ω-3 fatty acids may improve oxygenation and compliance, decrease duration of ventilation, and protect the lungs from systemic inflammation.[9] Traumatic injury and major surgery lead to an increase in production of arginase, causing a relative arginine deficiency, which can adversely affect T-cell function causing immune suppression.[15] Arginase is eventually converted to ornithine to aid in wound healing.[36]

Though there are limited studies in children, one conducted by Briassoulis et al[37] found that delivery of an immune-enhancing formula (compared with standard formula) to children with severe head injury led to an improvement in nitrogen balance, lower interleukin-8 levels, and less positive gastric cultures. There was no difference in nosocomial infections, length of stay, length of mechanical ventilation, and survival.

Similar interest is given to other potential immune modulators. For example, in adults, very high doses of vitamin C, selenium, and vitamin E are reported to attenuate traumatic brain injury. Similarly, enteric supplementation with N-acetylcysteine (a potent inhibitor of the Nuclear Factor kB (NFkB) inflammatory pathway) and other additives have garnered interest. But as of this writing, none of these supplements carries strong evidence of beneficial effect. Omega 3 fatty acids and other additives may be found in pediatric formulas, but their doses and real effects remain to be delineated. Currently use of immunonutrition is not recommended in pediatric patients.

▶ Peculiar Surgical Constraints

Volume Limits and Advancements
Gastric Capacity

Gastric capacity should be a determinant of appropriate feeding regimens and becomes particularly important in infants and children who suffer from altered gastrointestinal manifestations as a result of surgery. Strangely, no one really knows how big the human stomach is. However, we can tell some things empirically. First, like pulmonary tidal volume, bladder capacity, and total blood volume, gastric capacity appears to scale roughly linearly with body mass. Second, few authors have attempted to measure gastric volume (essentially the volume to discomfort, not the volume to failure) and the consensus measure is roughly 18–21 ml/kg. For example, Perrella et al[38] utilized ultrasound images to calculate gastric volume in infants, finding that post-feed volume had a strong positive correlation with delivered volumes of 18–21 mL/kg.

This value does not withstand perturbations to the stomach. For example, patients who have been fed for weeks or months via jejunal tubes seem to have smaller stomachs. Similarly, some surgical conditions in which there is fetal obstruction of the esophagus (e.g. pure esophageal atresia, cervical teratoma, etc.) can result in microgastria. But even fundoplication makes a functionally smaller stomach. We found that large bolus volumes between 20–27 mL/kg following fundoplasty caused retching in 28% of patients studied which had led us to recommend limiting bolus feeds to 15 mL/kg/day (and heuristically, overnight feeds to 8 mL/kg/hr) following fundoplication.[21] Anecdotally, using these small volumes has improved tolerance in those babies with congenital anomalies such as CDH, GO, and TEF/EA who suffer from GERD even without fundoplication. On the reverse side, the stomach may "act" larger in children who eat by mouth (compared with those receiving gastric tube feeds) because the accommodation reflex relaxes the stomach somewhat.

How Do You Advance?

Traditionally following surgery, the presence of bowel sounds and passage of stool or flatus is the clinical evidence for restoration of bowel function and initiation of nutrition, either oral or enteral. Studies have demonstrated that small bowel motility resumes within hours of operation followed by gastric and colonic function within 24 hours and 48–72 hours.[39] Early enteral nutrition not only maintains the intestinal mucosal barrier, improves blood flow, and decreases infectious complications but it may also have some direct anti-inflammatory effects on enterocytes.[39] Early enteral feeding following colostomy closure in children was shown to stimulate earlier passage of stool while decreasing hospital length of stay without any adverse complications[40] while early oral feeding (before the traditional markers of bowel function) in patients undergoing either elective or emergency surgery with anastomosis distal to the Ligament of Treitz without contamination was to be both safe and decrease hospital length of stay.[41] Multiple studies following gastrostomy placement have correlated early initiation of feeds with decreased hospital length of stay with no increased complications.[42,43]

Little has been published on post-operative feeding advancements in children. Implementation of a standardized feeding protocol in infants who underwent abdominal surgery for **necrotizing enterocolitis** (NEC), intestinal atresia, neonatal bowel obstruction, or gastroschisis which utilized weight at the time of initiation of feeds as well as calculating and categorizing the percentage of remaining small bowel in continuity with the colon was found to be both feasible and safe though it did not improve the time to achieve full enteral feeds nor length of stay or parenteral nutrition days.[44]

But the question remains, How to advance? The evidence is paltry, leaving clinicians to resort to heuristics and caution. Generally, a prudent strategy is: start early, go slow at first, accelerate, but then be careful when close to goal. Signs of advancing too fast include: distention, cramps, loose stools (water loss), sugar in the stools (positive reducing substances), or trace blood. Feeding imposes work on the gut, and the gut may require time for adaptation, allowing mucosal mass development and adequate oxygen delivery to the gut before the workload can be imposed. This is the root of the slow advance, especially in babies. Physiological scaling shows us that the smaller the child, the greater the workload imposed by full feeds on the gut. This workload becomes relatively even larger in any condition in which oxygen delivery to the gut is impaired, e.g. the pulmonary hypertension of CDH, the reduced systemic oxygenation of babies with single cardiac ventricles, or the poor vasculature of type 3b intestinal atresia. In any condition where the gut oxygen delivery may be restricted, extremely slow advances of feeds (and therefore of intestinal work) may be needed. By the same token, reckless advances or aggressive fortification of feedings can produce intolerance, necrotizing enterocolitis, and death.

Overgrowth

A number of surgical conditions produce circumstances in which it appears that the bowel becomes "overgrown" by bacteria. In particular, overgrowth is promoted by decreased motility and areas of stasis, alteration of the bacterial counts and content, and degradation of the mucosal immune barrier. So a classic patient exhibiting overgrowth might be a patient with gastroschisis (decreased motility) who had some bowel loss and compensatory gut dilatation (stasis), who was on chronic proton-pump inhibitors and had exposure to broad spectrum antibiotics (altered bacterial content) and extended time on parenteral rather than enteral nutrition (reduced mucosal barrier capability). Patients like this seem to become distended with even low volume feeds, have loose stools or sometimes constipation, and in extreme cases may even exhibit altered mental status from production of d-lactic acid by unfriendly bacteria.

Overgrowth, sometimes called "**small intestinal bacterial overgrowth**" (SIBO) is difficult to diagnose, and tricky to treat. While endoscopic sampling of enteric contents, radiolabeled hydrogen breath tests, and blood tests for d-lactate are available, none are easy or definitive, leaving SIBO often an empirical diagnosis. Mainstays of treatment include antibiotics (metronidazole, neomycin, etc.), reducing or eliminating acid blockade in the stomach, using formulas without fiber, and even surgical intervention to remove strictures or dilated areas of intestine. While no single intervention is guaranteed to work, occasionally remarkable improvement is exhibited. Regardless of intervention, no progress can be made if the diagnosis is not suspected, and clinicians should consider SIBO on any patient with the "setup" conditions described above.

▶ Conclusion

Surgical nutrition need not be ad hoc. Applying just a few principles in specific contexts can mean the difference between a surgical success and child who has been "broken" by clumsy intervention. Some principles to remember include:

- Nothing makes sense in pediatrics unless viewed through the lens of physiological scaling. The clinician must account for nonlinear and linear variations in parameters based on body mass in order to correctly calculate caloric needs, feeding volumes, and growth targets.
- Treat the gut gently. Absorption costs energy, and surgical patients commonly exist in states of diminished intestinal oxygen delivery. The gut can adapt, but it takes time to adapt.
- Mechanical constraints limit volumes that the gut can handle.
- The chemical composition of enteric feeds radically changes how the gut responds. Osmolarity, protein source, water content, and long-chain triglycerides profoundly change gut physiology, and these effects are magnified in patients with ostomies, fundoplications, and intestinal losses.
- Additives can divide success and failure. Chief among these is NaCl, but pectin, omega-3 fatty acids, and other additives (like selective antibiotics) support nutrition.

🔍 CASE STUDY

Two month old FT female with prenatally diagnosed left CDH, pulmonary hypertension, s/p patch repair of L CDH, GERD, s/p Ladd's, Toupet fundoplication, and gastrostomy tube (POD #1). Infant with no evidence of malnutrition and an admission weight of 4 kg. Before surgery, infant was receiving Similac Advance 24 kcal/oz at 29 mL/hr × 24 hrs via nasojejunal tube. Medications include, furosemide, chlorothiazide, spironolactone, KCl, NaCl, sildenafil, bosentan, ranitidine, bethanechol, and multivitamin.

Case Study Questions

1. Calculate the infant's nutrition needs using the parameters discussed in the chapter.
2. What is the most appropriate formula for this infant following surgery?
3. Design a feeding regimen that takes into account gastric mechanics following fundoplication.

Review Questions

1. What are the allometric calorie and fluid needs for a 6 kg infant with TEF/EA following Nissen fundoplication with gastrostomy?

2. A 3-year-old, 12 kg female is admitted to the PICU with gunshot wound (GSW) to the abdomen. She underwent damage control laparotomy with abdominal packing and placement of temporary abdominal closure. The wound VAC is putting out an average of 600 mL/day. How much additional protein will this patient require?

3. What facets of GO contribute to a propensity for GERD?

4. Based on studies discussed above, what is the sodium requirement of an infant with an ileostomy due to total colonic Hirschsprung's Disease?

5. What are the maximum recommended postfundoplasty bolus and overnight volumes?

References

1. Powis MR, Smith K, Rennie M, Halliday D, Pierro A. Effect of major abdominal operations on energy and protein metabolism in infants and children. *J Pediatr Surg.* 1998;33(1):49–53.

2. Jaksic T, Shew SB, Keshen TH, Dzakovic A, Jahoor F. Do critically ill surgical neonates have increased energy expenditure? *J Pediatr Surg.* 2001;36(1):63–67.

3. Mtaweh H, Smith R, Kochanek PM, et al. Energy expenditure in children after severe traumatic brain injury. *Pediatr Crit Care Med.* 2014;15(3):242–249.

4. Meyer R, Kulinskaya E, Briassoulis G, Taylor RM, Cooper M, Pathan N, Habibi P: The challenge of developing a new predictive formula to estimate energy requirements in ventilated critically ill children. *Nutr Clin Pract.* 2012;27(5):669–676.

5. Bechard L, Ziegler, J., Duggan, C. Is energy expenditure of infants predictable after surgery? *ICAN: Infant, Child, Adolesc Nutr.* 2010;2(3):170–176.

6. De Wit B, Meyer R, Desai A, Macrae D, Pathan N. Challenge of predicting resting energy expenditure in children undergoing surgery for congenital heart disease. *Pediatr Crit Care Med.* 2010;11(4):496–501.

7. Blinman T, Cook R. Allometric Prediction of Energy Expenditure in Infants and Children. *Infant Child Adolesc Nutr.* 2011;3(4):216–224.

8. Denne SC, Kalhan SC. Leucine metabolism in human newborns. *Am J Physiol.* 1987;253(6 Pt 1):E608–E615.

9. Cook AM, Peppard A, Magnuson B. Nutrition considerations in traumatic brain injury. *Nutr Clin Pract.* 2008; 23(6):608–620.

10. Fullerton BS, Sparks EA, Khan FA, et al. Whole Body Protein Turnover and Net Protein Balance After Pediatric Thoracic Surgery: A Noninvasive Single-Dose 15N Glycine Stable Isotope Protocol With End-Product Enrichment. *JPEN.* 2018;42(2):361–370.

11. Velazco CS, Zurakowski D, Fullerton BS, Bechard LJ, Jaksic T, Mehta NM: Nutrient delivery in mechanically ventilated surgical patients in the pediatric critical care unit. *J Pediatr Surg.* 2017;52(1):145–148.

12. Mehta NM, Skillman HE, Irving SY, et al. Guidelines for the Provision and Assessment of Nutrition Support Therapy in the Pediatric Critically Ill Patient: Society of Critical Care Medicine and American Society for Parenteral and Enteral Nutrition. *JPEN.* 2017;41(5):706–742.

13. Jaksic T: Effective and efficient nutritional support for the injured child. *Surg Clin North Am.* 2002;82(2):379–391.

14. Shew SB, Jaksic T: The metabolic needs of critically ill children and neonates. *Semin Pediatr Surg.* 1999;8(3):131–139.

15. McClave SA, Taylor BE, Martindale RG, et al. Guidelines for the Provision and Assessment of Nutrition Support Therapy in the Adult Critically Ill Patient: Society of Critical Care Medicine (SCCM) and American Society for Parenteral and Enteral Nutrition (A.S.P.E.N.). *JPEN.* 2016; 40(2):159–211.

16. Holliday MA, Segar WE. The maintenance need for water in parenteral fluid therapy. *Pediatrics.* 1957;19(5):823–832.

17. Meyer R, Foong RX, Thapar N, Kritas S, Shah N. Systematic review of the impact of feed protein type and degree of hydrolysis on gastric emptying in children. *BMC Gastroenterol.* 2015;15:137.

18. Adams RL, Broughton KS. Insulinotropic effects of whey: mechanisms of action, recent clinical trials, and clinical applications. *Ann Nutr Metab.* 2016;69(1):56–63.

19. Tolia V, Lin CH, Kuhns LR. Gastric emptying using three different formulas in infants with gastroesophageal reflux. *J Pediatr Gastroenterol Nutr.* 1992;15(3):297–301.

20. Savage K, Kritas S, Schwarzer A, Davidson G, Omari T. Whey- vs casein-based enteral formula and gastrointestinal function in children with cerebral palsy. *JPEN.* 2012;36(1 Suppl):118S–123S.

21. Cook RC, Blinman TA. Alleviation of retching and feeding intolerance after fundoplication. *Nutr Clin Pract.* 2014;29(3):386–396.

22. Croll A and Blinman T. The eccentricities of nourishing the infant with abdominal abnormalities. *Topics Clin Nutr.* 2012;27(3):218–230.

23. Friedmacher F, Kroneis B, Huber-Zeyringer A, et al. Postoperative complications and functional outcome after Esophageal Atresia Repair: results from Longitudinal Single-Center Follow-Up. *J Gastrointest Surg.* 2017;21(6):927–935.

24. Pearson F, Johnson MJ, Leaf AA. Milk osmolality: does it matter? *Arch Dis Child Fetal Neonatal Ed.* 2013;98(2):F166–F169.

25. Salvia G, De Vizia B, Manguso F, Iula VD, Terrin G, Spadaro R, Russo G, Cucchiara S. Effect of intragastric volume and osmolality on mechanisms of gastroesophageal reflux in children with gastroesophageal reflux disease. *Am J Gastroenterol.* 2001;96(6):1725–1732.

26. Kreissl A, Zwiauer V, Repa A, et al. Effect of fortifiers and additional protein on the osmolarity of human milk: is it still safe for the premature infant? *J Pediatr Gastroenterol Nutr.* 2013;57(4):432–437.

27. O'Neil M, Teitelbaum DH, Harris MB. Total body sodium depletion and poor weight gain in children and young adults with an ileostomy: a case series. *Nutr Clin Pract* 2014;29(3):397–401.

28. Bower TR, Pringle KC, Soper RT. Sodium deficit causing decreased weight gain and metabolic acidosis in infants with ileostomy. *J Pediatr Surg.* 1988;23(6):567–572.

29. Sacher P, Hirsig J, Gresser J, Spitz L. The importance of oral sodium replacement in ileostomy patients. *Prog Pediatr Surg.* 1989;24:226–231.

30. Van Citters GW, Lin HC. The ileal brake: a fifteen-year progress report. *Curr Gastroenterol Rep.* 1999;1(5):404–409.

31. Malcolm WF, Lenfestey RW, Rice HE, Rach E, Goldberg RN, Cotten CM. Dietary fat for infants with enterostomies. *J Pediatr Surg* 2007;42(11):1811–1815.

32. Barbera R, Peracchi M, Brighenti F, Cesana B, Bianchi PA, Basilisco G. Sensations induced by medium and long chain triglycerides: role of gastric tone and hormones. *Gut.* 2000, 46(1):32–36.

33. Atia A, Girard-Pipau F, Hebuterne X, Spies WG, Guardiola A, Ahn CW, Fryer J, Xue F, Rammohan M, Sumague M et al. Macronutrient absorption characteristics in humans with short bowel syndrome and jejunocolonic anastomosis: starch is the most important carbohydrate substrate, although pectin supplementation may modestly enhance short chain fatty acid production and fluid absorption. *JPEN.* 2011;35(2):229–240.

34. Musch MW, Bookstein C, Xie Y, Sellin JH, Chang EB. SCFA increase intestinal Na absorption by induction of NHE3 in rat colon and human intestinal C2/bbe cells. *Am J Physiol Gastrointest Liver Physiol.* 2001;280(4):G687–693.

35. Kocoshis SA. Medical management of pediatric intestinal failure. *Semin Pediatr Surg.* 2010;19(1):20–26.

36. Cook RC, Blinman TA. Nutritional support of the pediatric trauma patient. *Semin Pediatr Surg.* 2010;19(4):242–251.

37. Briassoulis G, Filippou O, Kanariou M, Papassotiriou I, Hatzis T. Temporal nutritional and inflammatory changes in children with severe head injury fed a regular or an immune-enhancing diet: A randomized, controlled trial. *Pediatr Crit Care Med.* 2006;7(1):56–62.

38. Perrella SL, Hepworth AR, Simmer KN, Hartmann PE, Geddes DT. Repeatability of gastric volume measurements and intragastric content using ultrasound in preterm infants. *J Pediatr Gastroenterol Nutr.* 2014;59(2):254–263.

39. Warren J, Bhalla V, Cresci G. Postoperative diet advancement: surgical dogma vs evidence-based medicine. *Nutr Clin Pract.* 2011;26(2):115–125.

40. Sangkhathat S, Patrapinyokul S, Tadyathikom K. Early enteral feeding after closure of colostomy in pediatric patients. *J Pediatr Surg.* 2003;38(10):1516–1519.

41. Mamatha B, Alladi A. Early Oral Feeding in Pediatric Intestinal Anastomosis. *Indian J Surg.* 2015;77(Suppl 2):670–672.

42. Rosenfeld EH, Mazzolini K, DeMello A, et al. Postoperative feeding regimens after Laparoscopic Gastrostomy Placement. *J Laparoendosc Adv Surg Tech A.* 2017;27(11):1203–1208.

43. Jensen AR, Renaud E, Drucker NA, et al. Why wait: early enteral feeding after pediatric gastrostomy tube placement. *J Pediatr Surg.* 2018;53(4):656–660.

44. Savoie KB, Bachier-Rodriguez M, Jones TL, et al. Standardization of feeding advancement after neonatal gastrointestinal surgery: does it improve outcomes? *Nutr Clin Pract* 2016;31(6):1–9.

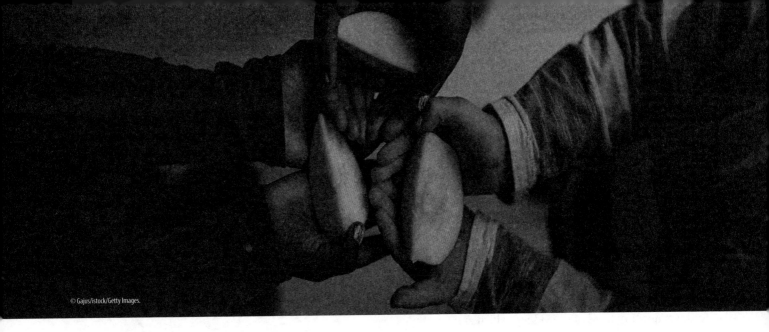

CHAPTER 18

Chronic Kidney Disease

Susan Tulley and Christine O'Connor

LEARNING OBJECTIVES

- Define the basic physiology of the kidney.
- Describe nutrition-related issues in CKD that affect weight gain and growth.
- Explain the nutritional needs corresponding with specific kidney dysfunction.
- Interpret the management of fluid and electrolytes in CKD.
- Describe mineral bone management in CKD.
- Restate health issues commonly found in CKD that need frequent monitoring.

▶ Introduction

Chronic kidney disease (CKD) is a rare condition in infants and children stemming from causes such as congenital malformations, genetic disorders, and acquired medical complications. Leading causes of pediatric CKD include renal aplasia/hypoplasia/dysplasia and congenital obstructive uropathy.[1] In children with CKD, dietary modifications are often required to ensure proper growth and development while preventing sometimes life-threatening electrolyte abnormalities.[2]

Additionally, depending on the severity of CKD, affected children often experience poor appetite and feeding intolerance while requiring dietary modifications that reduce or eliminate favorite childhood foods. This, along with the physical and emotional effects of chronic illness, can result in outcomes counterproductive to normal growth and development.[3] However, with improved understanding of the effects of CKD and individualized medical and nutritional management, historical negative outcomes of growth retardation and metabolic bone disease are no longer acceptable.

▶ Anatomy, Physiology, and Pathology of Condition

The kidneys are located in the retroperitoneal space on either side of the lumbar spine. The functional unit of the kidney is called the nephron, with each kidney containing over half a million to 1.5 million nephrons. Within each nephron, basic structures include the filtering unit of the kidney called the glomerulus, tubules consisting of the proximal tubule, the Loop of Henle, and the distal tubule where the exchange of solutes and fluids take place, and the collecting duct where electrolytes and pH are balanced.[4]

The physiology of the nephron corresponds directly to the major functions of the kidney, which are:

- **Excretory** – removal of excess fluid and waste
- **Acid-base balance** – removal and/or reabsorption of hydrogen and/or bicarbonate ions as well as other organic compounds in order to maintain the blood's pH at approximately 7.4
- **Endocrine function** – activation of vitamin D to its active form and production of erythropoietin, a hormone involved in production of red blood cells
- **Fluid and electrolyte balance** – regulation of blood volume, electrolyte homeostasis, and blood pressure maintenance via interaction with a series of hormonal pathways.[4]

Refer to anatomy and physiology of the kidneys for deeper understanding. The renal system is extremely complex and affects multiple bodily functions as outlined above. Kidneys may become damaged due to congenital anomalies or acquired conditions. Data collected on over 7,000 pediatric patients enrolled in the **North American Pediatric Renal Trials and Collaborative Studies** (NAPRTCS) registry were used to report the prevalence of underlying causes of CKD in children (see **TABLE 18.1**).[1] Significant kidney injury can occur before symptoms such as edema, low or excessive urine output, lack of appetite, nausea/vomiting, lethargy, osteodystrophy, stunted growth, and hypertension appear. Although symptoms may present in varying degrees of severity, progression invariably occurs as the nephrons become more diseased and dysfunctional.

CKD is a typically progressive, characterized by a permanent loss of **glomerular filtration rate** (GFR) occurring over a period of months to years. The National Kidney Foundation has defined stages of CKD to help identify the progression of the disease based on glomerular GFR, where normal GFR is >90 ml/min/m². GFR is defined as the amount of filtrate formed per minute normalized to the total body surface area, and is representative of the number of functioning glomeruli.

TABLE 18.1 Chronic Kidney Disease Primary Diagnosis		
Primary Diagnosis	**N**	**%**
Obstructive uropathy	14,541	20.7
Aplastic/hypoplastic/dysplastic kidney	220	17.3
Focal segmental glomerulosclerosis	613	8.7
Reflux nephropathy	594	8.4
Polycystic disease	278	4.0
Prune belly	193	2.7
Renal infarct	158	2.2
Hemolytic uremic syndrome	141	2.0
SLE (systemic lupus erythematosus) nephritis	114	1.6
Familial nephritis	111	1.6
Cystinosis	104	1.5
Pyelo/interstitial nephritis	99	1.4
Medullary cystic disease	90	1.3
Chronic glomerulonephritis	82	1.2
Congenital nephrotic syndrome	75	1.1
Membranoproliferative glomerulonephritis, type I	75	1.1
Berger's (IgA) nephritis	66	0.9
Idiopathic crescentic glomerulonephritis	47	0.7
Henoch-Schonlein nephritis	43	0.6
Membranous nephropathy	37	0.5
Wilms' tumor	32	0.5

Primary Diagnosis	N	%
Membranoproliferative glomerulonephritis, type II	30	0.4
Other systemic immunologic disease	26	0.4
Wegener's granulomatosis	25	0.4
Sickle cell nephropathy	14	0.2
Diabetic glomerulonephritis	11	0.2
Oxalosis	7	0.1
Drash's syndrome	6	0.1
Other	1110	15.8
Unknown	182	2.6

Percentages based on a total number of patients (N = 7037)
Modified from North American Pediatric Renal Trials and Collaborative Studies. NAPRTCS 2008 Annual Report. Available at: www.naprtcs.org. Accessed October 2017.[1]

These stages progress from mild CKD (stages 1 and 2), to moderate (stage 3), to severe (stage 4), and finally to end stage (stage 5). See **TABLE 18.2** for GFR ranges corresponding to each CKD stage. Usually when CKD has progressed to CKD stage 5, complications of renal failure necessitate the initiation of renal replacement therapy, the options of which are dialysis (stage 5D) and transplant (stage 5T).[5] CKD staging is useful in estimating the degree of medical nutrition therapy necessary for controlling uremia, managing electrolyte balance, and setting goals for calorie, protein, and other nutrients. Main nutritional goals for infants and children with CKD are normal growth and bone health, which are often difficult to achieve in those with more advanced CKD (CKD stages 3–5).[6]

▶ Condition-specific Nutrition Screening

CKD and its underlying cause can remain asymptomatic for many years and may therefore go undiagnosed until significant kidney damage and disease progression has already occurred. It is not uncommon for some cases of pediatric CKD to be diagnosed through routine medical check-ups required for school entry or sports participation. In the general population, appropriate and thorough general nutritional screening should be conducted, including carefully obtained anthropometric measurements, appetite and food intake, presence of nausea/vomiting, urine output volume and stooling pattern. In children with CKD, a problem in one or many of these areas is often identified and may require specific nutritional interventions. In children with chronic health conditions, routine surveillance occurs. This generally includes obtaining routine blood work, vital signs, and anthropometric measurements. This allows the pediatric dietitian to screen the child for conditions specific to nutrition risk.

TABLE 18.2 NKF KDOQI Classifications Stages of Chronic Kidney Disease

Stage	Description	GFR (mL/min/1.73 m)	Treatment
1	Kidney damage with normal Or ↑ GFR	≥ 90	
2	Kidney damage with mild ↓ GFR	60–89	
3	Moderate ↓ GFR	30–59	1-5T if kidney transplant recipient
4	Severe ↓ GFR	15–29	
5	Kidney failure	< 15 (or dialysis)	5D if dialysis (HD or PD)

Abbreviations: CKD, chronic kidney disease; HD, hemodialysis; GFR, glomerular filtration rate; PD, peritoneal dialysis; ↑ increased, ↓ decreased
Data from National Kidney Foundation. K/DOQI clinical practice guidelines for chronic kidney disease; evaluation, classification, and stratification. *Am J Kidney Dis.* 2002;3 (2 suppl 1):S1–S164.[7]

Nutritional screening can include clinical information specific to kidney disease, such as the presence of edema, medication use, vitamin/mineral supplementation, electrolyte values – sodium, potassium, bicarbonate; bone health lab values – serum calcium, serum phosphorus, PTH level, 25-OH Vitamin D level; protein status – serum albumin, proteinuria; and anemia status – hemoglobin, hematocrit, iron, MCV level.[8]

▶ Nutrition Assessment

Intake: A detailed assessment should include a focused history of nutrient intake, frequency of meals and snacks, volume, and feeding intolerance. CKD symptoms often include inadequate intake, frequent vomiting, and altered taste and oral aversions. Oral intake often decreases with CKD progression and many children with CKD require dietary restrictions that often limit or eliminate favorite and typical childhood foods such as milk, cheese, potatoes, peanut butter, and bananas. Children with CKD frequently have delayed or abnormal eating skills that started in infancy. Healthy infants are developmentally ready for solids by 4–6 months of age. This progresses to include increased textures and tastes until they are able to self-feed table food.[9] Infants born with CKD often have poor appetite and frequent vomiting that takes place as infants are developing vital feeding skills. This alteration in the natural progression of eating can cause oral aversions and impact learned behaviors that are difficult to overcome without early and consistent feeding therapy.[8] Regardless of age, compromised dietary intake can lead to a need for oral nutritional supplementation or nutrition support in order to maintain weight gain and growth.[10] A 3-day food diary is very useful in assessing the adequacy of intake and assists the **registered dietitian nutritionist** (RDN) with interventions.[8]

Linear growth: The physical exam of a child with CKD will often reveal short stature where the child appears much younger than chronological age. It is helpful to determine the height age of the child for nutritional assessment purposes. Height age is easily obtained by using the child's current height to determine the age point at which this height intersects the 50th percentile on the growth chart. The corresponding age is the child's height age. Poor linear growth is often multifactorial and may be secondary to decreased nutritional intake, uncorrected acidosis, osteodystrophy, and excessive urinary sodium losses. Some children with congenital abnormalities are born small for gestational age and/or have comorbidities that can affect growth. If steroids have been used as part of medical therapy, this too must be taken into consideration when assessing linear growth due to its negative impact on linear growth velocity.[11]

In larger medical centers, many children with CKD are seen by medical teams in various clinics and will have multiple anthropometric measurements. If these measurements are not carefully obtained and entered into the electronic medical record, their computerized growth chart can be inaccurate and confusing to clinicians and can prevent or delay proper intervention. Therefore, a helpful tip for RDNs who frequently follow CKD patients is to keep a paper copy of an age-appropriate growth chart for each CKD patient with carefully obtained anthropometric measurements plotted in order to ensure accuracy and to assist with assessing and decision-making. For infants under 2 years of age, the **World Health Organization** (WHO) growth charts are recommended and for children over 2 years of age, the **Centers for Disease Control and Prevention** (CDC) growth charts are appropriate. Currently, z-scores should also be utilized for assessment and are especially helpful in this patient population since linear growth is so often below normal growth distribution.[12]

In all cases of inadequate linear growth in a child with CKD whose height is < −1.88 SDS or height for age <3rd percentile, adequacy of nutritional status (BMI or weight for length >50th percentile and z-score >0 SD) as well as correction of any and all other factors affecting growth must be achieved before considering growth hormone therapy due to its cost and required delivery mode, which is daily injections.[12] Medical insurance coverage for growth hormone therapy is difficult to obtain due to the high cost of the medication. Requirements for insurance coverage includes a wrist X-ray to observe the epiphyseal plate, which helps to determine bone age in order to assure the child still has growth potential.[13] Poor growth is often a deciding factor for many pediatric nephrologists to initiate renal replacement therapy, either dialysis or kidney transplant, since poor growth is associated with impaired quality of life, including increased hospitalizations and mortality.[14]

Weight: Weight should be monitored frequently in children with CKD and plotted on age-appropriate growth charts. However, weight is dependent on fluid status, which can be greatly affected depending on level of CKD and the underlying cause of CKD. For example, some conditions may cause oliguria and result in edema, while others are characterized by polyuria causing frequent dehydration. Not recognizing fluid overload is the most common error when assessing anthropometric data in the CKD population and can lead to inappropriate nutritional interventions such as a reduction in caloric intake due to mistakenly thinking that the weight gain is real and simply due to edema.[15] Because of this, determining the patient's correct "euvolemic" weight is essential. Competent RDNs who keep accurate growth curves on patients can provide valuable assistance to the nephrologist in determining the etiology of medical complications such as elevated blood pressure and electrolyte abnormalities. Rapid weight gain indicating fluid retention can become more problematic in later stages of CKD, sometimes leading to the decision to initiate **renal replacement therapy** (RRT).

Weight-for-length/BMI: Weight for length is used for children 24 months and under and is plotted on WHO growth charts. BMI should be accurately calculated and plotted on CDC growth charts for children greater than 2 years of age. The patient's dry weight should be determined and used. Because stunted linear growth is common in children with CKD, using BMI at the child's "height age" is recommended in order to determine the child's ideal weight to avoid overestimation due to their stunted height.[16]

Head Circumference: Accurate measurement of each child's head should be obtained and plotted on a WHO head circumference growth curve at regular intervals up to the age of three. Variances in head circumference that are not otherwise explained by co-morbidities, such as hydrocephalus, should be noted and brought to the attention of the pediatric nephrologist.[8] It is important to monitor the incremental growth and curve of head circumference growth in all infants.

Serum Albumin: Serum albumin has historically been used as a marker for nutritional status. However, serum albumin is affected by systemic inflammation and fluid retention, both conditions that are common in CKD. Therefore, albumin is not a reliable marker for nutritional status in children with CKD. Hypoalbuminemia can be used as a flag to assess for fluid status, protein losses in urine, and potential causes of inflammation.[8]

Nutrition Focused Physical Assessment (NFPA): Nutrition Focused Physical Assessment (NFPA) is a thorough systematic examination by a RDN of a patient's physical appearance and functionality in order to uncover nutritional issues that may be difficult to determine in patients with CKD using only traditional methods of assessment. NFPA is a relatively new assessment tool that can greatly enhance standard nutritional assessment.[17] The use of NFPA in children with CKD can be helpful in assessing this population for malnutrition. For further details, see the chapter on Nutrition Focused Physical Exam.

▶ Nutrition Diagnosis

Sample PES statements used in CKD include:

- Altered nutrition-related labs related to decreased kidney function as evidenced by elevated serum phosphorus level.
- Excessive fluid intake related to knowledge deficit as evidenced by 3 kg weight gain between dialysis treatments.
- Altered nutrition-related labs related to excessive dietary potassium in CKD as evidenced by elevated serum potassium level.
- Altered nutrition-related labs related to inappropriate formula in CKD as evidenced by elevated serum potassium level.

- Suboptimal oral intake related to advancing CKD as evidenced by 3-day food record.
- Altered nutrient utilization related to excessive sodium intake in CKD as evidenced by elevated blood pressure percentile.
- Inadequate intake of enteral nutrition related to hyperemesis as evidenced by poor weight gain and parental report.

▶ Nutrition Intervention

Nutritional Requirements

The following nutritional requirements are only an overview. For more in-depth discussion, please refer to the National Kidney Foundation's Kidney Disease Outcomes Quality Initiative (KDOQI) Clinical Practice Guideline for Nutrition in Children with CKD, 2008 Update.[6]

Macronutrients

Caloric needs: Caloric needs of children with CKD have not been found to vary from caloric requirements for healthy children, and no evidence exists that show excessive caloric intake improves linear growth in children with CKD.[18] Please refer to **TABLE 18.3** for estimated energy requirements and **TABLE 18.4** for determining physical activity level.

TABLE 18.3	Equations to Estimate Energy Requirements for Children at Healthy Weights
Age	Estimated Energy Requirement (EER) (kcal/d) = Total Energy Expenditure + Energy Deposition
0–3 mo.	EER = [89 × weight (kg) – 100] + 175
4–6 mo.	EER = [89 × weight (kg) – 100] + 56
7–12 mo.	EER = [89 × weight (kg) – 100] + 22
13–35 mo.	EER = [89 × weight (kg) –100] + 20
3–8 y	Boys: EER = 88.5 – 61.9 × age (y) + PA × [26.7 × weight (kg) + 903 × height (m)] + 20 Girls: EER = 135.3 – 30.8 × age (y) + PA × [10 × weight (kg) + 934 × height (m)] + 20
9–18 y	Boys: EER = 88.5 – 61.9 × age (y) + PA × [26.7 × weight (kg) + 903 × height (m)] + 25 Girls: EER = 135.3 – 30.8 × age (y) + PA × [10 × weight (kg) + 934 × height (m)] + 25

Modified from Institute of Medicine. Food and Nutrition Board. Dietary reference intakes for energy, carbohydrate, fiber, fat, fatty acids, cholesterol, protein, and amino acids (macronutrients). Washington, DC; National Academics: 2005.[18]

TABLE 18.4 Physical Activity (PA) Coefficients for Determination of Energy Requirements in Children Ages 3 to 18 Years for EER.

Gender	Sedentary	Low Active	Active	Very Active
	Typical activities of daily living (ADL) only	ADL + 30–60 min of daily moderate activity (eg, walking at 5–7 km/h)	ADL + ≥60 min of daily moderate activity	ADL + ≥60 min of daily moderate activity + or 120 min of moderate activity
Boys	1.0	1.18	1.26	1.42
Girls	1.0	1.16	1.31	1.56

Modified from Institute of Medicine. Food and Nutrition Board. Dietary reference intakes for energy, carbohydrate, fiber, fat, fatty acids, cholesterol, protein, and amino acids (macronutrients). Washington, DC; National Academics: 2005.[18]

It should be noted that children who are underweight may require additional calories to gain weight at a faster rate in order to correct pre-existing energy-malnutrition.[12] As noted above, children with CKD often require a specific and individualized intervention in order to obtain adequate energy needs. Keep in mind the "height age" to determine ideal weight as explained above when determining energy needs in order to prevent overestimation of calorie needs. **TABLE 18.3 and 18.4** may be used for guidance when assessing energy needs. However, this is only a guide. The whole clinical picture of the CKD patient needs to be taken into account and individualized for the most accurate assessment of energy needs.

If nutritional supplementation and other methods of increasing caloric and protein oral intake have been ineffective, nutrition support, typically enteral nutrition, is often required for children with CKD. This requires either a nasogastric feeding tube or a more permanent surgically-placed gastric feeding tube for longer term nutrition support. Having a gastric feeding tube may sound like a drastic measure to some; however, many parents and caregivers express relief once their child has had a gastric tube placed. A gastric feeding tube often helps to alleviate concerns regarding their child's poor intake and helps to more effectively administer medications that are sometimes not tolerated orally. Commercially available infant and adult formulas with low renal solute load are typically used for enteral feedings. However, human milk for infants and other non-renal specific formulas may be used in certain cases.

Protein needs: Due to issues such as proteinuria (loss of protein in urine), use of corticosteroids and acidosis, many children with CKD require more protein than their healthy counterparts while the same time avoiding excessive protein intake to prevent uremia and limiting

phosphorus in the diet (which is further explained in Bone Health section).[19] Excessive azotemia when consuming only the recommended amount of protein is a consideration for starting dialysis since uremia can have deleterious effects such as poor appetite, increased vomiting, increased lethargy, poor attention span, and decreased ability to learn.[8] Please refer to **TABLE 18.5** for recommended protein intake in children with CKD.

Fat needs: Fat is a vital energy source for children due to its concentrated calorie load, however increased fat intake can supplant other nutrients and is associated with higher risk of coronary heart disease, diabetes mellitus, and obesity.[20] Using fat for calories in undernourished children with CKD in order to prevent an excess of

TABLE 18.5 Recommended Dietary Protein Intake in Children with CKD Stages 3 to 5

Age	DRI (g/kg/d)	Recommended for CKD Stage 3 (g/kg/d) (100%–140% DRI)	Recommended for CKD Stages 4–5 (g/kg/d) (100%–120% DRI)
0–6 mo.	1.5	1.5–2.1	1.5–1.8
7–12 mo.	1.2	1.2–1.5	1.05–1.25
1–3 y	1.05	1.05–1.5	1.05–1.25
4–13 y	0.95	0.95–1.35	0.95–1.15
1418 y	0.85	0.85–1.2	0.85–1.05

Data from National Kidney Foundation, KDOQI Clinical Practice Guidelines for Nutrition in Children with CKD: 2008 Update. *Am J Kidney Dis.* 2009;53(Suppl 2):S1–S124.[6]

more acutely harmful potassium and phosphorus found in protein and carbohydrate sources is an acceptable practice, but it should be used with thought and care since CKD is a life-long and progressive disease with a high correlation to cardiovascular disease.[21] Especially in children with CKD, it is never too early to promote healthful dietary habits.

Micronutrients

Pediatric CKD patients are at increased risk for developing micronutrient deficiencies due to inadequate intake, kidney metabolism dysfunction, abnormal absorption, and drug-nutrient interactions. Risk for malnutrition, including poor growth, is increased if children with CKD are not supplemented with water-soluble vitamins in cases of inadequate dietary intake or if clinical signs of deficiency are present. A water-soluble pediatric multivitamin taken is usually sufficient for supplementing marginal dietary intake.[12]

Close attention should be paid to fat-soluble vitamins in children with CKD as metabolism of these vitamins may differ from healthy children. Retinol-binding protein levels tend to be elevated in children with CKD leading to elevated retinol levels. Therefore, supplemental vitamin A in both retinol and beta carotene forms is not recommended due to risk of toxicity that could lead to liver damage.[22]

Much interest and research is currently being conducted on 25-hydroxyvitamin D. This inactive form of vitamin D has been found to be particularly deficient in children with CKD, and current recommendations include checking serum levels at least yearly and supplementing with ergocalciferol (vitamin D_2) or cholecalciferol (vitamin D_3) if serum levels are under 30 ng/ml. Specific monitoring and dosing guidelines are available from the National Kidney Foundation.[8] The active form of vitamin D – 1, 25 hydroxyvitamin D - will be discussed in the Bone Health section.

Vitamin E has known anti-oxidative properties and has been shown to be beneficial in treating anemia in children with CKD. Modest vitamin E supplementation may be helpful for CKD patients with anemia but excessive dosing should be avoided due to poor renal clearance.[23] Vitamin K, the final fat-soluble vitamin, is synthesized in the intestinal tract and should not have any further consideration in children with CKD unless other health issues are present requiring long-term antibiotic use or other conditions affecting the gastrointestinal system.[8]

The minerals zinc, copper, selenium and iron in CKD deserve specific attention. Zinc, known for benefiting skin integrity, taste enhancement and growth, and preventing anemia, may become deficient in children with CKD due to poor intake and dietary restrictions.

Copper levels have also been shown to be deficient for the same reasons. It is recommended to check zinc and copper serum levels and to supplement according to the **daily referenced intake** (DRI).[8] Selenium plays a role in thyroid function and has been shown to be deficient in CKD patients. However, no recommendations on supplementation of selenium in children with CKD exist currently.[8] Anemia is a commonly occurring problem in children with CKD due to the impaired production of erythropoietin, a hormone produced by the kidneys and needed to utilize iron in the production of red blood cells. Iron deficiency can be due to poor dietary intake and is often supplemented by prescription to ensure accuracy in quality and quantity. Of note, iron deficiency has been associated with pica, the practice of eating non-food substances such ice, clay, corn starch, ashes, paper, etc.[12] Asking parents/caregivers if they notice the practice of pica in their children is recommended in routine nutritional screening.

Fluid and Electrolytes

Managing fluid, sodium, and potassium varies widely among children with CKD and is dependent on the amount of urine output, dietary intake of sodium and potassium, underlying disease, CKD stage and blood pressure control.[8]

Sodium is routinely restricted in order to prevent fluid retention and to control blood pressure and should be individualized based on fluid gain, blood pressure, and dietary intake. Since most dietary sodium is obtained by consuming processed foods, increasing intake of freshly prepared foods seasoned with herbs and spices is recommended. Adherence to low-salt diets is often difficult[12] but can be improved through creative plans. For example, rather than restrict all processed foods high in sodium, it may be more acceptable to give a daily sodium allowance that the child can "spend" in a day that will allow one or two high sodium items. For example, in order for the child to attend a pizza party after school, breakfast and lunch should be extremely low sodium. Allowing some leeway with dietary restrictions will improve the child's quality of life and overall adherence. Patients and parents/caregivers should be educated on low sodium foods to enjoy and high sodium foods to avoid as well as tips on seasoning without the use of table salt and other high sodium sauces and condiments. They should learn to read nutrition fact labels. "Lite" salt or salt substitutes are not recommended due to the use of potassium in place of sodium in many of these products, which could lead to dangerous levels of serum potassium in those with kidney dysfunction.[12]

Some patients with CKD have excessive urination or "polyuria," which is a condition that may be accompanied by increased urinary sodium losses. These patients must be adequately hydrated and supplemented with sodium to prevent growth failure. Pediatric patients with polyuric CKD old enough to self-feed often crave high sodium foods and drink water excessively.[12]

The ability to excrete potassium often decreases as CKD advances, leading to hyperkalemia (high potassium in the serum), which can cause cardiac muscle dysfunction and death. It is imperative to restrict foods high in potassium and to check serum levels routinely. Knowing the drug-nutrient interactions of the medications each patient is on is very important since some medications can result in high serum potassium. If dietary management is insufficient to control serum potassium levels, certain medications and medical treatments may be necessary to reduce the serum potassium in order to prevent serious consequences.[8] For those on enteral formulas, including infants, potassium can be removed from formula by treating with a medication called *sodium polystyrene sulfonate*, which exchanges formula-contained potassium ions for sodium ions and allows the potassium ions to precipitate from the formula. This is an effective method of reducing potassium intake for children who are not able to excrete potassium normally.[23]

Bone Health

Bone and mineral metabolism abnormalities are a serious consequence in CKD that can have long-lasting effects on skeletal growth and cardiovascular health.[20] When CKD becomes more advanced, usually stage 3 and above, the kidneys are often incapable of excreting dietary phosphorus effectively and/or active vitamin D is too low for adequate calcium absorption, driving up the **parathyroid hormone** (PTH) level. Elevated PTH levels can cause increased bone turnover, increased calcium loss from bones, and consequently, calcification of organs and small blood vessels. Elevated PTH level is also another factor associated with poor growth.[24] Treatment goals are to maintain normal serum levels of calcium and phosphorus and to prevent secondary hyperparathyroidism. The latter is typically achieved in more advanced stages of CKD by providing the active-form of vitamin D–1, 25 di-hydroxy vitamin D–in order to suppress excessive PTH secretion. Paradoxically, the vitamin D therapy can also increase gastrointestinal absorption of phosphorus, making adherence to a low phosphorus diet more imperative.

Additional dietary phosphate management can be achieved by using phosphate binders, usually a calcium-containing medication taken with food to bind phosphorus in the GI tract and prevent absorption of

TABLE 18.6 Suggested Maximal Calcium Intake from Oral, Enteral and Phosphate Binder

Age	DRI mg/d	Maximal Intake, mg/d
0–6 mo.	200	≤ 400
7–12 mo.	260	≤ 520
1–3 years	700	≤ 1400
4–8 years	1,000	≤ 2000
9–18 years	1,300	≤ 2500

Data from KDOQI clinical practice guidelines for nutrition in children with CKD: 2008 update. *Am J Kidney Dis.* 2009;53(suppl 2):S1–S124.[6]

phosphorus. Other medications, specifically calcimimetic drugs (cinacalcet), to control high PTH levels have been successfully used in adult CKD patients to treat secondary hyperparathyroidism refractory to traditional management. However, cinacalcet must be used with extreme caution with careful monitoring of serum calcium levels, as life-threatening hypocalcemia can occur (see **TABLE 18.6** for maximal calcium levels). For this reason, the FDA has not approved the use of cinacalcet in children, and more research is still required before this medication is deemed safe for pediatric patients.[12]

Hypophosphatemia may also occur in children with CKD due to urinary wasting of phosphorus and/or over-treatment for high phosphorus levels. This condition is associated with poor bone mineralization and impaired growth and should be addressed and corrected promptly. Some infants and toddlers often require supplemental phosphorus due to the increased phosphorus need for age. See **TABLE 18.7** for details.

Nutrition interventions for patients with CKD become more complex as the disease progresses. RDN managing CKD patients should always obtain and plot accurate anthropometric measurements and track weight gain and growth as these clinical markers are very important in nutritional and medical management.[8] In earlier stages, intervention may be as simple as dietary counseling in order to prevent high serum levels of electrolytes or changing an infant formula to a renal-specific formula that lowers the renal solute load. As CKD progresses, attention should be given to weight gain, growth, intake of macro- and micronutrients, fluid and electrolyte balance and mineral bone health all while taking into account any co-morbidities and/or underlying

TABLE 18.7 Suggested Maximal Oral and /or Enteral Phosphorus Intake, mg/d			
Age	**Phosphorus DRI, mg/d**	**If PTH is High and Phosphorus Normal**	**If Both PTH and Phosphorus are High**
0–6 mo.	100	≤ 100	≤ 80
7–12 mo.	275	≤ 275	≤ 220
1–3 y	460	≤ 460	≤ 400
4–8 y	500	≤ 500	≤ 400
9–18 y	1,250	≤ 1200	≤ 1000

*DRI, dietary reference intake; PTH parathyroid hormone
Data from Dietary Reference Intakes Definitions, Health Canada http://www.hc-sc.gc.ca/fn-an/alt_formats/hpfb-dgpsa/pdf/nutrition/dri_tables-eng.pdf.[6]

Nutrition Monitoring and Evaluation

More frequent monitoring is required as CKD progresses to higher stages. Providing optimal care for CKD patients requires a multidisciplinary approach, and the RDN often works closely with the nephrologist and other team members to ensure comprehensive care and achieve the best outcomes. There are at least five corresponding health issues found in CKD that the RDN needs to be aware of and monitor in order to improve the health status and quality of life for CKD patients. Weight gain and growth need to be carefully monitored on a regular basis by obtaining and plotting anthropometrics for each pediatric CKD patient. This information should be shared with the nephrologist in order to help with decision-making. To optimize bone health, serum calcium, and phosphorus as well as PTH and 25-hydroxy, Vitamin D levels should be tracked and appropriate action taken that could entail medications, supplementation and education. PTH levels will often become elevated, especially if dietary phosphorus intake is not limited. If so, then the active form of vitamin D (1, 25 dihydroxy vitamin D) will need to be prescribed to help decrease PTH levels and to prevent excessive bone turnover. Anemia is another common problem in children with CKD but is rarely caused by a lack of dietary iron. Instead, anemia in CKD is usually due to the kidneys' inability to produce erythropoietin, a hormone involved in production of red blood cells.[4] The development of recombinant human erythropoietin has greatly improved anemia management and the quality of life for people with CKD. The nephrologist typically prescribes erythropoietin that is administered subcutaneously and pharmaceutical grade ferrous sulfate for most CKD patients.

conditions. Please refer to **TABLE 18.8** for recommended diet modifications to help address electrolyte-induced symptoms of CKD. Proper nutritional intervention must be executed in partnership with a pediatric nephrologist since many nutritional interventions cannot be accomplished if the medical management is inadequate or inappropriate. For example, if a child is acidotic (low bicarbonate levels in blood), growth will not be optimized no matter how adequate the nutritional intake. The nephrologist will need to order an alkalizing agent to correct this condition, which will then allow improved utilization of nutritional intake.

Sodium Bicarb

TABLE 18.8 Electrolyte/mineral Management		
Nutrient	**Indication for Treatment**	**Modification**
Sodium	Hypertension	No added salt, may need a fluid restriction.
	Daily steroid therapy	No added salt diet.
	Increased urine losses (which can indicate sodium wasting)	May be sodium wasting and so will require sodium supplement along with increased fluid.
Potassium	Hyperkalemia	Low potassium diet. If dependent on enteral nutrition, may need to change to a low renal solute formula or treat the formula with medication called *sodium polystyrene sulfonate*.
	Diuretic therapy; diarrhea; other reasons leading to hypokalemia	Encourage foods high in potassium or give supplementation.

(continues)

TABLE 18.8 Electrolyte/mineral Management *(continued)*

Nutrient	Indication for Treatment	Modification
Calcium	Hypercalcemia	If on calcium-containing phosphate binder, change to non-calcium phosphate binder.
		For children eating orally, give only DRI for calcium – may need to give alternative "milk" such as rice milk. Refer to Table 18.7.
		If dependent on enteral nutrition, may need to manipulate formula by giving less calcium-containing formula and adding in calcium-free nutritional modular products.
		May need to stop Vitamin D supplementation temporarily.
	Hypocalcemia	If albumin is low, this may cause serum calcium to appear low. Obtain an ionized calcium to determine accurate level of serum calcium. If truly low, ensure child is receiving at least DRI for calcium intake. See Table 18.7. If not, give calcium supplementation.
		May need to be started on Vitamin D (cholecalciferol or ergocalciferol) to increase absorption from the gut.
Phosphorus	Hyperphosphatemia	Phosphate binders and/or low phosphate diet (refer to Table 18.6.)
	Hypophosphatemia (seen more in infants and toddlers)	Sodium phosphate supplement
	Elevated parathyroid hormone level, with or without hyperphosphatemia	25-OH Vitamin D supplement (cholecalciferol or ergocalciferol) and active form 1,25 OH Vitamin D (calcitriol).

[handwritten annotation: has Ca^{2+}?]

The RDN still monitors hemoglobin, hematocrit and mean corpuscular volume and other iron studies if available and makes appropriate recommendations such as folic acid and/or vitamin B_{12} supplementation in the cases of macrocytic anemia. Blood pressure control often requires medications, however RDNs assist with monitoring dietary sodium and fluid intake and providing dietary education as needed. As stated above, cardiovascular disease is a major cause of death of patients with CKD and is a life-long health consideration through every stage of kidney disease, including post-kidney transplant.[12] Therefore, the RDN should routinely monitor serum lipid profiles and provide dietary education to support a heart-healthy diet and lifestyle for each patient with CKD. The RDN plays a large role in educating CKD patients about their disease and helps to empower them to self-management and better adherence.

▶ Conclusion

In summary, nutritional intervention is dependent on a comprehensive and integrated understanding of all aspects of medical management, including age-specific nutritional needs, growth trends, stage of CKD, underlying diseases and conditions, amount of urination, serum levels of electrolytes, bone health lab values, cholesterol, and triglyceride levels, the presence of proteinuria, medications and drug-nutrient interactions, and psychosocial aspects of the patient and family.[8] Because of the often intense and extreme complexity of CKD, interventions should be individualized and frequently monitored as outlined above, usually corresponding with stage of CKD. Managing CKD is not constant and changes with age and development of patient and progression of disease. Once CKD has progressed to end-stage renal disease (ESRD), the nutritional care management changes and is dependent on the form of renal replacement therapy chosen. In the case of CKD stage 5D, a dialysis modality is chosen that will greatly affect nutritional management depending on if the patient initiates hemodialysis or peritoneal dialysis. In the event of CKD stage 5T or kidney transplant, nutritional management will usually become less cumbersome and a large majority of children will experience improved appetite and growth following transplantation. However, nutritional management in ESRD exceeds the scope of this text. Interested practitioners should refer to the National Kidney Foundation's Kidney Disease Outcomes Quality Initiative (NKF-KDOQI) Clinical Practice Guidelines for more information and guidance in providing nutrition care in kidney disease.

🔍 CASE STUDY

17 year old female AB scheduled in nephrology clinic post findings from a ruptured right tendon.

AB reported falling on leg as result of ruptured tendon. Per guidance from orthopedics, AB underwent a MRI which revealed hyperparathyroidism including diffuse abnormalities of bone in the right femur.

Pt prior to this clinic visit had no medical history other than ear infections. Pt parents also reported no family history of renal disease on either side.

Physician contacts the dietitian to assess patient nutritional status and to provide diet counseling.

Lab Results

Na 142, K 3.2, CO_2 11, albumin 3.1, calcium 8.9, phosphorus 8.6, Vitamin D 25 OH 19.8, PTH 2,000, GFR Calculated 40.

Anthropometrics

Weight: 49.75 kg (23rd percentile)
Height: 151.1 cm (3rd percentile)
BMI: 21.79 kg/m² (59th percentile)
Mid-parental height of 164 cm plotting at the 50th percentile.
Physical Assessment:
Pt appearing short stature, yellow toned skin, and thinning hair and brace on right leg, sitting in wheel chair.
Medications: none currently

24 Hour Diet Recall

Breakfast- sausage biscuit
Lunch- Spagetti O's with Franks
Dinner- Chicken baked, vegetables, and macaroni and cheese
Pt reports will eat carrots, and a variety of fruits. Drinks lemonade and 2–3 cans of Coke per day.

Assessment: low GFR (between 30-59) stage 3 CKD. Patient with poor linear growth, not meeting genetic growth potential. Metabolic bone disease due to bone demineralization – vitamin D3 deficiency due to inadequate intake and inability to metabolize vitamin D2 to vitamin D3 and inadequate sun exposure.

Diagnosis: Altered nutrition-related labs related to stage 3 CKD as evidenced by hyperphosphatemia, ↑ PTH, vitamin D3 deficiency.

Intervention:
1. Calcium supplementation: 1300-2000 mg per day
2. Low phosphorus diet (<1000 mg per day)
3. Vit D supplementation 2000 units per day

Questions:
1. What food recommendations would you make for this family?
2. What foods would be restricted on a low phosphorus diet?
3. What other advice might be helpful to help support bone health?
4. Would you restrict protein for this child?

Study Questions

1. What are the most common two underlying diagnoses that cause CKD in children?

2. Once CKD has progressed to stage 5, what are the available options to address the kidney failure?

3. When performing a nutritional screening for a patient with CKD, what are some relevant questions to ask?

4. What underlying reasons affect linear growth in children with CKD?

5. Why may children with CKD require more protein than their healthy counterparts? Why should they avoid excessive protein?

6. Why should vitamin A supplement be avoided in children with later stages of kidney disease?

7. Which main two nutrients affect blood pressure? What nutritional intervention is often warranted?

8. What are side-effects of elevated PTH? How is elevated PTH medically and nutritionally treated?

9. What condition is a major cause of death for people with CKD and requires life-long health consideration? What interventions should the RDN take regarding this potential condition for these patients?

10. What is the National Kidney Foundation's practice guidelines resource for management of CKD?

References

1. North American Pediatric Renal Trials and Collaborative Studies. NAPRTCS 2008 Annual Report. Available at: www.naprtcs.org. Accessed October 2017.

2. National Kidney Foundation: K/DOQI clinical practice guidelines on hypertension and antihypertensive agents in chronic kidney disease. *Am J Kidney Dis.* 2004; 43(suppl 1):S1–S290.

3. Flynn JT, Mitsnefes M, Pierce C, et al; Chronic Kidney Disease in Children Study Group. Blood pressure in children with chronic kidney disease: report from the Chronic Kidney Disease in Children Study. *Hypertension.* 2009;52(4):631–637.

4. Skorecki K, Chertow GM, Marsden PA, Taal MW, Alan You ASL. *Brenner & Rector's The Kidney.* 10th ed. Elsevier Inc. Publishing: 2016.

5. Karlberg J, Schaefer F, Hennicke M, Wingen AM, Rigden S, Mehls O: Early age-dependent growth impairment in chronic renal failure. European Study Group for Nutritional Treatment of Chronic Renal Failure in Childhood. *Pediatr Nephrol.* 10:283–287.

6. National Kidney Foundation. KDOQI clinical practice guideline for nutrition in children with CKD: 2008 update. *Am J Kidney Dis.* 2009;53(Suppl 2):S1–S124.

7. National Kidney Foundation. K/DOQI clinical practice guidelines for chronic kidney disease; evaluation, classification, and stratification. *Am J Kidney Dis.* 2002;39 (2 suppl 1):S1–S164.

8. Akers S, Groh-Wargo S. Normal nutrition during infancy. In: Queen Samour P, King K, eds. *Handbook of Pediatric Nutrition.* 3rd ed. Lake Dallas TX: Helm Publishing: 2005.

9. Tom A, McCauley L, Bell L, et al. Growth during maintenance hemodialysis: impact of enhanced nutrition and clearance. *J Pediatr.* 1999;134:464–471.

10. Rees L, Shaw V. Nutrition in children with CRF and on dialysis. *Pediatr Nephrol.* 2007;22:1689–1702.

11. Nelms C, Juarez M, Warady B. *Renal Disease.* 2015 A.S.P.E.N. Available at: www.nutritioncare.org. Accessed October 2017.

12. Mahan JD, Warady BA. Assessment and treatment of short stature in pediatric patients with chronic kidney disease: a consensus statement. *Pediatr Nephrol.* 2006;21:917–930.

13. Fischbach M, Fothergill H, Seuge L, Saloszyc A. Dialysis strategies to improve growth in children with chronic kidney disease. *J Ren Nutr.* 2011;21(1):43–46.

14. Baumgartner RN, Roche AF, Himes JH. Incremental growth tables: supplementary to previously published charts. *Am J Clin Nutr.* 1986;43:711–722.

15. Foster BJ, Leonard MB. Measuring nutritional status in children with chronic kidney disease. *Am J Clin Nutr.* 2004;80:801–814.

16. Scollard T. Malnutrition and Nutrition-Focused Physical Assessment: Practical Methods to Start and Move Your Clinical Practice Forward. Utah Academy of Nutrition and Dietetics Annual Meeting, Provo, UT. Available at: http://www.eatrightutah.org/docs/AM15-Speaker2-04b.pdf. Accessed October 2017.

17. Shapiro A, Bandini L, Kurtin P. Estimating energy requirements for children with renal disease: a comparison of methods. *J Am Diet Assoc.* 1992;92:571–573.

18. IOM. Food and Nutrition Board: *Dietary Reference Intakes for Energy, Carbohydrate, Fiber, Fat, Fatty Acids, Cholesterol, Protein, and Amino Acids (Macronutrients).* Food and Nutrition Board. Washington, DC; National Academics: 2005.

19. Foreman JW, Abitbol CL, Trachtman H, et al. Nutritional intake in children with renal insufficiency: a report of the growth failure in children with renal disease study. *J Am Coll Nutr.* 1996;15:579–585.

20. National Kidney Foundation. KDOQI clinical practice guidelines for cardiovascular disease in dialysis patients. *Am J Kidney Dis.* 2005;45(suppl 3):S1–S154.

21. Vannucchi MTI, Vannucchi H, Humphreys M. Serum levels of vitamin A and ertinol binding protein in chronic renal patients treated by continuous ambulatorial peritoneal dialysis. *Int J Vitam Nutr Res.* 1992;62:107–112.

22. Mason NA, Boyd SM. Drug nutrient interactions in renal failure. *J Ren Nutr.* 1995;5:214–222.
23. Bunchman, T, Wood E, Schenck M, Weaver K, Klein B, Lynch R. Pretreatment of formula with sodium polystyrene sulfonate to reduce dietary potassium intake. *Pediatr Nephrol.* 1991;5:29–32.
24. Wesseling K, Bakkaloglu S, Salusky I. Chronic kidney disease mineral and bone disorder in children. *Pediatr Nephrol.* 2008;23:195–207.

Alternate Study Questions

1. Give an example of a PES of this initial assessment of AB.

2. Identify lab values that indicate bone disease.

3. Would you consider growth hormone for a 17 year old female?

4. What stage does AB fall into of Chronic Kidney Disease (CKD)?

5. What food/beverages in AB's diet indicate excessive phosphorus intake?

6. What medication along with diet counseling would help in lowering AB's phosphorus level?

7. What vitamin or minerals would you recommend for supplementation?

8. How would you identify if the dietary interventions were working? What monitoring and evaluation would you recommend?

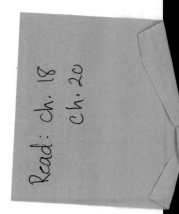

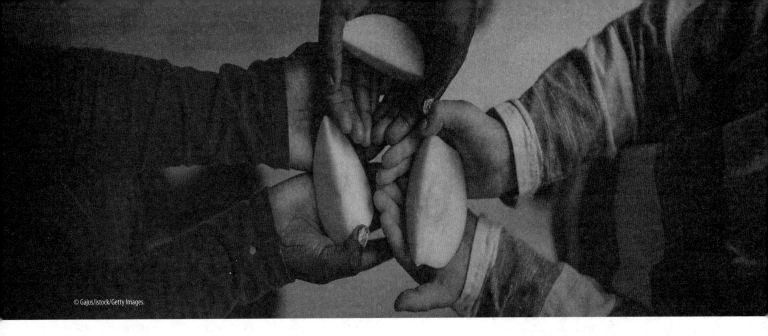

© Gajus/istock/Getty Images.

CHAPTER 19

Nutrition for Burned Pediatric Patients

Michele Morath Gottschlich and Christina A. Sunderman

LEARNING OBJECTIVES

- Review the pathophyisiologic response to a burn injury and its nutritional implications.
- Discuss the methods for determining energy needs along with macro and micronutrient requirements.
- Identify the optimal methods for feeding a pediatric burn patient and nutritional monitoring to assess tolerance and adequacy.

▶ Introduction

Burn injuries are one of the most common and devastating forms of trauma and are a major cause of mortality in children. They are also the most hypermetabolic of all traumatic injuries and pose a complex nutritional challenge. As such, an important determinant of outcome is adequacy of energy and nutrient provision. If nutriture becomes impaired, wound healing and organ function will suffer, along with the deterioration of immune defenses and profound catabolism of lean body mass and bone tissue.

The purpose of this chapter is to discuss metabolic changes, physiologic deficiencies, and nutritional requirements of burned infants and children. Because the common denominator to which all nutrients are related is adequacy of energy intake, methods for evaluating caloric requirements will be emphasized. The optimal profile of macro and micronutrients to meet burn-specific needs will be reviewed, along with the safest and most efficacious methods of providing nutrition support to meet those needs. Nutritional assessment and monitoring practices of the pediatric burn patient will be addressed as well as modifications to the nutrition care plan that occur with convalescence into the rehabilitative phase of care.

▶ Anatomic and Physiologic Considerations

Pediatric burn injury has a high mortality rate, compared with that of adults with equivalent burns,[1,2] although outcome has clearly improved with advancements in burn care.[3] The higher incidence of complications in pediatric burn patients is partially attributable to the fact that the unique physical and metabolic features of infants and children are frequently overlooked. It is important to recognize that providing medical nutrition therapy to a pediatric burn patient often presents a separate and much more complex therapeutic problem than does his or her adult counterpart.

Although the older child rapidly approaches the physical and metabolic makeup of the adult and responds to injury and treatment in a corresponding fashion, specialized nutritional care is required by younger age groups due to their anatomic and physiologic immaturity (**TABLE 19.1**). It is a special challenge to meet obligatory growth needs because of the unique catabolic state of a burn injury. Bone growth is slowed during the acute phase postburn[4] and height and weight gain velocities have not demonstrated significant catch-up growth during the first 3 years following a burn injury.[5,6]

A burned child, with more limited endogenous reserves and greater caloric and protein requirements than an adult, quickly reaches negative nitrogen balance with a smaller area of burn. Furthermore, the functional immaturity of the infant's gastrointestinal tract and renal system[6–8] poses a unique challenge to his or her ability to tolerate nonvolitional feeding regimens and nutrient-dense products. These functional limitations can make infants extremely susceptible to diarrhea, dehydration, and malnutrition, which can only worsen the degree of catabolism.

Metabolic Manifestations of Thermal Injury

Extensive burn injury initiates the most marked alterations in body metabolism that can be associated with any other type of illness or trauma. The pattern of physiologic events following a thermal injury falls into two phases: the ebb response and the flow response.[9,10] The initial, or ebb, response of the burn syndrome is short, lasting 3 to 5 days postinjury. This phase is characterized by general hypometabolism and is manifested by reductions in oxygen consumption, cardiac output, blood pressure, and body temperature (**TABLE 19.2**). Fluid resuscitation is conducted during this time in response to the tremendous integumentary fluid losses that occur during the early postburn period.

With the resuscitative restoration of circulatory blood volume, the body advances to a prolonged state of hypermetabolism and increased nutrient turnover,

TABLE 19.1 Anatomic and Physiologic Immaturities of Children of Various Ages

System	Deficit	Clinical Implications	Age of Maturation
Renal	Glomerular immaturity Young kidneys inefficient in excretion of sodium chloride and other ions, as well as in water resorption	Renal concentrating ability low; therefore, more water required to excrete the renal solute load produced by the metabolism of protein and electrolytes	1–2 years
Gastrointestinal	Immature tract Limited surface area of the small intestinal mucosa Decreased gastric volume capacity	Limited capacity to digest or assimilate some nutrients Prone to antigen absorption High incidence of diarrhea	1–2 years
Temperature regulation	Labile system Surface area/body weight ratio greatly increased	Increased radiant and evaporative heat loss Increased metabolic rate in an attempt to maintain core temperature	10–12 years
Integument	Thin skin	Heat penetrates more rapidly, with resultant deeper burn	16–18 years

TABLE 19.2 Metabolic Alterations Following Burns

| | | Flow Response | |
	Ebb Response	**Acute Phase**	**Adaptive Phase**
Dominant changes	Reduced plasma volume Shock Low plasma insulin Elevating stress hormone levels	Elevated catecholamines Elevated glucagon Elevated glucocorticoids Normal or elevated insulin High glucagon-to-insulin ratio	Stress hormone levels subsiding Hypermetabolism resolving
Clinical signs	Hypovolemia Hyperglycemia Reduced oxygen consumption Tissue hypoxia Depressed resting energy expenditure Decreased cardiac output Impaired glucose tolerance Decreased body temperature	Catabolism Hypermetabolism Hyperglycemia Mobilization of metabolic reserves Accelerated gluconeogenesis Mobilization of metabolic reserves Accelerated gluconeogenesis Elevated respiratory rate Increased oxygen consumption Increased body temperature Increased cardiac output Redistribution of polyvalent cations, such as zinc and iron Increased urinary excretion of nitrogen, sulphur, magnesium, phosphorus, and potassium Immunosuppression	Anabolism Restoration of endogenous protein stores Normoglycemia Wound healing Convalescence

termed the flow phase. This second phase is influenced by elevations in circulating levels of catecholamines,[11,12] glucocorticoids,[13–15] and glucagon.[16–20] Insulin levels are usually in the normal range or even elevated. The rise in the glucagon/insulin ratio,[15–18] in combination with other hormonal derangements, initiates gluconeogenesis, lipolysis, and protein degradation. Hypermetabolism and hypercatabolism have been shown to vary with the time postburn.[19] The classic studies of Wilmore and colleagues [15] demonstrated that, following the ebb phase, catabolic hormone production and oxygen consumption increase dramatically, peaking between the 6th and 10th day postburn[16–19] Thereafter, the metabolic rate slowly begins to decrease, and a gradual recession of catabolism occurs. These metabolic and hormonal sequelae have important implications from a nutritional perspective.

Fluid Requirements

Altered capillary permeability results in the escape of fluid, electrolytes, and protein from the vascular compartment to the interstitial area surrounding the burn wound. The injured area also loses its ability to act as a barrier to water evaporation. In children, with their relatively larger surface area per weight, the insensible water loss is of critical magnitude. Infants and young children are particularly susceptible to dehydration because of their considerably higher obligatory urinary and insensible water losses, compared with those of adults. Children also require more fluid per square meter of body surface area than do adults with burns.[20]

Hemodynamic dysfunction as a consequence of fluid shifts necessitates prompt provision of intravenous fluid resuscitation in order to restore tissue blood flow and to prevent shock following a burn injury.[20,21]

The most commonly used pediatric fluid replacement formula is the Parkland formula,[21] modified for children (**TABLE 19.3**). The modified Parkland formula includes a factor for basal fluid needs, in addition to compensation for losses from the burn wound. The application of this formula should be used in conjunction with assessment

---

TABLE 19.3 Pediatric Fluid Calculations for Resuscitation and Maintenance

I. Resuscitation

   A. Calculated resuscitation + basal requirement (less than 2 yrs: 2000 cc/m^2 BSA)

      1. (4 cc × _____ kg × _____ % burn) + (1500 cc × _____ m^2 BSA)

        (_____) + (_____) = _____ cc/24 hours

   B. Resuscitation fluid per 8 hours

      1. 1st 8 hours: give ½ of total calculated cc/24 hours

      2. 2nd 8 hours: give ¼ of total calculated cc/24 hours

      3. 3rd 8 hours: give ¼ of total calculated cc/24 hours

II. Maintenance Fluids

   A. Basal fluid requirement: 1500 cc/m^2 BSA (less than 2 yrs: 2000 cc/m^2 BSA)

      1. Total body surface area _____ m^2 BSA

      2. 24 hours _____ cc

   B. Evaporative water loss

      1. Adults: (25 + % burn) m^2 BSA = cc/hr

        Children: (35 + % burn) m^2 BSA = cc/hr

      2. Calculated evaporative water loss

        a. (_____ + _____ % burn) _____ m^2 BSA = _____ cc/hr;

        _____ cc/24 hours

   C. Total maintenance fluids = basal requirement + evaporate water loss

      1. 24 hours _____ cc

      2. Hourly _____ cc

Example calculation for a 7-year-old patient weighing 25kg, with a 45% TBSA burn, 0.95 m^2 BSA

I. Resuscitation

   A. Calculated resuscitation + basal requirement

      1. (4 cc × 25 kg × 45% burn) + (1500 cc × 0.95 m^2 BSA)

        (4500 cc) + (1425 cc) = 5925 cc/24 hours

   B. Resuscitation fluid per 8 hours

      1. 1st 8 hours: give ½ of total calculated cc/24 hours = 2962 cc, 370 cc/hr

      2. 2nd 8 hours: give ¼ of total calculated cc/24 hours = 1481 cc, 185 cc/hr

      3. 3rd 8 hours: give ¼ of total calculated cc/24 hours = 1481 cc, 185 cc/hr

II. Maintenance Fluids

   A. Basal fluid requirement: 1500 cc/m^2 BSA

      1. Total body surface area 0.95 m^2 BSA

      2. 24 hours 1425 cc

   B. Evaporative water loss

      1. Adults: (25 + % burn) × m^2 BSA = cc/hr

        Children: (35 + % burn) × m^2 BSA = cc/hr

      2. Calculated evaporative water loss

        a. (35 + 45% burn) × 0.95 m^2 BSA = 76 cc/hr; 1824 cc/24 hours

   C. Total maintenance fluids = basal requirement + evaporate water loss

      1. 24 hours: 1425 cc + 1824 cc = 3249 cc/24 hours

      2. Hourly: 3249 cc/24 hours = 135 cc/hr

Abbreviations: BSA, body surface area; TBSA, total body surface area.
Data from Courtesy of the Shriners Hospitals for Children, Cincinnati, Ohio.

of the patient's vital signs, blood pressure, and urinary output to determine adequacy of fluid replacement.

Caloric Requirements

Burn injuries create a pathophysiological stress response that results in a hypermetabolic state that can persist for years. The degree of hypermetabolism is generally related to the size of the burn,[19,22] with a peak in energy expenditure at approximately 50% total body surface area (TBSA). The root cause of hypermetabolism continues to be an active area of investigation, however, a number of studies support the role of cytokines in postburn metabolism.[22-25] Following injury, cytokines appear to produce neuromediators that activate endocrine organs to produce higher concentrations of catecholamines, epinephrine, glucagon, and cortisol, which can lead to the breakdown and depletion of endogenous reserves and inhibit protein synthesis.[13,22-25]

Sleep pattern disturbance has also been suggested as a factor contributing to increased metabolism following burn injury.[26] Elevations in catabolic hormones have been reported following sleep deprivation.[27,28] Furthermore, specific to burns, Gottschlich et al. report an inverse correlation between epinephrine and norepinephrine levels and rapid eye movement stage of sleep, suggesting a neuroendocrine response to lack of sleep as a contributor to postburn hypermetabolism and hypercatabolism.[29] As a metabolic correlation with sleep is increasingly established, nightly promotion of uninterrupted sleep, with attention to duration and quality, should be viewed as an intricate component of the care plan.

Wound coverage and infection control[30] are currently the primary means of decreasing metabolic rate. However, sufficient pain and anxiety control are crucial means of reducing metabolism in the pediatric population as well. The application of a reliable pain scale index is vital so that severity of pain is understood and therefore treated appropriately. Age-appropriate explanations of procedures before performance may appear trivial, but can be extremely beneficial in the reduction of anxiety.

The provision of sufficient calories to meet the increased metabolic expenditure is a critical factor in managing the burned child. Studies support increased energy demands in this population,[31-35] and it has been demonstrated that during stress there is a shift in energy expenditure for growth to that needed for acute illness and healing. The hypermetabolic demand and increase in energy requirements result in the mobilization of carbohydrate, protein, and fat stores. Endogenous reserves can quickly become depleted which leads to delayed wound healing, immune dysfunction, and malnutrition. Estimation of energy needs to determine that the appropriate nutrition regimen is imperative in the pediatric burn patient.

A number of pediatric energy equations have been applied successfully in the pediatric burn population. (**TABLE 19.4**).

The wide range of formulas for calculating energy needs indicates the uncertainties of this approach. Most mathematic derivations utilize body weight, age, and burn size as the only determinants of caloric requirements. Although these three factors represent significant effectors of metabolic rate, energy expenditure is also influenced by surgery, pain, anxiety, sepsis, body composition, gender, thermal effect of food, sleep deprivation, and physical activity. Therefore, mathematic formulas could derive fairly inaccurate caloric goals, considering the variability among individuals.[31,33-35] If caloric needs are underestimated, both endogenous reserves and exogenous substrates will be consumed for energy. Although it is important to provide pediatric burn patients with the energy needed to compensate for hypermetabolism,

TABLE 19.4 Formulas for Calculating Energy Requirements of Burned Children			
Reference	**Age**	**%TBSA Burned**	**Calories/Day**
Curreri[36]	0–1 yr	< 50	Basal + (15 × % BSAB)
	1–3 yr	< 50	Basal + (25 × % BSAB)
	4–15 yr	< 50	Basal + (40 × % BSAB)
Davies and Liljedal[37]	Child	Any	60W + (35 × % BSAB)
Hildreth[31-33]	< 15 yr	> 30	(1800/m² BSA) + (2200/m² burn)
Hildreth[34]	< 12 yr		(1800/m² BSA) + (1300/m² burn)
Mayes[35]	0–3 yr	10–50	108 + 68W + (3.9 × % BSAB)
			818 + 37.4W + (9.3 × % BSAB)

Abbreviations: W, weight in kg; BSA, body surface area burn; TBSA, total body surface area.

as well as for growth and development, caution must also be taken against the delivery of an overabundance of calories. Administering a surfeit of calories has been associated with increased metabolic rate, hyperglycemia, liver abnormalities and an increase in carbon dioxide production which can compromise respiratory function.[38-40]

Indirect calorimetry is considered the gold standard in assessing energy expenditure in pediatric burn patients. Using indirect calorimetry in burn care has been extensively reviewed elsewhere.[38] The patient's caloric goal should be calculated at 120–130% of the **measured resting energy expenditure** (MREE).[40-42] Although some degree of error is possible with this extrapolation, it is more accurate than mathematical formulas based solely on weight, age, and burn size. To ensure the clinical validity of this goal, tests must be repeated regularly and because hypermetabolism undergoes transient variation during the acute phase, it is recommended that indirect calorimetry be conducted twice weekly, at minimum, for proper adjustment of the nutritional support regimen.[9]

Carbohydrate Requirements

Metabolic changes that accompany a thermal injury include deranged carbohydrate metabolism characterized by glycolysis, glycogenolysis, and impaired tissue uptake.[9,10] In the acute phase post burn, hyperglycemia is primarily caused by decreased peripheral tissue utilization in lieu of impaired tissue perfusion and low insulin levels.[43-46] Glucose intolerance typically persists as a result of enhanced hepatic glucose production and gluconeogenesis.[44,45]

Carbohydrate plays an important role in the nutritional support of the burned child. It appears to be the most important nonprotein calorie source in terms of nitrogen retention in burned patients,[47] although a limit exists to its effectiveness as an energy source.[43,48] Carbohydrates stimulate endogenous insulin production, which can have an anabolic effect on muscle and burn wounds. However, excessive glucose loads can have detrimental effects such as an increase in carbon dioxide production, heightened glucose intolerance, and induced hepatic fat deposition.[49,50] Therefore, the maximum rate at which glucose should be utilized is 5mg/kg/min in pediatric burn patients, with close monitoring for hypercapnia and hyperglycemia.[51,52]

Exogenous insulin administration is often necessary to improve blood glucose levels and to achieve maximal glucose utilization. Intensive insulin therapy that maintains blood glucose levels significantly below previous thresholds has been correlated with reduced morbidity and mortality in critical care.[53-61] As a result, insulin protocols are increasingly supported in the burn intensive care unit and have been associated with improved outcomes.[56-59]

Protein Requirements

Amino acid metabolism after a burn injury is characterized by extreme proteolysis and urea synthesis.[9,19] Protein is an important substrate necessary for wound healing, immune function, and to minimize the loss of lean body mass.[8,62-66] The protein requirements of the burned infant and child are elevated because of accelerated tissue breakdown and exudative losses during a period of rapid repair and growth.[63] Additionally, alterations in skeletal muscle protein catabolism can persist for up to a year post burn[62] Failure to meet heightened protein needs can yield suboptimal clinical results in terms of wound healing and resistance to infection.[46,63] The infant and child further adapt to inadequate protein intake by curtailing growth of cells, conceivably sacrificing genetic potential.

Studies have shown that enteral fortification using large quantities of protein can accelerate the synthesis of visceral proteins and promote positive nitrogen balance and host defense factors.[43,63-65] Alexander and colleagues[63] demonstrated that severely burned children on enteral diets containing approximately 22% of calories as protein had higher levels of total serum protein, retinol-binding protein, prealbumin, transferrin, C3, and immunoglobulin G (IgG), and better nitrogen balance than patients receiving 15% of calories as protein. Additionally, the high-protein group had improved survival and fewer episodes of bacteremia. Therefore, it is imperative that a high protein diet or nutrition support regimen be an integral component of the pediatric burn patient's medical nutrition therapy plan.

Patients greater than 6 months of age with burns in excess of 30% TBSA should receive 20–23% of calories as protein. This translates to 2.5–4.0g/kg, for a nonprotein calorie/nitrogen ratio of 80:1. The safe provision of this level of protein in those less than 3 years of age has been documented with evidence correlating decreased length of stay.[8,9,43,63,65] Protein repletion, assuming an adequate intake of energy can be further optimized by utilizing high-quality, intact whey protein.

Close monitoring of protein intake is necessary because excessive protein loads or amino acid imbalances may result in azotemia, hyperammonemia, or acidosis. Particular care must be taken when administering high-protein feedings to children younger than 12 months of age because large amounts can have adverse effects on immature or compromised kidneys. Ongoing assessment of fluid status, **blood urea nitrogen** (BUN), plasma proteins, and nitrogen balance is recommended for individual evaluation of tolerance and adequacy. However, when fluid intake is adequate, pathways of intermediary metabolism are relatively mature and renal or hepatic dysfunction does not exist, a high-protein diet is usually tolerated well.

Glutamine & Arginine Skeletal muscle and organ efflux of arginine and glutamine are increased after a burn injury.

Glutamine is a conditionally essential amino acid that is rapidly exhausted from muscle and serum postburn. It serves as a direct fuel to the lymphocyte and enterocytes and is essential for maintaining small bowel integrity and preserving gut associated immune function.[67-69] Glutamine has also been shown to promote protein synthesis and wound healing and help modulate the degree of immunosuppression.[69] There is not a current consensus on the dose, route, and administration of glutamine; however, a number of studies have shown a therapeutic range between 0.3–0.5g/kg/day for >3–5days.[51,70] Arginine is another important conditionally essential amino acid because it stimulates T lymphocytes and accelerates nitric oxide synthesis which may help improve resistance to infection.[71-73] There is also some evidence that supplementation of arginine in burn patients can lead to an improvement in wound healing and immunosuppression[72,73]; however, there are not any current guidelines on dosage and administration at this time.

Fat Requirements

Burn-mediated increases in catecholamine and glucagon levels stimulate an accelerated rate of fat mobilization and oxidation.[9,10] Lipid is an important fuel in the diet of the burned child because of its high caloric density, its role in the myelination of nerve cells and brain development and its action in the transport of fat soluble vitamins.[19,74-77] Additionally, fat in the form of the essential fatty acid linoleate provides vital components for cellular membranes and is a precursor for dienoic prostaglandin synthesis[74-76]

An overabundance of exogenous lipid can be detrimental to recovery from burns.[74] Complications ascribed to excessive fat intake include lipemia, fatty liver, diarrhea, and decreased resistance to infection.[74-79] Furthermore, lipid appears to represent an inefficient source of calories for maintaining nitrogen equilibrium and lean body mass following major injury.[74,75,79] Therefore, conservative administration of fat, particularly linoleic acid, given its immunosuppressive metabolites, is recommended for burned children greater than 6 months of age.[9,43,74] The minimimum requirement for linoleic acid needed to prevent omega-6 fatty acid deficiency is considered to be approximately 2–3% of calories consumed.

This requirement is usually not difficult to accomplish because most enteral feeding supplements and intravenous fat emulsions contain high levels of fat and linoleic acid.[43,76,78,79]

Given its competitive effects on the down-regulation of linoleic acid, provision of omega-3 fatty acid, a proven anti-inflammatory and immune-enhancing agent, is recommended.[76-79]

Micronutrient Requirements

The post burn inflammatory response can result in heightened oxidative stress and depletion of antioxidant defenses, which are dependant on micronutrients. Vitamin and mineral requirements escalate with the severity of thermal injury and are related to increased protein catabolism, enhanced energy expenditure and increased losses via the wounds.[80,81] Decreased levels of Vitamins A, C, D, and Fe, Cu, Se, and Zn have been identified to impair wound healing and immune function.[80-83] The specific functions of each vitamin and trace element pertinent to burn injury have been summarized elsewhere.[73,86,87]

A deficiency of vitamins and minerals can compromise reparative processes, and oral, tube feeding, and intravenous hyperalimentation regimens frequently do not meet these heightened needs for certain micronutrients. Thus, it is recommended that additional supplementation be provided,[80-83] especially of those vitamins and trace elements associated with energy expenditure, wound healing, immune function, bone mineral density, coagulation, and those likely to have enhanced urinary and wound losses. Thiamine, riboflavin, niacin, folate, biotin, vitamin K, magnesium, phosphorus, chromium, and manganese are all cofactors for energy-dependent processes. The requirement for pyridoxine is closely related to dietary protein intake and protein metabolism. Furthermore, inadequacy of many micronutrients, particularly vitamins A, C, E, and zinc, copper, and iron can adversely affect immune function.[81-83] Iron supplementation, however, remains controversial because excessive iron administration may enhance susceptibility to infection.[88] Optimal vitamin and mineral intake for the burned child remains to be determined because requirements vary based on size and degree of burn and also on the patient's preburn status. Daily intakes of a multivitamin and supplemental vitamins A, C, D, and zinc (**TABLE 19.5**) are often recommended because of their important roles in the wound healing process. Vitamin A decreases time of wound healing via increased epithelial growth and vitamin C aids in the creation and cross-linking of collagen.[80,81] Zinc is also important for its role in protein synthesis and lymphocyte function.[89,90] Intravenous vitamin K can be used as a therapeutic agent to help control excessive bleeding following burns and burn surgeries in the post-operative period.[91] Although select vitamin and mineral replacement in excess of RDAs appears to be justified in burned children, some micronutrients, particularly fat-soluble vitamins, can be toxic in large amounts. Thus, all micronutrients should be administered judiciously.

Vitamin D A high incidence of hypovitaminosis D has been demonstrated in pediatric burn patients.[4,85-87] Evidence also suggests a high rate of bone demineralization and increased risk of fractures in the acute postburn phase.[85] Burn patients are at risk for bone disease for a variety of reasons including extended bedrest, institutionalization, increased glucocorticoids, decreased growth hormone, and reduced serum cholesterol, a precursor of vitamin D.[84-87,91] Vitamin D depletion is an

TABLE 19.5 Vitamin and Trace Mineral Recommendations

Children and adolescents (3 years or older)

1. Major burn (> 20% TBSA)
   - One multivitamin daily
   - 500mg ascorbic acid twice daily*
   - 220mg zinc sulfate daily*
   - 1600IU vitamin D$_3$ daily
2. Minor burn (< 20%) or reconstructive patient
   - One multivitamin daily

Children (less than 3 years of age)

1. Major burn (> 20% TBSA)
   - One children's multivitamin daily
   - 250mg ascorbic acid twice daily*
   - 100mg zinc sulfate daily*
   - 800IU vitamin D$_3$ daily
2. Minor burn (< 20%) or reconstructive patient
   - One multivitamin daily

*Delivery should be in suspension for tube feeding because oral vitamin C and zinc in large doses may precipitate nausea or vomiting.

Data from Gottschlich MM, Warden GD. Vitamin supplementation in the burn patient. *J Burn Care Rehabil*. 1990;11:275–279.[80]

Hein GL, Rodriguez NA, Branksi K, Herndon D. Vitamin and trace element homeostasis following severe burn injury. In Herndon DN, ed. *Total Burn Care*. London:WB Saunders. 2012:321–324.[81]

Berger MM. Antioxidant micronutrients in major trauma and burns: evidence and practice. *Nutr Clin Practice*. 2006;21(5):438–439.[82]

Berger MM, Binnert C, Chiolero RL, et al. Trace element supplementation after major burns increases burned skin trace element concentrations and modulates local protein metabolism, but not whole-body substrate metabolism. *Am J Clin Nutr*. 2007;85(5):1301–1306.[83]

Caldis-Courtis N, Gawaziuk J, Logsetty S. Zinc supplementation in burn patients. *J Burn Care Res*. 2012;33(5):678–682.[89]

Khorasani G, Hosseinimehr S, Kaghazi Z. The alteration of plasma's zinc and copper levels in patients with burn injuries and the relationship to time after burn injuries. *Singapore Med J*. 2008;49(8):627–630.[90]

additional causative factor and the most effective means to treat this acute deficiency appears to be supplemental vitamin D$_3$; however, the effects of such treatment on outcomes is unknown.[87,91-93] Additionally, vitamin D depletion has been reported well into convalescence, potentially impacting long-term bone growth and development in pediatric burns.[85,93-95]

Nutritional Intervention Strategies

The goal of nutritional support for the pediatric burn patient is to provide adequate calories and nutrients to facilitate wound healing, maximize immunocompetence, maintain or improve organ function, and prevent loss of lean body mass. Specific objectives vary, according to the underlying metabolic and nutritional status of each patient and special considerations are indicated whenever fluid restriction, organ failure, septicemia, mechanical ventilation, or any other presenting comorbidities limit the ability to administer vital nutrients.

Small Burn Area (Less Than 20%)

Small burns (less than 20% surface area) not complicated by facial injury, psychologic problems, inhalation injury, or preburn malnutrition can usually be supported by an oral high-protein, high-calorie diet. Between-meal snacks should be encouraged and commercial high calorie/high protein oral supplements or the addition of nutrient modules to menu selections may be helpful in optimizing the marginal intake of calories and protein.

Larger Surface Burns (More Than 20%)

Children with burns covering a larger surface area (20% or more) generally cannot meet their nutrient requirements by oral intake alone. In these cases, alternative forms of supplemental nutrition are warranted. For those patients who are able to tolerate an oral diet, but unable to meet their increased nutrient needs, a post-pyloric feeding tube should be placed with an enteral nutrition regimen to supplement their nutritional intake. Strict monitoring of intake and outputs and daily calorie counts can serve as useful tools in assessing the adequacy of both oral intake and nutrition support. As the patient's oral intake improves and nutrient needs decrease with wound healing and closure, the child can gradually be weaned from the tube feeding regimen. Initially, tube feedings can be held for two hours around mealtime to stimulate appetite; however, once the patient demonstrates the ability to consume 25–50% of caloric needs by mouth, the enteral regimen program may changed to a nocturnal cycle to run for 10–12 hours. When the patient is able to meet approximately 75% or greater of their caloric needs orally, tube feedings can then be discontinued and full reliance on an oral diet can commence.

Enteral Nutrition

Enteral nutrition is the preferred route of support because it helps to maintain the structural and functional integrity of the gastrointestinal tract,[9,43,51,64,67,96,97] thus minimizing the risk of bacterial translocation.[43,51,96-98] Enteral alimentation that bypasses the stomach and uses the functional small intestine is desirable because it can decrease the risk of aspiration. Small bowel feedings also minimize potential interruptions of the nutrition regimen, thereby maximizing nutrient intake. Feeding tube placement into the third portion of the duodenum is recommended and can be a safe means of enteral nutritional support, even during critical periods such as resuscitation, surgery, anesthesia for major dressing changes, or septic ileus.[98-100]

Gastric feedings are not supported for a number of reasons in burn patients, including the fact that postburn gastric ileus can inhibit the initial advancement and full-volume delivery of enteral feedings. Additionally, the multiple position changes (for example, prone and neck hyperextension) that patients undergo for dressing changes, physical therapy, and operative procedures increase the aspiration risk when they are fed nasogastrically. Gastric feedings also potentiate limited oral intake because the patient minimally experiences hunger.

Once a small bowel feeding tube is placed, determining the correct time to initiate a tube feeding regimen requires great consideration. Enteral nutrition support should commence as soon as possible, ideally within the first 24 hours post-burn.[51] Significant nutrient deficits can develop when alimentation is delayed following thermal injury, which can have a direct bearing on morbidity and mortality. Early and aggressive enteral support has been associated with improved tube feeding tolerance and sustained bowel mucosal integrity[96,97,101–105] When tube feeding is initiated within the first few hours postburn, the hypermetabolic response can be partially suppressed, as evidenced by decreased energy expenditure and improvements in measurements of nitrogen balance, visceral proteins, and catabolic hormones.[63,101–104]

Gottschlich and colleagues evaluated the effects of early versus delayed enteral feeding on various outcomes postburn.[105] Patients were randomized to receive enteral feedings within 24 hours (study group) or 48 hours (control group) of burn injury. Results indicated that early feeding reduced cumulative caloric deficits and potentially stimulated insulin secretion while conserving lean body mass. Feeding within 24 hours of injury did not limit postburn hypermetabolism, nor did it improve nutritional status, reduce infection, or decrease hospital stay. Some question the definition of early feeding (initiated within 24 hours) applied in this study. Perhaps benefit would have been increasingly apparent if nutrition support was initiated within a few hours of insult or if the control group delayed feeds for a greater period of time. Nevertheless, this is the only prospective clinical feeding trial of its nature in pediatric burns. Additional studies are recommended to establish feeding times that maximize clinical benefit and minimize morbid outcomes.

Providing early enteral nutrition during burn shock rescuscitation continues to be controversial and warrants close monitoring of hemodynamic parameters and gastrointestinal tolerance. Riegel and associates examined the effects of fluid resuscitation, inotrope use, and early feeding on the development of bowel necrosis.[106] He found that patients who sustained bowel necrosis required more fluid resuscitation during burn shock and tended to have prolonged (greater than 24 to 48 hours) burn shock. This subgroup of patients required higher doses of dopamine and tended to receive dopamine more frequently during burn shock rescuscitation. Initiation of enteral feeds within 24 hours of insult did not

increase the incidence of bowel necrosis; however, it did demonstrate that patients who are underresuscitated and require inotropic support greater than renal dose dopamine should be monitored for bowel necrosis during the postresuscitation phase. Additionally, there is some evidence that supports trophic enteral feeds are safe and shoud be employed for this subpopulation until fluid rescuscitation is complete and hemodynamic stability is achieved.[107]

Because burn patients usually have unscathed digestive and absorptive capabilities, products containing intact nutrients should be used. Elemental or dipeptide formulations are unnecessary, unless dictated by concomitant disease or anatomic anomalies, and appear to yield less favorable results in burns.[108–110] Most tube feedings can be started at full strength and the initial hourly infusion rate should begin at approximately half of the final desired volume and be increased by 5mL/hour in the infant and toddler, 10mL/hour in the school-age child, and 20mL/hour in the teenager, as tolerated, until the final hourly goal rate is achieved. Enteral nutrition support should be continued until positive wound healing progression is demonstrated and/or they are able to meet estimated nutrient needs with an oral diet alone.

The composition of the enteral infusate should take into account the unique metabolic and age-related alterations in nutrient utilization that accompany an extensive burn injury. Suggested tube feeding regimens for pediatric burn patients can be divided into two major categories: (1) formulas appropriate for children younger than 6 months of age and (2) formulas for patients 6 months of age or older.

Enteral protocols for infants less than 6 months of age are generally conservative, relying on commercial infant formulas. The normal dilution of infant formula is 20kcal/oz (0.66 kcal/mL). To better meet the increased calorie and protein needs of a burn injury, the concentration of the infant formula can be gradually advanced to 22–24kcal/oz. Further progression to 27–30 kcal/oz to meet the infant's energy needs must be monitored carefully, due to the resulting increased renal solute load. Additionally, nutritional support regimens containing significantly reduced fat content are likewise not routinely recommended during infancy (<6mos) because fat is an extremely important nutrient during the period of central nervous system maturation.

The protein content of infant formulas ranges from 9% to 12% of total calories. This level is sometimes insufficient for those with larger (>20% TBSA) burns, so adding a protein module to the infant formula may be indicated in such cases if biochemical indices are carefully monitored. Infant formulas derived from soy protein should not be used unless casein or whey intolerances have been confirmed, because the biologic value of soy protein is less than that of animal protein.

Tube feeding products for children over 6 months of age can generally be selected from formularies established for adults. The coincident fluid needs and energy requirements normally result in utilizing a tube feeding concentration of 30kcal/oz or 1kcal/mL. According to established guidelines, if the tube feeding formula is low in protein, it should be enriched with modular protein to yield 20–25% of total calories.[8,9,51,63,67,73,105]

Specialized enteral nutrition formulas continue to be developed in order to meet the nutrient demands of critical illness and disease; however, to date, there aren't any that specifically address the unique needs of a burn injury. The burn patient population has atypical nutritional needs that transcend traditional recommendations for a high-calorie, high-protein solution. Modular tube feeding recipes have been developed that not only take into consideration energy and quantitative protein guidelines, but also currently offer the only means of incorporating findings regarding unique fat, amino acid, vitamin, and mineral requirements.[43,74,100,105] Employment of modular tube feeding prescriptions has been correlated with statistically significant reductions in infection rates and length of hospital stay.[43] However, because complex recipes are not feasible at many institutions, due to the labor intense preparation procedures involved, careful scrutiny of the formulary for a low residue, high-protein, low-fat, omega-3 fatty acid–enriched product is recommended as a practical alternative.[110]

Parenteral Nutrition

During the 1960s and 70s, parenteral nutrition (PN) was routinely used for all burn patients, however, over time, studies have shown that it can be associated wth overfeeding, liver dysfunction, decreased immune response and increased mortality. Additionally, PN has more mechanical and infectious complications of catheters and PN solutions are significantly more expensive than EN formulas.[111-113] As described earlier, utilizing the gastrointestinal tract with EN is the preferred route of nutrition, however, under certain circumstances intravenous feeding can become a necessary, and even lifesaving, part of burn management.

Appropriate indications for intravenous feeding in burns are listed in **TABLE 19.6**. There are two general categories of pediatric patients for whom parenteral nutrition is indicated. The first major category includes youngsters with tube feeding intolerance, protracted diarrhea or malabsorptive issues resulting in significant caloric deficits. Children with gastrointestinal disease or injury form the second group that may require PN. Attempts should be made to administer at least some nutrients enterally via trophic feeds during episodes of diarrhea to help maintain the integrity of the gastrointestinal tract.

Peripheral parenteral support does not provide adequate calories and nitrogen, and the delivery of intravenous nutrients via a central line is necessary in order to promote anabolism in the presence of burns.[112] Standard

TABLE 19.6 Indications for Total Parenteral Nutrition in Burns

- Gastrointestinal trauma
- Curling's ulcer
- Severe pancreatitis
- Superior mesenteric artery syndrome
- Obstructions of the gastrointestinal tract
- Severe vomiting or abdominal distention
- Intractable diarrhea
- Adjunct to insufficient enteral support
- Necrotic bowel

central venous regimens for the thermally injured patient usually consist of a final concentration of 25% dextrose and 5% crystalline amino acids, although individualized balancing is often warranted to avoid overfeeding carbohydrates and underfeeding protein.[52]

If essential fatty acid requirements are being met with trophic enteral feeds, then additional intravenous fat is not warranted. Patients receiving 100% of their energy needs via the parenteral route require administrating modest amounts of intravenous fat. Five hundred milliliters of 10% lipid emulsion (or 250mL of 20% lipid emulsion) infused two to three times weekly will assist in meeting essential fatty acid requirements for patients >6 months of age. The metabolic and mechanical complications of providing parenteral hyperalimentation warrant adherence to strict protocols of infection control, along with continuous monitoring of tolerance. As soon as the gastrointestinal tract can be fed and nutrition advanced to goal, PN should be weaned off in order to minimize the immunosuppression concomitant with its use.[112,113,114]

▶ Nutritional Assessment

Nutritional assessment is the process of identifying an individual's energy and nutrient requirements and evaluating the adequacy of an oral diet or a nutrition support program in meeting these needs. Clinical nutrition protocols for the care of burned children have been published; however, there is little specific information regarding their precise nutritional requirements.[114-116] Therefore, assessing and monitoring patient response to their medical nutrition therapy regimen is especially important, so that the clinician can react to alterations in metabolism that occur over time and reduce the opportunity for complications. Commonly measured variables in this population include anthropometrics, nitrogen balance, lean body mass imaging, and measurement of serum visceral proteins and specific vitamins and minerals.[115] **FIGURES 1** and **2** summarize the nutrition assessment program successfully employed at the Cincinnati Shriners Hospital for Children.

1. Review clinical data
- Age, gender, ethnic background
- Percent of: body surface area that has been burned and thickness of the burn
- Burned body area
- Determine the inhalation injury and the ventilatory status
- Determine the anthropometric data including: weight, height/length, body mass index / weight for length, head circumference (< 3 years)

2. Review Histories
- Medical history, other conditions or illness, gastrointestinal issues
- Social history
- Regularly used medications, vitamin/mineral supplementation
- Concomitant injuries, referring hospital course

3. Review Nutritional Status
- Diet history, food restrictions-allergies, dentition, appetite
- Assess growth parameters, evaluate anthropometric z-scores, nutrition focused physical findings

4. Calculate and assess needs and goals
- Calorie and protein needs
- Vitamin/mineral supplementation recommendations
- Nutrition support goals

5. Determine Intervention
- Oral, enteral, parenteral

6. Initiate Assessment Tool
- Obtain measured resting energy expenditure (Indirect calorimetry) within 24 hours of admission.
- A 24-hour urinary urea collection must be obtained and tested to determine kidney functionality.
- The following must be acquired: renal panel, serum prealbumin, C-Reactive Protein, and serum Vitamin D level
- Take note of the caloric and protein intake of the patient.

Daily:
- Analysis of nutrient intake
- Labs
- BUN/creatinine
- Blood glucose
- Electrolytes
- GI tolerance: nausea, vomiting, diarrhea, constipation, abdominal distention
- Hydration status

Weekly:
- Weight/height/growth assessment
- Labs:
- Vitamin D
- Albumin/pre-albumin
- C-reactive protein
- Nitrogen balance studies
- Measured energy expenditure/metabolic cart studies
- Wound healing assessment

At discharge:
- Follow up nutrition care
- Home going medical nutrition therapy
- Vitamin/mineral supplementation
- Home nutrition education

▶ Conclusion

Nutrition assessment and support are critical aspects of the pediatric burn patient treatment plan. The metabolic dysfunction, physiologic immaturity, and heightened macro and micronutrient needs make feeding this population a nutritional challenge. Burned infants and children present separate and much more complex diet therapy problems compared with their adult counterparts because requirements for growth and development must be considered along with the increased nutrient demands of a burn. Early and aggressive nutrition intervention is of paramount importance in burned children to prevent malnutrition, delayed wound healing and immunoincompetence. Additionally, establishing nutritional assessment and monitoring protocols can help the clinician complete a thorough nutritional review and ensure individualized nutritional needs are being met to support wound healing and growth. Further research and the development of more definitive guidelines are warranted in order to better assist in tailoring medial nutrition therapy regimens to the pediatric burn population.

🔍 CASE STUDY

Nutrition Assessment

TD is a previously healthy 11-month-old female admitted to the intensive care unit. She suffered 40% total body surface area (TBSA) burns, 35% full thickness, when she pulled on the electric cord of a frying pot, tipping the container. The hot liquid splattered over her face, head, neck, and right side of her upper body and thigh.

In anticipation of face and neck swelling over the course of the next few hours, TD is sedated and intubated to maintain oxygen and airway. A nasogastric tube is placed to low wall suction. Her abdomen is soft and nondistended. She is 9kg in weight and 74cm in length. Her intravenous resuscitative fluids are infusing to maintain a urine output of approximately 1.0mL/kg/hour. Past medical history is noncontributory. Labs are initially monitored every 6 hours and electrolyte adjustment, glucose management, blood product replacement, and ventilator therapies are coordinated with respective panel results. A nutrition history from the mother indicated the baby is beginning to wean from the bottle and increasing her intake of baby foods and soft table foods. She accepts a pacifier at afternoon nap and bedtimes. The patient has no known food allergies or intolerances.

Nutrition Intervention

TD's initial goals for calorie, protein, and micronutrients were established. Within 6 hours of admission to the unit, feeding tube placement is confirmed in the upper portion of the duodenum. Given her adequate hydration status and hemodynamic stability (i.e., lack of vasopressor use), tube feeding (TF) rate is initiated at 5mL per hour and advanced every 2 hours by 5mL to a goal of 35mL per hour. The goal TF rate provides 95% of kcal and 103% of protein goals.

TD undergoes surgery six times. Each excision procedure is followed by a 24-hour period of stabilization before donor site harvest and skin grafting over the burned areas. Enteral feeds are continued through surgery to ensure adequate nutritional support throughout the perioperative period.[98-100]

While on mechanical ventilatory support, oral stimulation is provided during physical therapy sessions. As TD progresses and sedation is weaned, a pacifier is provided for comfort as well as oral stimulation. Given her young age, she maintains a high risk for subsequent oral feeding coordination deficiencies due to prolonged NPO status. The pacifier supports skills necessary for eventual oral feeding coordination.

The patient's endotracheal tube is uncuffed so indirect calorimetry is not possible initially; however, once extubated, indirect calorimetry is performed biweekly. The tube feeding rate is adjusted based upon a 30% addition to the resting energy expenditure. This ensures sufficient calories to cover additional metabolic influences such as fever spikes, pain, anxiety, dressing changes, therapy sessions, and the like that are not an inherent component of the test.

Following extubation on postburn day 10, TD is permitted an oral diet. Clear liquids are provided via bottle and accepted well. Gastrointestinal tolerance is deemed appropriate and the diet therefore advanced to regular, age-appropriate provision. As wounds are increasingly covered, appetite improves and tube feedings are tapered. When TD is consuming 20% of the calorie goal consistently for a period of 2 days, feeds are tapered to be held 2 hours at meal times. When her wounds are 95% covered, and she is accepting 80% of her nutrition goal orally, the feeding tube is discontinued.

Monitoring and Evaluation

The enteral regimen is assessed daily for calorie and protein intake and gastrointestinal tolerance. TD's clinical course is evaluated daily for parameters related to nutritional status and regimen tolerance. These include surgery, labs including fluid and electrolytes, infection, antibiotic use, respiratory status, physical therapy gains (e.g., head control, sitting up independently in a high chair, feeding self), and wound status. BUN/creatinine levels are assessed daily to ensure proper balance of fluids/hydration status. Glucose levels and need for insulin supplementation are monitored daily; however, the enteral regimen is not changed when insulin needs are increased. The preference for carbohydrate versus fat calories for wound healing supersedes a regimen change to a higher fat formula in an effort to assist glucose management. As TD's clinical course progresses, the appropriateness of an enteral feeding taper is evaluated daily.

Discharge

On postburn day 39, TD is discharged to home. She has 98% wound coverage. TD is at 95% of her preburn weight. She is eating well, having improved to 90% of her estimated goal, and including a diet similar to that consumed before injury. TD does not require any nutritional supplementation at this time.

Questions for the Reader

1. What are the patient's energy, protein, and micronutrient supplementation needs upon admission to the burn unit (weight 9kg)?
2. What are TD's weight and height percentiles on the WHO growth chart upon admission?
3. Complete a PES statement for this patient.
4. What type of tube feeding product was recommended for TD?
5. What other weekly assessment parameters were closely monitored in TD?
6. What type of nutritional follow-up will TD receive in the outpatient clinic?

Study Questions

1. What are the hallmark physiologic responses of the body during the EBB and FLOW response after a burn injury?

2. What formula is used for fluid resuscitation in pediatric burn patients? What other parameters should be monitored to ensure that hydration needs are being met?

3. What are the drivers of the hypermetabolic response after a burn injury?

4. List the ways to assess a pediatric burn patient's energy needs.

5. Describe the metabolic dysfunction of carbohydrates, protein, and fat after a burn injury.

6. What are the common micronutrients supplemented after a burn injury?

7. What is the role of Vitamin D after a burn injury and why is additional supplementation warranted?

8. What are the perceived benefits of providing early enteral nutrition support?

9. Name three indications for the use of parenteral nutrition support in pediatric burn patients.

10. Name some of the components of a nutrition assessment and monitoring program for pediatric burn patients.

References

1. Kraft R, Herndon DN, Al-Mousawi AM, Williams F, Finnerty C, Jeschke M. Burn size and survival probability in pediatric patients in modern burn care. *Lancet.* 2012;379(9820):1013–1021.

2. Erickson EJ, Merrell SW, Saffle JR, Sullivan JJ. Differences in mortality from thermal injury between pediatric and adult patients. *J Pediatr Surg.* 1991;26:821–825.

3. Sheridan RL, Remensnyder JP, Schnitzer JJ, et al. Current expectations for survival in pediatric burns. *Arch Pediatr Adolesc Med.* 2000;154:245–249.

4. Klein GL. Burn induced bone loss: importance, mechanisms and management. *J Burns Wounds.* 2006;5:e5.

5. Rutan RL, Herndon DN. Growth delay in postburn pediatric patients. *Arch Surg.* 1990;125:392–395.

6. Prelack K, Ming Y, Sheridan RL. Nutrition and metabolism in the rehabilitative phase of recovery in burn children: a review of clinical and research findings in a specialty burn hospital. *Burns Trauma.* 2015;3:7.

7. Commare C, Tappenden K. Development of the infant intestine: implications for nutrition support. *Nutr Clin Pract.*2007;22(2):159–173.

8. Coss-Bu J, Hamilton-Reeves J, Patel J, Morris C, Hurt R. Protein requirement of the critically ill patient. *Nutr Clin Pract.*2017;32(Suppl):128S–141S.

9. Gottschlich M, Mayes T. Burns and Wound Healing. In Cresci G. *Nutrition Support for the Critically Ill Patient: A Guide to Practice*. Florida: CRC Press; 2005: 435–452.

10. Cuthbertson DP, Zagreb H. The metabolic response to injury and its nutritional implications: retrospect and prospect. *JPEN*. 1979;3:108–130.

11. Wilmore DW, Long JM, Mason AD, et al. Catecholamines: mediators of the hypermetabolic response to thermal injury. *Ann Surg*.1974;180:653–669.

12. Bane JW, McCaa RE, McCaa CS. The pattern of aldosterone and cortisone blood levels in thermal burn patients. *J Trauma*.1974;14:605–611.

13. Jeshke MG, Chinkes D, Finnerty C, et al. Pathophysiologic response to severe burn injury. *Ann Surg*. 2008;248: 387–401.

14. Vaughn GM, Becker RA, Allen JP, et al. Cortisol and corticotrophin in burned patients. *J Trauma*.1982;22:263–273.

15. Wilmore DW, Lindsey CA, Moylan JA, et al. Hyperglucagonemia after burns. *Lancet*. 1974;1:73–75.

16. Johoor F, Herndon DH, Wolfe RR. Role of insulin and glucagon in the response of glucose and alanine kinetics in burn-injured patients. *J Clin Invest*.1986;78:807–814.

17. Nygren J, Sammann M, Malm M, et al. Disturbed anabolic hormonal patterns in burned patients: the relation to glucagon. *Clin Endocrinol*. 2008;43:491–500.

18. Nair KS, Halliday D, Matthews DE, Welle SL. Hyperglucagonemia during insulin deficiency accelerates protein catabolism. *Am J Physiol Endocrinol Metab*. 1987;253:E208–E213.

19. Porter C, Tompkins RG, Finnerty CC, Sidossis LS, Suman OE, Herndon DN. The metabolic response to burn trauma: current understanding and therapies. *Lancet*. 2016;388(10052):1417–1426.

20. Barrow RE, Jeschke MG, Herndon DN. Early fluid resuscitation improves outcomes in severely burned children. *Resuscitation*. 2000;45:91–96.

21. Baxter CR, Shires T. Physiological response to crystalloid resuscitation of severe burns. *Ann NY Acad Sci*.1968;150:874–894.

22. Finnerty CC, Herndon DN, Przkora R, et al. Cytokine expression profile overtime in severely burned pediatric patients. *Shock*. 2006;26:13–19.

23. Tracey KJ. TNF and other cytokines in the metabolism of septic shock and cachexia. *Clin Nutr*. 1992;11:1–11.

24. Tredgett EE, Yu YM, Zhong S, et al. Role of interleukin-1 and tumor necrosis factor on energy metabolism in rabbits. *Am J Physiol*. 1988;255:E760–E768.

25. Warren RS, Starnes HF, Gabrilove JL. The acute metabolic effects of tumor necrosis factor administration. *Arch Surg*.1987;122:1396–1400.

26. Gottschlich MM, Jenkins ME, Mayes T, et al. A prospective clinical study of the polysomnographic stages of sleep following burn injury. *J Burn Care Rehabil*. 1994;15: 486–492.

27. Copinschi, G. Metabolic and endocrine effects of sleep deprivation. *Essent Psychopharmacol*. 2005;6:341–347.

28. Van Cauter E, Homback U, Knutson K, et al. Impact of sleep and sleep loss on neuroendocrine and metabolic function. *Horm Res*. 2007;67(suppl1):2–9.

29. Gottschlich MM, Khoury J, Warden GD, Kagan RJ. An evaluation of the neuroendocrine response to sleep in pediatric burn patients. *JPEN*. 2009;33:317–326.

30. Barret JP, Herndon DN. Modulation of inflammatory and catabolic responses in severely burned children by early wound excision in the first twenty four hours. *Arch Surg*. 2003;138(2):127–132.

31. Hildreth M, Caravajal HF. Caloric requirements in burned children: a simple formula to estimate daily caloric requirements. *J Burn Care Rehabil*. 1982;3:78–80.

32. Hildreth MA, Herndon DN, Desai MH, Duke MA. Calorie needs of adolescent patients with burns. *J Burn Care Rehabil*. 1989;10:523–526.

33. Hildreth MA, Herndon DN, Parks DH, et al. Evaluation of a caloric requirement formula in burned children treated with early excision. *J Trauma*. 1987;27:188–189.

34. Hildreth MA, Herndon DN, Desai MH, Broemeling LD. Current treatment reduces calories required to maintain weight in pediatric patients with burns. *J Burn Care Rehabil*. 1990;11:405–409.

35. Mayes TM, Gottschlich MM, Khoury J, Warden GD. An evaluation of predicted and measured energy requirements in burned children. *J Am Diet Assoc*. 1996;96: 24–29.

36. Curreri PW, Luterman A, Braun DW, et al. Burn injury: analysis of survival and hospitalization time for 937 patients. *Ann Surg*. 1980;192:472–478.

37. Davies JWL, Liljedahl SL. Metabolic consequences of an extensive burn. In: Polk HC, Stone HH, eds. *Contemporary Burn Management*. Boston:Little Brown;1971:151–169.

38. Klein CJ, Stanek GS, Wiles CE. Overfeeding macronutrients to critically ill adults. *Metab Complications*. 1998;98: 795–806.

39. Hart DW, Wolf SE, Herndon DN, Chinkes DL, Lal S, Obenk MK et al. Energy expenditure and caloric balance post burn: increased feeding leads to fat rather than lean mass accretion. *Ann Surg*. 2002;235(1):152–161.

40. Sion-Sarid R, Cohen J, Houri Z, Singer P. Indirect calorimetry: a guide for optimized nutrition support in the critically ill child. *Nutrition*. 2013;29(9):1094–1099.

41. Mlcak RP, Jeschke MG, Barrow RE, Herndon DN. The influence of age and gender on REE in severely burned children. *Ann Surg*. 2006;244:121–130.

42. Suman O, Mlcak R, Chinkes D, Herndon D. Resting energy expenditure in severely burned children: analysis of agreement between indirect calorimetry and predictive equations using the Bland-Altman Method. *Burns*. 2006;32(3):335–342.

43. Gottschlich MM, Jenkins M, Warden GD, et al. Differential effects of three enteral regimens on selected outcome parameters. *JPEN*. 1990;14:225–236.

44. Wilmore DW, Goodwin CW, Aulick LH, et al. Effect of injury and infection on visceral metabolism and circulation. *Ann Surg*. 1980;192:491–500.

45. Gauglitz GG, Herndon DN, Jeschke MG. Insulin resistance postburn: underlying mechanisms and current therapeutic strategies. *J Burn Care Res*. 2008;29:683–694.

46. McGowen KC, Malhotra A, Bistrian BR. Stress-induced hyperglycemia. *Crit Care Clin*. 2001;17:107–124.

47. Hart DW, Wolf SE, Zhang X-J, et al. Efficacy of a high-carbohydrate diet in catabolic illness. *Crit Care Med*. 2001;29:1318–1324.

48. Gore DC, Chinkes DL Hart DW, et al. Hyperglycemia exacerbates muscle protein catabolism in burn injured patients. *Crit Care Med*. 2002;30:2438–2442.

49. Barrocas A, Tretola R, Alonso A. Nutrition and the critically ill pulmonary patient. *Respir Care.* 1983;28:50–61.

50. Askanazi J, Rosenbaum SH, Hyman AI, et al. Respiratory changes induced by large glucose loads of total parenteral nutrition. *JAMA.* 1980;243:1444–1447.

51. Rousseau, A, Looser M, Ichai C, Berger M. ESPEN endorsed recommendations : Nutritional therapy in major burns. *Clin Nutr.* 2013;21:297–302.

52. Sheridan RL, Yu YM, Prelak K, Young VR, Burke JF, Tompkins RG. Maximal parenteral glucose oxidation in hypermetabolic young children. *JPEN.*1998;22:212–216.

53. Van den Berghe G, Wouters P, Weekers F, et al. Intensive insulin therapy in critically ill patients. *N Engl J Med.* 2001;345:1359–1367.

54. Van den Berghe G, Wouters P, Bouillion R, et al. Outcomes benefit of intensive insulin therapy in the critically ill: insulin dose versus glycemic control. *Crit Care Med.* 2003;31:359–366.

55. Van den Berghe C, Wilmer A, Hermans G, et al. Intensive insulin therapy in the medical ICU. *N Engl J Med.* 2006;354:449–461.

56. Collier BC, Diaz J, Forbes R, et al. The impact of a normoglycemic management protocol on clinical outcomes in the trauma intensive care unit. *JPEN.* 2005;29:353–359.

57. Cochran A, Davis L, Morris SE, Saffle JE. Safety and efficacy of an intensive insulin protocol in a burn-trauma intensive care unit. *J Burn Care Res.* 2008;29:187–191.

58. Hemmila MR, Taddonio MA, Arbabi S, et al. Intensive insulin therapy is associated with reduced infectious complications in burn patients. *Surg.* 2008;144:629–635.

59. Pham TN, Warren AJ, Phan HH, et al. Impact of tight glycemic control in severely burned children. *J Trauma.* 2005;59:1148–1154.

60. Thomas SJ, Morimoto K, Herndon DN, et al. The effect of prolonged euglycemic hyperinsulinemia on lean body mass after severe burn. *Surg.* 2002;132:341–347.

61. Jeschke MG, Klein D, Herndon DN. Insulin treatment improves the systemic inflammatory reaction to severe trauma. *Ann Surg.* 2004;239:553–560.

62. Chao T, Herndon D, Porter C, et al. Skeletal muscle protein breakdown remains elevated in pediatric burn survivors up to one year post injury. *Shock.* 2015;44(5):397–401.

63. Alexander JW, MacMillan BG, Stinnett JD, et al. Beneficial effects of aggressive protein feeding in severely burned children. *Ann Surg.* 1980;192:505–517.

64. Dominioni L, Trocki O, Mochizuki H, et al. Prevention of severe postburn hypermetabolism and catabolism by immediate intragastric feeding. *J Burn Care Rehabil.* 1984;5:106–112.

65. Serog P, Baigts F, Apfelbaum M, et al. Energy and nitrogen balances in 24 severely burned patients receiving 4 isocaloric diets of about 10 MJ/m²/day (2392 kcal/m²/day). *Burns.* 1983;9:422–427.

66. Dominioni L, Trocki O, Fang CH, et al. Enteral feeding in burn hypermetabolism: nutritional and metabolic effects of different levels of calorie and protein intake. *JPEN.* 1985;9:269–279.

67. Peng X, Yan H, You Z, Wang P, Wang S. Effects of enteral supplementation with glutamine granules on intestinal mucosal barrier function in severe burned patients. *Burns.* 2004;30:135–139.

68. Peng X, Yan H, You Z, Wang P, Wang S. Glutamine granule-supplemented enteral nutrition maintains immunological function in severely burned patients. *Burns.* 2006;32:589–563.

69. Zhou YP, Jiang ZM, Sun YH, Wang XR, Ma El, Wilmore D. The effect of supplemental enteral glutamine on plasma levels, gut function, and outcome in severe burns: a randomized double-blind controlled clinical trial. *JPEN.* 2003;27:241–245.

70. Windle EM. Glutamine supplementation in critical illness: evidence, recommendations and implications for clinical practice in burn care. *J Burn Care Res.* 2006;27(6):764–772.

71. Yu YM, Ryan CM, Castillo L, Lu XM, Beaumier L, Tompkins RG et al. Arginine and ornithine kinetics in severely burned patients: increased rate of arginine disposal. *Am J Physiol Endocrin Metab.* 2001;28(3):E509–E517.

72. Marin VB, Rodriguez-Osiac L, Schlessinger L, Villegas J, Lopez M, Castillo-Duran C. Controlled study of arginine supplementation in burned children: impact on immunologic and metabolic status. *Nutrition.* 2006;22(78): 705–712.

73. Yu M, Sheridan RL, Burke JF, Chapman TE, Tompkins RG, Young VR. Kinetics of plasma and arginine and leucine in pediatric burn patients. *Am J Clin Nutr.* 1996;64(1):60–66.

74. Gottschlich MM, Warden GD, Michel MA, et al. Diarrhea in tube-fed burn patients: incidence, etiology, nutritional impact and prevention. *JPEN.* 1988;12:338–345.

75. Mochizuki H, Trocki O, Dominioni L, et al. Optimal lipid content for enteral diets following thermal injury. *JPEN.* 1984;8:638–646.

76. Gottschlich MM, Alexander JW. Fat kinetics and recommended dietary intake in burns. *JPEN.* 1987;11:85–89.

77. Clark A, Imran J, Madni T, Wolf S. Nutrition metabolism in burn patients. *Burns Trauma.* 2017;5(11):1–12.

78. Garrel D, Razi M, Larivire F et al. Improved clinical status and length of care with low fat nutrition support in burn patients. *JPEN.* 1995;19(6):482.

79. Freund H, Yoshimura N, Fisher JE. Does intravenous fat spare nitrogen in the injured rat? *Am J Surg,* 1980;140: 377–383.

80. Gottschlich MM, Warden GD. Vitamin supplementation in the burn patient. *J Burn Care Rehabil.* 1990;11:275–279.

81. Hein GL, Rodriguez NA, Branksi K, Herndon D. Vitamin and trace element homeostasis following severe burn injury. In Herndon DN, ed. *Total Burn Care.* London. England: WB Saunders; 2012:321–324.

82. Berger MM. Antioxidant micronutrients in major trauma and burns: evidence and practice. *Nutr Clin Practice.* 2006;21(5):438–439.

83. Berger MM, Binnert C, Chiolero RL, Taylor W, Raffoul W, Cayeux et al. Trace element supplementation after major burns increases burned skin trace element concentrations and modulates local protein metabolism, but not whole-body substrate metabolism. *Am J Clin Nutr.* 2007;85(5):1301–1306.

84. Gottschlich MM, Mayes T, Khoury J, Warden GD. Hypovitaminosis D in acutely injured pediatric burn patients. *J Am Diet Assoc.*2004;104:931–941.

85. Klein GL, Langman CB, Herndon DN. Vitamin D depletion following burn injury in children: a possible factor in post-burn osteopenia. *J Trauma.*2002;52:346–350.

86. Klein GL, Herndon DN, Langman CB, et al. Long term reduction in bone mass after severe burn injury in children. *J Pediatr.*1995;126:252–256.

87. Mayes T, Gottschlich MM, Scanlon J, Warden GD. Four year review of burns as an etiologic factor in the development of long bone fractures in pediatric patients. *J Burn Care Rehabil.* 2003;24:279–284.

88. Cassat J, Skaar E. Iron in infection and immunity. *Cell Host & Microbe.* 2013;13(5):509–519.

89. Caldis-Courtis N, Gawaziuk J, Logsetty S. Zinc supplementation in burn patients. *J Burn Care Res.* 2012;33(5): 678–682.

90. Khorasani G, Hosseinimehr S, Kaghazi Z. The alteration of plasma's zinc and copper levels in patients with burn injuries and the relationship to time after burn injuries. *Singapore Med J,* 2008;49(8):627–630.

91. Jenkins ME, Gottschlich MM, Kopcha R, et al. A prospective analysis of serum vitamin K and dietary intake in severely burned pediatric patients. *J Burn Care Rehabil.* 1998;19:75

92. Gottschlich MM, Mayes T, Allgeier C, et al. Clinical trial of vitamin D_2 vs D_3 supplementation in critically ill pediatric burn patients. *JPEN.* 2015;41(3): 412–421.

93. Mayes T, Gottschlich MM, Khoury J, Kagan RJ. Investigation of bone health subsequent to vitamin D supplementation in children following burn injury. *Nutr Clin Practice.* 2015;30(6):830–837.

94. Klein GL. The interaction between burn injury and vitamin D metabolism and consequences for the patient. *Curr Clin Pharmacol.* 2008;3:204–210.

95. Klein GL, Chen TC, Holick MF, et al. Synthesis of vitamin D in skin after burns. *Lancet.* 2004;363:291–292.

96. Saito H, Trocki O, Alexander JW, et al. The effect of route of nutrient administration on the nutritional state, catabolic hormone secretion, and gut mucosal integrity after burn injury. *JPEN.* 1987;11:1–7.

97. Saito H, Trocki O, Alexander JW. Comparison of immediate postburn enteral versus parenteral nutrition. *JPEN.* 1985;9:115.

98. Jenkins M, Gottschlich M, Baumer T, et al. Enteral feeding during operative procedures. *J Burn Care Rehabil.* 1994;15:199–205.

99. Sunderman C, Gottschlich MM, Allgeier C, James L, Warden GD. Safety and efficacy of intraoperative nutrition support in a pediatric burn unit. Proceedings of the American Burn Association. *J Burn Care Res.* 2016;37(1):S92.

100. Varon D, Freitas G, Neha M, Wall J, Bharadia D, Sisk E, et al. Intraoperative feeding improves calories and protein delivery in acute burn patients. *J Burn Care Res.* 2017;38(5):299–303.

101. Mochizuki H, Trocki O, Dominioni L, et al. Mechanism of prevention of postburn hypermetabolism and catabolism by early enteral feeding. *Ann Surg.* 1984;200:297–310.

102. Jenkins M, Gottschlich M, Waymack JP, et al. An evaluation of the effect of immediate enteral feeding on the hypermetabolic response following severe burn injury. *Proc Am Burn Assoc.* 1988;112.

103. Venter M, Rode H, Sive A. Visser M. Enteral rescuscitation and early enteral feeding in children with major burns-effect on McFarlane response to stress. *Burns.* 2007;33(4):464–471.

104. Khorsani E, Mansouri F. Effect of early enteral nutrition on morbidity and mortality in children with burns. *Burns.* 2010;36(7):1067–1071.

105. Gottschlich MM, Jenkins MJ, Mayes T, et al. An evaluation of the safety of early versus delayed enteral support and effects on clinical, nutritional and endocrine outcomes after severe burns. *J Burn Care Rehabil.* 2002;23:401–415.

106. Riegel T, Allgeier C, Gottschlich M, et al. Fluid resuscitation, inotropic agents and early feeding: is there a relationship to bowel necrosis? *J Burn Care Rehabil.* 2003;24:S61.

107. Sunderman C, Gottschlich M, Allgeier C, Kagan RJ. Translating research into clinical practice: modification of an early enteral nutrition support algorithm improves safety in pediatric burn patients. *Support Line.* 2017;39(1):20–24.

108. Trocki O, Mochizuki H, Dominioni L, et al. Intact protein versus free amino acids in the nutritional support of thermally injured animals. *JPEN.* 1986;10:139–145.

109. Bell SJ, Molnar JA, Carey M, et al. Adequacy of a modular tube feeding diet for burned patients. *J Am Diet Assoc.* 1986;86:1386–1391.

110. Bower RH, Cerra FB, Bershadsky B, Licari JJ, Hoyt DB, Jensen GL et al. Early enteral administration of a formula (Impact) supplemented with arginine nucleotides and fish oil in intensive care unit patients: results of a multicenter prospective randomized clinical trial. *Crit Care Med.* 1995;23(3):436–439.

111. Barrett JP, Jeschke MG, Herndon DN. Fatty infiltration of the liver in severely burned pediatric patients. *J Am Diet Assoc.* 1986;86:1386–1391.

112. ASPEN Board of Directors and the Clinical Guidelines Task Force. Guideliess for the use of parenteral and enteral nutrition in adult and pediatric patients. *JPEN.* 2002;26:1SA–138SA.

113. Chen Z, Wang S, Yu B. Li A. A comparison study between early enteral nutrition and parenteral nutrition in severe burn patients. *Burns.* 2007;33(6):708–712.

114. Mayes T, Gottschlich MM, Warden GD. Clinical nutrition protocols for continuous quality improvements in the outcomes of patients with burns. *J Burn Care Rehabil.* 1997;18:365–368.

115. Graves C, Saffle J. Cochran A. Actual burn nutrition care practices: an update. *J Burn Care Res.* 2009;30(1):77–82.

116. Prelack K, Dylewski M, Sheridan RL. Practical guidelines for nutritional management of burn injury and recovery. *Burns.* 2007;33:14–24.

117. Mayes T, Gottschlich MM. Burns and wound healing. In: *The Science and Practice of Nutrition Support: A Case-Based Core Curriculum.* Silver Spring, MD: A.S.P.E.N.; 2001:402.

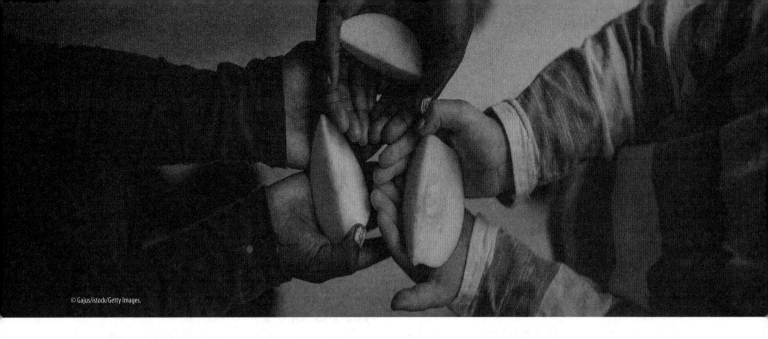

© Gajus/istock/Getty Images.

CHAPTER 20

Diabetes

Kasey Metz and Megan Robinson

▶ Introduction

The incidence of both Type 1 and Type 2 diabetes (T1D and T2D) remains on the rise among children and adolescents, however T1D continues to be the most prevalent in this population.[1] It is important for **registered dietitian nutritionists** (RDNs) to distinguish the needs of these patients based on their diagnoses (patients diagnoses is plural) and to provide individualized nutritional care plans. T1D and T2D have different characteristics and therefore different treatment goals.

Through considerable research and new technologies, the knowledge base regarding childhood diabetes has been extended, giving healthcare professionals new tools to help this population balance and improve their diabetes management. These tools include intensive insulin therapy, new medications, **self-monitoring blood glucose** (SMBG) devices, **continuous glucose monitoring** (CGM) (continuous glucose monitoring will be described in more detail later in the chapter), psychological intervention, inclusion and education for family and support persons, insulin/food adjustment for exercise, and state-of-the-art **medical nutrition therapy** (MNT). The challenge to the RDN on the diabetes team is to support the family's efforts and to help promote healthy eating habits by using information gained from current research coupled with insight into family dynamics.

Empowering parents to care for their child with T1D is the ultimate challenge for many healthcare professionals working with pediatric patients. Families already faced with altering their lifestyle to include insulin injections, **blood glucose** (BG) monitoring, and scheduled meals must face these challenges in combination with feelings of anger, fear, denial, and guilt. It is critical for families and caregivers to realize the importance of their role in caring for their child with diabetes, while also providing the balance of allowing the child to take part in their own self-care with the appropriate amount of supervision. When children are included in the responsibility for some of their own care, it better equips them to transition and manage their diabetes as they enter adulthood.

MNT has proven to be a powerful tool in the management of diabetes. Reviews in the literature have shown a 1%–2% lowering in **hemoglobin A1C** (A1C) values if dietary and lifestyle changes are made and followed.[2] Educators on the diabetes team must not lose sight of the fact that food provides more than nutrients, especially for children. Changes in eating should not be viewed as restrictions and losses, but rather as a healthful way for the entire family to eat. To be successful, meals must not only meet nutritional requirements, but also be realistic and workable without requiring major routine changes for those involved. Every attempt should be made to establish a meal plan that reflects the youth's food preferences and the family's social and cultural attitudes. Flexibility and graduated goal setting are important keys to success, increasing the chances of children and adolescents achieving optimal management and decreasing the development of complications. The goals for MNT are listed in **FIGURE 20.1**.

> - To provide adequate nutrition to maintain normal growth and development based on the child's appetite, food preferences, and family lifestyle
> - To maintain near-normal BG levels and reduce/prevent the risks of acute and chronic diabetes complications
> - To achieve optimal serum lipid levels
> - To preserve social and psychological well-being
> - To improve overall health through optimal nutrition
> - To provide a level of information that meets the interest and ability of the family, and
> - To provide information on current research to help the family make appropriate nutrition decisions

FIGURE 20.1 Goals of Medical Nutrition Therapy (MNT) for Children and Adolescents

▶ Anatomy, Physiology, Pathology of Condition

Diagnosing pediatric diabetes is not straightforward. Types of diabetes can differ by gene mutations or the presence of antibodies. Diabetes can also present itself after years of poor diet and lifestyle choices, such as in T2D. Relatives or friends of children with diabetes may have a type of diabetes that differs from that of the child and the treatment can be vastly different; therefore, it is critical to know the exact diagnosis of a child to be able to provide a proper treatment plan and MNT.

Type 1 Diabetes

T1D is an autoimmune disease defined by hyperglycemia and the need for insulin. T1D was previously referred to as juvenile or insulin-dependent diabetes. Most cases of T1D are diagnosed after the age of 5 and into adolescence; however, diagnosis can occur at any age in life.[3,4] Genetic factors are known to play a role in the incidence of T1D. However, a child's environment, including viral and bacterial infections, or deficiencies of vitamins and nutrients, can be the triggers to elicit an autoimmune response.[4]

T1D can fall into two different categories, the most prominent being classified by pancreatic beta cell destruction, which usually leads to a total lack of insulin production. Autoantibodies are tested to determine the degree of destruction of the beta cells and therefore the ability of the pancreas to produce insulin.[3] It may not be common practice for a facility to test a child for all five antibodies, since only 2 positive tests are needed for a diagnosis; however, the antibodies that may be tested include glutamic acid decarboxylase (GAD), islet cell antibodies (ICA), insulin autoantibodies (IAA), protein tyrosine phosphatase antibodies (ICA512 or IA2A), and zinc transporter protein (ZnT8).[5] A child may test positive for autoantibodies months to years before becoming symptomatic, or the child may be genetically predisposed to T1D without the presence of autoantibodies.[4]

The other, much less common form of T1D, is idiopathic with no known etiologies. Most patients that fall into this category are of African or Asian ancestry.[6] There is no evidence of autoimmunity in these patients, and some tend to be more prone to ketoacidosis, requiring varying degrees of insulin between DKA episodes. There may or may not be a continuous daily need for exogenous insulin therapy in these patients.[3]

Type 2 Diabetes

T2D is increasing in our population, especially in high-risk ethnic groups such as African American, Hispanic, Native American, and Pacific Island populations.[4,7] T2D was previously thought of as non-insulin dependent diabetes or a disease amongst older individuals.

There are trends around the world towards increased consumption of processed, calorically dense foods and beverages, and a lifestyle trend towards decreases in physical activity, which are leading factors towards weight gain and obesity. RDN's and healthcare professionals across the country are seeing an increased incidence of T2D in children which is proportional to the increased incidence of childhood obesity. A child or adolescent who is overweight (BMI at or above the 85th percentile and below the 95th percentile), or obese (BMI at or above the 95th percentile) places them at an increased risk for insulin resistance.[4]

T2D in children, as in adults, is due to the combination of insulin resistance and beta-cell failure. Over time, insulin secretion eventually becomes deficient and the body is unable to keep up with the greater insulin demands that are required to compensate for the insulin resistance.[3]

Along with poor diet and lifestyle, genetics and family history are also to blame for the spike in the incidence of T2D. At diagnosis, children and adolescents with T2D often have other disorders present including: polycystic ovarian syndrome and acanthosis nigricans which is secondary to their insulin resistance and obesity.[1,8] Children are encouraged to make diet and lifestyle changes often including: decreased caloric and carbohydrate intake, increased physical activity, and gradual weight loss if needed; however, they also may require insulin or oral Glucophage (Metformin) for management. Per the US Department of Health and Human Services, Metformin is presently the only oral diabetes medication approved by the Food and Drug Administration (FDA) for pediatric use.[9]

Types of Monogenic Diabetes

Monogenic diabetes (MD) consists of a group of different types of diabetes including **maturity onset diabetes of the young** (MODY) and **neonatal diabetes mellitus** (NDM). MD results from a defect in the beta cells and typically includes: a diagnosis at an age of 25 or under, mild fasting hyperglycemia (100–150mg/dL [5.5–8.5mmol/L]), strong family history of diabetes, and negative diabetes autoantibodies.[4,10]

MODY is a heterogeneous group of disorders with defects in several different genes. MODY is defined by impaired insulin secretion with little or no defect in insulin action.[10] There is generally a strong family history of diabetes with abnormal characteristics, and therefore MODY can often be misdiagnosed as T1D or T2D. The diagnosing, naming and specific type of MODY is based on the gene that is involved - diagnosis can only be completed through genetic testing.[4] Dependent on the stage or type of disease, treatment may not be required; however, when treatment is necessitated, sulfonylureas or insulin will typically be used.[4]

Neonatal diabetes mellitus (NDM) is diagnosed with onset before 6 months of age and is likely non-autoimmune,

and the result of a gene defect in the beta cell.[1,4] NDM may be misdiagnosed as T1D. However, T1D is rarely present before 6 months of life. The exact gene involvement will determine the treatment method which may be either sulfonylureas or insulin[10]

Cystic Fibrosis Related Diabetes

Cystic Fibrosis Related Diabetes (CFRD) results from damage to the pancreas due to large amounts of pancreatic secretions and ductal obstruction. Annual screening for diabetes with **oral glucose tolerance testing** (OGTT) begins after the age of 10 in all patients with CF.[10] Patients will experience a loss in beta cells resulting in decreased insulin secretion along with insulin resistance from CF associated illnesses[11] and may eventually require exogenous insulin therapy for the treatment of their hyperglycemia.[1,4] The CF Foundation recommends patients with CFRD need to continue eating a high calorie, high protein, high fat, high salt diet to achieve and maintain a healthy weight; however, if they require insulin therapy, they will need to count carbohydrates to determine the appropriate amount of insulin to take with their meals and snacks.[12]

▶ Condition Specific Nutrition Screening

It is recommended that the pediatric patient with diabetes be in the care of a team of specialists who focus in pediatric diabetes.[10] The child will need quarterly and annual follow-up to assess the family's individualized needs, comply with treatment recommendations, and monitor glycemic control. Along with assessing BG history and A1C levels it is important to regularly screen for other common diabetes related autoimmune diseases including cardiovascular disease, nutrient deficiencies, or the presence of eating disorders.[10] **TABLE 20.1** – (adapted from Chiang & Associates[5]) includes a list of the clinical evaluations and laboratory assessments that will be performed by the diabetes specialist at most annual and quarterly medical appointments.

Further condition specific nutrition screening may be warranted; however, it is uncommon to see nephropathy, neuropathy, and retinopathy in young children with diabetes, or those who have been diagnosed only 1–2 years. Following puberty, or 5–10 years after initial diagnosis of diabetes, nephropathy, neuropathy and retinopathy have a greater chance of occurrence and regular screening should be performed into and throughout adulthood.[5]

Thyroid Disease

Thyroid Disease is the most common autoimmune disease associated with T1D as approximately 25% of children have positive thyroid antibodies at the time of diabetes diagnosis.[10] Antithyroid peroxidase and

TABLE 20.1 Clinical Evaluation and Laboratory Assessment Criteria

Upon Initial Diagnosis:

- Retinal Exam by Eye Care Specialist (at age ≥10 years, or after puberty has started, whichever is earlier, once the youth has had diabetes for 3–5 years) and every 2 years
- Assess clinically relevant issues (e.g., alcohol, drug and tobacco use; use of contraception; driving)
- Query for evidence of other autoimmune diseases
- Immunizations as recommended by CDC (and annually)
- Antithyroid Antibodies
- Celiac Antibody Panel
- TSH (and as needed based on symptoms or treatment)
- Creatinine Clearance/Estimated Glomerular Filtration Rate (and annually)
- GAD/ICA/IA2A/IAA/ZnT8
- C-peptide levels

Upon Initial Diagnosis, Quarterly and Annually:

- Height
- Weight
- BMI percentile
- General Physical Exam
- Thyroid Exam
- Injection/Infusion Sites
- Depression Screen
- Hypoglycemia Assessment
- Diabetes Self-Management Skills
- A1C
- Nutrition Knowledge

Annually and as Needed:

- Comprehensive Foot Exam
- Visual Foot Exam (and quarterly as needed)
- Lipid Panel (and as needed based on treatment)
- Urine Albumin-to-Creatinine Ratio (beginning five years after diagnosis)

Modified from Chiang JL, Kirkman MS, Laffel LM, et al. Type 1 diabetes through the life span: a position statement of the American Diabetes Association. *Diabetes Care.* 2014;37:2034–2054.[5]

antithyroglobulin antibodies should be tested soon after T1D diagnosis.[10] The presence of these antibodies is most often associated with hypothyroidism[13] Decreases in linear growth and increased instances of hypoglycemia can be a result of hypothyroidism.[13] Once glycemic control has been established, thyroid stimulating hormone levels should be monitored every 1–2 years or if the patient becomes symptomatic.[10]

Celiac Disease

Celiac disease (CD) is an immune mediated disease affected by both genetics and the environment. Children with T1D are at a greater risk for CD (6%) when compared with the general population (1%).[14] Testing of tissue transglutaminase antibodies (anti-tTG) is often performed at diagnosis of T1D in order to determine

if there is a presence of CD.[14] Most cases of CD will be diagnosed within the first 5 years of T1D diagnosis and therefore screening should be repeated every 2–5 years after initial testing.[10] If a positive result for anti-tTG is confirmed, the patient should immediately begin a gluten free diet.[10] Failure to follow a gluten free diet may cause more incidence of hypoglycemic events.[15]

Cardiovascular Disease

Cardiovascular disease risk factors are higher in children and adolescents with diabetes compared with the general population. The **American Heart Association** (AHA) places children with diabetes in the highest tier for cardiovascular risk.[10] Evidence shows that glucose control is directly related to the levels of several plasma lipids.[16]

Routine blood pressure monitoring should be performed at all clinic visits. The **American Diabetes Association** (ADA) recommends children with high-normal blood pressure (systolic blood pressure or diastolic blood pressure >90th percentile for age, sex, and height) or hypertension (systolic blood pressure or diastolic blood pressure >95th percentile for age, sex, and height) be initially treated with a heart healthy diet, exercise, and weight management.[10]

Fasting lipids should be obtained in children >10 years of age following diabetes diagnosis and once blood glucose control has been achieved.[10] If initial labs are abnormal, a fasting lipid panel should be performed annually; however, if labs are normal, they may then only need repeating every 3–5 years.[10] Elevated lipids should be treated with glucose control and an AHA heart healthy diet focused on lowering saturated fats and dietary cholesterol.[10]

Weight Control and Disordered Eating

Weight control can become an important issue to children prior to, and when entering, adolescence. Parents and the health care team must take concerns about body image seriously. Some weight gain is usually seen before growth spurts. If a child's weight is disproportionate to height, the weight should be kept stable until the height fits the weight. The child should be encouraged to become involved in active play and physical exercise and to incorporate more fresh fruits and vegetables into his or her daily intake.

Children and adolescents who are overly concerned about weight gain but who find it hard to reduce their intake may choose to skip insulin injections to promote quick weight loss. Eating disorders in pediatric diabetes can include anorexia nervosa, bulimia nervosa, and diabulimia. Diabulimia is an eating disorder specific to persons with T1D and is characterized by limiting and/or skipping insulin dosing to directly affect weight control.[17] Early identification of eating disorders by the diabetes team can help the individual get the treatment necessary. Some of the signs are:[18]

- Deterioration of psychosocial functions (school, work, interpersonal)
- Weight fluctuations of 10 pounds or more
- High glycosylated hemoglobin (A1C) (A1C >7.5%)
- Controlled diabetes only when hospitalized
- Unexplained diabetic ketoacidosis
- Reluctance or refusal to take more insulin or other medications
- Not checking blood glucose (BG)
- Blaming insulin for weight problems
- Preoccupation with body image
- Engaging in excessive exercise
- Bingeing

- Restricting food
- Depression with low self-esteem

Referral to a RDN or **certified diabetes educator** (CDE) is the first line of defense when a child or adolescent exhibits weight dissatisfaction but does not exhibit clinical eating pathology. Strict guidelines regarding food and blood glucose should not be implemented because this may promote binge eating or weight gain. Adolescents should be advised that glucose fluctuations could create increased hunger and result in weight gain. Education should also be provided about serious short and long-term consequences of destructive food behaviors. Referral to a mental health professional, who is knowledgeable about diabetes and disordered eating, or hospitalization, is often necessary to break the disordered eating cycle.

▶ Nutrition Assessment

The initial visit in the outpatient setting should lay the groundwork in nutrition basics and serve to develop a sound and trusting relationship with the child and family. The Children's Checklist (**FIGURE 20.2**) offers a detailed analysis of the child's and family's eating habits and behaviors, food preferences, and family lifestyle, and will assist the RDN in producing a realistic and workable meal plan for this very important population.

Growth

Anthropometrics are obtained at the first visit and all subsequent visits. It is important to maintain records of height and weight and to monitor the child's growth. Assessing growth will assist the RDN in creating the meal plan and providing adequate nutrition for growing and gaining at an age appropriate rate.

Biochemical Indices

The child and their family are responsible for daily BG monitoring with a minimum goal of 4 blood glucose checks per day (before meals and at bedtime). Studies have shown that frequency of blood glucose monitoring is directly related to improved blood glucose control and statistically significant decreases in A1C levels.[19] The diabetes care providers will review BG history from glucose meters or CGM's in order to determine trends and adjust the child's insulin doses or treatment plan.

A1C or **estimated average glucose** (eAG) will also be checked at the initial visit and routinely at follow-up appointments. A1C reflects average glycemia over several months and has strong predictive value for diabetes complications[10] A1C can be a better indicator of blood glucose history than blood glucose results alone, particularly when a child is suspected of having manipulated

Growth (Anthropometrics):
- Height
- Weight
- BMI % (BMI z-score) or weight-for-height % (z-score)
- History of growth pattern
- Recent weight changes

Biochemical Indices:
- Blood glucose
- Glycosylated hemoglobin (A1C) and estimated average glucose (eAG) or fructosamine
- Lipid profile
- Albuminuria
- Ketones

Psychosocial Information:
- Identify the family unit at home (two parents, separated parents, single parent, divorced, siblings, other family, friends, or caretakers)
- Evaluate emotional state of parents, child, siblings (anger, fear, guilt, denial, anxiety)
- Assess child's interactions with parents and siblings
- Identify person(s) responsible for shopping/cooking
- Evaluate knowledge/comprehension levels and literacy
- Identify cultural/religious systems that influence attitudes
- Identify family members or friends with diabetes
- Assess parents and family beliefs about the "diabetic diet"

Child's Usual Food Intake Before Symptoms of Diabetes
Home
- Eats scheduled meals/snacks
- Includes a variety of foods daily
- Eats meats, fruit, and vegetables on a regular basis
- Consumes beverages at meals/snacks other than milk
- Drinks soda/juice/water for thirst
- Follows special diet
- Food allergies or intolerances

School:
- Eats breakfast at home or eats at school
- Brings lunch from home or has school lunch
- Beverage at lunch/snacks
- Scheduled snacks are part of regular class activities
- Obtains snack at school or snack sent from home
- Frequency, length, and time of day of gym class
- Participates in school sports or activities after school

Weekends:
- Evaluate meals prepared or eaten with others on weekends
- Identify meal schedule if different from weekdays
- Determine restaurant eating habits on weekends
- Assess sports/activities scheduled on weekends

Eating Behaviors
Child:
- Overeats or under-eats
- Relies on convenience and fast foods
- Experiences food jags often
- Refuses many of the family foods offered
- Finishes meals in reasonable amount of time
- Respects limits set for acceptable eating behavior at the table
- Location where meals and snacks are consumed
- Food allergies or intolerances

Family:
- Evaluate parents as role models
- Healthy eaters, structured meals, planned meals, limit junk food in home
- Unhealthy eaters, overweight, chronic dieters
- Identify supervision at meals/snacks
- Evaluate limit-setting around food choices
- Assess cultural/religious eating behaviors
- Identify whether food is used as a reward

FIGURE 20.2 Children's Checklist: Assessing the Child Newly Diagnosed with Diabetes

values in their blood glucose meter, or are unable to provide blood glucose history information at their appointment. The ADA recommends that A1C for children and adolescents (<18 years) be <7.5%.[10]

Lipids will be monitored annually, but may be assessed every 3–5 years if within normal limits.[10]

Albuminuria and ketones can both be checked by a urine sample. Protein in the urine can suggest kidney dysfunction. Exercise in the last 24 hours, infection, fever, and marked hyperglycemia may cause elevated urine albumin levels. If levels are above normal, they will need to be re-checked 2–3 times over a 3–6-month period to determine true renal function or damage.[20]

Ketones are a result of fat metabolism for energy and often occur in children with poorly controlled diabetes. A positive test for ketones will require additional insulin to normalize blood glucose levels and treat ketones. Ketones and marked hyperglycemia are a concern for **diabetic ketoacidosis (DKA)**. **TABLE 20.2** lists diagnostic criteria of DKA and **Hyperosmolar Hyperglycemia (HHS)**

Psychosocial Information

It is important for a RDN to analyze the entire family dynamic. How the parents or caregivers and child interact, who resides in the household and the acceptance of the disease diagnosis will all be vital to the nutrition

TABLE 20.2 Diagnostic Criteria for Diabetic Ketoacidosis (DKA) and Hyperosmolar Hyperglycemia State (HHS)

Criteria	DKA	HHS
Plasma glucose (mg/dL)	>250	>600
Arterial pH	<7.30	>7.30
Serum bicarbonate (mmol/L)	≤15	>15
Urine ketones	Positive	Small
Serum ketones	Positive	Small

Modified from Academy of Nutrition and Dietetics. Nutrition terminology reference manual (eNCPT): dietetics language for nutrition care. Available at:http://ncpt .webauthor.com. Accessed November 13, 2017.[20]

assessment. The RDN needs to assess a family's literacy and education level to verify the type of learner they are and to determine if further resources are needed, including determining who in the household is responsible for grocery shopping and food preparation. Many children are left to fend for themselves with little supervision, therefore diet and nutrition education needs to be provided to all members of the family.

Child's Usual Food Intake Prior to Symptoms of Diabetes

Obtaining a diet recall or a food history should be completed as part of the nutrition assessment. The food history will be assessed to determine that it meets the child's needs for all nutrients and with adequate intake from all food groups. Also, the types of beverages and snacks the child is consuming along with their timing will be important when making future diet recommendations.

It is important for the RDN to determine where the child eats most their meals and what food choices they have. It may be at home, a grandparent's house, school or a friend's house.

School

Frequently, a child will eat both breakfast and lunch at school. In these cases, when a highly restrictive diet is essential, an RDN can provide a meal plan to the school to help ensure the child's diet is meeting their needs. The RDN can work with the school food service staff to determine what types of foods and beverages are available to the child and provide information on the carbohydrate gram amount in these foods. Children with diabetes often will require scheduled snacks during the school day or before or after physical activity. Working with the school schedule and staff and determining the timing of meals, snacks and physical activity will help to develop meal plan recommendations.

Weekends

When obtaining a diet recall, this should include a weekend day. A child's schedule on the weekend is often vastly different from that of the week day, and their dietary intake will be different as well. They may sleep in and skip breakfast or the family may eat only two meals per day versus the three the child is used to when in school. There may be sports and activities on the weekends that leave very little time for family meals and more meals may be eaten at restaurants. Advanced planning will be essential to ensure that the child is getting the meals and snacks they need and at the appropriate times.

Eating Behaviors – Child

A child with diabetes requires a well-rounded diet with adequate intake of all macronutrients. Working with a child who is a picky eater can pose many challenges. Questions to ask may include: What are the eating and mealtime behaviors of the child? Do they tend to over or under eat, refuse to try new foods, or eat meals within a reasonable time frame? These are all topics that need to be discussed when assessing dietary intake. Also, a child may have food allergies or restrictions which are imperative to know when developing the meal plan. Allergies or restrictions may make a child more likely to refuse new foods and make them more insistent on eating convenience or known foods.

Eating Behaviors – Family

Evaluate parents as role models. Do they provide healthy structured meals or allow "junk" foods for snacks? Identifying the diet of the parent is often a good insight to the diet of the child. A parent may have beliefs about foods and impose their un-healthy choices and dietary restrictions on their child. It is the job of the RDN to analyze a family's cultural and religious needs and determine how food is used in the household. Foods may be used as reward and punishment. There may be no limits as to how much, what and when a child may eat. Dietary recommendations and MNT will be provided based on the child's behaviors with and towards food.

Nutrition-Focused Physical Findings

One of the most prominent physical observations in diabetes is unintentional weight loss. Prolonged hyperglycemia, elevated A1C and ketones will occur because of inadequate insulin or purposeful omission of insulin leading to weight loss. In children and adolescents with diabetes, growth should be on par with that of the general population.[5]

An obese child with T2D may often have a very characteristic skin condition referred to as **acanthosis nigricans** (AN). AN is easily identified by a darkening and thickening of the skin on the neck and may be seen on other areas of the body as well. Per the American Academy of Dermatology, studies have shown that patients who lose a significant amount of weight will often see a clearing of their skin.[21]

▶ Nutrition Diagnosis

T1D can be diagnosed utilizing 4 criteria including: signs and symptoms, fasting blood glucose levels, OGTT and A1C.[1] Although these signs and/or symptoms may not be present at the time of diagnosis, the onset of T1D typically occurs with the classic symptoms of hyperglycemia, polyuria, polydipsia, and weight loss.[1]

It is important to properly diagnose the correct form of diabetes to provide the appropriate treatment. Overweight and obesity may make it difficult for a provider to distinguish between T1D and T2D. Testing for autoantibodies is the only proper way to correctly classify the exact type of diabetes.[1] **TABLE 20.3** lists diagnostic criteria for diabetes adapted from the ADA.

T2D in children is typically diagnosed after the age of 10 and during middle to late puberty.[8] Obese children, who have a family history of diabetes and physical characteristics of insulin resistance such as acanthosis nigricans, should be tested for T2D.

- Altered nutrition-related laboratory values (specify) (NC-2.2)
- Underweight (NC-3.1)
- Unintended weight loss (NC-3.2)
- Overweight/obesity (NC-3.3.2)
- Unintended weight gain (NC-3.4)
- Growth rate below expected (NC-3.5)
- Excessive growth rate (NC-3.6)
- Increased nutrient needs (NI-5.1)
- Decreased nutrient needs (NI-5.4)
- Inadequate fat intake (NI-5.6.1)
- Excessive fat intake (NI-5.6.2)
- Intake of types of fats inconsistent with needs (NI-5.6.3)
- Excessive carbohydrate intake (NI-5.8.2)
- Inadequate carbohydrate intake (NI-5.8.1)
- Intakes of types of carbohydrates inconsistent with needs (NI-5.8.3)
- Inconsistent carbohydrate intake (NI-5.8.4)
- Inadequate fiber intake (NI-5.8.5)
- Inadequate intake of vitamin D (NI-5.9.1.3)
- Inadequate intake of calcium (NI-5.10.1.1)
- Food- and nutrition-related knowledge deficit (NB-1.1)
- Not ready for diet/lifestyle change (NB-1.3)
- Disordered eating pattern (NB-1.5)
- Limited adherence to nutrition-related recommendations (NB-1.6)
- Physical inactivity (NB-2.1)
- Inability or lack of desire to manage self-care (NB-2.3)
- Impaired ability to prepare foods/meals (NB-2.4)

Modified from Academy of Nutrition and Dietetics. Nutrition terminology reference manual (eNCPT): dietetics language for nutrition care. Available at:http://ncpt.webauthor.com. Accessed November 13, 2017.[20]
Academy of Nutrition and Dietetics. Nutrition Care Manual®. Conditions, Diabetes Mellitus Type 1, Nutrition Diagnosis. Available at: https://nutritioncaremanual.org. Accessed October 18, 2017.[22]

FIGURE 20.3 Nutrition Diagnosis

After thorough review and analysis of the nutrition assessment, a nutrition diagnosis can be made. The eNCPT: Nutrition Terminology Reference Manual, the source of the Dietetics Language for Nutrition Care, provides a list of nutrition diagnosis (**FIGURE 20.3**) that may be used when working with the child with diabetes. This list is not conclusive and other diagnoses may be used as well.

Once a nutrition diagnosis has been determined a nutrition diagnostic statement can be made. The following are examples of nutrition diagnostic statements using the **Problem, Etiology, Signs and Symptoms (PES)** format:

- Excessive carbohydrate intake related to picky eating and poor dietary choices as evidenced by 3-day diet recall

TABLE 20.3 Diagnostic Criteria for Diabetes

Signs and Symptoms	Polyuria, polydipsia, polyphagia, weight loss
	Blood glucose concentration ≥200mg/dL.
	Nausea, vomiting, abdominal pain, rapid breathing, dehydration, altered mental status.
Fasting Blood Glucose:	≥126mg/dL on 2 separate occasions
Oral Glucose Tolerance Test:	75g of anhydrous carbohydrates are administered with a 2-hr blood glucose level ≥200mg/dL
Hemoglobin A1C:	≥ 6.5% (blood glucose of 139.85mg/dL)

Data from Beck JK, Cogen FR. Outpatient Management of Pediatric Type 1 Diabetes. *J Pediatr Pharmacol Ther.* 2015;20(5): 344–357.[1]

- Inability or lack of desire to manage self-care related to denial of T2D diagnosis and its potential health complications as evidenced by continued poor diet and lifestyle changes and weight gain
- Altered nutrition-related laboratory values (blood glucose) related to excessive carbohydrate intake between meals as evidence BG meter results frequently >200mg/dL.
- Limited adherence to nutrition-related recommendations related to continued intake of sugary beverages as evidenced by patient and family report on 24-hour dietary recall

▶ Nutrition Intervention

Managing diabetes requires three main components: MNT, exercise, and medication. MNT is an important part of diabetes management in children and adolescents with diabetes. The goals of MNT include normalizing glucose, blood pressure, lipids and promoting healthy weight and growth.[1] A positive approach to meal planning is to encourage family members and other support persons to follow the same lifestyle recommendations as the child with diabetes.

It is important that the nutrition recommendations promote "normal" healthy eating and prevent isolating the child from the family in their food choices. Research suggests that the nutrition needs of children with diabetes are no different than those of children without diabetes and should follow the Dietary Guidelines for Americans.[23] The nutrition prescription should be based on the child's nutrition assessment, individual treatment goals, and health outcomes.

TABLE 20.4 provides information on percent of calories from the major macronutrient categories.

Calories

The meal plan should include enough calories (kcal) to maintain a consistent growth and to achieve and/or maintain a desirable body weight. In growing children, caloric intake should not be restricted, and should be the same as for children without diabetes, unless the child is overweight or obese.[25] Energy needs vary during periods of growth, so calorie needs should be compared and validated based on age, height, ideal body weight (IBW), activity, average energy allowance per day, and environmental factors such as the type and availability of food.[26] **FIGURE 20.4** provides common equations for estimating energy needs.

TABLE 20.5 provided Physical Activity Coefficients (PA Values) for Use in EER Equations (abbreviation: PA, physical activity.)

Insulin Therapy

Intensive management using a basal/bolus insulin regimen is the standard of care for managing diabetes in

TABLE 20.4 Nutrition Recommendations Redistributed the Calories from Macronutrients

Acceptable Macronutrient Distribution Range (% of energy)			
	Children 1–3 Years	**Children 4–18 Years**	**Adults**
Protein	5–20%	10–30%	10–35%
Carbohydrate	45–65%	45–65%	45–65%
Fat	30–40%	25–35%	20–35%
Saturated Fat	<10%	<10%	<10%
Added Sugars	<10%	<10%	<10%
Calories	Requirements for growth, based on nutrition assessment		

Modified from Institute of Medicine of the National Academies. *Dietary Reference Intakes: The Essential Guide to Nutrient Requirements.* Washington, DC: National Academies Press;2006. Available at: https://www.nap.edu/read/11537/chapter/7#73. Accessed September 15, 2017.[24]

children. Intensive insulin therapy can include **multiple daily injections** (MDI) using rapid-acting insulin with either an intermediate or long-acting insulin or CSII (**continuous subcutaneous insulin infusion**) pump therapy. A basal/bolus regimen increases flexibility in meal or snack schedules and allows children to eat based on hunger rather than when the insulin is peaking. The insulin action (onset, peak, and duration) of the insulin available is listed in **TABLE 20.6**.[29] It is important to consider that insulin action will vary from person to person and can be affected by the injection site, activity level before and after the injection is given, and time of day.

Conventional insulin therapy is no longer the standard of care but is still used in practice. This therapy may include two daily injections of intermediate-acting insulin (NPH) or one injection of NPH with a long-acting/basal insulin (glargine [Lantus] or detemir [Levemir]), possibly combined with a small amount of rapid-acting insulin (lispro [Humalog], aspart [Novolog], and glulisine [Apidra]). Children who have difficulty with taking multiple insulin shots using basal/bolus insulin, may benefit from conventional therapy. Advantages of split-mixed insulin therapy include the following: less insulin injections; no lunchtime injections at school; simpler insulin regimen; and less self-monitoring of BG (4 times/day). However, since NPH is a fixed insulin dose, children need to eat at consistent times and eat a consistent amount of carbohydrates at each meal and snack to achieve optimal BG control.[1] This may be difficult to achieve due to the nature of unpredictable eating patterns of children and adolescents.

Based on nutrition assessment and typical day recall. Validate caloric estimation.

Method 1: Dietary Reference Intakes: Estimated Energy Requirements (EER)

Infants and Young Children

0–3 months EER = (89 × weight [kg] − 100) + 175

4–6 months EER = (89 × weight [kg] − 100) + 56

7–12 months EER = (89 × weight [kg] − 100) + 22

13–35 months EER = (89 × weight [kg] − 100) + 20

Children and Adolescents 3–18 Years

Boys

3–8 yrs EER = 88.5–(61.9 × age [y]) + PA × [(26.7 × weight [kg]) + (903 × height [m])] + 20

9–18 yrs EER = 88.5–(61.9 × age [y]) + PA × [(26.7 × weight [kg]) + (903 × height [m])] + 25

Girls

3–8 yrs EER = 135.3–(30.8 × age [yr] + PA × [(10.0 × weight [kg]) + (934 × height [m])] + 20

9–18 yrs EER = 135.3–(30.8 × age [yr] + PA × [(10.0 × weight [kg]) + (934 × height [m])] + 25

Weight Maintenance TEE in overweight boys Ages 3–18 Years:

TEE = 114 – (50.9 × age [y] + PA × (19.5 × weight [kg] + 1,164 × height [m])

Weight Maintenance TEE in overweight girls Ages 3–18 Years:

TEE = 389 – (41.2 × age[y] + PA × (15 × weight [kg] + 701.6 × height [m])

Adults 19 Years and Older

Men EER = 662 – (9.53 × age [yr]) + PA × [(15.91 × weight [kg]) + (539.6 × height [m])

Women EER = 354 – (6.91 × age [yr]) + PA × [(9.36 × weight [kg]) + (726 × height [m])

Method 2: Schofield Equation for Calculating Basal Metabolic Rate in Children

Males

0–3 years REE = 0.167W + 15.174H – 617.6

3–10 years REE = 19.59W + 1.303H + 414.9

10–18 years REE = 16.25W + 1.372H + 515.5

> 18 years REE = 15.057W + 1.004H + 705.8

Females

0–3 years REE = 16.252W + 10.232H – 413.5

3–10 years REE = 16.969W + 1.618H + 371.2

10–18 years REE = 8.365W + 4.65H + 200

> 18 years REE = 13.623W + 23.8H + 98.2

REE × activity

Method 3: WHO Equations

WHO	Male	Female
0–3 y	60.9W – 54	61.0W – 51
3–10 y	22.7W + 495	22.5W + 499
10–18 y	17.5W + 651	12.2W + 746
18–30 y	15.3W + 679	14.7W + 496

WHO Activity/Stress Factors		
Type of Stress	**Multiply REE by**	
Starvation	0.70–0.85	
Surgery	1.05–1.5	
Sepsis	1.2–1.6	
Closed head injury	1.30	
Trauma	1.1–1.8	
Growth failure	1.5–2.0	
Burn	1.5–2.5	

Data from National Academy of Sciences, Institutes of Medicine, Food and Nutrition Board. Dietary reference intakes for energy, carbohydrate, fiber, fat, fatty acids, cholesterol, protein, and amino acids (macronutrients). 2005. Available at: https://www.nap.edu/read/10490/chapter/2#5. Accessed:September 10, 2017.[27]
World Health Organization. Energy and protein requirements. report of a joint FAQ/WHO/UNU Expert Consultation. Technical Report Series 724. Geneva, Switzerland:World Health Organization;1985. Avaialble at: http://www.fao.org/docrep/003/AA040E/AA040E00.HTM#TOC. Accessed:October 2, 2017.[28]

FIGURE 20.4 Estimating Caloric Requirements

Many circumstances require permanent or temporary insulin adjustments to be made. As a child grows and food intake increases, the total daily dose (TDD) of insulin also increases.[30] Young children may require 0.25 to 0.5 units/kg/d; whereas during puberty, the TDD may increase from 0.75 to 1.5 units/kg/d.[1] During brief periods of illness, times of stress, or changes with activity, insulin needs may also vary. A change in the child's level of activity, which may be especially dramatic at the beginning and end of the

TABLE 20.5 Physical Activity Coefficients (PA Values) for Use in EER Equations

	Sedentary (PAL 1.0–1.39)	Low Active (PAL 1.4–1.59)	Active (PAL 1.6–1.89)	Very Active (PAL 1.9–2.5)
	Typical daily living activities (e.g., household tasks, walking to the bus)	Typical daily living activities *plus* 30–60 minutes of daily moderate activity (e.g., walking 5–7 km/h)	Typical daily living activities *plus* At least 60 minutes of moderate activity	Typical daily living activities *plus* At least 60 minutes of moderate activity *plus* An additional 60 minutes of vigorous activity or 120 minutes of moderate activity
Boys 3–18 yrs	1.00	1.13	1.26	1.42
Girls 3–18 yrs	1.00	1.16	1.31	1.56
Men 19+ yrs	1.00	1.11	1.25	1.48
Women 19+ yrs	1.00	1.12	1.27	1.45

Abbreviation: PAL, physical activity level.

Modified from Institute of Medicine of the National Academies. *Dietary Reference Intakes: The Essential Guide to Nutrient Requirements.* Washington, DC: National Academies Press; 2006. Available at: https://www.nap.edu/read/11537/chapter/7#73. Accessed September 15, 2017.[24]

TABLE 20.6 Insulin Actions

Insulin	When to Take	Onset	Peak	Effective Duration	Maximum Duration
Rapid Acting: Lispro (Humalog)	10–20 minutes before the meal or snack	15–30 minutes	30–90 minutes	3–4 hours	4–6 hours
Aspart (Novolog)	10–20 minutes before meal or snack	15–30 minutes	30–75 minutes	3–4 hours	4–6 hours
Glulisine (Apidra)	10–20 minutes before meal or snack	15–30 minutes	30–75 minutes	3–4 hours	4–6 hours
Short Acting: Regular (R)	30 minutes before the meal	30–60 minutes	2–3 hours	3–6 hours	6–8 hours
Intermediate Acting: NPH	Does not need to be given with food	2–4 hours	6–10 hours	10–16 hours	14–16 hours
Long Acting: Glargine (Lantus)	Does not need to be given with food	30–90 minutes	8–16 hours	18–20 hours	20–24 hours
Glargine U-300 (Toujeo)	Does not need to be given with food	30–90 minutes	none	24 hours	30 hours
Detemir (Levemir)	Does not need to be given with food	30–90 minutes	6–8 hours	14 hours	20 hours
Degludec (Tresiba)	Does not need to be given with food	30–90 minutes	none	24 hours	40 hours

Modified from Chiang JL, Kirkman MS, Laffel LM, et al. Type 1 diabetes through the life span: a position statement of the American Diabetes Association. *Diabetes Care.* 2014;37:2034–2054.[5]

school year, usually requires an adjustment in the insulin dosage. When these events resolve or change, the child's insulin dose will need to be readjusted. Otherwise, an increase of food in response to the higher insulin levels may result in inappropriate weight gain or hypoglycemia, whereas too little insulin may result in hyperglycemia.

Since the introduction of CSII in the 1970s, pump therapy has become very popular in patients with T1D. Diabetes centers around the country started using the pump on pediatric patients in the 1980s. Pump therapy demonstrated benefits such as improved glycemic control[31] reduced episodes of hypoglycemia, improved linear growth, and decreased episodes of recurrent DKA. Pumps are becoming more widely used even in children as young as 1 to 2 years of age. The advantage of the pump for the young child is that it offers the parents the ability to dose a very small amount of insulin and provide multiple doses throughout the day without having to give the child injections by syringe or pen.

Pump therapy provides only a rapid-acting insulin (Humalog, Novolog, or Apidra), which eliminates the unpredictable action of the longer-acting insulins. The pump delivers a small amount of insulin continuously (basal) and can be programmed to deliver boluses when eating a meal or snack, or for correcting hyperglycemia. There are pros and cons of pump therapy, which should be considered very carefully before putting any child or adolescent on an insulin pump.

Long-acting insulins (basal) are popular in school-age children, adolescents, and young adults in place of the intermediate insulin NPH. They allow the child the flexibility of the insulin pump without the additional equipment required. Long-acting insulin is given in one or two injections daily to meet the child's background or basal insulin needs. Additional injections of rapid insulin are given at meals and snacks in order to cover the carbohydrate and to correct hyperglycemia. Long-acting insulin typically lasts up to 24 hours and is usually started with one injection a day, typically given at dinner or bedtime for consistency. Younger children have benefited from splitting the dose, due to the insulin possibly not lasting a full 24 hours or having some peaking action. Ultra-long acting basal insulin, degludec, recently has been available, which provides a longer half-life and duration of action up to 40 hours.[29]

Before a family or child starts CSII or MDI, the child and the family must master advanced skills, including having a good understanding of advanced carbohydrate counting, which includes using insulin-to-carbohydrate ratios (ICR); understanding the sensitivity or correction factor (CF) to determine each insulin dose; and having the necessary math skills needed to calculate dosage.[1]

Hybrid Closed-Loop Automated Insulin Pumps

The hybrid closed-loop automated insulin pump, also known as the Artificial Pancreas System, was recently approved by the FDA for patients with T1D aged 14 years and older. This new system uses CGM and a closed loop algorithm built into the pump to automatically adjust basal insulin in order to keep glucose levels within a target range. Bolusing for the carbohydrate grams consumed remains required; however, it does recommend correction doses based on fingerstick results. The closed-loop pump provides two modes, a manual mode and auto mode. During the manual mode, the user programs a pre-programed basal insulin dose which will automatically suspend and resumes insulin delivery to maintain euglycemia. Basal insulin during the auto mode is automatically adjusted based on sensor BG readings which differs from the manual mode where the basal rate is delivered at a constant rate. Even though the auto mode adjusts basal rates automatically, boluses for carbohydrates continue to be done manually.[29,32]

▶ Carbohydrate and Sweeteners

Amount and Type of Carbohydrate

Carbohydrates are nutrients in foods and beverages that have the greatest impact on blood glucose (BG) levels. Carbohydrate-rich foods such as whole grains, legumes, fruit, vegetables, milk and yogurt should be encouraged daily to provide adequate dietary fiber and essential vitamins and minerals in children's and adolescent's diets. Carbohydrates should not be restricted in children with diabetes, but the percentage of calories ingested from carbohydrate will vary and is individualized based on nutritional assessment and treatment goals. For example, a young athlete with T1D may require a higher percentage of total kcal from carbohydrates to maintain muscle glycogen stores, enhance sports performance, and promote growth and development; whereas, an adolescent with T2D may require less kcal from carbohydrates to prevent excessive weight gain and to help manage BG.[8,33,34]

Many factors influence the glycemic response to foods, including the total amount of carbohydrate, type of carbohydrate (glucose, sucrose, fructose, lactose, or starch), degree of processing, glycemic index, glycemic load, and combination with other foods and ingredients. One of the most common misconceptions about carbohydrate is the belief that sugars are more rapidly digested and absorbed than are starches and therefore sugar contributes significantly to hyperglycemia. However, published research found little or no scientific evidence that supports this theory.[2]

Studies show a strong relationship between the total carbohydrate intake and the pre-meal insulin dose; therefore, adjustment of the pre-meal insulin dose can allow children and adolescents with diabetes to incorporate most carbohydrates into the meal plan and still maintain appropriate blood glucose control. Matching rapid-acting insulin to carbohydrate gram intake is a common practice for children with both T1D and T2D in order to allow for flexibility with the amount and timing of meals and snacks.[26] It is common practice to encourage the family whenever possible to provide rapid insulin 10–20 minutes before the meal when the pre-meal blood sugar is in range. If pre-meal BG is above the child's target range, rapid-acting insulin should be given 20–30 minutes before the meal or snack. If the pre-meal BG is below the target range, pre-meal insulin should be delayed until after carbohydrates have been consumed.[29] Administering rapid-acting insulin pre-meal has been shown to reduce postprandial BG spikes by 50mg/dL. However, dosing insulin postprandial (post-dosing) is often recommended for infants and toddlers with T1D to prevent hypoglycemia and to allow them to dose based on what was eaten rather than "forcing" them to eat an unrealistic amount of carbohydrates to match the insulin. Post meal dosing may not achieve tight BG control, but does give parents and caregivers a more normalized approach to eating.[30]

Snacks

Snacks can be part of a healthy eating plan, and depending on the age of the child and type of insulin regimen, might be necessary. Snacks can help maintain the BG and provide adequate calories during the day for growth and development. Eating snacks one to three times daily may eliminate hunger in the evening hours, especially in young children. Snacks before bedtime are not necessary if the child is on basal/bolus insulin, unless the BG is lower than 100mg/dl or if the child is hungry. Children on conventional insulin therapy may require snacks between meals and at bedtime to prevent hypoglycemia. Typically, a snack containing 15 to 20g of carbohydrate, one to three times daily, is recommended for young children and a snack of 30g of carbohydrate or more is recommended for adolescents, to promote adequate calories for growth and development. Snacking could also be necessary depending on activity, length of time at recess, physical education (PE) classes, and/or sports at after-school activities. For example, if PE is offered only on Monday and Wednesday at 10:00 am, a larger snack may be required before class on those days in order to prevent hypoglycemia. For inactive, overweight, or obese children, choosing smaller snacks and/or limiting snacks to less than 30 grams of carbohydrate may be necessary to prevent excessive weight gain.[25]

Carbohydrate Counting

The standard of care for children with T1D is to manage their diabetes on MDI or CSII using pump therapy. Advanced carbohydrate (carb) counting allows users greater flexibility in the timing of meals, the amount of food eaten at the meal, and the selection of specific foods. The meal-planning objective is to coordinate food intake (carbohydrate) by matching the peak activity of insulin with the peak levels of glucose resulting from the digestion and absorption of food. Only the carbohydrate value of the food is counted, which allows more accurate adjustment of pre-meal, rapid-acting insulin using an ICR. The ICR assumes that carbohydrate intake is the main consideration in determining meal related insulin requirements together with SMBG values. Targeted blood glucose values are set by the diabetes team, the child, and his or her family. A general rule is that approximately 1 unit of rapid-acting insulin will be needed for every 10 to 15 grams of carbohydrate. The child's insulin-to-carb ratio should be individually determined by the diabetes team based on the child's present insulin needs and meal plan. A child's ratio can range from 0.5–1 unit of insulin for every 5 to 40 grams of carbohydrate depending on age, activity, and insulin needs. Younger children benefit from using 0.5 unit marking and pens with 0.5-unit dosing to better match insulin to the carbohydrate gram amount consumed.[35]

In addition to covering the carbs at a meal, children and adolescents are given a sensitivity factor (SF) and a target BG. This allows them to adjust the dose based on their BG before the meal or snack. If their BG is higher than target they will add some additional insulin, and if BG is lower than target subtract some insulin using the SF.

Special care must be given to prevent overeating because increased availability of insulin and food may promote unwanted weight gain. A good understanding of how carbohydrate affects blood glucose, what food groups contain carbohydrates, and the importance of portion control is necessary for carbohydrate counting to be effective. Reference books, apps and websites providing the carbohydrate content of specific foods are also helpful. Continuous reinforcement of healthy eating habits is advisable, because many young people tend to omit food groups as well as meals to accommodate busy schedules or to manage weight.

Since the amount of carbohydrate and available insulin is a crucial factor in the postprandial BG, carbohydrate counting continues to be a common practice for both T1D and T2D. Benefits of carbohydrate counting include a reduced hemoglobin A1c (A1C) and improved quality of life by allowing increased diet flexibility.[26] The DCCT provided important insight into the role of nutrition intervention in intensive diabetes management and stated that registered dietitian nutritionists (RDN) are best qualified to match appropriate meal-planning approaches to the needs of the patient. Today, there are several effective methods for teaching patients about food. Any method can be equally effective when geared to the patient's intellectual level, repeated frequently, and evaluated. There is no one method of carbohydrate counting that has been proven to be more effective than another, but accurate measurement of carbohydrates rather than estimating or guessing the amount can achieve improved BG control.

Common types of carbohydrate counting include:

1. Consistent carbohydrate intake for individuals with diabetes taking fixed insulin regimens or with T2D requiring a set amount of carbohydrates eaten at meals and snacks. This type of eating may use exchange or portions of carbohydrates, using tools such as The Plate Method.[36]

2. ICR is more common in pediatric diabetes for those taking MDI of basal/bolus insulin and/or using continuous insulin infusion pumps. This approach involves adjusting preprandial insulin based on the carbohydrates consumed.

Choose Your Food List

The lists of food choices are based on the following food groups:

- *The carbohydrate group:* Starches (breads, cereals, grains, starchy vegetables, etc.), fruit, milk, non-starchy vegetables, sweets, desserts, and other carbohydrates
- *The meat and meat substitute group:* Protein (meat, poultry, fish, dried peas, and beans)
- *The fat group:* Vegetable oils, avocado, and regular salad dressings

Examples of the specific amount of carbohydrate, protein, fat, or combination of these nutrients in each food group are found in **TABLE 20.7** Choose Your Foods Lists are used to achieve a consistent timing and intake of carbohydrate, protein, and fat and provide needed variety when planning meals. Choose Your Foods Lists and a meal plan can be a starting point for those patients on intensive insulin management and can help them to understand and learn the carbohydrate content of foods.

Glycemic Index and Glycemic Load

The **glycemic index** (GI) and the **glycemic load** (GL) categorize individual food items by their postprandial glucose response, which continues to be a controversy. GI rankings are determined by the glucose response after ingesting a 50-gram portion of carbohydrate of a food and comparing it with the glucose response of an index food.[38] The GI measures the relative area under the glucose curve; not how quickly BG levels are affected by different carbohydrates.[2] The glycemic index is not a precise tool because the exact effect of foods on BG differs significantly among individuals and is affected by many factors such as processing, preparation, and digestion.[39] On the other hand, the glycemic index can be used as an indicator of the general glucose response of an individual food. Choosing lower GI foods may be a helpful tool to encourage eating more whole-grain foods, fresh fruits, and vegetables to lower the postprandial glucose response.[38]

The GL takes the GI into account but also uses the quantity of the carbohydrate eaten. This again can be used as a teaching tool to educate the youth and their family that when choosing a food with a high GI, the GL can be decreased by choosing a smaller portion of that food to reduce the postprandial response.[26]

Sucrose

Sucrose has not been shown to increase BG more than isocaloric amounts found in starches. It is advisable to substitute sucrose and sucrose-containing foods for other carbohydrates in the diet, and not simply to add these foods to the meal plan. Most added sugars in the diet can be found in fruit juices, regular soda, energy/sports drinks, and in foods such as desserts, breads/muffins and sweetened milk/yogurt, which are considered empty calorie foods with low nutrient density.[40,41] However, flexibility in allowing some sucrose into the meal plan may lead to better adherence. Sucrose can be incorporated into children's meal plans on a regular basis, assuming their intake is adequate and consists of foods from all of the essential food groups. The most recent recommendations of added sugars range from less than 5% up to 25% of total kcal daily.[23,40] The AHA recommends reducing the intake of added sugars to less than 25 grams daily to decrease the risk of cardiovascular disease.[41]

Nutritive Sweeteners

Sweeteners other than sucrose also contain large amounts of carbohydrate and calories that impact glycemic control. Common sweeteners such as fructose, corn syrup, honey, molasses, carob, dextrose, lactose, and maltose do not decrease calories or carbohydrate and offer no significant advantage over foods sweetened with sucrose.[40,41] Although fructose has been shown to produce a somewhat smaller rise in blood glucose compared with the other sweeteners listed, research suggests potential negative effects of consuming large amounts of fructose (not naturally occurring in fruit) on serum triglycerides. Fructose should also not be added as a sweetening agent to foods.[42]

TABLE 20.7 Choose Your Foods: Food List for Diabetes

Foods List	Carbohydrates (grams)	Protein (grams)	Fat (grams)	Calories
Carbohydrate				
Starch: breads, cereals and grains, starchy vegetables, crackers, snacks, beans, peas, and lentils	15	0–3	0–1	80
Fruits	15	—	—	60
Milk				
Fat-free, low-fat, 1%	12	8	0–3	100
Reduced-fat, 2%	12	8	5	120
Whole	12	8	8	150
Sweets, Desserts, and Other Carbohydrates	15	Varies	Varies	Varies
Non starchy Vegetables	5	2	—	25
Meat and Meat Substitutes				
Lean	—	7	0–3	45
Medium-fat	—	7	4–7	75
High-fat	—	7	8+	100
Plant-based proteins	Varies	7	Varies	Varies
Fats	—	—	5	45
Alcohol	Varies	—	—	100

Modified from Geil, PB. Choose your foods: exchange lists for diabetes: The 2008 revision for exchange lists for meal planning. *Diabetes Spectrum.* 2008;21(4):281–283.[37]

High-fructose corn syrup (HFCS) is a mixture of glucose and fructose and is a less expensive sugar replacement in many foods and beverages. HFCS has been proven safe by the FDA and contains 4 calories per gram, similar to table sugar.[43] Research continues to be mixed on whether HFCS is correlated with an increased risk of obesity and diabetes.[44,45]

Hypocaloric Sweeteners

Commonly used sugar alcohols such as sorbitol, mannitol, xylitol, erythritol, lactitol, isomalt, maltitol, and hydrogenated starch hydrolysate may produce less of a glycemic response and average about 0.2 to 2.7kcal/g, compared with 4kcal/g from other carbohydrates.[46] However, gastrointestinal side effects such as stomach distress or diarrhea are noted when sugar alcohols are ingested in large amounts (50g/day for sorbitol, 20g/day for mannitol, ≥30g/day for lacitol, isomalt, and xylitol); whereas, erythritol does not appear to have a laxative effect.[43,47] Children may be more sensitive and have been shown to have diarrhea with intake as low as 0.5 or less g/kg body weight.

Nonnutritive Sweeteners (NNS)

Aspartame, acesulfame K, neotame saccharin, sucralose, and steviol glycosides are the most common noncaloric sweeteners used in the United States and have been approved by the FDA. The FDA determines an **acceptable daily intake** (ADI) for these sweeteners. ADI is defined as the amount of a food additive that can be safely consumed daily over a person's lifetime without any adverse effects, and includes a 100-fold safety factor (**TABLE 20.8**). Despite the ADI limits for safe consumption, the **Institutes of Medicine** (IOM) does not support the use of NNS in children since they may displace drinking healthier beverages such as milk and 100% fruit juice.[48] In addition, the **American Academy of Pediatrics** (AAP) states that NNS have not been extensively studied in children and should be limited in their diet. Per the

Academy of Nutrition and Dietetics (AND), studies have determined that NNS do not influence glycemic control and can reduce calorie and carbohydrate intake; however, studies are mixed on whether the use of NNS are beneficial for weight control in overweight or obese children.[42,48]

Aspartame contains 4kcal/g but is 160 to 220 times sweeter than sucrose; therefore, aspartame provides negligible calories. Aspartame is rapidly metabolized in the gastrointestinal tract and does not accumulate in the system at recommended intakes. Aspartame is not heat stable and may decompose on long exposure to high temperatures.

TABLE 20.8 FDA ADI Guidelines for Non-Nutritive Sweeteners

	ADI (mg/kg body wt)	Average Amount (mg) in 12-oz. Can of Soda*	Cans of Soda to Reach ADI for 45-kg (100-lb.) Child	Amount (mg) in a Packet of Sweetener	Packets to Reach ADI for a 45-kg (100-lb.) Child
Acesulfame K *Sweet One®, Sunett®*	15	40+	17	50	13
Aspartame *Nutrasweet®, Equal®, Sugar Twin®*	50	200	11	35	63
Neotame *Newtame®*	18	6a	135	N/A	N/A
Saccharin *Sweet and Low®, Sweet Twin®, Necta Sweet®*	15	140*	1.6	36	6.25
Sucralose *Splenda®*	5	70	3.2	5	45
Stevioside (steviol glycosides) *Truvia®, PureVia®,*	4b	56	10	28	20
Luo Han Guo Fruit Extracts *Nectresse® Monk Fruit in the Raw® PureLo®*	NS***	NS	NS	NS	NS

These recommendations are set by the Food and Drug Administration (FDA) for Acceptable Daily Intake (ADI) and include a 100-fold safety factor. The World Health Organization's Joint Expert Committee of Food Additives has set the ADI for saccharin. Use these as guidelines.18

*This number represents an average; different brand names and fountain drinks may have varied amounts of sweeteners.

+Based on the most common blend with 90 mg aspartame.

ahttp://www.neotame.com/pdf/neotame_science_brochure_US.pdf

bADI is translated to 12 mg/kg/day for Rubiana (Truvia) and RebA (PureVia)

***Not specific

Data from US FDA. Additional information about high-intensity sweeteners permitted for use in the United States. 2015. Available at: https://www.fda.gov/Food/IngredientsPackagingLabeling/FoodAdditivesIngredients/ucm397725.htm#Aspartame. Accessed: September 10, 2017.[49]

Aspartame safety data have been evaluated by regulatory agencies and expert committees[49], including the FDA, the EU **Scientific Committee for Food** (SCF), and the **Joint FAO/WHO Expert Committee on Food Additives** (JECFA), which have deemed it safe for its intended use. Aspartame was first approved by the FDA in 1981 for dry products and was expanded in 1983 to include carbonated beverages. Aspartame is presently approved in many countries and has been widely used by hundreds of millions of people over the last 20 years with no adverse effects. However, because aspartame is composed of phenylalanine and aspartic acid, it should be restricted in those with **phenylketonuria** (PKU), a homozygous recessive inborn error of metabolism in which persons are unable to metabolize the amino acid phenylalanine. The FDA requires all products containing aspartame to display the words "Phenylketonurics: Contains Phenylalanine."[43]

Acesulfame K has no caloric value and is 200 times sweeter than sucrose. It is not metabolized by the body and is eliminated unchanged in the urine. Acesulfame K is heat stable and blends well with other sweeteners. The amount of potassium (K) in this sweetener is minimal, with only 10 mg of potassium in one packet. No safety concerns have been raised about acesulfame K and it has been reported safe for all individuals.[49]

Saccharin is 200 to 700 times sweeter than sucrose and has no caloric value. Saccharin is heat stable, is not metabolized by the body, and is excreted unchanged in the urine. Parents often question whether it's safe for their child to ingest it, based on highly publicized research results in the 1970s suggesting a possible causal relationship between saccharin and bladder tumors in laboratory rats. It has been documented that the saccharin samples used in the studies were impure and the results were incorrectly interpreted.[49]

Sucralose is 600 times sweeter than sugar, is the only low-calorie sweetener made from sugar, and is excreted in the urine essentially unchanged. Sucralose is not recognized by the body as either sugar or carbohydrate because it is not broken down or metabolized by the body. Furthermore, it does not affect blood glucose levels. Sucralose is marketed as Splenda, which contains a small amount of maltodextrin or dextrose and does provide some carbohydrate and calories. Individual packages contain less than 1 gram of carbohydrate, but 1 cup of Splenda granular contains 96 calories and 24 grams of carbohydrate. Sucralose is heat stable and may be used during cooking and baking. The FDA states that no adverse or carcinogenic effects are associated with sucralose consumption.[49]

Neotame is 7000 to 13,000 times sweeter than sugar, partially digested in the small intestine, and excreted in the urine and the feces. Neotame does have a small amount of phenylalanine, but even when consumed at 90% of the estimated daily intake, it was clinically not significant for individuals with PKU. It is marketed as

having a clean, sweet taste without the aftertaste associated with other noncaloric sweeteners, and is used in beverages and a variety of other foods. It is heat stable and can be used in a variety of products such as beverages, dairy products, and baked goods.[49]

Stevioside is 200–400 times sweeter than sucrose and comes from the stevia plant. It is extracted from the leaf of the plant and is used as a noncaloric sweetener. The JECFA (Joint Expert Committee on Food Additives) established an ADI for steviol glycosides and is being used in a variety of foods.[50] Steviosides are marketed as Rubiana (Truvia) and RebA (PureVia), both of which have zero calories per serving.

Lo Han Guo also known as Monk Fruit, is a fruit sweetener derived from removing the juice from the small fruit grown in Southeast Asia. The fruit extract is 150–200 times sweeter than sucrose and contains zero calories per serving. Monk fruit is considered safe for the general population, including children, and does not affect glucose control; however, an ADI has not been established due to the lack of studies.[49,51]

Dietary Fiber

Total dietary fiber consists of structural and storage polysaccharides and lignin in plants that are not well digested in humans.[53] These can include plant nonstarch polysaccharides: cellulose, pectin, gums, hemicelluloses, β-glucans, and fibers in oat and wheat bran; plant carbohydrates such as inulin, oligosaccharides, and fructan; lignan, and resistant starch. Functional fibers are considered fibers that are added to foods or supplements which have health benefits. Even though the Nutrition Facts label continues to divide dietary fiber as soluble and insoluble, the IOM classifies fiber as fermentable and viscous, which is based on their physiological function.

Dietary fiber recommendations for children do not specify the type or function of fiber to consume, but the 2015–2020 Dietary Guidelines for Americans suggests consuming 14g dietary fiber/1000kcal/day in children.[23] Fiber recommendations for children with diabetes are the same as for children without diabetes which include to increase both types of fiber from a wide variety of food sources and base this increase upon the child's usual eating habits, glucose, and lipid goals (**TABLE 20.9**).

Research has been mixed on the benefits of consuming dietary fiber to reduce hyperglycemia. Choosing low GI foods and increasing dietary fiber may reduce the risk of T2D in adults, but data are lacking in children. Few studies have shown the benefits of consuming a high fiber diet to reduce hyperglycemia; however, recent findings have shown that glycemic control may be improved by eating a high-fiber, low glycemic-index diet in children with T1D.[53]

TABLE 20.9 Dietary Fiber Recommendations

Ages	Total Dietary Fiber grams/day
Children 1 to 3 y	19
Children 4 to 8 y	25
Boys 9 to 13 y	26
Girls 9 to 18 y	26
Boys 14 to 18 y	31

Modified from Institute of Medicine of the National Academies. *Dietary Reference Intakes: The Essential Guide to Nutrient Requirements*. Washington, DC: National Academies Press; 2006.[24]

Dietary fiber, specifically soluble viscous fiber, additionally has been shown to reduce cholesterol. The **Cardiovascular Health Integrated Lifestyle Diet** (CHILD) intervention recommends treating dyslipidemia by adding psyllium fiber 6g/d for children 2–12 years old and 12g/d for those 12 years and older to lower LDL-cholesterol by approximately 7%.[54,55]

Protein

Protein intake in children and adolescents should be sufficient to support adequate growth and development. At this time, there are no data to support children with diabetes requiring a higher or lower protein intake than the RDA. It is estimated that the average protein intake in the United States for all ages is about 15–20% of total daily calories, including sources from legumes, fish, lean cuts of meat and low-fat dairy products.[26] For children with diabetes related kidney disease, protein should not be restricted. Reducing protein intake below the RDA is not recommended since it does not improve the **glomerular filtration rate** (GFR) decline.[42] Children engaging in consistent competitive exercise may need some additional protein due to increased muscle tissue support needs, which can be met by increasing consumption of protein-rich foods.

Because most protein sources are low in carbohydrate, families sometimes consider these foods as a free option because they do not require insulin. Foods such as cheese, lean meats, and eggs are healthy protein-rich foods and should be eaten throughout the day, but should not be eaten in excess and considered a free food.

Effect of Protein on Blood Glucose

Previously, it was believed that eating protein with carbohydrates was helpful to prevent hypoglycemia[2]; however, gluconeogenesis increases after eating protein causing delayed postprandial hyperglycemia, requiring additional insulin and prolonging insulin delivery for those individuals using intensive insulin therapy.[31,42,56] Studies have shown different effects on glycemia when protein is consumed alone versus consumed with carbohydrates and/or fat. Consuming 30g protein in a mixed meal or, consuming 75g protein alone, will delay hyperglycemia (approximately 100 minutes).[57] There is no consensus on the amount of insulin required for high protein meals; but changing the delivery of insulin through the insulin pump by either using a dual-wave, combination, or square-wave bolus, or by splitting the bolus dose has been beneficial to prevent delayed hyperglycemia.[31,56]

Dietary Fat

The primary dietary fat goal in children with diabetes is to promote a healthy fat intake, sufficient to optimize growth and development. Intakes of 30–40% and 25–35% of total fat are recommended in children ages 1 to 3 years and ages 4 to 18 years respectively.[23] Careful consideration should be given to providing enough fat in the diet for children less than 2 years of age, because the development of the brain and central nervous system are dependent upon an adequate intake of fats.

Screening for dyslipidemia entails measuring a lipoprotein profile after an overnight fast, including **total cholesterol** (TC), **triglyceride** (TG), **low-density lipoprotein-cholesterol** (LDL-C), **high-density lipoprotein-cholesterol** (HDL-C), and non-HDL-C. Non-HDL-C can be measured non-fasting (subtracting HDL-C from TC) and may be a more advantageous screening tool for pediatric patients.[58] However, treatment algorithms are based on fasting LDL-C.

T1D and T2D are both considered the highest possible risk classification for cardiovascular disease (CVD).[54] Evidence suggests that insulin deficiency increases hepatic release of VLDL, leading to elevated TG and LDL-C. Furthermore, blood glucose control may directly influence the levels of TG and LDL-C worsening endothelial dysfunction. The ADA has published guidelines for managing dyslipidemia in children with diabetes.[38]

Screening

- Obtain a fasting lipid profile in children ≥10 years (at puberty) of age soon after the diagnosis (after glucose control has been established) in those without a history of hypercholesterolemia or early CVD; those with a family history or known cardiovascular risk factors, lipid screening should be performed in all children after the age of 2 years. See **TABLE 20.10** for cholesterol screening guidelines.
- If lipids are abnormal, annual monitoring is reasonable. If LDL cholesterol values are within the accepted risk level (<100mg/dL), a lipid profile repeated every 3–5 years is reasonable

TABLE 20.10 NHLBI Cholesterol Screening Guidelines and Cut Points for Children and Adolescents with Diabetes (Adapted from AAP Cardiovascular Guidelines)

Category	Acceptable (mg/dL)	Borderline* (mg/dL)	Abnormal ** (mg/dL)
TC	<170	170–199	≥200
LDL-C	<100	100–129	≥130
Non-HDL-C	<120	120–144	≥145
TG 0–9 years 10–19 years	 <75 <90	 75–99 90–129	 ≥100 ≥130
HDL-C	>45	40–45	<40

*Borderline values represent the 75th percentile, except for HDL-C, which represents the 25th percentile.

**Abnormal values represent the 95th percentile, except for the HDL-C, which represents the 10th percentile.

Modified from American Academy of Pediatrics. Expert Panel on Integrated Guidelines for Cardiovascular Health in Risk Reduction in Children and Adolescents: Summary Report. Pediatr. 2011;128 (Suppl5):S213–S256.[59]

MNT Treatment Strategies

- Maximize glycemic control
- Weight reduction, if necessary
- Initiate Cardiovascular Health Integrated Lifestyle Diet CHILD-1 Diet Intervention for 6 months to lower LDL-C
  - Total fat 30% of daily kcal/d
  - 8–10% of total kcal from saturated fat
  - Avoid *trans* fat as much as possible
  - Monounsaturated fat (MUFA) and polyunsaturated fat (PUFA) fat up to 20% of daily kcal
  - Cholesterol <300mg/d
  - Limit/avoid sugar-sweetened beverages, encourage water
  - Encourage dietary fiber from foods
- Medication in collaboration with a physician
- Manage other cardiac disease risk factors:
  - Blood pressure
  - Smoking
  - Obesity
  - Inactivity
- RDN should initiate CHILD-2 Diet MNT if CHILD-1 diet does not result in lowering LDL-C to goal level:
  - 25–30% of total kcal from fat
  - ≤7% of total kcal from saturated fat
  - 10% of total kcal from MUFA
  - <200 mg/d of cholesterol
  - Avoid *trans* fat as much as possible
  - Add 2g/d plant sterol esters and/or plant stanol esters in children older than 2 y of age
  - Add water-soluble fiber psyllium: 6g/d for children 2–12 y of age and 12g/d for those ≥12 y of age

- To lower TG or non-HDL-C RDN should initiate CHILD-2 TG MNT:
  - Decrease sugar intake
  - Replace simple with complex carbohydrates
  - No sugar-sweetened beverages
  - Increase dietary fish to increase ω-3 fatty acids

If LDL-C remains elevated (>160mg/dL or >130mg/dL with one or more CVD risk factors) despite MNT and lifestyle changes, a statin may be suggested in children 10 years and older.[38]

Effect of Dietary Fat on Blood Glucose

Dietary fat reduces insulin sensitivity, increases hepatic glucose production, and delays gastric emptying, all contributing to delayed postprandial glycemia. Meals containing carbohydrates and high in dietary fat, can cause hyperglycemia more than 3 hours later. Traditional preprandial bolusing for high fat meals may cause initial hypoglycemia with subsequent delayed hyperglycemia; therefore, those on intensive insulin therapy are advised to use extended dual-wave or square-wave bolusing when using insulin pumps or to split the bolus dose to maintain euglycemia.[57,60,61]

Vitamins and Minerals

Vitamins and minerals are necessary for normal growth and development. Most children with diabetes do not need additional vitamin and mineral supplements if their food intake is adequate and well balanced. However, a child's normal eating habits throughout the growth cycle may exclude or severely limit foods or food groups; thus nutrient supplementation may be needed. The response to vitamin and mineral supplements will be favorable only when deficiencies are present; therefore, micronutrient adequacy should be evaluated periodically as a youth's food preferences change. There has not been substantial evidence to support supplementation with chromium, magnesium, and vitamin D, as well as herbs such as cinnamon, to improve glycemic control.[2,39] Individuals taking metformin (glucophage) may experience vitamin B_{12} deficiency, therefore it is suggested to test periodically in those with anemia or peripheral neuropathy. Routine supplementation is not recommended by the ADA because of lack of evidence and concern related to long-term safety of antioxidant supplements, such as vitamins E and C and carotene.[26,38] It is important that children with diabetes annually meet with a RDN to ensure their diet is nutritionally sound and no further recommendation is necessary. Children who lack a varied diet, eliminate certain food groups, strict vegetarians (vegans), take medications known to alter certain micronutrients, or who have consistently poor glycemic control, are at risk for nutrient deficiencies and may benefit from a multivitamin supplement.

Vitamin D

Evidence suggests that low vitamin D (25OHD) levels are associated with insulin resistance and may be a risk factor for both T1D and T2D. Recent studies suggest that vitamin D deficiency and insufficiency is common in children in the US; however, children and adolescents with diabetes have a lower level of serum 25OHD compared with healthy controls.[62–64] Low levels may be attributed to drinking less milk, obesity, and wearing sun protection. The Endocrine Society defines vitamin D deficiency as a 25OHD<20ng/mL; insufficiency as 21–29ng/mL and sufficiency as at least 30ng/mL.[65] The AAP has increased its recommendation to 400IU/d for infants and 600IU/d for children and adolescents. Tolerable upper limits include 1000IU/d (0–6 months), 1500IU/d (6–12 months), 2500IU/d (1–3 y), 3000IU/d (4–8 y) and 4000IU/d (9–18 y).[66] If a child is not consuming adequate fortified milk or milk substitute, supplementation might be necessary in order to meet the new recommendations, especially during the winter months in northern areas.

Sodium

Sodium recommendations in children and adolescents with diabetes vary from less than 2.3g/day, like the general population, to less than 1.5g/day for children >9 years of age.[26,38] Whereas, it has been found that US children ages 6–8 years eat an average of about 3.3g of sodium a day.[67]

Reduced sodium intake lowers blood pressure (BP) in children and may have a significant impact on reducing cardiovascular morbidity and mortality.[68] Furthermore, it has been shown that dietary sodium intake is related to vascular dysfunction in children with T1D.[69] This relationship between sodium intake and vascular smooth muscle is independent of glycemic control and blood pressure. Routine monitoring of BP and dietary advice to reduce sodium is important for all children and adolescents with diabetes, to reduce the prevalence of BP-related cardiovascular disease in adults.[68]

Alcohol

Alcohol use and abuse should be discussed with the adolescent in an objective manner. Although consuming alcohol is illegal and is always discouraged for teens, early screening for alcohol use and facts about how alcohol affects BG levels should be available to teens who express an interest in drinking. Alcohol lowers the BG level and increases the risk of hypoglycemia (up to 10–12 hours) by blocking gluconeogenesis, reducing counter-regulatory hormones, leading to erratic behavior, loss of consciousness, or seizures, particularly if food is not consumed with the alcohol.[26,70] Additionally, the teen should understand that glucagon is not effective in the treatment of alcohol-induced hypoglycemia since alcohol depletes glycogen stores.

Pointing out that alcohol alters the ability to think clearly may help the teen to be more cautious about drinking alcohol or, to avoid it altogether. It is important that those who choose to drink, don't drink alone and make sure that they always wear diabetes identification since intoxication and symptoms of hypoglycemia can often be confused for one another. Eating a carbohydrate snack before bedtime is also encouraged to prevent nocturnal hypoglycemia. Insulin doses may need to be adjusted for food when drinking to prevent hypoglycemia as well.[26] Frequent BG monitoring through fingersticks and/or CGM are helpful tools for teens to identify the effects alcohol has on glucose levels and insulin adjustments required to avoid complications.[70] If alcohol is consumed, it should be consumed in moderate amounts (no more than one drink per day for most females and no more than two drinks a day for most males) and only if diabetes is well managed. One drink or alcohol portion is defined as 12 oz. of beer, 5 oz. of wine, or 1.5 oz. of 80-proof distilled spirits. Each of these portions provides about 15 g. of alcohol.

Nutrition and Insulin Management During Exercise and Activity

Regular exercise or activity is an important element in reducing cardiovascular disease risk, lowering A1c, improving insulin sensitivity, lowering lipid levels, improving cardiorespiratory fitness, and maintaining appropriate body weight.[71,72] Exercise recommendations for children with diabetes do not differ than that of the general population: exercise 60 minutes or more daily, including muscle-strengthening activities three days a week.[73] Children with well-controlled T1D can have similar exercise capacity and optimal athletic performance compared to those without diabetes; whereas children with T2D may have impaired exercise capacity, related insulin resistance and increased free fatty acid production.[74] However, children with diabetes tend to be less active compared to children without diabetes related to the fear of hypoglycemia, the inconvenience of checking BG levels frequently, as well as feeling different than their peers.[74]

Exercise is classified as either aerobic or anaerobic. Aerobic exercise involves longer duration, low-to-moderate intensity walking, jogging, or swimming, by using large muscle groups dependent on using the aerobic energy systems. Aerobic exercise can reduce BG levels 50–100 mg/dL within 20–60 minutes after starting the activity, but hypoglycemia most likely occurs within 45 minutes of starting the activity. Anaerobic exercise involves resistance strength training which is often performed at a higher intensity and shorter duration. High intensity training, including sprint intervals, increases the breakdown of glycogen and can reduce the risk of hypoglycemia. Additionally, resistance training may cause a rise in blood glucose levels for 30–60 minutes after the activity due to counter-regulatory hormone increases (adrenal response); however, this may be transient, resulting in hypoglycemia hours later.[72,75]

Delayed hypoglycemia may continue 4 to 24 hours after intense exercise or after a very active day due to increased insulin sensitivity, decreased glycogen stores, and decreased counter-regulatory response.[74,76,77] Additionally, the risk of nocturnal hypoglycemia is heightened after exercising in the late afternoon. Reducing insulin doses as well as eating a snack or meal containing carbohydrate plus protein within 30–60 minutes after intense exercise, is advised to replenish glycogen stores and to prevent delayed hypoglycemia.

Before exercise begins, blood glucose levels should be greater than 90mg/dL.[72,74] If levels are less than 90mg/dL, children should consume enough carbohydrates necessary to achieve a pre-exercise blood glucose goal. Blood glucose goals ranging between 126–180mg/dL should be established before exercise in order to prevent hypoglycemia and can vary depending on the type of exercise and duration. Exercising with unexplained hyperglycemia (>240mg/dL) related to insulin deficiency increases the risk of blood ketones and DKA; therefore, it is recommended for children and adolescents with diabetes to avoid exercising when ketones are present. In contrast, exercising with severe hypoglycemia (BG <50mg/dL) or having a previous hypoglycemic event 24 hours before exercise, increases the risk of a more serious hypoglycemic episode. To maintain healthy blood glucose levels during and after exercise, additional blood glucose monitoring every 30 minutes of activity, nutrition, and insulin adjustments are required to effectively manage diabetes.[72]

Nutrition Adjustments for Exercise

Exercise lasting less than 30 minutes may not require eating additional carbohydrates unless BG levels are less than 90mg/dL before exercise.[72] To prevent hypoglycemia during activity, food intake may need to be increased.

Food adjustments will depend on the duration and intensity of the exercise and on the BG level before the activity. If the pre-exercise insulin dose is not decreased and exercise is longer than 30 minutes, a general rule is to add 10 to 15g of carbohydrate for every 30 minutes of activity without insulin coverage if on basal/bolus insulin regimens. Prolonged activity (longer than 60 minutes) may utilize most glucose stores in the muscle and require additional carbohydrates, 30–60 grams/hour. Carbohydrate taken in smaller amounts, 10–20 grams every 20 minutes, may be helpful to prevent gastrointestinal upset and maintain blood glucose control, instead of larger amounts of carbohydrate every hour.[75]

The type of carbohydrate may play a role in effective management of diabetes and exercise. High GI foods and beverages, such as sports drinks, gels, and carbohydrate chews will provide a faster release of glucose to prevent and/or treat hypoglycemia when exercising. They may also be advantageous after exercise to promote recovery and restore muscle glycogen more quickly. Eating lower GI foods before exercise may be helpful to maintain euglycemia, especially for long endurance type sports; however, research is not conclusive to support using the GI to enhance exercise performance or maintain glucose control.[72,75]

Insulin Adjustments for Exercise

For planned exercise or weight management, adjusting insulin dosages to prevent hypoglycemia may be more desirable than increasing carbohydrate intake, unless the activity is greater than one hour. It is advantageous to avoid exercise when insulin is peaking, but it is not always preventable. The amount of insulin reduction depends upon the results of BG checks done before, during, and after the activity. When on a basal/bolus insulin regimen, it is important to reduce fast-acting insulin when the dose is given within 40–90 minutes before exercise.[75] It is advisable to start decreasing the fast-acting insulin dose by 20% for the meal or snack before exercise if exercising 30 minutes or longer; however, insulin reductions may be greater than 50% of the bolus dose depending upon blood glucose results.[77]

Long-acting insulin doses should be reduced by 20% the night before the day of heavy and extended exercise or activity. This includes an all-day sports camp or an all-day sports tournament. Children and adolescents on an insulin pump have the advantage of using a reduced temporary bolus rate set for exercise to maintain euglycemia. However, it is important to not disconnect from the insulin pump for more than hour to prevent hyperglycemia. Basal rate reductions 60–90 minutes before exercise is more effective to reduce hypoglycemia during exercise and post exercise hyperglycemia rather than disconnecting or suspending insulin.[72]

Absorption of insulin may influence the blood glucose result during exercise. Warm temperatures can increase insulin absorption, whereas colder temperatures cause decreased insulin absorption. Furthermore, it is advisable to avoid injecting insulin in the exercising limb to prevent insulin absorption increases resulting in hypoglycemia.[75]

Children and adolescents with T2D continue to have some beta cell function and insulin resistance. Oral medications, such as metformin, are provided to enhance insulin sensitivity, but do not increase the risk of exercise induced hypoglycemia. The risk of hypoglycemia increases for those individuals taking metformin combined with insulin therapy.[74] Decreases in metformin as well as insulin may be necessary if weight loss and regular training improves insulin sensitivity.[76]

▸ Designing the Meal Plan

The ultimate goals when designing a meal plan for a child who has been recently diagnosed with T1D are to:

- Provide healthy eating guidelines for the youth and family
- Promote positive behavioral changes
- Provide healthy meals and snacks
- Focus on healthy eating habits for the entire family

The amount of time required by the family to learn meal planning depends on multiple factors such as family dynamics, emotional status, extended support system, preconceived ideas about the "diabetic diet," and the family's social and cultural attitudes. The child should participate in the initial visit and be reassured that he or she will not be put on a "diet" or have many favorite foods taken away. Rather, healthy guidelines (a meal plan) will be provided based on the child's usual eating pattern to help promote healthy food choices. To avoid isolating the child and dividing the family, it should be emphasized that meal planning is simply a heart-healthy eating plan for both the child and the entire family. Eating the same foods provides a sense of unity within the family.

Nutrition Counseling

At the time of diagnosis, the parent and/or child may be asked to keep a record of what is eaten at each meal and snack. This helps establish the amount of food that is currently needed to satisfy the child's appetite. An accurate measurement of weight and height (or length), information on recent weight loss, and a calculation of IBW are needed to estimate the child's current nutrient and caloric needs. Determining the percentile of the height (length), weight, body mass index (BMI), and the range for IBW will identify the child's initial nutrition status and help guide the development of the meal plan. A newly diagnosed child is more likely to experience increased hunger due to glycosuria. It is important to respond to this stimulated appetite by providing sufficient food so that hunger and restriction are not associated with having diabetes. The appetite of most children will stabilize within the first few weeks after diagnosis, though it could take longer. If the youth has lost weight or not grown to their potential, their appetite may be greater than estimated needs. Within reason, the meal plan should reflect the amount of food the child desires and be readjusted once the appetite resumes to normal. The family should be told that the meal plan might need to be adjusted two or three weeks after diagnosis once the child has returned to his or her growth potential.

Nutrition intervention at diagnosis should be based on the family's ability, interest, and readiness to learn. Attempts to present all concepts upon initial diagnosis may result in confusion and the family members' loss of confidence in their ability as caretakers. Provide only general guidelines such as consistency with timing, amount and types of foods, and the relationship among food, insulin, and exercise, and their effect on BG. The initial education might be in a hospital or an outpatient setting; routine follow-up visits or contact by phone may be beneficial. Many questions will arise when the child returns home and normal activity resumes. Above all, it should be stressed that:

- Parents should not limit carbohydrates to maintain BG control.
- Any changes associated with food choices should be made slowly.
- Ranges for food choices should be used with young children (i.e., 1–2 oz. protein, ½–1 fruit), offering smaller amounts first and using the larger end of the range if more food is requested.
- During initial education the length of time required to achieve nutrition management survival skills varies considerably between families and may require 2 to 4 hours of education in addition to time for menu writing and food selection using the meal plan.
- After the initial education, additional outpatient nutrition visits will be necessary to achieve ultimate nutrition education goals.

General guidelines to help develop a positive working relationship with the youth and their caretakers include:

- Include children and adolescents in the interview to allow them to be part of the decision-making process. The child or adolescent will dictate the amount of food based on hunger and the parent will dictate the food choices.
- Do not refer to or label the child or adolescent as a diabetic but as a child or adolescent with diabetes.
- Interview the pre-pubertal child separately and then together with family to stimulate self-management.
- Provide reassurance that many of the child's or adolescent's usual foods can be included in his or her meal plan.
- Describe the meal plan as a guideline for healthy eating rather than a diet.
- Stress healthy eating practices for the entire family rather than just focusing on the child or adolescent with diabetes.
- Avoid negative words when explaining meal planning such as *cannot, do not, never, should not, bad, restrict*, and especially the word *diet*. In a child's mind, *diet* connotes deprivation or a short-term process, rather than an ongoing process.
- Avoid using the terms *good* or *bad* for foods. Instead, use *healthy* and *not as healthy* to describe individual foods.
- Ask about favorite foods and avoid eliminating these foods. Instead, stress balance, moderation, and variety.
- Review the reality of special treats for birthday parties, holidays, and special occasions
- Encourage the caregiver to include the child or adolescent in shopping and meal preparation.
- Revise or draft a realistic and workable meal plan with input from the parent and/or child or adolescent.
- Encourage the parents to always keep the lines of communication open so the child or adolescent can request special foods that he or she wants to eat and that can be worked into the meal plan. Avoid being the "food police." If the youth is always told "no," he or she may start to sneak food, which will cause unexplained high blood glucose levels.
- Advise the caregivers that it is not advisable to omit foods from the meal plan because of a single high BG reading. An elevated BG level caused by stress

may decrease rapidly when the stress is reduced, and hypoglycemia may occur if food is omitted.

- Continued nutrition follow-up and education are required every 6 months to 1 year as the child grows and develops and as the family works to gain expertise in the nutrition management of diabetes.

Nutrition Monitoring and Evaluation
Monitoring Blood Glucose

Glycosylated hemoglobin (A1C) measures the weighted average amount of glucose in the blood over a 2- to 3-month period and is recommended to measure four times a year.[78] Used in conjunction with regularly SMBG, the A1C can help evaluate the level of control. However, it reflects an average amount of glucose in the blood and can be the result of very high and low BG levels, which is not indicative of good control. Although "excellent control" for an adult with diabetes is 6% or less, the activity levels and eating habits of children and adolescents vary, so even a level under 7% can be difficult to achieve in children. A1C goals should be set by the child's diabetes team and tailored to each individual case. A1C goals are shown in **TABLE 20.11**.

Key Concepts in Setting Glycemic Goals

Goals should be individualized and lower goals may be reasonable based on a benefit-risk assessment. Blood glucose goals should be modified in children with frequent hypoglycemia or hypoglycemia unawareness. Postprandial blood glucose values should be measured when there is a discrepancy between preprandial blood glucose values and A1C levels and to assess preprandial insulin doses in those on basal-bolus or pump regimens.

Fructosamine is an alternative measurement that reflects the BG levels over the preceding three to four weeks. It measures the glycation of serum proteins (albumin) and replaces using the A1C in children and adolescents with red blood cell disorders such as sickle cell or hemolytic anemia.[78]

Home SMBG meters provide the child and family with immediate feedback on the effects of food, exercise, insulin, and stress on blood glucose levels, allowing

TABLE 20.11	Blood Glucose and A1C Goals for Pediatric Type 1 Diabetes			
Before Meals	**Bedtime**	**A1C**	**Rationale**	
90–130 mg/dL	90–150 mg/dL	<7.5%	A goal <7.0% is reasonable if it can be achieved without excessive hypoglycemia	

Modified from American Diabetes Association. Standards of medical care in diabetes- children and adolescents. *Diabetes Care.* 2017;40(Suppl1):S105–S113.[38]

for more flexibility in lifestyle and food intake. SMBG should be performed four to six times daily, before each meal, and before bedtime. Additional checks should be done before and throughout physical activity, if there is suspicion of hypoglycemia or hyperglycemia, or if the child is ill. Blood glucose checks can also be performed 2 hours after the start of meals or snacks to determine if the insulin-to-carbohydrate ratio or if carbohydrate counting is accurate. This should only be performed if the pre-meal BG level is within a healthy range and a correction or sensitivity factor is not required to correct for hyperglycemia.

A child or adolescent with diabetes has many self-care responsibilities. Checking and recording the BG levels may be one of the most bothersome responsibilities because it must be done so often and because others may inappropriately evaluate and judge the results. Blood glucose results are not totally reliable as a monitor of adherence to carbohydrate counting. If, by reporting a high BG reading, a child risks accusations of sneaking food or overeating, and they may choose to record a more acceptable but false level. This practice may result in poor diabetes management. Establishing a nonjudgmental and honest atmosphere for the exchange of information is imperative for the parent, the RDN, and other healthcare providers. When monitoring BG, use the word "check" rather than "test" and use positive words to describe the results, such as "high" or "low" rather than "good" or "bad." Any information received from monitoring provides information with positive feedback, regardless of the number.[79]

High or low BG levels will still occur in most children even when insulin, exercise schedules, and carbohydrate counting are followed closely. When a high or low level occurs, it is useful to review the day's activities to see if there is an obvious explanation. Looking for BG patterns is more important when making insulin adjustments rather than a single abnormal glucose level. The extent to which children should monitor BG levels is variable, depending on many factors such as the type of insulin therapy, increased activity or exercise, sickness or infection, new food choices, change in lifestyle, increased stress, change in insulin type or dose, episodes of hypoglycemia, or overall control. A general guideline is to achieve at least 50% of BG within a healthy range (70–180 mg/dL) and less than 10% below the range.[78]

Continuous Glucose Monitoring

CGM is now widely available for the consumer and provides a complete picture of blood glucose activity in real time. The system is made of three components: the sensor, transmitter, and receiver. The sensor is a small flexible electrode that sits under the skin in the interstitial fluid, which is the liquid that surrounds our cells. The

sensor catheter is introduced by a needle, but the needle is removed, and the sensor can be worn 3–7 days depending on the CGM. The transmitter is a tiny computer attached to the sensor that sends the information from the sensor to a wireless receiver. The receiver is the size of a beeper or cell phone and it will collect the information and display it on a screen. It will display the BG reading every 1–5 minutes and provide a directional trend of where the glucose is going. There is a lag time in the reading, so a finger stick remains the gold standard when treating hypoglycemia. The devices display arrows and alarms that can be set to warn if the BG is rising or dropping rapidly so treatment can be administered quickly. This technology is very helpful to families and children with diabetes so educators can teach them how to cover meals with adequate insulin (such as pizza, fast food, and Chinese food) that have been challenging in the past. Once the effect of the meal on the BG is viewed, the diabetes educator can help the youth determine the best way to cover the meal.

Glucose Downloads

Downloading blood glucose reports is a common practice for families and diabetes providers to interpret data trends, especially when hand written reports are difficult to maintain.[78] Disadvantages of using downloads include the expense, proper insurance coverage, intrusive to wear, and inaccurate loading of date and time of the glucose meters which make it difficult to interpret data.[29,78]

Hypoglycemia

Hypoglycemia is a common acute complication in diabetes. It has several causes, including excess insulin, missed meals, alcohol intake, and exercise. Severe prolonged hypoglycemia is defined in pediatrics as an event that results in coma or seizures.[38]

For a child treated with insulin, hypoglycemia is defined as less than 70mg/dL.[38,80] Adrenergic symptoms, such as shaking and sweating, may occur when blood glucose levels are dropping rapidly even when the level is still in the normal range.

Neuroglycopenic symptoms may include drowsiness and headache, but young children may experience behavioral changes such as irritability and tantrums. Compromised counter-regulatory hormone increases the risk of hypoglycemia and can lead to impaired hypoglycemia awareness. Children and adolescents with diabetes should be instructed to wear medical alert identification always to ensure proper treatment of hypoglycemic reactions, which may render the child unable to communicate.

Treating mild hypoglycemia involves the 15-15 rule: Treat the low BG with 15 grams of fast-acting carbohydrate, wait 15 minutes, and then recheck the blood glucose. If glucose levels remain low, the treatment should be repeated until euglycemia is reached. One gram of carbohydrate raises an average adult's BG up ~3mg/dL; young children tend to be more sensitive, so 1 gram could raise their BG up 3–5mg/dL. Therefore, it is recommended that families and diabetes providers use 0.3 g/kg of a fast-acting carbohydrate to prevent over-treating hypoglycemia.[80] Those caring for children may want to use sweets to treat hypoglycemia; however, foods and beverages that contain dietary fat are absorbed more slowly and delay the BG rise and should be avoided.[80] The counter-regulatory hormone, glucagon should available for injection in case fast acting carbohydrates cannot be ingested.[80]

TABLE 20.12 provides information on foods recommended to treat hypoglycemia.

Age-Specific Developmental Considerations

The most important psychosocial issues facing families with children with diabetes are:

- Defining responsibilities and support for diabetes management within the family
- Sharing treatment responsibilities among family members
- How and when these responsibilities are transferred from parent to child as the child develops

As the child with diabetes progresses through the different stages of development, it is important to address how these changes affect the parents and/or the child and focus on the normal developmental issues of each stage. Encouraging parental involvement throughout childhood and early adulthood can be beneficial in the child's diabetes management. See **TABLE 20.13** for some of the development stages and how they relate to T1D.

TABLE 20.12 Recommended Foods for Treating Hypoglycemia

Food item	1–5 Years	6–10 Years	10+ Years
Amount recommended	5–10 g carbohydrate	10–15 g carbohydrate	15–20 g carbohydrate
Regular soda 1 fl oz = 3–4g carb	2–3 fl oz	4–5 fl oz	5–6 fl oz
Cane sugar 1 tsp = 4g	2 tsp	3 tsp	4–5 tsp
Jelly beans 5 beans = 5g	5–10 beans	10–15 beans	15–20 beans
Orange juice ½ cup = 13–15g carb	¼–½ cup	½–3/4 cup	3/4–1 cup
Apple juice ½ cup = 15g carb	1/6–1/3 cup	1/3–½ cup	½–2/3 cup
Honey, pancake, or Corn syrup 1 tsp = 4–5g carb	2 tsp	3 tsp	4–5 tsp
Jolly Ranchers 1 piece = 5g	2–3 candies	4–5 candies	5–6 candies
Marshmallows, Mini (2 = 5g)	2–4	4–6	6–8
Marshmallows Large (1 = 5g)	1–2	2–3	3–4
Raisins 1 Tbsp. = 7.5g	1 Tbsp	1½–2 Tbsp	2½ Tbsp
Glucose tablets 4–5g carb/each	1–2 tablets	2–3 tablets	3–4 tablets
Insta-glucose 2 g carb/tube	1/3–½ tube	½–2/3 tube	2/3–1 tube
Glucose 45 45g/tube	1/6–¼ tube	¼–1/3 tube	1/3–½ tube

Data from Laffel LMB, Butler DA, Higgins LA, Lawlor MT, Pasquarello CA, eds. *Joslin's Guide to Managing Childhood Diabetes: A Family Teamwork Approach.* Boston, MA: Joslin Diabetes Center; 2009.[81]

Silverstein J, Klingensmith G, Copeland K, et al. Care of children and adolescents with type 1 diabetes: a statement of the American Diabetes Association. *Diabetes Care.* 2005;28(1):186–212.[82]

TABLE 20.13 Major Development Issues and Their Effect on Diabetes in Children and Adolescents

Developmental Stage (Approximate Ages)	Normal Developmental Tasks	T1D Management Priorities	Family Issues in T1D Management
Infancy (0–12 months)	Developing a trusting relationship/"bonding" with primary caretakers	■ Preventing and treating hypoglycemia ■ Avoiding extreme fluctuations in the BG levels	■ Coping with stress ■ Sharing the "burden of care" to avoid parent burnout
Toddler (13–36 months)	Developing a sense of mastery and autonomy	■ Preventing and treating hypoglycemia ■ Avoiding extreme fluctuations in the BG levels due to irregular food intake	■ Establishing a schedule ■ Managing the picky eater ■ Setting limits and coping with toddlers' lack of cooperation with regimen ■ Sharing the burden of care
Preschooler and early elementary age (3–7 years)	Developing initiative in activities and confidence in self	■ Preventing and treating hypoglycemia ■ Unpredictable appetite and activity ■ Positive reinforcement for cooperation with regimen ■ Trusting other caretakers with diabetes management	■ Reassuring the child that diabetes is no one's fault ■ Educating other caretakers about diabetes management
Older elementary school age (8–11 years)	■ Developing skills in athletic, cognitive, artistic, and social areas ■ Consolidating self-esteem with respect to the peer group	■ Making diabetes regimen flexible to allow for participation in school/peer activities ■ Child learning short- and long-term benefits of optimal control	■ Maintaining parental involvement in insulin and BG monitoring tasks while allowing for independent self-care for "special occasions" ■ Continuing to educate school and other caretakers
Early adolescence (12–15 years)	Managing body changes Developing a strong sense of self-identity	■ Managing increased insulin requirements during puberty ■ Diabetes management and blood glucose control become more difficult ■ Weight and body image concerns	■ Renegotiating parents' and teen's role in diabetes management to be accepted by both ■ Learning coping skills to enhance ability to self-manage ■ Preventing and intervening with diabetes-related family conflict ■ Monitoring for signs of depression, eating disorders, and risky behaviors
Later adolescence (16–19 years)	Establishing a sense of identity after high school (decision about location, social issues, work, education)	■ Begin discussion of transition to new diabetes team ■ Integrating diabetes into new lifestyle	■ Supporting the transition to independence ■ Learning coping skills to enhance ability to self-manage ■ Preventing and intervening with diabetes-related family conflict ■ Monitoring for signs of depression, eating disorders, or risky behavior

Birth to 12 Months of Age

Initially, most infants consume 100% of their calories as breast milk or formula, eating every 3 to 4 hours. The AAP recommends that all babies are breastfed exclusively for the first 6 months and to continue nursing until the infant's first year of life or longer depending on the desires of the mother and infant;[83] iron-fortified infant formula is the only acceptable substitute. Solids are typically introduced at 6 months but should not be before 4 months. Parents should introduce one new food each week and start with rice cereal to fruits, meat, vegetables, and/or vegetable-meat dinners. 100% fruit juice should also not be introduced in infants before the age of 12 months.[84] Infants with diabetes do well following the same schedule to manage insulin and BG levels more effectively.[35] Eventually when the infant begins eating 2 to 3 tablespoons of baby foods and/ or table food (other than low-calorie vegetables), basic carbohydrate counting can be introduced as a guideline. It is recommended to establish a feeding schedule despite somewhat erratic eating behaviors in the infant.

One to 4 Years of Age

A 1992 report in the *New England Journal of Medicine* proposed a possible link between drinking cow's milk as an infant and the development of T1D. Upon further inspection, the association of exposure to cow's milk and T1D is unlikely.[85,86] Although whole cow's milk should not be given during the child's first year, after the first year, cow's milk should not be removed from the diets of infants who have a family history of T1D.

Between 12 and 15 months of age, breastmilk (or formula) intake may begin to decrease and the intake of solid food increases. A total revision of the meal plan is needed at this time. During this time, a child may begin to be more accepting of meat and cheese, which can be added to the meal plan. Although fruits are included in the meal plan, 100% fruit juice should be limited to less than 4 ounces or avoided due to its effect on appetite, weight, and BG.[84]

As the toddler develops more mobility, interest in the environment also increases, and interest in food may wane. In some instances, getting a toddler to eat anything at a meal is an accomplishment. Erratic eating behaviors as well as grazing in toddlers require careful monitoring and make it difficult to dose insulin. Pre-meal dosing is always suggested to achieve euglycemia; however, in some cases, insulin is given after the meal (post-dosing), based on what the toddler ate rather than dosing on an estimated intake. Post-dosing helps to avoid forced eating and food battles between the toddler and caregiver; however, post-dosing can become a habit which should gradually be transitioned to pre-meal dosing as the toddler grows older.[35] This is also a very popular time for parents to transition their child to CSII, which will give them flexibility to split the insulin dose and provide small doses of insulin to bolus for small amounts of carbohydrate eaten. For instance, they can give the amount of insulin to correct the BG if higher than desired and some of the insulin to cover the food as much as they feel comfortable giving and then make up the difference at the end of the meal. Using a combination bolus when eating small amounts of food over an extended period, as well as suspending a bolus, can help manage BG levels when toddlers stop eating after the meal is completed. Food-behavior guidelines for this young group, with or without diabetes, should be firmly established by caregivers at the time the child begins solid foods. Young children with T1D learn quickly how important it is for them to eat and it is very easy for parents to fall into behaviors of short order cooking or letting the child choose the foods.

School-Age Children

Children with diabetes are in school for most the day and require appropriate supervision and assistance in managing their diabetes. Older elementary school students can perform their own BG checks and, with supervision, administer their own insulin. School nurses, as well as teachers, bus drivers and other school staff need to be educated on the signs and symptoms of abnormal BG levels and to keep the child safe while at school.[87] Adjusting diabetes around the school schedule rather than changing physical education classes or lunch periods in order to accommodate an insulin regimen communicates to the child that the child is more important than the diabetes. It is possible to arrange snacks and injections around most school schedules. Parents should be encouraged to address food and diabetes treatment issues with school personnel; however, some parents may require assistance from their diabetes care team. School-age children will ordinarily eat three meals and two to three snacks a day, scheduled according to their insulin regimen. However, some children can omit the morning snack without creating a problem as long as lunch is not delayed. Children using basal/bolus insulin regimens have increased flexibility with their eating and should eat based on their hunger rather than having to eat dictated by when their insulin is peaking. Children should be instructed to carry a fast-acting carbohydrate with them always in case of emergency to treat or prevent hypoglycemia. Most schools will offer lunch items appropriate to the needs of children following a meal plan, such as low-fat milk and fresh fruit. If school personnel are unwilling to cooperate, reference can be made to Section 504 of the Rehabilitation Act of 1973 and the Individuals with Disabilities Education Act of 1991 (originally the Education for All Handicapped Children Act of 1975), Public Law No. 94–142, which mandates that handicapped students, including children with diabetes, have access to all services necessary to assist in full participation in school.[87]

Adolescents

During adolescence, glycemic control is affected by increased insulin resistance, inconsistent eating patterns, risk-taking behaviors, eating disorders, and noncompliance with taking insulin and BG checks. The advent of adolescence may bring a great deal of conflict into the lives of family members. Adolescents strive for independence and expect parents to trust them to manage their own diabetes; whereas parents may expect their teen to manage their diabetes on their own, leading to early burnout and poor diabetes control.[88] During the adolescent period, they may vent their anger for the first time about having diabetes. The key to working successfully with adolescents is for the parents and the diabetes team to make every effort to provide positive reinforcement, negotiated support, and develop a sense of trust. Parents should continue their involvement and supervision of monitoring blood glucose and insulin administration at home. It is often more effective for team members to see adolescents and their parents individually, while at the same time respecting their confidentiality. More flexibility in food choices and increasing calorie needs during this period of growth is usually necessary. Food choices may improve in a nonjudgmental atmosphere and with assistance for the teen to work favorite foods into the meal plan. In clinic visits, teens should be routinely asked if they have any questions about their food choices. Focusing on the positive choices the adolescents are making and what they are doing right can lead to open discussion and follow-up visits.

Growth Maintenance

Routine charting of a child's height, weight, and BMI is an excellent way to monitor their growth pattern. Deviating from the child's normal growth curve (except for increased height or decreasing weight in a child who has reached full height potential) needs close monitoring. In a child whose diabetes is poorly controlled, weight percentile will often remain stationary or decrease. After about 6 months of little or no weight gain, height velocity may also begin to slow. Achieving optimal height potential can be used to motivate boys and girls to strive for better blood glucose control. Adolescents are more likely to be interested in improved self-care when they understand the relationship between good control, appropriate weight gain, consistent height increase, and/or normal menses.

Illness

Illness in the child with diabetes always presents a challenge increasing the risk of developing ketoacidosis, dehydration, hyperglycemia, and hypoglycemia.[89] Insulin must always be given and may need to be increased during these periods even during times of decreased food intake. The BG should be monitored frequently, every 3 to 4 hours during illness. Parents need to know when to call the doctor or diabetes provider for assistance in managing illness because certain symptoms, such as prolonged vomiting and fever, can lead to rapid dehydration and DKA. During a brief illness, the child's normal eating pattern should be maintained as much as possible by using foods that can be well tolerated. Drinking 6–8 oz. of sugar-free fluids every 1–2 hours can prevent dehydration, but if the child cannot tolerate food or if BG levels are falling, it is important to replace the carbohydrate missed with sugar-containing liquids that the body can easily use for energy. Some examples of easily tolerated liquids that contain 15g of carbohydrate include, 8 ounces of a regular carbonated beverage (with sugar), 8 ounces of sports drink, 4 ounces of fruit juice, a frozen fruit bar, or ½ cup of regular flavored gelatin. It is recommended to sip on room temperature liquids at a rate of about 15g of carbohydrate per hour. Sick-day guidelines should include increasing BG checks and ketone testing, continuing insulin administration, maintaining adequate hydration, treating the illness, and adjusting insulin to prevent DKA and/or hypoglycemia.[89] Parents and caregivers should be well educated on sick-day rules and notify their diabetes provider if ketones are present during illness that cannot be managed at home.

▶ Special Considerations

Obesity in T1D: Double Diabetes

Obesity is not only seen in T2D, but the prevalence of overweight and obesity in children and adolescents with T1D has increased to 22.1% and 12.6% respectively. Children and adolescents with T1D are more likely to be overweight but less likely to be obese than their peers without diabetes, placing them at even higher risk for cardiovascular disease.[25,90,91] Intensive insulin therapy combined with reduced physical activity, increased screen time, and poor diet, are common reasons for weight gain in T1D.[25] Furthermore, excessive weight gain may play a part in increased incidence of T1D called the "accelerated hypothesis". This theory concludes that increased insulin resistance accelerates beta-cell destruction coupled with genetics, increasing the rate of developing diabetes.[90]

Diagnosing diabetes in children may not be as straightforward, especially in those who are obese. Obese and overweight children with T1D may show signs of T2D, such as insulin resistance, but clinically are diagnosed with T1D (positive autoantibodies), called double diabetes. Characteristics such as being overweight (BMI>85th percentile) or obese (BMI>95th percentile), insulin resistance, acanthosis nigricans, hyperlipidemia, hypertension and family history of T2D, are found in children and adolescents with double diabetes.[92] Clinical markers used to diagnose double diabetes include autoantibodies, C-peptide, and insulin levels. Children diagnosed with double diabetes tend to have a slower beta-cell decline, but require insulin and may add insulin sensitizers such as Biguanides (metformin) to manage their diabetes and insulin resistance.

MNT for children and adolescents with double diabetes should focus on lifestyle changes in order to reduce the risks of developing cardiovascular disease, hypertension, and polycystic ovary syndrome (PCOS).[90,92] Lifestyle changes include: weight management; eating a heart healthy diet, reducing saturated and trans fats, increasing dietary fiber, and replacing refined carbohydrates with unsaturated fats; as well as, increasing physical activity.[25,38] Furthermore, the DASH (**Dietary Approaches to Stop Hypertension**) and the Mediterranean diets have been found to be effective to reduce body weight, improve lipids, and increase insulin sensitivity. Even though there have been no specific macronutrient recommendations to achieve weight loss, the RDN should individualize the diet plan in order to reduce cardiovascular risk and weight, as well as to maintain euglycemia.[38]

▶ Conclusion

Nutrition management of the child and adolescent with diabetes is one of the most important factors in attaining and maintaining metabolic control. Devising meal plans that provide flexibility while conforming to guidelines based on current research can be challenging for the RDN. A thorough understanding of all the components of diabetes management will help the family adapt diabetes into their lifestyle instead of fitting their lifestyle into the diabetes. It is the role of the diabetes team members to empower the family and child with the knowledge to make healthy decisions in the management of diabetes.

🔍 CASE STUDIES

Nutrition Assessment

Patient History

JH is an 11-year-old male who's in the pediatrician's office for a sick visit. The parents noticed that JH was going to the bathroom frequently and had nocturnal enuresis the last two nights. They also reported that he had not been eating very well, had been drinking a lot of water, and had decreased energy. In the pediatrician's office, it was noted that he had lost 5 lbs (6% weight loss) since his last well visit 4 months ago. His urinalysis was positive for glucose and negative for ketones. The pediatrician checked his BG, which was > 500 mg/dL. The family was referred to the local diabetes outpatient clinic for education. Additional lab work was done and it was determined JH was not in diabetic ketoacidosis (DKA).

Family History

No family history for diabetes, autoimmune diseases, hyperlipidemia, hypertension, cardiac disease, or renal disease. Mom's family has history of breast cancer.

Nutrition History

JH has no food allergies or intolerances. He typically eats breakfast at home, brings his lunch to school, and eats his afternoon snack and dinner at home. JH and his parents provided a typical day dietary recall and daily schedule.

Activity History

JH plays intramural soccer twice/week in the fall and baseball in the spring (three times/week); JH has gym class twice weekly before lunch
Breakfast: 7–7:30 am on weekdays: 1½ cups cold cereal (Fruit Loops, Multigrain Cheerios), ½ cup 1% milk, and lately 6–8 oz. orange juice
Weekends, 8–8:30 am: bagel (large), scrambled egg, and milk (6–8 oz.)
Morning snack at school: 11 am: Kellogg's blueberry bar
Lunch: 12 pm: usually brings—raisin bagel, grape juice pouch, raisins or a piece of fresh fruit (does not like school milk)
School lunch: usually once a week: Domino's pizza (1 slice), juice box
Afternoon snack: 3 pm: apple or grilled cheese sandwich or frozen pizza, water or milk to drink
Dinner: 5:30–6:30 pm: 3 oz. chicken, ¼–½ cup green beans, ¾–1 cup rice, pasta, or mashed potato. Mom tries to have 1–2 nights a week vegetarian, which is usually pasta 1¼ cup with cheese, milk, or water, ½–¾ cup of chopped fruit or ice cream
Evening snack: usually none

Anthropometric Measurements
Weight: 30.2kg
Height: 143.4 cm
BMI: 14.66
BMI Goal: 17.01
Other Labs: A1C 10.8, Cholesterol 133, HDL 34, LDL 39, Trig 501
Insulin Plan
Basal insulin: 7 units at 9 pm
Insulin-to-carbohydrate ratio (ICR): 1:30g
Sensitivity factor (SF): 1:75mg/dL
Target BG: 100mg/dL

Nutrition Diagnosis/Problem

1. Weight loss >5%- acute mild-malnutrition related to hyperglycemia and new onset T1D diagnosis
2. Food and nutrition-related knowledge deficit related to new diagnosis of T1D

Nutrition Interventions

1. Comprehensive nutrition education.
   a. Review advanced carbohydrate counting.
   b. Review label reading.
      i. Weighing and measuring food
   c. Introduce calculating insulin doses using insulin-to-carbohydrate ratio
   d. Review diabetes and exercise guidelines to prevent hypoglycemia
2. Provide basic meal plan for weekend for family to use as a guide until they return at their next nutrition visit.
3. Reinforce education at following visit and build on the survival skills.
4. Goals of nutrition therapy:
   a. Advanced carb count
   b. Gain back lost weight and continue to grow along growth parameters
   c. Maintain blood glucose between 70 and 150 mg/dL
   d. Reinforce healthy eating

Questions for the Reader

1. What percentile on a growth chart are his weight, height, and BMI?
2. What are JH's estimated energy needs per day?
3. Write one PES statement.
4. What survival skills does must the family learn to get them through the first weekend of diabetes?
5. Does the child need any further vitamin or mineral supplementation?
6. What guidelines should the family follow to prevent hypoglycemia with exercise?

Study Questions

1. List at least one of the common signs or symptoms of Type 1 diabetes (T1D) at diagnosis?

2. Type 1 diabetes (T1D) is an autoimmune disease defined by **X** and the need for **X**.

3. What is the most common autoimmune disease associated with T1D?

4. What are other types of diabetes that may be present in childhood, besides TID?

5. T/F: Children with diabetes have higher energy needs than those children without diabetes.

6. What lifestyle changes may require adjustments to be made to total daily dose (TDD) of insulin?

7. Insulin pumps utilize rapid acting insulin, long acting insulin or both?

8. What is the recommended range for percent of dietary calories from added sugar for children with T1D?

9. What can be a negative side effect from consuming hypocaloric sweeteners or sugar alcohols?

10. What are the benefits of regular exercise or activity on individuals with diabetes?

References

1. Beck JK, Cogen FR. Outpatient management of Pediatric Type 1 Diabetes. *J Pediatr Pharmacol Ther.* 2015;20(5):344–357.

2. Franz MJ, Boucher JL, Evert AB. Evidence-based diabetes nutrition therapy recommendations are effective: the key is individualization. *Diabetes, Metabolic Syndrome and Obesity: Targets and Therapy.* 2014;Volume 7:65–72.

3. American Diabetes Association. Diagnosis and classification of Diabetes Mellitus. *Diabetes Care.* 2014;37(suppl1):S81–S90.

4. Unnikrishnan R, Shah VN, Mohan, V. Challenges in diagnosis and management of diabetes in the young. *Clin Diabetes Endocrinol.* 2016;2(18).

5. Chiang JL, Kirkman MS, Laffel LM, et al. Type 1 Diabetes through the life span: a Position Statement of the American Diabetes Association. *Diabetes Care.* 2014;37:2034–2054.

6. American Diabetes Association. Diagnosis and classification of Diabetes Mellitus. *Diabetes Care.* 2012;35(suppl1):S64–S71.

7. Hamman RF, Bell RA, Dabelea D, et al. The SEARCH for diabetes in youth study: rationale, findings, and future directions. *Diabetes Care.* 2014;37:3336–3344.

8. Zeitler P, Fu J, Tandon N, et al. Type 2 diabetes in the child and adolescent. *Pediatr Diabetes.* 2014;15(20):26–46.

9. U.S. Department of Health and Human Services, U.S. Food and Drug Administration. Consumer Updates: How is Diabetes Treated in Children? Available at: https://www.fda.gov/ForConsumers/ConsumerUpdates/ucm276191.htm. Updated July, 25, 2015. Accessed October 23, 2017.

10. American Diabetes Association. Standards of medical care in Diabetes – 2016. *Diabetes Care.* 2016;39 (1):.

11. Moran A, Brunzell C, Cohen RC, et al. (2010). Clinical Care Guidelines for Cystic Fibrosis-Related Diabetes. *Diabetes Care.* 2010; 33(12):2697–2708.

12. Cystic Fibrosis Foundation Website. Available at: https://www.cff.org/Life-With-CF/Daily-Life/Cystic-Fibrosis-Related-Diabetes/. Accessed September 18, 2017.

13. Orzan A, Novac C, Mihu M, Tirgoviste C, Balgradean M. Type 1 Diabetes and Thyroid Autoimmunity in children. *Maedica – a Journal of Clinical Medicine.* 2016;11(4):308–312.

14. Parkkola A, Harkonen T, Ryhanen SJ, Uibo R, Ilonen J, Knip M. Transglutaminase antibodies and celiac disease in children with type 1 diabetes and in their family members. *Pediatr Diabetes.* 2017;19(2)305–313.

15. Singh P, Seth A, Kumar P, Saijan S. Coexistence of celiac disease & type 1 diabetes mellitus in children. *Indian J Med Res.* 2017;145(1):28–32.

16. Maahs DM, Dabelea D, D'Agostino RB, Andrews JS, Shah AS, Crimmins N, et al. Glucose control predicts 2-year change in lipid profile in youth with Type 1 Diabetes. *J Pediatr.* 2013;162(1):101–107.

17. Falcoão MA, Francisco R. Diabetes, eating disorders and body image in young adults: an exploratory study about "diabulimia". *Eating and Weight Disord.* 2017;22(4):675–682.

18. Colton P, Rodin G, Berenstal R, Parkin C. Eating disorders and diabetes: introduction and overview. *Diabetes Spectrum.* 2009;22(3):138–142.

19. Bailey TS, Grunberger G, Bode B, Hirsch I, Roberts VL, Rodbard D, et al. American Association of Clinical Endocrinologists and American College of Endocrinology 2016 Outpatient Glucose Monitoring Consensus Statement. 2016; Endocr Pract.22(2):231–261.

20. Academy of Nutrition and Dietetics. Nutrition terminology reference manual (eNCPT): dietetics language for nutrition care. Available at:http://ncpt.webauthor.com. Accessed November 13, 2017.

21. American Academy of Dermatology. Acanthosis Nigricans. Available at: https://www.aad.org/public/diseases/color-problems/acanthosis-nigricans. Accessed October 18, 2017.

22. Academy of Nutrition and Dietetics. Nutrition Care Manual®. Conditions, Diabetes Mellitus Type 1, Nutrition Diagnosis. Available at: https://nutritioncaremanual.org. Accessed October 18, 2017.

23. U.S. Department of Health and Human Services and U.S. Department of Agriculture. 2015–2020 Dietary Guidelines for Americans. 8th ed. December 2015. Available at: https://health.gov/dietaryguidelines/2015/guidelines/. Accessed: September 28, 2017.

24. Institute of Medicine of the National Academies. *Dietary Reference Intakes: The Essential Guide to Nutrient Requirements.* Washington, DC: National Academies Press; 2006. Available at: https://www.nap.edu/read/11537/chapter/7#73. Accessed September 15, 2017.

25. Mottalib A, Kasetty M, Mar J, Elseaidy T, Ashrafzadeh S, Hamdy O. Weight management in patients with Type 1 Diabetes and Obesity. Curr Diab Rep. 2017;;17(10):92.

26. Smart C, Annan F, Bruno L, Higgins L, Acerini C. Nutritional management in children and adolescents with diabetes. Pediatr Diabetes. 2014;15(suppl20):135–153.

27. National Academy of Sciences, Institutes of Medicine, Food and Nutrition Board. Dietary reference intakes for energy, carbohydrate, fiber, fat, fatty acids, cholesterol, protein, and amino acids (macronutrients). 2005. Available at: https://www.nap.edu/read/10490/chapter/2#5. Accessed September 10, 2017.

28. World Health Organization. Energy and protein requirements. report of a joint FAQ/WHO/UNU Expert Consultation. Technical Report Series 724. Geneva, Switzerland:World Health Organization;1985. Available at: http://www.fao.org/docrep/003/AA040E/AA040E00.HTM#TOC. Accessed: October 2, 2017.

29. Subramanian S, Baidal D, Syker J, Hirsch I. The management of Type 1 Diabetes. NCBI Bookshelf; November 16, 2016. Available at: https://www.ncbi.nlm.nih.gov/books/NBK279114/. Accessed September 10, 2017.

30. Cemeroglu AP, Thomas JP, Zande LV, et al. Basal and bolus insulin requirements in children, adolescents, and young adults with Type 1 Diabetes Mellitus on Continuous Subcutaneous Insulin Infusion (CSII): effects of age and puberty. *Endocr Pract.* 2013;19:805–811.

31. Peichowiak K, Dzygato K, Szypowska A. The additional dose of insulin for high-protein mixed meal provides better glycemic control in children with type 1 diabetes on insulin pumps: randomized cross-over study. Pediatr Diabetes. 2017;1–8. doi 10.1111/pwis.12500.

32. Giani E, Scaramuzza AE, Zuccotti GV. Impact of new technologies on diabetes care. *World J Diabetes.* 2015;6(8):999–1004.

33. Robertson K, Riddell MC, Guinhouya BC, Adofsson P, Hanas R. Exercise in children and adolescents with diabetes. Pediatr Diabetes. 2014;15(20):203–223.

34. Spinks J, Guest S. Dietary Management of children with type 1 diabetes. Paediatrics and Child Health. 2017;27(4):176–180.

35. Sundberg F, Barnard K, Cato A, et al. Managing diabetes in preschool children. Pediatric Diabetes. 2017.;18(7):499–517.

36. Bowen, M, Cavanaugh KL, Wolff K, et al. The diabetes nutrition education study randomized controlled trial: A comparative effectiveness study of approaches to nutrition in diabetes self-management education. *Patient Education and Counseling.* 2016;99:1368–1376.

37. Geil, PB. Choose your foods: exchange lists for diabetes: the 2008 revision for exchange lists for meal planning. *Diabetes Spectrum.* 2008;21(4):281–283.

38. American Diabetes Association. Standards of medical care in Diabetes- children and adolescents. *Diabetes Care.* 2017;40(suppl1):S105–S113.

39. MacLeod J, Franz MJ, Handu D, et al. Academy of Nutrition and Dietetics Nutrition Practice Guideline for Type 1 and Type 2 Diabetes in Adults: Nutrition Intervention Evidence Reviews and Recommendations. *J Acad Nutr Dietetics.* 2017:1–22.

40. Erikson J, Slavin J. Total, added, and free sugars: are restrictive guidelines science-based or achievable? *Nutrients.* 2015;7: 2866–2878.

41. Vos MB, Kaar JL, Welsh JA, et al. AHA Scientific Statement: added sugars and Cardiovascular Disease Risk in children. *Circulation.* 2016;135(19):e1017–e1034.:

42. Evert AB, Boucher JL, Cypress M, et al. Nutrition therapy recommendations for the management of adults with Diabetes. *Diabetes Care.* 2014;37(suppl1):S120–S143.

43. Academy of Nutrition and Dietetics. Position of the Academy of Nutrition and Dietetics: Use of Nutritive and Nonnutritive Sweeteners. *J Acad Nutr Diet.* 2012;112:739–758.

44. Johnson RJ, Sanchez-Lozada, LG, Andrews P, Lanaspa MA. Perspective: A historical and scientific perspective of sugar and its relation with Obesity and Diabetes. Adv Nutr. 2017;8:412–422.

45. Schorin M, Sollid K, Smith EM, Bouchoux A. A closer look at sugars. Nutr. Today. 2012;47(3):96–101.

46. Grembecka M. Sugar alcohols-their role in the modern world of sweeteners: a review. *Eur Food Res Technol.* 2014;241:1–14.

47. Makinen, KK. Gastrointestinal disturbances associated with the consumption of sugar alcohols with special consideration of Xylitol: scientific review and instructions for dentists and other health-care professionals. *Int J Dentistry.* 2016:1–16.http://dx.doi.org/10.1155/2016/5967907.

48. Sylvetsky A, Rother KI, Brown R. Artificial sweetener use among children: epidemiology, recommendations, metabolic outcomes, and future directions. *Pediatr Clin North Am.* 2011; 58(6):1467–1480.

49. U.S. FDA: Additional information about high-intensity sweeteners permitted for use in the United States. Available at: https://www.fda.gov/Food/IngredientsPackaging Labeling/FoodAdditivesIngredients/ucm397725.htm #Aspartame. Accessed: September 10, 2017.

50. Shannon M, Rehfeld A, Frizzell C, et al. *In vitro* bioassay investigations of the endocrine disrupting potential of steviol glycosides and their metabolite steviol, components of the natural sweetener *Stevia. Mol Cell Endocrinol.* 2016;427: 65–72.

51. IFIC Foundation: Everything you need to know about Monk Fruit Sweeteners. Available at: http://www.foodinsight.org/print/8560. Accessed: September 25, 2017.

52. Academy of Nutrition and Dietetics. Position of the Academy of Nutrition and Dietetics: health implications of Dietary Fiber. *J Acad Nutr Diet.* 2015;115:1861–1870.

53. Nansel TR, Lipsky LM, Liu A. Greater diet quality is associated with more optimal glycemia control in a longitudinal study of youth with type 1 diabetes. *Am J Clin Nutr.* 2016;104: 81–87.

54. Bamba V. Update on screening, etiology, and treatment of Dyslipidemia in children. *J Clin Endocrinol Metab.* 2014;99(9):3093–3102.

55. Kranz S, Brauchia M, Slavin JL, Miller KB. What do we know about dietary fiber intake in children and health? The effects of fiber intake on constipation, obesity, and diabetes in children. *Adv. Nutr.* 2012;3:47–53.

56. Smart CE, Evans M, O'Connell SM, et al. Both dietary protein and fat increases postprandial glucose excursions in children with Type 1 Diabetes, and the effect is additive. *Diabetes Care.* 2013;36:3897–3902.

57. Bell KJ, Smart CE, Steil GM, Brand-Miller JC, King B, Wolpert HA. Impact of fat, protein, and Glycemic Index on Postprandial Glucose Control in Type 1 Diabetes: implications for intensive diabetes management in the Continuous Glucose Monitoring Era. *Diabetes Care.* 2015;38:1008–1015.

58. Kwiterovich PO. Recognition and management of Dyslipidemia in children and adolescents. *J Clin Endocrinol Metab.* 2008;93:4200–4209.

59. American Academy of Pediatrics. Expert Panel on Integrated Guidelines for Cardiovascular Health in Risk Reduction in Children and Adolescents: Summary Report. *Pediatrics.* 2011;128 (suppl5):S213–S256.

60. Kordonouri O, Hartmann R, Remus K, Blasig S, Sadeghian E, Danne T. Benefit of supplementary fat plus protein counting as compared with conventional carbohydrate counting for insulin bolus calculation in children with pump therapy. *Pediatr Diabetes,* 2012;13:540–544.

61. Wolpert HA, Atakov-Castillo A, Smith SA, Steil GM. Dietary fat acutely increases glucose concentrations and insulin requirements in patients with Type 1 Diabetes. *Diabetes Care.* 2013;36:810–816.

62. Feng R, Li Y, Li G, et al. Lower serum 25 (OH) D concentrations in Type 1 Diabetes: a meta-analysis. *Diabetes Res Clin Prac.* 2015;108:e71–e75.

63. Savastio A, Cadario F, Genoni G, et al. Vitamin D deficiency and glycemia status in children and adolescents with Type 1 Diabetes Mellitus. *Plos One.* 2016:1–13.

64. Kelly A, Brooks LJ, Dougherty S, Carlow DC, Zemel BS. A cross-sectional study of vitamin D resistance in children. *Arch Dis Child.* 2011;96:447–452.

65. Holick MF. The vitamin D deficiency pandemic: Approaches for diagnosis, treatment and prevention. *Rev Endocr Metab Disord.* 2017;18:153–165.

66. Abrams SA. Dietary guidelines for calcium and Vitamin D: a new era. Pediatr. 2011;127(3):566–568.

67. Centers for Disease Control and Prevention. Reducing sodium in children's diets. Available at: https://www.cdc.gov/vitalsigns/children-sodium/index.html. Accessed October 2, 2017.

68. Appel LJ, Lichtenstein AH, Callahan EA, Sinaiko A, Van Horn L, Whitsel L. Reducing sodium intake in children: a public health investment. J Clin Hypertens. 2015;17(9):657–661.

69. Anderson J, Couper JJ, Toome S, et al. Dietary sodium intake relates to vascular health in children with type 1 diabetes. Pediatr Diabetes. 2017;0:1–5.

70. Pastor A, Conn J, Teng J, et al. Alcohol and recreational drug use in young adults with type 1 diabetes. *Diabetes Res Clin Prac.* 2017;130:186–195.

71. Francescato MP, Stel G, Stenner E, Geat M. Prolonged exercise in Type 1 Diabetes: performance of a customizable algorithm to estimate the carbohydrate supplements to minimize glycemic imbalances. *Plos One.* 2015;1–14. https://doi.org/10.1371/journal.pone.0125220.

72. Riddell MC, Gallen IW, Smart CE, et al. Exercise management in Type 1 Diabetes: a consensus statement. Lancet Diabetes Endocrinol. 2017;1–14

73. U.S. Department of Health and Human Services and U.S. Department of Agriculture. 2015–2020 Dietary Guidelines for Americans: Appendix 1. Physical Activity Guidelines for Americans. 8th ed. December 2015. Available at: http://health.gov/dietaryguidelines/2015/guidelines/appendix-1/

74. Nadella S, Indyk JA, Kamboj MK. Management of diabetes mellitus in children and adolescents: engaging in physical activity. *Transl Pediatr.* 2017;6(3):215–224.

75. Robertson K, Riddell MC, Guinhouya BC, Adolfsson P, Hanas R. ISPAD Clinical Practice Consensus Guidelines 2014; Exercise in children and adolescents with diabetes. *Pediatr Diabetes.* 2014;15(suppl20):203–223.

76. Harris GD, White RD. Diabetes in the competitive athlete. *Curr Sports Med Rep.* 2012;11(6):309–315.

77. Roberts AJ, Taplin CE. Exercise in youth with Type 1 Diabetes. *Curr Pediatr Rev.* 2015;11:120–125.

78. Rewers MJ, Pillay K, de Beaufort C, et al. Assessment and monitoring of glycemic control in children and adolescents with diabetes. *Pediatr Diabetes.* 2014;15(Suppl.20):102–114.

79. Lawlor MT, Anderson B, Laffel L. *Blood Sugar Monitoring Owner's Manual Booklet.* Boston, MA: Joslin Diabetes Center;2007.

80. Ly TT, Maahs DM, Rewers A, Dunger D, Oduwole A, Jones TW. Assessment and management of hypoglycemia in children and adolescents with diabetes. *Pediatr Diabetes.* 2014;15(suppl20):180–192.

81. Laffel LMB, Butler DA, Higgins LA, Lawlor MT, Pasquarello CA, eds. *Joslin's Guide to Managing Childhood Diabetes: A Family Teamwork Approach.* Boston, MA: Joslin Diabetes Center;2009.

82. Silverstein J, Klingensmith G, Copeland K, et al. Care of children and adolescents with Type 1 Diabetes: a statement of the American Diabetes Association. *Diabetes Care.* 2005;28(1):186–212.

83. American Academy of Pediatrics. Infant Food and Feeding. Available at: https://www.aap.org/en-us/advocacy-and-policy/aap-health-initiatives/HALF-Implementation-Guide/Age-Specific-Content/Pages/Infant-Food-and-Feeding.aspx. Accessed September 25, 2017.

84. Heyman MB, Abrams SA. Fruit juice in infants, children, and adolescents: current recommendations. *Pediatri.* 2017;136(6): e20170967.

85. Couper JJ, Steele C, Beresford S, et al. Lack of association between duration of breast-feeding or introduction of cow's milk and development of islet autoimmunity. *Diabetes.* 1999;48(11):2145–2149.

86. Kimpimaki T, Erkkola M, Korhonen S, et al. Short-term exclusive breastfeeding predisposes young children with increased genetic risk of type I diabetes to progressive beta-cell autoimmunity. *Diabetologia.* 2001;44(1):63–69.

87. Jackson, CC, Ablanese-O'Neill A, Butler KL, et al. Diabetes care in the school setting: A Position Statement of the American Diabetes Association. *Diabetes Care.* 2015;38(10:1958–1963).

88. Cameron FJ, Amin R, deBeaufort C, Coder E, Acerini CL. Diabetes in adolescence. *Pediatr Diabetes.* 2014;15 (suppl20):245–256.

89. Brink S, Joel D, Laffel L, et al. Sick day management in children and adolescents with diabetes. *Pediatr Diabetes.* 2014;15(suppl20):193–202.

90. Minges KE, Whittemore R, Grey M. Overweight and Obesity in youth with Type 1 Diabetes. *Annu Rev Nurs Res.* 2013;31:47–69.

91. Liu LL, Lawerence JM, Davis C, et al. Prevalence of overweight and obesity in youth with diabetes in USA: the search for diabetes in youth study. *Pediatr Diabetes.* 2010;11:4–11.

92. Robinson M, Estell K. Defining double diabetes in youth. *Top Clin Nutr.* 2012;27(3):277–290.

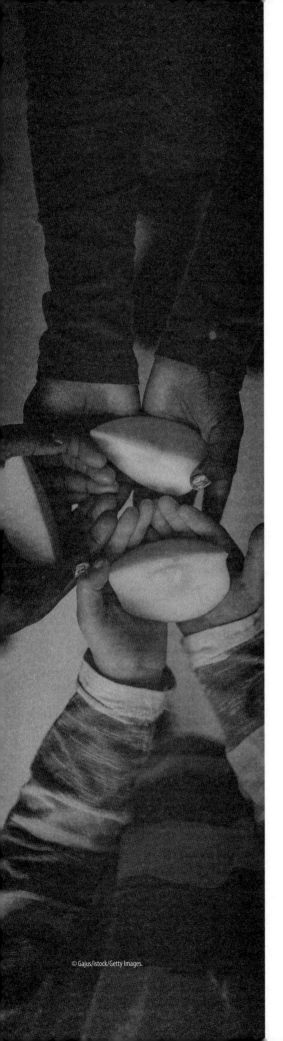

SECTION VI

Special Considerations

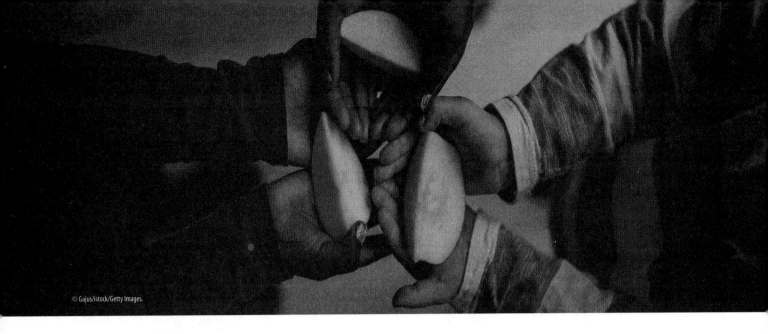

© Gajus/istock/Getty Images.

CHAPTER 21

Obesity and Weight Management

Mary Mullens

LEARNING OBJECTIVES

- Define the current pediatric definitions of overweight and obesity.
- Describe the health consequences related to pediatric overweight and obesity.
- Apply the recommendations for assessing children and adolescents identified as overweight or obese.
- Develop a care plan applying the recommendations for pediatric overweight and obesity intervention.

▶ Introduction

It has been well documented that the growing epidemic of childhood overweight and obesity is one of the most significant public health concerns facing the United States today. The percentage of children with obesity (ages 6–19) in the United States has more than tripled since the 1970s.[1] Childhood obesity has immediate and long term impacts on physical, social, and emotional health.[2,3] Current medical and scientific evidence suggests that excessive weight gain is a result of several factors including genetic predisposition and biological issues related to weight regulation, environmental, and behavioral influences such as dietary and exercise habits and sociocultural influences.

In a culture that glorifies being thin, many youth become overly preoccupied with their physical appearance and, in an effort to achieve or maintain a thin body, begin to diet obsessively. A minority of these youth eventually develops an eating disorder such as anorexia nervosa, bulimia nervosa, or eating disorders not otherwise specified.

Adults and health professionals should take it seriously when children or adolescents express concerns about their body weight. Health professionals can help children and their parents understand the importance of

TABLE 21.1 Obesity Prevalence/Trends

Age	NHANES 1988–1994	NHANES 1999–2000	NHANES 2003–2006	NHANES 2007–2008	NHANES 2011–2014
2- to 5-year-olds	7.2%	10.4%	12.4%	10.4%	8.9%
6- to 11-year-olds	11.3%	15.3%	17.0%	19.6%	17%
12- to 19-year-olds	10.5%	15.5%	17.6%	18.1%	20%

Data from Ogden CL, Carroll MD, Lawman HG, Fryer CD, Moran D, Kit BK, Flegal KM. Trends in obesity prevalence among children and adolescents in the United States, 1988–1994 through 2013–2014., *JAMA* 2016;315(12):2292–2299.[1]
Ogden CL, Carroll MD, Curtin LR, Lamb MM, Flegal KM. Prevalence of high body mass index in US children and adolescents, 2007–2008. *JAMA*. 2010;303(3):242–249.[4]
Ogden CL, Carroll MD, Flegal KM. High body mass index for age among US children and adolescents, 2003–2006. *JAMA*. 2008;299(20):2401–2405.[5]

physical activity and appropriate nutrition for maintaining health. In doing so, it is important to keep in mind the family's resources and their cultural background, both of which may influence the family's ability to make changes.

This chapter reviews the literature about overweight and obesity and provides the reader with an overview of current assessment and intervention recommendations that can help providers address and treat these medical issues and concerns.

Prevalence and Trends of Overweight/Obesity

Childhood obesity has become the most prevalent pediatric nutritional problem in the United States. The most recent data from the National Health and Nutrition Examination Study show that an estimated 17.2% of US children and adolescents aged 2–19 years are obese and another 16.2% are overweight.[1]

The increases are occurring in both boys and girls, across all states and socioeconomic lines as well as among all racial and ethnic groups; however, African American and Hispanic children and adolescents are disproportionately affected.[1] **TABLE 21.1** shows changes in obesity rates over time. More detailed statistics on the prevalence of obesity including specifics on ethnic and racial differences updated approximaetely every 2 years can be found on the Centers for Disease Control and Prevention National Center for Health Statistics website (www.cdc.gov).

▶ Defining Overweight and Obesity

In 2007, 14 professional organizations met to develop a set of evidence-based recommendations for preventing, assessing, and managing pediatric overweight and obesity. All recommendations were endorsed by these professional organizations.[6,7,8] The **American Academy of Pediatric** (AAP) Expert Committee on Assessment recommended that BMI be used as the preferred measure for evaluating obesity in children and adolescents 2 to 19 years of age. Weight-for-length is still recommended to assess children less than 2 years of age. BMI expresses the weight-for-height relationship as a ratio: weight (kg)/height (m²). BMI is recommended because it is easily obtained, is highly correlated with body fat percentage, and can correctly identify the obese individuals with acceptable accuracy (e.g., greater than 95th percentile).[6] For children and teens, age- and sex-specific percentiles are used to interpret the BMI because the amount of body fat changes with age and differs between girls and boys. The **Centers for Disease Control and Prevention** (CDC) growth charts take into account these differences and allow the BMI number to be translated into a percentile for a child's sex and age. A BMI in the 85th to 94th percentile defines overweight. Children and adolescents with BMI in this range often have excess body fat and health risks, although for some, the BMI category will reflect high lean body mass rather than fat. A BMI ≥ 95th percentile defines obesity.[8] Almost all children and adolescents with BMI in this range are likely to have excess body fat and associated health risks.[6,9]

Children and adolescents with extreme or severe obesity are increasing in prevalence. The Expert Committee on the Prevention, Assessment and Treatment of Childhood Obesity suggested using 99th percentile defined by Freedman using NHANES data to define severe obesity. More recent recommendations by the American Heart Association Atherosclerosis Hypertension, and Obesity in Youth Committee recommended defining severe obesity in children age 2 years and older and in adolescents as having a BMI greater or equal to 120% of the 95th percentile or absolute BMI greater than or equal to 35, whichever is lower based on age and sex.[9] Children and adolescents with BMI at or above the 99th percentile have a higher health risk, and therefore intervention is more urgent.[9]

Excess weight in infants is defined by weight-for-recumbant lengh. The CDC recommends using WHO growth standards to monitor growth in children under age 2 in the United States. The recommended definitions of excess weight in children under age 2 is +2 z-scores (corresponding to the 97%) on the WHO weight-for-recumbant growth charts. Some analyses use the 95% on the CDC growth charts for excess weight.[10]

▸ Anatomy, Physiology, Pathology of Condition

Obesity is associated with significant health problems in children and is a risk factor for much of adult morbidity and mortality. Medical problems are common in obese children and adolescents and can affect cardiovascular health, the pulmonary system, the musculoskeletal system, the endocrine system, gastrointestinal system and mental health.[11–13]

Research raises increased concerns for children and adolescents who experience rapid weight gain, for increased risk of carrying obesity into adulthood along with serious obesity related complications.[11,13]

Cardiovascular Concerns

The cardiovascular complications associated with obesity include hypertension, dyslipidemia, left ventricular hypertrophy, and pulmonary hypertension. Cardiovascular risk factors tend to cluster in obese and overweight children.[14,15] Data from the Bogalusa Heart Study showed that children who were obese (BMI ≥95th percentile) had a higher rate of cardiovascular risk factors than their peers,[9] increasing from 27% (nonobese) to 61% (obese).[16] Obese children also had increased rates of dyslipidemia. More than 50% of children with obesity have lipid abnormalities as measured by fasting lipid profiles.[17]

Rises in the rate of hypertension in childhood are now found to be more commonly associated with obesity than with renal disease. Blood pressure tends to track with BMI; as BMI increases, so does blood pressure. It has been shown that the risk for elevated blood pressure in children is three times greater in obese children compared with nonobese children. The correlation of BMI and hypertension has been reported independently of race, gender, or age.[12,18,19]

Pulmonary Concerns

Childhood obesity has been shown to be related to increases in childhood pulmonary complications, such as sleep apnea, exercise intolerance, and asthma. A relationship between asthma and obesity has been shown in the pediatric population. The prevalence of obesity is reported to be significantly higher in youth with asthma than peers without asthma, although studies have shown that the severity of asthma was not related to obesity.[20,21] For many children, exercise can be a trigger for asthma. Weight loss has been shown to improve lung function in individuals who have asthma and obesity. Physical activity should be a part of the care plan for treating overweight/obesity in children. Exercise in children with asthma should be managed under the care of the medical team to allow for including physical activity in nutrition intervention.

Obstructive sleep apnea (OSA) is the most common type of sleep apnea and is caused by complete or partial obstructions of the upper airway. It is characterized by repetitive episodes of shallow or paused breathing during sleep, despite the effort to breathe, and is usually associated with a reduction in blood oxygen saturation.[22–24]

Loud snoring, mouth breathing, daytime sleepiness, depression, and hyperactive behavior in children are all indicators of possible OSA. The diagnosis of obstructive sleep apnea should be confirmed by polysomnography (sleep study). Consequences of untreated OSA include delayed growth, bedwetting, behavior problems, poor academic performance, and cardiopulmonary disease. Studies show a strong association between pediatric sleep apnea and childhood obesity. Daytime sleepiness and fatigue secondary to obstructive sleep apnea may impair the ability of a child to get adequate physical activity, which in turn may worsen obesity.[22–24]

Musculoskeletal Concerns

Obesity and overweight in children has been found to be associated with an increased incidence of slipped capital femoral epiphysis, the most common hip disorder among young teenagers. Slipped capital femoral epiphysis happens when the cartilage plate (epiphysis) at the top of the thighbone (femur) slips out of place. The classic patient is an obese, early pubertal boy with delayed bone age. Symptoms include a limp, and hip or knee pain. This can only happen during growth, before the epiphysis plates fuse.[25,26]

Blount's disease, also known as tibia vera, presents as a bowing of the tibia and femur, affecting one or both knees. Patients usually present with a limp with or without pain. Obesity has been reported in two-thirds of the patients with Blount disease. It is unclear whether this abnormality is caused by excess weight placed on the joint at a critical stage in development or whether it is an underlying condition aggravated by excessive weight.[27]

Endocrine Concerns

The American Diabetes Association reported that Type 2 Diabetes now accounts for up to 45–50% of newly diagnosed cases of diabetes in children and adolescents, especially minority teens.[28] This increase in adolescent diabetes is almost completely attributable to childhood obesity. Family history is strongly associated with Type 2 Diabetes in children. The frequency of a history of Type 2 Diabetes in a first- or second-degree relative of obese teens ranges from 74% to 100%.[29,30]

Acanthosis nigricans is often associated with insulin resistance and Type 2 Diabetes. It is seen in 90% of individuals with insulin resistance.[28] This condition is characterized by hyperpigmentation and velvety thickening that occurs in the skin of the neck, axillae, and groin. Skin tags are seen in more severe cases. Many patients present with complaints of a dirty neck that they cannot get clean with soap and water.

Polycystic ovarian syndrome is one of the most common endocrine problems in females.[31,32] Patients usually present with menstrual irregularities. It is characterized by insulin resistance in the presence of elevated androgens. Patients present with irregular menstrual periods or amenorrhea, hirsutism, acne, polycystic ovaries, and obesity. Hair usually forms mid-line with hair on face, chest, abdomen, and back. Adolescents who are obese are becoming increasingly linked to PCOS.[31,32] Weight loss will improve symptoms, but treatment with hormones will often help in the short-term.[32]

Metabolic Syndrome

In 1988, the metabolic syndrome was first described in adults. It is defined as a link between insulin resistance and hypertension, dyslipidemia, Type 2 Diabetes, and other metabolic abnormities and is associated with an increased risk of atherosclerotic cardiovascular disease.[9,12,33] Obesity is the most common cause of insulin resistance in children and is associated with dyslipidemia, Type 2 Diabetes, and long-term vascular complications. Currently, there is a lack of consensus on how to define metabolic syndrome in children. In adults, metabolic syndrome is defined as three or more of the following risk factors: elevated waist circumference, triglyceride levels, blood pressure and/or fasting blood glucose.

Results of a study by Weiss and others have suggested that the metabolic syndrome was more common among children and adolescents than previously reported and that its prevalence increased directly with the degree of obesity. Insulin resistance in obese children was found to be strongly associated with specific adverse metabolic factors. Preliminary follow-up of the subjects suggested that the metabolic syndrome persists over time and tends to progress clinically. Many of the children diagnosed with metabolic syndrome developed Type 2 Diabetes in a very short period of time.[33]

Gastrointestinal Concerns

Obesity is associated with several gastrointestinal concerns including constipation, GERD, gallstones, and nonalchoholic fatty liver disease.[12] **Nonalcoholic fatty liver disease** (NAFLD) has increased with the increased rate of childhood obesity. The exact prevalence is hard to determine and although it can occur in young children, it is more prevalent in adolescents. Like adults, most children with NAFLD are obese. NAFLD is the early stages of hepatic steatosis and is associated with the degree of obesity, elevated triglycerides, and insulin resistance. Patients with NAFLD usually have no symptoms, although some may present with right upper quadrant abdominal pain or tenderness. Serum **alanine aminotransferase** (ALT) and **aspartate aminotransferase** (AST) levels are usually elevated and can be used as good screening tests for NAFLD.[34–36]

Neurological Concerns

Obesity occurs in 30–80% of children diagnosed with pseudotumor cerebri. This is often diagnosed due to elevated intracranial pressure, but no tumor or other abnormalities are seen. Pseudotumor cerebri presents with headache, dizziness, diploplia, and mild unsteadiness, and generally has a gradual onset. Neck, shoulder, and back pain have also been reported. Weight loss is recognized as the best treatment.[37,38]

Psychological Concerns

Children and adolescents are at risk of developing psychosocial problems related to being obese in a society that values thinness.[39–41] The likelihood of a severely obese child or adolescent having impaired health-related quality of life was 5.5 times greater than a healthy child or adolescent, and similar to a child diagnosed as having cancer.[42] Overweight children and youth with decreased levels of self-esteem reported increased rates of loneliness, sadness, and nervousness. Overweight adolescents also are more likely to be socially isolated than normal weight adolescents. Additionally, obese children and adolescents are four times more likely than healthy children to report impaired school function. Psychological effects may also contribute to worsening obesity.[39–41]

▶ Condition Specific Screening and Assessment

Screening for obesity risk is an ongoing process. It starts with a BMI evaluation, and then incorporates evaluations of medical conditions and risks, current behaviors, family attitudes, and psychosocial situations.[6,43] Based on this information, clinicians can provide obesity prevention or obesity treatment. Generally, children with a BMI below the 85th percentile will benefit from prevention counseling, which will guide them toward healthier behaviors or reinforce current healthy behaviors. This counseling should be framed as growing healthy bodies rather than achieving a specific weight.[6]

Children whose BMI is in the overweight category (85th–95th percentile), but just above the 85th percentile category, are unlikely to have excess body fat; however, they should receive standard obesity prevention counseling without necessarily a goal of a lower BMI percentile. These children and adolescents should be seen more frequently to ensure that the BMI is remaining stable and not increasing. If BMI begins to increase, these children would need more in-depth intervention.[6]

Assessing an obese child or adolescent is critical in the treatment of childhood obesity. The assessment is based on a wide variety of factors, including age, sex, family history, developmental stage, ethnicity, and social environment. Each of these factors will influence the treatment goal, the selection of type of treatment, and the course of therapy.[6,43] Obesity is a complex disease, and even with excellent adherence to treatment recommendations, progress may be slow. Because of the extended time that children may need to be in treatment, the assessment must include a careful review of family lifestyle patterns and the child's social environment.

Factors in the screening/assessment include:[44,45]

1. Anthropometric Measures
   a. **BMI Assessment:** It is recommended that physicians and other allied health professionals assess the weight status of children and adolescents yearly which includes height, weight, and BMI and plotting these on standard growth charts.
   b. **BMI z-scores:** Athough mainly used in research, practitioners have started to use in clinical practice. BMI z-scores, like percentiles allow comparing weight changes across different age and sex but are more sensitive to quantified changes in weight status.[46]
   c. **Other Anthropometric Measures:** Many clinicians and researchers use other measures of body composition including skinfold measures and waist circumferences to assess children. The AAP Expert Committee on Assessment[6] reviewed using these measures to determine whether they provide important clinical information beyond just using the BMI. Although skinfold measurements are predictive of total body fat in children and adolescents, the expert committee did not recommend their use in routine clinical assessment because they are often difficult to measure, require expertise in assessment techniques, and therefore are not feasible in routine medical care. Waist circumference measures assess visceral adiposity and can track with cardiovascular disease and metabolic risk factors. They are easier to assess than skinfold measurements. They are used when assessing obesity in adults; however, reference values for children and adolescents are not available. It was the opinion of the expert committee that waist circumference measurements do not provide additional information for identifying risk that is not identified by BMI percentiles. In the future, once reference values become available for children and adolescents, waist circumference values may be useful in providing an adjunct to identify children who are at increased risk for metabolic co-morbidities.
   d. **BMI Rebound:** BMI changes substantially with age. After about 1 year of age, BMI-for-age begins to decline, and it continues falling during the preschool years until it reaches a minimum around 4 to 6 years of age. After 4 to 6 years of age, BMI-for-age begins a gradual increase through adolescence and most of adulthood. The rebound or increase in BMI that occurs after it reaches its lowest point is referred to as *BMI rebound.* This is a normal pattern of growth that occurs in all children. The age when the BMI rebound occurs may be a critical period in childhood for the development of obesity as an adolescent or adult. An early BMI rebound, occurring before ages 4 to 6, has been cited as a risk factor for the development of obesity.[42] However, studies have yet to determine whether the higher BMI in childhood is truly adipose tissue versus lean body mass or bone. Additional research is needed to further understand the impact of early BMI rebound on adult obesity.

2. Screening
   In addition to BMI, screening and assessment of risk factors and characteristics associated with childhood and adolescent obesity include:
   a. **Parental Obesity:** Parental obesity is one of the strongest risk factors in childhood obesity that persists into adulthood.
   b. **Family Medical History:** A positive family history includes a history of

early cardiovascular disease, parental hypercholesterolemia, parental hypertension, or a first- or second-generation relative with Type 2 Diabetes (siblings, parents, aunts, uncles, and grandparents). Providers should regularly review and update family history, especially for at-risk children.

c. **Blood Pressure:** Elevated systolic blood pressure is seen in 13% of obese children. Blood pressure should be checked at all health supervision visits. Children's and adolescents' blood pressure evaluation should be based on age, gender, and height. Blood pressure greater than the 90th percentile for age/gender/height is considered at risk; blood pressure greater than the 95th percentile for age/gender/height is considered high if elevated on three or more occasions.[14]

3. Assessment of Weight-related Problems
A review of systems through a detailed family and patient history as well as a physical examination for current obesity-related conditions should be performed. The provider should be aware that even with a thorough history, some of the co-morbidities have no symptoms or signs.[6] Laboratory assessment may be necessary to complete the assessment.

4. Laboratory Assessment/Testing
History and physical examination cannot effectively screen for abnormal lipid profile, NAFLD, and Type 2 Diabetes mellitus; therefore, these conditions must be identified by laboratory tests. The expert committee recommended that children with BMI between the 85th and 94th percentiles have a lipid panel performed. If risk factors are present, then a fasting glucose and ALT and AST should also be measured every 2 years for individuals age 10 years or older. When the BMI is 95th percentile, the expert committee suggests a fasting glucose and ALT and AST every 2 years starting at age 10 years, regardless of other risk factors.[6] The National Heart, Lung, and Blood Institiute have published acceptable, borderline, and high or low concentrations for lipoproteins for children and adolescents.[47] The American Diabetes Association has developed screening recommendations for Type 2 Diabetes.[48] Elevation of ALT or AST on two occasions may indicate the need for further evaluation, probably with guidance from a pediatric gastroenterology/hepatology expert.[43]

5. Behavior Assessment
Providers often find it helpful for parents and/or the child (depending on age) to complete a quick screening form online or in the waiting room before being seen for their first visit. This allows the provider to target the assessment and counseling to potential problem areas. Behavior assessment includes:

a. **Dietary:** A brief assessment of foods and beverages typically consumed and the pattern of consumption can uncover modifiable behaviors associated with excess caloric intake. Not all areas can be assessed or addressed at one visit. The following questions are areas that should be assessed during subsequent visits:

   - Frequency of eating food prepared outside the home, including restaurants, school and work cafeterias, fast food establishments, and food purchased for take-out
   - Amount of sugar-sweetened beverages consumed each day
   - Amount of 100% juice consumed each day
   - Frequency and quality of breakfast
   - Energy density in the diet, such as high-fat foods
   - Number of fruit and vegetable servings each day
   - Number of meals and snacks each day, including frequency and quality of snacks
   - Number of meals eaten together as a family
   - Portion sizes
   - Number of calcium sources
   - Number of fiber sources
   - History of breastfeeding, especially if the child was breastfed to age 6 months and if breastfeeding was continued after introduction of solids to age 12 months and beyond

b. **Physical Activity:** It is important to assess age-appropriate vigorous activity, both structured and unstructured, and routine activity. Areas to be addressed include the following:

   - Time spent in moderate to vigorous physical activity each day, to estimate whether the goal of 60 minutes of activity daily is met. One hour or more should be vigorous intensity at least 3 days per week.[49]

- Frequency of participating in muscle- and bone-strengthening activities. This should be occurring at least 3 days per week. These include climbing, jumping, running, and hanging/climbing on playground equipment.
  - Barriers to physical activity.

c. **Physical Inactivity:** Asking about hours of television viewing and other "screen time" will uncover a very important opportunity to modify behavior for improved energy balance. A large number of hours of screen time each day has been associated with increased risk of obesity. Reducing the number of hours can improve weight. Therefore, hours of television, video/DVD, and video game viewing, and non-homework computer use should be limited to less than 2 hours per day, with no television for children less than 2 years of age.[50]

d. **Sleep and Obesity:** It is also important to ask about sleep habits. Counseling to ensure adequate amounts of sleep may be helpful in preventing and treating obesity.

It has been found that children and adolescents who do not get enough sleep are twice as likely to be overweight or obese. Additionally, going to bed later has also been shown to be associated with a higher BMI in children and adolescents.[51,52] Unfortunately, poor quality and insufficient quantity of sleep are common problems in children. It is estimated that 80% of adolescents get less than the recommended sleep on school nights. Recommended sleep time for school age children is 9 to 11 hours and for teeneagers is 8 to 10 hours of sleep per night, but teens average only 7 hours per night.[53] Many factors impact teens' sleep time, including school, jobs, sports, friends, TV, phones, and computers.

6. Attitude Assessment

The complexity of obesity prevention and intervention lies less in identifying target health behaviors and much more in the process of influencing families to change behaviors when habits, culture, and environment promote less physical activity and more energy intake. Before providing counseling about new behaviors, clinicians should assess attitude, capacity, and motivation for change of the parents and child.[6,42]

▶ Nutrition Assessment

If a child or adolescent is identified as obese or overwight with health risks, an in depth nutrition assessment should be completed to individualize treatment. A nutrition assessment will help determine what areas needed to be addressed in the intervention.[44,54] Some of the data needed can be obtained from the universal screening and assessment, observations and measurements, interviews, and medical record. Dietary intake data can be obtained from 24 hour recall, food record or **food frequency questionnaire** (FFQ). Examples of nutrition assessment data include:[55,56]

1. Client History – personal information such as age, race/ethnicity and grade level, personal family medical history such as diabetes or hypertension and social history such as socioeconomic factors
2. Food/Nutrition related History – examples include diet experience, mealtime behavior, eating environments, total energy intake, food/beverage intake and food intake
3. Anthropometrics – height/length, weight, BMI, BMI z-score, weight change and growth patterns
4. Nutrition Focused Physical Finding – examples include cardiovascular (shortness of breath), digestive (constipation or heartburn), vitals (blood pressure) and skin (ancanthosis)
5. Biomedical or Medical tests and procedures – examples include lipid profile, fasting glucose or Hemoglobin A1C and liver enzymes

▶ Nutrition Diagnosis

The nutrition assessment will provide data needed to make a nutrion diagnosis. Each diagnosis written as a **problem, etiology, and signs and symptoms** (PES) statement.

Appropriate nutrition diagnosis for children includes:

- Excessive energy intake: NI 1.3
- Excessive oral intake: NI .2.2
- Excessive fat intake NI 5.5.2
- Excessive carbohydrate intake NI 5.8.2
- Overweight/obesity NC 3.1
- Overweight adult or pediatric NC 3.3.1
- Obese pediatric NC 3.3.2
- Unintended weight gain NC 3.4
- Excessive growth rate NC 3.6
- Examples of etiology may include healthful food choices not provided as an option by caregiver or parent, lack of appetite awareness or excessive energy intake

- Examples of signs and symptoms may include report of overconsumption of high-fat or calorically dense foods or beverages, weight gain in excess or normal growth patterns or parents report constant hunger[55,56]

▶ Nutrition Intervention

Treating children who are overweight or obese seems easy—just counsel children and their families to eat less and exercise more. In practice, however, treating childhood obesity is often time-consuming, frustrating, difficult, and expensive. Choosing the most effective methods for treating overweight and obesity in children is complex, especially for healthcare providers who have limited resources to offer interventions.[7,57] It's also complicated by the lack of third-party reimbursement for healthcare services related to obesity.[58]

The US Preventative Services Task Force recommends that clinicians screen for obesity in children and adolescents 6 years and older and offer or refer them to comprehensive, intense behavioral interventions to promote improvements in weight.[7] Comprehensive interventions that include behavioral therapy along with changes in nutrition and physical activity are the most closely studied and appear to be the most successful approaches to improving long-term weight and health status. The USPSTF found that comprehensive, behavioral interventions (> or equal to 26 contact hours) can result in improvements in weight status for up to 12 months.[7] Ultimately, children and adolescents become overweight or obese because of an imbalance between energy intake and expenditure. Dietary patterns, media/screen time and other sedentary activities, and an overall lack of physical activity play key roles in creating this imbalance, and therefore represent opportunities for intervention. Interventions should focus on improving these eating and activity behaviors. Components of a successful weight management program include:[6]

- Nutrition/dietary
- Increasing physical activity
- Reducing sedentary behavior
- Behavioral modification

Nutrition/Dietary Component

It is often difficult to determine which part of the nutritional intervention is responsible for the greatest behavioral change in treating obesity. In fact, the majority of studies that show a positive effect are comprehensive and include physical activity and behavioral counseling. Although comprehensive approaches that provide intervention in diet, physical activity, family behavior, and the social and physical environment are undoubtedly needed, studies involving multiple modalities cannot assess the efficacy of any specific component (e.g., diet).[6,8]

After a nutrition assessment, the family and patient can identify dietary factors that may be contributing to weight concerns, such as consumption of sweetened beverages or large portion sizes. The RDN should work with the child or teen and family to choose goals based on readiness to change and dietary factors. Several dietary factors have been targeted as important in preventing and treating pediatric overweight and obesity and include:[6,8]

- *Fruits and Vegetables:* Fruits and vegetables have been promoted for preventing childhood obesity due to their low energy density, high fiber content, and satiety value. The AAP endorses a modestly positive effect of fruit and vegetable consumption on preventing overweight and obesity in children.[58] According to USDA, children and adolescents should eat at least 5 combined servings of fruits and vegetables a day.[59] Unfortunately, many children do not consume enough fruits and vegetables. **The National Youth Risk Behavior Survey** (YRBS) is conducted every 2 years and surveys students in grades 7–12.[60] The YRBS provides data on dietary intakes, physical activity, and nutrition behaviors. The most recent findings indicated that 7% did not eat vegetables during a 7 day period and 5% did not eat fruit.
- *Fruit Juice:* The AAP recommends that maximum daily intakes of 100% juice products should be 4 ounces for children ages 1–3 years, 4–6 ounces for children ages 4–6 years and 8 ounces for those 7 and older.[61]
  - Unfortunately, many patients and families cannot distinguish between 100% fruit juice and fruit drinks, which are high in sugar and low in nutrients. It is often helpful for interventions to educate about the difference between fruit drinks and 100% fruit juice and ways to limit 100% juice in children who drink excessive amounts.
- *Sugar Sweetened Beverages:* Consuming excessive quantities of low nutrient energy density foods such as sugar sweetened beverages are a risk factor for obesity. Sugar sweetened beverages have become substitutes for healthier options such as low-fat milk, water, or 100% fruit juices. Although the rate of soda consumption is decreasing, it still remains elevated with 20.4% of students consuming a serving of **sugar-sweetened beverages** (SSB) at least once a day.[62] According to the YRBS, SSB were accounting for 9.3% of the total daily caloric intake for boys aged 12–19 and 9.7% of total calories from girls aged 12–19.[63] The Dietary Guidelines for Americans recommend reducing SSB to reduce the intake of added sugars to less than 10% of calories per day.[59]
- *Portion Size*: Research indicates that portion size may contribute to obesity because larger than recommended portions provide excessive energy intake.[64] A study of preschool children 4 to 6 years of age

found that the most powerful determinant of the amount of food consumed at meals was the amount served. Reducing food portion sizes may be an effective strategy for decreasing energy intake when eating out or in the home.[65]

- *Breakfast:* Obese children are more likely to skip breakfast or eat smaller breakfasts than leaner children. The evidence seems to suggest that breakfast skipping may be a risk factor for increased obesity, particularly among older children or adolescents.[66] Population-based surveys have revealed that many children, particularly adolescents, skip breakfast and other meals, but consume more food later in the day, and that this pattern has increased in recent years. In addition to having a poorer nutritional intake, children who skip breakfast have been shown to have a decrease in academic performance.[67]

- *Snacking:* Choosing healthy snacks should be encouraged for obesity prevention and intervention. Snacking frequency seems to have increased concurrently with the prevalence of overweight and obesity.

  According to national surveys, although the average size of snacks and the energy content of snacks have remained relatively constant, only when the frequency of snacking increases (greater than two or three per day) does snacking become a risk factor among children of all age groups. Reportedly, between one-fourth and one-third of the energy intake of adolescents is derived from snacks.[68] Snack foods tend to have higher energy density and fat content than meals, and frequent snacking has been associated with high intakes of fat, sugar, and calories. The primary snacks selected by teens include potato chips, ice cream, candy, cookies, breakfast cereal, popcorn, crackers, soup, cake, and carbonated beverages. It is important not to eliminate snacks, but to help children choose healthy snacks and watch portion sizes.

- *Eating Out:* Interventions should target education in eating out and increases in family meals. Eating out can negatively impact the diets of children, and consumption of foods away from home has increased considerably in recent years. This increase may be associated with obesity, especially among adolescents.[69] The frequency of eating foods away from home has been associated with greater intakes of total energy, sugar-sweetened beverages, and trans fats as well as lower consumption of low-fat dairy foods and fruits and vegetables.[70] Adding to this, portion sizes have increased in restaurants. Portion sizes can significantly influence energy intake. Additionally, children and adolescents who consumed fast food more frequently had higher energy intakes, poorer diet quality, and higher BMIs. In 2011–2012, 34.3% children consumed fast food on a given day. Almost 12% of children and adoelescents obtained fewer than 25% of their daily calories from fast food, 10.7% obtained 25–40% and 12% obtained more than 40% of their daily calories from fast food.[71] The currently available evidence suggests that frequent eating at fast food restaurants may be a risk factor for obesity in children, and fast food ingestion year after year may accumulate to larger weight gains that can be clinically significant.[72]

- *Dairy Foods and Calcium:* Increasing fat-free or low-fat dairy products to three to four servings a day while consuming a lower calorie diet may assist with weight loss. However, more research in this area is needed.[73]

- *Dietary Fiber:* Dietary fiber may be related to regulation of body weight in children. Increasing fiber increases satiety, causing the child to eat less. Additionally, high fiber foods such as vegetables, fruits, and whole grains tend to be lower calorie foods and high in nutrients (high nutrient density), which also contributes to weight loss.[73]

Increasing Physical Activity

Along with diet, physical activity is the other key factor in maintaining energy balance. In addition to helping to control weight, physical activity provides numerous mental and physical benefits to health including reduction in the risk of cardiovascular disease, hypertension, diabetes, depression, and cancer. The greatest benefits of physical activity are gained from regular participation. The 2008 Physical Activity Recommendations for Americans state that children and adolescents should participate in 60 minutes or more of physical activity every day.[49] Unfortunately, the trend is for children to spend less and less time engaging in physical activity, with approximately 75% US children not meeting the recommendations.[74] Physically active children are also more likely to remain physically active throughout adolescence and possibly into adulthood. However, measuring physical activity in children is challenging because children often have difficulty understanding the concepts of time, duration, and intensity of activity. The nature, context, and practice of physical activity vary with age.[74]

Particular individuals are at increased risk of having low levels of physical activity, including children from ethnic minorities, those living in poverty, children with disabilities, those residing in apartments or public housing, and children living in neighborhoods where outdoor physical activity is restricted by climate or safety concerns. Many barriers exist that may prevent children and youth from getting the recommended 60 minutes of daily physical activity. Communities and neighborhoods where inadequate after-school programs exist, lack of community recreation facilities, inadequate access to quality daily physical activity, and lack of discretionary income may contribute to the high obesity rates in these populations. Additionally, safety concerns such as heavy traffic, high crime rate, lack of equipment, lack of space, and urban development that favors cars are significant barriers to outside play. Walking or biking to and from school can help students meet their physical activity needs. However, heavy traffic, lack of bicycle lanes, unmarked intersections, and other obstacles have reduced the number of children who transport themselves to school today compared to previous generations.[75]

The 2008 Physical Activity Guidelines for Americans recommends the following for children and adolescents ages 6–17.[49]

- Aerobic activity should make up most of the child's 60 or more minutes of physical activity each day. This can include either moderate-intensity aerobic activity, such as brisk walking, or vigorous-intensity activity, such as running. Include vigorous-intensity aerobic activity on at least 3 days per week
- Muscle strengthening activities should be included at least 3 days per week.
- Bone strengthening activities, such as jumping rope or running, should be included at least 3 days per week as part of the 60 minute activity per day.

Reducing Physical Inactivity

Reducing television viewing and sedentary behaviors may be more important in obesity reduction than physical activity. Increasing time spent on physical activities, especially electronic media, constributes to the levels of physical activity among young people. Everyday, 8 to 18 year olds spend on average, more than 7.5 hours using electronic media.[76]

Behavioral Modification

Behavior intervention for pediatric obesity uses a number of techniques that modify and control children's food and activity environment to bring about weight loss. These interventions include removing unhealthy foods from the home, monitoring behavior by asking children or parents to keep logs of behavioral components (e.g., food consumed, TV time, physical activity amounts), setting goals for nutrient intake and physical activity, and rewarding children's and sometimes parents' successful changes in diet and physical activity.[6,73,77]

▶ Motivational Interviewing

Most healthcare professionals, such as nurses, dietitians, and physicians have not been adequately trained in behavioral counseling and have even less experience in counseling children and adolescents with obesity. In order to successfully treat obesity, providers must address not only diet and exercise, but also behavior change. Often healthcare professionals provide information they think the patient needs to know without finding out what the person wants to know or what changes the client thinks would be most helpful to them. Understanding behavioral interviewing and counseling is critical to successfully working with overweight and obese children and adolescents.

Motivational interviewing (MI) can be defined as a directive, client-centered counseling style for eliciting behavioral change by helping clients explore and resolve ambivalence.[78,79] The resolution of ambivalence is one of the central purposes of MI and is particularly effective for individuals who are initially not ready to make changes. The tone of MI is nonjudgmental, empathetic, and encouraging. It provides a supportive environment where clients feel comfortable expressing both positive and negative aspects of their current behaviors.[78,79] Traditional models of counseling for nutrition rely on information exchange and counselor insight on what should be done. In contrast, the MI approach has the patient do much of the psychological work. In other words, the client is responsible for making the change. MI encourages clients to make fully informed and contemplated life choices, even if the decision is not to change.

MI operates under the premise that behavior change is affected more by motivation than information. There are specific techniques and strategies that, when used effectively, help ensure that the spirit of MI is evoked.[78,79] MI counselors rely heavily on reflective listening and positive affirmations. Clients make changes when they assign value to the change. In other words, clients are motivated to change what they value as important. Other core MI techniques include setting an agenda, rolling with resistance, building discrepancy, and eliciting self-motivation statements.

▶ Staged Approach to Treating Childhood Obesity

The AAP Expert Committee on Childhood Obesity Treatment provided guidance for treating childhood and adolescent overweight and obesity. These gudelines have been used as the framework for more recent recommendations. The Expert Committee used available evidence to propose a comprehensive staged approach to treatment. The recommendations suggest that providers should counsel patients on healthy behaviors, utilize MI techniques to motivate patients and families, establish office systems that help providers monitor and care for these children, and implement a staged approach to intervention that is tailored to the individual child and family. **TABLE 21.2** provides an overview of the staged approach.

TABLE 21.2 Staged Approach for Treatment of Childhood and Adolescent Obesity			
Stage	**Stage Recommendations**	**Setting and Staff**	**Frequency of Visits**
Stage 1: Prevention Plus	<ul><li>5+ fruits and vegetables a day</li><li>< 2hours/day screen time</li><li>≥ 1 hour/day physical activity</li><li>Reduce/eliminate sugar-sweetened beverages</li><li>Modify eating behaviors (e.g., three meals a day, family meals, limit eating out)</li><li>Family-based change</li></ul>	Primary care office–based Ensure scheduled follow-up visits	Frequency of visits based on readiness to change/behavioral counseling. Reevaluate in 3 to 6 months. Advance to next level if no improvement.
Stage 2: Structured Weight Management	Develop a plan for the family and/or adolescent to include:<ul><li>More structure (timing and content) of daily meals and snacks</li><li>Balanced macronutrient diet</li><li>Reduced screen time (< 1 hour/day)</li><li>Increased time spent in physical activity</li><li>Monitoring to improve success (e.g., logs of screen time, physical activity, dietary intake, or dietary patterns)</li></ul>	Office-based (dietitian, physician, nurse) trained in motivational interviewing/behavioral counseling	Monthly visits tailored to child/adolescent and family. Advance if needed or if no improvement after 3 to 6 months.
Stage 3: Comprehensive Multidisciplinary Intervention	<ul><li>Structured behavioral program (e.g., food monitoring, goal setting, contingency management)</li><li>Improved home food environment</li><li>Structured dietary and physical activity interventions designed to result in negative energy balance</li><li>Strong parental/family involvement, especially for children under 12 years of age</li></ul>	Multidisciplinary team (includes dietitian and counselor or behavioralist, with medical oversight)	Weekly for 8–12 weeks, then monthly for 6–12 months. Consider stage 4 if no improvement for children ages 12–18.
Stage 4: Tertiary Care Intervention	Continued diet and activity behavioral counseling plus consider more aggressive approaches, such as medication, surgery, or meal replacement	Pediatric weight management center operating under established protocols Multidisciplinary team	According to protocol.

Adapted from Barlow SE. Expert committee recommendations regarding the prevention, assessment and treatment of child and adolescent overweight and obesity: summary report. *Pediatrics.* 2007;120(suppl 4):S164–S192.[6]

Spear BA, Barlow SE, Ervin C, et al. Recommendations for treatment of child and adolescent overweight and obesity. *Pediatrics.* 2007;120:S254–S288.[73]

Stage 1: Prevention Plus

All children should receive prevention counseling in the form of healthy lifestyle eating and activity habit. For children ages 2 to 18 years who are above the 85th percentile, stage 1 (Prevention Plus) should be implemented. This differs from basic prevention counseling by recommending that providers spend more time and intensity while providing closer follow-up every 3–6 months.

All intervention in this stage should be based on the family's and/or child's readiness to change. Intervention should focus on basic prevention behavior strategies. The outcome goal for this stage is based on the age of the child and improving the BMI status of the child or adolescent. Positive outcomes can be maintaining weight until the BMI is less than the 85th percentile or gradual weight loss until the BMI is less than the 85th percentile. Specific behavioral components to address in this stage include:

Eating Behaviors:

- Minimize or eliminate sugar-sweetened beverages, such as soda, sports drinks, and punches. If sweetened beverages cannot be eliminated, children who consume large amounts will benefit from a reduction to one serving a day.
- Consume at least five servings of fruits and vegetables daily. Families may subsequently increase to nine servings a day, as recommended by the USDA dietary guidelines.
- Limit eating out and purchasing restaurant food.
- Eat at the table as a family (family meals).
- Consume a healthy breakfast daily.
- Involve the whole family in lifestyle changes.

Physical Activity Behaviors:

- Decrease television viewing as well as other forms of nonhomework screen time to 2 or fewer hours a day. If the child is less than 2 years of age the committee recommends no television viewing. Removing the television from the bedroom will help reduce TV viewing time.
- Engage in 1 hour or more of physical activity per day. It is important to gradually increase physical activity for sedentary children. Initially, children may be unable to achieve 1 hour per day, but can gradually increase activity to reach 1 hour or more per day. Unstructured play is most appropriate for young children; older children may enjoy sports, dance, martial arts, bike riding, and walking. Physical activity can be done all at one time or in several shorter periods of activity over an entire day.

Follow-up visit frequency will be tailored to the individual family, and MI techniques may be useful to set the frequency. After 3 to 6 months, if the child has not made appropriate improvement, the provider can offer the next level of obesity care, Structured Weight Management.

Stage 2: Structured Weight Management

This stage targets the same behaviors as the Prevention Plus stage (food consumption, activity, and screen time), and offers additional support and structure to help the child and family achieve healthy behaviors in eating and physical activity. This stage requires the primary provider to have additional training in behavioral counseling. The eating plan requires a dietitian or a clinician who has received additional training in creating this kind of eating plan for children. Additionally, this stage requires the ability to add monitoring to the recommendations. Patients who monitor behavior change through such things as behavior logs, food diaries, or exercise logs have greater success in weight changes. This stage is characterized by closer follow-up,

more structure, and the monitoring of activities. The outcome goal for this stage is based on the age of the child and improving the BMI status of the child or adolescent. Positive outcomes can be maintaining weight until BMI is less than the 85th percentile or gradual weight loss until BMI is less than the 85th percentile. Specific behavioral components to address in this stage include:

Eating behaviors:

- Planned and structured daily meals and snacks (breakfast, lunch, dinner, with one or two snacks) with the following characteristics:
  - Balanced macronutrients based on the US Dietary Guidelines
  - Emphasis on foods low in energy density, such as those with high fiber or water content
  - Mild energy (caloric) deficit
  - Behavioral monitoring such as the use of food, activity, and screen time logs
  - Planned reinforcement for achieving targeted behavior goals

Physical Activity Behaviors:

- Planned and supervised physical activity or active play for 60 minutes daily
- Reducing screen time for leisure to 60 minutes or less each day (not including time dedicated to schoolwork). For example, the patient or family can record the minutes spent watching television, and they can keep a 3-day recording of foods and beverages consumed.

Ideally, monthly office visits are most effective at this level. After 3 to 6 months, if the child has not made significant improvement based on age and BMI level, the provider can offer the next level of obesity care, Comprehensive Multidisciplinary Intervention.

Stage 3: Comprehensive Multidisciplinary Intervention

The eating and activity goals associated with the Comprehensive Multidisciplinary Intervention stage are generally the same as those of the other treatment stages. The distinguishing characteristics of this stage are an increased intensity of behavioral change strategies, greater frequency of patient–provider contact, and an increase in the number of disciplines/specialists involved. The need for formalized behavioral therapy and a multidisciplinary treatment team exceeds the capacity of services that most primary care offices can provide. Specific behavioral components to address in this stage include:

Eating Behaviors:

- Negative energy balance achieved through structured diet and physical activity (e.g., lower calorie diets that will help with weight reduction, decreasing high intake of sugar-sweetened beverages in children who have excessive consumption, or decreased TV viewing in children who watch greater than 2 hours per day)

- Planned and structured daily meals and snacks (breakfast, lunch, dinner, and one or two snacks) with the following characteristics:
  - Balanced macronutrients based on US Dietary Guidelines.
  - Emphasis on foods low in energy density, such as those with high fiber or water content.
  - Behavioral monitoring such as the use of food, activity, and screen time logs. For example, the patient or family can record the minutes spent watching television, and they can keep a 3-day recording of foods and beverages consumed.
- Planned reinforcement for achieving targeted behavior goals
- Education for parents to improve home environment

Physical Activity Behaviors:

- Planned and supervised physical activity or active play for at least 60 minutes daily
- Planned and supervised muscle-strengthening and bone-strengthening activity at least 3 days per week[17]
- Reduction in screen time for leisure to 60 minutes or less each day

Frequent office visits, weekly for a minimum of 8–12 weeks, appears most efficacious. Subsequently, monthly visits will help maintain new behaviors. Patients ages 6 to 18 years old who do not show improvement in weight after participating in stage 3 for 3 to 6 months may benefit from a referral to a tertiary care center. However, when these centers are not available or if families are motivated they may achieve success with longer implementation of components in Stage 3 with closer follow-up by healthcare providers.

Stage 4: Tertiary Care Intervention

The intensive interventions in this category have been used only to a limited extent in the pediatric population but may be an option for some severely obese youth who have significant co-morbidities. These interventions are more intensive and need more supervision than recommendations in the other stages. Candidates being considered for this stage should have attempted weight loss at the level of stage 3, Comprehensive Multidisciplinary Intervention; have the maturity to understand possible risks associated with stage 4 interventions; and be willing to maintain physical activity, follow a prescribed diet, and participate in behavior monitoring. However, lack of success with stage 3 is not by itself a qualification for stage 4 treatment. It is recommended that programs that provide these intensive treatments operate under established protocols to

evaluate patients, implement the program, and monitor patients.

Although the interventions included in this stage have been used in adolescents, careful consideration should be made in implementing the components of this stage. The appropriateness of each of these interventions depends on the patient, family resources, age, and the geographic area's resources. Interventions to consider include the following:

- *Very-low-calorie diet/meal replacement:* There are few reports on the use of highly restrictive diets in children or adolescents. A restrictive diet has been employed as the first step in a childhood weight management program, followed by a mildly restrictive diet.[11] Long-term outcome data have not been reported.
- *Pharmacotherapy/medication:* The only current drug approved by the US Food and Drug Adminsitration (FDA) is orlistat for children over 12 years of age. Medication should only be used in conjunction with nutrition, physical activity, and behavioral counseling.[9]
- *Weight control surgery:* Because of the increasing number of children with severe obesity who are not responsive to behavioral intervention, weight loss surgery is a possible option for adolescents.[6,80,81]

▶ Recommended Weight Change Goals

The general goal for all ages is for the BMI to deflect downwards until it is less than the 85th percentile. This may be done by maintaining weight while height increases. In other cases, a gradual weight loss may be needed in order to reach a BMI less than the 85th percentile. However, realizing that some children will be healthy between the 85th and 95th percentiles, clinical judgment will play a critical role in weight recommendations. Although monitoring BMI over the long term is ideal, in the short term (3 months), weight changes may be an easier parameter to measure.[6]

Bariatric Surgery

Often, severe obesity is persistent even when treated through diet and lifestyle change and weight management medications. For some very obese adolescents bariatric surgery may be a justifiable treatment option.[6,80,81] Although weight loss surgery has resulted in substantial weight loss and medical conditions, pre and post operative risks as well as the necessity of lifelong commitment make this a difficult option for adolescents.[82] Stringent guidelines for using bariatric surgery in physically mature adolescents has been developed that include strict qualification criteria for the patients and the centers performing the surgery, and to take into account the noncompliant nature of adolescents. They cover the specific nutritional and developmental needs for adolescents.[80,81]

To be eligible for bariatric surgery, the patient must:

- Have reached physical maturity. Tanner stage 4 or 5, age > or equal 13 years for girls and > or equal for boys, exceptions made be made for more severe comorbidities)
- Have a BMI ≥ 35 with serious obesity related conditions eg, (type 2 diabets, moderate or severe sleep apnea or pseudotumor cerebi)
- Have a BMI ≥ 40 with a minor co-morbidities (eg, hypertension, insulin resistence, dyslipidemia, glucose intolerance)
- Have failed a formal 6-month or longer weight loss program
- Be capable of adhering to the long-term lifestyle changes that are required postoperatively by demonstrating commitment to comprehensive medical and psychological evaluations before and after surgery
- Capable of making his or her own decisions
- Has a supportive family environment
- Be aware of the known risks and possible side effects of the surgery and provide informed consent
- Agrees to avoid pregnancy for at least 18 months postoperatively
- Undergo preoperative testing focusing on identifying co-morbidities associated with obesity and routine lab screenings including:
  - Fasting insulin and glucose
  - Oral glucose tolerance test
  - Lipid profile
  - Liver profile
  - Complete blood count
  - Vitamin B_1, B_{12}, and folate levels

Success in maintaining weight loss long term depends on the patient's ability to adhere to behavior changes and a reduced calorie diet. Taking into account the developmental behaviors of adolescents and their propensity to rebel against strict regimens, it is important to provide consistent support and follow-up postoperatively. Meticulous, lifelong medical supervision of patients who undergo bariatric procedures during adolescence is essential to ensure optimal postoperative weight loss, eventual weight maintenance, and overall health. This is particularly important for adolescents, given the fact that the long-term effects of bariatric surgery in younger, reproductively active populations have not been well characterized.[81,82] Postoperative vitamin and mineral supplementation is critical in a reduced calorie diet, and usually consists of a chewable adult multivitamin, calcium supplement, B-complex vitamins, and folic acid in females.[81,82]

▶ Nutrition Monitoring and Evaluation

Follow-up is an essential component of treating overweight or obese children and adolescents in order to monitor and evaluate behavior changes. The AAP Expert Committee on Assessment, Prevention and Treatment provided recommendations for frequency of follow-up.[6] See **TABLE 18.2**. A greater frequency of follow-up may lead to more successful weight loss and maintenance.

Follow-up should include monitoring progress, measuring outcomes and nutrition care indicators against comparative standards. Examples of outcome data include food and nutrition (amount and type of food, total energy intake, self-monitoing, behavior change goal attainment), anthropometrics (decrease or increase in weight), change in BMI or BMI z-score,[55] biomedical/medical (improvement in hemoglobin A1C, improvement in liver enzymes, decrease in cholesterol), and nutrition focused physical findings (decrease in blood pressure, decrease in acanthosis, improvement in shortness of breath).[55]

Prevention/Intervention programs are few and program cost may prevent many from being able to participate in or integrate into school curriculums. As we continue to intervene with already-at-risk children and adolescents, we also need to increase our preventative measures.[57,58,83] Below is a list of recommendations for prevention from the Institute of Medicine and the World Health Organization:[57,84]

- Implement comprehensive programs that promote the intake of healthy foods and decrease the intake of unhealthy foods.
- Create healthy food and beverage environments that ensure healthy food and beverage options.
- Implement comprehensive programs that promote physical activity and decrease physical inactivity.
- Make healthy messages about physical activity and nutrition.
- Make school a national point for obesity prevention.
- Implement comprehensive programs that promote healthy school environments, health and nutrition literacy, and physical activity among school age children.
- Provide guidance and support for preconception and prenatal care to reduce the risk of childhood obesity.
- Provide guidance and support for healthy diet, sleep, and physical activity in early childhood.

Prevention is the responsibility of the health care provider, the family, the child, the school, and the community as well as the insurer and government agencies.[57,58,84] The following provides an overview of prevention activities for each segment.

Primary Care Provider

- Early recognition of overweight/obesity. Plot BMI routinely, and if the BMI percentile increases, address this before it reaches more than 95%.
- Identify those at risk. Risk factors can include:
  - Parents are overweight
  - Sibling is overweight
  - Lower socioeconomic status
  - Children with less cognitive stimulation
- Provide anticipatory guidance in nutrition and physical activity. Anticipatory guidance is information and counseling that helps patients and families understand what to expect during a child or adolescent's current and/or approaching stage of development (e.g., growth spurts, increased/decreased energy needs, ways to prevent obesity through exercise and nutrition). Healthcare professionals can provide anticipatory guidance on nutrition and physical activity to help with obesity and eating disorder prevention as well as provide information to families.
- Promote water and milk consumption over juice and soda.
- Eat as a family.
- Encourage nonsedentary family activities.
- Do not use food as a reward.
- Limit TV/computer/video games to 1–2 hours per day.
- Do not eat in front of the TV.
- Do not put a TV in the child's room.

Family

- Parents act as a role model
- Nutrition
- Physical activity
- Limit eating out
- Eat family meals
- "Special times" do not have to involve food or sedentary activities

School

- Promote physical activity.
- Provide nutritious meals.
- Have recess before lunch when possible.
- Control vending machines/healthy vending.
- Have nutrition and activity education integrated into the school curriculum.
- Encourage children to walk or bike to school when safe.

Community

- Have safe playgrounds.
- Provide safe places for bike riding and walking.
- Promote physical activity outside of school.

Insurance and Government

- Acknowledge obesity as a medical condition for which one can be reimbursed.
- Provide reimbursement for anticipatory guidance on nutrition and physical activity.

▶ Eating Disorders Related to Obesity

Eating disorders (ED) are the third most common chronic illness in adolescents behind obesity and asthma. The prevalence of eating disorders in children and adolescents has increased dramatically over the past three decades, especially in females. They remain a serious cause of morbidity in children, adolescents, and young adults.

Defining Eating Disorders

Eating disorders are considered medical illnesses with diagnostic criteria based on psychological, behavioral, and physiologic characteristics.[85,86] Generally, these illnesses are characterized by abnormal eating patterns and cognitive distortions related to food and weight, which in turn result in adverse effects on nutrition status, medical complications, and impaired health status and mental function.[87-89] Eating disorders that can result in overweight and obesity include binge eating disorder and night eating syndrome.

Diagnostic Criteria

Diagnostic criteria for binge eating disorder and night eating syndrome are identified in the fifth edition of the *Diagnostic and Statistical Manual of Mental Disorders* (DSM-5).[90] These clinical diagnoses are based on psychological, behavioral, and physiologic characteristics.

Binge Eating Disorder (Diagnostic Code 307.51)

A. Recurrent episodes of binge eating, characterized by both of the following:
  1. Eating, in a discrete period of time (e.g., within any 2-hour period), and amount of food that is definitely larger than what people would eat in a similar period of time under similar curcumstances.
  2. A sense of lack of control over eating during the episode (e.g., a feeling that one cannot stop eating or control what or how much one is eating).

B.   The Binge-eating episodes are associated with three (or more) of the following:
1.   Eating much more rapidly than normal
2.   Eating until feeling uncomfortably full
3.   Eating large amounts of food when not physically hungry
4.   Eating alone because of feeling embarrassed by how much one is eating
5.   Feeling disgusted with oneself, depressed, or very guilty afterward.

C.   Marked distress regarding binge eating present.

D.   The binge eating occurs, on average, at least once a week for 3 months.

E.   The binge eating is not associated with the recurrent use of inappropriate compensatory behaviors as in bulimia nervosa and does not occur exclusively during the course of bulimia nervosa or anorexia nervosa.

F.   Night Eating Syndrome
Recurrent episodes of night eating, as manifested by eating after awakening from sleep or by excessive food consumption after the evening meal. There is awareness and recall of the eating. The night eating is not better explained by external influences such as changes in the individual's sleep-wake cycle or by social norms. The night eating causes significant distress and/or impairment in functioning. The disordered pattern of eating is not better explained by binge-eating disorder or another mental disorder, including substance abuse, and is not attributable to another medical disorder or to an effect of medication.[90]

Nutrition Intervention Binge Eating Disorder In Binge Eating Disorder the patient has binging behavior without the compensatory purging seen in BN. Binge episodes must occur at least twice a week and have occurred for at least 6 months. Most patients diagnosed with BED are overweight and suffer the same medical problems faced by the nonbingeing obese population, such as diabetes, high blood pressure, high blood cholesterol levels, gallbladder disease, heart disease, and certain types of cancer.

The patient with BED often presents with weight management concerns rather than eating disorder concerns. Although researchers are still trying to find the treatment that is most helpful in controlling binge eating disorder, many treatment manuals exist utilizing the CBT model shown effective for BN.[91,92]

Nutrition Monitoring and Evaluation The frequency which patients are monitored will depend on several factors such as Joint Commission Standards, set policies and protocol, severity of complications and patient goals. Examples include monitoring nutrient intake and adjustments as necessary, rate of weight gain, and once weight is restored, adjusting food intake to maintain weight and changes in laboratory values. It is essential that communication and updates are provided to the healthcare team.[93,94]

▶ Conclusion

The causes of overweight and obesity in children are multifactorial, therefore the solutions must also be. The staged approach to the treatment of overweight and obesity is supported by many of the professional, regulatory, and governmental organizations who care for children.

Multi-level interventions show the greatest impact for prevention; thus, early childhood and school-based interventions should include behavioral and environmental approaches that focus on dietary intake and physical activity using a systems-wide approach. Secondary prevention and tertiary prevention/treatment should emphasize sustained family-based, age appropriate approaches that include nutrition education, dietary counseling, parenting skills, behavioral strategies, and physical-activity promotion.[46]

This family centered, team approach to care for childhood overweight/obesity is highly recommended.

This chapter provides information and resources for the management and treatment of childhood overweight and obesity.

🔍 CASE STUDY

Nutrition Assessment

Patient and Family History

Adam is a 12-year-old white male who presents in clinic today with complaints of stomach pain for 6 months. Family history reveals that his parents have been divorced for approximately 1 year and he is not able to see his father as often as he would like. Because of the divorce, mom and Adam have moved to a new neighborhood and mom often works late and is unable to prepare home-cooked meals on a regular basis. Adam is not allowed to cook when mom is not at home. Mother has just recently been diagnosed with diabetes and his father is overweight and has hypertension. His mother is concerned about Adam's rapid weight gain but feels the new neighborhood is not safe and does not allow Adam to be outdoors unsupervised. He watches TV or plays video games after school. Adam's main concern is stomach pain, although he does identify concerns about his weight gain.

Food/Nutrition-Related History

Diet history shows an average intake of 3100 kcal (range 2900–3400). Average protein intake is 90 g/day (range 60–120 g/day). Fat intake is approximately 37% of total kcal. Fiber intake is approximately 14 g/day. Average intake of calcium is approximately 1000 mg/day, iron 14mg/day, and sodium 3800 mg/day from food. Estimated beverage intake is ~40 oz/day of sweetened beverages. Physical activity history reveals TV viewing/computer games 3–4 hours/day.

Anthropometric Measurements

Height: 64.5 inches (156 cm)
Weight: 130 lbs (59 kg)
BMI: 21.9 (85th–90th percentile)

One year ago, Adam was 62 inches (157.5 cm) and 100 lbs (45.45 kg). His BMI was 18.2 (50th–75th percentile). Patient has had a 30-pound weight gain over the past year. Sexual Maturity Rating or Tanner State 2. Blood pressure and heart rate are normal for age and height. Bowel history shows two bowel movements per week.

Nutrition Diagnoses

There could be many nutrition diagnoses which may include lack of physical activity, high level of physical inactivity, unhealthy snacking, high intake of sugar sweetened beverages.

Intervention Goals

The overall goal of treatment is to decrease overall caloric intake and increase activity to maintain current weight until appropriate height for weight is achieved. Increasing fluid and fiber intake will address the patient's concern of constipation.

Monitoring and Evaluation

The expert committee recommends monthly follow-up for children in stage 2 treatment. The patient and his mother should be encouraged to monitor suggestions and return for weight checks and nutrition counseling to ensure BMI maintenance or BMI trending downward during growth spurt. Weight loss is not necessarily recommended.

Questions for the Reader

1. What does Adam's BMI percentile mean? Where was he 1 year ago?
2. What are Adam's energy needs and protein needs?
3. What factors are affecting nutrient and physical activity requirements?
4. Write at least one PES statement for this patient.
5. Identify interventions in at least two domains of nutrition intervention to use in counseling Adam and his mother.

NUTRITION DOCUMENTATION FORM

ASSESSMENT: Summary of Subjective and Objective Data from Chart Review and Interview.

Age: 12   **Sex:** Male   **Family health hx:** Mother has diabetes, father overweight and hypertensive
Ht: 64.5″ (156 cm)   **Wt:** 130 lb (59 kg)   **BMI:** 85th to 90th percentile—overweight; 1 year ago in normal weight range

Estimated Nutritional Needs

Energy: 2200–2500 kcal/day; protein: ~45–55 g/day; calcium: 1300 mg/day; fiber: 20–30 g/day. SMR level of 2 indicates that growth spurt has not yet started; opportune time to affect BMI as height changes.

Intake

Average of 3100 kcal per day, 90 g protein, 37% of calories from fat, 14 g fiber, 1000 mg calcium, 14 mg iron, 3800 mg sodium. Fast food two times/week; sweetened beverages (~40 oz per day) and two or less servings of fruit and vegetables/day; no whole grain servings/day. Access to fresh fruits and vegetables and ability to prepare foods is minimal during after school hours before mother arrives home, limited availability of home-prepared meals. Symptoms of constipation may be affected by fiber intake and lack of physical activity.

(continues)

NUTRITION DOCUMENTATION FORM (continued)

Physical Activity

PE at school; greater than 3 hours TV/video games per day; after-school activities limited by mother's perception of lack of safety in neighborhood.

Food allergies or intolerances: None   **Medications/supplements:** None

Nutrition Diagnosis	Signs and Symptoms (As Evidenced By)	Etiology (Related to)	Goals	Planned Interventions
Excessive energy intake	Weight gain of 30 pounds over past year, 500–700kcal/day above EER	Undesirable food choices and physical inactivity	Decrease daily calorie intake approximately 400–500kcal/day; BMI maintenance or trending downward.	Provide meal plan to include healthier snacks and lower caloric beverages, and increase fruits and vegetables to five a day.
Physical inactivity	Greater than 3 hours/day of TV/video game use	Unsafe neighborhood and mother's increased work hours	Decrease physical inactivity.	Limit television viewing/computer games to 1–2 hours per day.
Undesirable food choices	Consuming greater than 40 oz sweetened beverages/day	Limited intake of foods consistent with Dietary Guidelines	Limit sweetened beverages to 6–8 oz juice/day.	Work with patient and mom to provide sugar-free drinks and water.
Inadequate fiber intake	Constipation (bowel movements two times per week)	Limited intake of fruits and vegetables and whole grain foods	Increase intake of fiber-rich foods: fruits, vegetables, and whole grains.	Develop with patient a meal plan that includes at least five fruits and vegetables per day, increase high fiber foods, whole grain foods, and healthy snacks.

PESS: Excessive energy intake (NI 1.3) related to unhealthy snacking and high intake of SSB as evidenced by a BMI for age between 85%ile and 90%ile.

Unintended weight gain (NC 3.3.2) or Excessive growth rate (NC 3.6) related to excessive energy intake as evidenced by 30 lb. weight gain/increase in BMI for age from 50–75%ile to the 85–90%ile.

Follow-up in one month

Date: _____   Dietitian _____ Nutrition Provider #_____

_____

_____

References

1. Odgen LO, Carroll MD, Lawman HG, et al. Trends in obesity prevalence among children and adolescents in the United States, 1988–1994 through 2013–2014. *JAMA*;2016:315(21):2292–2299.

2. Centers for Disease Control and Prevention. Childhood obesity causes & consequences. Updated June 19, 2015. Available at: http://www.cdc.gov/obesity/childhood/causes.html. Accessed October 15, 2017.

3. Centers for Disease Control and Prevention. Childhood obesity facts. Updated August 27, 2016. Available at: http://www.cdc.gov/healthyyouth/obesity/facts.htm. Accessed October 15, 2017.

4. Ogden CL, Carroll MD, Curtin LR, Lamb MM, Flegal KM. Prevalence of high body mass index in U.S. children and adolescents, 2007–2008. *JAMA*. 2010;303(3):242–249.

5. Ogden CL, Carroll MD, Flegal KM. High body mass index for age among U.S. children and adolescents, 2003–2006. *JAMA*. 2008;299(20):2401–2405.

6. Barlow SE, Expert Committee recommendations regarding the prevention, assessment, and treatment of child and adolescent overweight and obesity: summary report. *Pediatr*. 2007;120(suppl4):S164–S192.

7. U.S. Preventive Task Force. Recommendations Statement. Screening for obesity in children and adolescents U.S. Preventive Services Task Force Recommendation Statement. *JAMA*. 2017:317(23):2417–2426.

8. Academy of Nutrition and Dietetics. Pediatric Weight Management (PWM) Guideline 2015. Available at: http://www.andeal.org/topic.cfm?menu=5296&cat=5632. Accessed February 20, 2016.

9. Kelly AS, Barlow SE, Rao G, et al on behalf of the American Heart Association Atherosclerosis, Hypertension, and Obesity in the Youth Committee Council on Cardiovascular Disease in the Young, Council on Nutrition, Physical Activity and Metabolism, and Council on Clinical Cardiology. Severe obesity in children and adolescents: identification, associated health risks, and treatment approaches: a scientific statement from the American Heart Association. Circ. 2013;128(15):1689–1712.

10. Centers for Disease Control and Prevention. Use and interpretation of the WHO and CDC Growth Charts for Children from Birth to 20 years in the United States. Available at http://www.growthcharts/nccdphp/resources/growthcharts.pdf. Accessed November 10, 2017.

11. Biro FM, Wien M. Childhood obesity and adult morbidities. *Am J Clin Nutr*. 2010;91(suppl):1499S–1505S.

12. Gumani M, Birken C, Hamilton J. Childhood obesity: causes, consequences, and management. *Pediatr Clin North Am*. 2015;62(4):821–840.

13. Daniels SR. Complications of obesity in children and adolescents. *Int J Obes*. 2009;38;560–565.

14. May AL, Kuklina EV, Yoon PW. Prevalence of Cardiovascular disease risk factors among U.S. adolescents, 1999–2008. *Pediatr*. 2012:129(6):1035–1041.

15. National Heart, Lung, and Blood Institute. Expert Panel on integrated guidelines for Cardiovascular Health and risk reduction in Children and Adolescents: Summary Report. 2012. Available at: www.nhlbi.nih.gov/ files/docs/guidelines/peds_guidelines_full.pdf.

16. Freedman DS, Mei Z, Srinivasan R, Berenson GS, Dietz WH. Cardiovascular risk factors and excess adiposity among overweight children and adolescents: the Bogalusa Heart Study. *J Pediatr*. 2007;150(1):12–17.

17. Daniels SR, Green FR. Committee on Nutrition, Lipids amd Cardiovascular Health in Childhood. *Pediatr*.2008; 122(1):198–208.

18. Parker ED, Sinaiko AR, Kharbanda EO, et al. Change in weight status and development of hypertension. *Pediatr*. 2016;137(3):1–9.

19. Luma GB, Spiotta RT. Hypertension in children and adolescents. *Am Fam Physician*. 2006;73(9):1558–1568.

20. Sutherland ER. Obesity and asthma. *Immunol Allergy Clin North Am*. 2008;28(3):589–602.

21. Gilland FD, Berhane K, Islam T, et al. Obesity and the risk of newly diagnosed asthma in school-age children. *Am J Epidemiol*. 2003;158(5):406–415.

22. Marcus CL, Brooks LJ, Draper KA, et al. Diagnosis and management of childhood obstructive sleep apnea syndrome. *Pediatr*. 2012;150(3):577–584.

23. Narang I, Mathew JL. Childhood obesity and obstructive sleep apnea. *J Nutr Metab*. 2012;2012:134202.

24. National Heart, Lung, and Blood Institute. What causes Sleep Apnea? Updated July 10, 2012. Available at: http://www.nhlbi.nih.gov/health/health-topics/topics/sleepapnea/causes. Accessed August 15, 2017.

25. Murray AW, Wilson NI. Changing incidence of slipped capital femoral epiphysis: a relationship with obesity. *J Bone Joint Surg Br*. 2008;90(1):92–94.

26. Manoff EM, Banify MB, Winell JJ. Relationship between body mass index and slipped capital femoral epiphysis. *J Pediatr Orthop*. 2005;25(6):744–746.

27. Dietz WH, Gross WL, Kirkpatrick JA. Blount disease (tibia vara): another skeletal disorder associated with childhood obesity. *J Pediatr*. 1982;101(5):735–737.

28. Centers for Disease Control and Prevention. National diabetes fact sheet: national estimates and general information on diabetes and prediabetes in the United States, 2011. Available at: https://www.cdc.gov/diabetes/pubs/pdf/ndfs_2011.pdf. Accessed November 2 2017.

29. Springer SC, Silverstein J, Copeland K, et al. Management of type 2 diabetes mellitus in children and adolescents. *Pediatr*. 2013:131(2)648–684.

30. American Diabetes Association. Classification and diagnosis of diabetes. In: Standards of Medical of Medical Care in Diabetes—2015. *Diabetes Care*. 2015:38(suppl1):S8–S16.

31. Office on Women's Health. U.S. Department of Health and Human Services. Polycystic ovary syndrome. Fact Sheet. Available at: http://womenshealth.gov/publications/our-publications/fact-sheet/polycystic-ovary-syndrome. html#c. Accessed August 20, 2016.

32. Rosenfield R. Polycystic ovary syndrome in adolescence associated with obesity. *AAP News*. 2007;28(4):20.

33. Weiss R, Dziura J, Burget TS, et al. Obesity and the metabolic syndrome in children and adolescents. *N Engl J Med*. 2004;350:2362–2374.

34. Bozic MA, Subbarao G, Molleston JP. Pediatric nonalcoholic fatty liver disease. *Nutr Clin Pract*. 2013;28(4):448–458.

35. Giorgio V, Prono F, Granziano F, Nobilli V. Pediatric non alcoholic fatty liver disease: old and new concepts on development, progression, metabolic insight and potential targets. *BMC Pediatr*. 2013;25(13). 10.1186/1471-2431-13-40.

36. Chalasani N, Younossi Z, Lavine JE, et al. The diagnosis and management of non-alcoholic fatty liver disease: practice guideline by the American Association for the Study of Liver Diseases, American College of Gastroenterology, and the American Gastroenterologist Association. *Hepatol*. 2012;55(6):2005–2023.

37. Bozic MA, Subbarao G, Molleston JP. Pediatric nonalcoholic fatty liver disease. *Nutr Clin Pract*. 2013;28(4):448–458.

38. Scott HG, DeMaia EJ, Felton WL III, Nakatsuka M, Sismanis A. Increased intra-abdominal pressure and cardiac filling pressure in obesity-associated pseudotumor cerebri. *Neurol*. 1997;49(2):507–511.

39. Duncan FJ, Corbett JJ, Wall M. Incidence of pseudotumor cerebri population studies in Iowa and Louisiana. *Arch Neurol*. 1988;45(8):875–877.

40. Morrison KM, Shin S, Tarnopolsky M, Taylor VH. Association of depression and health related quality of life with body composition and youth with obesity. *J Affect Disord*. 2015;172:18–23.

41. Halfon N, Larson K. Slusser W. Associations between obesity and comorbid mental health, developmental, and physical health conditions in a nationally representative

sample of U.S. children aged 10 to 17. *Academic Pediatr.* 2013:13:6–13.

42. Schwimmer JB, Burwinkle TM, Varni JW. Health-related quality of life of severely obese children and adolescents. *JAMA.* 2003;289(14):1813–1819.

43. Krebs NF, Himes JH, Jackson D, Nicklas TA, Guilday P, Styne D. Assessment of child and adolescent overweight and obesity. *Pediatr.* 2007;120(suppl4):S193–S228.

44. Mullen MC, Shield J. The Academy of Nutrition and Dietetics Pocket Guide to Pediatric Weight Management, 2nd Ed. 2017.

45. Academy of Nutrition and Dietetics. Weight management. Pediatric Nutrition Care Manual. Available at: www. nutritioncaremanual.org/pncd. Accessed November 2, 2017.

46. Hoelscher DM, Kirk S, Ritchie L, et al. Position of the Academy of Nutrition and Dietetics: interventions for the prevention and treatment of pediatric overweight and obesity. *J Acad Nutr Diet.* 2013;113(10):1375–1394.

47. National Heart, Lung, and Blood Institute. National High Blood Pressure Education Program Working Group on High Blood Pressure in Children and Adolescents. The fourth report on the diagnostic evaluation and treatment of high blood pressure in children and adolescents. Available at: www.nhlbi.nih.gov/files/ docs/resources/heart /hbp_ped.pdf. Accessed November 8, 2017.

48. American Diabetes Association. Classification and diagnosis of Diabetes. In: Standards of Medical of Medical Care in Diabetes—2015. *Diabetes Care* 2015:38(suppl1):S8–S16.

49. U.S. Department of Health and Human Services. *Physical Activity Guidelines for Americans.* Washington, DC: Government Printing Office; 2008.

50. American Academy of Pediatrics. Children, adolescents, and the media. *Pediatr.* 2013;132(5):958–964.

51. Center for Disease Control and Prevention. Insufficient sleep is a public health concern. Available at: https://www.cdc.gov /features/dssleep/index.html. Accessed November 10, 2017.

52. Fatima Y, Doi SA, Manun AA. Longitudinal impact on sleep and obesity in children and adolescents: a systemic review and bias-adjusted meta-analysis. *Obes. Rev.* 2015;16:137–149.

53. Hirshkowitz M, Whiton K, Albert SM, et al. National Sleep Foundation's updated sleep duration recommendations: final report. *Sleep Health.* 2015;1(4):233–243.

54. Leonberg BL. *ADA Pocket Guide to Pediatric Nutrition Assessment.* Chicago, IL: Academy of Nutrition and Dietetics; 2013.

55. Academy of Nutrition and Dietetics. eNCPT: Nutrition Terminology Reference Manual. Published August 5, 2015. Available at: https://www.ncpro.org. website (login required).

56. Academy of Nutrition and Dietetics. *Nutrition Care Process in Pediatric Management.* Chicago, IL: Academy of Nutrition and Dietetics; 2014.

57. World Health Organization. *Report of the Commission on Ending Childhood Obesity.* 2016. http://apps.who. int/iris/ bitstream/10665/204176/1/9789241510066_ eng.pdf?ua=. Accessed November 2, 2017.

58. Daniels SR, Hassinik SG, and Committee on Nutrition. The role of the pediatrician in primary prevention of obesity. *Pediatr.* 2015;135:275–292.

59. U.S. Department of Health and Human Services and U.S. Department of Agriculture. Dietary Guidelines for Americans 2015–2020. 8th ed. Available at: http://

health.gov/dietaryguidelines/2015/guidelines/. Accessed November 15, 2017.

60. Ambrosini GL, Emmett PM, Northstone K, Jebb SA. Tracking a dietary pattern associated with increased adiposity in childhood and adolescence. Obesity. 2014;22(2):458-465.

61. Heymann MB, Abrahams SA, Section on Gastroenetrology, Hepatology, and Nutrition and Committee on Nutrition. Fruit juice in Infants, children, and adolescents: Current recommendations. *Pediatr.* 2017;139:DOI:10.154/ peds.2017–0967.

62. Han E, Powell LM. Consumption patterns of sugar sweetened beverages in the United States. *J Acad Nutr Diet.* 2013;113:43–53.

63. Miller G, Merlo C, Demissie Z, Sliwa S, Park S. Trends in beverage consumption among high school students - United States, 2007–2015. *MMWR Morb Mortal Wkly Rep.* 2017;66(4):112–116.

64. Piernas C, Popkin BM. Food portion patterns and trends among U.S. children and the relationship to total eating occasion size, 1977–2006. *J Nutr.* 2011;141:1159–1164.

65. Portion sizes and school-aged children. Available at: https:// www.fns.usda.gov/cacfp/meals-and-snacks. Updated 2003. Accessed November 16, 2017.

66. Deshmukh-Taskar PR, Nicklas TA, O'Neil CE, Keast DR, Radcliffe JD, Cho S. The relationship of breakfast skipping and type of breakfast consumption with nutrient intake and weight status in children and adolescents: the national health and nutrition examination survey 1999–2006. *J Am Diet Assoc.* 2010;110:869–878.

67. Jackson LW. The most important meal of the day: why children skip breakfast and what can be done about it. *Ped Ann.* 2013;42:184–187.

68. Piernas C, Popkin BM. Trends in snacking among U.S. children. *Health Affairs.* 2010;9:398–404.

69. Centers for Disease Control and Prevention. Child and Nutrition Facts. Available at: https://www.cdc.gov/healthy schools/nutrition/facts.htm. Accessed November 17, 2017.

70. Vikraman S, Fryar CD, Odgen CL. *Caloric Intake From Fast Food Among Children and Adolescents in the United States, 2011–2012. NCHS Data Brief, no 213.* Hyattsville, MD:National Center for Health Statistics; 2015.

71. Powell LM, Nguyen BT. Fast-food and full-service restaurant consumption among children and adolescents: Effect on energy, beverage, and nutrient intake. *JAMA Pediatr* 167(1):14–20.

72. Poti JM, Popkin BM. Trends in energy intake among U.S. children by eating location and food source, 1977–2006. *J Am Diet Assoc.* 2011;11(8):1156–1164.

73. Spear BA, Barlow SE, Ervin, et al. Recommendations for treatment of child and adolescent overweight and obesity. Pediatr. 2007;120:S254–S288.

74. Centers for Disease Control and Prevention. Physical activity facts. Available at: https://www.cdc.gov/healthyschools /physicalactivity/facts.htm. Accessed November 10, 2017.

75. National Physical Activity Play Alliance. 2016. U.S. report card on physical activity for children and youth. Columbia, SC;2016.

76. American Academy of Pediatrics. Policy Statement Media and Children, 2016.

77. Shield J, Mullen MC. *The Complete Counseling Kit for Pediatric Weight Management.* Chicago, IL: Academy of Nutrition and Dietetics; 2016.

78. Schwartz RP. Motivational interviewing (patient-centered counseling) to address childhood obesity. *Pediatr Annals.* 2010;39(3):154–158.

79. Resnicow K, Davis R, Rollnick S. Motivational interviewing for pediatric obesity: conceptual issues and evidence review. *J Am Diet Assoc.* 2006;106:2024–2033.

80. Michalsky M, Reichard K, Inge T, Pratt K, Lenders, C. ASMBS pediatric committee practice guidelines. *Surg Obes Relat Dis.* 2012;8(1):1–7.

81. Weight Management Practice Group. *Pocket Guide to Bariatric Surgery.* Chicago, IL: Academy of Nutrition and Dietetics; 2016.

82. Inge TH, Courcoulas AP, Jenkins TH, et al. Weight loss and health status 3 years after bariatric surgery in adolescents. *N Engl J Med.* 2016:374(2);113–123.

83. National Association of Anorexia Nervosa and Associated Disorder. Eating Disorder Statistics. Available at: http://www.anad.org/get-information/about-eating-disorders/eating-disorders-statistics/. Accessed November 10, 2017.

84. Institute of Medicine. *Accelerating Progress in Obesity Prevention: Solving the Weight of the Nation.* Washington, DC: National Academies Press; 2012.

85. American Dietetic Association. Position of the American Dietetic Association: nutrition intervention in the treatment of eating disorders. *J Am Diet Assoc.* 2011;111(8):1236–1241.

86. Reiter CS, Graves L. Nutrition therapy for eating disorders. *Nutr Clin Pract.* 2010;25:122–136.

87. The Society of Adolescent Health and Medicine. Position paper of the society for adolescent health and medicine: medical management of restrictive eating disorders in adolescents and young adults. *J Adolesc Health* 2015; 56(1):121–125.

88. Westmoreland P, Krantz MJ, Mehler P. Medical complications of anorexia and bulimia. *Am J Med.* 2016:129(1); 30–37.

89. Academy for Eating Disorders' Medical Care Standards Committee. AED Report 2016, Eating Disorders: a Guide to Medical Care. 2016, 3rd ed. Available at http://www.massgeneral.org/psychiatry/assets/pdfs/EDCRP/eating-disorders-medical-guide-aed-report-2016.pdf. Accessed October 15, 2017.

90. American Psychiatric Association. *The Diagnostic and Statistical Manual of Mental Disorders.* 5th ed. Arlington, VA. American Psychiatric Association; 2013.

91. Williamson DA, Martin CK, Binge eating disorder: a review of the literature after publication of the DSM_IV. *Eating Weight Disord Stud Anorexia Bulimai Obes.* 1999;4(3):103–114.

92. Goldfein JA, Devlin JH, Spitzer RL. Cognitive behavioral therapy for the treatment of binge eating disorder: what constitutes success? *Int J Eating Disord.* 2000;157(7): 1051–1056.

93. Setnick J. *Academy of Nutrition and Dietetics Pocket Guide to Eating Disorders.* 2nd ed. Academy of Nutrition and Dietetics, Chicago, Il: 2017.

94. Academy of Nutrition and Dietetics. *eNCPT Nutrition Care Process Terminology.* Chicago, IL: Academy of Nutrition and Dieteics;2014. https://www.ncpro.org/nutrition-care-process.

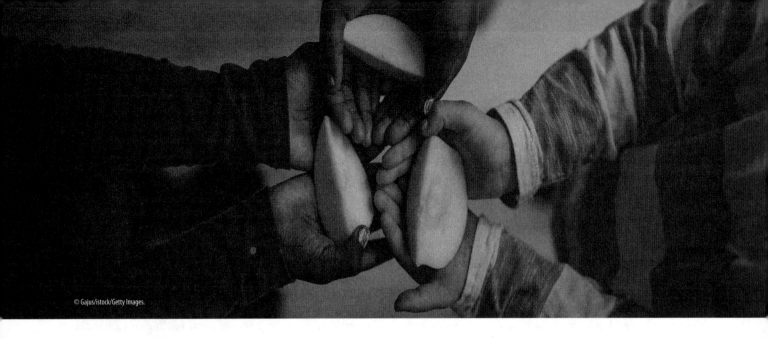

© Gajus/istock/Getty Images.

CHAPTER 22
Eating and Feeding Disorders

Rashelle Berry, Julie Cooper and Kerri Heckert

LEARNING OBJECTIVES

- Identify elements of clinical presentations of disordered eating and criteria for diagnosis
- Describe best practices for nutrition screening and assessing patients with established or suspected disordered eating
- Develop appropriate nutrition plan of care for patients with disordered eating diagnosis including understanding caloric needs and weight goals
- Explain the main principals of standard approaches to care of patients with disordered eating

▶ Introduction

Eating and feeding disorders as covered in this chapter are psychological disorders that have nutritional implications and can result in adverse physical signs and symptoms. Children and adolescents are especially vulnerable to these disorders as the consequences of disordered eating include growth and pubertal stunting, cardiovascular complications, abnormal lab values, and other physical and mental changes.[1] An estimated 1–3% of adolescents meet the criteria for diagnosis of eating or feeding disorder.[2–4] Health practitioners who care for children and teens should therefore be familiar with common characteristics and presentation of these conditions.

▶ Defining and Diagnosing Feeding and Eating Disorders

Psychological diagnoses are standardized by the American Psychiatric Association in the Diagnostic and Statistical Manual of Mental Disorders, commonly called the DSM. The fifth and most recent edition, DSM-5, was published in 2013.[5] While a variety of healthcare professionals contribute to assessing a patient with a suspected eating disorder, diagnosis and coding are made by qualified medical and mental health professionals. Registered Dietitians cannot diagnose eating disorders.[5,6]

Using the previous edition, DSM-IV, many individuals did not qualify for **anorexia nervosa** (AN) or **bulimia nervosa** (BN) diagnoses and by default were diagnosed with the heterogeneous residual category of **eating disorder not otherwise specified** (EDNOS).[7,8] Early identification, diagnosis, and intervention is associated with improved prognosis in eating disorders. Any nutritional disturbance or malnutrition during adolescence, a period of profound brain and physical development, prolongs the presence of medical complications and cognitive deficits associated with starvation.[9-11] While patients with EDNOS could experience the same degree of medical severity as patients with AN or BN, treatment options were limited without a more definitive diagnosis.[8,12,13] By expanding the diagnostic criteria for AN and BN, more patients are receiving the appropriate diagnosis and accompanying treatment, especially given the growing prevalence of eating disorders in males and young children.[14]

The publication of DSM-5 eliminated the section titled "Feeding and Eating Disorders of Infancy or Early Childhood" which included the diagnoses of pica, rumination disorder, and feeding disorder of infancy or early childhood. Feeding disorder of infancy or early childhood was renamed **avoidant/restrictive food intake disorder**, or ARFID. ARFID, along with pica and rumination disorder, were all moved to be included in the chapter "Feeding and Eating Disorders." These diagnoses are now in the same section as anorexia nervosa, bulimia nervosa, binge-eating disorder, other specific feeding

or eating disorder, and unspecified feeding or eating disorder.[5] **TABLE 22.1** provides an overview of the revisions to classification between the DSM-IV and DSM-5. Specific diagnostic criteria for individual feeding and eating disorders will be reviewed later in this chapter.

Per the DSM-5, "Feeding and eating disorders are characterized as persistent disturbance of eating or eating-related behavior that results in the altered consumption or absorption of food and that significantly impairs physical health or psychosocial functioning." All of the conditions listed in the DSM-5 with the exception of pica are written to be mutually exclusive. This means that at one point in time, a patient can only have one diagnosis. Pica, however, can occur concurrently with other feeding and eating disorders. Of note, while there cannot be simultaneous diagnoses of most feeding or eating disorders, it is not uncommon for patients to meet criteria for more than one disorder over the course of illness.[16,17]

From a nutrition perspective, feeding and eating disorders generally result in an imbalance of caloric intake compared with expenditure and/or inadequate intake of macro and/or micronutrients. This can lead to physical and cognitive disturbances in affected patients. Patients do not need to qualify for a DSM diagnosis in order to elicit concern about eating practices; however, nontraditional disordered eating patterns could potentially fall into the DSM diagnostic category of unspecified feeding or eating disorder.

TABLE 22.1 Overview of Revision in DSM

DSM-IV	DSM-5
Diagnostic category: "Feeding and Eating Disorders of Infancy or Early Childhood" <ul><li>Feeding disorder of Infancy or Early Childhood</li><li>Pica</li><li>Rumination Disorder</li></ul> Diagnostic category: "Eating Disorders" <ul><li>Anorexia nervosa</li><li>Restricting type</li><li>Binge-eating/purging type</li><li>Bulimia nervosa</li><li>Purging type</li><li>Non-purging type</li><li>Eating disorder not otherwise specified (EDNOS)</li></ul>	Diagnostic category: "Feeding and Eating Disorders" <ul><li>Anorexia nervosa*</li><li>Restricting type</li><li>Binge-eating/purging type</li><li>Avoidant/restrictive food intake disorder (ARFID)**</li><li>Binge-eating disorder**</li><li>Bulimia nervosa*</li><li>Other specified feeding or eating disorder (OSFED)*</li><li>Atypical anorexia nervosa</li><li>Bulimia nervosa (of low frequency and/or limited duration)</li><li>Binge-eating disorder (of low frequency and/or limited duration)</li><li>Purging disorder</li><li>Pica</li><li>Rumination disorder</li><li>Unspecified feeding or eating disorder**</li></ul>

*Revisions to prior diagnostic criteria introduced in DSM-5
**New diagnosis introduced in DSM-5
Data from Association AP. *Diagnostic and Statistical Manual of Mental Disorders.* 5th ed. Washington, DC: American Psychiatric Publishing; 2013.[5]
Association AP. *Diagnostic and Statistical Manual of Mental Disorders: DSM-IV.* 4th ed. Washington, DC: American Psychiatric Publishing; 1994.[15]

▶ Anatomy, Physiology, Pathology of Condition

Etiology and Risk Factors

The etiology of feeding and eating disorders is not yet clearly defined. These conditions are often multifactorial, and the history and presentation vary from patient to patient. There are, however, some common biological and environmental risk factors for developing disordered eating conditions.

Many of the biological risk factors outlined below highlight the importance of a thorough medical work-up in a child or adolescent presenting with disordered eating to identify the presence of concurrent organic causes of growth concerns or food aversion. On a similar note, practitioners should remain vigilant and screen as appropriate for disordered eating behaviors in patients with existing medical conditions.

Biological Factors

Family History and Genetics There is evidence for a component of heritability in disordered eating with data showing association between prior diagnoses in family members, and research is emerging on the potential for specific genetic links to etiology.[18–22]

Of interest to the pediatric and adolescent population, initial research has shown some support that stronger genetic effects are seen in pubertal versus prepubertal populations, indicating that transition to puberty could activate predisposing factors to development of an eating disorder. This is therefore, a key time to be vigilant for emerging disordered eating behaviors.[23]

Gastrointestinal and Autoimmune Conditions Conditions associated with gastrointestinal (GI) discomfort such as **gastroesophageal reflux** (GERD) or life-threatening reactions such as food allergies can create unpleasant associations with eating and delay acceptance of new foods and textures.[24,25] This can lead to developing maladaptive feeding behaviors in both children and in parents who adjust feeding practices in an effort to improve intake. Food refusal is significantly higher in children diagnosed with GERD compared with those who do not have the condition.[26] Anorexia nervosa has been found to be associated with the presence of food allergies in children.[25]

Within the class of autoimmune diseases, a significant risk association has been shown between **type 1 diabetes mellitus** (T1DM) and disordered eating.[27–30] Patients with disordered eating have been shown to have poorer glucose management.[27,31] An extremely concerning behavior would be the withholding of insulin to induce weight loss. Commonly called "diabulimia," this practice does not meet criteria for the DSM diagnosis for bulimia nervosa, nor is it a stand-alone diagnosis at this time. Theoretically, it could fall under a sub-diagnosis of purging disorder under the DSM category of other specified feeding or eating disorder. Purging disorder is defined as "recurrent purging behavior to influence weight or shape (e.g., self-induced vomiting, misuse of laxatives, diuretics, or other medications) in the absence of binge eating."[5] The incidence of insulin omission has been varied thus far in available literature, and remains an important topic for further research.[32]

Historically not a typical disease of childhood, **type 2 diabetes mellitus** (T2DM) is now more prevalent in pediatric and adolescent populations in the setting of increased obesity.[33] Of note, obesity has independently been associated with increased eating disorder risk.[34,35] Within a sample of adolescents with T2DM, 26% qualified for "clinical or subclinical" binge eating. This study took place before the diagnosis of binge-eating disorder was made official in DSM-5.[36] A different sample of youth ages 10 to 21 years old showed that patients with T2DM were more likely than those with T1DM to report using unhealthy weight-loss practices, and females exhibited a higher prevalence of unhealthy practices than males.[31]

Finally, functional GI disorders are a class of diagnosis that present as chronic or recurrent GI symptoms, but do not have an identified underlying pathophysiology. One example of a functional diagnosis is irritable bowel syndrome. A strong association between functional GI disorders and feeding and eating disorders has been seen. Though a cause and effect relationship has not been defined, the two categories of diagnoses often seem to perpetuate one another.[37]

Fetal and Early Development Some association has been suggested between elements of fetal development and psychiatric diagnoses in later life. In children with early-onset eating disorders, 21% had a history of feeding concerns or fussy eating during early development.[38] Feeding problems in both infancy and later childhood have been associated with significantly increased odds of later anorexia nervosa diagnosis.[39] Factors that have been associated with the development of bulimia nervosa or anorexia diagnosis included both low birth weight and high birth weight for gestational age, twin or triplet status, fetal dysmaturity, and prematurity.[40,41]

Psychological Risk Factors Youth diagnosed with disordered eating often have a reported family history of psychiatric conditions, most commonly anxiety and depression, but also **obsessive-compulsive disorder** (OCD), psychosis, substance abuse and neurodevelopmental disorders.[38,39] Behavioral health diagnoses in children or adolescents with or without family history, can also be associated with disordered eating or feeding. Such diagnoses can include those already mentioned such as anxiety, depression, and OCD, in addition to autism and attention-deficit/hyperactivity disorder.[42–48]

Environmental Factors

Body Dissatisfaction Body dissatisfaction, perceived pressure to be thin or weight concerns in early adolescence have been found to be related to later eating disorder diagnosis.[49,50] Of note, higher media usage and messaging activity is associated with increased body image dissatisfaction.[51,52] Encouragingly, high self-esteem is reported to be a protective factor against AN, and therefore should be an important area of focus for child and adolescent practitioners.[39]

Socioeconomic Factors Outdated stereotypes of eating disorders predominantly characterized these diagnoses as those of wealthy, Caucasian females. More recent research has indicated that eating disorders occur across the population spectrum.[53,54] Emphasis should therefore be made on creating the availability of quality care for eating difficulties across socioeconomic and demographic groups.

Trauma or Abuse History Developing disordered eating behaviors such as body and weight dissatisfaction, restricting, and purging have been linked to history of sexual abuse during early adolescence.[55] Also of note, patients with eating disorder diagnosis and history of emotional, physical, or sexual abuse are more likely to have increased severity of illness, earlier age of onset, and increased binge-purge behaviors compared with eating disorder patients with no abuse history.[56] Details of abuse history are most appropriately addressed by a behavioral health practitioner, though sensitivity to personal history is a valuable skill for all members of a treatment team.

▶ Physical Presentation: Signs & Symptoms

There are typical physiological signs and symptoms that result from disordered feeding or eating.

Cardiovascular Function

The cardiovascular system is likely the most acutely impacted by disordered eating. The most common cardiovascular changes seen with significant weight loss and malnutrition are bradycardia (low heart rate) and hypotension (low blood pressure). This is a result of loss of cardiac muscle mass leading to reduced cardiac output. These changes can further present as fatigue, exercise intolerance, potential arrhythmias, and even sudden death.[1,57] Decreased blood perfusion can result in cold extremities.[14] Defined parameters for bradycardia vary across pediatric care, but accepted guidelines suggest concern for patients 18 years and under who present with a waking heart rate of <50 beats per minute (BPM).[58]

Heart rate and blood pressure changes affect orthostatic vital signs, which are often used during the assessment of cardiovascular status in eating disorders. Both heart rate and blood pressure should be obtained in supine and upright positions. A significant rise in heart rate called orthostatic tachycardia (>20 BPM) or drop in blood pressure called orthostatic hypotension (>10 mm Hg) with upright postural changes can indicate cardiovascular compromise and increase risk of syncope.[14] Dizziness may or may not accompany positive orthostatic vital signs.

Electrolyte derangements can also be associated with cardiac risks, specifically arrhythmias. Increased losses through self-induced vomiting or laxative abuse can lead to electrolyte abnormalities such as low potassium (hypokalemia) or low magnesium (hypomagnesemia). An excessive intake of water, often called "water-loading" is sometimes seen in disordered eating, and can lead to irregular electrolyte results, specifically low serum sodium (hyponatremia).[59]

Endocrine Function

Several areas of endocrine function can be altered in the setting of disordered eating and especially in malnutrition associated with anorexia nervosa. Abnormal hormone levels can impact metabolic rate, appetite regulation, growth, and development.

One of the most commonly discussed endocrine alterations in eating disorders is that of the sex hormones in both females and males, since changes to this axis can have repercussions on pubertal development and bone health. In the setting of malnutrition, lower levels of estrogen in females and testosterone in males can slow progression through puberty or delay onset of puberty altogether. The most common manifestation of this hormonal change in females will be irregular or absent menses. If menses are missed for three months or more after the establishment of regular cycling, this is defined as amenorrhea. Low testosterone in adolescent males with anorexia nervosa has been associated with alterations in body composition and lean body mass.[60]

Thyroid hormone levels, which regulate the body's rate of metabolism, can also be altered in the setting of disordered eating. Abnormal levels of thyroid hormones are likely due to adaptation of the body to conserve energy and down-regulate metabolism in the setting of restricted caloric intake.[61] Levels will generally normalize with renourishment.[1]

Levels of growth hormone and related **insulin-like growth factor 1** (IGF-1) can be abnormal in the setting of malnutrition related to disordered eating. IGF-1 plays an important role in cartilage and bone development. One of the most significant results of abnormal endocrine function in eating disorders is the impact on bone health.

Bone Health

Bone density can be negatively impacted due to inadequate bone accrual from insufficient nutrition, as well as endocrine abnormalities from malnutrition.[62] As noted previously, impaired endocrine function often presents as amenorrhea. Bone density is highly reliant on estrogen levels associated with normal menses, therefore amenorrhea can be associated with low bone mineral density in adolescents.[63] Impaired bone health leads to a higher risk for fracture and stunted height.[62,64] Renourishment, resulting in weight gain, has been shown to normalize bone formation activity and turnover in adolescents, though the long term impact of insult to bone accrual during formative years is still unclear.[65] Bone mineral density can be evaluated using **dual energy X-ray** (DEXA) in female patients with three months of amenorrhea in the setting of six months of weight loss, or in males who have had low weight for six months or more.[1]

Gastrointestinal System

Changes in GI function and related symptoms are common in the setting of disordered eating and feeding. As previously discussed, patients often present with gastroesophageal reflux, GI-related autoimmune disorders and functional GI diagnoses. Common symptoms often include sensation of bloating or fullness, nausea, and constipation.

Very frequently, these complaints are related to the occurrence of gastroparesis, or delayed stomach emptying, and slowed GI motility that can occur with irregular or inadequate nutrition intake. Just as altered intake can result in gastroparesis, the discomfort with eating caused by slowed motility can subsequently hinder efforts to normalize eating patterns. A structured approach to increasing nutrition and symptom management with non-stimulant stool softeners can help address discomfort during the refeeding process.[14] Gastric motility and related symptoms can improve over time with renourishment and weight gain.[66]

In the setting of self-induced vomiting, symptoms of reflux can be exacerbated by the weakening of the gastroesophageal sphincter, which can increase contact of stomach acid with esophageal tissue.[67,68] Though rare, the risks of repeated vomiting can also include upper GI bleeding, and theoretically higher long-term risk of cellular changes of the esophagus.[14,69,70] Additional physical signs of vomiting behaviors can include knuckle abrasion from manually-induced purging (i.e. Russell's sign) and enlargement of parotid salivary glands. Purging via laxative abuse can result in diarrhea and fluid or electrolyte disturbance via increased GI losses. Effects of long-term stimulant laxative abuse, such as permanently impaired peristalsis and bowel evacuation, are more commonly seen in adults with eating disorders; however providers should be mindful of such future risks for younger patients.[68]

Laboratory Values

Previously discussed physical complications of eating and feeding disorders are closely associated with a variety of potential derangements of laboratory values. The most acute risk comes from electrolyte disturbances that can result from disordered eating behaviors such as purging, or from initial reintroduction of caloric intake leading to refeeding syndrome. Refeeding syndrome is discussed in more detail later in this chapter. Other common alterations in lab values with disordered eating-related causes are outlined in **TABLE 22.2**. Abnormal lab results can also occur in the setting of other disease states, and should be evaluated with this in mind.

TABLE 22.2 Common Potential Alterations in Laboratory Values Related to Eating and Feeding Disorders

Laboratory Value (only commonly altered values included)	Potential Cause(s) of Altered Value (Note: Table includes eating disorder-related causes. Lab alterations could also be due to unrelated medical conditions.)
Metabolic Panel: ■ ↓ Potassium (hypokalemia) ■ ↓ Sodium (hyponatremia) ■ ↑ Carbon Dioxide ■ ↓ Chloride ■ ↑ Urea Nitrogen (BUN) ■ ↑ Creatinine ■ ↓ Glucose ■ ↑ Liver enzymes	 ■ Vomiting, laxative abuse, diuretic abuse, refeeding syndrome ■ Consider disordered behavior such as water-loading, diuretic abuse, excessive losses from vomiting or diarrhea ■ Vomiting, diuretic abuse ■ Vomiting, diuretic abuse ■ Dehydration ■ Dehydration, muscle breakdown ■ Starvation ■ Malnutrition or during refeeding process

(continues)

TABLE 22.2 Common Potential Alterations in Laboratory Values Related to Eating and Feeding Disorders   (*continued*)

Laboratory Value (only commonly altered values included)	Potential Cause(s) of Altered Value (Note: Table includes eating disorder-related causes. Lab alterations could also be due to unrelated medical conditions.)
Additional Electrolytes (not included in Basic Metabolic Panel): ■ ↓ Phosphorus (hypophosphatemia) ■ ↓ Magnesium (hypomagnesemia)	 ■ Refeeding syndrome, starvation ■ Refeeding syndrome
Hematology: ■ ↓ or ↑ Hemoglobin ■ ↓ or ↑ Hematocrit ■ ↓ Mean Corpuscular Volume ■ ↓ White Blood Cell count	 ■ Anemia, fluid status ■ Anemia, fluid status ■ Anemia (consider iron deficiency) ■ Malnutrition
Endocrinology: ■ ↓ Thyroid function (T_3, T_4) ■ ↓ Gonadal hormones	 ■ Malnutrition ■ Malnutrition
Other: ■ ↑ Cholesterol ■ ↑ Amylase ■ ↓ Ferritin (low iron stores) ■ ↓ Vitamin D 25OH ■ ↑ Methylmalonic acid ■ ↓ Prealbumin ■ ↑ Hemoglobin A1c	 ■ Malnutrition ■ Chronic vomiting ■ Malnutrition ■ Malnutrition ■ Low vitamin B_{12} (vegans at higher risk) ■ Acute malnutrition ■ In patients with prior diagnosed diabetes, consider insulin withholding for weight loss

▶ Psychological and Cognitive Presentation

As previously discussed, psychiatric comorbidities are commonly associated with eating disorders. Presentation of an eating disorder can coincide with diagnoses of depression, anxiety, or obsessive-compulsive disorder.[14,71]

Social anxiety as well as impairments in social function and interaction have also been seen in adolescent and young adult female patients with anorexia nervosa.[72-74] Patients might also demonstrate cognitive rigidity or an inability to adapt to unexpected situations, which can pose challenges in the setting of eating disorder treatment.[75] Impulsivity can also be seen, and has been found to be more prevalent in bulimia nervosa versus anorexia nervosa.[76,77]

▶ Condition-Specific Nutrition Screening

Several tools exist for the initial screening of pediatric and adolescent populations for feeding and eating disorders. Compared to a full assessment, screening is meant to provide an initial level of insight into food-related thoughts and behaviors. If concern is raised after screening, a full assessment is warranted.

The most concise screening tool is the five-question SCOFF questionnaire. Developed by Morgan, et al, it evaluates basic markers of anorexia nervosa and bulimia nervosa. Two or more affirmative answers suggest an increased likelihood of having an eating disorder.[78] Details of the questionnaire can be found in **TABLE 22.3**. The SCOFF questionnaire has successfully been used in adolescent populations.[79]

A longer but commonly used screening tool used in behavioral health or research settings is the **Eating Disorder Examination Questionnaire** (EDE-Q). It is adapted from the original **Eating Disorder Examination** (EDE), which is a longer tool used in interview format for eating disorder evaluation.[80] The EDE-Q is a thirty-six item self-administered questionnaire that covers psychopathology of disordered eating behavior. It has shown consistency in results with the EDE in an adolescent population.[81]

Similar in length to the EDE-Q is the Eating Attitudes Test, or EAT-26, named as such because it consists of 26 self-administered questions.[82] The EAT-26 evaluates the frequency of disordered thoughts and behaviors

TABLE 22.3 Disordered Eating Screen

The SCOFF questions*
Do you make yourself **S**ick because you feel uncomfortably full?
Do you worry you have lost **C**ontrol over how much you eat?
Have you recently lost more than **15 pounds** in a 3-month period?**
Do you believe yourself to be **F**at when others say you are too thin?
Would you say that **F**ood dominates your life?

*One point for every "yes"; a score of ≥2 indicates a likely case of anorexia nervosa or bulimia nervosa
The original questionnaire was developed in the United Kingdom and questioned weight loss of **One stone over a 3-month period.
Reproduced from Morgan JF, Reid F, Lacey JH. The SCOFF questionnaire: assessment of a new screening tool for eating disorders. BMJ. 1999;319(7223):1467–1468.[78]

around eating and provides a score value from which the likelihood of disorder can be evaluated. While the EDE-Q and EAT-26 have shown somewhat more validity compared to SCOFF, the benefits of the short format of SCOFF should be considered in the often hectic pace of patient care.[83,84]

Finally, Bright Futures, published by the American Academy of Pediatrics, provides publicly-accessible questionnaires for use in pediatric and adolescent populations that can help identify potential factors of nutrition risk related to disordered weight and body image. These questionnaires cover a broader scope of subject matter than screening tools focused only on disordered eating, but they can be a simple tool for use in direct care settings.[85]

▶ Nutrition Assessment

If a child or adolescent appears to meet screening parameters as described previously, or if behavior related to eating or physical activity becomes atypical, a more detailed assessment is indicated. Concurrent with a nutrition assessment, if not already completed, a full medical evaluation for organic causes of these changes should be completed by a physician. A diagnosis of medical condition, however, does not necessarily rule out the possibility of an eating disorder.

A comprehensive nutrition assessment should include a standard nutrition evaluation, as well as focused questions related to disordered feeding behavior. This would include objective data from a medical record such as current anthropometrics (e.g. height, weight, body mass index [BMI]), growth curve history and trends, stage of puberty, family history, vital signs (e.g. pulse and blood pressure) and

laboratory values. Additional questions should elicit information about eating pattern and adequacy, activity level, and disordered eating behaviors (e.g. restricting, purging).

Typically, an initial indicator for concern is acute or gradual decline of height, weight, or BMI from usual trends as plotted on age- and gender- appropriate growth curves (Centers for Disease Control, 2 to 20 years). While very common, this will not always be seen in patients with feeding disorders. For example, patients with autism will often exhibit limited variety based on food type and texture, though they might consume adequate calories via accepted foods. In this case, macro- and micronutrient balance could be of more concern, but growth curves could appear normal.[86]

While weight loss can be a short-term indicator of inadequate nutrition, height stunting can appear in the setting of chronic malnutrition. Practitioners should be familiar with typical growth patterns before and during puberty in order to best assess trends. Pending stage of puberty, girls and boys have varying potential for additional height growth. A complete detail of pubertal development (e.g. Tanner Staging) is beyond the scope of this chapter; however, it is important to note that girls tend to grow no more than 2 to 3 inches after their first menses (menarche), while boys can grow taller for longer and until later in puberty. If a patient displays linear stunting in the setting of malnutrition and is within the pubertal window of growth, he or she could have the potential for catch-up growth with improved nourishment. This information can be crucial in both initial assessment and setting of goal weights for patients with disordered eating.

An accurate typical dietary recall of food and fluid intake is a critical part of a comprehensive nutrition assessment. Diet histories can be obtained via several methods including a 24-hour recall, 3-day food record, or verbal recall of a typical eating pattern guided by a nutrition professional. A pitfall to a 24-hour recall or 3-day food record is that these methods provide information for a 'snapshot' in time that might not be representative of recent eating patterns. In adolescents, both age and disordered eating patterns can be associated with inaccurate or untruthful data about typical intake and portion sizes.[87,88] Parental input can therefore often be of great help when assessing typical food intake.

In children with feeding disorders marked by significantly reduced acceptance of food adequacy and variety, proportion of nutrient intake from supportive enteral feeds, if applicable, is important data in a nutrition assessment. Also helpful can be an evaluation of over-reliance on specific textures or beverages such as milk and juice instead of other solid food.

A comprehensive overview of elements of an initial nutrition assessment for disordered eating is outlined in **TABLE 22.4**.

Criteria for inpatient medical stabilization can vary between practitioners, but suggested guidelines are available from the Society for Adolescent Health and Medicine. Though the decision for admission is most often made by a physician, eating disorder care is a heavily interdisciplinary practice. Allied health practitioners should be equally familiar with these guidelines.

TABLE 22.4 Elements of Initial Nutrition Assessment for Children or Adolescents with Disordered Eating	
General	▪ Age (including date of birth to help correctly plot on growth curves) ▪ Grade or level of schooling
Diet and Physical Activity	▪ Food allergies and/or intolerances ▪ Typical recent intake of food and beverage (via 24-hour diet recall, 3-day food record or other) ▪ Meals eaten inside vs. outside the home ▪ Vitamin/mineral/supplement intake ▪ Cultural or religious dietary needs ▪ Adherence to a diet (e.g. vegetarianism, veganism, calorie counting) ▪ Physical activity and competitive sports ▪ Intake of liquid nutrition supplements ▪ Enteral nutrition regimen (if applicable) ▪ Texture and variety acceptance
Anthropometrics	▪ Height (note any stunting) ▪ Weight ▪ BMI ▪ Growth curve history of the above ▪ Biological parents' heights to calculate mid-parental height
Medical History	▪ Disease(s) that might affect intake, growth or mobility ▪ Surgery or injury that could affect intake or mobility ▪ Psychological conditions ▪ Sexual Maturity Rating ▪ Menstrual history (girls) ▪ Age at menarche ▪ Regularity ▪ Biological mother's age at menarche
Pertinent Family History	▪ History of underweight, overweight or obesity ▪ History of nutrition-related disease states (e.g. cardiac, diabetes, eating disorder) ▪ Menstrual difficulties (women)
Nutrition-Focused Physical Findings	▪ Constipation ▪ Diarrhea ▪ Nausea ▪ Vomiting ▪ Dizziness or blurry vision upon standing ▪ Feeling cold more often (associated with underweight) ▪ Cold or blue appearance of extremities ▪ Fatigue or weakness ▪ Hair loss or thinning ▪ Abdominal pain ▪ Headache ▪ Temporal wasting ▪ Presence of lanugo ▪ Russell's sign (knuckle abrasion due to self-induced vomiting) ▪ Enlarged parotid glands (can be associated with repeated vomiting)

Laboratory Values and Vital Signs	▪ Cholesterol panel ▪ Iron studies ▪ Vitamin levels if suspicion for deficiency (e.g. vitamin D 25OH) ▪ Electrolytes (especially with report of diarrhea or suspicion of disordered eating) ▪ Blood pressure ▪ Biopsy results (e.g. celiac disease)
Social History (if appropriate)	▪ Members of household ▪ Food insecurity ▪ Extracurricular activities ▪ Alcohol intake

Data from M B. *Adolescent Nutrition. Nutrition Across the Life Stages* 1st ed. Burlington, MA: Jones & Bartlett Learning; 2018.[89]

Indications supporting hospitalization in an adolescent with an eating disorder[58]

- One or more of the following justify hospital admission:
- ≤ 75% median BMI for age and gender
- Dehydration
- Electrolyte abnormality
- EKG abnormality
- Physiologic instability/hypotension-bradycardia-hypothermia-ortostatic hypotension or heart rate
- Arrested growth/development
- Failed outpatient treatment
- Acute food refusal
- Acute comorbid psychiatric or medical condition that limits outpatient treatment

▶ Nutrition Diagnosis

Anorexia Nervosa

AN is characterized by restricted caloric intake, refusal to reach or maintain an appropriate weight, or persistent behavior that interferes with weight gain. Children and adolescents may not experience weight loss, but rather experience failure to maintain normal developmental trajectory, such as expected weight gain or linear growth.[5,14] Patients with AN typically display an intense fear of weight gain or becoming fat, which is exacerbated by further weight loss.[5,90] AN is accompanied by body image distortion, seeing the body as overweight when the body is a healthy weight or underweight as well as self-esteem that is linked tightly to the perception of body shape and weight. A patient may view themselves as globally "fat" or be unhappy with specific body parts. Patients are also often unable to recognize the presence or seriousness of their illness and the medical complications associated with starvation (anosognosia).[5,91] Many patients with AN engage in excessive exercise, both for weight control and mood regulation.[92,93] The semi-starvation associated with AN can result in significant and potentially lethal medical complications, including amenorrhea, hypotension, bradycardia, hypothermia, electrolyte derangements, and bone mineral loss. Malnutrition may also lead to depression, obsessive-compulsive features, social withdrawal, irritability, and insomnia.[94,95] Patients may have a high degree of preoccupation with food, rigid thinking, limited social spontaneity, and concern about eating in public.[5]

There are two sub-types of AN – restricting type and binge-eating/purge type. Restricting type AN describes weight loss through dieting, fasting, and/or exercise. Binge-eating/purge type involves recurrent episodes of binge eating or purging behavior, which presents with self-induced vomiting or abuse of laxatives, diuretics, or enemas.[5]

In the DSM-5, the amenorrhea requirement was removed, improving inclusion for females with irregular periods or taking birth control as well as males and premenarchal females. The explicit weight criteria was removed, allowing for diagnosis of malnourished patients either following a significant weight loss or failure to maintain normal growth trajectory during developmental years, regardless of their weight at presentation.[5,14] Many patients will not express fear of gaining weight when they are at a dangerously low weight, and resistance may only arise as weight gain occurs. Young patients, especially, may not be able to recognize, acknowledge, or express fear of weight gain.[96] The DSM-5 diagnostic language was modified with less of an emphasis on cognitive symptoms and self-report, allowing for a diagnosis based on persistent behaviors that interfere with weight gain rather than verbalized fear.[5,97]

PES Statement: Inadequate energy intake related to disordered eating as evidenced by x% weight loss in y months.

Bulimia Nervosa (BN)

BN is characterized by recurrent episodes of eating a significantly large amount of food (binging) in a relatively short time frame of less than 2 hours. During these eating episodes, individuals with BN feel a lack of self-control with regards to eating. The eating episode is then followed by compensatory behavior intended to prevent weight gain.[5] Compensatory behaviors include vomiting, inappropriate use of laxatives, diuretics, or enemas, excessive exercise, or fasting.[98]

Individuals with BN must have these behaviors of binging and then purging at least once a month for three months in order to be diagnosed. BN does not necessarily occur within the context of AN. Like individuals with AN, individuals with BN are preoccupied by self-evaluation of body shape and weight.[5] Individuals with BN may appear healthy due to a healthy weight or a slightly higher than healthy weight. There is often shame and secrecy associated with this condition. Providers need to be aware of clues such as electrolyte imbalances and behaviors that may indicate BN.[99]

In the DSM-5, the frequency of binge episodes was decreased from twice per week for three months to once per week for three months. The types of BN by compensatory behavior (purging vs. non-purging) was also removed in the DSM-5, primarily because treating both types is very similar if not the same. Lastly, the DSM-5 includes severity of disease based on frequency of compensatory behavior; mild: one to three episodes per week; moderate: four to seven episodes per week; severe: eight to thirteen episodes per week; and extreme: more than fourteen episodes per week.[5]

PES Statement: Disordered eating patterns related to weight regulation/preoccupation as evidenced by eating 4000 calories within 2 hours followed by self-induced vomiting.

Binge Eating Disorder

BED is characterized by consuming a significantly large amount of food compared with what someone would normally eat in similar situations in a discrete period of time (typically less than 2 hours) at least once per week for three months. Unlike BN, there are no compensatory behaviors following the binge episode. A sense of lack of control will accompany the excessive consumption and the person will be unable to stop eating. Patients with BED must experience at least three of the following features: eating more rapidly than normal; feeling uncomfortably full after eating; eating large amounts of food despite not feeling physically hungry; eating alone due to embarrassment by how much one is eating; or feeling disgusted, guilty, or depressed after eating. Binge eating typically occurs in secrecy as

patients are often ashamed of their behavior. Triggers for bingeing include interpersonal stressors, restrictive intake, boredom, and negative feelings about body shape, weight, or food.[5]

BED is associated with overweight and obesity, but is distinct when considering psychopathology, weight and shape concerns, and quality of life.[5,100–102] BED affects approximately 2.8% of Americans in their lifetime.[100] Comorbid mood conditions and anxiety disorders, as well as substance abuse (usually alcohol), are commonly associated with BED.[103] While BED appears to be at least as chronic as AN or BN, there is little cross-over from BED to other eating disorders and remission rates are higher for BED than AN or BN.[5,104,105]

PES Statement: Excessive energy intake related to binge eating disorder as evidenced by sense of lack of control over eating and feeling guilty after eating.

OSFED

Other specified feeding and eating disorders (OSFED) applies to clinical presentations that cause clinically significant distress, but do not meet full criteria for any of the other feeding and eating disorders. Atypical anorexia nervosa is appropriate for a patient who meets all the criteria for AN, except that despite significant weight loss, the patient's weight is within or above normal range. Low frequency or limited duration BN or BED is present when all the diagnostic criteria for BN or BED are met, except they happen less than once a week and/or for less than 3 months. Purging disorder involves recurrent purging e.g., self-induced vomiting, misuse of laxatives, diuretics, or other medications without the presence of binge eating. Night eating syndrome is diagnosed by the presence of recurrent episodes of night eating that causes significant distress and cannot be attributed to external influences, schedule change, societal norms, or another mental disorder such as BED or substance abuse.[5]

PES Statement: Disordered eating patterns related to weight regulation/preoccupation as evidenced by unable or unwilling to eat sufficient energy/protein to maintain a healthy body weight.

Female Athlete Triad

Prevalence of disordered eating among athletes varies from 1%–62% in female athletes and 1%–57% in male athletes.[106] Eating disorders are common in athletes, possibly because the traits that make them successful in sport, perfectionism, competitiveness, and concern for performance are also risk factors for developing eating disorders. Participation in sports that emphasize leanness, low body weight, body building, or body appearance also increase the risk of eating disorders. These included gymnastics, running, wrestling, dance, and modeling. There is also a possibility that individuals with pre-existing eating disorders gravitate towards sports that support their desire to achieve a specific physique.[6,107–109] Although sport-specific dietary and weight control practices are common, they may pose a threat to both performance and health.[109,110]

The Female Athlete Triad is not a clinical diagnosis in the DSM-5, but often exists in athletic young women whose energy intake is inadequate to support normal growth and development in addition to the high energy output. The term "Female Athlete Triad" was introduced in 1992 and the first position stand was released by the American College of Sports Medicine in 1997.[111,112] A revised position stand was published in 2007 and in 2014, a comprehensive consensus paper on the diagnosis, treatment and return to play was published by the Female Athlete Triad Coalition.[113,114]

The triad is a medical condition that involves the interrelationship among energy availability, menstrual function, and bone mineral density. With proper nutrition, these relationships support total health. Low energy availability which is defined as dietary energy intake minus exercise energy expenditure, with or without disordered eating, leads to menstrual dysfunction and low bone mineral density. The presence of symptoms exists along a spectrum of severity and female athletes may present with one or more of the three triad components. Without prevention and early intervention, energy deficiency, whether intentional or unintentional, may progress to the clinical end points of the triad – eating disorder, amenorrhea, and/or osteoporosis. Chronic low energy availability leads to health consequences that negatively impact the entire body, including effects on the musculoskeletal, cardiovascular, endocrine, gastrointestinal, and neuropsychiatric systems.[113,114] A useful tool for assessing children for risk of this disorder includes the Triad consensus panel screening questions. Positive responses to these questions suggests that a child athlete is at risk for this condition.

The Triad Consensus Panel Screening Questions: [113]

1. Have you ever missed a menstrual period?
2. How old were you when you had your first menstrual period?
3. When was your last menstrual period?
4. Are you taking any female hormone medication?
5. Do you worry about your weight?
6. Are you trying to gain or lose weight?
7. Has anyone told you to gain or lose weight?
8. Have you ever had a bone fracture or stress fracture?
9. Do you have low bone mineral density?
10. Have you ever had an eating disorder?

In 2014, the **International Olympic Committee** (IOC) introduced the term "**Relative Energy Deficit in Sport**" (RED-S) with hopes of being more inclusive and comprehensive. The IOC defined RED-S as impaired physiological function including, but not limited to, metabolic rate, menstrual function, bone health, immunity, protein synthesis, and cardiovascular health caused by relative energy deficiency.[115]

Avoidant/Restrictive Food Intake Disorder

Avoidant/restrictive food intake disorder, or ARFID, is defined as a disturbance to eating or feeding that leads to an inability to meet nutritional and/or energy needs. This disturbance then results in at least one of the following outcomes: significant weight loss and/or poor growth, nutritional deficiency, dependency on supplementation (either via enteral feeding or oral supplementation), and/or problems with psychosocial functioning. This condition is distinct from other eating disorders in that sufferers of this condition specifically do not fear weight gain nor do they experience a preoccupation with body shape. This condition and its associated symptoms can also not be explained by a lack of available food, dietary restriction, or a different medical, or mental condition.[5]

This diagnosis was previously referred to as "feeding disorder of infancy or early childhood" in the DSM-IV and was defined as occurring exclusively in children younger than the age of 6. (American Psychiatric Association, 2000)[130] The current definition for ARFID does not have any age limitations; however, it is most often diagnosed in children and adolescents.[116]

Patients with ARFID have a variety of eating characteristics, ranging from the complete refusal of food resulting in feeding tube dependence to a high degree of food selectivity resulting in significant nutritional deficiencies. The range of precipitants to this disorder are equally as broad, including generalized anxiety, history/fear of vomiting or choking, gastrointestinal symptoms, and food allergies.[117] Similar to other eating disorders, this condition requires management by a multidisciplinary team for effective treatment. **FIGURE 22.1** describes the diagnostic criteria for eating and feeding disorders.

PES Statement #1: Inadequate oral intake related to complete refusal of food as evidenced by dependence on enteral nutrition to meet caloric needs.

Anorexia Nervosa

- Restriction of energy intake relative to requirements leading to a significantly low body weight in the context of age, sex, developmental trajectory and physical health
- Intense fear of gaining weight or of becoming fat, or persistent behavior that interferes with weight gain, even though the individual is at a significantly low weight
- Disturbance in the way in which one's body weight or shape is experienced, undue influence of body weight or shape on self-evaluation, or persistent lack of recognition of the seriousness of the current low body weight

AN subtypes:

- Restricting type: No binge/purge behavior in the last 3 months. Weight loss accomplished primarily through dieting, fasting, and/or excessive exercise
- Binge-eating/purging type: Recurrent episodes of binge eating or purging behaviors in the last 3 months

Bulimia Nervosa

Recurrent episodes of binge eating, with an episode of binge eating being characterized by the following:

- Eating, in a discrete period (e.g. within a two-hour period), an amount of food that is larger than most people would eat during a similar period and under similar circumstances
- A sense of lack of control over eating during the episode
- Recurrent inappropriate compensatory behaviors to prevent weight gain, such as self-induced vomiting, fasting, excessive exercise or misuse of laxatives, diuretics, or other medications
- Binge eating and inappropriate compensatory behaviors that both occur, on average, at least once a week for three months
- Self-evaluation that is unduly influenced by body shape and weight

Binge-Eating Disorder

Recurrent episodes of binge eating, with an episode of binge eating being characterized by the following:

- Eating, in a discrete period (e.g. within a two-hour period), an amount of food that is larger than most people would eat during a similar period and under similar circumstances
- A sense of lack of control over eating during the episode

The binge-eating episodes are associated with three (or more) of the following:

- Eating much more rapidly than normal
- Eating until uncomfortably full
- Eating large amounts of food when not feeling physically hungry
- Eating alone because of being embarrassed by the amount of eating
- Feeling disgusted with oneself, depressed, or very guilty afterward
- Marked distress regarding binge eating
- Binge eating occurs, on average, at least once a week for three months
- Binge eating that is not associated with recurrent use of inappropriate compensatory behavior

Avoidant/Restrictive Food Intake Disorder

An eating or feeding disturbance (e.g., apparent lack of interest in eating or food, avoidance based on the sensory characteristics of food, concern about aversive consequences of eating) as manifested by persistent failure to meet appropriate nutrition and/or energy needs associated with one (or more) of the following:

- Significant weight loss (or failure to achieve expected weight gain or faltering growth in children)
- Significant nutritional deficiency
- Dependence on enteral feeding or oral nutritional supplements
- Marked interference with psychosocial functioning
- No evidence of a disturbance in the way in which one's body weight or shape is experienced
- An eating disturbance not attributable to a concurrent medical condition, mental disorder, food unavailability, or associated culturally sanctioned practice

Other Specified Feeding or Eating Disorder

OSFED signs and symptoms cause clinically significant distress or impairment in social, occupational, or other important areas of functioning but do not meet the full criteria for another specified disorder.

- Atypical Anorexia Nervosa: All of the criteria for AN are met, except that despite significant weight loss, the individual's weight is within or above the normal range.

FIGURE 22.1 Diagnostic Criteria for Eating and Feeding Disorders

- Bulimia Nervosa (of low frequency and/or limited duration): All of the criteria for BN are met, except that the binge eating and inappropriate compensatory behaviors occur, on average, less than once a week and/or for less than three months.
- Binge-eating disorder (of low frequency and/or limited duration): All of the criteria for BED are met, except that the binge eating occurs, on average, less than once a week and/or for less than three months.
- Purging disorder: Recurrent purging behavior to influence weight or shape (e.g., self-induced vomiting or misuse of laxatives, diuretics, or other medications) occur in the absence of binge eating.
- Night eating syndrome: Recurrent episodes of night eating, as manifested by eating after awakening from sleep or by excessive food consumption after the evening meal, with awareness and recall of the eating.

Modified from Association AP. *Diagnostic and Statistical Manual of Mental Disorders*. 5th ed. Washington, DC: American Psychiatric Publishing; 2013.[5]

FIGURE 22.1 (continued)

▶ Nutrition Intervention

Goals for nutrition intervention in the treatment of feeding and eating disorders are multifactorial: Normalize eating patterns, restore appropriate weight and hunger cues, and correct physical and psychological complications of malnutrition.[6,58,118,119] Registered dietitians are uniquely qualified to provide nutrition therapy across the full continuum of disordered eating and at various levels of care and should assist with medical monitoring, understand medications and pharmacological therapies, and utilize medical nutrition protocols in order to optimize nutrition and stabilize eating.[6,120] Nutrition intervention will vary based on diagnosis and severity of disease as determined by the patient's multidisciplinary team, including medical, behavioral, health, and nutrition professionals.[6,121,122] Given the resistance associated with the malnourished brain, forced treatment and refeeding should be considered a "life-saving rescue effort."[6,123,124]

The RD should assess dietary intake, determine energy needs, and address specific food questions, family preferences, food allergies, or intolerances. RDs may be responsible for developing meal plans, with or without patients, as well as calculating enteral or parenteral feeding requirements as necessary.[122] RDs are often consulted to recommend treatment goal weight ranges for patients, which should be based on historical growth curves, stage of pubertal development, menstrual history, hormone levels and growth potential.[6,125-127] The RD may provide nutrition therapy by assisting the patient in recognizing disordered eating behaviors then setting realistic nutrition-related goals including those related to food intake, supplement use, compensatory behaviors, physical activity, and the patient's relationship with his/her body.[6,128] Nutrition education is not recommended in isolation when treating eating disorders. Patients who are extremely malnourished may lack the cognition necessary to comprehend information discussed during nutrition education, so teaching may need to be provided to caregivers.[122]

Determining energy needs for patients with eating disorders presents a challenge. For patients with eating disorders, attempts to correlate energy requirements using equations typically used for determining energy expenditure in hospitalized patients and general populations have been unsuccessful.[64-66] Indirect calorimetry is the most accurate method for determining energy requirements in patients with AN and BN.[64,67,68]

However, most clinicians do not use indirect calorimetry. The cost, availability, and portability of state-of-the-art equipment limit its use in many settings. Lower cost, handheld, indirect calorimeters offer an affordable option, but research in a healthy population is very limited,[69] and these units have not been studied in an eating-disorder population.

Indirect calorimetry is the Gold Standard for determining energy needs. It is the most accurate method for determining individual energy requirements, and should be utilized when available. Its use among RDNs who work with children with eating disorders is often limited due to availability.[6] Therefore, predictive equations like the FAO/WHO and Schofield equations are widely used to estimate energy needs.[129]

Micronutrients

Children with feeding and eating disorders, especially restrictive disorders, are often deficient in micronutrients.[6,130,131] It is common to supplement patients with a complete multivitamin/mineral supplement during treatment and to check serum levels of thiamine, methylmalonic acid (a more sensitive and specific marker for assessing B_{12} deficiency), zinc, 25-OH vitamin D, calcium, and folic acid and supplement in the case of deficiency.[6,132] Consensus amongst researchers is that a target level of vitamin D is 35–40 ng/mL, and levels below that should be supplemented for deficiency or insufficiency.[133] Elevated ferritin may serve as an indicator of starvation in children with AN, though iron-deficiency, with or without anemia, may also be present and patients should be supplemented accordingly.[134] Prophylactic zinc supplementation in children with AN may decrease the levels of anxiety and depression and enhance recovery by increasing weight gain and BMI, though there is no clinical consensus on dosage.[135-137] Prophylactic thiamine supplementation may be helpful in preventing deficiency associated with the initiation of refeeding, but if levels are drawn to assess for deficiency, whole blood rather than serum levels should be drawn.[138,139] Micronutrient deficiencies are increasingly being seen in patients with ARFID, specifically patients with a high degree of food selectivity. Scurvy, rickets, and hypovitaminosis A have been diagnosed due to complete refusal of fruits, vegetables, and dairy products.[140–142]

Anorexia Nervosa

The primary goal of nutrition intervention in AN is weight restoration. While loss of lean body mass during starvation causes hypometabolism, a slowing of the resting metabolic rate, the refeeding process drastically accelerates metabolic rate causing hypermetabolism, which elevates caloric requirements for both weight restoration and weight maintenance.[6,129] The hypermetabolic effect is related to a delay in normalization of endocrine and metabolic systems, energy required for digestion and absorption of nutrients as well as psychological challenges of anxiety, depression, and fear of weight gain.[6,143] Studies have shown that some patients require REE multiplied by an activity factor range of 2.5–3.5, or 70 to 100 kcal/kg or more to promote weight gain.[6,144] Patients with restricting-type AN need more calories than patients with binge-purge type AN to gain the same amount of weight.[145] Patients who engage in excessive exercise have increased caloric requirements.[145,146]

A high calorie diet that incorporates a wide variety of calorie dense foods is recommended, including foods that have recently been eliminated.[122,147,148] Underfeeding malnourished patients can slow treatment progress, prolong downregulation of metabolic rate, limit growth, impair endocrine function, and limit ability to engage in psychotherapy.[6] Several programs utilize meal-based approaches to refeeding – the caloric prescription is divided among meals and snacks, a liquid nutrition supplement is taken orally for unconsumed calories, and nasogastric feeds are only used for acute food refusal. Other programs begin with a combination of supplemental nasogastric feeding and oral intake immediately upon admission. Parenteral nutrition is uncommon in patients with AN, since there have been several reported complications including transaminitis, lower extremity edema, and hypophosphatemia.[149]

Refeeding Syndrome

Malnourished patients whose bodies have down-regulated in response to undereating are at risk for refeeding syndrome, a potentially lethal derangement of electrolytes that can lead to cardiac arrhythmia, muscle weakness, immune dysfunction, or sudden death, especially during the first week of refeeding.[11,150,151] Patients at risk for refeeding syndrome may require hospitalization for medical monitoring and stabilization.[122] Body stores of phosphorus are often depleted during starvation, and as carbohydrate intake increases with refeeding, the demand for phosphorus increases in order to meet the demands of glycolysis and for the production of **adenosine triphosphate** (ATP). This shift of phosphate from intracellular to extracellular spaces causes hypophosphatemia, the hallmark of refeeding syndrome. Patients may also experience hypokalemia, hypomagnesemia, hypocalcemia, thiamine deficiency, and fluid retention.[6]

A conservative "start low, go slow" approach has been recommended for initiating and advancing calories in malnourished patients in order to prevent refeeding syndrome; however, recent studies have found that refeeding hypophosphatemia is associated with a degree of malnutrition rather than initial calorie level or rate of caloric advancement.[144,149,152] Current guidelines are also based on adults and are not specific for patients with AN.[153–155] There is concern that hypocaloric diets with slow advancement may be insufficient to meet the needs of hypermetabolic, malnourished patients, and "underfeeding syndrome" has been associated with further weight loss, lengthier hospitalization, and lower discharge weights.[11,149]

Since one of the best predictors of remission from AN is a high discharge weight, optimizing rate of weight gain during hospitalization is ideal.[153,155–157] There is a growing interest in higher calorie refeeding in clinical practice and research. **TABLE 22.5** provides nutrition recommendations to prevent complications of refeeding syndrome.

TABLE 22.5 Nutrition Recommendations to Prevent Refeeding Syndrome

	Caloric Initiation	Caloric Advancement
Academy of Nutrition and Dietetics[120]	1000–1200 calories per day	200 calories every other day
American Psychiatric Association[130]	1000–1600 calories per day	"advance progressively" to as high as 70–100 kcal/kg/day
National Institute for Health and Care Excellence[160]	5–10 calories/kg/day	Increase levels slowly with a goal of meeting or exceeding full needs by 4–7 days

While there is no clinical consensus in treatment recommendation at this time, more aggressive nutrition intervention is recommended for mildly to moderately malnourished patients hospitalized with AN as long as there is close monitoring of cardiac status and electrolyte levels.[11,58] Lower initial caloric prescription may be beneficial for severely malnourished patients (i.e. <70% ideal body weight/average weight).[158,159]

Psychological Treatment

Family-based treatment (FBT), or the Maudsley approach, is the gold standard and most evidence-based treatment for medically stable adolescents who have been ill for less than three years.[121,161–163] FBT supports the caregiver(s) in their effort to refeed their child at home, providing a successful alternative to costly inpatient or residential options and limiting disruption of the adolescents' lives.[162,164]

FBT typically involves 15 to 20 therapeutic treatment sessions over 9 to 12 months and progresses through three phases.[165] Phase I focuses on early and complete weight restoration, viewing it as the cornerstone of this treatment method with the rationale that psychological recovery is achieved through weight gain.[161] Phase II slowly transitions age-appropriate control back to the adolescent, and Phase III addresses any remaining psychological issues that might interfere with achieving or maintaining recovery.[121,165] Discussing co-occurring psychological symptoms specifically occurs in later stages of FBT after weight restoration has been completed and the brain is better nourished.[161] Approximately two thirds of adolescents with AN reach recovery upon completion of FBT, and 75–90% are fully weight restored at 5-year follow up.[166] Rates of hospitalization and relapse are both lower in FBT compared with individual therapy.[121,162,167]

Adolescent-focused therapy (AFT) is an individualized psychotherapy approach in which adolescents with AN are viewed as using food and weight to avoid distressing environmental situations, thus arresting psychological development. Therapy guides the adolescent towards using more constructive coping strategies in order to improve self-efficacy and identify, define, and tolerate emotions.[121,167]Although FBT has better outcomes than AFT, AFT is a valuable alternative when FBT is not an option.[167]

Medication

Psychotropic medications are widely prescribed in the treatment of AN with the aim of reducing anxiety, obsessional thinking, and enhancing weight gain; however, there is insufficient evidence to support this practice.[121]

Bulimia Nervosa

Nutrition therapy for BN involves stabilization of weight, normalization of eating patterns, and cessation of disordered behaviors (i.e., bingeing, purging, restricting).[6] Despite compensatory behaviors, patients with BN are often at a normal weight or overweight and their condition may go undetected by family members or medical providers.[98] They may have normal or slower metabolic rates, so their caloric needs may be less than normal adolescent needs and should be determined based on their diet history and clinical judgment.[6,121,168] Bingeing followed by purging or periods of restriction have been proposed as causative factors in the hypometabolic state seen in BN.[168–170] The majority of patients with BN can be treated outpatient; however, hospitalization may be warranted for electrolyte instabilities from vomiting or laxative abuse, dehydration, bradycardia, orthostatic hypotension, cardiac arrhythmias, and seizures.[98] The recovery rate for BN is around 40% after six to twelve months of treatment with a remission rate of about 50% at 5 years.[121]

Psychological Treatment

The evidence base for treating BN in adolescence is limited. FBT is an effective treatment modality for adolescents with BN, with similar effectiveness to **cognitive behavioral therapy** (CBT).[121,163,171–173] CBT-A (adapted for adolescents) focuses on the relationship between thoughts, feelings, and behaviors and has been adapted for adolescents based on its successful use in adults.[172] CBT-guided self-care and enhanced cognitive behavioral therapy for eating disorders (CBT-E) have also shown good outcomes for treating BN.[121,171,174] **Dialectical behavioral therapy** (DBT) uses emotional regulation to reduce eating disordered behaviors in BN by teaching patients to recognize emotional triggers and develop appropriate coping strategies.[175]

Medication

CBT is considered to be more effective as the first line approach to treatment. There is research to support using fluoxetine in adults, but limited studies to support its usage in adolescents.[176,177]

Binge Eating Disorder

Most patients with BED are treated outpatient, and CBT-E is effective for adolescents who are not underweight.[174] **Interpersonal psychotherapy** (IPT), a type of psychotherapy that focuses on how unsatisfactory interpersonal interactions affect psychological distress, reduces loss-of-control eating, objective binge eating, anxiety, depression, and BMI.[178] Most patients with BED will not develop another ED and rates of improvement and remission are better for BED than BN, though chronicity is similar to BN. No medications have been studied in adolescents with BED.[121]

Avoidant/Restrictive Food Intake Disorder

To date, there is no evidence-based treatment approach for ARFID and intervention is generally individualized based on the type of feeding difficulty (e.g. choking phobia, nasogastric tube dependence, pain associated with food allergy).[121]

In addition to the multidisciplinary team, an occupational therapist skilled in chewing and swallowing or a medical subspecialist with expertise in symptom-related food avoidance may be indicated.[179,180] Severity of disorder will determine level of care, which ranges from outpatient to day program to inpatient hospitalization.[180] Malnourished children may require hospitalization, and children with ARFID have higher rates of remission at follow up and often require longer hospitalizations due to an increased need for nutritional support.[181]

For anxiety or fear-based food avoidance ARFID subtypes, CBT is appropriate. A more behavioral approach is ideal for sensory selectivity or lack of interest in eating. The tenants of FBT have been extended to ARFID treatment with a focus on psychoeducation, parental empowerment, and uniting the family to focus on eating. Systematic desensitization, exposure therapy, relaxation training, behavioral incentives, and scheduled eating are all suggested management tools. Caregivers may be coached on various techniques to create more positive mealtime interactions. Liquid supplements or tube feeds may be required to prevent further weight loss while progressing food acceptance.[121,180]

Though there is no evidence-based pharmacological recommendation for ARFID, atypical antipsychotics, anxiolytics, and selective serotonin reuptake inhibitors have been used to address anxiety.[121,179,180] Cyproheptadine, an antihistamine with an appetite stimulant side effect, may be considered for children with low appetite and poor growth for whom psychological and nutritional interventions have been ineffective.[182]

▶ Nutrition Monitoring and Evaluation

The primary goals of nutrition monitoring and evaluation in feeding and eating disorders are to monitor vital signs, monitor anthropometrics, monitor laboratory values, and adjust energy requirements as needed based on weight gain and activity level.[122] Within this framework, the unique aspects of monitoring and evaluation in each disorder are discussed in the next sections.

Anorexia Nervosa

The main nutrition goal for treating AN is that the patient consumes an adequate amount of calories to restore weight and correct malnutrition.[183] For hospitalized patients, higher calorie diets are associated with a reduced length of stay.[157] Exact energy needs are unique to each individual patient, but patients should receive "as much energy as they require to reverse their malnourished state."[122,184] Some patients might throw away, hide, or purge foods, so supervision during eating occasions and immediately following is recommended.[122] Caloric needs should be adjusted as necessary for patients with AN to ensure continued progress towards treatment goals.

Weight should be monitored and tracked by the dietitian so that adjustments to the meal plan can be made accordingly. The recommended rate of weight gain has historically been 2–3 pounds per week for hospitalized patients and 0.5–1 pound per week in outpatient treatment.[123,130,160] However, weight gain, particularly early in treatment, is predictive of greater reduction in eating disorder psychopathology.[161,185] Recent studies have had success with rates of weight gain of up to 4.4 pounds per week inpatient and up to 10 pounds per week outpatient.[144,185,186]

Vital signs, specifically orthostatic tachycardia, orthostatic hypotension, bradycardia, hypotension, and hypothermia will be monitored routinely by the medical team.[122] Studies have shown that vital signs normalize as weight increases.[187] Exercise and physical activity should be limited in the presence of bradycardia and hypotension.[188]

Laboratory values, specifically those used to monitor for refeeding syndrome (potassium, magnesium, phosphorus, sodium), should be monitored regularly for patients hospitalized with AN.[183]

Bulimia Nervosa

As stated previously, the primary goals for nutrition therapy in BN include weight stabilization, establishing a normal eating pattern, and cessation of disordered eating behaviors.[6] The dietitian will need to monitor the structured meal plan in order to reduce the risk of bingeing patterns as a response to normal hunger cues. This structured meal plan is designed to normalize weight and to help quell the patient's anxiety over gaining weight in the absence of compensatory behaviors.[98] Energy needs might need to be reassessed and reset due to the potential for slower metabolic rates.[121]

Electrolyte levels should continue to be monitored in patients with BN. Some patients with BN appear to be at a higher risk of hypokalemia and might need blood tests as frequently as two to three times per week.[98]

Dietitians, as a part of the treatment team, should continue to monitor patients for the use of compensatory behaviors as these affect the patients' overall health and nutrition.

Binge Eating Disorder

As stated previously, there is a lack of research on BED, seen in both the psychology and nutrition literature. While the relationship between obesity and BED remains unclear, it is reasonable to assume that many patients with BED will present as overweight or obese.[55] For children and adolescents presenting with the concurrent diagnoses of BED and overweight/obesity, the dietitian may need to work with mental health practitioners to set reasonable weight loss or weight management goals as appropriate in the context of therapy. Weight management has been found to be critical during adolescence.[189] Patients with BED have been found in numerous studies to consume a greater number of calories than patients without BED.[100] Nutrition monitoring of the patient with BED might include continued evaluation of caloric consumption within the context of behavioral therapy.

Avoidant/Restrictive Food Intake Disorder

Currently there are no evidenced-based guidelines for the nutrition monitoring of children diagnosed with ARFID.[116,190] The dietitian working with the child with ARFID should monitor nutrition based on the presenting nutrition diagnosis. As part of the multidisciplinary team treating the child, the dietitian should be in frequent contact with the other clinicians to make updates to the nutrition plan as progress is made. If the patient is dependent on enteral nutrition due to a refusal to eat or inadequate oral intake, the dietitian should monitor tube feedings as oral intake increases with therapy. This will include decreasing tube feedings as oral intake increases. Nutrition monitoring will also include evaluating formula tolerance, reviewing and modifying tube feeding schedules (bolus versus continuous), and monitoring energy balance.[122] For children diagnosed with ARFID due to extreme food selectivity, nutrition monitoring will include monitoring for inadequate intake of macronutrients and micronutrients, as well as ensuring that supplementation is being used in cases of deficiency. Weight and BMI should be monitored as well, as is the case for nutrition monitoring for all children.[191]

▶ Special Considerations

Mortality and Comorbidities

Mortality risk is increased in all eating disorder diagnoses, with the highest rates seen in patients with AN.[192] Causes of death can include medical outcomes such as cardiac complications or psychological outcomes such as suicide. Eating disorder diagnoses, specifically anorexia nervosa and bulimia nervosa, place patients at increased risk of suicidal ideation and attempts compared with the general population.[193-195] Estimates place the rates of suicide as high as 20% of deaths from AN and 23% of deaths related to BN.[101,196] Adolescents with eating disorders are also more likely to engage in self-harm without the intent of committing suicide as well as substance abuse.[197-199]

While assessing suicidality and substance abuse does not fall under the typical practice of nutrition professionals, these risk factors highlight the importance of working with an interdisciplinary team in treating eating disorders that includes behavioral health and medical colleagues.

Gender and Sexuality

The separate issues of gender identification and sexuality are both associated with an increased risk of disordered eating behaviors. In a transgender college student population, greater odds were found for an eating disorder diagnosis or a self-report of compensatory behaviors such as vomiting, diet pill use, or laxative abuse.[200] A higher prevalence of eating disorder diagnosis has also been estimated in homosexual and bisexual adolescents and young adults.[201,202] Practitioners should have a low threshold for screening for disordered eating in these high-risk populations.

▶ Conclusion

Eating and feeding disorders are complex biopsychosocial diseases with significant medical complications and high mortality rates. Despite their high prevalence, they are often underdiagnosed and untreated. Though the exact etiology is unknown, genetic predisposition, psychological traits, and environmental and sociocultural influences are all contributing factors. Malnourished patients have improved prognosis when treatment prioritizes weight restoration which then allows for cognitive improvement. Since childhood and adolescence are critical periods for growth and development, and also a prime window for onset of eating disorders, early identification and intervention is essential.

The 5th edition of the Diagnostic and Statistical Manual of Mental Disorders (DSM-5) was updated in 2013 to better represent the symptoms and behaviors of patients dealing with eating and feeding disorders. Some of the updates in the DSM-5 include revised diagnostic criteria for Anorexia Nervosa and Bulimia Nervosa, renaming EDNOS as OSFED and introducing the terms ARFID and BED. More inclusive criteria enable appropriate diagnoses and treatment resulting in improved prognosis.

Nutrition intervention will vary based on the diagnosis and severity of disease as determined by the patient's multidisciplinary team, which includes medical, behavioral health, and nutrition professionals. Registered Dietitians may be responsible for nutrition assessment, nutrition intervention recommendations, goal weight calculations, and nutrition therapy and/or education.

🔍 CASE STUDIES

Case Study #1

History

Madison is a 16 year-old female with a history of anxiety and OCD, admitted to the hospital in the setting of restrictive eating and excessive exercise. She is a high-achieving student, and she and her family are very athletic. Currently, Madison dances three days per week and plays on the varsity soccer team. She was sent to the emergency department by her pediatrician after a well-check visit where she was found to have a bradycardic heart rate of 42 bpm and 11 kg weight loss in six months.

Madison reports she started trying to "eat healthy" a few months ago in an effort to improve her running speed. She became a vegetarian and cut out soda, butter, dessert, and fast food from her diet. Her parents reported that her portion sizes have become increasingly smaller, she eats slowly and picks apart her foods. Madison will argue with her parents about what they serve her, so she has started making her own meals. She endorses minimal appetite and early satiety. She also hasn't had a bowel movement in about a week and has skipped her menses for the past four months. Recently, she has felt like her dance and soccer practices have not been sufficient to keep her body "toned" so she has added a daily exercise routine in her bedroom before going to sleep.

Typical Daily Diet Recall

Breakfast: 8 oz hot green tea with zero calorie sweetener, banana sprinkled with cinnamon
Lunch: 6 oz plain Greek non-fat yogurt, ½ apple
Dinner: ½ cup whole wheat pasta, 1 cup broccoli
Evening: 8 oz hot green tea with zero calorie sweetener

Anthropometrics

Weight: 44 kg
Height: 165 cm
Usual body weight (six months ago): 55 kg

Nutrition-focused Physical Findings

Dizziness with standing up, difficulty concentrating, feeling cold all of the time, constipation, temporal wasting, lanugo

Pertinent Lab Values

- BMP within normal limits
- Thyroid function below normal range
- Hormone levels below normal range
- Cholesterol above desired range
- Ferritin within normal range
- Celiac panel negative
- Vitamin D 25OH below desired range

Estimated Needs

Calories: REE (WHO equation) 1283 kcals/day x 2–3 (activity factor for 2+ pounds of gain/week) = 2566–3849 kcals/day
Protein: 1+ g/kg
Fluid: 1980 mL/day (maintenance needs)

Assessment

Weight loss percent from usual trend: 20%
Calorie intake (estimate): 360 kcals/day (14% low end of estimated kcals for weight gain)
Protein intake (estimate): 22 g (0.5 g/kg) (≤50% estimated needs)
Fluid intake (estimate): 480 mL/day (24% estimated maintenance needs)

Nutrition Diagnosis/PES Statement

Inadequate energy intake related to disordered eating as evidenced by 20% weight loss from usual trend and diet recall

Nutrition Intervention

- Gradual increase toward estimated goal calories for consistent weight gain toward usual trend
- Structured and supervised meal plan (3 meals, 2–3 snacks/day) with support from Behavioral Health expert as needed
- Wide food variety; calorically-dense options can help reduce volume. Include typical foods from before eating disorder (e.g. meat).
- Encourage fluid intake to meet maintenance needs (~2L/day)
- Age-appropriate multivitamin with minerals; consider vitamin D supplementation
- Limit activity

Monitoring and Evaluation

Immediate:

- Monitor refeeding labs regularly and replete electrolytes if needed
- Daily weight monitoring (Consider "blind weights" for patient)
- Fluid status

Over weeks to months:

- Return to usual growth trends followed by age-appropriate growth and gain
- Eventual return of menses
- Evaluate severity of eating disordered cognitions
- Follow up thyroid studies, hormone studies, vitamin labs as patient is renourished

Nutrition Education

As appropriate, provide guidance for caregivers and/or patient on meal plan structure and nutritional adequacy. Consider if inappropriate to counsel patient directly at this time given severity of illness.

Questions for the Reader

1. What interdisciplinary professionals should be on the treatment team for this patient?
2. Madison is upset that she has been told she cannot exercise at this time; she says she is able to run for miles and feels great. Why is it important that she rests her body?
3. Madison is upset about not being able to choose own meals. She cries and complains that it is too much food and says this is making her more depressed. What might you say to her and her family?

Case Study #2

History

Sam is an 11-year-old male with a history of autism spectrum disorder (ASD). He is nonverbal. Sam presented to the emergency department (ED) refusing to walk due to left leg pain. Symptoms began 2 weeks before the ED visit. X-rays revealed no broken bones in the lower extremities. He was subsequently admitted to the hospital.

Nutrition was consulted after MRI findings revealed the potential for scurvy. Caregivers reported a restrictive diet history in which Sam would only eat Goldfish crackers, Pop tarts, pepperoni, bread, water, and soda. He occasionally drank apple juice. Sam refused all multivitamins. When caregivers tried to put liquid vitamins into Sam's drink he began refusing all beverages that were unsealed.

Anthropometrics

Weight: 34 kg
Height: 136.5 cm
BMI: 18.76

Nutrition-focused Physical Findings

Dizziness with standing up, difficulty concentrating, feeling cold all of the time, constipation, temporal wasting, lanugo

(continues)

🔍 *CASE STUDIES* (continued)

Pertinent Lab Values

	Ref. Range	Results
IRON	Latest Range: 30–150 ug/dL	84
IRON BINDING (TOTAL)	Latest Range: 250–450 ug/dL	288
IRON % SATURATION	Latest Units: %	29
VITAMIN B$_{12}$	Latest Range: 180–914 ng/L	265
FOLATE SERUM	Latest Range: >=4.0 mcg/L	10.8
VITAMIN C, PLASMA	Latest Range: 23–114 umol/L	<5 (L)
25-HYDROXYVITAMIN D TOTAL	Latest Units: ng/mL	<13.0
ZINC	Latest Range: 0.60–1.20 mcg/mL	0.60
COPPER	Latest Range: 0.80–1.80 mcg/mL	2.10 (H)

Estimated Needs

Calories: 1700 kcal/day (49 kcal/kg)
Protein: 0.8–1g/kg
Fluid: 1798 mL/day (maintenance needs)

Assessment

This child has a severe nutritional deficiency resulting from ARFID. In the process of diagnosing Sam with scurvy he was admitted to the hospital and had an X-ray and MRI. The dietary recall ultimately yielded the most information towards positively identifying his diagnosis. When assessing a child with ASD, it is important to consider the potential for ARFID.

Weight: 60th percentile, z-score = 0.25
Height: 29th percentile, z-score = 0.56
BMI: 78th percentile, z-score = 0.76

Nutrition Diagnosis/PES Statement

Inadequate vitamin C intake related to complete refusal of fruits, vegetables, and multivitamin supplements as evidenced by diet recall analysis.

Nutrition Intervention

The patient was provided with samples of a variety of nutritional supplement drinks. He found one to be acceptable. Caregivers were educated to provide 2 bottles per day to Sam. A referral was made to a local feeding program that specializes in the treatment of ARFID in children with ASD.

Monitoring and Evaluation

Sam's dietary intake and vitamin levels were monitored post discharge. Ultimately, treatment included an intensive behavioral feeding program to address underlying refusal behaviors secondary to ARFID and expand Sam's diet to include all food groups.

Questions for the Reader

1. What would Sam's short-term nutrition goals be?
2. What would his long-term nutrition goals be? Should his long-term plan include continued oral nutrition supplementation?
3. How could hospital policy be changed to identify nutrient deficiency syndromes such as scurvy more quickly? How could this have been identified in the pediatrician's office?

References

1. Mehler PS AA. *Eating Disorders: A Guide to Medical Care and Complications.* 2nd ed. Baltimore, MD: The Johns Hopkins University Press; 2010.

2. Hammerle F, Huss M, Ernst V, Burger A. Thinking dimensional: prevalence of DSM-5 early adolescent full syndrome, partial and subthreshold eating disorders in a cross-sectional survey in German schools. *BMJ Open.* 2016;6(5):e010843.

3. Smink FR, van Hoeken D, Oldehinkel AJ, Hoek HW. Prevalence and severity of DSM-5 eating disorders in a community cohort of adolescents. *Int J Eat Disord.* 2014;47(6):610–619.

4. Stice E, Marti CN, Rohde P. Prevalence, incidence, impairment, and course of the proposed DSM-5 eating disorder diagnoses in an 8-year prospective community study of young women. *J Abnorm Psychol.* 2013;122(2):445–457.

5. Association AP. *Diagnostic and Statistical Manual of Mental Disorders.* 5th ed. Washington, DC: American Psychiatric Publishing; 2013.

6. Reiter CS, Graves L. Nutrition therapy for eating disorders. *Nutr Clin Pract.* 2010;25(2):122–136.

7. Call C, Walsh BT, Attia E. From DSM-IV to DSM-5: changes to eating disorder diagnoses. *Curr Opin Psychiatry.* 2013;26(6):532–536.

8. Chamay-Weber C, Narring F, Michaud PA. Partial eating disorders among adolescents: a review. *J Adolesc Health.* 2005;37(5):417–427.

9. Bravender T, Bryant-Waugh R, Herzog D, et al. Classification of child and adolescent eating disturbances. Workgroup for Classification of Eating Disorders in Children and Adolescents (WCEDCA). *Int J Eat Disord.* 2007;40 (suppl):S117–S122.

10. Casey BJ, Getz S, Galvan A. The adolescent brain. *Dev Rev.* 2008;28(1):62–77.

11. Katzman DK. Refeeding hospitalized adolescents with anorexia nervosa: is "start low, advance slow" urban legend or evidence based? *J Adolesc Health.* 2012;50(1):1–2.

12. Eddy KT, Celio Doyle A, Hoste RR, Herzog DB, le Grange D. Eating disorder not otherwise specified in adolescents. *J Am Acad Child Adolesc Psychiatry.* 2008;47(2):156–164.

13. Peebles R, Hardy KK, Wilson JL, Lock JD. Are diagnostic criteria for eating disorders markers of medical severity? *Pediatr.* 2010;125(5):e1193–e1201.

14. Rosen DS, American Academy of Pediatrics Committee on A. Identification and management of eating disorders in children and adolescents. *Pediatr.* 2010;126(6):1240–1253.

15. Association AP. *Diagnostic and Statistical Manual of Mental Disorders: DSM-IV.* 4th ed. Washington, DC: American Psychiatric Publishing; 1994.

16. Eddy KT, Dorer DJ, Franko DL, Tahilani K, Thompson-Brenner H, Herzog DB. Diagnostic crossover in anorexia nervosa and bulimia nervosa: implications for DSM-V. *Am J Psychiatry.* 2008;165(2):245–250.

17. Tozzi F, Thornton LM, Klump KL, et al. Symptom fluctuation in eating disorders: correlates of diagnostic crossover. *Am J Psychiatry.* 2005;162(4):732–740.

18. Davis C. The epidemiology and genetics of binge eating disorder (BED). *CNS Spectr.* 2015;20(6):522–529.

19. Hinney A, Volckmar AL. Genetics of eating disorders. *Curr Psychiatry Rep.* 2013;15(12):423.

20. Scherag S, Hebebrand J, Hinney A. Eating disorders: the current status of molecular genetic research. *Eur Child Adolesc Psychiatry.* 2010;19(3):211–226.

21. Strober M, Freeman R, Lampert C, Diamond J, Kaye W. Controlled family study of anorexia nervosa and bulimia nervosa: evidence of shared liability and transmission of partial syndromes. *Am J Psychiatry.* 2000;157(3):393–401.

22. Trace SE, Baker JH, Penas-Lledo E, Bulik CM. The genetics of eating disorders. *Annu Rev Clin Psychol.* 2013;9:589–620.

23. Culbert KM, Burt SA, McGue M, Iacono WG, Klump KL. Puberty and the genetic diathesis of disordered eating attitudes and behaviors. *J Abnorm Psychol.* 2009;118(4):788–796.

24. Haas AM. Feeding disorders in food allergic children. *Curr Allergy Asthma Rep.* 2010;10(4):258–264.

25. Shanahan L, Zucker N, Copeland WE, Costello EJ, Angold A. Are children and adolescents with food allergies at increased risk for psychopathology? *J Psychosom Res.* 2014;77(6):468–473.

26. Field D, Garland M, Williams K. Correlates of specific childhood feeding problems. *J Paediatr Child Health.* 2003;39(4):299–304.

27. d'Emden H, Holden L, McDermott B, et al. Disturbed eating behaviours and thoughts in Australian adolescents with type 1 diabetes. *J Paediatr Child Health.* 2013;49(4):E317–E323.

28. Raevuori A, Haukka J, Vaarala O, et al. The increased risk for autoimmune diseases in patients with eating disorders. *PLoS One.* 2014;9(8):e104845.

29. Smith FM, Latchford GJ, Hall RM, Dickson RA. Do chronic medical conditions increase the risk of eating disorder? A cross-sectional investigation of eating pathology in adolescent females with scoliosis and diabetes. *J Adolesc Health.* 2008;42(1):58–63.

30. Wotton CJ, James A, Goldacre MJ. Coexistence of eating disorders and autoimmune diseases: Record linkage cohort study, UK. *Int J Eat Disord.* 2016;49(7):663–672.

31. Lawrence JM, Liese AD, Liu L, et al. Weight-loss practices and weight-related issues among youth with type 1 or type 2 diabetes. *Diabetes Care.* 2008;31(12):2251–2257.

32. Gottesman K. Insulin omission for weight control in adolescents with type 1 diabetes mellitus. *Top Clin Nutr.* 2015;30(4):314–323.

33. Pinhas-Hamiel O, Zeitler P. The global spread of type 2 diabetes mellitus in children and adolescents. *J Pediatr.* 2005;146(5):693–700.

34. Eddy KT, Tanofsky-Kraff M, Thompson-Brenner H, Herzog DB, Brown TA, Ludwig DS. Eating disorder pathology among overweight treatment-seeking youth: clinical correlates and cross-sectional risk modeling. *Behav Res Ther.* 2007;45(10):2360–2371.

35. Rancourt D, McCullough MB. Overlap in Eating Disorders and Obesity in Adolescence. *Curr Diab Rep.* 2015;15(10):78.

36. Group TS, Wilfley D, Berkowitz R, et al. Binge eating, mood, and quality of life in youth with type 2 diabetes: baseline data from the today study. *Diabetes Care.* 2011;34(4):858–860.

37. Boyd C, Abraham S, Kellow J. Appearance and disappearance of functional gastrointestinal disorders in patients with eating disorders. *Neurogastroenterol Motil.* 2010;22(12):1279–1283.

38. Nicholls DE, Lynn R, Viner RM. Childhood eating disorders: British national surveillance study. *Br J Psychiatry.* 2011;198(4):295–301.

39. Nicholls DE, Viner RM. Childhood risk factors for lifetime anorexia nervosa by age 30 years in a national birth cohort. *J Am Acad Child Adolesc Psychiatry.* 2009;48(8):791–799.

40. Goodman A, Heshmati A, Malki N, Koupil I. Associations between birth characteristics and eating disorders across the life course: findings from 2 million males and females born in Sweden, 1975–1998. *Am J Epidemiol.* 2014;179(7):852–863.

41. Tenconi E, Santonastaso P, Monaco F, Favaro A. Obstetric complications and eating disorders: a replication study. *Int J Eat Disord.* 2015;48(4):424–430.

42. Bandini LG, Anderson SE, Curtin C, et al. Food selectivity in children with autism spectrum disorders and typically developing children. *J Pediatr.* 2010;157(2):259–264.

43. Cederlof M, Thornton LM, Baker J, et al. Etiological overlap between obsessive-compulsive disorder and anorexia nervosa: a longitudinal cohort, multigenerational family and twin study. *World Psychiatry.* 2015;14(3):333–338.

44. Ferreiro F, Wichstrom L, Seoane G, Senra C. Reciprocal associations between depressive symptoms and disordered eating among adolescent girls and boys: a multiwave, prospective study. *J Abnorm Child Psychol.* 2014;42(5):803–812.

45. Haynos AF, Watts AW, Loth KA, Pearson CM, Neumark-Stzainer D. Factors predicting an escalation of restrictive eating during adolescence. *J Adolesc Health.* 2016;59(4):391–396.

46. Kaisari P, Dourish CT, Higgs S. Attention Deficit Hyperactivity Disorder (ADHD) and disordered eating behaviour: A systematic review and a framework for future research. *Clin Psychol Rev.* 2017;53:109–121.

47. Mas S, Plana MT, Castro-Fornieles J, et al. Common genetic background in anorexia nervosa and obsessive compulsive disorder: preliminary results from an association study. *J Psychiatr Res.* 2013;47(6):747–754.

48. Zucker N, Copeland W, Franz L, et al. Psychological and psychosocial impairment in preschoolers with selective eating. *Pediatr.* 2015;136(3):e582–e590.

49. Loth KA, MacLehose R, Bucchianeri M, Crow S, Neumark-Stzainer D. Predictors of dieting and disordered eating behaviors from adolescence to young adulthood. *J Adolesc Health.* 2014;55(5):705–712.

50. Rohde P, Stice E, Marti CN. Development and predictive effects of eating disorder risk factors during adolescence: Implications for prevention efforts. *Int J Eat Disord.* 2015;48(2):187–198.

51. Benowitz-Fredericks CA, Garcia K, Massey M, Vasagar B, Borzekowski DL. Body image, eating disorders, and the relationship to adolescent media use. *Pediatr Clin North Am.* 2012;59(3):693–704.

52. Dakanalis A, Carra G, Calogero R, et al. The developmental effects of media-ideal internalization and self-objectification processes on adolescents' negative body-feelings, dietary restraint, and binge eating. *Eur Child Adolesc Psychiatry.* 2015;24(8):997–1010.

53. Mitchison D, Hay P, Slewa-Younan S, Mond J. The changing demographic profile of eating disorder behaviors in the community. *BMC Public Health.* 2014;14:943.

54. Mulders-Jones B, Mitchison D, Girosi F, Hay P. Socioeconomic correlates of eating disorder symptoms in an Australian Population-Based Sample. *PLoS One.* 2017;12(1):e0170603.

55. Wonderlich SA, Crosby RD, Mitchell JE, et al. Relationship of childhood sexual abuse and eating disturbance in children. *J Am Acad Child Adolesc Psychiatry.* 2000;39(10):1277–1283.

56. Molendijk ML, Hoek HW, Brewerton TD, Elzinga BM. Childhood maltreatment and eating disorder pathology: a systematic review and dose-response meta-analysis. *Psychol Med.* 2017:1–15.

57. Olivares JL, Vazquez M, Fleta J, Moreno LA, Perez-Gonzalez JM, Bueno M. Cardiac findings in adolescents with anorexia nervosa at diagnosis and after weight restoration. *Eur J Pediatr.* 2005;164(6):383–386.

58. Society for Adolescent H, Medicine, Golden NH, et al. Position Paper of the Society for Adolescent Health and Medicine: medical management of restrictive eating disorders in adolescents and young adults. *J Adolesc Health.* 2015;56(1):121–125.

59. NNIfHaCE. Eating disorders: Recognition and treatment. NICE guideline. Available at: https://www.nice.org.uk /guidance/ng69. Accessed December 3, 2017.

60. Misra M, Katzman DK, Cord J, et al. Percentage extremity fat, but not percentage trunk fat, is lower in adolescent boys with anorexia nervosa than in healthy adolescents. *Am J Clin Nutr.* 2008;88(6):1478–1484.

61. Misra M, Klibanski A. Endocrine consequences of anorexia nervosa. *Lancet Diabetes Endocrinol.* 2014;2(7):581–592.

62. Munoz MT, Argente J. Anorexia nervosa in female adolescents: endocrine and bone mineral density disturbances. *Eur J Endocrinol.* 2002;147(3):275–286.

63. Gordon CM, Nelson LM. Amenorrhea and bone health in adolescents and young women. *Curr Opin Obstet Gynecol.* 2003;15(5):377–384.

64. Faje AT, Fazeli PK, Miller KK, et al. Fracture risk and areal bone mineral density in adolescent females with anorexia nervosa. *Int J Eat Disord.* 2014;47(5):458–466.

65. Mika C, Holtkamp K, Heer M, Gunther RW, Herpertz-Dahlmann B. A 2-year prospective study of bone metabolism and bone mineral density in adolescents with anorexia nervosa. *J Neural Transm (Vienna).* 2007;114(12):1611–1618.

66. Benini L, Todesco T, Dalle Grave R, Deiorio F, Salandini L, Vantini I. Gastric emptying in patients with restricting and binge/purging subtypes of anorexia nervosa. *Am J Gastroenterol.* 2004;99(8):1448–1454.

67. Brown CA, Mehler PS. Medical complications of self-induced vomiting. *Eat Disord.* 2013;21(4):287–294.

68. Sachs K, Mehler PS. Medical complications of bulimia nervosa and their treatments. *Eat Weight Disord.* 2016;21(1):13–18.

69. Pacciardi B, Cargioli C, Mauri M. Barrett's esophagus in anorexia nervosa: a case report. *Int J Eat Disord.* 2015;48(1):147–150.

70. Shinohara ET, Swisher-McClure S, Husson M, Sun W, Metz JM. Esophageal cancer in a young woman with bulimia nervosa: a case report. *J Med Case Rep.* 2007;1:160.

71. Puccio F, Fuller-Tyszkiewicz M, Ong D, Krug I. A systematic review and meta-analysis on the longitudinal relationship between eating pathology and depression. *Int J Eat Disord.* 2016;49(5):439–454.

72. Bentz M, Jepsen JR, Pedersen T, et al. Impairment of social function in young females With recent-onset anorexia nervosa and recovered individuals. *J Adolesc Health.* 2017;60(1):23–32.

73. Menatti AR, DeBoer LB, Weeks JW, Heimberg RG. Social anxiety and associations with eating psychopathology: Mediating effects of fears of evaluation. *Body Image.* 2015;14:20–28.

74. Swinbourne J, Hunt C, Abbott M, Russell J, St Clare T, Touyz S. The comorbidity between eating disorders and anxiety disorders: prevalence in an eating disorder sample and anxiety disorder sample. *Aust N Z J Psychiatry.* 2012;46(2):118–131.

75. Arlt J, Yiu A, Eneva K, Taylor Dryman M, Heimberg RG, Chen EY. Contributions of cognitive inflexibility to eating disorder and social anxiety symptoms. *Eat Behav.* 2016;21:30–32.

76. Boisseau CL, Thompson-Brenner H, Eddy KT, Satir DA. Impulsivity and personality variables in adolescents with eating disorders. *J Nerv Ment Dis.* 2009;197(4): 251–259.

77. Fischer S, Smith GT, Anderson KG. Clarifying the role of impulsivity in bulimia nervosa. *Int J Eat Disord.* 2003;33(4):406–411.

78. Morgan JF, Reid F, Lacey JH. The SCOFF questionnaire: assessment of a new screening tool for eating disorders. *BMJ.* 1999;319(7223):1467–1468.

79. Hautala L, Junnila J, Alin J, et al. Uncovering hidden eating disorders using the SCOFF questionnaire: cross-sectional survey of adolescents and comparison with nurse assessments. *Int J Nurs Stud.* 2009;46(11):1439–1447.

80. Fairburn CG, Beglin SJ. Assessment of eating disorders: interview or self-report questionnaire? *Int J Eat Disord.* 1994;16(4):363–370.

81. Binford RB, Le Grange D, Jellar CC. Eating Disorders Examination versus Eating Disorders Examination-Questionnaire in adolescents with full and partial-syndrome Bulimia Nervosa and anorexia nervosa. *Int J Eat Disord.* 2005;37(1):44–49.

82. Garner DM, Olmsted MP, Bohr Y, Garfinkel PE. The eating attitudes test: psychometric features and clinical correlates. *Psychol Med.* 1982;12(4):871–878.

83. Berger U, Wick K, Holling H, et al. [Screening of disordered eating in 12-Year-old girls and boys: psychometric analysis of the German versions of SCOFF and EAT-26]. *Psychother Psychosom Med Psychol.* 2011;61(7):311–318.

84. Mond JM, Myers TC, Crosby RD, et al. Screening for eating disorders in primary care: EDE-Q versus SCOFF. *Behav Res Ther.* 2008;46(5):612–622.

85. Pediatrics AAo. Bright Futures: Nutrition 3rd ed. Nutrition Tools. Available at: https://brightfutures.aap.org/Bright %20Futures%20Documents/BFNutrition3rdEdition _tools.pdf. Accessed December 14, 2017.

86. Cermak SA, Curtin C, Bandini LG. Food selectivity and sensory sensitivity in children with autism spectrum disorders. *J Am Diet Assoc.* 2010;110(2):238–246.

87. Schap TE, Six BL, Delp EJ, Ebert DS, Kerr DA, Boushey CJ. Adolescents in the United States can identify familiar foods at the time of consumption and when prompted with an image 14 h postprandial, but poorly estimate portions. *Public Health Nutr.* 2011;14(7):1184–1191.

88. Wolkoff LE, Tanofsky-Kraff M, Shomaker LB, et al. Self-reported vs. actual energy intake in youth with and without loss of control eating. *Eat Behav.* 2011;12(1):15–20.

89. M B. *Adolescent Nutrition. Nutrition Across the Life Stages* 1st ed. Burlington, MA: Jones & Bartlett Learning; 2018.

90. Yucel B, Ozbey N, Demir K, Polat A, Yager J. Eating disorders and celiac disease: a case report. *Int J Eat Disord.* 2006;39(6):530–532.

91. Kaye W. Neurobiology of anorexia and bulimia nervosa. *Physiol Behav.* 2008;94(1):121–135.

92. Klein DA, Mayer LE, Schebendach JE, Walsh BT. Physical activity and cortisol in anorexia nervosa. *Psychoneuroendocrinol.* 2007;32(5):539–547.

93. Renz JA, Fisher M, Vidair HB, et al. Excessive exercise among adolescents with eating disorders: examination of psychological and demographic variables. *Int J Adolesc Med Health.* 2017. doi: 10.1515/ijamh-2017-0032.

94. Attia E, Walsh BT. Anorexia nervosa. *Am J Psychiatry.* 2007;164(12):18051810.

95. Keys A. *The Biology of Human Starvation.* Minneapolis, MN: University of Minnesota Press;1950.

96. Becker AE, Thomas JJ, Pike KM. Should non-fat-phobic anorexia nervosa be included in DSM-V? *Int J Eat Disord.* 2009;42(7):620–635.

97. Ornstein RM, Rosen DS, Mammel KA, et al. Distribution of eating disorders in children and adolescents using the proposed DSM-5 criteria for feeding and eating disorders. *J Adolesc Health.* 2013;53(2):303–305.

98. Castillo M, Weiselberg E. Bulimia Nervosa/Purging Disorder. *Curr Probl Pediatr Adolesc Health Care.* 2017;47(4): 85–94.

99. Kruger D. Bulimia nervosa: easy to hide but essential to recognize. *JAAPA.* 2008;21(1):48–52.

100. Hudson JI, Hiripi E, Pope HG, Jr., Kessler RC. The prevalence and correlates of eating disorders in the National Comorbidity Survey Replication. *Biol Psychiatry.* 2007;61(3): 348–358.

101. Smink FR, van Hoeken D, Hoek HW. Epidemiology of eating disorders: incidence, prevalence and mortality rates. *Curr Psychiatry Rep.* 2012;14(4):406–414.

102. Wonderlich SA, Gordon KH, Mitchell JE, Crosby RD, Engel SG. The validity and clinical utility of binge eating disorder. *Int J Eat Disord.* 2009;42(8):687–705.

103. Ulfvebrand S, Birgegard A, Norring C, Hogdahl L, von Hausswolff-Juhlin Y. Psychiatric comorbidity in women and men with eating disorders results from a large clinical database. *Psychiatry Res.* 2015;230(2):294–299.

104. Agras WS, Crow S, Mitchell JE, Halmi KA, Bryson S. A 4-year prospective study of eating disorder NOS compared with full eating disorder syndromes. *Int J Eat Disord.* 2009;42(6):565–570.

105. Pope HG, Jr., Lalonde JK, Pindyck LJ, et al. Binge eating disorder: a stable syndrome. *Am J Psychiatry.* 2006;163(12):2181–2183.

106. Beals KA, Meyer NL. Female athlete triad update. *Clin Sports Med.* 2007;26(1):69–89.

107. Glazer JL. Eating disorders among male athletes. *Curr Sports Med Rep.* 2008;7(6):332–337.

108. Nichols JF, Rauh MJ, Lawson MJ, Ji M, Barkai HS. Prevalence of the female athlete triad syndrome among high school athletes. *Arch Pediatr Adolesc Med.* 2006;160(2): 137–142.

109. Sundgot-Borgen J, Meyer NL, Lohman TG, et al. How to minimise the health risks to athletes who compete in weight-sensitive sports review and position statement on behalf of the Ad Hoc Research Working Group on Body Composition, Health and Performance, under the auspices of the IOC Medical Commission. *Br J Sports Med.* 2013;47(16):1012–1022.

110. Bonci CM, Bonci LJ, Granger LR, et al. National athletic trainers' association position statement: preventing, detecting, and managing disordered eating in athletes. *J Athl Train.* 2008;43(1):80–108.

111. Otis CL, Drinkwater B, Johnson M, Loucks A, Wilmore J. American College of Sports Medicine position stand. The Female Athlete Triad. *Med Sci Sports Exerc.* 1997;29(5):i–ix.

112. Yeager KK, Agostini R, Nattiv A, Drinkwater B. The female athlete triad: disordered eating, amenorrhea, osteoporosis. *Med Sci Sports Exerc.* 1993;25(7):775–777.

113. Joy E, De Souza MJ, Nattiv A, et al. 2014 female athlete triad coalition consensus statement on treatment and return to play of the female athlete triad. *Curr Sports Med Rep.* 2014;13(4):219–232.

114. Nattiv A, Loucks AB, Manore MM, et al. American College of Sports Medicine position stand. The female athlete triad. *Med Sci Sports Exerc.* 2007;39(10):1867–1882.

115. Mountjoy M, Sundgot-Borgen J, Burke L, et al. The IOC consensus statement: beyond the Female Athlete Triad—Relative Energy Deficiency in Sport (RED-S). *Br J Sports Med.* 2014;48(7):491–497.

116. Zimmerman J, Fisher M. Avoidant/Restrictive Food Intake Disorder (ARFID). *Curr Probl Pediatr Adolesc Health Care.* 2017;47(4):95–103.

117. Fisher MM, Rosen DS, Ornstein RM, et al. Characteristics of avoidant/restrictive food intake disorder in children and adolescents: a "new disorder" in DSM-5. *J Adolesc Health.* 2014;55(1):49–52.

118. Ozier AD, Henry BW, American Dietetic A. Position of the American Dietetic Association: nutrition intervention in the treatment of eating disorders. *J Am Diet Assoc.* 2011;111(8):1236–1241.

119. Rome ES, Ammerman S, Rosen DS, et al. Children and adolescents with eating disorders: the state of the art. *Pediatrics.* 2003;111(1):e98–e108.

120. American Dietetic A. Position of the American Dietetic Association: Nutrition intervention in the treatment of anorexia nervosa, bulimia nervosa, and other eating disorders. *J Am Diet Assoc.* 2006;106(12):2073–2082.

121. Mairs R, Nicholls D. Assessment and treatment of eating disorders in children and adolescents. *Arch Dis Child.* 2016;101(12):1168–1175.

122. Group PNDP. Pediatric Nutrition Care Manual: Eating Disorders. https://www.nutritioncaremanual.org/topic.cfm?ncm_category_id=13&lv1=144633&lv2=144778&ncm_toc_id=144778&ncm_heading=NutritionCarehomepage Accessed 09/30/2018

123. Cockfield A, Philpot U. Feeding size 0: the challenges of anorexia nervosa. Managing anorexia from a dietitian's perspective. *Proc Nutr Soc.* 2009;68(3):281–288.

124. Excellence NIfC. Eating Disorders: Core Interventions in the Treatment and Management of Anorexia Nervosa, Bulimia Nervosa and Related Eating Disorders (Clinical Guideline 9). 2004.

125. Golden NH, Jacobson MS, Schebendach J, Solanto MV, Hertz SM, Shenker IR. Resumption of menses in anorexia nervosa. *Arch Pediatr Adolesc Med.* 1997;151(1):16–21.

126. Golden NH, Jacobson MS, Sterling WM, Hertz S. Treatment goal weight in adolescents with anorexia nervosa: use of BMI percentiles. *Int J Eat Disord.* 2008;41(4):301–306.

127. Le Grange D, Doyle PM, Swanson SA, Ludwig K, Glunz C, Kreipe RE. Calculation of expected body weight in adolescents with eating disorders. *Pediatr.* 2012;129(2):e438–e446.

128. King K KB. *Nutrition Therapy: Advanced Counseling Skills* Philadelphia, PA: Lippincott Williams & Wilkins;2007.

129. Becker P, Carney LN, Corkins MR, et al. Consensus statement of the Academy of Nutrition and Dietetics/American Society for Parenteral and Enteral Nutrition: indicators recommended for the identification and documentation of pediatric malnutrition (undernutrition). *Nutr Clin Pract.* 2015;30(1):147–161.

130. American Psychiatric A. Treatment of patients with eating disorders,third edition. American Psychiatric Association. *Am J Psychiatry.* 2006;163(suppl7):4–54.

131. Ross CC. The importance of nutrition as the best medicine for eating disorders. *Explore (NY).* 2007;3(2):153–157.

132. Stabler SP. Clinical practice. Vitamin B_{12} deficiency. *N Engl J Med.* 2013;368(2):149–160.

133. Moyad MA. Vitamin D: a rapid review. *Dermatol Nurs.* 2009;21(1):25–30.

134. Wanby P, Berglund J, Brudin L, Hedberg D, Carlsson M. Increased ferritin levels in patients with anorexia nervosa: impact of weight gain. *Eat Weight Disord.* 2016;21(3):411–417.

135. Birmingham CL, Gritzner S. How does zinc supplementation benefit anorexia nervosa? *Eat Weight Disord.* 2006;11(4):e109–e111.

136. Katz RL, Keen CL, Litt IF, Hurley LS, Kellams-Harrison KM, Glader LJ. Zinc deficiency in anorexia nervosa. *J Adolesc Health Care.* 1987;8(5):400–406.

137. Su JC, Birmingham CL. Zinc supplementation in the treatment of anorexia nervosa. *Eat Weight Disord.* 2002;7(1):20–22.

138. Crook MA, Hally V, Panteli JV. The importance of the refeeding syndrome. *Nutr.* 2001;17(7–8):632–637.

139. Mehanna H, Nankivell PC, Moledina J, Travis J. Refeeding syndrome—awareness, prevention and management. *Head Neck Oncol.* 2009;1:4.

140. Duignan E, Kenna P, Watson R, Fitzsimon S, Brosnahan D. Ophthalmic manifestations of vitamin A and D deficiency in two autistic teenagers: case reports and a review of the literature. *Case Rep Ophthalmol.* 2015;6(1):24–29.

141. Ma NS, Thompson C, Weston S. Brief Report: Scurvy as a Manifestation of Food Selectivity in Children with Autism. *J Autism Dev Disord.* 2016;46(4):1464–1470.

142. Stewart C, Latif A. Symptomatic nutritional rickets in a teenager with autistic spectrum disorder. *Child Care Health Dev.* 2008;34(2):276–278.

143. Garber AK, Michihata N, Hetnal K, Shafer MA, Moscicki AB. A prospective examination of weight gain in hospitalized adolescents with anorexia nervosa on a recommended refeeding protocol. *J Adolesc Health.* 2012;50(1):24–29.

144. Peebles R, Lesser A, Park CC, et al. Outcomes of an inpatient medical nutritional rehabilitation protocol in children and adolescents with eating disorders. *J Eat Disord.* 2017;5:7.

145. Marzola E, Nasser JA, Hashim SA, Shih PA, Kaye WH. Nutritional rehabilitation in anorexia nervosa: review of the literature and implications for treatment. *BMC Psychiatry.* 2013;13:290.

146. Kaye WH, Gwirtsman HE, Obarzanek E, George DT. Relative importance of calorie intake needed to gain weight and level of physical activity in anorexia nervosa. *Am J Clin Nutr.* 1988;47(6):989–994.

147. Schebendach JE, Mayer LE, Devlin MJ, et al. Dietary energy density and diet variety as predictors of outcome in anorexia nervosa. *Am J Clin Nutr.* 2008;87(4):810–816.

148. Schebendach J, Mayer LE, Devlin MJ, Attia E, Walsh BT. Dietary energy density and diet variety as risk factors for relapse in anorexia nervosa: a replication. *Int J Eat Disord.* 2012;45(1):79–84.

149. Garber AK, Sawyer SM, Golden NH, et al. A systematic review of approaches to refeeding in patients with anorexia nervosa. *Int J Eat Disord.* 2016;49(3):293–310.

150. O'Connor G, Goldin J. The refeeding syndrome and glucose load. *Int J Eat Disord.* 2011;44(2):182–185.

151. Solomon SM, Kirby DF. The refeeding syndrome: a review. *JPEN.* 1990;14(1):90–97.

152. Maginot TR, Kumar MM, Shiels J, Kaye W, Rhee KE. Outcomes of an inpatient refeeding protocol in youth with anorexia nervosa: Rady Children's Hospital San Diego/University of California, San Diego. *J Eat Disord.* 2017;5:1.

153. Katzman DK. Medical complications in adolescents with anorexia nervosa: a review of the literature. *Int J Eat Disord.* 2005;37 (suppl):S52–S59; discussion S87–S59.

154. Mehanna HM, Moledina J, Travis J. Refeeding syndrome: what it is, and how to prevent and treat it. *BMJ.* 2008;336(7659):1495–1498.

155. Ornstein RM, Golden NH, Jacobson MS, Shenker IR. Hypophosphatemia during nutritional rehabilitation in anorexia nervosa: implications for refeeding and monitoring. *J Adolesc Health.* 2003;32(1):83–88.

156. Gentile MG, Pastorelli P, Ciceri R, Manna GM, Collimedaglia S. Specialized refeeding treatment for anorexia nervosa patients suffering from extreme undernutrition. *Clin Nutr.* 2010;29(5):627–632.

157. Golden NH, Keane-Miller C, Sainani KL, Kapphahn CJ. Higher caloric intake in hospitalized adolescents with anorexia nervosa is associated with reduced length of stay and no increased rate of refeeding syndrome. *J Adolesc Health.* 2013;53(5):573–578.

158. Sylvester CJ, Forman SF. Clinical practice guidelines for treating restrictive eating disorder patients during medical hospitalization. *Curr Opin Pediatr.* 2008;20(4):390–397.

159. Whitelaw M, Gilbertson H, Lam PY, Sawyer SM. Does aggressive refeeding in hospitalized adolescents with anorexia nervosa result in increased hypophosphatemia? *J Adolesc Health.* 2010;46(6):577–582.

160. (NICE) NIfHaCE. Nutritoin support for adults: oral nutrition, enteral tube feeding and parenteral nutritoin. Guidance and guidelines. 2006. Available at: https://www.nice .org.uk/guidance/cg32/chapter/1-Guidance#what-to -give-in-hospital-and-the-community.

161. Accurso EC, Ciao AC, Fitzsimmons-Craft EE, Lock JD, Le Grange D. Is weight gain really a catalyst for broader recovery? The impact of weight gain on psychological symptoms in the treatment of adolescent anorexia nervosa. *Behav Res Ther.* 2014;56:1–6.

162. Couturier J, Isserlin L, Lock J. Family-based treatment for adolescents with anorexia nervosa: a dissemination study. *Eat Disord.* 2010;18(3):199–209.

163. Lock J. Evaluation of family treatment models for eating disorders. *Curr Opin Psychiatry.* 2011;24(4):274–279.

164. Lock J LGD. *Help Your Teenager Beat an Eating Disorder.* New York, NY: The Guilford Press; 2005.

165. Lock J LGD. *Treatment Manual for Anorexia Nervosa: A Family Based Approach.* New York, NY: The Guilford Press; 2001.

166. Eisler I, Simic M, Russell GF, Dare C. A randomised controlled treatment trial of two forms of family therapy in adolescent anorexia nervosa: a five-year follow-up. *J Child Psychol Psychiatry.* 2007;48(6):552–560.

167. Lock J, Le Grange D, Agras WS, Moye A, Bryson SW, Jo B. Randomized clinical trial comparing family-based treatment with adolescent-focused individual therapy for adolescents with anorexia nervosa. *Arch Gen Psychiatry.* 2010;67(10):1025–1032.

168. Schebendach J, Golden NH, Jacobson MS, et al. Indirect calorimetry in the nutritional management of eating disorders. *Int J Eat Disord.* 1995;17(1):59–66.

169. Devlin MJ, Walsh BT, Kral JG, Heymsfield SB, Pi-Sunyer FX, Dantzic S. Metabolic abnormalities in bulimia nervosa. *Arch Gen Psychiatry.* 1990;47(2):144–148.

170. Sedlet KL, Ireton-Jones CS. Energy expenditure and the abnormal eating pattern of a bulimic: a case report. *J Am Diet Assoc.* 1989;89(1):74–77.

171. Schmidt U, Lee S, Beecham J, et al. A randomized controlled trial of family therapy and cognitive behavior therapy guided self-care for adolescents with bulimia nervosa and related disorders. *Am J Psychiatry.* 2007;164(4):591–598.

172. Le Grange D, Lock J, Agras WS, Bryson SW, Jo B. Randomized Clinical Trial of Family-Based Treatment and Cognitive-Behavioral Therapy for Adolescent Bulimia Nervosa. *J Am Acad Child Adolesc Psychiatry.* 2015;54(11):886–894.

173. le Grange D, Crosby RD, Rathouz PJ, Leventhal BL. A randomized controlled comparison of family-based treatment and supportive psychotherapy for adolescent bulimia nervosa. *Arch Gen Psychiatry.* 2007;64(9):1049–1056.

174. Dalle Grave R, Calugi S, Sartirana M, Fairburn CG. Transdiagnostic cognitive behaviour therapy for adolescents with an eating disorder who are not underweight. *Behav Res Ther.* 2015;73:79–82.

175. Fischer S, Peterson C. Dialectical behavior therapy for adolescent binge eating, purging, suicidal behavior, and non-suicidal self-injury: a pilot study. *Psychotherapy (Chic).* 2015;52(1):78–92.

176. Kotler LA, Devlin MJ, Davies M, Walsh BT. An open trial of fluoxetine for adolescents with bulimia nervosa. *J Child Adolesc Psychopharmacol.* 2003;13(3):329–335.

177. Fluoxetine in the treatment of bulimia nervosa. A multicenter, placebo-controlled, double-blind trial. Fluoxetine Bulimia Nervosa Collaborative Study Group. *Arch Gen Psychiatry.* 1992;49(2):139–147.

178. Tanofsky-Kraff M, Shomaker LB, Wilfley DE, et al. Targeted prevention of excess weight gain and eating disorders in high-risk adolescent girls: a randomized controlled trial. *Am J Clin Nutr.* 2014;100(4):1010–1018.

179. Kelly NR, Shank LM, Bakalar JL, Tanofsky-Kraff M. Pediatric feeding and eating disorders: current state of diagnosis and treatment. *Curr Psychiatry Rep.* 2014;16(5):446.

180. Mammel KA, Ornstein RM. Avoidant/restrictive food intake disorder: a new eating disorder diagnosis in the diagnostic and statistical manual 5. *Curr Opin Pediatr.* 2017;29(4):407–413.

181. Strandjord SE, Sieke EH, Richmond M, Rome ES. Avoidant/Restrictive Food Intake Disorder: Illness and Hospital Course in Patients Hospitalized for Nutritional Insufficiency. *J Adolesc Health.* 2015;57(6):673–678.

182. Sant'Anna AM, Hammes PS, Porporino M, Martel C, Zygmuntowicz C, Ramsay M. Use of cyproheptadine in young children with feeding difficulties and poor growth in a pediatric feeding program. *J Pediatr Gastroenterol Nutr.* 2014;59(5):674–678.

183. Moskowitz L, Weiselberg E. Anorexia Nervosa/Atypical Anorexia Nervosa. *Curr Probl Pediatr Adolesc Health Care.* 2017;47(4):70–84.

184. Katzman DK, Peebles R, Sawyer SM, Lock J, Le Grange D. The role of the pediatrician in family-based treatment for adolescent eating disorders: opportunities and challenges. *J Adolesc Health.* 2013;53(4):433–440.

185. Redgrave GW, Coughlin JW, Schreyer CC, et al. Refeeding and weight restoration outcomes in anorexia nervosa: Challenging current guidelines. *Int J Eat Disord*. 2015;48(7):866–873.

186. Garber AK, Mauldin K, Michihata N, Buckelew SM, Shafer MA, Moscicki AB. Higher calorie diets increase rate of weight gain and shorten hospital stay in hospitalized adolescents with anorexia nervosa. *J Adolesc Health*. 2013;53(5):579–584.

187. Shamim T, Golden NH, Arden M, Filiberto L, Shenker IR. Resolution of vital sign instability: an objective measure of medical stability in anorexia nervosa. *J Adolesc Health*. 2003;32(1):73–77.

188. Lock J. An Update on Evidence-based psychosocial treatments for eating disorders in children and adolescents. *J Clin Child Adolesc Psychol*. 2015;44(5):707–721.

189. Barlow SE, Expert C. Expert committee recommendations regarding the prevention, assessment, and treatment of child and adolescent overweight and obesity: summary report. *Pediatrics*. 2007;120 (suppl4):S164–S192.

190. Norris ML, Spettigue WJ, Katzman DK. Update on eating disorders: current perspectives on avoidant/restrictive food intake disorder in children and youth. *Neuropsychiatr Dis Treat*. 2016;12:213–218.

191. Hyman SL, Stewart PA, Schmidt B, et al. Nutrient intake from food in children with autism. *Pediatrics*. 2012;130 Suppl 2:S145–153.

192. Arcelus J, Mitchell AJ, Wales J, Nielsen S. Mortality rates in patients with anorexia nervosa and other eating disorders. A meta-analysis of 36 studies. *Arch Gen Psychiatry*. 2011;68(7):724–731.

193. Suokas JT, Suvisaari JM, Grainger M, Raevuori A, Gissler M, Haukka J. Suicide attempts and mortality in eating disorders: a follow-up study of eating disorder patients. *Gen Hosp Psychiatry*. 2014;36(3):355–357.

194. Wade TD, Fairweather-Schmidt AK, Zhu G, Martin NG. Does shared genetic risk contribute to the co-occurrence of eating disorders and suicidality? *Int J Eat Disord*. 2015;48(6):684–691.

195. Zerwas S, Larsen JT, Petersen L, Thornton LM, Mortensen PB, Bulik CM. The incidence of eating disorders in a Danish register study: Associations with suicide risk and mortality. *J Psychiatr Res*. 2015;65:16–22.

196. Bodell LP, Joiner TE, Keel PK. Comorbidity-independent risk for suicidality increases with bulimia nervosa but not with anorexia nervosa. *J Psychiatr Res*. 2013;47(5):617–621.

197. Mann AP, Accurso EC, Stiles-Shields C, et al. Factors associated with substance use in adolescents with eating disorders. *J Adolesc Health*. 2014;55(2):182–187.

198. Micali N, Solmi F, Horton NJ, et al. Adolescent eating disorders predict psychiatric, high-risk behaviors and weight outcomes in young adulthood. *J Am Acad Child Adolesc Psychiatry*. 2015;54(8):652–659.

199. Peebles R, Wilson JL, Lock JD. Self-injury in adolescents with eating disorders: correlates and provider bias. *J Adolesc Health*. 2011;48(3):310–313.

200. Diemer EW, Grant JD, Munn-Chernoff MA, Patterson DA, Duncan AE. Gender Identity, Sexual Orientation, and Eating-Related Pathology in a National Sample of College Students. *J Adolesc Health*. 2015;57(2):144–149.

201. Feldman MB, Meyer IH. Eating disorders in diverse lesbian, gay, and bisexual populations. *Int J Eat Disord*. 2007;40(3):218–226.

202. Shearer A, Russon J, Herres J, Atte T, Kodish T, Diamond G. The relationship between disordered eating and sexuality amongst adolescents and young adults. *Eat Behav*. 2015;19:115–119.

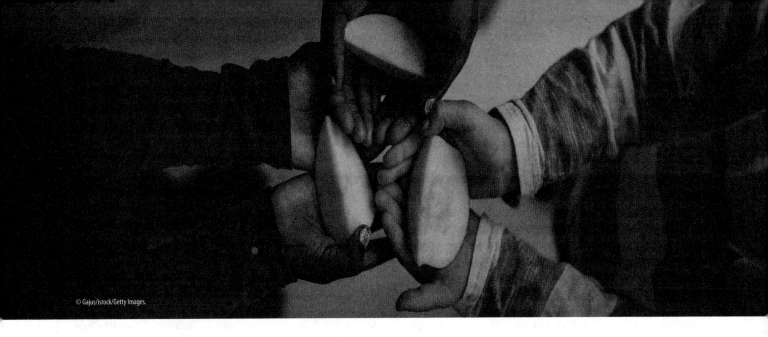

© Gajus/istock/Getty Images.

CHAPTER 23

Pediatric Sports Nutrition

Britt Schuman-Humbert

LEARNING OBJECTIVES

- Learn to appropriately assess energy and macronutrient requirements in highly active children, adolescents, and young adults in order to optimize performance and body composition.
- Understand the increased macronutrient and micronutrients required for vegan athletes.
- Understand the signs of the female athlete triad and provide appropriate intervention.

▶ Introduction

In addition to physical fitness, regular and appropriate exercise provides multiple benefits to children and adolescents, including both psychological and social advantages.[1]

The US Department of Health and Human Services recommends 1 hour of physical activity for children ages 6–17 years each day.[2] However, the number of young athletes who participate in serious training and competition continues to increase annually. The age at which children initiate serious training with a single sport becomes younger every year.[1,3] Overuse injuries, such as stress fractures, were once considered unheard of in children and are now a common occurrence.[3] The cost of participation in sports to families has gone up significantly as

well. This is true particularly for children who participate in elite youth sports.[4] In a desire to help children succeed, parents and coaches often turn to the internet to find nutrition information in order to give young athletes a competitive edge. The intensity of the environment and prevalence of misinformation creates an urgency for qualified dietitians to provide evidenced-based information to prevent injury, promote growth, and optimize athletic performance in young athletes. Providing sound nutrition information to parents, coaches, and young athletes provides the pediatric dietitian with an opportunity to improve both the health and performance of the child.

This chapter will provide the basics to pediatric sports nutrition and the optimal equations needed to provide a basic nutrition therapy for a young athlete.

Growth and Development

Preschoolers and young children's primary source of activity should be unstructured play, experimentation, exploration, and having fun. Child athletes should be encouraged to participate in a variety of sports until puberty, waiting until older ages for sport specialization.[5] Young children who spend hours practicing every day will not develop into better athletes but will increase their risk for injury and potentially create emotional or other psychological issues as well.[5] The AAP Council on Sports Medicine and Medical Fitness clearly states that they do not support premature specialization due to the increased risk of injury related to repetitive stress injury.[4-6] While the typical pediatric athlete usually is healthy, has an adequate support system, and food security, determining nutrient needs can be complex because they are related to multiple variables. Physical performance, growth, and pubertal development must be taken into consideration with the nutrition assessment.

Body Composition

Body composition before puberty is fairly similar between boys and girls. Growth during the adolescent phases is extremely variable and should be individualized. The Tanner Stages of Development is a tool developed by Professor James Tanner that divides puberty into 5 stages including not only biological changes, but psychosocial and cognitive changes as well. Delayed puberty within an age group can be indicative of inadequate energy intake.[6,7]

As part of the nutrition assessment either via client interview, health record review, or nutrition focused physical findings, knowing the child's Tanner Stage can be helpful. This information may be determined via questionnaire, visual observation, and/or data obtained from a physician as to where a young athlete is in relation to pubertal development and it will be helpful in providing appropriate nutrition interventions.[6,7]

While BMI for age on growth curves between 5th and 85th percentile is considered normal growth in pediatrics, it fails to differentiate between lean body mass and adipose tissue. Many young athletes can inaccurately be classified as obese with a BMI > 85%ile for increased muscle mass and bone density. Inversely, BMI values can provide a false sense of security for young athletes with eating disorders, resulting in a failure to diagnose and/or underestimation of malnutrition.[7]

Body composition measurements can be routinely obtained by using 3 point or 7 point measures of skinfold thickness, **air displacement plethysmography** (BOD POD), or **dual X-ray absorptiometry** (DEXA). Skinfold thickness technique is completed by using hand held calipers with either a 3 or 7 skinfold measure using the right side of the body. This technique is inexpensive and convenient and it continues to be widely used to determine lean body mass vs. body fat composition in athletes. It can be extremely useful to determine the effectiveness of a program with data routinely taken over time instead of a specific estimate of body fat percentage.

Both BOD and POD use air displacement in a sealed capsule. This test can determine slight changes in body composition. A person wears minimal clothing and is sealed in a capsule for 3 minutes. This testing is fairly quick and reliable but possibly underestimates body fat by 2–3%.[8]

DXA is the highest in expense and can be difficult to obtain. DXA remains the most accurate of all methodologies.[8] There is also a small amount of radiation exposure which provides additional drawbacks for some athletes.

Regardless of the methodology of body composition assessment, athletes need to be educated on their limitations and prevent the promotion of unhealthy practices. Body composition goals should be expressed as ranges versus a specific body fat percentage.

Generally, body composition goals are sport dependent and need to be individualized to the child, taking into consideration the age, activity level, and nutrient needs for growth and development. As with all children, every young athlete requires individualized assessment and interventions due to the variability in puberty, activity, and growth. Pediatric dietitians generally focus on improvements in the nutrition profile in order to promote improvement in athletic ability over the alteration of body composition in young athletes.

Energy

Child athletes need to support increased energy expenditure, as well as the increased needs required for growth. The **Institute of Medicine** (IOM) recommends indirect calorimetry as the preferred method for determining energy needs in this population. When indirect calorimetry is not available, predictive equations such as the **Estimated Energy Requirements** (EER) equations developed by the IOM are recommended.[9,10] These equations take into account not just height, weight, and age, but also physical activity level. The physical activity coefficients used for most young athletes are either active or very active. See **TABLE 23.1** and **TABLE 23.2**.

Determining EER from the IOM remains the preferred method for determining daily energy needs in young athletes. Additional estimated energy expenditures of specific activities can also be determined in older adolescents and adults by using **Metabolic Equivalents** (MET).[11] This can be a particularly useful

TABLE 23.1 Estimated Energy Requirement Equations

Boys 3–8 years old	EER (kcal/day) = 88.5 – (61.9 × Age [y]) + PA × (26.7 × Wt. (kg) + 903 × Ht [M]) + 20 kcal
Girls 3–8 years old	EER (kcal/day) = 135.3 – (30.8 × age [y]) + PA × (10 × weight [kg]) + 934 × Ht [m]) + 20 kcal
Boys 9–18 years old	EER (kcal/day) = 88.5 – 61.9 × Age [y] + PA × (26.7 × Wt. [kg] + 903 × Ht [m]) + 25
Girls 9–18 years old	EER (kcal/day) = 135.3 – (30.8 × age [y] + PA × {(10 × weight [kg]) + (934 × height [m])} + 25
Men 19 years and older	EER (kcal/day) = 662 – (9.53 × age [y]) + PA × {(15.91 × weight [kg]) + (539.6 × height [m])}
Women 19 years and older	EER (kcal/day) = 354 – (6.91 × age [y]) + PA × {(9.36 × weight [kg]) + (726 × height [m])}

Modified from Institute of Medicine of the National Academies. *Dietary Reference Intakes For Energy, Carbohydrate, Fiber, Fat, Fatty acids, Cholesterol, Protein, and Amino Acids.* Washington, DC: The National Academies Press;2005.[9]

TABLE 23.3 Physical Activity Using METs

Activity	Intensity METs	Activity	METs
Aerobic Dance	6.0	Ice skating general	7.0
Running, team practice	10.0	Soccer competitive	10
Rowing ergometer-general	9.5	Soccer general	7
Jogging general	7.0	Basketball general	6
Swimming general	7.0	Basketball game	8
Swimming vigorous effort	10	Football competitive	9

Modified from Ainsworth B, Haskell W, Whitt M, et al. Compendium of physical activities: an update of activity codes and MET intensities. *Med Sci Sports Exerc.* 2000;32 (suppl9):S498–S504.[11]

tool if their resting metabolic rate is known from indirect calorimetry. A MET is defined as the ratio of a work to the standard resting metabolic rate of sitting quietly. Testing, which was determined on adults and defined as 1 MET, requires 3.5 ml of oxygen/kg body weight per minute (ml/kg/min).[11]

See **TABLE 23.3** for examples of Physical Activity using METs.

TABLE 23.2 Physical Activity (PA) Values

| Boys age 3 to 18 years of age | PA = 1.0 (sedentary) PA = 1.13 (low active) PA = 1.26 (active) PA = 1.42 (very active) |
| Girls 3 to 18 years of age | PA = 1.0 (sedentary) PA = 1.16 (low active) PA = 1.31 (active) PA = 1.56 (very active) |

Modified from Institute of Medicine of the National Academies. *Dietary Reference Intakes for Energy, Carbohydrate, Fiber, Fat, Fatty Acids, Cholesterol, Protein, and Amino Acids.* Washington, DC: The National Academies Press; 2005.[9]

Here is an example of calculating estimated energy expenditure using METs and known RMR. A 17 year old female weighing 65 kg with an RMR of 1578 kcals/day determined by indirect calorimetry rowing for 45 minutes on an ergometer (rowing machine):

1578/1440 = 1.09 kcals/min (RMR) × 9.5 (MET ergometer general) = 10.4 kcals/min × 45 minutes = 468 kcals of energy expended during her 45 minute session on the rowing machine.

METs can be calculated using just the weight of the athlete in kg × MET × hours (minutes/60); however, this does not take growth into account or body composition, significantly limiting accuracy. EER calculations may be preferred for accuracy; however, this may be useful as general guidelines or if limited information is available on an athlete.

An example of this calculation with the same athlete listed above would be 65 (kg) × 9.5 (MET for rowing) 0.75 hours performed = 463 kcals expended during that exercise.

While every attempt must be made to accurately determine energy requirements in young athletes, growth, athletic ability, and body composition will always vary from day to day and season to season. Therefore, providing a range of energy needs or minimum calorie goal combined with best clinical judgement continues to be a prudent practice with this population.

▶ Protein

Increased protein needs above the DRI for age are required for muscle protein synthesis; however, most young athletes and non-athletes routinely eat above the DRI for this macronutrient.

A protein intake of 1.0–1.5 grams/kg/day protein is indicated, using the higher values for those activities that would require higher levels of muscle turnover.[10] Examples include gymnastics, crew, or weight training. A child engaged in endurance sport such as soccer, biking, or running may require the lower end of the range.[10]

Young endurance athletes who routinely train require 1.2–1.4 grams/kg/day.[10] This is easily consumed as part of a usual meal plan as the increased energy requirements for endurance athletes and is therefore not usually an issue.

Elite young athletes who train regularly could require even higher levels of protein of 1.5–2 gm/kg/day.[10] Also, a young athlete's energy intake while training may need a protein intake above 1.7 gm/kg/day in order to preserve lean body mass.[10]

Protein needs can also be prescribed as a percentage of total energy intake. Children and teens aged 4 to 18 years of age require 10–30% of energy from protein.[9,10] Special attention to adequate protein intake will be indicated for athletes who consume exclusively vegan or predominantly plant based diets. These diets may require increased protein intakes of 10–20% in order to meet protein needs.[8]

▶ Carbohydrate

Next to energy intake, optimal carbohydrate intake is a key component to optimizing an athlete's performance through nutrition.[8,10,12] Carbohydrate recommendations vary based on sport, sex, and environmental conditions. Carbohydrates are required to maintain blood glucose levels during exercise and replace muscle glycogen stores.[8,10,12] Compared with protein or energy restricted diets, carbohydrate restricting appears to be the most detrimental to athletes.[8] Ideally, providing a combination of complex and simple carbohydrate sources is best in order to promote rapid repletion of glycogen stores and support aerobic activity.

The recommended ranges for carbohydrate are from 6 to 10 grams/kg/day depending on the athlete and duration of time before a competition. Younger athletes

typically fall in the lower end and older adolescent typically require the higher end of the range.[10] The intensity of the exercise, the higher the amount of carbohydrate required for optimal performance. Zero to light intensity activity requires 3–5 grams of carbohydrate per kilogram per day.[8,10,12] Moderate to heavy activity requires 5–8 grams per kilogram per day.

To promote increased glycogen storage, fueling before an event generally requires 8–9 grams/kg/day of carbohydrates for the 24 hours before an event. Repletion of glycogen stores after an event requires 0.8–1.0 grams/kg/hour for the remainder of the day.[8,10,12]

The timing of carbohydrate with moderate amounts of protein can help a young athlete perform and recover from intense physical activity. Meals should be approximately 4–6 hours before an event to allow optimal storage of fuel and digestion to occur.[8,10,12] Meals should be well balanced including a mix of simple and complex carbohydrates combined with quality protein. A light snack can be provided within 1 hour of exercise that includes ~50 grams of carbohydrate and 5–10 grams of protein.[10]

During exercise, most children and young athletes do not require additional carbohydrates since most activities are less than 1 hour in duration. If there are multiple events in one day, light snacks between events with complex and simple carbohydrates are preferred along with some protein sources. A high carbohydrate meal should be provided within 2 hours after exercise. Chocolate milk with 23 grams of carbohydrate and 8 grams of protein per 8 oz. serving is typically considered high in sugar for non-athletic children and remains an optimal suggested light snack for young athletes which is widely accepted and consumed.

If an athletic event lasts longer than 1 hour duration a 6% carbohydrate solution can be consumed at the rate of 0.7 gram/kg/hour.[8,10,12] However, athletes should be encouraged to rinse with water after consuming sports beverages. Sports drinks are considered extremely corrosive to teeth and increase the risk of dental caries.[13] While sports drinks can prevent hyponatremia from hypervolemia, discussed later in the chapter, it remains uncertain if carbohydrate or fat is the preferred nutrient for prolonged exercises since children have higher rates of fatty acid oxidation than adults.[14]

▶ Fat

Fat calories can be considered the protein sparing calories that provide additional energy to prevent the use of protein as a fuel source. Once estimated needs for carbohydrate and protein have been met, additional calories in the form of fats are required to meet estimated energy requirements. Children ages 4–18 years of age should consume a range between 25–35% of calories from fat.[9,10]

Fat calories are nutrient dense at 9 kcals per gram which allow for greater calorie intake with decreased volume. This is extremely useful for athletes with extremely high energy requirements. Higher fat foods prolong gastric emptying and are not encouraged as part of the meal before exercise or meet, therefore are more typically consumed early in the morning or after athletic events have concluded for the day. Encouraging healthy fats such as avocado, olive oil, nuts, and nut butters are excellent ways to increase calories without increasing volume.

▶ Fiber

Fiber remains part of a healthy diet for young athletes. Current recommendations are 14 grams per 1000 calories.[8,10] It's commonly understood that high fiber diets remain helpful for lowering cholesterol, blood pressure, and enhance insulin sensitivity.[8] A high fiber intake delays gastric emptying and can promote feelings of satiety.[10] A high fiber diet rich in fruits and vegetables has been shown to promote weight loss and weight maintenance.[8] In athletes with high calorie needs, a high fiber diet may result in delayed gastric emptying and premature feelings of fullness that can make meeting their energy goals difficult.

If an athlete requires a high carbohydrate and high energy diet, consuming mostly whole grains and fruits can be potentially too high in fiber for a young athlete to perform optimally. This can cause GI distress particularly with prolonged or stressful competitive events. Encourage whole grains and whole fruits and vegetables in combination with some 100% fruit juices and lower fiber foods to allow for a balanced diet. It's important that athletes know how their bodies react with particular foods and adopting the "nothing new on competition day" is good advice. Working with a young athlete to determine which foods provide the best nutrients and which foods to avoid so they may perform at their best is a significant part of a sports dietitian's role in training young athletes.

▶ Hydration, Heat and Electrolyte Management

Recent research shows that young athletes are just as effective at thermoregulation and exercise heat tolerance as adults if adequate hydration is maintained.[10,15,16] However, according to the American Academy of Pediatrics, exertional heat stroke is the leading cause of preventable death in youth sports.[16] There is greater emphasis on acclimatization of young athletes in sport, which means allowing young athletes to develop a tolerance to the environment over time. Exercise intensity should be increased in increments as well as the addition of protective equipment in stages, which may prevent evaporation

TABLE 23.4 Sweat Rates of Young Athletes Based on Age	
Prepubescent children	<400 ml/hr.
9–12 year old boys and girls	300–700 ml/hr.
Young adolescents	1000 ml/hr.
Older adolescents	2.5 L or more/hour with intense exercise in heat

Data from Bergeron M F, Hargreaves M. Haymes E. et al. Exercise and fluid replacement. American College of Sports Medicine Position Stand. *Med Sci Sports Exerc.* 2007;39(2):377–390.[15]
Bergeron MF. Reducing sports heat illness risk. *Pediatr Rev.* 2013;34(6):270–279.[16]

of sweat (cooling mechanisms in the body).[16] **TABLE 23.4** provides information on sweat rates for young athletes. Young athletes are at high risk for fluid and sodium deficits during exercise and competition.[15,16] As little as 2% of body weight loss can decrease aerobic capacity and performance.[12,15,16] There is also evidence that this impairs mental acuity and cognition.[12,15,16] Meal consumption 8 to 12 hours before exercise promotes euhydration.[16]

If sodium and electrolyte loss is expected as part of the day's events, meal consumption should also be higher in sodium. Pizza, commonly limited in most healthy diets, can be appropriate for young athletes before an event. Pizza tends to be readily accepted by young athletes, high in sodium, carbohydrates, nutrient dense, generally well tolerated and is easily obtained during travel events. A high sodium intake the night before an event is commonly referred to "front loading-salt." Occasional use of jargon appropriate to the activity may help promote participation with a skeptical teen athlete during a counseling session.

The 5–7 ml/kg of fluid 4 hours before exercise has been recommended for adults. Customized fluid replacement programs will always remain preferred and are most effective with young athletes. If additional hydration is determined to be required 2 hours before an event, an additional 3–5 ml/kg of fluid can be consumed slowly.[17]

▶ During Exercise

One of the biggest challenges for young athletes is to maintain hydration during exercise. The goal of any athlete is to prevent dehydration and electrolyte changes that may impair athletic performance with excessive

TABLE 23.5 Fluid Replacement During Exercise		
100–250 ml	Every 20 minutes	9–12 year olds during exercise
1.5–2 liters	Per hour	Older adolescents

Modified from Bergeron MF. Reducing sports heat illness risk. *Pediatr Rev.* 2013;34(6):270–279.[16]

dehydration of > 2% of body weight lost during exercise.[17] Frequent water breaks are needed to prevent 1–2 % loss of body weight during exercise. (See **TABLE 23.5**) Both flavored and unflavored beverages should be offered to promote intake. Although sports drinks have not been shown to be more beneficial than just water in most activities, flavored beverages tend to have increased acceptance by young athletes over plain water.[18] Since preventing dehydration is of primary concern, both should be offered for those young athletes who may not drink enough water.

▸ Post Exercise

The goal is to replace fluids and electrolytes lost during exercise. Typically this can be accomplished with regularly scheduled meals and beverages.[16] Consuming sodium in foods and in fluids help promote thirst and increase retention of fluids. Offering salty foods such as soups, pretzels, vegetable juice, and pickles can be a useful tool to increase fluid and electrolyte intake.[16]

▸ Hyperhydration

Under specific conditions, such as in very hot weather, if an athlete is only drinking water this can cause dilutional hyponatremia. Dehydration tends to be very common, however, dilutional hyponatremia is more dangerous. When visceral sodium levels fall extremely low, dangerous swelling of the brain can result in seizures, coma, and death.[10,14–16] Women appear to be more at risk for dilutional hyponatremia than men.[17]

Sweat rates for children vary greatly. Prepubescent children have lower sweat rates, while adolescent boys have significantly higher sweat rates (see Table 23.4). Pediatric health care providers and dietitians should tailor their fluid and electrolyte recommendations using clinical judgement regarding fluids and sodium intake via food or electrolyte beverages.

Additionally, an interesting symptom often described by athletes in need of more electrolytes is a change in the taste of water. If water suddenly does not taste good in extremely hot weather, it is possible more sodium is indicated. Therefore, providing athletes, and in particular young children, with frequent breaks, salty snacks, and flavored beverages as well as water is recommended.

▸ Energy Drinks and Sports Drinks

By definition, a sports drink contains carbohydrates, minerals, electrolytes, and flavoring that are intended for replacing fluid and electrolytes during exercise. Energy drinks contain stimulants such as caffeine, guarana, taurine, ginseng, l- carnitine, and creatine for the purported purpose of performance enhancing effects.[18]

Dental erosion is one of the harmful effects of both sports and energy drinks. Most of these beverages have a pH between 3–4. Citric acid is a frequent additive that contributes to dental erosion even after pH has been neutralized.[13,18]

Sports drinks might have a specific role for some young athletes engaged in extensive activity or tournaments in order to help with hydration and electrolyte repletion. For most children and adolescents, sports drinks, as with other sugar sweetened beverages, potentially increase the risk of obesity.[18] Energy drinks, on the other hand, have no benefit at all and have potential health risks. Energy drinks routinely contain large quantities of caffeine, which can be harmful to children. Energy drinks and the use of caffeine should be discouraged in all children.[18] **TABLE 23.6** describes energy vs. sports drinks.

TABLE 23.6 Examples of Sports Drinks vs Energy Drinks (Common Brand Names)	
Sports Drinks	**Energy Drinks**
Gatorade	Java Monster
Gatorade Propel	Monster Energy
Gatorade Endurance	Monster Low Carb
Gatorade G2	Red Bull
PowerAde	Full Throttle
PowerAde Zero	Rock Star

Modified from Bergeron MF. Reducing sports heat illness risk. *Pediatr Rev.* 2013;34(6): 270–279.[16]

Marketing

The impacts of marketing on children and unhealthy food choices, brand choices, and purchase intentions are well understood. According to a one study with over 100 professional athletes' endorsements of energy-dense, nutrient-poor food products, both adolescents and their parents are more likely to perceive them as being healthier than non-endorsed products.[19] Parents as well as young athletes can fall prey to clever marketing.

Ergogenic Aids and Supplements

Adolescents in particular are more prone to try new diets or supplements in order to improve their performance or change their body composition. Many psychological factors are motivation for these risk taking behaviors.[20] Society and social media tend to reward success in sports with favoritism in social circles.[20] This dangerous fact remains concerning to health care professionals regarding habits or supplements that have not been adequately studied in young athletes. A clinical dietitian should be aware of the supplements and fad diets, their purported advantages, and discourage any harmful behaviors.

A performance-enhancing substance is any substance that is taken for the purpose of improving athletic performance by altering body composition, speed, strength, or causing changes in behavior and pain sensitivity.[20]

The American Academy of Pediatrics has made a 3-point statement on performance enhancing substances[20]:

1. The intentional use of any substance for performance enhancement is unfair and, therefore, morally and ethically indefensible.[20]

2. Using any substance for the purpose of enhancing sports performance, including over-the-counter supplements, the composition and quality of which are not under federal regulation, may pose a significant health risk to the young person.[20]

3. Using and promoting performance-enhancing substances tends to devalue the principles of a balanced diet, good coaching, and sound physical training.[20]

Young athletes will not usually volunteer information regarding the use of performance enhancing substances. Therefore, it can be difficult to determine their use. Pediatric dietitians and health care providers are encouraged to ask about performance enhancing substances. **TABLE 23.7** provides information on these ergogenic aids and supplements. Adolescent male athletes

TABLE 23.7 List of Common Ergogenic Aids and Supplements

Category		Purported Intended Use	Suggested Response
Free amino acid supplements	Amino acid powders under many names	Purported to boost muscle growth	Can be obtained from high protein foods particularly cottage cheese and Greek yogurt
Creatine monohydrate	The most popular supplement used for strength training	Purported to increase strength and power	Not studied in children and notable weight gain of 10 pounds or more if found to be a responder. Major sources of creatine can be found in beef and fish
Protein shakes	Marketed under a variety of names.	More protein builds muscle faster.	Chocolate milk is preferable with two types of protein and 23 grams of carbohydrate to make a 4:1 carb to protein ratio
Caffeine	Found in energy drinks as well as coffee tea and colas	Purported to decrease perception of exertion in athletes	Caffeine should be avoided with children and adolescents. Increased risk of cardiovascular and neurological risks.
Bicarbonate citrate	3 grams/kg/body weight	Purported use in high intensity events of anaerobic system. Bicarbonate is used as an extra buffering system.	Children have limited anaerobic capacity below a certain age. There is also a risk that any supplement can be potentially contaminated with banned substances.

Data from Rodriguez NR, DiMarco NM, Langley S, et al. Position of the Academy of Nutrition and Dietetics, Dietitians of Canada, and the American College of Sports Medicine: Nutrition and athletic performance. *J Amer Diet Assoc.* 2009;109(3)509–527.[8]
Academy of Nutrition and Dietetics. Sports nutrition manual. Available at: www.nutritioncaremanual.org. Accessed January 13, 2018.[10]

involved in activities in which strength, power, and size are of value are known to be at higher risk for using anabolic or androgenic compounds, so teens involved in these types of sports are at greatest risk.[20] Also, those that are involved in lean sports are more likely to use performance-enhancing compounds over non lean sports.[20]

The World Anti-Doping Agency and the NCAA provide updated annual lists of substances banned both in and out of competition. These lists include anabolic agents, growth hormones, beta-2 agonists, diuretics and masking agents, blood products, stimulants, steroids and more. Young athletes with future plans of participating in sports in college or beyond should be made aware of the dangers when taking any supplement for fear of disqualification. Regardless of rationale or intent, athletes are responsible for everything they consume including vitamins or protein supplements. They need to be prepared for the consequences of testing positive which would likely lead to disqualification and lose their eligibility.

The USP verification (United States Pharmacopeia) might test for purity, quality, and potency, however, they do not check for banned substances found in sport. Therefore they are not the best certification to determine safety if a supplement is required. Better certification choices to find sport approved supplements can be found with Aegis Shield Certification, **Banned Substances Control Group** (BSCG certified drug free logo), Informed Choice, and NSF Certified for Sport www.nsfsport.com.[10]

▶ Vegetarian Athlete

Many young athletes choose to avoid animal and animal products in their diet. Lacto-ovo vegetarians and pesco-vegetarians typically can have fairly balanced diets meeting most of their nutrient requirements. In young athletes who receive the majority of their protein intake from vegetarian sources such as beans, whole grain cereals may need to have their estimated protein needs determined at a higher level.[8,10,21] These incomplete amino acid proteins have a low **Digestible Indispensable Amino Acid Score** (DIAAS) or **Protein Digestibility Corrected Amino Acid Score** (PDCAAS).[21] If animal protein has scores closer to 1.0 maximum score, many nuts, grains, and cereals, including soy, have scores 10 to 30 percent lower on average.[21] Milk has a PDCAA score of 100%, soy 91% and wheat of 42%.[21]

For example an active young vegan athlete with a high protein need of 1.5 grams/kg/day, would need a goal of 1.8 grams/kg/day since their protein sources are

plant based. This might also apply to non-vegetarian athletes who have food preferences that tend to be from a majority of plant-based protein sources as well. It is also recommended that when calorie intake is reduced for weight management, that protein intake be increased to as high as 2.2 gm/kg/day.[22]

While recent research shows combining foods during each meal is no longer required.[10,21] Vegetarian athletes tend to be have lower intakes of lysine, threonine, tryptophan, and methionine.[8] It remains beneficial to consume a recovery snack including a complete amino acid profile to optimize muscle synthesis.[21]

Vegan athletes are at higher risk for both macronutrient deficiencies, low protein, and fat intake while having adequate or high carbohydrate and fiber intakes. **TABLE 23.8** provides information on high protein food choices for vegetarian athletes. There is some evidence that vegans appear to have a lower intake of n-3 fatty acids with the omission of seafood,[21] therefore emphasis on high in ALA such as flax seeds, chia seeds, and walnuts should be encouraged. Particular focus on micronutrients such as Vitamin D, iron, zinc, calcium, iodine and vitamin B_{12} become significantly important in young athletes to support daily requirements and growth, and the increased need related to muscle development.[23]

TABLE 23.8 High Protein Vegetarian Food Choices

Mixed nuts lightly salted	1 oz.	5.68 grams protein
Tofu	½ cup	10.3 grams protein
Black beans	1 cup cooked	15.24 grams
High protein cereals (kashi GO lean crisp)?	3/4 cup	11.27 grams protein
Egg noodles	1 cup cooked	7.25 grams protein
Peanut butter	1 tablespoon	7.11 grams protein
Quinoa	1 cup cooked	8.14 grams

Modified list from United States Department of Agriculture. USDA branded food products database. Available at: https://ndb.nal.usda.gov/ndb/foods Accessed: June 1, 2018.[24]

Special Consideration of Micronutrients Specific to Athletes

There is no research to show additional vitamins above DRI for age enhanced athletic performance. If a young athlete is taking in an adequate number of calories to meet their needs and eating a variety of foods, they can easily meet their micronutrient requirements for vitamins and minerals. However particular attention should be paid to iron, calcium, and vitamin D as both athletes and non-athletes are more likely to be deficient as determined to be under consumed relative to the **estimated average requirement** (EAR).[25]

Iron

Iron in food occurs in both heme and non heme foods. The major sources of heme iron occur from consuming hemoglobin and myoglobin beef, fish, chicken, and eggs. Nonheme iron in foods occurs from plant based foods such as green leafy vegetables, beans, cereals, and grains. Heme iron is more readily available at 15–35% versus nonheme iron of 2–20%.[26] The DRI for iron in children ages 4–8 years is 10 mg per day. At 8 to 13 years the DRI decreases to 8 mg per day for both sexes. Girls ages 14–18 require 15 mg of iron per day and boys ages 14–18 require 11 mg per day.[25] Iron supplementation may be required if a young athlete consumes a limited diet low in heme iron. Biochemical data to determine iron deficiency include Hematocrit, hemoglobin, low mean corpuscular volume, transferrin saturation, and increased total iron-binding capacity and decreased ferritin levels are of particular interest.[10]

Calcium

Calcium is an essential mineral for bone development. Young athletes typically have an increased bone mineral density (BMD) of 5–15% from non-athletes which implies that calcium intake requirement might be higher; however, no evidence has proven that increased calcium above DRI enhances athletic performance.[8,25] The DRI for calcium for children ages 4–8 years old is 1000 mg per day and increases to 1300 for both boys and girls ages 9–18 years of age.[25]

Vitamin D

There has been considerable interest in vitamins in recent years related to the increased rate and magnitude of Vitamin D deficiency and its importance in many functions beyond bone mineralization and health. In the last 30 years, over 77% of Americans are now considered to have vitamin D insufficiency.[27,28] For adult and young athletes alike, the discovery of vitamin D receptors in other tissue in the body, particularly muscle, has become a particular interest with physical performance and injury.[27] Studies have indicated that low vitamin D levels show signs of atrophy in muscle fibers.[28] There is potential that those athletes with low vitamin D levels might have improved muscle strength when supplementation is initiated.[27]

Athletes that are at high risk for vitamin D deficiency are those who practice indoors, wear large quantities of padding/helmets, or any scenario with limited UVB sun exposure.[27] A pediatric health care practitioner should ensure adequate vitamin D intake in order to meet DRI for age and possible recommendations to check vitamin D levels in the event additional supplementation is required. Vitamin D deficiency treatment has two phases:

1. Restoration of vitamin D levels to acceptable limits based on lab tests
2. Maintenance supplementation dose to support levels within acceptable range.

Adult indoor athletes who are deficient or insufficient, can require up to 5,000 IU of vitamin D per day for eight weeks in order to reach normal levels; then 1,000 IU per day for maintenance with a plan to recheck vitamin D levels to ensure that levels remain within acceptable limits.[29]

Weight Management and Lean Sports

Prepubertal young athletes should not be encouraged to lose weight for the sole purpose of improving athletic performance.[30] While physique itself has not been shown to improve athletic performance, some athletes that carry excessive amounts of body fat have increased heat sensitivity, decreased speed, and endurance moving the additional weight through space. Young athletes with the desire to lose body fat must continue to consume enough energy to support growth, muscle, and the energy expended with sport. Fat loss should be gradual: about ½ pound per week is preferred; however, other methods determining fat loss are preferred. Maximum allowable weight loss for young athletes is 1.5% per week.[10] Beyond this, most athletes start to lose lean body mass. As stated earlier in this chapter, the using BMI in athletes is not recommended since they tend to weight more with increased muscle and bone.[31] Most athletes have a BMI between the 50th and 75%ile for age.[31] DEXA scans used to determine BMD (as described later in this chapter) will also provide **fat free muscle mass** (FFM) data for estimated calculations. For practical

TABLE 23.9 Adolescent Reference Ranges for Body Fat		
Male body fat of 12.7–17.2%	Female 21.5–25.4%	Reference ranges for adolescents
10–13% for males	17–20% for females	Low fat body composition
7–10% for male – very low fat	14–17% for female	Very low fat *Female must be eumenorrheic to meet considered meeting energy requirement

Data from American Academy of Pediatrics Committee on Sports Medicine and Fitness. Promotion of healthy weight-control practices in young athletes. *Pediatrics.* 2005;116(6):1557–1564.[31]

TABLE 23.10 Lean vs. Non Lean Sports	
Lean Sports	**Non Lean Sports**
Gymnastics, dance, cheerleading, diving, skating (aesthetic sports)	swimming
Rowing, Horse racing, (weight-class sports)	baseball
Wrestling, weight lifting (weight-class sports)	football
Bodybuilding (weight-class and aesthetic)	soccer
Triathlon, cycling, distance running (endurance sports)	hockey

Modified from Thompson R. Sherman R T. *Eating Disorders in Sport.* New York, NY: Routledge Taylor & Francis Group; 2010:33–51.[32]

purposes, a simple waist circumference measure can be used to determine a gradual loss of body fat if needed in athletes. However, if body composition is available in a young athlete, a single target number should be avoided and should be expressed as a range that is realistic and appropriate. (**TABLE 23.9**) Regardless of the measure used for determining progress, practitioners and clinicians should reinforce how an athlete feels, the rate of recovery, their performance and ensure that growth continues. Generally speaking, calorie deficits for weight loss would be only 200–300 less than originally estimated to provide enough of a deficit to decrease body fat and conserve muscle mass. Protein intake should remain the same or increase to 1.8–2 grams/kg/day as previously described in the chapter under protein.[8,10]

The type of sport a child participates in can impact intake or increase risk for disordered eating and unhealthy weight related practices. Children who engage in lean sport vs. non-lean sports are at greater risk. Lean sports are defined by an advantage in performance based on a low weight or lower body fat provides an advantage or improved scoring by judges.[31] See **TABLE 23.10**.

Dehydration is a common practice used by athletes in weight classed sports such as wrestling. These practices include fluid restriction, spitting, using laxatives, diuretics, rubber suits, steam baths, and saunas.[31] **Lowest allowable weight** (LAW) was developed as part of preventing dehydration and rapid weight loss related to wrestlers as part of the National College Athletic Association.[33] This is a combination of calculations using a urine specific gravity that must be less than or equal to 1.020. The sample is taken to determine euhydration. Body composition is then obtained in order to determine

FFM, with an additional 5% for body fat to calculate the lowest possible weight of the athlete. Lowest allowable weight for an athlete must have 5% body fat.[33]

Weight gain in athletes most often involves an increase in desired muscle mass and avoiding additional body fat. EER using calculation previously described in this chapter should be determined, and then add additional energy that the young athlete can tolerate. Nutrient dense foods with a variety of nutrients should be encouraged. Many young athletes have significant energy requirements making it difficult to meet based on time and scheduling limitations. Meeting energy needs can sometimes be a challenge:

- Encourage 6–8 meals per day
- Stress the importance of eating frequently
- Encourage the consumption of high calorie beverages such as full fat chocolate milk, smoothies, and shakes
- Encourage snacks that include carbohydrates, proteins, and fats

Weight gain in athletes generally involves a change in body composition with an increase in desired muscle mass and avoiding additional body fat. (EER using the calculation previously described in this chapter should be determined, and then add additional energy that the young athlete can tolerate. Nutrient dense foods with a variety of nutrients should be encouraged. Many young athletes have significant energy requirements making it difficult to meet based on time and scheduling limitations. Since athletes are typically very regimented, it is easier to add nutrient dense foods to established meal plans by the athlete versus creating new meals entirely.

TABLE 23.11 Nutrient Rich Add-ons to Meals	
	Examples of Supplemental Calories that Can be Added to Meals
Breakfast	16 oz. 100% fruit juice
Snack	12 oz. chocolate milk, ½ cup salted nuts
Lunch	2 sandwiches with banana, peanut butter, and 16 oz. chocolate milk
Snack	Whole wheat bagel with cream cheese and nut based granola bar
Snack	Protein shake with protein powder, Greek yogurt, banana, chocolate syrup, and nut butter
Supper	16 oz. low fat milk or juice, 2 tablespoons flavored olive oil and 2 oz. whole grain bread for dipping
Bedtime Snack	2 Peanut butter and jelly sandwich and 16 oz. glass of milk and large piece of fruit

Additionally, stress the importance of meals and snacks as part of the training program and avoid skipping as them as much as possible. See **TABLE 23.11**.

▶ Female Athlete Triad

The Female Athlete Triad was developed as part of a combination of symptoms noted in female athletes in 1992.[17] The components of the female athlete triad are **low energy availability** (EA) with or without an **eating disorder** (ED), low BMD, and functional hypothalamic amenorrhea.[17,34,35] These symptoms can occur in combination or in isolation.

In 2007 the **Academy of Sports Medicine** (ACSM) went further to describe the Female Athlete Triad as a part of 3 interrelated spectrums; energy availability, menstrual function, and bone density. Menstrual function ranges from eumenorrhea to amenorrhea (cycle >90 days), including oligo menorrhea (cycle of >35 days).[17]

Incidence and prevalence since the ACSM position paper was published shows that only a small percentage of athletes actually have all 3 Triad conditions of either low estimated availability or disordered eating in combination with menstrual imbalance and measured low BMD of 0–15.9%.[35] However, the incidence of having only one or two of the conditions appears to be considerably higher in recent studies.[35] More recent studies focusing on adolescents show that BMD based on participation in certain sports such as endurance running have a higher prevalence of low BMD with a z-score of <1.0.[35] Additionally, studies that show low BMD as young adults might be contributing from low BMD as adolescents and the inability to accumulate adequate bone mass verses increased bone loss.[35]

Diagnosis

Early diagnosis and treatment of any disordered eating is a priority. Typically, athletes will not disclose disordered eating.[31] Attitudes and food habits should be routinely incorporated into medical portions of participation examinations.[36] While no "gold standard" questionnaire exists, the RED-S Risk Assessment Model and the Low Energy Availability in Females Questionnaire are a few examples.

It is understood than young athletes have higher BMI scores compared with their non-athletes of the same age due to the increased amount of muscle and bone thereby limiting the ability to screen for obesity in athletes. BMI can still be a useful tool to determine changes for the monitoring of under feeding and inadequate energy intake. Delayed onset of puberty can also be an indicator of inadequate energy availability, therefore assessing maturity levels (Tanner Stages of Puberty) is required.[17] As a dietitian working with any athlete, if there is a situation where disordered eating is suspected, referrals to a supervising physician should be made and an interdisciplinary team should be assembled as soon a feasible.

BMD should also be tested after a stress or low impact fracture and after a total of 6 months of menstrual dysfunction and disordered eating.[17] Diagnosis via DEXA for athletes less than 20 years of age, posterior-anterior spine, and whole body are the preferred sites for testing.[17] The **International Society for Clinical Densitometry** (ISCD) recommends avoiding the terms osteopenia and osteoporosis in adolescents.[34] BMD is to be expressed in terms of z-scores instead of T-scores as is done with postmenopausal women. z-scores of <-2.0 is considered "low bone mineral density" for chronological age for adolescents and premenopausal females.[34] However, a z-score of <-1 might be indicative of lower than expected BMD in athletes as they have between 5–15% more bone density than non-athletes. Any z-score of <-1 in athletes, indicates further evaluation is necessary.[34,36]

Recommended laboratory tests include chemistry profiles, complete blood counts, thyroid function tests, and urinalysis. Normal values can still be found in severely undernourished individuals. No tests exist for hypothalamic amenorrhea which is a diagnosis of exclusion of other causes of amenorrhea.

Intervention

The treatment requires a multidisciplinary approach including physician, psychologist or psychiatrist, a registered dietitian, physical therapist, athletic trainer, coach, family, and patient.

The initial and crucial first step in treatment is to restore positive energy balance and or reduce energy expenditure by decreasing activity.[17,35,37] Athletes are often able to continue to practice provided they can increase their intake to meet estimated energy requirements and promote participation in treatment.[17,34,35]

Providing adequate energy availability in the treatment of low BMD by either increasing energy intake or decreasing energy expenditure is crucial. Increased calorie intake is more effective in improving BMD with weight gain and hypothalamic amenorrhea than with medication.[17,34–37] Increasing energy intake to >30 kcals/kg of FFM per day has been found to restore menses however > 45 kcals/kg/day of FFM is considered optimal.[34]

Estimation of FFM can be obtained with the results of DEXA determination of BMD. This can be done using bioelectrical impedance or triceps skinfold calipers. It is recommended that the same healthcare provider obtain the serial measurements over time for the sake of accuracy.[36] Determining energy needs can be complex; additional recommendations of 200–600 kcals increase in daily intake along with reducing training 1 day per week can also be implemented when indicated by clinical judgement.[36]

Additionally, 1300 mg of calcium, and 600 IU of vitamin D should be either incorporated into the diet or supplemented. Vitamin D levels should be obtained with the next available blood draw along with routine lab work to determine if additional deficiencies are present.

Oral contraceptives should only be prescribed for the purpose of contraception and not for correcting amenorrhea in women of child-bearing age.[34] Bisphosphonates for bone mineral density used for treating osteoporosis in postmenopausal women should be avoided due to their teratogenic effects and long half-life in athletes of childbearing age.[34]

▶ Male Athletes

Males have also been known to have decreased energy availability potentially causing decreased bone mineral density and negatively impacting the endocrine system.[35] Low testosterone and estradiol levels have been documented in adolescent males with anorexia nervosa.[36] Recently, the IOC consensus group has introduced a new term, **Relative Energy Deficiency in Sport** (RED-S), to describe a variety of physiological implications from decreased energy availability for both men and women in 2014.[38] However, it appears much more research needs to be done in this area before this terminology is routinely adopted.[39]

▶ Conclusion

In conclusion, there is no one particular factor in opitmizing nutrition in young athletes. It remains a constant balance of assessing nutrient utilization related to nutrient intake. Determining macronutrient and micronutrient needs to optimize growth and performance remains a combination of clinical judgement with evidence based nutrition in with extremely active young athletes. Adequate hydration continues to be one of the most frequent and significant factors in ensuring optimal performance. Insufficient energy intake related to energy expenditure cannot only lead to decreased performance and suboptimal growth but possible other metabolic complications as described in the female athlete triad. While protein recommendations and supplements remain ubiquitous on the internet, young athletes tend to easily reach these increased goals in their diet. It is crucial that pediatric clinical dietitians provide evidenced based nutrition information to young athletes to protect them from false and potentially harmful practices frequently promoted on the web and on social media.

🔍 CASE STUDIES

Case Study #1
Nutrition Assessment

CJ is a 15-year-old female figure skater. She is 5'2" (1.57 m) tall and weighs 138 pounds (62.7 kg). She was instructed by her coach to lose weight for competition. She started a low carbohydrate diet avoiding all grains, cereals, and starches. She eats protein and vegetables for most meals. Her mother expresses concern that she has a hard time waking up in the morning. CJ also complains of constant fatigue. She has been logging her calories in a dieting app on her phone. Per her log, she consumes 1400–1600 kcals per day and 80 to 120 grams of protein. She practices on the ice 5 days a week for 2 hours. She teaches skating to children on Saturdays for 3 hours and does two high intensity cardio classes per week for 1 hour and an additional yoga class on Sunday. Per CJ's mother, her pediatrician has said she is nearly done growing, but her menstrual cycle is sporadic. She has not had any weight loss success since starting the low carbohydrate low calorie diet. No medical tests are available.

Estimated Needs

EER = 135.3 – (30.8 × 15 years) + (1.56 very active PA) × (10 × 62.7 + 934 × 1.57 m) + 25

EER = 135 – 462 + 3,265 + 25

EER = 2963 kcals per day

Estimated protein intake of 1.8 grams/kg/day = 113 grams per day

Minimum carbohydrate intake to be above 5 grams/kg/day = 314 grams per day

Medical tests: CBC with iron stores including ferritin level and Vitamin D level

Nutrition Diagnosis

(NI-1.2) inadequate energy intake related to inappropriate diet information as evidenced by reported intake significantly below EER and decrease in athletic performance.

(NB1.2) unsupported beliefs/attitudes about food or nutrition related topics related to low carbohydrate, low calorie diet to lose weight with intense training days.

Intervention Goals

1. Increase calories to 2,600 to 2,700 calories per day providing a 300 calorie deficit for fat loss. Provide 50% of calories from carbohydrate = 325–338 grams per day 20% of calorie from protein = 130–135 grams/day 30% of calories from fat = 80–90 grams per day.
2. Provide a meal plan with 6 meals per day of a combination of carbohydrate, protein, and fats including grains, dairy, fruit, and vegetables.
3. Recommend CBC, Ferritin, Vitamin D levels and basic metabolic panel be obtained in light of poor intake and variable menses.
4. Use waist circumference measurement to determine changes in body composition as weight can fluctuate with increased muscle and bone development.
5. Suggest one day of rest to repair muscles and regain strength.

Follow-up appointment 3 months later: CJ's weight has remained stable; however, her waist circumference has declined 1.5 inches. She is on 5,000 IU's of vitamin D daily for repletion of vitamin D deficiency. Other labs are within normal limits and her menses are more regular.

Most importantly is that her energy and stamina have improved greatly and she has expressed satisfaction with her athletic performance.

Discussion

CJ was on a low calorie diet but had no success with weight loss. If CJ had continued to have difficulty reaching her goals with the follow up appointment, the next recommendation might have been from further testing with Metabolic Efficiency (ME) to determine what type of fuel source she is using with training. ME testing is similar to indirect calorimetry involving oxygen and carbon dioxide exchange however this test goes further to determine if she is burning fat or carbohydrate during exercise at a specific heart rate. ME testing is often used by endurance runners to optimize the use of body fat over carbohydrate during races to reduce the amount of additional carbohydrate required during a race.

Case Study #2

Nutrition Assessment

17-year-old TL is a baseball player that has been instructed by his coach to gain weight in the hope of increasing interest of college baseball coaches and possible athletic scholarship. His current practice schedule includes baseball practice Monday - Friday after school from 3:30 to 5:30. He also weight trains at the local gym 4 days per week after dinner and on weekends when he doesn't have a game. Based on 24 hour recall and normal diet with TL's mother's input, he consumes ~2400–2500 kcals per day and 150–200 grams of protein. He eats a variety of foods, fruit, vegetables, whole grains. He avoids dairy and uses almond milk vs regular milk based on information he read on the internet regarding inflammation and protein powders.

Ht 5'11" Weight 177 pounds (80.5 kg)   Goal weight: 190–200 pounds (LBM)

Estimated Needs

EER = 88.5 – (30.8 × 17) + 1.42 × (26.7 × 80.5 + 903 × 1.8) + 25

EER = 5,012 kcals/day + 500 calories for weight gain = 5,000–5,500 kcals per day

Estimated protein needs of 145 grams/kg/day (1.8 gm/kg/day)

(continues)

CASE STUDIES

Nutrition Diagnosis

(NB-2.2) Excessive physical activity related to high intensity exercise of more than 3 hours per day most days per week as evidenced by inability to gain weight.

(NB1.1) Food and nutrition related knowledge deficit related to avoidance of milk products and use of almond milk causing inflammation.

Interventions/Goals

1. Provide a meal plan with 8 meals per day including high calorie foods to meet estimated needs of 5,000–5,500 kcals per day and a macronutrient breakdown of 50% of calories as carbohydrate 625 grams – 688 grams per day (7 grams/kg/day), 15 % of calorie from protein 187 grams– 206 grams per day and 35% of calories from fat 195 grams – 214 grams per day
2. Vitamin D level with next blood draw and physician's office
3. Reintroduce dairy products such as yogurt, milk, chocolate milk and cheeses
4. Provide education regarding NCAA regulations on supplements, testing and potential risks of disqualification
5. Allow one day of rest minimum for muscle repair
6. Eat both whole grains and some refined carbohydrates with unsaturated fats such as avocados, olive oils, nuts and seeds to high nutrition and moderate to low volume

Follow-up Appointment 3 Months Later

TL complains of constant hunger now even though he is eating constantly. He has gained 10 pounds and is happy with the progress he has made. He is very careful to avoid any supplements that could potentially disqualify him next year in college.

Discussion

Additional testing such as skin calipers or bio-impedance data would have been helpful to obtain to ensure that TL's weight gain was lean body mass or muscle mass. Note TL's protein at 15% of energy needs to continue to be at or above estimated needs to lean body mass.

Additionally his constant hunger indicates a need to reevaluate his EER as he likely needs a further increase in his calories.

Study Questions

1. A mother inquires about how much water she should encourage her 10 year old son to drink during a soccer game in hot weather. What is the most appropriate response to her question?

2. A 16 year old female gymnast has made an appointment to see you with her mother because her coach has instructed her to lose 10 pounds. What would the optimal methods to determining body composition be?

3. A 15 year old male long distance runner is complaining of weight loss and fatigue. He weighs 68 kg and 5'10" tall. What percentage of calories should come from carbohydrates?

4. A young 13 year old female soccer player is vegetarian but consumes limited dairy. What are her estimated protein requirements?

References

1. Healthychildren.orgv. Sports goals and applications–preschoolers American Academy of Pediatrics. Available at: https://www.healthychildren.org/English/ages-stages/preschool/Pages/default.aspx. Accessed July 18, 2017.
2. Physical Activity Guidelines Midcourse Report Subcommittee, 2012. PA guidelines for Americans midcourse report: Strategies to increase physical activity among youth. U.S. Department of Health and Human Services, 2012. Available at: http://www.health.gov/paguidelines/. Accessed January 6, 2018.
3. Stricker PR. *Sports Success Rx: Your Child's Prescription for the Best Experience.* American Academy of Pediatrics Department of Marketing and Publications:2006.
4. Shell, Adam: Why families stretch their budgets for high-priced youth sports. *USA Today* Sept 5th 2017.
5. Mutz M, Albrecht, P. Parents social status and children's daily physical activity: the role of familial socialization and support. *J Child Fam Stud.* 2017;26(11):3026–3035.
6. Intensive training and sports specialization in young athletes. American Academy of Pediatrics Committee on Sports Medicine and Fitness. *Pediatr.* 2000;106(1 Pt 1):154–157.

7. Sundgot-Borgen J, Torstveit MK. Prevalence of eating disorders in athletes is higher than in the general population. *Clin J Sport Med.* 2004;14(1):25–32.

8. Rodriguez NR, DiMarco NM, Langley S, et al. Position of the Academy of Nutrition and Dietetics, Dietitians of Canada, and the American College of Sports Medicine. Nutrition and athletic performance. *Journ Amer Dietetic Assoc.* 2009:109(3)509–527.

9. Institute of Medicine of the National Academies. *Dietary Reference Intakes for Energy, Carbohydrate, Fiber, Fat, Fatty Acids, Cholesterol, Protein, and Amino Acids.* Washington, DC: The National Academies Press; 2005. www.nap.edu.

10. Academy of Nutrition and Dietetics. Sports nutrition manual. Available at: www.nutritioncaremanual.org 2017. Accessed: January 13, 2018.

11. Ainsworth B, Haskell W, Whitt M, et al. Compendium of physical activities: an update of activity codes and MET intensities. *Med Sci Sports Exerc.* 2000;32 (suppl 9): S498–S504.

12. Kreider B. et al ISSN exercise and Sport nutrition review: research and recommendations. *J Int Soc. Sports Nutr.* 2010;7:7.8–211.

13. Reddy A. Norris D. Momeni S. Waldo B. Ruby J. The Ph of beverages in the United States. *J Am Dental Assoc.* 2016;147(4):255–263.

14. Montfort-Steiger V. Williams C. Carbohydrate intake considerations for young athletes. *J Sports Sci Med* 2007;6:342–352.

15. Bergeron M F. Hargreaves M. Haymes E. et al. Exercise and fluid replacement. American College of Sports Medicine Position Stand. *Med Sci Sports Exerc.* 2007;39(2):377–390.

16. Bergeron M F. Reducing sports heat illness risk. *Pediatr Rev.* 2013;34(6):270–279.

17. Nattiv A. Loucks AB. Manore M. Sanborn CF. Sundgot-Borgen J. Warren M. American College of Sports Medicine. Position of the American College of Sports Medicine: Female Athlete Triad. *Medi Sci Sports Exer.* 2007;39(10)1867–1882.

18. Committee on Nutrition and the Council on Sports Medicine and Fitness. Sports drinks and energy drinks for children and adolescents: are they appropriate?. *Pediatr.* 2011;127(6):1182–1189.

19. Bragg MA, Yanamadala S, Roberto CA, Brownell H, Brownell KD. Athlete endorsements in food and marketing. *Pediatr.* 2013;132(5):805–810.

20. Gomez J, American Academy of Pediatrics Committee on Sports Medicine and Fitness. Use of performance-enhancing substances. *Pediatr.* 2005; 115(4):1103–1106.

21. World Health Organization (WHO) Food and Agriculture Organization (FAO) of the United Nations, United Nations University. *Protein and Amino Acid Requirements in Human Nutrition: Report of a Joint FAO/WHO/UNU Expert Consultation.* Geneva, Switzerland: *World Health Organization*; 2002. WHO Technical Report Series No. 935.

22. Kniskern MA, Johnston CS. Protein dietary reference intakes may be inadequate for vegetarians if low amounts of animal protein are consumed. *Nutr.* 2001;27(6):727–730.

23. Rogerson, D. Vegan diets: practical advice for athletes and exercisers. *J Int Soc Sports Nutr.* (2017) 14:36 DOI 10.1186 /s12970-017-0192-931.

24. United States Department of Agriculture. USDA branded food products database. Available at: https://ndb.nal.usda .gov/ndb/foods. Accessed June 1, 2018.

25. U.S. Dietary Guidelines Scientific Report of the U.S. Dietary Guidelines Advisory Committee. Available at: https://health .gov/dietaryguidelines/2015-scientific-report/06-chapter-1 /d1-2.asp. Accessed: January 9, 2018.

26. Abbaspour N. Hurrell R. Kelishadi R. Review on iron and its importance in human health. *J Res Med Sci.* 2014;19(2):164–174.

27. Ginde A. Liu MC. Carmargo C. Demographic differences and trends of vitamin D insufficiency in the U.S. population, 1988–2004. *Arch Intern Med.* 2009;169:626–632.

28. Villacis D. Yi A. Jahn R. et al Prevalence of abnormal Vitamin D levels among Division 1 NCAA Athletes. *Sports Health.* 2014;6(4):340–347.

29. Ogan D. Pritchett K. Vitamin D and the athlete, recommendations and benefits. *Nutrients* 2013;5(6):1856–1868.

30. Carl RL, Johnson MD, Martin TJ, Council on Sports Medicine and Fitness. Promotion of Healthy Weight-Control Practices in Young Athletes. *Pediatrics.* 2017;140(3): e2017187. Available at: http://pediatrics.aappublications .org/content/140/3/e20171871.long

31. American Academy of Pediatrics Committee on Sports Medicine and Fitness. Promotion of healthy weight-control practices in young athletes *Pediatr.* 2005;116(6):1557–1564.

32. Thompson R. Sherman RT. *Eating Disorders in Sport.* New York, NY: Routledge Taylor & Francis Group; 2010:33–51.

33. Beashler RST. The National Collegiate Athletic Association Wrestling 2013–2014 Rules and Interpretations. Indianapolis, IN:National Collegiate Athletic Association;2013.

34. Thein-Nissenbaum J, Hammer E. Treatment strategies for the female athlete triad in the adolescent athlete: current perspectives. *Open Access J Sports Med.* 2017;8:85–95. Available at: https://www.ncbi.nlm.nih.gov/pmc/articles /PMC5388220/pdf/oajsm-8-085.pdf

35. Barrack MT. Ackerman KE. Gibbs JC. Update on the Female Athlete Triad. *Curr Rev Musculoskelet Med.* 2013 6(2):195–204.

36. KA. Weiss K. Hecht S. and Council on Sports Medicine and Fitness. The Female Athlete Triad. *Pediatr.* 2016;138(2): DOI:10.1542/peds.2016-0922.

37. Bonci CM. Bonci LJ. Granger LR. Johnson CL. et al. National Athletic Trainers Association Position Statement: preventing, detecting, and managing disordered eating in athletes. *J Athl Train.* (2008);43(1):80–108.

38. Mountjoy M. Sundgot-Borgen J. Burke L. et al. The IOC consensus statement: beyond the female athlete triad-relative energy deficiency in sport (RED-S). *Br J Sports Med.* 2014;48:491–497.

39. De Souza MJ, Williams N. Nattiv A. et al Misunderstanding the Female Athlete Triad; Refuting the IOC Consensus Statement on Relative Energy Deficiency in Sport (RED-S) *Br J Sports Med.* 2014;48(20):1461–1465.

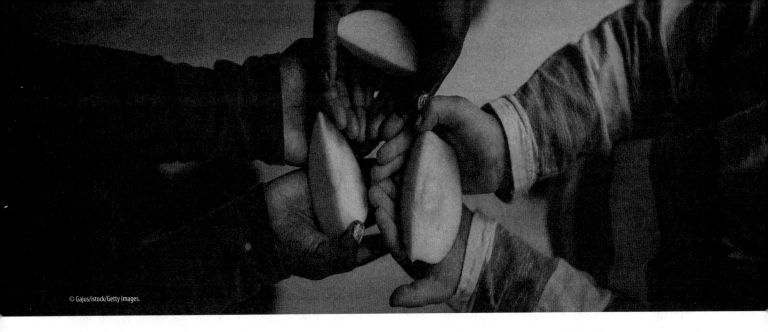

© Gajus/istock/Getty Images.

CHAPTER 24

Children with Special Needs

Harriet H. Cloud

LEARNING OBJECTIVES

- To review the definitions of the terms encompassed by special needs such as developmental disabilities and special health care needs
- To identify the etiology and prevalence of various conditions covered by special needs
- To review the evidence based practice for nutrition problems associated with selected syndromes and disabilities
- To review community resources and legislation for children with special needs

▶ Introduction

The term children with special needs includes children with special health care needs and developmental disabilities. These children often need care from multiple systems involving health care, public health, special education, mental health and social services, physical therapy, occupational therapy, speech pathology, and nutrition services. The nutritional needs of children with special needs vary and primarily involve energy, growth, regulation of the biochemical processes, and repair of cells and body tissue. Nutritional risk factors often include growth deficiency, obesity, gastrointestinal disorders, metabolic problems, feeding problems, and drug–nutrient interaction problems. The Centers

for Disease Control and Prevention have reported that 20% of children under age 18 have some type of special health care needs which includes intellectual and developmental disabilities.[1]

▶ Definition of Developmental Disabilities

A developmental disability was defined in Public Law 99–101–496 ed. (1990, revised in 2000 to PL 106–402), the Developmental Disabilities Assistance and Bill of Rights Act,[2] as a severe chronic disability of a person that is attributable to a mental or physical impairment or a combination of mental and physical impairments with the following characteristics:

- Manifests before the person attains age 22
- Likely to continue indefinitely
- Results in substantial functional limitations in three or more areas of major life activity (self-care, receptive and expressive language, learning, mobility, self-direction, capacity for independent living, and economic self-sufficiency)
- Reflects the person's need for a combination of special interdisciplinary or generic care, treatments, or other services that are lifelong or of extended duration and are individually planned and coordinated

Intellectual disability starts at any time before a child turns 18 and is characterized with problems involving intellectual functioning or intelligence and adaptive behavior which includes every day social and life skills. Current terminology combines developmental disability and intellectual disability as **Intellectual and Developmental Disabilities** (IDD).[2]

Children with special healthcare needs were defined in 1998 as those children who have or are at increased risk for a chronic physical, developmental, behavioral, or emotional condition and who require health and related services of a type or amount beyond that required by children generally.[3]

The etiology of developmental disabilities has been traced to chromosomal aberrations such as Down syndrome (trisomy 21) and Prader-Willi syndrome, neurologic insults in the prenatal period, prematurity, cerebral palsy, infectious diseases, trauma, congenital defects such as cleft lip and palate, neural tube defects such as spina bifida, untreated inherited disorders of metabolism, and other syndromes of lesser incidence.[4]

Nutrition Considerations

Nutrition considerations that involve the child with special needs include assessing growth, feeding difficulties, and the problems surrounding energy balance, biochemical measures, and dietary intake. Growth assessment may reveal a failure to thrive, obesity, or slow growth rate in height. The second major consideration includes feeding from the standpoint of oral motor problems, developmental delays in feeding skills, inability to self-feed, behavioral problems, and tube feedings. Other areas for nutritional consideration include drug–nutrient interaction, constipation, dental caries, urinary tract infections, and allergies. One additional concern involves food or nutrition misinformation the parent has received related to hyperactivity, attention deficit disorders, and treating disorders such as Down syndrome and autism with alternative or complementary medicine. **TABLE 24.1** includes a list of selected developmental disorders and their nutrition considerations.[5]

TABLE 24.1 Developmental Disorders and Corresponding Nutrition Considerations

Syndrome or Developmental Disability	Nutrition Diagnostic Terms	Indicators of this Nutrition Diagnosis
Autism spectrum disorders (ASD) Characterized by delayed speech and language development, ritualistic or repetitive behaviors, and impairments in social interactions.	Inadequate energy intake Excessive energy intake Food-medication interactions Underweight	Limited or restricted food choices High intake of food (kcal) due to food obsessions or use of food by behavioral interventions Potential interactions between food and a variety of medications used for individuals with ASD Inadequate energy intake Body mass index (BMI) <5th percentile for children 2–19 y Refusal to eat Restricted or limited food choices that result in low energy intake
	Overweight	BMI >85th percentile for children 2–19 y Excessive energy intake Infrequent, low duration, and/or low intensity physical activity Large amounts of sedentary activities Limited food choices that result in excessive energy intake

Syndrome or Developmental Disability	Nutrition Diagnostic Terms	Indicators of this Nutrition Diagnosis
	Harmful beliefs/attitudes about food	Eating behavior serves a purpose other than nourishment Pica Food fetish
	Undesirable food choices	Intake that reflects an imbalance of nutrients/food groups Avoidance of foods/food groups Complementary and alternative medicine treatments, often nutrition-based (vitamin B-6 supplements, gluten-free casein-free diet) may place child at risk for nutrient deficiencies Intake inconsistent with Dietary Reference Intakes, US Dietary Guidelines, MyPlate, or other methods of measuring diet quality Inability, unwillingness, or disinterest in selecting food consistent with the guidelines Condition associated with diagnosis, ASD–food selectivity, rigid eating patterns
Cerebral palsy A disorder of muscle control or coordination resulting from an injury to the brain during early fetal, perinatal, and early childhood development. There may be associated problems with intellectual, visual or other system functions. CP is often classified as Mild (child can move without assistance, daily activities not limited; Moderate (child will need braces, medications, and adaptive technology); Severe (child will require a wheelchair and will have significant challenges in daily activities), No CP: child has CP signs but disorder was acquired after completion of brain development, and is classified under the incident that caused the CP such as traumatic brain injury or encephalopathy)	Increased energy expenditure	Unintentional weight loss Evidence of need for accelerated or catch-up growth or weight gain; absence of normal growth Condition associated with a diagnosis (eg. cerebral palsy)
	Inadequate energy intake	Failure to gain or maintain appropriate weight Insufficient energy intake from diet compared with needs Inability to independently consume foods/fluids
	Excessive energy intake	Increased body adiposity Weight gain greater than expected Enteral nutrition more than measured/estimated energy expenditure
	Swallowing difficulty	Abnormal swallow study Prolonged feeding time Coughing, choking, prolonged chewing, pouching of food, regurgitation, facial expression changes during eating Decreased food intake Avoidance of food Mealtime resistance

(continues)

TABLE 24.1 Developmental Disorders and Corresponding Nutrition Considerations   *(continued)*

Syndrome or Developmental Disability	Nutrition Diagnostic Terms	Indicators of this Nutrition Diagnosis
	Altered gastrointestinal (GI) function Food-medication interactions Underweight	Constipation Condition associated with diagnoses: internal muscle tone in cerebral palsy can be affected as well as more visible external muscle tone Seizure medications: food and medication interactions Inadequate energy intake BMI <5th percentile for children 2–19 years Decreased muscle mass, muscle wasting Inadequate intake of food compared with estimated or measured needs
	Overweight	History of physical disability or malnutrition BMI at or above 85th percentile for children 2–19 years Excessive energy intake Infrequent, low duration and/or low-intensity physical activity Large amounts of sedentary activities
Cystic fibrosis An inherited disorder of the exocrine glands, primarily the pancreas, pulmonary system, and sweat glands, characterized by abnormally thick luminal secretions.	Increased energy expenditure	Unintentional weight loss Evidence of need for accelerated or catch-up growth or weight gain; absence of normal growth Condition associated with a diagnosis (eg. cystic fibrosis)
	Altered gastrointestinal function	Abnormal digestive enzyme and fecal fat studies Malabsorption Steatorrhea
	Impaired nutrient utilization	Abnormal digestive enzyme and fecal fat studies Growth stunting or failure Evidence of vitamin and/or mineral deficiency Steatorrhea Condition associated with diagnoses: cystic fibrosis
Down syndrome A genetic disorder that results from an extra no. 21 chromosome, causing developmental problems such as congenital heart disease, mental retardation, short stature, and decreased muscle tone	Excessive energy intake	Increased body adiposity Energy intake higher than estimated need Reduced energy needs related to short stature, low muscle tone
	Breastfeeding difficulty Feeding problems	Poor sucking ability as an infant (due to low tone) Poor weight gain

Syndrome or Developmental Disability	Nutrition Diagnostic Terms	Indicators of this Nutrition Diagnosis
Incidence-1/600-1/800 live births.	Altered GI function	Constipation (related to low muscle tone, low activity, and/or low fiber intake) Celiac disease (higher incidence in Down syndrome)
Prader-Willi syndrome (PWS) A genetic disorder marked by poor feeding skills in infancy, hypotonia, short stature hyperphagia, and cognitive impairment. When not carefully managed, hyperphagia leads to obesity. May be treated with growth hormone. Incidence—1/10,000–1/25,000 live births.	Excessive energy intake	Increased body adiposity Energy intake higher than estimated need Condition associated with diagnosis (eg. hyperphagia and PWS) Reduced energy needs related to short stature, low muscle tone
	Breastfeeding difficulty	Poor sucking ability as an infant (due to low tone) Poor weight gain
	Harmful beliefs/attitudes about food	Eating behavior serves a purpose other than nourishment Pica Food obsession
	Undesirable food choices	Intake inconsistent with diet quality guidelines Unable to select foods, independently, that are consistent with food quality, kcal controlled guidelines Condition associated with diagnosis, PWS-food hyperphagia, obsession with food
Spina bifida (myeolomeningocele) results from a midline defect of the skin, spinal column and spinal cord. It is characterized by hydrocephalus, lack of muscular control, and mental retardation Incidence—2.7–2.8 per 10,000 live births.	Excessive energy intake	Increased body adiposity Energy intake higher than estimated need Reduced energy needs related to altered body composition, short stature
	Swallowing difficulty	Abnormal swallow study Noisy wet upper airway sounds Condition associated with diagnosis of Arnold Chiari malformation of the brain
	Altered gastrointestinal function	Constipation Condition associated with diagnosis: neurogenic bowel

Modified from Van Riper C, Wallace L, American Dietetic Association. Position of the America Dietetic Association: Providing Nutrition Services for Infants, Children and Adults with Developmental Disabilities. J. Am Diet Assoc. 2010;110(2): 296–307.[5]

▶ Nutritional Needs of the Child with Special Needs

Energy needs for children with special needs vary as they do for all children; very little specific information is available for either. A decreased energy need is most apparent in chromosomal aberrations such as Down syndrome, conditions accompanied by limited gross motor activity such as in spina bifida, and syndromes characterized by low muscle tone such as is found in Prader-Willi syndrome, Rubinstein-Tabyi syndrome, Williams syndrome, and Turner's syndrome.

Energy needs of infants and children with other special needs such as cerebral palsy and Rett syndrome are highly individualized and vary widely.[4]

TABLE 24.2 Criteria and Dietary Reference Intake Values for Energy by Active Individuals in the Pediatric Age Group[a]

Life Stage Group	Criterion	Active PAL[b] EER (kcal/d)	
		Male	Female
0 through 6 months	Energy expenditure plus energy deposition	570	520 (3 mo)
7 through 12 months	Energy expenditure plus energy deposition	743	676 (9 mo)
1 through 2 years	Energy expenditure plus energy deposition	1046	992 (24 mo)
3 through 8 years	Energy expenditure plus energy deposition	1742	1642 (6 years)
9 through 13 years	Energy expenditure plus energy deposition	2279	2071 (11 years)
14 through 18 years	Energy expenditure plus energy deposition	3152	2368 (16 years)
Over 18 years	Energy expenditure plus energy deposition	3067[c]	2403 (19 years)

[a]For healthy, moderately active Americans and Canadians.
[b]PAL 5 physical activity level, EER 5 estimated energy requirement, TEE 5 total energy expenditure.
[c]Subtract 10 kcal per day for males and 7 kcal per day for females for each year of age over 19 years.
Data from Institute of Medicine of the National Academies. *Dietary Reference Intakes for Energy, Carbohydrate, Fiber, Fat, Fatty Acids, Cholesterol, Protein and Amino Acids (Macronutrients)*. Washington, DC: The National Academies Press; 2005.[6]

The **dietary reference intakes** (DRIs) are a set of nutrient-based reference values that have replaced the **recommended dietary allowances** (RDAs) www.nap.edu.[6] (see Resources). They were developed in response to a need for a more precise and customized approach to defining nutrient requirements. Criteria and dietary reference intake values for energy in the pediatric age group are shown in **TABLE 24.2**. The adaptability of these reference sets to the special needs population requires further research.

Lowered Energy Needs

Children with Down syndrome, Prader-Willi syndrome, or spina bifida have been found to have a slower growth rate, and lower basal energy needs. Additionally, they often have low muscle tone, leading to diminished motor activity.[7] Not to be forgotten is a familial predisposition to obesity. As a result of these factors, children with these conditions tend to become overweight and obese when fed according to normal standards. Recent studies have shown that children with disorders such as Down syndrome are frequently provided food intake greater than the DRI.[7,8] Monitoring the growth of these children is essential in order to prevent excessive weight gain or becoming overweight. One method of determining the energy needs of several conditions of special needs is to determine the kilo-calorie needs per centimeter of height as shown in **TABLE 24.3**.

Higher Energy Needs

Children with **cerebral palsy** (CP) often tend to be seriously underweight for height. There are three types of cerebral palsy with differing energy needs. The three types include Spastic CP, Ataxic CP, and Athetoid or Dyskinetic CP.[10] One study found that poor growth was associated with increased occurrence of health problems.[11] Studies have been conducted to estimate the energy needs of the child with cerebral palsy and have utilized indirect calorimetry and the doubly labeled water method. A study by Bandini and colleagues[12] found that the **resting energy expenditure** (REE) of adolescents with cerebral palsy was lower than in adolescent controls. Stallings and associates[13] completed a study of children ages 2 to 12 with spastic quadriplegia cerebral palsy compared with a normal control group. The conclusion was that growth failure and an abnormal pattern of REE are related to inadequate energy intake.[14] Many factors contribute to the inadequate energy intake including feeding issues, swallowing, oral motor issues, and positioning. Often the total energy needs are not greater than normal, but meeting those needs may require more concentration of formulas or foods provided.

Two other methods for determining the energy needs of this population include using a nomogram for calculating body surface area and standards based on kcal/m²/hour.[15] This method can be used for males and females who are 6 years of age and older. Indirect

TABLE 24.3 Methods to Determine Energy Needs for Special Needs Conditions

Condition	Kcal. Per Cm /Ht.	Comments
Normal Child	Average 16	
Prader Willi	Maintain growth 10–11 kcal/cm height Promote weight loss 8–9 kcal/cm/height	For all children and adolescents.
Cerebral Palsy		
Mild Severe limited mobility Athetoid C P	13.9 kcal/height, ambulatory 11.1 kcal/height, non-ambulatory 10 kcal /height Up to 6000 kcal per day (adolescence)	For children ages 5–11 yrs. For children ages 5–11 yrs.
Down Syndrome	Girls 14.3 Boys 16.1	For children ages 5–11 yrs.
Motor Dysfunction Non-ambulatory Ambulatory	7–11 14	For children ages 5–12 yrs. For children ages 5–12 yrs.
Spina Bifida	Maintain weight 9–11 kcal/cm height Promote weight loss 7 kcal/cm height	For all children older than 8 years of age and minimally active.

Modified from Weston S, Murray P. Alternative methods of estimating daily energy requirements based on health condition. In: Devore J, Shotton A, eds: *Pocket Guide to Children with Special Health Care Needs*. Chicago,IL: Academy of Nutrition and Dietetics;2012.[9]

calorimetry is generally considered to be the most accurate method of determining energy requirements. However, access to the equipment may be limited and its use impractical in this population.

The information in determining the basal energy need must be modified for growth and activity level. The DRIs are generally not appropriate to use in determining the energy levels of children with certain types of developmental disabilities. A more appropriate strategy would be to utilize basal energy needs with an individualized percentage added for growth rates and energy levels, which encompasses slower growth rates and lowered motor activity. The dearth of research in this area makes it difficult to develop standards and requires that the registered dietitian and physician evaluate the child's nutritional needs individually.

Protein, Carbohydrates, and Fats

Careful monitoring of protein intake is essential in the child with special needs. It is generally recommended that 15–20% of the total calories come from protein, which may be difficult for a child with an oral motor feeding problem

such as a child with cerebral palsy. These children often suffer from serious malnutrition manifested by little or no weight gain and limited growth in height. A recent study completed by the Vanderbilt Evidence based Practice Center examined the effects of available interventions for feeding and nutrition problems that have been evaluated in individuals with cerebral palsy. The studies compared surgical (enteral feeding) and non-surgical intervention which included positioning and oral motor intervention. All studies showed greater improvement in growth with gastrostomy feeding.[16] More research of a comprehensive longitudinal design is needed.[16]

Carbohydrates are the primary source of energy for all individuals. According to the usual pediatric dietary recommendations, at least 50% of calories should come from carbohydrates with no more than 10% coming from sucrose. Surveys have shown that children special needs often have a high percentage of their carbohydrate calories coming from foods highly concentrated in sucrose, such as candy, carbonated beverages, cookies, and so forth.[17] Dietary counseling related to better choices of carbohydrate foods is frequently required, just as it is for all children.

Fats should provide 30–35% of the total caloric intake, increasing palatability and satiety, as well as providing a supply of the essential fatty acids. For the child who tends to be overweight or obese, fat intake should be carefully evaluated and controlled. For the underweight child, fat can provide an important source of supplemental calories. Infant formulas are now modified to include a higher percentage of the fatty acids **arachidonic acid** (ARA) and **docosahexanoeic acid** (DHA) based upon research indicating improvement in visual acuity and cognitive development. These formulas should be used for the infant with special needs when the infant is not breastfed.

Vitamins, Minerals, and Botanicals

Research findings do not indicate that children with special needs have higher than normal vitamin and mineral needs. Historically, studies have addressed the vitamin needs of children with Down syndrome, spina bifida, fragile X syndrome, and autism.[18,19] Children on anticonvulsant medications (such as phenobarbital, Dilantin, Depakote, Topamax, and others) may experience poor absorption of both vitamins and minerals.

Numerous studies[18,19] have searched for nutritional deficiencies as causative factors in Down syndrome. Traditionally, the studies have included numerous vitamins, minerals, fatty acids, digestive enzymes, lipotropic nutrients, and drugs. Media coverage has promoted using antioxidants (vitamins A, C, and E and minerals such as zinc, copper, manganese, and selenium) along with the amino acids glucosamine, tyrosine, and tryptophan. The expected outcomes are improved growth; increased cognition, alertness, and attention span; and changed facial features. The key concept in the nutritional intervention is metabolic correction of genetic overexpression. It is reported that presence of the third chromosome 21 causes overproduction of superoxide dismutase and cystathionine beta synthase, which disrupt active methylation pathways. Vitamin supplements of antioxidants are considered key to the treatment. Although these studies are of interest, at this point, nutritional supplements are considered an expensive, questionable approach, and do not result in improvements in IQ, physical appearance, or general health.[20]

Additionally, parents of children with ADHD report that omitting sugar from the diet decreases hyperactivity. Historically this was reported, but is not found in the current literature.[21]

A variety of therapies have been proposed to help children with special health care needs, including the following: Blue green algae has been promoted for children with Down syndrome and other developmental disabilities, purportedly to increase attention span and concentration. Of concern is that little monitoring is part of the initiation of these treatments. High-dose supplementation of vitamin B$_6$ and magnesium has been proposed for autism to diminish tantrums and self-stimulation activities, and improve attention and speech.[20] Other proposed treatments include **dimethyl glycine** (DMG), and gluten- and casein-free diets.[22] Limited research is available to substantiate anything other than subjective reports that the child is helped.[22]

Diminished bone density and a propensity to fracture with minimal trauma are common in children and adolescents with moderate to severe cerebral palsy. A recent study demonstrated that 77% of the children with CP had osteopenia correlated with medication, feeding problems, and lower triceps skinfold measures.[23]

Studies involving children with spina bifida have involved ascorbic acid saturation and the impact of supplementation of ascorbic acid for producing an acidic urinary pH, designed to prevent urinary tract infections. Concern was shown in recent studies related to the effect of supplemental ascorbic acid on serum vitamin B$_{12}$ levels. No evident B$_{12}$ deficiency developed in one study of 40 children receiving long-term vitamin C supplementation.[24]

Since 1980, the literature has reflected the growing interest in vitamin supplementation in the prevention of spina bifida.[25] Nutritional deficiencies identified as possible etiologic factors include folic acid, multivitamins, and zinc.[25] A British study[24] supplemented 234 mothers with a multivitamin/iron preparation 1 month before conception. Vitamins included were A, D, thiamine, riboflavin, pyridoxine, niacin, ascorbic acid, and folic acid. Supplemented mothers had a recurrence rate of 0.9% compared with 5.1% of the 219 mothers without supplementation. Homocysteine-methionine metabolism appears to be altered in women with pregnancies affected by neural tube defects; however, the specific mechanisms of causation are not yet known.

As a result of these studies, the US Public Health Service recommends that all women between the ages of 14 and 45 get an extra 400 mcg of folate daily.[25] Recent data demonstrate that this public health action is associated with increased folate blood levels among US women of childbearing age and that the national rate of spina bifida has decreased by 20%. The Food and Drug Administration approved fortification of all enriched cereal grain products with folic acid in 1998, although at a level that still requires folic acid supplementation.[26]

An additional concern related to children with spina bifida has been their allergic reaction to latex brought about by multiple surgeries.[27] For those children affected, it has been recommended that they avoid certain foods: bananas, water chestnuts, kiwi, and avocados. Mild reactions can occur from apples, carrots, celery, tomatoes, papaya, and melons.[27] The foods listed were identified as having a protein with a cross reactivity to the proteins found in latex.

A special concern regarding adequacy of vitamin and mineral intake is the effect of certain medications commonly prescribed to children with special needs. Among these medications are antibiotics, anticonvulsants, antihypertensives, cathartics, corticosteroids, stimulants, sulfonamides, and tranquilizers (see **TABLE 24.4**). Their nutritional effects can include nausea and vomiting, gastric distress, constipation, and interference with the absorption of vitamins and minerals. In some cases, vitamin and mineral supplements are recommended.[28]

TABLE 24.4 Drug–Nutrient Interaction

Generic Name	Brand Name	Drug–Nutrient Interaction
Cardiovascular Disease		
Digoxin	Lanoxin	Anorexia Nausea
Furosemide	Lasix	Hyponatremia Hypokalemia Hypomagnesemia Calcium loss
Respiratory Disease		
Prednisone	Deltisone Orasone Liquid Prednisone	Weight gain due to drug-induced appetite increase or edema Stunting of growth in children Hyperglycemia
Trimethaprim	Bactrim	Can cause folate depletion Sulfa in the product can cause anemia
Amoxicillin	Amoxil	Absorption provided by increased fluids
Gastrointestinal Disease		
Ranitidine	Zantac	May cause nausea/diarrhea Constipation
Metoclopramide	Reglan	Nausea and diarrhea
Seizure Disorders		
Carbamazepine	Tegretol	Unpleasant taste Anorexia Sore mouth

Phenobarbital	Phenobarbital	Can induce folate deficiency
		   vitamin D deficiency
		   vitamin K deficiency
		High intake of folic acid (.5 mg per day) can interfere with seizure control
		Folate depletion can lead to megaloblastic anemia

Phenytoin	Dilantin	Same as phenobarbital
Primidone	Mysoline	Folate depletion leading to megaloblastic anemia

(continues)

TABLE 24.4 Drug–Nutrient Interaction		(*continued*)
Generic Name	**Brand Name**	**Drug–Nutrient Interaction**
Seizure Disorders		
Valproic Acid	Depakene and Depakote	Carnitine deficiency Coagulating defects may occur with risk of bleeding and anemia
Hyperactivity		
Methylphenidate	Ritalin	Anorexia when given before a meal

Modified from Pronsky ZM, Redfern CM, Crowe J, Epstein J, Young V. *Food Medication Interactions*. 13th ed. Birchrunville, PA: Food-Medication Interactions; 2007.[28]

▶ Nutrition Assessment

Assessing the child with special needs includes all components of nutrition assessment for normal children plus including an evaluation of feeding skills and development. Taking anthropometric measurements of children who are unable to stand and who have gross motor handicaps will require some ingenuity. Weights may be difficult to obtain on standing calibrated balance beam scales for the child with spina bifida or CP. Chair and bucket scales are available for use in both clinics and schools, and bed scales are indicated for the severely affected. Recumbent boards can be constructed or commercially obtained. Alternate measures for height measurements include arm span, knee-to-ankle height, or sitting height.[29]

Standards for comparison of weight, height, and head circumference are found on the 2000 Centers for Disease Control and Prevention (CDC) growth charts and the WHO charts: https://www.cdc.gov/growthcharts/index.htm.[30] Because these standards were developed using a normal population, the child with developmental disabilities may plot as short, especially when length or height for age is considered. This is particularly true for children with chromosomal aberrations such as Down syndrome[30] or those with a neural tube defect such as spina bifida. Growth charts have been developed for children with a number of disabilities (see **TABLE 24.5**), but for the most part the CDC charts and the WHO charts are recommended. Copies of the Down syndrome growth curves are Resource C. Proper interpretation is needed.

Weight-for-age, interpreted for the child with special needs is also an important indicator of nutritional status and requires comparison with height-for-age. Again, it is the child with Down syndrome, spina bifida, CP, Cornelia de Lange syndrome, Prader-Willi, or chromosomal aberrations in general whose height/weight relationship should be carefully monitored. Early identification of inappropriate relationships is critical so that nutrition counseling related to energy balance can be given. The CDC charts include the **body mass index** (BMI) as an indicator of overweight or risk for overweight. Using the BMI for age can be very helpful for the child with developmental disabilities; however, it may not always identify overweight in children who are overfat because of decreased muscle mass. Skinfold measures also should be used. Growth velocity is also an important anthropometric measurement as growth velocity information assists the registered dietitian in evaluating changes in rate of growth over a specified period of time. Incremental growth curves are available for plotting growth velocity.[32] Mid upper arm (tricep) skinfold thickness is a useful measurement for estimating body fat and is recommended along with arm circumference.[33] Z-scores can be determined from the CDC and WHO curves; however interpretation of the z-score to parents is necessary.

Biochemical measures for the child with special needs should include at minimum hemoglobin and hematocrit levels, complete blood count, urinalysis, and semiquantitative amino acid screening. Including this test in an assessment would depend upon biochemical testing the child received in the primary healthcare facility. Other tests may be indicated for children on an anticonvulsant medication who may have low serum levels of folic acid, carnitine, ascorbic acid, calcium, vitamin D, alkaline phosphatase, phosphorus, and pyridoxine. A glucose tolerance test is recommended for individuals with Prader-Willi syndrome.[34] Thyroid levels are part of the protocol for children with Down syndrome. After an initial screening, thyroid levels should be checked annually.[34]

Dietary Assessment

The methods used to obtain dietary information about a child with special needs are identical to those used with a non-affected child. The parent must be interviewed for the infant and young child. Often it is difficult to obtain the food intake for an older child who has a degree of cognitive impairment. It is highly recommended that written dietary records be analyzed with computer software.

TABLE 24.5 List of Some Special Growth Charts

Condition	Reference(s)	Printed Copies Available
Achondroplasia	Horton WA, Rotter JI, Rimoin DL, Scott CI, Hall JG. Standard growth curves for achondroplasia. *J Pediatr*. 1978;93(3):435–438.	Cedars-Sinai Medical Center Birth Defects Center 444 S. San Vincente Blvd., Los Angeles, CA 90048 (213) 855–2211 Camera-ready copies
Brachmann-(Cornelia) de Lange syndrome	Kline AD, Stanley C, Belevich J, Brodsky K, Barr M, Jackson LG. Developmental data on individuals with the Brachmann-de Lange syndrome. *Am J Med Genet*. 1993;47(7):1053–1058.	
Cerebral palsy (quadriplegia)	Krick J, Murphy-Miller P, Zeger S, Wright E. Pattern of growth in children with cerebral palsy. *J Am Diet Assoc*. 1996;96:680–685. Brooks J, Day S, Shavelle R, Strauss D. Low weight, morbidity and mortality in children with cerebral palsy: new clinical growth charts. *Pediatr*. 2011;128 (2. E299–307.	Kennedy Krieger Institute 707 N. Broadway, Baltimore, MD 21205 www.kennedykrieger.org
Down syndrome	Zemel BS, Pipan M, Stallings VA, Hall W, Schadt K, Freedman D and Thorpe P. Growth charts for children with Down Syndrome in United States. *Pediatr*. 2015;136 (5)1652[31]	
Marfan syndrome	Pyeritz RE, Marfan Syndrome and related disorders. In: Emery AH, Rimoirn LD, eds; *Principles and Practice of Medical Genetics*. New York, NY: Churchill Livingstone;1983:3579–3624. Pyeritz RE, Murphy EA, Lin SJ, Rosell EM. Growth and anthropometrics in the Marfan syndrome. *Prog Clin Biol Res*. 1985;200:355–366.	Camera-ready copies in article
Myelomeningocele	Ekvall S, ed. *Ped Nutrition in Chronic Disease and Developmental Disorders: Prevention, Assessment and Treatment*. New York, NY:Oxford Press;1993: Appendix 2.	
Noonan syndrome	Witt DR, Keena BA, Hall JG, Allanson JE. Growth curves for height in Noonan syndrome. *Clin Genet*. 1986;30(3):150–153.	Camera-ready copies in article
Prader-Willi syndrome	Greenswag L, Alexander R. *Management of Prader-Willi Syndrome*, 2nd ed. New York, NY: Springer-Verlag; 1995: Appendix B growth chart.	
Sickle cell disease	Phebus CK, Gloninger MF, Maciak BJ. Growth patterns by age and sex in children with sickle cell disease. *J Pediatr*. 1984;105:28–33. Tanner JM, Davies PS. Clinical longitudinal standards for height and height velocity for North American children. *J Pediatr*. 1985;107:317–329.	

In addition to dietary information, assessing feeding skills and identifying feeding problems that influence the child's food intake is indicated. This part of the evaluation may include such members of the healthcare team as the physical therapist, occupational therapist, dentist, speech therapist, registered dietitian/nutritionist, and psychologist. Each specialist will bring their expertise to the evaluation. Observation of an actual feeding session is critical and may utilize an evaluation tool such as the **Developmental Feeding Tool** (DFT) from the Boling Center for Developmental Disabilities, University of Tennessee, which provides a checklist of factors involved in the feeding of a specific child.[35] **FIGURE 24.1** provides a sample of this evaluation tool.

Parent/Guardian _____   Date _____

Address_____   Staff member _____

City _____ State _____ Zip _____   Child's name_____

County _____ Telephone _____ Birth date _____ Age ____ Sex ____ Race _____

Head circumference (cm) _____ (%ile CDC) _____ Hand dominance _____

Height (cm) _____ (%ile CDC)_____ Weight (kg)_____ (%ile CDC)_____

Height for height (%ile CDC) _____ Hematocrit _____ Urine screen _____

PHYSICAL

Yes   No   Size

____ ____ 1. Weight (Avg. %ile CDC)
____ ____ 2. Underweight
____ ____ 3. Overweight
____ ____ 4. Stature (Avg. %ile CDC)
____ ____ 5. Short (Below 5th %ile for ht. CDC)
____ ____ 6. Tall (Above 95th %ile for ht. CDC)
____ ____ 7. Abnormal body proportions*
____ ____ 8. Head circumference (Avg. %ile CDC)
____ ____ 9. Microcephalic
____ ____ 10. Macrocephalic

Laboratory

____ ____ 11. Hematocrit (Normal)
____ ____ 12. Urine screen (Normal)*

Health Status

____ ____ 13. Bowel problems*
____ ____ 14. Diabetes
____ ____ 15. Vomiting
____ ____ 16. Dental caries
____ ____ 17. Anemia
____ ____ 18. Food allergies/intolerance*
____ ____ 19. Medications*
____ ____ 20. Vitamin/mineral supplements*
____ ____ 21. Ingests nonfood items
____ ____ 22. Therapeutic diet*
____ ____ 23. General appearance (Normal)*
____ ____ 24. Head (Normal)*
____ ____ 25. Eyes (Normal)*
____ ____ 26. Ears (Normal)*
____ ____ 27. Nose (Normal)*

____ ____ 28. Teeth/gums (Normal)*
____ ____ 29. Palate (Normal)*
____ ____ 30. Skin (Normal)*
____ ____ 31. Muscles (Normal)*
____ ____ 32. Arms/hands (Normal)*
____ ____ 33. Legs/feet (Normal)*

NEUROMOTOR/MUSCULAR

Yes   No   Tonicity

____ ____ 34. Body tone (Normal)*

Head and Trunk Control

____ ____ 35. Head control (Normal)*
____ ____ 36. Lifts head in prone
____ ____ 37. Head lags when pulled to sitting
____ ____ 38. Head drops forward
____ ____ 39. Head drops backward
____ ____ 40. Trunk control (Normal)*

Upper Extremity Control

____ ____ 41. Range of motion (Normal)*
____ ____ 42. Approach to object (Normal)*
____ ____ 43. Grasp of object (Normal)*
____ ____ 44. Release of object (Normal)*
____ ____ 45. Brings hand to mouth
____ ____ 46. Dominance established

Reflexes

____ ____ 47. Grossly normal
____ ____ 48. Asymmetrical tonic neck reflex*
____ ____ 49. Symmetrical tonic neck reflex*
____ ____ 50. Moro reflex*
____ ____ 51. Grasp reflex*

Body Alignment

____ ____ 52. Scoliosis
____ ____ 53. Kyphosis

FIGURE 24.1 Developmental Feeding Tool

____ ____ 54. Lordosis

____ ____ 55. Hip subluxation or dislocation suspected

Position in Feeding

____ ____ 56. Mother's lap

____ ____ 57. Infant seat

____ ____ 58. High chair

____ ____ 59. Table and chair

____ ____ 60. Wheelchair

____ ____ 61. Other adaptive chair*

ORAL/MOTOR

Yes   No   Facial Expression

____ ____ 62. Symmetrical structure/function*

____ ____ 63. Muscle tone lips/cheeks (Normal)

____ ____ 64. Hypertonic muscle tone of lips

____ ____ 65. Hypotonic muscle tone of lips

Oral Reflexes

____ ____ 66. Gag (Normal)*

____ ____ 67. Bite (Normal)*

____ ____ 68. Rooting (Normal)*

____ ____ 69. Suck/swallow (Normal)*

Respiration

____ ____ 70. Mouth

____ ____ 71. Nose

____ ____ 72. Thoracic

____ ____ 73. Abdominal

____ ____ 74. Regular rhythm*

Oral Sensitivity

____ ____ 75. Inside mouth (Normal)*

____ ____ 76. Outside mouth (Normal)*

____ ____ 77. Hypersensitivity*

____ ____ 78. Hyposensitivity*

____ ____ 79. Intolerance to brushing teeth

FEEDING PATTERNS

Yes   No   Bottle-Feeding

____ ____ 80. Suckling tongue movements

____ ____ 81. Sucking tongue movements

____ ____ 82. Firm lip seal*

____ ____ 83. Coordinated suck-swallow-breathing

____ ____ 84. Difficulty swallowing*

Cup-Drinking

____ ____ 85. Adequate lip closure*

____ ____ 86. Loses less than ½ total amount*

____ ____ 87. Wide up-and-down jaw movements

____ ____ 88. Stabilizes jaw by biting edge of cup

____ ____ 89. Stabilizes jaw through muscle control

____ ____ 90. Drinks through a straw

Feeding Patterns—Spoon-Feeding

____ ____ 91. Suckles as food approaches

____ ____ 92. Cleans food off lower lip

____ ____ 93. Cleans food off spoon with upper lip

____ ____ 94. Munching pattern

Lateralizes Tongue

____ ____ 95. When food placed between molars

____ ____ 96. When food placed center of tongue

____ ____ 97. To move food from side to side

____ ____ 98. Vertical jaw movements

____ ____ 99. Rotary jaw movements

Feeding Patterns—Chewing

____ ____ 100. Lip closure during chewing*

Isolated, Voluntary Tongue Movements

____ ____ 101. Protrudes/retracts tongue

____ ____ 102. Elevates tongue outside mouth

____ ____ 103. Elevates tongue inside mouth

____ ____ 104. Depresses tongue outside mouth

____ ____ 105. Depresses tongue inside mouth

____ ____ 106. Lateralizes tongue outside mouth

____ ____ 107. Lateralizes tongue inside mouth

Special Oral Problems

____ ____ 108. Drools*

____ ____ 109. Thrusts tongue when utensil placed in mouth*

____ ____ 110. Thrusts tongue during chewing/ swallowing*

____ ____ 111. Other oral-motor problem*

NUTRITION HISTORY

Yes   No   Past Status

____ ____ 112. Feeding problems birth–1 year*

____ ____ 113. Breast-fed

____ ____ 114. Bottle-fed

____ ____ 115. Weaned

____ ____ 116. Eats blended food

____ ____ 117. Eats limited texture

____ ____ 118. Eats chopped table foods

____ ____ 119. Eats table foods

____ ____ 120. Feeds unassisted

____ ____ 121. Feeds with partial guidance

____ ____ 122. Feeds with complete guidance

____ ____ 123. Drinks from a cup unassisted

____ ____ 124. Drinks from a cup assisted

____ ____ 125. Finger feeds

____ ____ 126. Uses a spoon

____ ____ 127. Uses a fork

____ ____ 128. Uses a knife

____ ____ 129. Average rate of eating

____ ____ 130. Fast rate of eating

____ ____ 131. Slow rate of eating

Diet Review

____ ____ 132. Appetite normal

FIGURE 24.1 (*continued*)

____ ____	133.	Eats 3 meals/day
____ ____	134.	Snacks daily

Dietary Intake, Current

____ ____	135.	Milk/dairy products, 3–4/day
____ ____	136.	Vegetables, 2–3/day
____ ____	137.	Fruit, 2–3/day
____ ____	138.	Meat/meat substitute, 2–3/day
____ ____	139.	Bread/cereal, 3–4/day
____ ____	140.	Sweets/snacks, 1–2/day
____ ____	141.	Liquids, 2 cups/day

SOCIAL/BEHAVIORAL

Yes	No		Child–Caregiver Relationship
____	____	142.	Child responds to caregiver
____	____	143.	Caregiver affectionate to child

Social Skills

____ ____	144.	Eye contact
____ ____	145.	Smiles
____ ____	146.	Gestures, i.e., waves bye-bye

____ ____	147.	Clings to caregiver
____ ____	148.	Interacts with examiner
____ ____	149.	Responds to simple directions
____ ____	150.	Seeks approval
____ ____	151.	Toilet trained
____ ____	152.	Knows own sex

Behavior Problems

____ ____	153.	Self-abusive
____ ____	154.	Hyperactive
____ ____	155.	Aggressive
____ ____	156.	Withdrawn
____ ____	157.	Other*

Play

____ ____	158.	Plays infant games, i.e., pat-a-cake
____ ____	159.	Solitary play
____ ____	160.	Parallel play
____ ____	161.	Cooperative play
____ ____	162.	Additional comments*

COMMENTS

Reproduced from Smith MAH, Connolly B, McFadden S, et al. Developmental feeding tool. In: Smith MAH. *Feeding Management for a Child with a Handicap*. Memphis, TN: Boling Child Development Center, University of Tennessee Center for Health Sciences; 1982:69. Used with permission.[35]

FIGURE 24.1 (*continued*) Developmental Feeding Tool

The feeding evaluation should include assessing the oral mechanism, neuromuscular development, head and trunk control, eye–hand coordination, position for feeding, and social-behavioral components, which include the interaction between child and caregiver. Children with developmental disabilities frequently have oral motor feeding problems and positioning problems and tend to be very easily distracted.[36]

Nutrition Intervention

Once the nutritional problems have been identified for the child with developmental disabilities and special needs, various types of intervention programs may be implemented. First, however, the motivation level and degree of understanding of the parents and the family must be taken into consideration. Indeed, the guidelines for intervention provided in the surgeon general's report[37] on case management for children with developmental disabilities specify that all approaches should be family-centered, community-based, comprehensive, and culturally competent. Intervention should include all aspects of a child's treatment program to avoid issuing an isolated set of instructions relevant only to the treatment goals of one discipline among the many involved in a child's care. This is an important consideration for the registered dietitian working with this particular population.[38,39] A parent or other designated family member may be the individual's case manager, or another healthcare professional may be the case manager. Nutrition intervention would then become a part of the total intervention package rather than standing alone.

Another important consideration is whether the family gives a high priority to a particular intervention procedure. This applies to any discipline, but in this case particularly to nutrition. For example, consider an obese child with spina bifida who has frequent urinary tract infections and a major problem with constipation. The family of this child may give a lower priority to weight management until they take care of the other problems. If that is the case, then suggestions should be provided when the family is ready. When suggestions are given, the coping and educational level of the family should be considered. Often parents have difficulty accepting the fact that they have a child with a developmental disability and may not be able to deal with too many suggestions at once. Cultural competence requires sensitivity to expectations and perspectives related to childcare within a given culture. Increasing numbers of diverse populations are moving into this country and often are non-English-speaking. This requires an interpreter to ensure that the family understands and accepts the intervention suggested.[39]

It is better to give one or two specific nutrition activities for a parent to work on at first. More evaluation and suggestions can be given at frequent follow-up visits. Also, it is important to communicate with the parent or caregiver by telephone for reinterpretation of what was said during the visit. This is particularly true when parents are distraught and find it difficult to follow through on several suggestions given at once. As a result, they may not attempt anything. Additionally, increasing numbers of parents have computer access to the Internet, a new avenue for communication; however, misinformation often is provided online.

An important consideration for this particular population is the cost of some of the nutrition intervention suggestions. The nutritionist should determine whether there is a community resource or insurance available for support. Variability in state coverage requires research on the part of the nutritionist.

The general principle in the management of nutritional concerns is the importance of the interdisciplinary team approach.[39] Again, it has been the author's experience that most children with developmental disabilities have problems that require input from the parent, physician, physical therapist, occupational therapist, speech pathologist, social worker, psychologist, and nurse, in addition to the nutritionist. Pulling that team together is important in order to have successful nutrition intervention. Some examples of the interdisciplinary approach include working with the occupational therapist or speech pathologist in control of oral motor problems and the positioning of the child with a feeding problem or working with a psychologist on behavioral problems. These problems influence how nutrition is addressed. Communication is a key element in the success of the interdisciplinary approach; group discussions, correspondence between groups, and good documentation are vital. The success of an interdisciplinary effort can be significant and bring about positive changes in the nutritional problems, so it is worth the effort to ensure lines of communication are maintained.

▶ Nutritional Problems

Many infants and children with special needs develop other problems such as obesity, malnutrition, constipation, and dental diseases.

Obesity

Weight management of the child with special needs is indicated for any child who tends to plot higher than the 75th percentile for BMI. Conditions that predispose a child to obesity are low muscle tone, limited physical activity, isolation, lack of knowledge about food, and slow growth in height, all of which are found in children with Down syndrome, Prader-Willi syndrome, spina bifida, Turner's syndrome, Myelomeningocele, and Cerebral Palsy.[40] The energy needs of such children were outlined previously in Table 24.3.

Prevention is the best way to avoid obesity. Counseling in appropriate feeding practices, increasing physical activity, and frequent monitoring of height and weight are essential in a prevention program. Important topics to cover in counseling the parent for preventive weight management include:

- Assessing growth curves and growth rates
- Identifying true hunger cues
- Increasing activity
- Selecting nutritious low-calorie foods
- Identifying food preparation practices
- Placing emphasis on food in the family
- Estimating serving sizes
- Having mealtime structure

Successful programs for the obese child should be individually planned and include a written meal plan. For the school-age child, successful management will require contact with the child's school in order to determine which foods are available through the school food service.[4] Often the family is unaware that Section 504 of the 1973 Rehabilitation Act provides for modified school lunches when a prescription is submitted for a child with special needs. Dietary modification of the school meal can be ordered by the physician or a registered dietitian/nutritionist and may address calories, protein, carbohydrates, consistency, and allergy/food intolerances. The prescription is generally submitted on a form that can be provided by the school or state child nutrition program.

Childhood weight management must be carefully planned in order to avoid poor growth or nutritional deficiencies. In the school setting, it should become a part of the individualized education plan. Dietary records maintained by the parent and others caring for the child such as teachers, day care workers, family, and friends are useful for monitoring intake. The diet plan for the older special needs child who is also cognitively delayed must be presented in a way the child can understand. The interdisciplinary approach of working with a special education teacher to present written or pictorial information in an understandable format is helpful for success in this area.

Lack of exercise is often common in the child or adolescent with developmental disabilities. The availability of exercise programs for such children varies from school system to school system, as does the availability of general community-based programs of exercise. Exploring and coordinating community exercise resources are an important part of the registered dietitian's role in providing good nutritional care. Special Olympics events exist in almost all states and are associated with school sports in which the child with special needs can participate and compete.

Behavioral considerations are also an important aspect of weight management programs for the child with developmental disabilities. Important behavioral assessments to make include:

- Speed of eating
- Meal frequency
- Length of time spent eating
- Where meals are eaten

Frequently used behavior strategies include establishing a reward system for compliance with diet, increasing exercise, and targeting eating behaviors to change.

Prader-Willi Syndrome

Intervention for obesity for the child with Prader-Willi syndrome requires special involvement of both the family and healthcare providers.[41] Total environmental control of food access plus a low-calorie diet combined with consistent behavior management techniques and physical exercise are necessary. Environmental control may include locking the refrigerator, cupboards, and kitchen. Individuals with Prader-Willi syndrome often hide and hoard food and exhibit emotional outbursts when food is withheld. Physical exercise is challenging due to the hypotonia that is characteristic of the syndrome, a poor sense of balance, and a reluctance to exercise. The individual tires easily and often has limited gross motor skills. Early introduction of growth hormone treatment has been effective in treating short stature and prevention of obesity.[42]

It has been estimated that the caloric needs of the child with Prader-Willi syndrome are 37–77% of normal for weight maintenance, that weight loss occurs at 8 to 9 calories per centimeter of height, and that maintenance of appropriate weight can be accomplished at 10 to 11 calories per centimeter of height.[41]

Several hypocaloric regimens have been used in various centers with variable success. Using a modified diabetic exchange list has been successful along with a balanced low-calorie diet, a ketogenic diet, and a protein-sparing modified fast.[41]

Increasing physical activity and exercise are important strategies, and daily exercise routines should be begun early to prevent problems secondary to hypotonia. Adaptive physical education programs in the school should be used with the school-age child with Prader-Willi. Recent treatment has included growth hormone therapy to increase stature, lean body mass and mobility as well as decrease fat mass and improve movement and flexibility

from infancy through adulthood.[42] Advances in the early diagnosis of infants with Prader-Willi syndrome is an important factor in beginning an early intervention program that includes working with malnutrition and early feeding problems, followed by hyperphagia and weight management concerns.

Malnutrition/Failure to Thrive

Malnutrition, previously known as failure to thrive, defined as inadequate weight for height, is frequently found in the child with special needs. It may result from the following:

- Impaired oral motor function, dysphagia, texture issues and resultant feeding problems
- Excessive energy needs, such as those that occur in cerebral palsy, pulmonary problems, and heart disease
- Gastrointestinal problems such as reflux, diarrhea, and malabsorption
- Infections and frequent illnesses
- Medications that may affect appetite
- Pica consumption leading to lead intoxication or parasites such as giardia
- Parental/caretaker inadequacy related to feeding

Nutrition intervention must begin with a careful assessment, including a feeding evaluation with the opportunity for observation of parent/caregiver–child interaction and environmental concerns. Management strategies will be individualized, but will generally require increasing calories by providing concentrated formula for the infant, using supplemental formulas, or providing energy-dense foods through carbohydrate or fat supplements (see **TABLE 24.6**).

TABLE 24.6 Foods that Can Be Added to Pureed Foods to Increase Calories	
Food	**Calories**
Infant cereal	9/tbsp
Nonfat dry milk	25/tbsp
Cheese (melted)	120/oz
Butter or Margarine	101/tbsp
Evaporated milk	40/oz
Vegetable oils	110/tbsp
Strained infant meats	100–150/jar
Glucose polymers, powdered or liquid	30/tbsp

See Chapter 4 on Malnutrition for a complete overview of assessment, diagnosis, and interventions to treat malnutrition.

Some children with special needs and malnutrition require medical evaluations to determine the existence of gastroesophageal reflux and aspiration leading to a need for tube feeding or total parenteral nutrition on a temporary basis following a surgical procedure for a gastrointestinal disorder. Studies evaluating the effectiveness of a gastrostomy feeding versus oral feeds have been completed with the need for more research in this area recommended. All of the studies demonstrated significant weight gain when tube feeding was implemented.[16] Long term enteral nutrition is required to adequately nourish some children with special needs. In some cases and where medically indicated, oral diet may also be offered for pleasure.

Constipation

Constipation, defined as infrequent bowel movements of hard stools, often afflicts children with developmental disabilities due to a lack of activity, generalized hypotonia, or limited bowel muscle function. It can also result from insufficient fluid intake, lack of fiber in the diet, frequent vomiting, and medications. Parents frequently report using laxatives, mineral oil, and enemas on a regular basis to correct the problem. As a rule, laxatives and enemas are not recommended because they can lead to dependency, and mineral oil decreases the absorption of the fat-soluble vitamins A, D, E, and K.

Treatment includes adjusting the diet to increase fiber and fluid content. Usual recommendations are:

- Maintain adequate fluid intake, exceeding the daily requirement for age, including water and diluted fruit juice.
- Increase fiber content of the diet by replacing white bread and canned fruits with whole-grain breads and cereals, raw vegetables, fresh fruits, dried fruits, commercial fiber-rich beverages, and cereals fortified with 1 to 2 tablespoons of unprocessed bran. Fiber can also be increased successfully by adding fiber supplements. A variety of fiber supplements are available for consideration for individual children.
- Yogurt now manufactured with pre- and probiotics has been successful in improving the intestinal function of children.
- Increase daily exercise.

Feeding Problems

Feeding problems are defined as the inability or refusal to eat certain foods because of neuromotor dysfunction, obstructive lesions, or psychosocial factors. Most feeding problems are the result of oral motor difficulties (see **TABLE 24.7**) caused by neuromotor dysfunction,

TABLE 24.7 Oral Motor Problems and Effect on Food Intake

Problem	Description	
Tonic bite reflex	Strong jaw closure when teeth and gums are stimulated	Interferes with actual intake of food
Tongue thrust	Forceful and often repetitive protrusion of an often bunched or thick tongue in response to oral stimulation	Parent or care taker may misinterpret as child's dislike of food
Jaw thrust	Forceful opening of the jaw to the maximal extent during eating, drinking, attempts to speak, or general excitement	Interferes with acceptance of food and swallowing
Tongue retraction	Pulling back the tongue within the oral cavity at the presentation of food, spoon, or cup	Makes swallowing and chewing difficult along with cup drinking
Lip retraction	Pulling back the lips in a very tight, smile-like pattern at the approach of the spoon or cup toward the face	Makes food intake difficult and requires facilitation to relax the lips
Sensory defensiveness	A strong adverse reaction to sensory input (touch, sound, light)	Can lead to refusal to accept a variety of foods due to oral sensitivity

Reproduced from Cloud, Harriet. *Feeding a Priority for the Dietetic Professional*. 2009. Available at: Specialkidsnutrition.com. Accessed October 16, 2018.[43]

developmental delays, positioning problems, a poor mother–child relationship, or sensory defensiveness.[35] All of these problems may contribute to such behavioral problems as a refusal to eat, mealtime tantrums, resistance to texture changes, and the like.

Intervention for feeding problems lends itself best to the team approach, utilizing occupational therapy, physical therapy, speech, nursing, psychology, nutrition, and social work.[35] A single written care plan developed by the team, prioritized with the parent's assistance according to the child's needs, should be provided. Nutritional intervention may involve increasing calories, altering the texture of foods offered, and determining tube-feeding formulas. Additional nutrition education and counseling, oral motor therapy, and behavior management counseling are part of the feeding plan. Many children with feeding problems of an oral motor nature will benefit from a modified barium swallow in order to detect the possibility of aspiration. This will allow the team to determine the necessity of thickening liquids. A number of products have been developed for thickening and generally consist of a corn starch base, which has advantages over using cereal. New technology now exists allowing specially trained speech therapists to treat dysphagia with **neuromuscular electrical stimulation** (NMES) or Vital Stim Therapy.[44]

Dental Disease

Dental health care contributes to overall improved nutritional status, but is often an unmet need in children and adolescents who are developmentally disabled. Dental caries and gum disease are prevalent in this population and are caused by plaque formation, tooth susceptibility, sugar consumption, and medication. Prevention includes home care, professional treatment, and nutritional intervention.

Nutritional intervention involves decreasing the sucrose intake of the diet by eliminating candy, sugar-containing gum, sugar-containing carbonated beverages, cookies, cakes, and highly sweetened foods. Supplying adequate fluoride in the drinking water is helpful in preventing caries. In communities where the water supply is not fluoridated, toothpaste and topical application of fluoride can be used. Many families drink bottled water, which may not contain fluoride; however, some manufacturers are now adding fluoride and list it on the food label.

Gingival disease is often found where dental hygiene is poor. Children taking Dilantin for seizures may suffer gingival hyperplasia, a side effect of the drug. Nutrition counseling to increase the intake of raw fruits and vegetables and improve snacking practices, coupled with good dental hygiene instruction from the dentist and regular dental care, are important components of dental

intervention problems. One additional concern for the child with developmental disabilities is late weaning from the bottle and extended use of the "sippy" cup filled with juice, tea, or other sweetened beverages. Permitting a child to constantly drink from this cup can contribute to an increase in dental caries.

Seizures

The ketogenic diet has been developed and used in the treatment of epileptic seizures nonresponsive to anticonvulsants.[45] Traditionally, the diet is recommended for children under age 5 with myoclonic, absence, and atonic seizures that are medically nonresponsive. This diet is high in fat and very low in protein and carbohydrates, and is designed to increase the body's reliance on fatty acids rather than glucose for energy. The classic fat-to-carbohydrate ratio is 3:1 to 4:1. It is thought that the ketosis produced by the high fat to low carbohydrate ratio decreases the number and severity of the seizures. Typically, the diet provides 1 gram of protein per kilogram of body weight, although protein can be increased if linear growth slows unacceptably.[46] To achieve dehydration and reduce urinary loss of ketones, fluids were limited; however, this led to constipation and kidney stones and is no longer considered beneficial.[47] Historically, the diet is high in saturated fat content; however, in recent years, corn oil and MCT oil have been used, but protocols also contain whipping cream, bacon, butter, margarine, and mayonnaise.[48]

The child under 18 months of age, older than 12 years, or obese may be started on a 3:1 ratio. Other variants of the ketogenic diet include the MCT diet originated in 1970;[48] the modified Atkins diet; and the low glycemic index treatment, which stabilizes blood glucose and allows more carbohydrate than the classic ketogenic diet. Infants and children fed by either bottle or tube can be given the ketogenic diet as a liquid feeding. Powdered or liquid formulas are available in 3:1 and 4:1 ratios for use in children who are enterally fed. These are available from Ketocal and Ketovolve, to name two.[49]

Numerous studies have evaluated the effectiveness of the ketogenic diet. A large study, completed by Johns Hopkins Hospital, enrolled 150 children.[50] Results of this demonstrated the effectiveness of the diet in controlling seizures in 3–5 year follow-up although some of the children stopped the diet during the first year. Numerous other studies have found the diet effective when properly monitored.[48] Daily carbohydrate-free vitamin and mineral supplements are required because the diet is low in calcium, magnesium, iron, vitamin C, and other water-soluble vitamins and minerals. The expense of the diet, compliance problems, and lack of palatability have made its use controversial. Concerns also have been raised related to growth which should be monitored for both height and weight.

Like all children on metabolic diets, the child requires close monitoring and frequent follow-up visits. Routine laboratory studies are required at clinic visits following initiation on months 1, 2, 6, 9, and 12, including urinalysis, electrolytes, transaminases, bilirubin, glucose, serum calcium, lipid profile, and prealbumin. The diet may be discontinued for children who are seizure-free for 2 years. Although this diet is high in fat and low in protein and carbohydrates, it is different from the Atkins diet and parents should be so advised. Although the ketogenic diet is restrictive and requires continued effort, it completely controls epilepsy in 10–15% of the children whose seizures are otherwise uncontrollable.

▶ Autism, Attention Deficit Disorder, and Attention Deficit Hyperactivity Disorder

There is an increased frequency of children diagnosed with Autism, Attention Deficit Disorder and Attention Deficit Hyperactivity Disorder. In a recent report the CDC estimated that 1 in 68 children were identified with autism spectrum disorder, a 30% increase since 2012.[51]

Autism

Autism is one of five disorders under the category **pervasive developmental disorders** (PDD) and has grown in prevalence since 1980. All types of PDD are neurologic disorders that are usually evident by age 3. Generally, children who have one of the types of PDD have difficulty in talking, playing with other children, and relating to others including their family. The five types of PDD are autistic disorder, Rett's disorder, childhood disintegrative disorder, Asperger's syndrome, and pervasive developmental disorder not otherwise specified. PDDs are four times more common in boys, with the exception of Rett's disorder, which is more commonly found in girls.

Autistic disorders or **autism spectrum disorders** (ASD) affect 1 in 68 children per year.[51] Many children with autistic disorders also have intellectual compromise. The term *Asperger's syndrome* is most often used to describe children with the problems of ASD but who have normal to high cognitive levels.[51] Efforts to find the cause of ASD have led to many studies involving a toxic environment, toxic food, nutritional deficiencies, immune system problems, oxidative stress, gastrointestinal problems, allergies, and emotional stress. The definition of a toxic environment or toxic food when applied

to ASD includes air pollution, lead in the soil, manipulation of food production with chemical spraying, hormones added to meat, and so on. The role of nutrition has involved neurotransmitters; essential fatty acids; nutrients with antioxidant qualities such as vitamins A, C, E, and selenium; mineral supplementation with zinc, calcium, and magnesium; a mercury-free diet; or an allergy elimination diet. So many possible causes have led to many proposed diets but little research on the various therapies and their outcomes.

Nutrition and eating problems may affect up to three-quarters of children with ASD. Some of these problems include routine intake and refusal to try new foods; short attention span; increased sensitivity to food textures, color, taste, or temperature; food obsessions or ritual; eating nonfood items; compulsive eating or drinking; packing the mouth with food; vomiting; and gag reflex. For some children, gastrointestinal problems similar to celiac disease have occurred. GI problems include constipation, diarrhea, reflux, vomiting, bloating, pain, and feeding problems. Intolerance to gluten and casein has been identified as a contributor to inflammation of the intestine and the occurrence of brain opioids, but there has been little research to support these claims. Even so, the gluten-free, casein-free diet is considered a complementary and alternative therapy and has gained increasing popularity with parents of children with ASD.[52]

No one therapy works for all individuals with ASD. Medical nutrition therapy should be individualized and used along with behavior management, speech therapy, occupational therapy, and counseling. Various diets have been described on the Internet and include a gluten-free, casein-free diet; specific carbohydrate diets; and the body ecology diets.[52] Numerous Websites exist for ordering products for these diets. When these diets are chosen, a registered dietitian should be contacted to work with the parents to ensure that energy and other nutrient needs are being met. Additional help may be required in label reading, meal preparation, and shopping for food sources. Extensive research is needed to keep up with the many products appearing on the market, in order to effectively counsel the parent.

Attention Deficit Hyperactivity Disorder and Attention Deficit Disorder

Attention deficit hyperactivity disorder (ADHD) or ADD is a neurobehavioral problem being seen with increasing frequency in children. It has been associated with learning disorders, inappropriate degrees of impulsiveness, hyperactivity, and attention deficit. Causes of ADHD are unclear. There are three subtypes of ADHD developed by the American Psychiatric Association: (1) combined type of hyperactivity and attention deficit, (2) predominately inattentive type, and (3) predominately hyperactive-impulse behavior.[53] Many of these children are on medications that may affect their weight and growth in height. Medications used to treat these disorders often cause anorexia, so the child's nutrition assessment and follow-up should include anthropometric measures. If the child is on medications, the time of administration is important, generally after eating to allow for more appetite at meal times.

Many dietary treatments have been proposed to treat ADHD and ADD, starting in 1973 when Feingold proposed removing food coloring and naturally occurring salicylates from the diet. This was followed by eliminating sugar and caffeine and the addition of large doses of vitamins. Feingold's treatments have been discounted as lacking scientific validity and effectiveness. The need for additional research is indicated.

It has been suggested that a lack of **essential fatty acids** (EFAs) is a possible cause of hyperactivity in children. Some children given omega-3 fatty acids showed improvement in hyperactivity.[54] Various biochemical reasons for a deficiency of the fatty acids could be a lack of ability to metabolize linoleic acid normally, an inability to absorb EFAs effectively, or because EFA requirements for these children are higher than normal. The dosage for omega-3 supplementation ranges from 20 to 60 mg/kg.[54] Because the supplement is in capsule form it lends itself to research studies. One study in Germany of 810 children ages 5–12 provided a food supplement containing omega 3 and omega 5 fatty acids plus zinc and magnesium and it resulted in considerable reduction in attention deficit and hyperactivity in the children after 12 weeks of supplementation.[55]

The most effective treatment for the child with ADHD or ADD is a diet based on the Dietary Guidelines or My Plate, mealtime structure, small amounts of food followed by refills, a distraction-free environment, and no "grazing" on food or liquids throughout the day.

Community Resources and Cost

Several federal programs provide financial coverage for nutrition services for children with developmental disabilities and special healthcare needs. Title V of the Social Security Act provides funding for maternal and child health services including children with special healthcare needs. Title XIX of the Social Security Act funds Medicaid, which funds medical services for low income individuals and families. Additionally, Medicaid has funded tube feeding formulas, dietary supplements, eating devices, and in some states formulas for inherited disorders of metabolism. Nutrition services are included in the legislation passed in 1985 for early intervention programs serving infants and toddlers from birth to age 5. Project Head Start was created in 1965 to promote school readiness among preschool children from low income families, and is mandated to include children with special needs.[55] One of the programs that provides actual formulas and food for children from low income families is the Supplemental Program for **Women, Infants and Children** (WIC). Infants and children from birth to 5 years of age with inherited disorders of metabolism can receive dietary supplements and special formulas. Children with special needs and developmental disabilities of school age are eligible for meal modification under Section 504 of the Rehabilitation Act of 1973 and the Americans with Disabilities Act of 1990.

Other legislation that provides funding for children with developmental disabilities and funding of nutrition services includes the Child Health Act of 2000 and State Children's Health Insurance Programs. All of these programs are possible sources of dietary needs; however, programs vary from state to state.

▶ Conclusion

The nutritional needs of children with developmental disabilities and special health care needs are important considerations in treatment and program planning. The nutritional goal is to ensure intake adequate for growth and to provide enough energy for participation in therapy. Research is needed to better define the nutritional requirements of this population and the use of the DRIs to estimate energy requirements.

Registered dietitians in programs serving this population are challenged to defend the cost effectiveness of nutritional care and to develop nutrition education materials and programs specifically adapted for these children and adolescents in collaboration with special education professionals.

🔍 CASE STUDY

Nutrition Assessment

Patient history: A 14-year-old girl with Down syndrome was admitted to a mental health services facility for treatment of sleep apnea, prediabetes, and severe behavioral reactions. A contributing factor to the medical problems was her severe obesity. Before her admission to the facility she had been in public school in their special education programs, but her behavior was so difficult to control that the school transferred her to the mental health facility. She is the only individual in her family with Down syndrome and was born when her mother was 40. There is a history of diabetes in the family. Food has always been used as a reward. **Food-nutrition-related history:** This child's birth weight was 7 lb., 8 oz, birth length was 19 inches, and the pregnancy was full term. She was breastfed until 3 months of age, when she was transitioned to a standard iron fortified infant formula. There were no feeding problems reported other than her consuming over 36 oz. of milk daily and eating baby food in unusually large amounts. Her weaning to a cup was late, at 18 months, and her motor skill development was late with an inability to walk until 28 months of age. She also had low muscle tone.

By the time she was 12 months of age her weight was 28 lbs., placing her above the 95th percentile, and each subsequent year she remained between the 75th and 95th percentile for her weight, but at the 10th percentile for her height.

During her preschool and school years the child's intake was reported as very limited in variety with a heavy concentration of foods from fast food restaurants, and little intake of fruits and vegetables. She drank milk but preferred soft drinks and sweetened tea. She also consumed many sweetened desserts, cookies, and bakery products. Although her mother reported trying to control this behavior, a grandparent was very indulgent. She also developed behavioral problems with a great deal of acting out behavior both at home and at school. It was this behavior that led to her referral to the mental health facility.

Anthropometric Measurements
Weight: 247 pounds (112.2 kg), (+ 2.86 z-score)
Height: 56 inches (142 cm), (-2.82 z-score)
BMI: 97% (+2.93 z-score)
Estimated energy needs: 1716 kcal
Estimated energy intake at home: 3000 kcal (based on maternal report)
Estimated protein needs: 52 g

Biochemical Data
Hgb: 14 mg
Hct: 36 mg
Cholesterol: 210
Glucose: 120 mg
Medications: Topomax, Clonidine for seizures and behavioral problems
Diet order following physical examination: 1500 calories plus exercise

Nutrition-Focused Physical Findings
Excessive appetite
Dry skin
Inactivity with behavioral outbursts related to walking
Feeding problems—very rapid eating with possibility of choking
Low muscle tone
Constipation

Nutrition Diagnoses
Obesity as evidenced by BMI of +2.93 z-score
Excessive intake of carbohydrates as evidenced by excessive intake of sweets by diet history
Inadequate fluid intake as evidenced by results of nutrition-focused physical exam
Refusal to eat raw fruits, vegetables and whole grains as evidenced by diet history results.

Intervention Goals
- Weight loss and acceptance of more variety in foods provided
- Increase consumption of high fiber foods
- Limit between meal snacks to fruit and vegetables
- Counsel parents related to meal management and poor behavior related to food
- Increase physical activity at school and home

Nutrition Interventions
- Modify the meal plan to provide 1500 calories including snacks
- Provide copies of menu to group home staff and parents
- Increase availability of fresh fruit and raw vegetables for snacks
- Increase water intake

(continues)

🔍 *CASE STUDY* (continued)

Monitoring and Evaluation
- Weigh monthly and plot continuously with report to parents
- Counsel parents monthly or as necessary related to food intake and exercise at home
- Walking at school with teachers and other students

Questions for the Reader
1. Teachers report that student eats only part of the meal provided and refuses the snacks offered. What would be your response?
2. The parents report in their monthly conference that the student is very rebellious and refuses to participate in the family activities unless provided with a trip to a fast food restaurant for hamburgers and French fries. What could you suggest?
3. Monthly weights show a loss of 2–3 pounds each month. How would you suggest using the weight loss to increase motivation?

Review Questions

1. True or False: Children with Special Needs is a term which include the following disorders?
   A. Intellectual and Developmental Disability
   B. Inherited Disorders of Metabolism
   C. Children with Seizures

2. Nutrition Assessment of CSH should include which of the following?
   A. Growth velocity
   B. Laboratory results
   C. BMI
   D. Triceps skinfold
   E. Adequacy of diet

3. Children with Special Needs may require special tests. Which of the following is important for Down Syndrome?
   A. Hemoglobin and hematocrit
   B. Thyroid level
   C. Glucose tolerance
   D. Carnitine levels.

4. Hyperactive gag reflex and swallowing difficulty are feeding problems that may be found in the course of a nutrition assessment. True or False

5. Give some examples of growth curves that are used for children with Special Needs.

6. Autism Spectrum Disorder is a complex developmental and neurological condition affecting 1 in 68 children. What are the most important nutrition concerns?
   A. Limited food selection
   B. Poor growth
   C. Constipation
   D. Gluten intolerance
   E. Food texture sensitivity

7. Are WIC, Head Start, and SNAP federal programs that may help Children with Special Needs and their families? Describe these programs.

8. Energy needs may be lower for Children with Special Needs especially those with chromosomal aberrations. Select the reasons:
   A. Lower basal metabolic rate
   B. Low muscle tone
   C. Medications
   D. Hyperactivity

References

1. American Association on Intellectual and Developmental Disabilities. Available at: http://www.aaidd.org/content. Accessed May 18, 2018.
2. *Developmental Disabilities Assistance and Bill of Rights Act.* Public Law. 106–402; 2000.
3. McPherson M, Arango P, Fox H, et al. A new definition of children with special health care needs. *Pediatr.* 1998;102:137–140.
4. Cloud H. Medical nutrition therapy for intellectual and developmental disabilities. In: Mahan, K , Chapman, J.

Eds. *Krauses Food and Nutrition Care Process.* St. Louis MI:Elsivier; 2017:909–930.
5. Van Riper C, Wallace L, American Dietetic Association. Position of the American Dietetic Association: providing nutrition services for people with developmental disabilities and special health care needs. *J Am Diet Assoc.* 2010;110(2):296–307.
6. Institute of Medicine of the National Academies. *Dietary Reference Intakes for Energy, Carbohydrate, Fiber, Fat, Fatty*

Acids, Cholesterol, Protein and Amino Acids. Washington, DC: National Academies Press; 2005.

7. Irby MB, Kolbash S, Garner-Edwards D,Skelton JA. Pediatric obesity treatment in children with neurodevelopmental disabilities. A case series and review of the literature. ICAN. 2012;4(4)212–215.

8. Hill DL, Parks EP, Zemel BS, Shults J, Stallings VA, Stettler N; Resting energy expenditure and adiposity accretion among children with Down syndrome: a three year prospective study. *Eur.J Clin Nutr.* 2013 67(10):1087–1091.

9. Weston S, Murray P. Alternative methods of estimating daily energy requirements based on health condition. In: Devore J, Shotton A, eds: *Pocket Guide to Children with Special Health Care Needs.* Chicago,IL:Academy of Nutrition and Dietetics;2012.

10. Ferluga ED, Archer KR, Sathe NA, et al. Interventions for feeding and nutrition in cerebral palsy. Comparative Effectiveness Review No, 94. Prepared by the Vanderbilt Evidenced–based Practice Center AHRQ Publication March 2013.Available at: www.effectivehealthcare.ahrq.gov/reports/final.cfm.

11. Andrew MJ, Sullivan PB. Growth in Cerebral Palsy. *Nutr Clin Pract.* 2010;25:357.

12. Bandini LG, Schneller DA, Fukagana NK, Wykes L, Dietz WH. Body composition and energy expenditure in adolescents with cerebral palsy or myelodysplasia. *Pediatr Res.* 1991;29:70–77.

13. Stallings VA, Cronk CE, Zemme BS, Charney EB. Body composition in children with spastic quadriplegic cerebral palsy. *J Pediatr.* 1995;126(5):833–839.

14. Stallings VA, Zemel BS, Davies JC, Cronk CE, Charney EB. Energy expenditure of children and adolescents with severe disabilities: a cerebral palsy model. *Am J Clin Nutr.* 1996;64(4):627–634.

15. Walker WA, Hendricks KM. Estimation of energy needs. In: *Manual of Pediatric Nutrition.* Philadelphia, PA:WB Saunders;1985.

16. Gantasala S, Sullivan PB, Thomas AG. Gastrostomy feeding versus oral feeding alone for children with cerebral palsy. Cochrane Database Sys Rev. 2013;(7):. No CDoo3943. DOI.

17. Ekvall SW. Chronic diseases and developmental disabilities. In: Ekvall SW, Ekvall V Eds. *Pediatric And Adult Nutrition in Chronic Diseases, Developmental Disabilities and Hereditary Metabolic Disorders.* New York, NY:Oxford University Press;2017: 81–84.

18. Bennett FC, McClelland S, Kriegsmann E, Andrus L, Sells C. Vitamin and mineral supplementation in Down's syndrome. *Pediatr.* 1983;72:707–713.

19. Bidder RT, Gray P, Newcombe RG, Evans BK, Hughes M. The effects of multivitamins and minerals on children with Down syndrome. *Dev Med Child Neurol.* 1989; 31:532–537.

20. Bull MJ, Committee on Genetics. Health supervision for children with Down Syndrome. Pediatr. 2011;128:393.

21. American Academy of Pediatrics (AAP): Your child's diet: a cause and cure of ADHD? Available at: http://pediatrics.aappublications.org/content/129/2/330. Accessed Jan 5, 2015.

22. Elder, JH.The gluten free-casein free diet in an overview with clinical implications. *Nutr Clin Prac.*2008;23(6): 583–588.

23. Henderson RC, Kairalla JA, Barrington JW, Abbas A, Stevenson RD. Longitudinal changes in bone density in children and adolescents with moderate to severe cerebral palsy. *J Pediatr.* 2005;146:769–775.

24. Bergman KE, Makoseh J, Tews KH. Abnormalities of hair zinc concentrations in mothers of newborn infants with spina bifida. *Am J Clin Nutr.* 1980;33:2145–2150.

25. Smithells RN, Nevin NC, Seller MJ, et al. Further experience of vitamin supplementation for prevention of neural tube defect recurrences. *Lancet.* 1983;1:1027.

26. Das JK, et al. Micronutrient fortification of food and its impact on woman and child health; a systematic review. *Syst. Rev.*2013;2:67.

27. Blumchen K, et al. Effects of latex avoidance on latex sensitization, atopy, and allergic disease in children with spina bifida. *Allergy.* 2010;65:1585.

28. Pronsky ZM, Redfern CM, Crowe J, Epstein J, Young V. *Food Medication Interactions.* 13th ed. Birchrunville, PA: Food-Medication Interactions; 2007.

29. Hogan, SE. Knee height as a predictor of recumbent length for individuals with mobility impaired CP. *Am J Coll Nutr.* 199.18:12 201–205.

30. National Center for Health Statistics in collaboration with National Center for Chronic Disease Prevention and Health Promotion. CDC growth charts. 2000. Available at: http://www.cdc.gov/growthcharts. Accessed December 9, 2017.

31. Zemel BS, Pipan M, Stallings VA, et al. Growth charts for children with Down Syndrome in the U.S. *Pediatr.* 2015;136(5);81–102.

32. Roche AF, Hines JH. Incremental growth charts. *Am J Clin Nutr.* 1980;33:2041–2052.

33. Frisancho AR. New norms of upper limb fat and muscle areas for assessment of nutritional status. *Am J Clin Nutr.* 1981;34:2540–2545.

34. Cassidy SB, Schwartz S, Miller Jl, Driscoll DJ. Prader Willi Syndrome. *Gen Med.* 2012;14(1):10–26.

35. Smith MAH, Connolly B, McFadden S, et al. Developmental feeding tool. In: Smith MAH. *Feeding Management for a Child with a Handicap.* Memphis, TN: Boling Child Development Center, University of Tennessee Center for Health Sciences; 1982:69.

36. Spear D, Cushing P, Ekvall SW, Cloud H, Hicks L, Wahoff,J. Feeding and eating problems of the child and adult with intellectual developmental disabilities and special health care needs. In: Ekvall SW, Ekvall VK, eds. *Pediatric and Adult Nutrition in Chronic Diseases. Developmental Disabilities, and Hereditary Metabolic Disorders.* Oxford Univeristy Press, 2017.

37. U.S. Department of Health and Human Services, Public Health Service. *Surgeon General's Report: Children with Special Health Care Needs.* Chicago: DHHS publication no. (HRS) D/MC, 87–92.

38. American Dietetic Association. Providing nutrition services for infants, children and adults with developmental disabilities and special health care needs. *J Am Diet Assoc.* 2009;104(1):97–106.

39. Novaakofski, KC. Education and counselling: behavioral change. In: Mahan KL, Raymond, JL Eds. *Krause's Food and the Nutrition Care Process.* 14th ed. Elsevier, 2017. 227–237.

40. Megan B, Irby MS, Kolbash S, Garner-Edwards D, Shelton JA. Pediatric obesity treatment in Children with

neurodevelopmental disabilities. A case series and review of the literature. ICAN. 2012;4(4):215–221.

41. McCandless SE, Committee on Genetics. Clinical report-health supervision for children with Prader Willi syndrome. Pediatr. 2011;127: 195–254.

42. Carrel AL, et al. Long term growth hormone therapy changes the natural history of body composition and motor function in children with Prader Willi syndrome. *J Clin End Met*. 2010; 95:1131.

43. Cloud, Harriet. *Feeding a Priority for the Dietetic Professional*. 2009. Available at: Specialkidsnutrition.com. Accessed Ocotber 16, 2018.

44. Rice K. Neuromuscular Electrical Stimulation in the Early Intervention Population. A series of 5 case studies. The Internet J Allied Health Sci Prac. 2012;10(3). Available at: https://pdfs.semanticscholar.org/ca77/2cc96ceb73bdb4286a2d32b8d5a664131378.pdf.

45. Zupec-Kania BA, Neal E, Schultz R, Roan ME, Turner Z, Welborn M. An update on diets in clinical practice. *J Child Neuro*. 2013;28(8):1015–1026.

46. Patel A, Pyzik PL, Turner Z, Rubenstein JE, Kossoff EH. Long term outcomes of children treated with the ketogenic diet in the past. *Epilepsia*. 2010;51(7):1277–1282.

47. Sampath A, Kossoff EH, Furth SL, Pyzik PL, Vining EP. Kidney stones and the ketogenic diet: risk factors and prevention. *J Child Neurol*. 2007;4:375–378.

48. Freeman JM, Vining EP, Pillas DJ, Pyzik PL, Casey JC, Kelly LM. The efficacy of the ketogenic diet—1998: a prospective evaluation of intervention of 150 children. *Pediatr*. 1998;102:1358–1363.

49. Nutricia Ketocal Ketogenic Diet: Available at: https://myketocal.com/ourproducts.aspx. Accessed November 27, 2017.

50. Neal EG, Chaffe H, Schwartz RH, et al. The ketogenic diet for the treatment of childhood epilepsy: a randomized controlled trial. *Lancet Neurol*. 2008;7:500–506.

51. Centers for Disease Control and Prevention (CDC). Autism and developmental disabilities monitoring network. Available at: http://www.cdc.gov/ncdd/autism/addm.hrml.

52. Whitely P, Shattock P, Knivsberg AM, et al.M. Gluten and casein free dietary intervention for autism spectrum conditions. Front *Hum Neurosci*. 2013; 6:344.

53. American Psychiatric Association. Diagnostic and Statistical Manual of Mental Disorders (DSM-5). Arlington, VA: American Psychiatric; 2013.

54. Gillies D, Sinn JKh, Las SS, Leach MJ, Ross MJ. Polyunsaturated fatty acids (PUFA) for attention deficit hyperactivity disorder in children and adolescents. Cochran Database Syst Rev. 2012;11(7) :CD007986.

55. Office of Head Start, Administration for Children and Families, U.S. Department of Health and Human Services. About Head Start. Available at: http://eclkc.ohs.acf.hhs.gov. Accessed August 31, 2010.

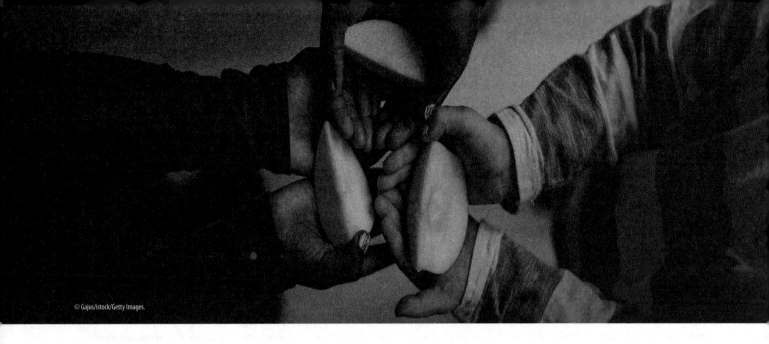

CHAPTER 25

Food Allergy

Alison Cassin

OBJECTIVES

- Describe types of food *allergy*, distinguishing them from *intolerances*, and explain nutritional management depending on the mechanism of reaction.
- Discuss appropriate food allergy management, including diagnosis, oral food challenges, and food allergen avoidance.
- Identify nutritional risks associated with removing common allergens from the diet.
- Discuss early introduction of peanut in infants at risk of peanut allergy.

▶ Introduction

Over the past few decades, mounting data suggests that food allergy is a growing problem, affecting up to 10% of individuals.[1] Yet accurate prevalence is difficult to ascertain. Self-reported food allergy rates are often higher than those confirmed by medically supervised food challenges.[2] Still, individual studies and systematic reviews estimate a food allergy prevalence between 2–10%[3] and are estimated to affect up to 8% of children in the Unites States.[4]

Ingested foods have the potential to induce adverse reactions in humans, yet not all adverse reactions are classified as food allergies. The **National Institutes of Allergy and Infectious Diseases** (NIAID) and the **American Academy of Allergy, Asthma, and Immunology** (AAAAI) define an *adverse food reaction*

as a clinically abnormal response to an ingested food or food additive. Adverse food reactions are categorized either as *food allergies* or as *intolerances*. Food allergy is caused by an *immunologic* reaction resulting from ingesting a food. Food intolerance is an *nonimmunologic* abnormal physiological response to an ingested food or a food additive.

Food allergy involves either **immunoglobulin E** (IgE)-mediated or non-IgE-mediated immune mechanisms. IgE-mediated reactions occur after ingesting a specific food, usually within 1 hour, and can be followed by a late-phase reaction. Non-IgE-mediated reactions such as **food protein–induced enterocolitis syndrome** (FPIES), proctocolitis, allergic eosinophilic gastrointestinal diseases, and gluten-sensitive enteropathy are cell-mediated, or non-IgE-mediated reactions. Food

TABLE 25.1 Food Allergic Disorders

IgE Mediated	Mixed (May Involve Both IgE-Mediated and Cell-Mediated Mechanisms)	Non-IgE Mediated
Anaphylaxis (immediate hives, angiodemia, pruritis, vomiting, diarrhea, hypotension) Food-dependent exercise-induced anaphylaxis (FDEIA) Pollen Food Syndrome (PFAS)/Oral allergy syndrome	Eosinophilic Gastrointestinal disorders (EGIDs) namely Eosinophilic Esophagitis (EoE) Atopic Dermatitis (AD)	Food protein induced enterocolitis syndrome (FPIES) Food protein-induced enteropathy (FPE) Food protein-induced allergic proctocolitis (FPIAP)

Modified from Panel NI-SE, Boyce JA, Assa'ad A, et al. Guidelines for the diagnosis and management of food allergy in the United States: report of the NIAID-sponsored expert panel. *J Allergy Clin Immunol.* 2010;126:S1–S58.[1]

allergies are further described in **TABLE 25.1** by their clinical manifestations and allergic mechanism. Milk, egg, peanut, soy, wheat, tree nuts, fish, and shellfish cause approximately 90% of food allergies in children in the United States.[1] Milk, egg, peanut, soy, and wheat are the primary foods responsible for allergy in children 3 years of age and younger.

Adverse food reactions that are not immunologic in nature are secondary to factors such as toxic contaminants, food-borne illness, pharmacological properties of foods, metabolic disorders, and idiosyncratic responses. For example, lactose intolerance produces symptoms of loose stools and abdominal pain, similar to non-IgE mediated cow's milk allergy. Toddler's diarrhea or chronic nonspecific diarrhea is aggravated by consuming simple sugars, especially sorbitol found in fruits (e.g., apple and pear juice), some sugar-free candies, and chewing gums. Unintentional consumption of food contaminants (infectious organisms and toxins) may result in symptoms similar to an allergic reaction.

Clinical Manifestations

Contact with an allergen is necessary before an IgE immunological response can occur. The skin, gastrointestinal tract, and respiratory tract can be involved with an allergic reaction. More severe, life-threatening reactions involve the cardiovascular system. Non-IgE mediated food allergies often involve the gastrointestinal tract. No matter the mechanism, avoiding ingesting the offending allergen is the basis of the medical management.

Pathophysiology

The allergic immune response begins with sensitization to a particular food antigen. The susceptible individual must come in contact with a food before becoming allergic. In a susceptible individual, plasma cells (mature B-cells) produce IgE to a particular food antigen. The food-specific IgE binds to mast cells and basophils, and then recurrent antigen exposure leads to a cross-linking of the food-specific IgE molecules, activating the mast cells and basophils. This activation causes the release of histamine, leukotrienes, and other mediators. These mediators produce the vasodilation, smooth muscle contraction, and mucous secretion resulting in the clinical symptoms detected in the skin, respiratory system, and gastrointestinal system. The immediate allergic reaction can occur within seconds and up to 2 hours after contact with the food allergen. This cross-linking can lead to the synthesis of proinflammatory cytokines and chemokines that are responsible for a late-phase reaction that might occur within 4 to 48 hours after the initial exposure. A chronic inflammatory response seen primarily with the skin and respiratory systems is thought to be due to the repetitive ingestion of a food allergen.[5]

▶ IgE-Mediated Food Allergies

The organ systems generally related to IgE-mediated allergic reactions are the skin, gastrointestinal (GI) tract, and respiratory tract. Once foods are ingested, there may be immediate oral symptoms such as itching mouth and swelling of the lips, palate, tongue, or throat. In the gastrointestinal tract, nausea, cramping, gas, distention, vomiting, abdominal pain, or diarrhea may be experienced. Once the antigen spreads through the bloodstream and lymphatics, degranulation of mast cells may occur in the skin, causing urticaria, angioedema, pruritis, or an erythematous macular rash. Respiratory symptoms include coughing, wheezing, profuse nasal rhinorrhea, sneezing, or laryngeal edema. The eyes may experience edema, tearing, excess mucus, itching, or burning.

Systemic anaphylaxis is an acute and potentially fatal reaction. Anaphylaxis can begin with any of the symptoms just mentioned plus cardiovascular symptoms including chest tightness, tachycardia, hypotension, and shock. A fatal reaction may begin with mild symptoms and progress to cardiorespiratory arrest and shock rapidly within 1 to 3 hours.

Risk factors for fatal or near-fatal allergy reactions include:

1. children with asthma;
2. allergies to peanuts, tree nuts, fish, and/or shellfish;
3. individuals who do not receive epinephrine immediately after the reaction begins; and
4. patients who had a previous allergic reaction to a food.[6] Milk, egg, and soy are less likely than the previously listed items to produce fatal reactions in children.[7]

Food-dependent exercise-induced anaphylaxis (FDEIA) is associated with ingesting a specific food before exercise. During or shortly after exercise, the individual experiences allergic symptoms that may progress to anaphylaxis.[8] The individual can usually exercise without any reaction as long as the specific food has not been ingested within the past 8 to 12 hours. Individuals with exercise-induced anaphylaxis typically have a positive skin prick test to foods that provoke symptoms. Wheat is most commonly associated with FDEIA, although reactions to tomato, peanut, soy, corn, and other foods have been reported. Management requires identifying the food through a food challenge that includes strenuous exercise after food ingestion and avoiding the food at least 8 to 12 hours before any expected exercise.

Pollen-food allergy syndrome (PFAS), also referred to as **oral allergy syndrome** (OAS), is another form of IgE-mediated food allergy.[9,10] PFAS occurs mainly in patients allergic to pollens. The proteins in the pollens that cause allergic rhinitis cross-react with the allergens in related raw fruits and vegetables. The reaction is limited to the lips, tongue, palate, and throat, and often resolves within minutes or an hour. In rare instances, systemic anaphylaxis can occur.[10] Individuals allergic to birch tree pollen may have PFAS symptoms when they eat raw carrots, celery, apples, pears, cherries, apricots, and kiwis. Those allergic to ragweed may react when they eat watermelon, cantaloupe, honeydew, and bananas. Generally, cooking fruits and vegetables denatures the relevant proteins, allowing symptom-free consumption.

▶ Non-IgE–Mediated Food Allergy

Food protein–induced enterocolitis syndrome, food protein–induced enteropathy, and food protein-induced allergic proctocolitis are immunologically mediated food allergic disorders, but are not IgE mediated.[11] Food protein–induced enterocolitis, enteropathy, and proctocolitis tend to be outgrown by 12 to 36 months of age. Diagnosis is usually made through clinical history and response to an elimination diet. Skin prick test to foods will be negative. Management involves avoiding the offending food(s).

Food protein–induced enterocolitis syndrome (FPIES) presents with profuse emesis followed by excessive diarrhea that can lead to dehydration, hypotension, and lethargy within 1–4 hours after ingesting the implicated food allergen.[12] Cow's milk, soy, grains such as rice and oat, are the most common offending foods.[13,14] New guidelines for the diagnosis and nutritional management of these patients was recently published.[12]

Food protein-induced enteropathy (FPE) presents within the first 1–2 months of life and can be seen as late as 9 months of age in the cow's milk formula–fed infant.[15] The onset of symptoms mimics acute enteritis with transient emesis, anorexia, and protracted diarrhea that leads to growth failure. While cow's milk is most commonly associated with FPE, reactions to soy, egg, wheat, and beef have also been reported.[16]

Food protein-induced allergic proctocolitis (FPIAP) presents as rectal bleeding within the first few weeks to months of life in well-nourished infants. These children do not typically have growth delay or poor weight gain. Cow's milk and soy proteins are the usual offending foods. Symptoms resolve with maternal milk and/or soy diet restriction in breastfed infants, or for formula fed infants, replacement with an extensively-hydrolysed casein formula or an amino acid based formula.[15]

Eosinophilic gastrointestinal disorders (EGID) involve eosinophilic inflammation in gastrointestinal tissues. **Eosinophilic esophagitis** (EoE) is the most common EGID, with symptoms that vary by age; young children present with vomiting and food refusal, school-aged children with abdominal pain, and adolescents and adults with complaints of dysphagia and sometimes food impaction.[17] Dietary allergen elimination induces remission in patients with EoE.[18] The most restrictive of elimination diets (the elemental diet) removes all possible food antigens while empiric elimination diets remove all (or a subset) of food antigens most commonly reported to cause esophageal eosinophilia and food allergies (milk, egg, wheat, soy, peanuts, tree nuts, fish, or legumes).[19] Eosinophilic disorders in the lower gastrointestinal tract, such as **eosinophilic gastritis/enteritis** (EoG) and **eosinophilic colitis** (EC) may be less responsive to diet therapy.

▶ Diagnosing Food Allergy

Food allergy evaluation requires a thorough medical history, physical examination, and various laboratory studies. Incomplete food allergy work-ups and unorthodox testing can erroneously label one with food allergies, resulting in incorrect diagnoses, nutrient deficiencies, and delay in treating disease.[20–25] For these reasons, pan-testing with food allergy panels is NOT recommended, as it can lead to misdiagnosis and unnecessary diet restriction.[26]

Clinical Reaction History

The medical history is useful in diagnosing food allergy in acute events (e.g., systemic anaphylaxis following the ingestion of peanuts).[27] The history may be helpful in distinguishing IgE-mediated food reactions from other forms of adverse food reactions.[28] The history should include:

- Food suspected to have provoked the reaction
- Quantity of the food ingested
- Length of time between ingestion and development of symptoms
- Description of the symptoms provoked
- What similar symptoms developed on other occasions when the food was eaten
- If other factors (e.g., exercise) are necessary for the reaction to occur
- Length of time since the last reaction

Physical Exam

Unless the patient is actively reacting to a food, no specific features of the physical examination will suggest IgE-mediated food allergy. The physical exam can identify other atopic conditions that increase the chance that the symptoms are related to food allergy, such as environmental allergy, asthma, allergic rhinitis, and atopic dermatitis. Anthropometrics, assessment of growth and development, and nutritional status should be performed.

Skin Testing and In Vitro Assays

If IgE-mediated food sensitivity is suspected, **skin prick testing** (SPT) with food extracts will help screen for the responsible food allergens. SPT is the first test used because of the ease of use, low cost, and immediate results. Glycerated food extracts, and positive (histamine) and negative (saline) controls are applied by a prick technique.[29,30] After 15–20 minutes, the diameter of the wheal is measured. If the wheal, defined as a localized area of edema not including erythema, is at least 3 mm greater than the negative control, it is considered positive; anything else is considered negative. A positive SPT indicates the presence of food-specific IgE, not necessarily that the child will have a clinical reaction to the food. Individuals may or may not be allergic to a specific food because the positive predictive accuracy of a SPT is less than 50%. A good history is critical when evaluating SPT results. If the SPT is negative, there is no detected food-specific IgE. With a negative history, it is highly unlikely that an IgE allergic reaction would occur to the tested food. The negative predictive value is greater than 95%, but severe reactions may occur in patients with negative test results.[31]

The mean diameter of the wheal can be used to predict whether an oral food challenge is indicated. **TABLE 25.2**

TABLE 25.2 Tests to Assess the Likelihood of Obtaining a Positive or Negative OFC in Children				
	Serum Food-IgE (kIU/L)*		**SPT Wheal (mm)***	
Food	**~95% Positive**	**~50% Negative†**	**~95% Positive**	**~50% Negative†**
Cow's milk	≥15 ≥5 if younger than 1 year	≤2	≥8	
Egg white	≥7 ≥2 if younger than 2 years	≤2	≥7	≤3
Peanut	≥14	≤2 with and ≤5 without history of peanut reaction	≥8	≤3
Fish	≥20			

A subset of patients with undetectable serum food-specific IgE antibody and negative SPT has been reported to have objective reactions confirmed by OFC.
*Phadia ImmunoCAP; SPT with commercial food extracts.
†In the authors' experience, children with about 50% chance of experiencing a negative challenge are the optimal candidates for an office-based OFC. However, serum levels of food-specific IgE antibodies and SPT wheal sizes are not absolute indications or contraindications to performing an OFC. Laboratory test results always have to be interpreted in the context of clinical history. For example, if a child had a recent anaphylactic reaction (past 6 mo) to a food, it is more prudent to defer an office OFC even if the test values are at 50% pass rate. In contrast, a child with peanut IgE of 20 kUA/L who recently tolerated an accidental ingestion of a product containing peanut butter may be a candidate for an OFC.
Adapted with permission from Nowak-Wegrzyn A, Assa'ad AH, Bahna SL, et al. Work Group report: oral food challenge testing. *J Allergy Clin Immunol.* 2009;123:S365–383.[32]

provides guidelines that can be used to determine the likelihood of a positive reaction with ingestion of milk, egg, or peanut.[32] If the SPT is ≤ 3 mm in response to egg or peanut, there is a 50% likelihood of a negative food challenge.

There are a few exceptions to the clinical findings to consider when interpreting the SPT results. A child less than 1 year of age may have an IgE-mediated food allergy without a positive SPT because of the lower concentration of IgE present in the skin; a child less than 2 years of age may have smaller wheals when tested by the SPT method.[33] Therefore, histories of strongly suspected foods for which the SPT is negative should not be discounted. Convsersely, patients may have a positive SPT long after they have outgrown the food allergy. A SPT is not indicated in patients with extensive skin disease, dermatographism, those who cannot be taken off antihistamines, or if prior exposure to minute amounts resulted in near-fatal anaphylaxis. In vitro tests for specific IgE would be indicated in these patients. Intradermal skin tests are not recommended because of the increased risk of inducing a systemic reaction.[29]

In vitro assays are available to detect and quantify food-specific serum IgE antibodies. Food-specific serum levels of IgE can predict a ≥ 95% probability of a reaction if that individual undergoes a food challenge to the specific food[32] (see Table 25.2). Such values for milk and egg are lower for younger children because of the less developed immune system.[34,35] Like SPT, the food-specific IgE tests for other foods has a false positive rate of less than 50%.

Monitoring food-specific serum IgE levels is clinically important in the follow-up of patients with food allergy. Pediatric food allergy is a dynamic process, with the majority of children developing oral tolerance. Patients destined to "outgrow" their allergies to milk or egg protein will demonstrate lowering levels of IgE antibodies to the food.[36] Food-specific serum IgE test results indicate an approximately 50% or better chance of tolerance with egg, milk, and peanut IgE[37] (Table 25.2). A diagnostic food challenge would be indicated when food-specific serum IgE values drop below these levels and if there is no known reaction to that food over the past 6 months. Again, these tests are to be viewed as guidelines rather than set diagnostic points. The food-specific serum IgE levels give no indication of the dose the patient may react to or predict the severity of the reaction.

Cross-reactivity can occur when an individual is allergic to more than one food in a food family. Clinical reactivity to more than one member of an animal species or botanical family is more common with fish, shellfish, tree nuts, and PFAS, as previously mentioned.[38,39] A significant amount of cross-reactivity is demonstrated through the food-specific positive SPTs and food-specific serum IgE because of the shared homologous proteins. However, SPT and food-specific serum IgE cannot determine the clinical relevance of cross-reactivity between foods because of the high rate of false-positive results. An example of test cross-reactivity is when the SPT or food-specific serum IgE is positive to environmental grasses and dietary wheat and the child suffers from allergic rhinitis. The child has always consumed and tolerated wheat products. The tests identified the common proteins found in grasses; wheat is part of this family. The positive wheat test was false positive. With a negative dietary history and a diagnosis of allergic rhinitis, dietary wheat should not be avoided.

Several alternative tests for food allergy have been developed but are not validated.[40,41] These alternatives include vega testing (electrodiagnostic devices),[42] applied kinesiology, hair analysis, pulse test, sublingual or subcutaneous provocative challenge, ELISA/ACT, IgG or IgG4 antibody food test, lymphocyte activation, and food antigen-antibody complexes.

Oral Food Challenges for IgE-Mediated Allergies

Oral food challenges (OFCs) determine whether an individual is, in fact, reactive to a food. There are three types of OFCs: (1) open, (2) single-blind, and (3) double-blind, placebo-controlled. The **double-blind, placebo-controlled food challenge** (DBPCFC) is considered the "gold standard" for accurately diagnosing food allergies and for examining a wide variety of food-related complaints.[32] However, open or single-blind food challenges are more practical in the medical practice setting in order to determine whether symptoms can be reproduced when a food is ingested. Challenges are labor intensive and require equipment to treat an anaphylactic reaction, therefore a challenge should be supervised by personnel appropriately trained to recognize and manage any severe food reaction.

Open Food Challenge

During an **open food challenge** (OFC), the patient eats a serving of the food in its traditional form (e.g., a cup of milk, a scrambled egg). Examples of good candidates for an open food challenge are patients who have had negative skin tests and doubtful histories and/or patients who have been "avoiding the food" yet ingest foods that contain the allergen (e.g., someone who eats cookies symptom-free that contain milk and eggs). Open challenges also are performed following a single-blind or double-blind OFC. A negative open challenge—no reaction within 2 hours after ingestion—will convince the individual that the food does not cause any symptoms.

Single-Blind Food Challenge

A single-blind OFC is where the patient and parent do not know what food is being challenged; therefore, it eliminates the bias of the subject and family. It is easily performed in an office setting to confirm objective symptoms. This challenge would be performed under the same conditions as a double-blind, placebo-controlled food challenge except the nurse, dietitian, or doctor performing the challenge would know which food is being challenged.

Double-Blind, Placebo-Controlled Food Challenge

The DBPCFC has the patient, parent, and medical personnel performing the challenge "blinded" to what substance is being administered. During the DBPCFC there are two servings of a food (vehicle)—one contains the food allergen (active arm) and the other contains a safe similar food (placebo arm). The active and placebo containing vehicles are randomized and fed to the patient in that order. The DBPCFC may be performed on one or two days. The DBPCFC is the most objective of the three tests and provides the most accurate information.

Certain medications (e.g., antihistamines and oral or injected steroids) may inhibit food allergy reactions. Recommended avoidance of medication before a food challenge may range from 36 hours to 1 month.[43] Children with atopic dermatitis may require aggressive skin care prior to food challenges.

Foods to be used in OFCs can be found locally. Powdered milk, individually packed flours, powdered egg, and baby foods are found in grocery and health food stores. Challenge substance and placebo material should be well mixed in a carrier food (vehicle). The vehicle should mask the smell, flavor, and texture of the food to be tested. Vehicles to use in food challenges include baby food fruits, hot cereals, applesauce, ice cream, mashed potatoes, fruit smoothies, and ground chicken or beef patties. Placebos can be safe foods not under suspicion, such as dextrose, cornstarch, or another grain.

The OFC is administered in a fasting state, starting with a dose unlikely to cause symptoms (10 to 100 mg of dry powder food, 0.1–1% of the total amount to be consumed). The dose is doubled every 10 to 60 minutes, depending on the type of reaction that might occur based on the history. Clinical reactivity is generally ruled out once the patient has tolerated 10 grams of a dried food, 100 mL of a wet food, or 30–60 g of meat/fish without symptoms. Following completion of the challenge, the individual should be observed for 2 hours for food allergic reactions and 4 to 8 hours for food intolerances, based upon the child's history. If the immediate onset of symptoms is suspected, the DBPCFC can be performed in a day. One series of challenges (active or placebo) is given in the morning. In the afternoon, a second series of challenges (the opposite of the earlier challenge) is performed. If the blinded challenge is negative, the food must be given openly in usual quantities, under observation, to rule out a rare false-negative challenge.[32]

Oral Food Challenges and Food Trials for Non IgE-Mediated Allergies

For children with FPIES, the OFC needs to be done in a hospital setting with placement of an IV to provide rehydration and anti-emetics in case of a reaction. Typically, FPIES challenges are useful in determining if a child has outgrown the allergy. Often times, FPIES diagnosis is made based on clinical history without requiring confirmatory challenge.[12] Consensus guidelines for FPIES challenges involve feeding 0.3 g of the food protein per kilogram of body weight, in 3 equal doses over 30 minutes, not to exceed a total of 3 g of protein or 10 g of total food (100 mL of liquid) for an initial feeding. The patient should be observed for for 4 to 6 hours.[32]

In the case of other non-IgE mediated food allergy, the child is placed on an elimination diet excluding the suspected food allergen(s) for 2 to 4 weeks. If there is no improvement, food allergy may not be the cause. If symptoms persist despite elimination, add the foods back and look for other causes. Elimination diets for EoE are often trialed for 6–12 weeks with a follow up endoscopy to assess esophageal inflammation.[19]

▶ Food Allergy Management

Avoidance and Education

Once properly diagnosed, food allergy management typically involves strict avoidance of the offending allergen(s). Education is the cornerstone for good compliance and a nutritionally adequate diet. This requires extensive education for the patient and family regarding all forms of the food to be avoided, how to read food labels, and alternative foods and/or supplements to replace foods and nutrients eliminated. If a child is allergic to a single food, such as peanuts or fish, the nutritional adequacy of the diet may not be compromised; however, eliminating milk, eggs, soy, or wheat can have a major impact on the quality of a diet. Most children outgrow milk, soy and egg allergies, therefore long-term follow-up involves repeated testing to determine if a child is still reactive to a food and to prevent unnecessary food avoidance.

Reading Labels

Foods in their natural state are often easy to identify, but most children consume a combination of whole and packaged foods. Allergen content may not be visually obvious in processed and packaged foods; thus label reading is an essential skill when following an allergy-restricted diet. The **Food Labeling and Consumer Protection**

Act of 2004 (FALCPA) requires disclosure of the top 8 common allergens in the United States (cow's milk, soy, egg, wheat, peanut, tree nuts, fish, crustacean shellfish).[44] FALCPA applies to all domestic and imported packaged food products and dietary supplements regulated by the **Food and Drug Administration** (FDA). The allergen must be clearly disclosed using its common name (such as MILK) within the ingredient list. Specific tree nut, fish species, or crustacean shellfish must be identified. Mollusks are not considered major allergens and will not be fully disclosed on the food label like crustacean shellfish. The allergen can be listed on the label in the following ways:

- Included in the ingredient list (e.g., milk, wheat)
- Parenthetically following a scientific term (e.g., whey, milk)
- Below the ingredient list in a "contains" statement (e.g., Contains: egg)

If a child is allergic to other foods (e.g., chicken or sesame), the family must contact manufacturers to determine if the food is allergen-free, especially if terms like *flavors* or *spices* are listed. Only intentional ingredients, not contaminants, are listed on the food product label. Other household products, including pet food, cosmetics, bath products, lotions, sunscreens, and so forth, are known to contain food allergens and may use creative terms for the ingredients on the label. It is advantageous for families to know specific terms for the allergens, such as casein or whey for milk. **TABLE 25.3** contains information from Food Allergy Research and Education group on how to read a label for the major allergens. Food labeling laws vary by country, therefore patients should take extra care when planning international travel.[45]

Some food packages bear advisory statements (such as "processed in the same facility" or "manufactured on shared equipment") with a particular allergen, complicating the patient or caregiver's ability to determine its allergen content. These statements are not mandatory; they are voluntarily placed on packaged by food manufacturers and in many cases, and the verbiage does not imply degree of risk. For example, a food bearing the statement "may contain" is not more likely to include the named allergen than a food label stating "processed in a shared facility."[46] Although most foods with advisory statements do *not* contain detectible levels of the stated allergen, it is important for highly allergic individuals to take caution. Certain foods are considered "high risk": dark chocolate, candies, cereal bars, and other confections have been found to be more likely to contain traces of milk and nuts

---

TABLE 25.3 How to Read Food Labels for the Major Allergens

How to Read a Label for a Milk–Free Diet

All FDA-regulated manufactured food products that contain milk as an ingredient are required by US law to list the word "milk" on the product label.

Avoid foods that contain milk or any of these ingredients

butter, butter fat, butter oil, butter acid, butter ester(s)	lactose
buttermilk	lactulose
casein	milk *(in all forms, including condensed, derivative, dry, evaporated, goat's milk and milk from other animals, low-fat, malted, milkfat, nonfat, powder, protein, skimmed, solids, whole)*
casein hydrolysate	
caseinates *(in all forms)*	
cheese	milk protein hydrolysate
cottage cheese	pudding
cream	Recaldent®
curds	rennet casein
custard	sour cream, sour cream solids
diacetyl	sour milk solids
ghee	tagatose
half-and-half	whey *(in all forms)*
lactalbumin, lactalbumin phosphate	whey protein hydrolysate
lactoferrin	yogurt

(continues)

TABLE 25.3 How to Read Food Labels for the Major Allergens (continued)

Milk is sometimes found in the following

artificial butter flavor	luncheon meat, hot dogs, sausages
baked goods	margarine
caramel candies	nisin
chocolate	nondairy products
lactic acid starter culture and other bacterial cultures	nougat

How to Read a Label for a Soy–Free Diet

All FDA-regulated manufactured food products that contain soy as an ingredient are required by US law to list the word "soy" on the product label.

Avoid foods that contain soy or any of these ingredients

edamame	soybean *(curd, granules)*
miso	soy protein *(concentrate, hydrolyzed, isolate)*
natto	soy sauce
shoyu	tamari
soy *(soy albumin, soy cheese, soy fiber, soy flour, soy grits, soy ice cream, soy milk, soy nuts, soy sprouts, soy yogurt)*	tempeh
	textured vegetable protein *(TVP)*
soya	tofu

Soy is sometimes found in the following

Asian cuisine	vegetable gum
vegetable broth	vegetable starch

Keep the following in mind

The FDA exempts highly refined soybean oil from being labeled as an allergen. Studies show most allergic individuals can safely eat soy oil that has been highly refined (*not* cold pressed, expeller pressed, or extruded soybean oil).

Most individuals allergic to soy can safely eat soy lecithin.

Follow your doctor's advice regarding these ingredients.

How to Read a Label for a Peanut–Free Diet

All FDA-regulated manufactured food products that contain peanut as an ingredient are required by US law to list the word "peanut" on the product label.

Avoid foods that contain peanuts or any of these ingredients

artificial nuts	goobers	monkey nuts	peanut butter
beer nuts	ground nuts	nut pieces	peanut flour
cold pressed, expeller pressed, or extruded peanut oil	mixed nuts	nutmeat	peanut protein hydrolysate

Peanut is sometimes found in the following

African, Asian (*especially Chinese, Indian, Indonesian, Thai, and Vietnamese*), and Mexican dishes	baked goods (*e.g., pastries, cookies*) candy (*including chocolate candy*)	chili egg rolls enchilada sauce	marzipan mole sauce nougat

Keep the following in mind

Mandelonas are peanuts soaked in almond flavoring.

The FDA exempts highly refined peanut oil from being labeled as an allergen. Studies show that most allergic individuals can safely eat peanut oil that has been highly refined (not cold pressed, expeller pressed, or extruded peanut oil). Follow your doctor's advice.

A study showed that unlike other legumes, there is a strong possibility of cross-reaction between peanuts and lupine.

Arachis oil is peanut oil.

How to Read a Label for a Wheat–Free Diet

All FDA-regulated manufactured food products that contain wheat as an ingredient are required by US law to list the word "wheat" on the product label. The law defines any species in the genus Triticum as wheat.

Avoid foods that contain wheat or any of these ingredients

bread crumbs	matzoh, matzoh meal (*also spelled as matzo, matzah, or matza*)
bulgur	pasta
cereal extract	seitan
club wheat	semolina
couscous	spelt
cracker meal	sprouted wheat
durum	triticale
einkorn	vital wheat gluten
emmer	wheat (*bran, durum, germ, gluten, grass, malt, sprouts, starch*)
farina	wheat bran hydrolysate
flour (*all purpose, bread, cake, durum, enriched, graham, high gluten, high protein, instant, pastry, self-rising, soft wheat, steel ground, stone ground, whole wheat*)	wheat germ oil
	wheat grass
	wheat protein isolate
hydrolyzed wheat proteins	whole wheat berries
kamut	

Wheat is sometimes found in the following

glucose syrup soy sauce	starch (*gelatinized starch, modified starch, modified food starch, vegetable starch*) surimi

How to Read a Label for a Shellfish–Free Diet

All FDA-regulated manufactured food products that contain a crustacean shellfish as an ingredient are required by US law to list the specific crustacean shellfish on the product label.

(continues)

TABLE 25.3 How to Read Food Labels for the Major Allergens (continued)

Avoid foods that contain shellfish or any of these ingredients

crab crawfish (crayfish, ecrevisse) lobster (langouste, langoustine, scampo, coral, tomalley) prawn shrimp (crevette)	Mollusks are not considered major allergens under food labeling laws and may not be fully disclosed on a product label.

Your doctor may advise you to avoid mollusks or these ingredients

abalone clams (cherrystone, littleneck, pismo, quahog) cockle (periwinkle, sea urchin) mussels	octopus oysters snails (escargot) squid (calamari)

Shellfish are sometimes found in the following

bouillabaisse cuttlefish ink fish stock	seafood flavoring (e.g., crab or clam extract) surimi

Keep the following in mind

- Any food served in a seafood restaurant may contain shellfish protein due to cross-contact.
- For some individuals, a reaction may occur from inhaling cooking vapors or from handling fish or shellfish.

How to Read a Label for an Egg–Free Diet

All FDA-regulated manufactured food products that contain egg as an ingredient are required by US law to list the word "egg" on the product label.

Avoid foods that contain eggs or any of these ingredients

albumin (also spelled albumen) egg (dried, powdered, solids, white, yolk)	eggnog lysozyme	mayonnaise meringue (meringue powder)	ovalbumin surimi

Egg is sometimes found in the following

baked goods egg substitutes	lecithin macaroni	marzipan marshmallows	nougat pasta

Keep the following in mind

- Individuals with egg allergy should also avoid eggs from duck, turkey, goose, quail, etc., as these are known to be cross-reactive with chicken egg.

How to Read a Label for a Tree Nut–Free Diet

All FDA-regulated manufactured food products that contain a tree nut as an ingredient are required by US law to list the specific tree nut on the product label.

Avoid foods that contain nuts or any of these ingredients			
almonds	filberts/hazelnuts	natural nut extract (*e.g., almond, walnut*)	pili nut
artificial nuts	gianduja (*a chocolate-nut mixture*)	nut butters (*e.g., cashew butter*)	pine nuts (*also referred to as Indian, pignoli, pigñolia, pignon, piñon, and pinyon nuts*)
beechnut	ginkgo nut	nut meal	
Brazil nuts	hickory nuts	nut paste (*e.g., almond paste*)	pistachios
butternut	litchi/lichee/lychee nut	nut pieces	praline
cashews	macadamia nuts	nutmeat	shea nut
chestnuts	marzipan/almond paste	pecans	walnuts
chinquapin	Nangai nuts	pesto	
coconut (not usually allergenic for individuals with tree nut allergy)			

Tree nuts are sometimes found in the following			
black walnut hull extract (*flavoring*)	natural nut extract nut distillates/alcoholic extracts	nut oils (*e.g., walnut oil, almond oil*)	walnut hull extract (*flavoring*)

Keep the following in mind
Mortadella may contain pistachios.
There is no evidence that coconut oil and shea nut oil/butter are allergenic.
Talk to your doctor if you find other nuts not listed here.

than are other foods bearing advisory statements.[47] This is a crucial detail for persons with IgE-mediated allergies. As a precaution, patients may choose to avoid foods bearing allergen advisory statements. However, depending on the patient and practioner, if a suitable alternative is not available, then such foods may be permissible to allow variety in the diet.[19]

Avoiding Common Allergens
Cow's Milk

Cow's milk avoidance excludes fluid milk, cheeses, yogurts, ice creams, butter, milk-based infant formulas, and all other food products containing traces of milk, such as baked goods and candies. Less obvious sources of milk include high-protein foods that use whey protein as an additive and "non-dairy" foods, that may contain the milk-protein casein. Goat's milk should not be used as an alternative to cow's milk because of the potential cross-reactivity with the beta-lactoglobulins in cow's milk.[48] Children with IgE-mediated milk allergy may tolerate small amounts of milk in extensively-heated, or baked goods,[49] which may, over time, hasten their tolerance to less-cooked forms of milk like cheese, yogurt, and fluid milk.[50] Plant-based milk alternatives, such as soy, rice, coconut, hemp, potato, flax, and sunflower seed

beverages are widely available, but are not to be considered nutritionally equivalent to cow's milk, especially in the diets of young children and toddlers. These alternative beverages are often enriched with calcium, vitamin D, and sometimes vitamin A, B vitamins, and phosphorus, but are poor sources of dietary fat and protein. While useful in baking and other cooking applications in place of fluid milk, plant-based milk alternatives should not be used as a primary beverages in children under 2 years of age.[51] Cow's milk often comprises a significant portion of the toddler diet, supplying much of the protein and fat needed for growth and for brain development. Children with cow's milk allergy should be prescribed a substitute formula such as extensively hydrolyzed casein formula or amino acid based formula until age 2.[51] The breastfed infants with IgE mediated allergies do not often require maternal diet restriction, but maternal diet restriction is often warranted for breastfed infants with non-IgE allergies. For formula fed infants, partially hydrolyzed milk-based formulas contain whole cow's milk allergens and will continue to cause allergic reactions in the milk-allergic child. 14% of children with IgE mediated cow's milk allergy cannot tolerate soy formulas[52] and 30–50% of those with non-IgE–mediated allergy are reactive to soy protein. Ten percent of infants or toddlers fail to tolerate an extensively hydrolyzed milk protein–based formula (Similac Alimentum, Nutramigen); therefore, an amino acid–based formula (Neocate, Elecare, PurAmino, Alfamino) is warranted in these cases.[53,54] Infant formulas will provide calcium, phosphorus, vitamin D, vitamin B_{12}, riboflavin, and pantothenic acid that would be otherwise supplied by milk in the diet.

For older children not using substitute formula or averse to drinking plant-based milk alternatives, calcium and vitamin D supplementation may be required to ensure providing these nutrients in the diet. Some ready-to-eat cereals, breads, and fruit juices are calcium fortified but may not be fortified with vitamin D. Check serum levels of 25(OH) vitamin D in infants and children with milk allergy if low intake is suspected.[55]

Milk provides a significant amount of protein in a child's diet. When a child avoids milk, they may need additional servings of protein-rich foods to ensure adequate intake for growth. Meats, poultry, fish, whole grains, legumes, and nuts can provide alternative sources of protein, but also phosphorus, riboflavin, and pantothenicc acid that are found in milk.

Egg Allergy

Eggs supply protein, biotin, choline, and selenium in the diet and act as a binding agent in baked goods that are favorite foods for many children. Nutrients in eggs are easily replaced by other high-protein foods and whole grains. However, eggs can be incorporated into breads, pastas, baking mixes, breaded or processed meats, custards, fat substitutes, salad dressings, sauces, candies, and other commercially prepared foods. It is the elimination of all of these other foods containing egg that causes problems in providing a nutritionally balanced diet. Similar to cow's milk allergy, children with IgE-mediated egg allergy may be able to tolerate extensively-heated or baked egg.[48,56]

Home recipes can be easily modified using substitutes for the binding and leavening properties of eggs. Equivalent to one egg:

- 1 tsp. baking powder, 1 Tbsp. water, 1 Tbsp. Vinegar
- ¼ cup applesauce or ¼ cup mashed banana
- 1 and ½ Tbsp. water, 1 and ½ Tbsp. oil, 1 tsp. baking powder
- 1 packet gelatin, 2 Tbsp. warm water (do not mix until ready to use)
- 1 Tbsp. flax or chia seed, 3 Tbsp. warm water, mix and let sit for 5 mins. until a gel forms
- Commercial Egg-replacer (follow directions on box): typically potato- or tapioca-based

Soy Allergy

Unless a child frequently consumes soy-based products such as tofu, edamame, tempeh or vegetarian meat analogs, or Asian cuisine, restricting soy from the diet is less troublesome, as heat-pressed soybean oil and soy lecithin,

the form of soy regularly present in packaged foods, is considered safe for individuals with soy allergy because the processing of the oil removes the protein portion.[57,58] The highly refined soybean oil is exempt from allergen labeling, but not soy lecithin. Products that contain soy lecithin may have a "contains soy" statement. To ensure that a product is safe, call the manufacturer to determine if any soy protein ingredients are included in the product.

Wheat Allergy

Wheat elimination includes avoiding all wheat-containing bread, pasta, crackers, breakfast cereals, and baked goods. This includes all-purpose flour and any food breaded, baked, or fried with wheat-based flour. Wheat flours are fortified with niacin, riboflavin, thiamin, and iron. If a child's diet is composed of very few whole grain products, they may be deficient in these and other nutrients. Encourage using fortified or 100% whole grains. Products made with the flours of amaranth, arrowroot, barley, buckwheat, corn, oats, potato, quinoa, rice, rye, soy, and tapioca are suitable wheat alternatives. Fortified and enriched corn and rice based breakfast cereals are readily available substitutes. Many substitutes for wheat products are corn-, rice- and potato-based, but ancient, whole grains such as quinoa, amaranth, and millet contain more fiber and trace minerals and are more nutrient-dense compared with corn, rice and potato. Gluten-free products used by individuals with celiac disease or gluten sensitivity may be good alternatives but often contain milk or egg products. Packaged gluten-free mixes or home baked recipes can be prepared with egg replacement and cow's milk substitute.

Peanut Allergy

Peanuts are legumes, but an allergy to peanuts does not automatically make one allergic to other legumes (soybeans, peas, beans, green beans, and lentils). However, there is a strong possibility of cross-reaction between peanuts and lupine,[59] a legume used predominantly in Europe but that may be found in high-protein and baked products manufactured in the United States. Peanuts can be found in pastries, candies, fruit-nut breads, salads, sauces, cereals, crackers, soups, and ethnic foods, particularly those of Africa, China, and Thailand. Highly-refined, heat-pressed peanut oil is considered safe for most individuals with peanut allergies,[60,61] but not crude peanut oil that has been cold pressed, expressed, extruded, or expelled. Nutrients such as vitamin E, niacin, magnesium, manganese, and chromium found in peanuts can also be found in legumes, whole grains, meats, and vegetable oils.

Tree Nut Allergy

Almond, brazil nut, cashew, chestnut, filbert/hazelnut, macadamia, pecan, pine nut, pistachio, and walnut are considered tree nuts. Tree nuts are used in cereals, crackers, ice cream, marinades, and sauces, and more recently, gluten-free foods (almond flour) and vegan foods (cashew cheese), making avoidance more difficult. Nut paste and nut butters are often made on shared equipment. Pure tree nut extracts, such as almond and walnut, may contain allergens; however, natural almond extract is often derived from peach pits and not allergenic.

Individuals allergic to any tree nut may be advised to avoid all tree nuts because of potential cross-reactivity.[62] Patients allergic to tree nuts frequently exhibit sensitization to peanuts and other tree nuts. For example, cashew–pistachio and walnut–pecan, co-sensitization is common.[63] Generally, only foods that have elicited reactions should be avoided, and in tree-nut-allergic individuals, previously tolerated individual tree nuts that were negative in skin test can likely be continued. Peanut and tree nut allergies have been reported to coexist in approximately 20–59% of nut allergic patients; however, data from studies using OFC indicate rates of co-allergy to be much lower. In special circumstances, such as for young children, it is not uncommon to suggest avoiding all peanuts and tree nuts in order to avoid accidental exposure. However, due to the growing use of tree nuts in packaged foods owing to reports on health benefits of nut consumption, there is some utility in following a targeted tree nut elimination based on testing, clinical history and cross-sensitivity. Coconut is not a tree nut and is safe for tree nut allergic individuals to consume.

Fish and Shellfish Allergy

An individual may be allergic to one fish and tolerate others,[38] but in the marketplace, substituting one fish for another is a common occurrence and is dangerous for the fish-allergic individual. Additionally, there is a 50% rate of cross-reactivity with fish allergies.[39] Cross-contamination occurs in restaurants because of shared equipment (frying oil, grill, and spatula). Those allergic to fish but not shellfish need to be aware of Surimi, an imitation shellfish made with fish. Nutrients in fish such as vitamin B_6, vitamin B_{12}, vitamin E, niacin, phosphorus, and selenium are also found in meats, grains, and oils.

If one is allergic to shellfish, all shellfish are typically avoided. The risk of cross-reactivity is 75% with shellfish.[39] Crustacean shellfish (crab, crawfish, shrimp, and lobster) are considered major allergens and listed on product labels. Mollusks (clams, mussels, oysters, scallops, and squid) are not considered major allergens under the food labeling laws. Therefore, the food company will need to be called in order to determine whether clams, for example, are used in a seafood flavoring. Shellfish are traditionally not hidden in foods, but beware of cross-contamination in seafood restaurants. Asian dishes use a number of fish and shellfish and should also be avoided.

Cross-Contact

Cross-contact occurs when an allergen-containing food comes in contact with a "safe" food.

This can happen in the home when other family members share the patient's restricted foods. Common sources of cross contact in the home include shared condiments (for example, as when double-dipping a knife transfers wheat crumbs into a jelly jar) as well as utensils that are hard to clean, such as colanders, slotted spatulas, and toaster appliances. Cross contact can occur in other settings, such as restaurants if staff members are not properly trained or inattentive to consumer requests. French fried potatoes cooked in the same fryers as breaded foods are contaminated with wheat and should be avoided. Cooking utensils, serving utensils, and containers may be shared on buffets, salad bars, and cafeteria lines, and in ice cream stores. Grills, marinades, cutting boards are all potential transferors of allergens. At supermarkets, the deli slicers, bulk bins, and salad bars all pose risk of cross contact.

▶ Nutritional Consequences of Food Allergy

Any degree of diet elimination has the potential to impact nutritional status and growth. Excluding major foods from the diet that significantly contribute to energy, protein, and micronutrient intake, such as milk and wheat can theoretically impact growth in children. Children with IgE-mediated food allergy have impaired growth[64-68] and weight gain[64-67,69] when compared to their peers, which cow's milk allergic children[68,70] and children with ≥ 3 avoided foods at greatest risk for lower weight.[65] The number of foods avoided due to IgE mediated allergy correlates with poor growth.[66,71] Although poor nutritional intake and growth failure are the primary nutritional concerns when managing children with food allergies, some children do experience excessive weight gain, even when several (≥ 3) foods are avoided, with up to 12% of children with IgE and non-IgE mediated food allergies identified as obese.[65]

▶ Other Principles of Management and Treatment

The registered dietitian plays a critical role in food allergy management, providing education on food avoidance, suggesting alternatives to the avoided foods, providing recipes and meal plans where necessary, evaluating compliance, and ensuring adequacy and enjoyment of the diet. Families need to be educated about new cooking techniques, how to eat away from home and at social events, and dealing with other family members' homes and schools where food is served.

Dining out and social gatherings where food is involved can be challenging for the food-allergic individual. Desserts are responsible for 43% of allergic reactions when eating out, followed by entrées (35%), appetizers (13%), and other foods (9%).[61] Individuals allergic to peanuts or tree nuts may choose to avoid Asian restaurants. "Chef Cards," stating a child's allergens can provide clearer communication for restaurant staff. For clearer communication, written information about one's food allergy can be shared with the manager or chef. To allow for the most attention to personal requirements, avoid the restaurant's busiest times.

A family's quality of life is impacted when a child is diagnosed with a food allergy.[72] Parents may be fearful of a life-threatening allergic reaction, giving rise to anxiety on their part. These families may feel that a situation is beyond their ability to manage and feel out of control, vulnerable, and helpless. This can be picked up by the child, leading to food fears. The more informed the family is about living with a food allergy, the more control they have, and the less stress they will experience.[73]

▶ Food Allergy Prevention

Recent studies suggest that certain strategies may be effective in the primary prevention of food allergy. Most compelling is the data from the **Learning Early About Peanut** (LEAP) trial, where infants at risk for peanut allergy (those with moderate/severe atopic dermatis or existing egg allergy) were randomized to consume peanut or avoid peanut for 5 years. Early consumption of peanut resulted in a 70% relative risk reduction of peanut allergy.[74] This lead to recommendations by an NIAID-sponsored expert panel to encourage early introduction of peanut in infants at moderate risk of developing peanut allergy.[75] This goes beyond recommendations by the American Academy of Pediatrics from 2008, which stated there was little evidence that delayed or early introduction of allergens had any affect on the development of atopic disorders.[76] The potential for prevention of other food allergens via early life exposure is less clear. There may be some evidence that early egg introduction prevents egg allergy,[77-79] but to date there are no current recommendations or guidelines for purposeful early introduction of egg in infancy. Data on milk is limited, but does suggest that delaying introduction may be associated with higher risk of milk allergy.[80]

A number of other factors, including maternal diet during pregnancy, breastfeeding, infant formula selection, vitamin D sufficiency, and the microbiome have been suspected of playing a role in preventing food allergy, however data on each of these points is inconclusive.[27]

▶ Conclusion

In summary, it is important to make an accurate diagnosis of food allergy. Nutrition assessment and education for avoidance diets is complex. Without appropriate education, the child is at risk of accidental reactions, persistent food allergies, growth problems, and impaired quality of life. New guidelines on early introduction of peanut in at-risk infants expand the role of the dietitian in food allergy management.

🔍 CASE STUDIES

Nutrition Assessment

Patient history: 16-month-old female was a term newborn with no perinatal complications. At 4 months of age she developed severe atopic dermatitis that was well managed with wet wraps and topical medication.

Family history: There is a family history of seasonal allergies in the child's mother.

Food/nutrition-related history: She was breastfed and weaned onto rice cereal, fruits, vegetables at 6 months of age. At 8 months old, she developed hives after eating a bite of scrambled eggs made with milk. She had not yet consumed any milk products, peanuts or tree nuts. The pediatrician referred the child to an allergy and immunology clinic. The allergist ordered skin prick tests for egg and milk because of the reported history of hives with ingestion of egg and butter. Because of her risk of peanut allergy due to moderate atopic dermatitis and possible egg allergy, the allergist also tested for peanut according to NIAID guidelines.[81]

She is not taking any vitamin/mineral supplements or infant formula.

Anthropometric Measurements

Weight: 9.8 kg (25th percentile)

Height: 78 cm (50th percentile)

Weight for length: (25th–50th percentile)

Estimated energy needs: 792 kcal [(89 3 wt (kg) – 100) 1 20]

Estimated protein needs: 11 grams [1.1 3 wt (kg)]

Medical test: Positive skin prick test to egg. Negative skin prick test to cow's milk, skin prick test to peanut was <2mm.

Nutrition Diagnoses

1. Food and nutrition-related knowledge deficit related to newly diagnosed food allergy as evidenced by positive egg allergy test.
2. Inadequate vitamin intake (vitamin D) related to breastfeeding without supplementation as evidenced by diet history.

Intervention Goals

1. Avoid all forms of egg.
2. Introduce peanut per NIAID guidelines for prevention of peanut allergy.

Nutrition Interventions

Comprehensive nutrition education:

- Egg Allergy
  - Instructed on strict avoidance of egg
  - Reviewed how to read labels
  - Discussed sources of cross-contact
  - Explained how to dine out
  - Instructed how to prepare safe foods at home
  - Provided sources of information on food allergies and day cares for the future
- Peanut Introduction
  - Feed 2 grams of peanut protein daily using textures safe and appropriate for infants, such as:
    - 2 tsp peanut butter thinned in 2–3 tsp warm water
    - 2 tsp peanut butter thinned in 2–3 tsp fruit or vegetable puree
    - 2 tsp peanut powder mixed in 2–3 tsp fruit or vegetable puree

Vitamin supplement:

- Begin Vitamin D drops, 400 IU daily

Monitoring and Evaluation

- Evaluate for accidental ingestions associated with allergens at follow-up clinic visits.
- Educate parents regarding possible food challenge to egg or baked egg in future.

Questions for the Reader

What will you do during the follow-up visit 2 months later:

1) If the child refuses to consume peanut regularly?
2) If the allergist feels that the child may now challenge baked egg?
3) If the child has not gained any weight since her last visit?

Study Questions

1. What type of food allergy puts children at the greatest risk for systemic anaphylaxis food reactions?
2. What foods are the most common trigger foods for **Food protein–induced enterocolitis syndrome (FPIES)**?
3. What is considered the "gold standard" for accurately diagnosing food allergies?
4. The **Food Labeling and Consumer Protection Act** of 2004 (FALCPA) requires disclosure of what food allergens?

Resources for Food Allergies

American Academy of Allergy, Asthma, and Immunology

To locate a board-certified allergist:
http://www.aaaai.org

American Partnership for Eosinophilic Disorders

http://www.apfed.org

Food Allergy Research & Education

http://www.foodallergy.org

Kids with Food Allergies

http://www.kidswithfoodallergies.org

Medline Plus: Food Allergy

http://www.nlm.nih.gov/medlineplus/foodallergy.html

References

1. Panel NI-SE, Boyce JA, Assa'ad A, et al. Guidelines for the diagnosis and management of food allergy in the United States: report of the NIAID-sponsored expert panel. *J Allergy Clin Immunol.* 2010;126:S1–58.

2. Nwaru BI, Hickstein L, Panesar SS, et al. The epidemiology of food allergy in Europe: a systematic review and meta-analysis. *Allergy.* 2014;69:62–75.

3. Savage J, Sicherer S, Wood R. The Natural History of Food Allergy. *J Allergy Clin Immunol Pract.* 2016;4:196–203.

4. Gupta RS, Springston EE, Warrier MR, et al. The prevalence, severity, and distribution of childhood food allergy in the United States. Pediatr. 2011;128:e9–e17.

5. Simons FE, Frew AJ, Ansotegui IJ, et al. Practical allergy (PRACTALL) report: risk assessment in anaphylaxis. Allergy. 2008;63:35–37.

6. Sicherer SH, Sampson HA. Food allergy: Epidemiology, pathogenesis, diagnosis, and treatment. *J Allergy Clin Immunol.* 2014;133:291–307.

7. Munoz-Furlong A, Weiss CC. Characteristics of food-allergic patients placing them at risk for a fatal anaphylactic episode. *Curr Allergy Asthma Rep.* 2009;9:57–63.

8. de Silva NR, Dasanayake WM, Karunatilleke C, Malavige GN. Food dependant exercise induced anaphylaxis a retrospective study from 2 allergy clinics in Colombo, Sri Lanka. *Allergy Asthma Clin Immunol.* 2015;11:22.

9. Price A, Ramachandran S, Smith GP, Stevenson ML, Pomeranz MK, Cohen DE. Oral allergy syndrome (pollen-food allergy syndrome). *Dermatitis.* 2015;26:78–88.

10. Tatachar P, Kumar S. Food-induced anaphylaxis and oral allergy syndrome. *Pediatr Rev.* 2008;29:e23–e27.

11. Nowak-Wegrzyn A, Katz Y, Mehr SS, Koletzko S. Non-IgE-mediated gastrointestinal food allergy. *J Allergy Clin Immunol.* 2015;135:1114–1124.

12. Nowak-Wegrzyn A, Chehade M, Groetch ME, et al. International consensus guidelines for the diagnosis and management of food protein-induced enterocolitis syndrome: Executive summary-Workgroup Report of the Adverse Reactions to Foods Committee, American Academy of Allergy, Asthma & Immunology. *J Allergy Clin Immunol.* 2017;139:1111–1126.

13. Hwang JB, Sohn SM, Kim AS. Prospective follow-up oral food challenge in food protein-induced enterocolitis syndrome. *Arch Dis Child.* 2009;94:425–428.

14. Katz Y, Goldberg MR. Natural history of food protein-induced enterocolitis syndrome. *Curr Opin Allergy Clin Immunol.* 2014;14:229–239.

15. Leonard SA. Non-IgE-mediated Adverse Food Reactions. *Curr Allergy Asthma Rep.* 2017;17:84.

16. Kuitunen P, Visakorpi JK, Savilahti E, Pelkonen P. Malabsorption syndrome with cow's milk intolerance. Clinical findings and course in 54 cases. *Arch Dis Child.* 1975;50:351–356.

17. Noel RJ, Putnam PE, Rothenberg ME. Eosinophilic esophagitis. *N Engl J Med.* 2004;351:940–941.

18. Liacouras CA, Furuta GT, Hirano I, et al. Eosinophilic esophagitis: updated consensus recommendations for children and adults. *J Allergy Clin Immunol.* 2011;128:3–20.

19. Groetch M, Venter C, Skypala I, et al. Dietary Therapy and Nutrition Management of Eosinophilic Esophagitis: A Work Group Report of the American Academy of Allergy, Asthma, and Immunology. *J Allergy Clin Immunol Pract.* 2017;5:312–324.

20. Hill ID, Fasano A, Guandalini S, et al. NASPGHAN Clinical Report on the Diagnosis and Treatment of Gluten Related Disorders. *J Pediatr Gastroenterol Nutr.* 2016;63(1):156–165.

21. Robertson DA, Ayres RC, Smith CL, Wright R. Adverse consequences arising from misdiagnosis of food allergy. *BMJ.* 1988;297:719–720.

22. Roesler TA, Barry PC, Bock SA. Factitious food allergy and failure to thrive. *Arch Pediatr Adolesc Med.* 1994;148: 1150–1155.

23. Noimark L, Cox HE. Nutritional problems related to food allergy in childhood. *Pediatr Allergy Immunol.* 2008;19:188–195.

24. Fortunato JE, Scheimann AO. Protein-energy malnutrition and feeding refusal secondary to food allergies. *Clin Pediatr (Phila).* 2008;47:496–499.

25. Carvalho NF, Kenney RD, Carrington PH, Hall DE. Severe nutritional deficiencies in toddlers resulting from health food milk alternatives. *Pediatr.* 2001;107:E46.

26. Bird JA, Lack G, Perry TT. Clinical management of food allergy. *J Allergy Clin Immunol Pract.* 2015;3:1–11.

27. Sicherer SH, Sampson HA. Food Allergy: A review and update on epidemiology, pathogenesis, diagnosis, prevention and management. *J Allergy Clin Immunol.* 2018;141(1):41–58.

28. Skypala IJ, Venter C, Meyer R, et al. The development of a standardised diet history tool to support the diagnosis of food allergy. *Clin Transl Allergy.* 2015;5:7.

29. Bock SA, Lee WY, Remigio L, Holst A, May CD. Appraisal of skin tests with food extracts for diagnosis of food hypersensitivity. *Clin Allergy.* 1978;8:559–564.

30. The use of standardized allergen extracts. American Academy of Allergy, Asthma and Immunology (AAAAI). *J Allergy Clin Immunol.* 1997;99:583–586.

31. Sampson HA. Utility of food-specific IgE concentrations in predicting symptomatic food allergy. *J Allergy Clin Immunol.* 2001;107:891–896.

32. Nowak-Wegrzyn A, Assa'ad AH, Bahna SL, et al. Work Group report: oral food challenge testing. *J Allergy Clin Immunol.* 2009;123:S365–S383.

33. Menardo JL, Bousquet J, Rodiere M, Astruc J, Michel FB. Skin test reactivity in infancy. *J Allergy Clin Immunol.* 1985;75:646–651.

34. Garcia-Ara C, Boyano-Martinez T, Diaz-Pena JM, Martin-Munoz F, Reche-Frutos M, Martin-Esteban M. Specific IgE levels in the diagnosis of immediate hypersensitivity to cows' milk protein in the infan. *J Allergy Clin Immunol.* 2001;107:185–190.

35. Boyano Martinez T, Garcia-Ara C, Diaz-Pena JM, Munoz FM, Garcia Sanchez G, Esteban MM. Validity of specific IgE antibodies in children with egg allergy. *Clin Exp Allergy.* 2001;31:1464–1469.

36. Shek LP, Soderstrom L, Ahlstedt S, Beyer K, Sampson HA. Determination of food specific IgE levels over time can predict the development of tolerance in cow's milk and hen's egg allergy. *J Allergy Clin Immunol.* 2004;114:387–391.

37. Perry TT, Matsui EC, Kay Conover-Walker M, Wood RA. The relationship of allergen-specific IgE levels and oral food challenge outcome. *J Allergy Clin Immunol.* 2004;114:144–149.

38. Bernhisel-Broadbent J, Scanlon SM, Sampson HA. Fish hypersensitivity. I. In vitro and oral challenge results in fish-allergic patients. *J Allergy Clin Immunol.* 1992;89:730–737.

39. Sicherer SH. Clinical implications of cross-reactive food allergens. *J Allergy Clin Immunol.* 2001;108:881–890.

40. Niggemann B, Gruber C. Unproven diagnostic procedures in IgE-mediated allergic diseases. *Allergy.* 2004;59:806–808.

41. Teuber SS, Beyer K. IgG to foods: a test not ready for prime time. *Curr Opin Allergy Clin Immunol.* 2007;7:257–258.

42. Krop J, Lewith GT, Gziut W, Radulescu C. A double blind, randomized, controlled investigation of electrodermal testing in the diagnosis of allergies. *J Altern Complement Med.* 1997;3:241–248.

43. Reibel S, Rohr C, Ziegert M, Sommerfeld C, Wahn U, Niggemann B. What safety measures need to be taken in oral food challenges in children? *Allergy.* 2000;55:940–944.

44. United States Food and Drug Administration CfFSaAN. Food Allergen Labeling and Consumer Protection Act of 2004 (Title II of Public Law 108e282). August 2004 ed2004.

45. Allen KJ, Turner PJ, Pawankar R, et al. Precautionary labelling of foods for allergen content: are we ready for a global framework? *World Allergy Organ J.* 2014;7:10.

46. Turner PJ, Kemp AS, Campbell DE. Advisory food labels: consumers with allergies need more than "traces" of information. *BMJ.* 2011;343:d6180.

47. Ford LS, Taylor SL, Pacenza R, Niemann LM, Lambrecht DM, Sicherer SH. Food allergen advisory labeling and product contamination with egg, milk, and peanut. *J Allergy Clin Immunol.* 2010;126:384–385.

48. Leonard SA, Sampson HA, Sicherer SH, et al. Dietary baked egg accelerates resolution of egg allergy in children. *J Allergy Clin Immunol.* 2012;130:473–480.

49. Nowak-Wegrzyn A, Bloom KA, Sicherer SH, et al. Tolerance to extensively heated milk in children with cow's milk allergy. *J Allergy Clin Immunol.* 2008;122:342–347.

50. Kim JS, Nowak-Wegrzyn A, Sicherer SH, Noone S, Moshier EL, Sampson HA. Dietary baked milk accelerates the resolution of cow's milk allergy in children. *J Allergy Clin Immunol.* 2011;128:125–131.

51. Fiocchi A, Schunemann HJ, Brozek J, et al. Diagnosis and Rationale for Action Against Cow's Milk Allergy (DRACMA): a summary report. *J Allergy Clin Immunol.* 2010;126:1119–128.

52. Zeiger RS, Sampson HA, Bock SA, et al. Soy allergy in infants and children with IgE-associated cow's milk allergy. *J Pediatr.* 1999;134:614–622.

53. Niggemann B, Binder C, Dupont C, Hadji S, Arvola T, Isolauri E. Prospective, controlled, multi-center study on the effect of an amino-acid-based formula in infants with cow's milk allergy/intolerance and atopic dermatitis. *Pediatr Allergy Immunol.* 2001;12:78–82.

54. Sicherer SH, Noone SA, Koerner CB, Christie L, Burks AW, Sampson HA. Hypoallergenicity and efficacy of an amino acid-based formula in children with cow's milk and multiple food hypersensitivities. *J Pediatr.* 2001;138:688–693.

55. Holick MF. The vitamin D deficiency pandemic: Approaches for diagnosis, treatment and prevention. *Rev Endocr Metab Disord.* 2017;18:153–165.

56. Lemon-Mule H, Sampson HA, Sicherer SH, Shreffler WG, Noone S, Nowak-Wegrzyn A. Immunologic changes in children with egg allergy ingesting extensively heated egg. *J Allergy Clin Immunol.* 2008;122:977–983.

57. Blom WM, Kruizinga AG, Rubingh CM, Remington BC, Crevel RWR, Houben GF. Assessing food allergy risks from residual peanut protein in highly refined vegetable oil. *Food Chem Toxicol.* 2017;106:306–313.

58. Crevel RW, Kerkhoff MA, Koning MM. Allergenicity of refined vegetable oils. *Food Chem Toxicol.* 2000;38:385–393.

59. Moneret-Vautrin DA, Guerin L, Kanny G, Flabbee J, Fremont S, Morisset M. Cross-allergenicity of peanut and lupine: the risk of lupine allergy in patients allergic to peanuts. *J Allergy Clin Immunol.* 1999;104:883–888.

60. Taylor SL, Busse WW, Sachs MI, Parker JL, Yunginger JW. Peanut oil is not allergenic to peanut-sensitive individuals. *J Allergy Clin Immunol.* 1981;68:372–375.

61. Furlong TJ, DeSimone J, Sicherer SH. Peanut and tree nut allergic reactions in restaurants and other food establishments. *J Allergy Clin Immunol.* 2001;108:867–870.

62. Sicherer SH, Sampson HA. Peanut and tree nut allergy. *Curr Opin Pediatr.* 2000;12:567–573.

63. Lomas JM, Jarvinen KM. Managing nut-induced anaphylaxis: challenges and solutions. *J Asthma Allergy.* 2015;8:115–123.

64. Berry MJ, Adams J, Voutilainen H, Feustel PJ, Celestin J, Jarvinen KM. Impact of elimination diets on growth and nutritional status in children with multiple food allergies. *Pediatr Allergy Immunol.* 2015;26:133–138.

65. Meyer R, De Koker C, Dziubak R, et al. Malnutrition in children with food allergies in the UK. *J Hum Nutr Diet.* 2014;27:227–235.

66. Flammarion S, Santos C, Guimber D, et al. Diet and nutritional status of children with food allergies. *Pediatr Allergy Immunol.* 2011;22:161–165.

67. Thomassen RA, Kvammen JA, Eskerud MB, Juliusson PB, Henriksen C, Rugtveit J. Iodine status and growth in 0-2-Year-Old Infants with Cow's Milk Protein Allergy. *J Pediatr Gastroenterol Nutr.* 2017;64:806–811.

68. Tuokkola J, Luukkainen P, Nevalainen J, et al. Eliminating cows' milk, but not wheat, barley or rye, increases the risk of growth deceleration and nutritional inadequacies. *Acta Paediatr.* 2017;106:1142–1149.

69. Berni Canani R, Leone L, D'Auria E, et al. The effects of dietary counseling on children with food allergy: a prospective, multicenter intervention study. *J Acad Nutr Diet.* 2014;114:1432–1439.

70. Robbins KA, Wood RA, Keet CA. Milk allergy is associated with decreased growth in U.S. children. *J Allergy Clin Immunol.* 2014;134:1466–1468 e6.

71. Christie L, Hine RJ, Parker JG, Burks W. Food allergies in children affect nutrient intake and growth. *J Am Diet Assoc.* 2002;102:1648–1651.

72. Greenhawt M. Food allergy quality of life and living with food allergy. *Curr Opin Allergy Clin Immunol.* 2016;16:284–290.

73. Baptist AP, Dever SI, Greenhawt MJ, Polmear-Swendris N, McMorris MS, Clark NM. A self-regulation intervention can improve quality of life for families with food allergy. *J Allergy Clin Immunol.* 2012;130:263–265 e6.

74. Du Toit G, Roberts G, Sayre PH, et al. Randomized trial of peanut consumption in infants at risk for peanut allergy. *N Engl J Med.* 2015;372:803–813.

75. Fleischer DM, Sicherer S, Greenhawt M, et al. Consensus communication on early peanut introduction and prevention of peanut allergy in high-risk infants. *Pediatr Dermatol.* 2016;33:103–106.

76. Greer FR, Sicherer SH, Burks AW, American Academy of Pediatrics Committee on N, American Academy of Pediatrics Section on A, Immunology. Effects of early nutritional interventions on the development of atopic disease in infants and children: the role of maternal dietary restriction, breastfeeding, timing of introduction of complementary foods, and hydrolyzed formulas. *Pediatr.* 2008;121:183–191.

77. Palmer DJ, Sullivan TR, Gold MS, Prescott SL, Makrides M. Randomized controlled trial of early regular egg intake to prevent egg allergy. *J Allergy Clin Immunol.* 2017;139: 1600–1607 e2.

78. Palmer DJ, Metcalfe J, Makrides M, et al. Early regular egg exposure in infants with eczema: A randomized controlled trial. *J Allergy Clin Immunol.* 2013;132:387–392.

79. Natsume O, Kabashima S, Nakazato J, et al. Two-step egg introduction for prevention of egg allergy in high-risk infants with eczema (PETIT): a randomised, double-blind, placebo-controlled trial. *Lancet.* 2017;389:276–286.

80. Onizawa Y, Noguchi E, Okada M, Sumazaki R, Hayashi D. The Association of the Delayed Introduction of Cow's Milk with IgE-Mediated Cow's Milk Allergies. *J Allergy Clin Immunol Pract.* 2016;4:481–488 e2.

81. Togias A, Cooper SF, Acebal ML, et al. Addendum guidelines for the prevention of peanut allergy in the United States: Report of the National Institute of Allergy and Infectious Diseases-sponsored expert panel. *Ann Allergy Asthma Immunol.* 2017;118:166–173 e7.

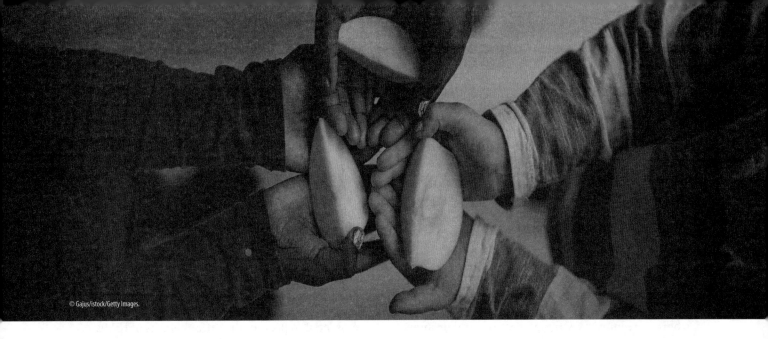

© Gajus/istock/Getty Images.

CHAPTER 26

Nutrition Management in Inborn Errors of Metabolism

Christine Hall

LEARNING OBJECTIVES

- Identify genetic conditions that require nutrition management
- Identify key nutrients that should be eliminated or limited in specific inborn errors of metabolism
- Compare disorder specific metabolic formulas

▶ Introduction

Inborn errors of metabolism (IEMs) consist of a large group of genetic disorders affecting amino acid, carbohydrate, or fat metabolism. Nutrition management of infants, children, and adults with inborn errors of metabolism requires an in-depth knowledge of biochemical processes, the pathophysiology of organ systems, as well as the science and application of nutrition, growth, and development. Providing nutrition management for patients with inborn errors requires individualized plans to meet the specific nutrient needs of each patient, based on genetic disorder and taking into consideration biochemical factors. Nutrient requirements established for normal populations[1] may not apply to individuals with

IEMs.[2] Some chemical compounds, normally not considered essential because they can be synthesized by the body, may not be synthesized in patients with a metabolic disorder. Consequently, dependent on the inborn error, the subsequent organ damage that accrues, and the rate of loss of specific chemicals from the body, several compounds become conditionally essential. Among these are the amino acids arginine,[3] carnitine,[4] cystine,[5] and tyrosine[6] and tetrahydrobiopterin (BH_4).[7] If these nutrient needs are not taken into consideration then metabolic crises, cognitive impairment, neurological crises, and growth failure are possiblities, and with some inborn errors, death may occur. Quality care is best achieved by an experienced genetic team that specializes in metabolic disorders.[8]

This chapter will address newborn screening for IEMs along with principles and practical considerations in nutrition support of IEMs identified by newborn screening[9,10] which include disorders of amino acid, carbohydrate, and fatty acid metabolism. For a detailed guide to nutrition support, see the *Nutrition Management of Patients with Inherited Metabolic Disorders.*[11]

▶ Newborn Screening

The American College of Medical Genetics recommends the core panel for screening newborns and includes tests for inherited metabolic disorders in which nutrition management is important (see **TABLE 26.1**). Newborn screening uses the process of **tandem mass spectrometry** (MS/MS) to analyze dried blood spots collected on filter paper.[9,10] Marker analytes for disorders recommended for newborn screening by mass spectrometry (MS/MS) are noted in Table 26.1.

Diseases in the secondary target are conditions essential in the differential diagnosis of a disorder in the core panel. Differential diagnosis by other analytes, enzymes, or mutation analysis is necessary for appropriate therapy, including nutrition management and preventing the serious effects of many IEMs.

Many other IEMs are known for which newborn screening does not occur. These may be diagnosed at a later age by clinical symptoms and diet therapy may be used to ameliorate or prevent worsening of symptoms.[11] However, early identification, diagnosis, and treatment are essential to prevent the serious effects of IEMs.

TABLE 26.1 Core and Secondary Targets of Inborn Errors of Metabolism Recommended for Newborn Screening and Marker Analytes Used with MS/MS Screening

Inborn Error	Marker Analyte
Core targets	
Amino Acid Disorders	
Argininosuccinic acidemia (ASA)	ASA, Citrulline (CIT)
Citrullinemia (CIT)	CIT
Homocystinuria (HCY)	Methionine (MET)
Maple syrup urine disease (MSUD)	Leucine (LEU) ± Valine (VAL)
Phenylketonuria (PKU)	Phenylalanine (PHE), PHE/Tyrosine (TYR)
Tyrosinemia type I (TYR I)	TYR
Fatty Acid Oxidation Disorders	
Carnitine uptake deficiency (CUD)	C^aO^b
Long-chain-hydroxy-acyl-CoA dehydrogenase deficiency (LCHAD)	C16-OH[c]; C^a18:1[d]-OH
Medium-chain acyl-CoA dehydrogenase deficiency (MCAD)	$C^a8/C^a10 ± C^a6$, $C^a10:1$, C8[a]
Trifunctional protein deficiency (TFP)	C^a16-OH, C^a18:1-OH
Very-long-chain acyl-CoA dehydrogenase deficiency (VLCAD)	C14:1, C14:1/C12:1 (± C14, C16, C18:1)
Organic Acid Disorders	
β-ketothiolase deficiency (BKT)[e]	$C^a5:1, ± C^a5OH$[c]
β-methylcrotonyl-CoA carboxylase deficiency (3MCC)[e]	C^a5-OH[c], ± [a]C5:1
Cobalamin A and B defects (Cbl A, B)[e]	$C^a3, C^a3/C^a2$
Glutaric acidemia type I (GA I)[e]	C^a5-DC[f]
HMG-CoA lyase deficiency (HMG)[e]	C^a5-OH, ± C^a6-DC[f]
Isovaleric acidemia (IVA)[e]	C^a5
Methylmalonic acidemia (MUT)[e]	$C^a3, C^a3/C^a2$
Multiple carboxylase deficiency (MCT)[e]	C^a5-OH, ± C^a3
Propionic acidemia (PROP)[e]	$C^a3, C^a3/C^a2$
Other Disorders	
Biotinidase deficiency (BIOT)[e]	± C^c5-OH[c], $C^a5:1$
Cystic fibrosis (CF)	
Galactose-1-phosphate uridyltransferase deficiency (GALT)[g]	

Inborn Error	Marker Analyte
Secondary targets	
Amino Acid Disorders	
Argininemia (ARG)	ARG
Biopterin regeneration deficiency (Biopt REG)	PHE, PHE/TYR
Biopterin synthesis defect (BS)	PHE, PHE/TYR
Citrin deficiency (CIT II)	CIT
Hypermethioninemia (MET)	MET
Hyperphenylalaninemia (Hyper-PHE)	PHE
Tyrosinemia type II (TYR II)	TYR
Tyrosinemia type III (TYR III)	TYR
Fatty Acid Oxidation Disorders	
Carnitine acylcarnitine transporter defect (CACT)	$C^a16{:}1$; $C^a18{:}1$
Carnitine palmitoyltransferase I defect (CPT IA)	Carnitine
Carnitine palmitoyltransferase II defect (CPT II)	$C^a16{:}1$, $C^a18{:}1$
Dienoyl-CoA reductase deficiency (DE RED)	
Glutaric acidemia type II (GA2)[e]	C^a4, C^a5, C^a5-DC^d, $C^a6, 8, 12, 14, 16$
Medium-chain ketoacyl-CoA thiolase deficiency (MCKAT)	C^a8, C^a8/C^a10, $\pm$ C^a6, $C^a10{:}1$
Medium-/short-chain hydroxy-acyl-CoA dehydrogenase deficiency (M/SCHAD)	C^a4-OH^c
Organic Acid Disorders	
α-methyl-β-hydroxy-butyric acidemia (2M3HBA)[e]	C^a5, $C^a5{:}1$, C^a5-OH^c
α-methylbutyryl-CoA dehydrogenase deficiency[e] (2MBG)	C^a5
β-methylglutaconyl hydratase deficiency (3MGA)[e]	C^a5-OH^c
Cobalamin C and D defects (Cbl C, D)[e]	C^a3/C^a2
Isobutyryl-CoA dehydrogenase deficiency (IBG)[e]	C^a4
Malonic acidemia (MAL)	C^a3
Other Disorders	
Galactokinase deficiency (GALK) [g]	
Galactose epimerase deficiency (GALE) [g]	

a. C = acyl group or carbon chain.

b. 0 = number of carbons: 0 to 18.

c. OH = hydroxy.

d. Colon (:) followed by number represents double bonds.

e. One or more amino acids involved in disorder.

f. DC = dicarboxyl.

g. Screened for by measuring blood galactose.

Data from Frazier DM. Newborn screening by mass spectrometry. In: Acosta PB, ed. *Nutrition Management of Patients with Inherited Metabolic Disorders.* Sudbury, MA: Jones and Bartlett Publishers; 2010:21–67.[9]

American College of Medical Genetics. Newborn screening: toward a uniform screening panel and system. *Genet Med.* 2006;8(suppl1):1S–252S.[10]

Chace DH, Lim T, Hansen CR, Adam BW, Hannon WH. Quantification of malonylcarnitine in dried blood spots by use of MS/MS varies by stable isotope internal standard composition. *Clin Chim Acta.* 2009;402(1–2):14–18.[12]

Gillingham MB. Nutrition management of patients with inherited disorders of mitochondrial fatty acid oxidation. In: Acosta PB, ed. *Nutrition Management of Patients with Inherited Metabolic Disorders.* Sudbury, MA: Jones and Bartlett Publishers; 2010:369–403.[13]

Korman SH. Inborn errors of isoleucine degradation. *Mol Genet Metab.* 2006;89:289–299.[14]

Matalon KM. Introduction to genetics and genetics of inherited metabolic disorders. In: Acosta PB, ed. *Nutrition Management of Patients with Inherited Metabolic Disorders.* Sudbury, MA: Jones and Bartlett Publishers; 2010:1–19.[15]

Miinalainen IJ, Schmitz W, Huotari A, et al. Mitochondrial 2, 4-dienoyl-CoA reductase deficiency in mice results in severe hypoglycemia with stress intolerance and unimpaired ketogenesis. *PLoS Genet.* 2009;5:e1000543.[16]

Molven A, Matre GE, Duran M, et al. Familial hyperinsulinemia and hypoglycemia caused by a defect in the SCHAD enzyme of mitochondrial fatty acid oxidation. *Diabetes.* 2004;53:221–227.[17]

Sim KG, Wiley V, Carpenter K, et al. Carnitine palmitoyltransferase I deficiency in neonate identified by dried blood spot free carnitine and acylcarnitine profile. *J Inherit Metab Dis.* 2001;24:51–59.[18]

▶ Principles and Practical Considerations in Nutrition Support

Principles

This section discusses a number of approaches to nutrition support of IEMs. The appropriate approach is dependent on the biochemistry and pathophysiology of disease expression. Several therapeutic strategies may be used simultaneously:[2]

- *Enhancing anabolism and depressing catabolism:* This involves using high-energy feeds including providing appropriate amounts of amino acids, carbohydrates, and fats. Fasting should be prevented to avoid catabolism.

- *Correcting the primary imbalance in metabolic relationships:* This correction reduces accumulated toxic substrate(s) through diet restriction. Examples for which this is used are phenylketonuria (PKU),[19] maple syrup urine disease (MSUD),[20] galactosemia,[21] and mitochondrial medium-chain, long-chain, and very-long-chain fatty acid oxidation[13] defects where phenylalanine; leucine, isoleucine, and valine; galactose; and long-chain fatty acids are limited, respectively.

- *Providing alternate metabolic pathways to decrease accumulated toxic precursors in blocked reaction sequences:* For example, isovalerylglycine is formed from accumulating isovaleric acid if supplemental glycine is provided to drive glycine-N-transacylase.[20] Isovalerylglycine is excreted in the urine.

- *Supplying products of blocked primary pathways:* Some examples are arginine in most disorders of the urea cycle,[3] cystine in homocystinuria,[5,16] tyrosine in PKU,[6,12] and BH$_4$[7] in biopterin synthesis defects.

- *Supplementing conditionally essential nutrients:* Examples are carnitine,[4] cystine,[5,22] and tyrosine[6] in secondary liver disease or with excess excretion of carnitine in organic acidemias.[23]

- *Stabilizing altered enzyme proteins:* The rate of biologic synthesis and degradation of holoenzymes (enzymes along with cofactors) is dependent on their structural conformation. In some holoenzymes, saturation by a coenzyme increases their biologic half-life and, thus, overall enzyme activity at the new equilibrium. This therapeutic mechanism is illustrated in homocystinuria and MSUD. Pharmacologic intake of pyridoxine in homocystinuria[22] and of thiamine in MSUD[2,20] increases intracellular pyridoxal phosphate and thiamine pyrophosphate, respectively, and increases the specific activity of any functional cystathionine β-synthase and branched-chain α-ketoacid dehydrogenase complex, respectively. BH$_4$ is available for use in patients with non-PKU hyperphenylalaninemia (HPA or mild PKU) to enhance phenylalanine hydroxylase activity.[24]

- *Replacing deficient coenzymes:* Many vitamin-dependent disorders are due to blocks in coenzyme production and are ameliorated by pharmacologic intake of a specific vitamin precursor. This mechanism presumably involves overcoming a partially impaired enzyme reaction by mass action. Impaired reactions required to produce methylcobalamin and adenosylcobalamin result in homocystinuria and methylmalonic aciduria/acidemia. Daily intakes of appropriate forms of milligram quantities of vitamin B$_{12}$ may ameliorate the disease.[25]

- *Inducing enzyme production:* If the structural gene or enzyme is intact but suppressor, enhancer, or promoter elements are not functional, abnormal amounts of enzyme may be produced. The structural gene may be "turned on" or "turned off" to enable normal enzymatic production to occur. In the acute porphyria of type I tyrosinemia, excessive δ-**aminolevulinic acid** (ALA) production may be reduced by suppressing transcription of the δ-ALA synthase gene with excess glucose.[2,26] Another suggested form of enzyme induction may be **phenylalanine hydroxylase** (PAH) where **phenylalanine** (PHE) loading with intact protein for 3 days induces a consistent decline in plasma PHE concentration in some patients.[27–31]

- *Supplementing nutrients that are inadequately absorbed or not released from their apoenzyme:* An example is biotin in biotinidase deficiency.[32]

- *Preventing absorption of a nutrient that may be toxic in excess:* Phenylalanine ammonia lyase, a plant enzyme that functions to catabolize PHE, is undergoing clinical studies for possible use in patients with mild PKU.[33] Norleucine, a structural analog of leucine, has been tried in mice with intermediate MSUD as a means of preventing leucine transport to the brain and brain injury.[34] **Large neutral amino acids** (LNAA) other than PHE are available for preventing the absorption of PHE from the intestinal tract and passage across the **blood–brain barrier** (BBB).[35] Long-term side effects of these high intakes of amino acids have not been studied.

Practical Considerations

The primary approach to therapy of patients with an IEM is with nutrition management.

Nutrients

The problem of ensuring adequate nutrition for infants and children with IEMs may be decreased by using a protocol or plan for treatment. Each patient requires individualized medical and nutrition care. Diet restrictions required to correct imbalances in some metabolic relationships usually require the use of elemental medical foods. These medical foods are normally supplemented with small amounts of intact protein that supply the restricted nutrient(s). These foods may supply up to 90%, but sometimes less, of the protein requirement of patients with disorders of amino acid or nitrogen metabolism. Other nitrogen-free foods that provide energy are limited in their range of nutrients. Consequently, care must be taken to provide nutrients previously considered to be food contaminants because their essentiality has been demonstrated through long-term use of total parenteral nutrition.[36] Thus, in addition to nutrients for which **dietary reference intakes** (DRIs)[1] are established, including fat, linoleic acid, and α-linolenic acid, other nutrients must be supplied in adequate amounts. These include minerals and vitamins. To ensure normal nutrition status indices, most mineral intakes must be greater than DRIs due to poor absorption by patients ingesting elemental diets; they also should be ingested in at least three meals per day for best absorption.[37]

Osmolality

Elemental medical foods and metabolic formulas used in amino acid disorders consist of small molecules that may result in an osmotic load greater than the physiologic tolerance of the patient. Abdominal cramping, diarrhea, distention, nausea, or vomiting may result from using hyperosmolar feeds. More serious consequences can occur in infants, such as hypertonic dehydration, hypovolemia, and hypernatremia.

▶ Changes in Nutrition Support Prescription

As soon as nutrition support is well established in an infant or child, the prescription should be adjusted frequently to account for weight gain and growth. The frequency depends on the age of the child. Infants require more frequent changes in prescription whereas older children who are growing more slowly may not require a diet change more than monthly or every 2 to 3 months depending on age. Small, frequent changes in prescription prevent drastic changes in plasma amino acid, glucose, organic acid, or ammonia concentrations and allow the intake to grow with the child.[38] These frequent adjustments are especially important in the preteen and teenage years to prevent inadequate intake of nutrients that result in poor linear growth. Pregnant women also require frequent diet changes based on biochemical indices.[38]

Monitoring

Successful management of IEMs requires frequent monitoring, which provides the physician and dietitian data that verify the adequacy of the nutrition support prescription. This data also can motivate patients/parents to be compliant with the prescription. Premature and full-term infants to at least 6 months of age require weekly to every other week monitoring. Monthly monitoring may be adequate if the patient is compliant with the diet prescription.

Some centers may wish to draw blood when the patient is fasting to monitor plasma analyte concentrations. Prolonged fasting (over 8 hours) may cause spurious elevations of plasma amino acid concentrations that could lead to unwarranted diet changes,[39] and blood drawn 15 minutes to 1 hour after a meal may also lead to falsely high values[40] in patients with amino acid disorders.

Nutrition Management of Aminoacidopathies

Inborn errors of amino acid metabolism are a group of disorders where the synthesis and degradation amino acids are impaired. These IMEs include **phenylketonuria** (PKU), tyrosinemia, **homocystinuria** (HCU), **maple syrup urine disease** (MSUD), and isovaleric acidemia. Dietary management of these disorders includes limiting the intake of the offending amino acid while avoiding deficiencies of certain essential amino acids. Most of these disorders require restriction of a branched-chain amino acid as part of the nutrition management, these are included in **TABLE 26.2**.

TABLE 26.2 Nutrition Support of Inborn Errors of Metabolism

Inborn Error and Defect	Nutrient(s) to Modify	Vitamin Responsive?	Medical Foods Available
Inborn errors of amino acid metabolism *Aromatic amino acids*[2,19]			
Phenylketonuria, classical (phenylalanine hydroxylase)	Restrict PHE, increase TYR, provide protein, mineral, and vitamin intakes greater than RDA.	No	See Table 26.5.

(continues)

TABLE 26.2 Nutrition Support of Inborn Errors of Metabolism *(continued)*

Inborn Error and Defect	Nutrient(s) to Modify	Vitamin Responsive?	Medical Foods Available
Inborn errors of amino acid metabolism *Aromatic amino acids*[2,19]			
Phenylketonuria, mild (phenylalanine hydroxylase)	Same as for PKU, classical.	±, Yes, BH$_4$ 10–20 mg/day	See Table 26.5.
Non-PKU hyperphenylalaninemia (phenylalanine hydroxylase)	Same as for PKU, if needed.	Yes, BH$_4$ 10–20 mg/day	See Table 26.5.
Hyperphenylalaninemia (dihydropteridine reductase)	Same as for PKU, if needed.	Yes, 1–10 mg/kg/day	See Table 26.5.
Tyrosinemia type I (fumarylacetoacetate hydrolyase)	Restrict PHE and TYR. Provide greater than RDA for protein, energy, mineral, and vitamin intakes. Drug: 2-(2-nitro-4-trifluromethylbenzyl)-1-3-cyclohexanedione.	No —	See Table 26.5.
Tyrosinemia type II (tyrosine aminotransferase)	Restrict PHE and TYR. Provide protein, mineral, and vitamin intakes greater than RDA.	No	See Table 26.5.
Tyrosinemia type III (phenylpyruvic acid dioxygenase)	Same as for tyrosinemia type II.	No	See Table 26.5.
Branched-chain amino acids[2,20]			
Maple syrup urine disease (branched-chain ketoacid dehydrogenase complex)	Restrict ILE, LEU, and VAL. Provide protein energy, mineral, and vitamin intakes above RDA.	Yes, thiamine-responsive if any residual enzyme activity. Response to thiamine inadequate to alleviate need for restriction of BCAAs.	See Table 26.5.
Isovaleric acidemia (isovaleryl-CoA dehydrogenase)	Restrict LEU; supplement with L-carnitine and GLY. Provide protein, energy, mineral, and vitamin intakes above RDA.	No	See Table 26.5.
β-methylglutaconic aciduria type I (β-methylglutaconyl-CoA hydratase)	Same as for isovaleric acidemia except no GLY supplement. Unknown if beneficial if started neonatally.	No	See Table 26.5.

Inborn Error and Defect	Nutrient(s) to Modify	Vitamin Responsive?	Medical Foods Available
Branched-chain amino acids[2,20]			
β-ketothiolase deficiency (mitochondrial acetoacetyl-CoA thiolase deficiency)	Restrict ILE, supplement L-carnitine. Provide protein, energy, vitamin, and mineral intakes above RDA. Supplement L-LEU and L-VAL.	No	See Table 26.5.
HMG-CoA lyase deficiency (β-hydroxy-β-methylglutaryl-CoA lyase deficiency)	Restrict LEU and fat; avoid fasting, supplement L-carnitine, provide protein, energy, minerals, and vitamins greater than RDA.	No	See Table 26.5.
Isobutyryl-CoA dehydrogenase deficiency	As yet unknown whether VAL should be restricted, L-carnitine supplemented, or protein, energy, minerals, and vitamins should be increased. If yes, supplement L-LEU and L-ILE.	No	See Table 26.5.
Sulfur amino acids[2,22]			
Homocystinuria, pyridoxine-nonresponsive (cystathionine-β-synthase)	Restrict MET, increase CYS, supplement folate, and betaine. Provide protein, energy, mineral, and vitamin intakes above RDA.	No	See Table 26.5.
Homocystinuria, pyridoxine-responsive (cystathionine-β-synthase)	None unless plasma homocystine remains elevated. If so, treat as B_6 nonresponsive.	Yes, vitamin B_6	See Table 26.5.
Hypermethioninemia I/III (methionine-s-adenosyltransferase deficiency)	Not treated by diet but with oral adenosylmethionine.	No	None
Other inborn errors of amino acid metabolism[2,23]			
Glutaric acidemia type I (glutaryl-CoA dehydrogenase)	Restrict LYS and TRP. Supplement L-carnitine. Provide protein, energy, mineral, and vitamin intakes above RDA.	Yes. Some patients have a partial response to oral riboflavin 100–300 mg daily. Administer 15–25 mg, with food, several times daily.	See Table 26.5.
Methylmalonic acidemia (methylmalonyl-CoA mutaseor mutase)	Restrict ILE, MET, THR, VAL, odd chain fatty acids, and long-chain unsaturated fatty acids. Supplement L-carnitine. Provide greater than RDA for protein, energy, mineral, and vitamin intakes.	No	See Table 26.5.

(continues)

TABLE 26.2 Nutrition Support of Inborn Errors of Metabolism   (*continued*)

Inborn Error and Defect	Nutrient(s) to Modify	Vitamin Responsive?	Medical Foods Available
Other inborn errors of amino acid metabolism[2,23]			
Methylmalonic acidemia (cobalamin reductase; adenosyltransferase)	Minimum restriction of ILE, MET, THR, and VAL. Supplement L-carnitine.	Yes, 1–2 mg hydroxycobalamin daily	See Table 26.5, if any used.
Propionic acidemia (propionyl-CoA carboxylase)	Restrict ILE, MET, THR, VAL, and long-chain fatty acids. Provide greater than RDA for protein, energy, mineral, and vitamin intakes. Supplement with L-carnitine daily.	Questionable. Some clinicians supplement D-biotin daily	See Table 26.5.
Cobalamin A and B	Vitamin B$_{12}$.	Yes, 1–2 mg hydroxycobalamin IM	
Cobalamin C and D	Supplement vitamin B$_{12}$, folate, betaine, and L-carnitine IM. Restrict ILE, MET, THR, VAL, if necessary.	Yes, hydroxycobalamin up to 20 mg as needed, and folate daily	
Inborn errors of nitrogen metabolism[2,41–44]			
Inborn Error and Defect	Nutrient(s) to Modify	No	See Table 26.5.
Carbamylphosphate synthetase deficiency; Ornithine transcarbamylase deficiency	Restrict protein. Add EAAs, L-carnitine, L-ARG, and L-CIT. Provide greater than RDA for energy, mineral, and vitamin intakes	No	See Table 26.5.
Citrullinemia (argininosuccinate synthetase deficiency)	Restrict protein. Add EAAs, L-carnitine, and L-ARG. Provide greater than RDA for energy, mineral, and vitamin intakes.	No	See Table 26.5.
Argininosuccinic aciduria (arginonosuccinate lyase)	Restrict protein. Add EAAs and L-ARG. Provide greater than RDA for energy, mineral, and vitamin intakes.	No	See Table 26.5.
Inborn errors of carbohydrate metabolism[2,21,4,45,4,62] *Galactosemias*			
Epimerase deficiency	Delete galactose. Add specific known amount of galactose. Provide RDA for protein, energy, minerals, and vitamins.	No	Isomil powder, ProSobee powder.
Galactokinase deficiency	Delete galactose. Provide RDA for protein, energy, mineral, and vitamin intakes.	No	Isomil powder, ProSobee powder.

Inborn Error and Defect	Nutrient(s) to Modify	Vitamin Responsive?	Medical Foods Available
Inborn errors of carbohydrate metabolism[2,21,4,45,4,62] **Galactosemias**			
Galactose-1-phosphate uridyl transferase deficiency	Delete galactose. Provide RDA for protein, energy, mineral, and vitamin intakes. Administer daily 750 mg calcium, 10 μg vitamin D, and 1 mg vitamin K₁ in addition to RDA. Unknown how strict diet should be in adults.	No	Isomil powder, ProSobee powder. *Do not use* formulas designed and marketed for lactase deficiency.
Inborn errors of fatty acid oxidation (mitochondrial)[15,47]			
Carnitine acylcarnitine translocase defect; Carnitine palmitoyltransferase II (CPT II) defect	Avoid fasting; use low-fat, MCT-supplemented diet. Administer linoleic and α-linolenic acids. Uncooked cornstarch for hypoglycemia. Water-miscible, fat-soluble vitamins.	L-carnitine therapy if plasma carnitine low	See Table 26.5.
Very-long-chain acyl-CoA dehydrogenase deficiency; Long-chain acyl-CoA dehydrogenase deficiency; Long-chain hydroxyacyl-CoA dehydrogenase deficiency; Trifunctional protein deficiency	Restrict long-chain fats, administer MCT, linoleic and α-linolenic acids. Uncooked cornstarch for hypoglycemia. Avoid fasting. Water-miscible fat-soluble vitamins. High-protein, moderate carbohydrates. Administer DHA for TFP.	No	See Table 26.5.
Medium-chain acyl-CoA dehydrogenase deficiency	Restrict long-chain and avoid medium-chain fats; administer linoleic and α-linolenic acids. Uncooked cornstarch for hypoglycemia. Avoid fasting.	Yes?	See Table 26.5.

Abbreviations: ALA, alanine; BCAAs, branched-chain amino acids; CYS, cystine; EAAs, essential amino acids (includes conditionally essential cystine and tyrosine); GLY, glycine; ILE, isoleucine; IM, intramuscular; LEU, leucine; LYS, lysine; MCT, medium-chain triglycerides; MET, methionine; MSUD, maple syrup urine disease; PHE, phenylalanine; THR, threonine; TRP, tryptophan; TYR, tyrosine; VAL, valine.

Data from Anderson HC, Marble M, Shapiro E. Long-term outcome in treated combined methylmalonic acidemia and homcystinuria. *Genet Med*. 1999;1:146–150.[48]

Carrillo-Carrasco J, Sloan J, Valle D, Hamosh A, Venditti CP. Hydroxocobalimin dose escalation improves metabolic control in cblC. *J Inherit Metab Dis*. 2009;52:728–731.[49]

Huemer M, Simma B, Fowler B, Suormala T, Bodamer OA, Sass JO. Prenatal and postnatal treatment in cobalamin C defect. *J Pediatr*. 2005;147:469–472.[50]

Urbon Artero A, Aldona Gomez J, Reig Del Moral C, Nieto Conde C, Merinero Cortes B. Neonatal onset methylmalonic aciduria and clinical improvement with betaine therapy. *An Esp Pediatr*. 2002;56:337–341.[51]

Singh RH. Nutrition management of patients with inherited disorders of urea cycle enzymes. In Acosta PB, ed. *Nutrition Management of Patients with Inherited Metabolic Disorders*. Sudbury, MA: Jones and Bartlett Publishers; 2010:405–429.[52]

Smith DL, Bodamer OA. Practical management of combined methylmalonic aciduria and homocystinuria. *J Child Neurol*. 2002;17:353–356.[53]

▶ Inborn Errors of Amino Acid Metabolism

Information in Table 26.2 describes various inborn errors, nutrients to modify, vitamin responsiveness, and medical foods available. Data in **TABLE 26.3** outline recommended nutrient intakes for beginning therapy. **TABLE 26.4**

describes information on nutrition support during acute illness, medication and nutrient interactions, and nutrition assessment parameters. Sources of medical foods, their ingredients, and their composition may be obtained from the information presented in **TABLE 26.5**.

Table 26.3 describes the amounts of amino acids with which to begin nutrition support. For some disorders in which the initial plasma concentration(s) of

TABLE 26.3 Recommended Nutrient Intakes for Initiating Therapy

Nutrients to Modify	Age (years)					
	0.0 <0.5	0.5 <1.0	1 <4	4 <7	7 <11	11 <19
Inborn errors of amino acid metabolism						
Aromatic amino acids						
Phenylketonuria and hyperphenylalaninemia[2,11,19,38]						
PHE (mg)	55 (70–20)/kg	30 (50–15)/kg	325 (230–450)/d	425 (225–625)/d	450 (250–650)/d	500 (300–750)/d
TYR (mg)	195 (210–180)/kg	185 (200–170)/kg	2800 (1400–4200)/d	3150 (1750–4550)/d	3500 (2100–4900)/d	3850 (2100–5600)/d
Protein (g)	3.5–3.0/kg	3.0–2.5/kg	≥ 30/d	≥ 35/d	≥ 40/d	≥ 50–65/d
Energy (kcal)	120/kg	110/kg	900–1300/d	1300–2300/d	1650–3300/d	1500–3300/d
Tyrosinemia type I[2,11,19,38]						
PHE (mg)	100 (125–65)/kg	80 (105–45)/kg	600 (500–700)/d	650 (550–750)/d	700 (600–800)/d	800 (700–900)/d
TYR (mg)	75 (95–45)/kg	55 (75–30)/kg	400 (300–500)/d	450 (350–550)/d	500 (400–600)/d	550 (450–650)/d
Protein (g)	3.5–3.0/kg	3.0–2.5/kg	≥ 30/d	≥ 35/d	≥ 40/d	≥ 50–65/d
Energy (kcal)	← 100–120% RDA →					
Tyrosinemia type II, III[2,11,19,38]						
PHE (mg)	100 (125–65)/kg	80 (105–45)/kg	450 (400–500)/d	500 (450–550)/d	550 (500–600)/d	600 (550–700)/d
TYR (gm)	75 (100–40)/kg	55 (80–20)/kg	400 (350–450)/d	450 (400–500)/d	500 (450–550)/d	475 (400–550)/d
Protein (g)	3.5–3.0/kg	3.0–2.5/kg	≥ 30/d	≥ 35/d	≥ 40/d	≥ 50–65/d
Energy (kcal)	120/kg	110/kg	900–1800/d	1300–2300/d	1650–3300/d	1500–3300/d

Branched-chain amino acids
Maple syrup urine disease[2,20,38]

Nutrient						
ILE (mg)	60 (90–30)/kg	50(70–30)/kg	50 (70–20)/kg		25 (30–20)/kg	25 (30–10)/kg
LEU (mg)	80 (100–40)/kg	55 (75–40)/kg	55 (70–40)/kg	50 (65–35)/kg	45 (60–30)/kg	40 (50–15)/kg
VAL (mg)	70 (95–40)/kg	55 (80–30)/kg	50 (70–30)/kg	40 (50–30)/kg	28 (30–25)/kg	22 (30–15)/kg
Protein (g)	3.5–3.0/kg	3.0–2.5/kg	≥ 30/d	≥ 35/d		≥ 50–65/d
Energy (kcal)	←————— 100–125% RDA —————→					

Isovaleric acidemia, β-methylglutaconyl hydratase deficiency type I[2,11,20,38]

Nutrient						
LEU (mg)	95 (110–65)/kg	75 (90–50)/kg	975 (800–1150)/d	1275 (1050–1500)/d	1445 (1190–1700)/d	1955 (1610–2300)/d
L-carnitine (mg)	←————— 300–100/kg —————→					
GLY (mg)	←————— 125 (150–100)/kg —————→					
Protein (g)	3.5–3.0/kg	3.0–2.5/kg	≥ 30/d	≥ 35/d	≥ 40/d	≥ 50–65/d
Energy (kcal)	←————— 100–125% RDA —————→					

HMG-CoA lyase deficiency[2,11,19,38]

Nutrient						
LEU (mg)	120 (140–100)/kg	110 (130–90)/kg	90 (100–80)/kg	80 (90–70)/kg	60 (80–40)/kg	50 (60–40)/kg
L-carnitine (mg)	←————— 50–100/kg —————→					
Protein (g)	3.5–3.0/kg	3.0–2.5/kg	≥ 30/d	≥ 35/d	≥ 40/d	≥ 50–65/d
Fat (g)	←————— 25–30% of energy —————→					
Energy (kcal)	←————— 100–125% of RDA —————→					
Avoid fasting	←————————————————→					

(continues)

TABLE 26.3 Recommended Nutrient Intakes for Initiating Therapy *(continued)*

Nutrients to Modify	Age (years)					
	0.0 <0.5	0.5 <1.0	1 <4	4 <7	7 <11	11 <19
β-ketothiolase deficiency[2,11,20,38]						
ILE (mg)	70 (80–60)/kg	65 (75–55)/kg	60 (70–50)/kg	55 (65–45)/kg	55 (65–45)/kg	45 (55–35)/kg
L-carnitine (mg)	← 100–200 mg/kg →					
Protein (g)	3.5–3.0/kg	3.0–2.5/kg	≥ 30/d	≥ 35/d	≥ 40/d	≥ 50–65/d
Fat (g)	← 25–30% of energy →					
Energy (kcal)	← 100–125% of RDA →					
Avoid fasting						
Supplemental L-LEU and L-VAL	← To maintain normal plasma concentrations →					
Isobutyryl-CoA dehydrogenase deficiency[20]						
ILE (mg)	70 (80–60)/kg	60 (70–50)/kg	55 (65–45)/kg	55 (65–45)/kg	50 (60–40)/kg	45 (55–35)/kg
GLY (mg)	← 100 (150–100)/kg →		← 125 (150–100)/kg →			
L-carnitine (mg)	← 100–300/kg →					
Protein (g)	3.5–3.0/kg	3.0–2.5/kg	≥ 30/d	≥ 35/d	≥ 40/d	≥ 50–65/d
Energy (kcal)	← 100–125% of RDA →					
Sulfur amino acids Homocystinuria, cystathionine-β-synthase deficiency (pyridoxine nonresponsive)[2,11,22,38]						
MET (mg)	35 (50–20)/kg	28 (40–15)/kg	20 (30–10)/kg	15 (20–10)/kg	15 (20–10)/kg	15 (20–10)/kg

CYS (mg)	300–250/kg	250–200/kg	150 (200–100)/kg	150 (200–100)/kg	150 (200–100)/kg	75 (60–50)/kg
Betaine (g)	←——— 1–3/d ———→		←——— 3–6/d ———→			
Folate (mg)	←—— 0.5–1.0/d ——→		←——— 1–3/d ———→			
Protein (g)	3.5–3.0/kg	3.0–2.5/kg	≥ 30/d	≥ 35/d	≥ 40/d	≥ 50–65/d
Energy (kcal)	120/kg	115/kg	900–1800/d	1300–2300/d	1650–3300/d	1500–3300/d

Other amino acids
Glutaric acidemia type I [2,11,23,38]

LYS (mg)	85 (100–70)/kg	65 (90–40)/kg	55 (80–30)/kg	50 (75–25)/kg	45 (65–25)/kg	40 (60–20)/kg
TRP (mg)	25 (40–10)/kg	15 (30–10)/kg	12 (16–8)/kg	12 (16–8)/kg	8 (10–5)/kg	6 (8–4)/kg
L-carnitine (mg)	←———————————— 300–100/kg ————————————→					
Riboflavin (mg)	←——— 300–100 d, administer in 25-mg doses orally with food ———→					
Protein (g)	3.5–3.0/kg	3.0–2.5/kg	≥ 30/d	≥ 35/d	≥ 40/d	≥ 50–65/d
Energy (kcal)	120/kg	115/kg	900–1800/d	1300–2300/d	1650–3300/d	1500–3300/d
Do not overrestrict TRP						

Propionic acidemia; Methylmalonic acidemia [2,11,23,38]

ILE (mg)	95 (120–60)/kg	70 (90–40)/kg	610 (485–735)/d	795 (630–960)/d	900 (715–1090)/d	1215 (956–1470)/d
MET (mg)	35 (50–15)/kg	25 (40–10)/kg	330 (275–390)/d	435 (360–510)/d	495 (410–580)/d	665 (550–780)/d
THR (mg)	90 (135–50)/kg	55 (75–20)/kg	505 (415–600)/d	660 (540–780)/d	745 (610–885)/d	1010 (830–1195)/d
VAL (mg)	85 (105–60)/kg	66 (75–30)/kg	690 (550–830)/d	900 (720–1080)/d	1020 (815–1225)/d	1380 (1105–1655)/d
D-biotin (mg)	←——————————— 5–10/d for propionic acidemia ———————————→					

(continues)

TABLE 26.3 Recommended Nutrient Intakes for Initiating Therapy

Nutrients to Modify	Age (years)					
	0.0<0.5	0.5<1.0	1<4	4<7	7<11	11<19
Propionic acidemia; Methylmalonic acidemia[2,11,23,38]						
Hydroxy-cobalamin (mg)	←————————— 1–2/d for cobalamin-responsive methylmalonic acidemia —————————→					
L-carnitine (mg)	←————————— 300–100/kg —————————→					
Protein (g)	3.5–3.0/kg	3.0–2.5/kg	≥ 30/d	≥ 35/d	≥ 40/d	≥ 50–65/d
Energy (kcal)	←————————— 100–125% of RDA —————————→					
Multiple carboxylase deficiency; Biotinidase deficiency[23]						
Biotin (mg)	←————————— 10–20/d —————————→					
Inborn errors of nitrogen metabolism *Citrullinemia; Argininosuccinic aciduria*[2,11,38,41,44]						
L-ARG (mg)	700–350/kg	700–350/kg	500–250/kg	500–250/kg	500–250/kg	400–200/kg
Protein (g)	2.5–1.10/kg	1.9–1.0/kg	1.8–0.7/kg	1.3–0.7/kg	1.7–0.9/kg	1.4–0.8/kg
Energy (kcal)	←————————— 125–150% of RDA —————————→					
Carbamylphosphate synthetase deficiency; Ornithine transcarbamylase deficiency[2,11,38,41,44]						
L-CIT (mg)	700–350/kg	700–350/kg	500–250/kg	500–250/kg	500–250/kg	400–200/kg
Protein (g)	2.5–1.7/kg	1.9–1.0/kg	1.8–0.7/kg	1.3–0.7/kg	1.7–0.9/kg	1.4–0.8/kg
Energy (kcal)	←————————— 125–150% of RDA —————————→					

(continued)

Argininemia[2,11,38,41,44]						
Protein (g)	2.5–1.0/kg	1.9–1.0/kg	1.8–0.7/kg	1.3–0.7/kg	1.7–0.9/kg	1.4–0.8/kg
Energy (kcal)	←———————————— 125–150% of RDA ————————————→					
Citrin deficiency[43]						
Protein (g)	4.5–4.0/kg		4.0–3.5/kg	3.5–3.0/kg	3.0–2.5/kg	2.5–2.0/kg
L-ARG (mg)	←———————————— 600–100/kg ————————————→					
Carbohydrate (g)	←———————————— Low ————————————→					
Energy (kcal)	←———————————— 100–125% RDA for age ————————————→					
Inborn errors of carbohydrate metabolism						
Galactosemias[2,11,21,45,46]						
Epimerase deficiency						
Galactose (mg)	←—— 1000–1500/d ——→		←—————— 500–1000/d ——————→			
Protein (g)	>2.2/kg	>2.0/kg	>23/d	>30/d	>35/d	>45–65/d
Energy (kcal)	120/kg	115/kg	900–1800/d	1300–2300/d	1650–3300/d	1500–3300/d
Galactokinase deficiency						
Protein (g)	>2.2/kg	>2.0/kg	>23/d	>30/d	>35/d	>45–65/d
Energy (kcal)	120/kg	115/kg	900–1800/d	1300–2300/d	1650–3300/d	>1500–3300/d

(continues)

TABLE 26.3 Recommended Nutrient Intakes for Initiating Therapy *(continued)*

Nutrients to Modify	Age (years)					
	0.0 <0.5	0.5 <1.0	1 <4	4 <7	7 <11	11 <19
Galactose-1-phosphate uridyltransferase deficiency						
Calcium (mg)[a]	360	540	800	800	800	1200
Vitamin D (μg)[b]	10	10	10	10	10	10
Vitamin K (μg)[c]	30	4	5	6	7	8
Protein (g)	>2.2/kg	>2.0/kg	>30/d	>35/d	>40/d	>45–65/d
Energy (kcal)	120/kg	115/kg	900–1800/d	1300–2300/d	1650–3300/d	1500–3300/d
Inborn errors of fatty acid oxidation[11,13,38,54] *Carnitine acylcarnitine translocase defect; Carnitine palmitoyltransferase defect*						
Avoid fasting						
Uncooked cornstarch			←——— To avoid hypoglycemia, 1 g/kg at bedtime ———→			
Protein (g)	←——— 15–20% of energy ———→					
Fat, long chain	←——— 10% of energy ———→					
Linoleic acid	←——— 3–4% of energy ———→					
α-linolenic acid	←——— 0.6–1% of energy ———→					
MCT oil	←——— 20% of energy ———→					

Nutrient	Recommendation
Energy	RDA for age. Avoid obesity
Glucose	As needed for hypoglycemia
Water-miscible fat-soluble vitamins	RDA for age
Very-long-chain acyl-CoA dehydrogenase deficiency; Long-chain acyl-CoA dehydrogenase deficiency; Long-chain hydroxy-acyl-CoA dehydrogenase deficiency; Trifunctional protein defect	
As above except protein	30% of energy
Add docosahexaenoic acid (DHA)	
Medium-chain acyl-CoA dehydrogenase deficiency; Short-chain acyl-CoA dehydrogenase deficiency; Short-chain β-hydroxyacyl-CoA dehydrogenase deficiency	
Avoid fasting	
Protein (g)	15–20% of energy
Fat	20–30% of energy
Linoleic acid	3–4% of energy
α-linolenic acid	0.6–1% of energy
Uncooked cornstarch	To prevent hypoglycemia, 1 g/kg at bedtime
Energy (kcal)	RDA, avoid obesity

a. In addition to 750 mg/day after 1 year of age, should be given in addition to recommendations for at least 2 years.

b. 10 μg vitamin D should be given for at least 2 years after 1 year of age in addition to recommendations.

c. 1 mg vitamin K should be given for 2 years after 1 year of age in addition to recommendations.

Abbreviations: ARG, arginine; CIT, citrulline; CYS, cystine; GLY, glycine; ILE, isoleucine; LEU, leucine; LYS, lysine; MET, methionine; PHE, phenylalanine; THR, threonine; TRP, tryptophan; TYR, tyrosine; VAL, valine.

TABLE 26.4 Nutrition Support During Acute Illness; Medications and Nutrient Interactions and Nutrition Assessment Parameters

Inborn Error and Nutrient Support During Acute Illness	Medication and Nutrient Interaction	Nutrition Assessment Parameters
Inborn errors of amino acid metabolism aromatic amino acids		
Phenylketonuria; Hyperphenylalaninemia[2,19,38]		
Delete dietary PHE 1–3 days *only*. For infant provide a PHE medical formula initially. Then add a prescribed amount of breast milk or standard infant formula to provide the desired amount of PHE to meet the individual patient PHE needs.	Usually no medication required with early and continuing therapy throughout life.	Plasma PHE, transthyretin, albumin, ferritin, and TYR; bone radiographs of lumbar vertebrae; dietary intakes of PHE, TYR, protein, energy, minerals, and vitamins, routine assessment parameters and standards.
Hyperphenylalaninemias		
Same as above.	Same as above.	Plasma PHE, TYR, transthyretin, albumin, and ferritin; dietary intake of PHE, TYR, protein, energy, minerals, vitamins.
Tyrosinemia type I[2,19,38]		
Delete dietary PHE and TYR, 1–3 days *only* using a TYR free formula. If necessary, give IV glucose and electrolytes at 150 mL/kg/24 hours to supply a glucose infusion rate of 10 mg/kg/min, and amino acids free of PHE and TYR to maintain anabolism. Return to oral medical food and complete diet as rapidly as tolerated.		Plasma PHE, TYR, transthyretin, albumin, ferritin, bicarbonate, phosphate, potassium, alkaline phosphatase, electrolytes, and liver enzymes; urinary succinylacetone; dietary intake of PHE, TYR, protein, energy, minerals, and vitamins. Growth. Liver imaging studies.
Tyrosinemia type II, III[2,19,38]		
Same as for tyrosinemia type I.		Plasma PHE, TYR, transthyretin, albumin, ferritin, urinary N-acetyl-tyrosine, p-tyramine, p-hydroxyphenyl organic acids; dietary intake of PHE, TYR, protein, energy, minerals, and vitamins.

Branched-chain amino acids

Maple syrup urine disease[2,20,38]

Delete dietary BCAAs 1–3 days only using a BCAA free medical formula. If necessary, give IV glucose and electrolytes at 150 mL/kg/24 hours to supply a glucose infusion rate of 10 mg/kg/min and amino acids free of BCAAs. Return to oral medical food and complete diet as rapidly as tolerated.	Anticonvulsants if seizures occur. Phenobarbital and phenytoin lead to accelerated metabolism of vitamin D and vitamin D deficiency that respond to 1,25-dihydroxyvitamin D. Valproate depresses appetite, and causes an increase in plasma GLY concentration and loss of carnitine.	Plasma BCAAs, ALA, ALLO, albumin, transthyretin, and ferritin; urine ketoacids of BCAAs. Bone radiographs of lumbar vertebrae, cation/anion gap; dietary intake of BCAAs, protein, energy, minerals, and vitamins.

Isovaleric acidemia; β-methylcrotonyl-glycinuria; β-methylglutaconic aciduria type I

Delete dietary LEU 1–3 days only. Increase GLY and L-carnitine. For infant, LEU free formula initially. If necessary, give IV glucose and electrolytes at 150 mL/kg/24 hours to supply a glucose infusion rate of 10 mg/kg/min, and amino acids free of LEU. Return to oral medical food and complete diet as rapidly as tolerated.	Benzoates and salicylates are contraindicated.	Plasma BCAAs. Carnitine, GLY, isovalerylglycine, transthyretin, albumin, ferritin; CBC/differential. Bone radiographs of lumbar vertebrae. Urinary isovalerylglycine, hydroxyisovaleric acid, cation/anion gap. Dietary intakes of LEU, protein, energy, minerals, and vitamins. See reference 55 (from this chapter) for other routine assessment parameters and standards. Growth.

HMG–CoA lyase deficiency[2,20,38]

Same as above.	Same as above.

Isobutyryl-CoA dehydrogenase deficiency[2,20,38]

Same as above except restrict VAL.	Same as isovaleric acidemia.

β-ketothiolase deficiency

Delete dietary ILE 1–3 days only, administer L-carnitine. For infant, ILE free formula initially, IV glucose and electrolytes at 150 mL/kg/24 hrs to supply a glucose infusion of 10 mg/kg/min, if required. Return to oral medical food and complete diet as rapidly as possible.	Same as isovaleric acidemia.

(continues)

TABLE 26.4 Nutrition Support During Acute Illness; Medications and Nutrient Interactions and Nutrition Assessment Parameters *(continued)*

Inborn Error and Nutrient Support During Acute Illness	Medication and Nutrient Interaction	Nutrition Assessment Parameters
Homocystinuria, pyridoxine nonresponsive[2,22,38]		
Delete dietary MET 1–3 days *only*. For infant MET formula initially. If necessary, give IV glucose, lipid, and amino acids free of MET. Return to oral medical food and complete diet as rapidly as tolerated.	Anticonvulsants if seizures occur. Phenobarbital and phenytoin lead to accelerated metabolism of vitamin D and cause vitamin D deficiency that responds to 1,25-dihydroxy- vitamin D. Valproate depresses appetite and causes an increase in plasma GLY.	Plasma MET, CYS, HOMOCYS; trans-thyretin; albumin, erythrocyte folate; bone radiographs of lumbar vertebrae; dietary intake of MET, CYS, protein, energy, minerals, and vitamins. See reference 55 (from this chapter) for other routine assessment parameters and standards. Growth.
Other inborn errors of amino acid metabolism		
Glutaric acidemia type I[23,38]		
Delete LYS and TRP 1–3 days *only*. For infant LYS and TRP free formula, adding a measured amount of MBM/standard formula back in when appropriate. If necessary, give IV glucose and electrolytes at 150 mL/kg/24 hours to supply a glucose infusion of 10 mg/kg/min, and amino acids free of LYS and TRP. Return to oral medical food and complete diet as rapidly as tolerated.	Baclofen-made by Geneva Generics, Inc. Valproate depresses appetite, and causes an increase in plasma GLY concentration and loss of carnitine.	Plasma LYS, TRP transthyretin, albumin, ferritin; free carnitine; urinary glutaric acid; dietary intake of LYS, TRP, protein, energy, minerals, and vitamins.
Propionic acidemia; Methylmalonic acidemia[2,23,38]		
Delete ILE, MET, THR, VAL 1–3 days *only*. Increase L-carnitine. If necessary, give IV glucose at 150 mL/kg, to supply 10 mg/kg/min, electrolytes and amino acids free of ILE, MET, THR, and VAL to maintain anabolism. Return to oral medical food and complete diet as rapidly as tolerated.	Supplement folate, pantothenate, pyridoxine, and vitamin B_{12} at 3 to 5 times RDA when phenylbutyrate is used. Valproate depresses appetite and causes an increase in plasma GLY concentration and loss of carnitine.	Plasma ILE, MET, THR, VAL, albumin, transthyretin, GLY, free carnitine, blood ammonia, and cation/anion gap. Urinary metabolites of propionate or methylmalonate, CBC/differential; plasma transthyretin, or RBP. Bone radiographs of lumbar vertebrae. Dietary intake of ILE, MET, THR, VAL, protein, energy, minerals, and vitamins.

Cobalamin A and B

Delete ILE, MET, THR, and VAL 1–3 days only. Return to usual diet as rapidly as possible.

Plasma ILE, MET, THR, VAL, albumin, transthyretin, GLY, free carnitine, blood ammonia, cation/anion gap. Urinary metabolites of propionate or methylmalonate, CBC/differential; plasma transthyretin or RBP. Bone radiographs of lumbar vertebrae. Dietary intake of ILE, MET, THR, VAL, protein, energy, minerals, and vitamins.

Multiple carboxylase deficiency; Biotinidase deficiency[2,23,38]

Biotin, 10–20 mg/day

Anticonvulsants if seizures occur. Phenobarbitol and phenytoin tend to accelerate metabolism of vitamin D and cause deficiency that responds to 1,25-dihydroxy-vitamin D. Valproate decreases appetite and causes loss of L-carnitine and an increase in plasma GLY.

Ketolactic acidosis, organic aciduria, hyperammonia, tachypnea and hyper-ventilation, skin rash, and alopecia. Growth.

Inborn errors of nitrogen metabolism

Urea cycle disorders[2,30,41–43]

Blood NH₃ > 200 μmol/L: Delete protein 1–3 days only. Increase L-ARG or L-CIT if not arginase deficient. Give Pedialyte and sugar-sweetened, caffeine-free soft drinks with added carbohydrate modular to maintain energy intake at 125–150% of RDA. If necessary give IV glucose, and electrolytes at 150 mL/kg/24 hours to supply 10 mg/kg/min. Return to oral medical food and complete diet as rapidly as tolerated.

Phenylbutyrate: folate, niacin pantothenate, pyridoxine, vitamin B₁₂ (administer at 3–5 times RDA). Anticonvulsants for seizures; phenobarbital and metabolism of vitamin D and vitamin D deficiency that responds to 1,25-dihydroxy vitamin D. Valproate depresses appetite and causes an increase in plasma GLY concentration and loss of carnitine.

Plasma amino acids, ammonia, albumin, transthyretin, and triglycerides; dietary intake of protein, energy, minerals, and vitamins.

(continues)

TABLE 26.4 Nutrition Support During Acute Illness; Medications and Nutrient Interactions and Nutrition Assessment Parameters *(continued)*

Inborn Error and Nutrient Support During Acute Illness	Medication and Nutrient Interaction	Nutrition Assessment Parameters
Inborn errors of carbohydrate metabolism Galactosemias[2,21,38]		
Epimerase deficiency		
Same as for normal infant. Avoid food and drugs containing galactose or lactose.		Albumin, transthyretin. Bone radiographs of lumbar vertebrae. Dietary intake of galactose, protein, energy, minerals, and vitamins.
Galactokinase deficiency		
Same as for normal infant. Avoid food and drugs containing galactose or lactose.		Urinary galactose; routine eye examinations for cataracts.
Galactose-1-phosphate uridyl transferase deficiency		
Same as for normal infant. Avoid drugs containing galactose or lactose.		Albumin, transthyretin. Erythrocyte galactose-1 phosphate; plasma or urine galactol; routine eye examinations for cataracts. Liver enzymes, bone radiographs. Dietary intake of galactose, protein, energy, minerals, and vitamins.
Inborn errors of fatty acid oxidation (mitochondrial)[13,38]		
Carnitine transporter deficiency; Carnitine translocase deficiency; Carnitine palmitoyl transferase I, II deficiency; Long-chain acyl-CoA dehydrogenase deficiency; Very-long-chain acyl-CoA dehydrogenase deficiency; Trifunctional protein deficiency; Medium-chain acyl-CoA dehydrogenase deficiency; Short-chain acyl-CoA dehydrogenase deficiency; Short-chain β-hydroxy acyl-CoA dehydrogenase deficiency		
Uncooked cornstarch as needed to help prevent hypoglycemia. If necessary, give IV glucose at 150 mL/kg to supply a glucose infusion rate of 10 mg/kg/min. At home, frequent feeds of fluids containing 2.5 g carbohydrate per fluid ounce. Return to usual diet as rapidly as possible.	Valproate depresses appetite and causes an increase in plasma GLY concentration and loss of carnitine.[11]	Plasma essential fatty acid and fat-soluble vitamins. Plasma glucose and blood gases during illness. Bone radiographs. Nutrient intake. Plasma acylcarnitines. See reference 55 (from this chapter) for other routine assessment parameters and standards. Growth.

Abbreviations: ARG, arginine; ALLO, alloisoleucine; BCAAs, branched-chain amino acids; CBC, complete blood count; CIT, citrulline; CYS, cystine; GLY, glycine; GTP, guanosine triphosphate; HOMOCYS, homocystine; ILE, isoleucine; IV, intravenous; LEU, leucine; LYS, lysine; MET, methionine; PHE, phenylalanine; RBP, retinol-binding protein; THR, threonine; TRP, tryptophan; TYR, tyrosine; UDP, uridine diphosphate; VAL, valine.

TABLE 26.5 Selected Nutrient Composition (Per 100 G Powder) and Sources of Medical Foods for Patients with Disorders of Amino Acid and Fatty Acid Metabolism

Disorder/ Medical Foods	Modified Nutrient(s) (mg/100 g, source)	Protein Equivalent[a] (g/100 g, source)	Fat (g/100 g, source)	Carbohydrate (g/100 g, source)	Energy (kcal/100 g)	Linoleic Acid/ α-Linolenic Acid (mg/100 g)	Minerals/ Vitamins Not Added
Phenylketonuria (PKU) Abbott nutrition[b]							
Phenex-[®]1	PHE 0, TYR 1500, L-carnitine 20, Taurine 40	15.0 Amino acids[c]	21.7 High oleic safflower, coconut, soy oils	53 Corn syrup solids	480	3500/350	None/none
Phenex-2 Unflavored	PHE 0, TYR 3000, L-carnitine 40, Taurine 50	30.0 Amino acids[c]	14.0 High oleic safflower, coconut, soy oils	35 Corn syrup solids	410	2200/225	None/none
Phenex-2 Vanilla	PHE 0, TYR 3000, L-carnitine 40, Taurine 50	30.0 Amino acids[c]	13.5 High oleic safflower, coconut, soy oils	36 Corn syrup solids	410	2200/225	None/none
Nutricia North america[d]							
Periflex Early Years	PHE 0, TYR 1440	13.5 Amino acids	23 High oleic sunflower, soy, canola	53 corn syrup solids	473	?	None/none
Periflex Jr Plus (plain/ flavored)	PHE 0	28 Amino acids	12.5 High oleic sunflower, canola, MCT	43/41	385/377	?	
Periflex Advance	PHE 0, TYR 3500	35 Amino acids	12.6	29	369	?	None/none
PhenylAde Essential Drink Mix	PHE 0, TYR 3000, L-carnitine 20, Taurine 80	25.0 Amino acids[c]	13 Safflower, canola, soybean, coconut, flaxseed oils	46 Sucrose, modified food starch, dextrin, corn syrup solids	393	2025/525	None/none

(continues)

TABLE 26.5 Selected Nutrient Composition (Per 100 G Powder) and Sources of Medical Foods for Patients with Disorders of Amino Acid and Fatty Acid Metabolism *(continued)*

Disorder/ Medical Foods	Modified Nutrient(s) (mg/100 g, source)	Protein Equivalent[a] (g/100 g, source)	Fat (g/100 g, source)	Carbohydrate (g/100 g, source)	Energy (kcal/100 g)	Linoleic Acid/ α-Linolenic Acid (mg/100 g)	Minerals/ Vitamins Not Added
Nutricia North america[d]							
PhenylAde 40 Drink Mix	PHE 0, TYR 3744, L-carnitine 20, Taurine 80	40.0 Amino acids[c]	2 Partially hydrogenated coconut oil	40 Sucrose, modified food starch	336	0/0	None/none
PhenylAde 60 Drink Mix	PHE 0, TYR 6990, L-carnitine added, Taurine added	60.0 Amino acids[c]	0	20 Sucrose, corn syrup solids, modified food starch	327	0/0	None/none
PhenylAde GMP Drink Mix	PHE 50, TYR 3700	80 Amino acids[c]	12 Refined vegetable oils	2.7 corn syrup solids	396	0/0	?
PhenylAde GMP Mix-In (per pouch)	PHE 15	10	0	0	42	-	-
Periflex LQ (per 250 ml)	PHE 0	15	High oleic sunflower oil	Sugar	160	-	-
PKU Lophlex LQ (per pouch)	PHE 0. TYR 1880	20	0.44	9.3	120	-	-
Lophlex Powder (1 sachet)	PHE 0	10	0.03	0.14	312	-	-
PhenylAde MTE Amino Acid Blend	PHE 0	81	0	0	323	-	-
XPhe Maxamum	PHE 0, TYR 4000	40	<1	34 Sugar	305	-	-

Mead Johnson Nutritionals[f]						
Phenyl-Free-1	PHE 0, TYR 1600	16 Amino acids	26	51	500	NA	None/none
Phenyl-Free-2	PHE 0, TYR 2200, L-carnitine 49, Taurine 49	22.0 Amino acids[c]	8.6 Soy oil	60 Sugar, corn syrup solids, modified cornstarch	410	4600/651	None/none
Phenyl-Free-2HP	PHE 0, TYR 4000, L-carnitine 36, Taurine 63	40.0 Amino acids[c]	6.3 Soy oil	44 Sugar, corn syrup solids, modified cornstarch	390	3200/453	None/none
Vitaflo US LLC[h]						
PKU Cooler (10, 15, 20) (per 100 ml)	PHE 0, TYR 1370	10/15/20 Amino acids[c]	0.44	9.3	120	0/0	None
PKU Express	PHE 0, TYR 6590, L-carnitine 65.1, Taurine 129.6	60.0 Amino acids[c]	<0.5	15 Sugar, dried glucose syrup	302	0/0	None
PKU Gel	PHE 0, TYR 4630, L-carnitine 45.8, Taurine 91.1	42.0 Amino acids[c]	< 0.5	43 Sugar, dried glucose syrup	342	0/0	None
Cambrooke						
Glytactin Original Bettermilk and Bettermilk Lite (per packet)	PHE 23,	15/20 Amino acids	4.5 Sunflower oil	Corn syrup solids, modified corn starch	160/150	NA	-
Glytactin Restore/ Restore Lite	PHE 15	10/10	0/0	31/7	170/70	-	-

(continues)

TABLE 26.5 Selected Nutrient Composition (Per 100 G Powder) and Sources of Medical Foods for Patients with Disorders of Amino Acid and Fatty Acid Metabolism *(continued)*

Disorder/ Medical Foods	Modified Nutrient(s) (mg/100 g, source)	Protein Equivalent[a] (g/100 g, source)	Fat (g/100 g, source)	Carbohydrate (g/100 g, source)	Energy (kcal/100 g)	Linoleic Acid/ α-Linolenic Acid (mg/100 g)	Minerals/ Vitamins Not Added
Tyrosinemia types I, II, III							
Abbott nutrition[b]							
Tyrex-1	PHE 0, TYR 0	15.0 Amino acids[c]	21.7 High oleic safflower, coconut, soy oils	53 Corn syrup solids	480		None/none
Tyrex-2	PHE 0, TYR 0, L-carnitine 40, Taurine 50	30.0 Amino acids[c]	14.0 High oleic safflower, coconut, soy oils	35 Corn syrup solids	410	2200/225	None/none
Mead Johnson Nutritionals[f]							
Tyros 1	PHE 0, TYR 0,	16.7 Amino acids[c]	26 Soy oil	51 Corn syrup solids, sugar, modified cornstarch	500	4500/-	None/none
Tyros 2	PHE 0, TYR 0, L-carnitine 49, Taurine 49	22.0 Amino acids[c]	8.5 Soy oil	60 Corn syrup solids, sugar, modified cornstarch	410	4600/651	None/none
Nutricia North America[g]							
TYR Anamix Early Years	PHE 0, TYR 0	13.5 Amino acids[c]	23 Refined vegetable oils	53 Corn syrup solids	473	None/none	None/none
TYR Anamix Next	PHE 0, TYR 0	28 Amino acids	12.5 Refined vegetable oils	43.2 Corn syrup solids	385	-	-
TYR Lophlex LQ	PHE 0, TYR 0	20	0.44	9.3	120	-	-

VitaFlo USA LLC[h]

Product	Amino acids	Amount	Fat	Carbohydrate			
TYR Cooler (per pouch)	PHE 0, TYR 0	11.5 Amino acids					None
TYR express	PHE 0, TYR 0,	60.0 Amino acids[c]	<0.5	15 Sugar, modified cornstarch, dried glucose syrup	302	0/0	None
TYR gel	PHE 0, TYR 0,	42.0 Amino acids[c]	<0.5	43 Sugar, modified cornstarch, dried glucose syrup	342	ND/ND	None

Cambrooke foods[e]

Product	Amino acids	Amount	Fat	Carbohydrate			
Tylactin RTD (per 250 ml)	PHE 25, TYR 3,	15.0 Amino acids	5	NA Sucrose	200	NA	None

Inborn errors of branched-chain amino acids
Branched-chain ketoaciduria (MSUD)
Abbott nutrition[b]

Product	Amino acids	Amount	Fat	Carbohydrate			
Ketonex-1	ILE 0, LEU 0, VAL 0, L-carnitine 100, Taurine 40	15.0 Amino acids[c]	21.7 High oleic safflower oil, coconut and soy oils	53 Corn syrup solids	480	3500/350	None
Ketonex-2	ILE 0, LEU 0, VAL 0, L-carnitine 200, Taurine 50	30 Amino acids[c]	14 High-oleic safflower, coconut, soy oils	35 Corn syrup solids	410	2200/230	None/none

Cambrooke foods[e]

Product	Amino acids	Amount	Fat	Carbohydrate			
Camino Pro MSUD (140 ml pouch)	LEU 0	15.0 Amino acids[c]	0	Sugar	140	NA	NA

(continues)

TABLE 26.5 Selected Nutrient Composition (Per 100 G Powder) and Sources of Medical Foods for Patients with Disorders of Amino Acid and Fatty Acid Metabolism   *(continued)*

Disorder/ Medical Foods	Modified Nutrient(s) (mg/100 g, source)	Protein Equivalent[a] (g/100 g, source)	Fat (g/100 g, source)	Carbohydrate (g/100 g, source)	Energy (kcal/100 g)	Linoleic Acid/ α-Linolenic Acid (mg/100 g)	Minerals/ Vitamins Not Added
Mead Johnson Nutritionals[f]							
BCAD 1	ILE 0, LEU 0, VAL 0, L-carnitine 50, Taurine added	16.2 Amino acids[c]	26 Soy oil	51 Corn syrup solids, sugar, modified cornstarch	500	4000/NA	None
BCAD 2	ILE 0, LEU 0, VAL 0, L-carnitine 49, Taurine added	24.0 Amino acids[c]	8.5 Soy oil	57 Corn syrup solids, sugar, modified cornstarch	410	4600/610	None/none
Nutricia North America[g]							
MSUD Anamix Early Years	ILE 0, LEU 0, VAL 0	13.5 Amino acids[c]	23 Refined vegetable oils	53 Corn syrup solids	473	3500/NA	None/none
Complex Junior MSD	ILE 0, LEU 0, VAL 0	13.0 Amino acids	29 Safflower oil, canola oil, coconut oi	46 Corn syrup solids, modified corn starch	494	4296/NA	None
Complex Essential MSD	ILE 0, LEU 0, VAL 0	25	12 Canola oil, Safflower oil	47 Sugar, modified cornstarch	380	1871/493	None
Complex MSD Amino Acid Blend	ILE 0, LEU 0, VAL 0	81	0	0	323	NA	None
MSUD Maxamum	ILE 0, LEU 0, VAL 0	40.0 Amino acids[c]	< 1	34 Sugar, corn syrup solids	305	0/0	None/none
MSUD Lophlex LQ (125 ml pouch)	ILE 0, LEU 0, VAL 0	20	0.44	9.3	120		

Vitaflo USLLC[h]

MSUD Gel	ILE 0, LEU 0, VAL 0	42.0 Amino acids[c]					
MSUD Express	ILE 0, LEU 0, VAL 0, L-carnitine 165.6, Taurine 129.6	60.0 Amino acids[c]	< 0.5	15 Dried glucose syrup	302	NA	None/inositol
MSUD Express Cooler (per 100 mL)	ILE 0, LEU 0, VAL 0, L-carnitine 0, Taurine NA	15.0 Amino acids[c]	< 0.1	7.8 Sugar	92	NA	None/inositol

Isovaleric acidemia
Abbott nutrition[b]

I-Valex-1	LEU 0, GLY 1000, L-carnitine 900	15.0 Amino acids[c]	High-oleic safflower, coconut, soy oils	Corn syrup solids	480	NA	None
I-Valex-2	LEU 0, GLY 2000, L-carnitine 1800	30.0 Amino acids[c]	14.0 High-oleic safflower, coconut, soy oils	35 Corn syrup solids	410	2200/230	None/none

Mead Johnson Nutritionals[f]

LMD	LEU 0, GLY 1100, L-carnitine 50	16.2 Amino acids[c]	26 Vegetable oil	51 Corn syrup solids	500	NA	None

Nutricia North America[g]

IVA Anamix Early Years	LEU 0	13.5 Amino acids	23 Refined vegetable oils	53 Corn syrup solids	473	NA	None
IVA Anamix Next	LEU 0	28	12.5 Refined vegetable oils	41.2 Corn syrup solids	377	NA	None
XLeu Maxamum	LEU 0	40.0 Amino acids[c]	< 1	34 Sugar, corn syrup solids	305	0/0	None/none

(continues)

TABLE 26.5 Selected Nutrient Composition (Per 100 G Powder) and Sources of Medical Foods for Patients with Disorders of Amino Acid and Fatty Acid Metabolism *(continued)*

Disorder/ Medical Foods	Modified Nutrient(s) (mg/100 g, source)	Protein Equivalent[a] (g/100 g, source)	Fat (g/100 g, source)	Carbohydrate (g/100 g, source)	Energy (kcal/100 g)	Linoleic Acid/ α-Linolenic Acid (mg/100 g)	Minerals/ Vitamins Not Added
Cambrooke foods[e]							
Isovactin AA Plus (per 250 ml)	LEU 0	20 Amino acids	6 Canola oil	NA sugar	146	NA	None
Homocystinuria Abbott nutrition[b]							
Hominex-1	MET 0	15.0 Amino acids	27 High oleic safflower, coconut, soy oils	53 Corn syrup solids	480	3500/350	None
Hominex-2	MET 0, CYS 900, L-carnitine 40, Taurine 50	30.0 Amino acids[c]	14.0 High oleic safflower, coconut, soy oils	35 Corn syrup solids	410	2200/225	None/none
Mead Johnson Nutritionals[f]							
HCY 1	MET 0	15 Amino acids[c]	22 High oleic safflower oil	53 Corn syrup solids	480	3500/350	None
HCY 2	MET 0, CYS 810, L-carnitine added, Taurine 57	22.0 Amino acids[c]	8.5 Soy oil	61 Sucrose, corn syrup solids	410	4600/610	None/none
Nutricia North America[g]							
HCU Anamix Early Years	MET 0	13.5 Amino acids	23 Refined vegetable oils	53 Corn syrup solids	473	3500/NA	None
HCU Anamix Next	MET 0	28 Amino acids	12.5 Refined vegetable oils	43.2 Corn syrup solids	385	NA	None
XMET Maxamum	MET 0	40.0 Amino acids[c]	< 1.0	34 Sugar	305	0/0	None/none

HCU Lophlex LQ (per 120 ml pouch)	MET 0	20 Amino acids	0.44	9.3	120	NA	None
Vitaflo US LLC[h]							
HCU Cooler (per 130 mL pouch)	MET 0	15 Amino acids[c]	0.4	4.5	92	NA	None
HCU Express	MET 0	60.0 Amino acids[c]	<0.5	15 Sugar, starch, dried glucose syrup	302	0/0	None
HCU Gel	MET 0	42.0 Amino acids[c]	<0.5	43 Sugar, starch, dried glucose syrup	342	0/0	None
Cambrooke foods[e]							
Homactin AA Plus	MET 0	20	6.0 Canola oil	Sugar	186	NA	None
Propionic/Methylmalonic acidemia Abbott nutrition[b]							
Propimex-1	MET 0, VAL 0	15.0 Amino acids[c]	22 High oleic safflower, coconut, soy oils	53 Corn syrup solids	480	3500/350	None
Propimex-2	MET 0, VAL 0	30.0 Amino acids[c]	14.0 High oleic safflower, coconut, soy oils	35.0 Corn syrup solids	410	2200/225	None/none
Mead Johnson Nutritionals[f]							
OA1	MET 0, VAL 0	15.7 Amino acids[c]	26 Vegetable oils	51 Corn syrup solids	500	4000/NA	None
OA2	MET 0, VAL 0	21.0 Amino acids[c]	9.0 Soy oil	59.0 Corn syrup solids, sugar, modified cornstarch, maltodextrin	410	4600/608	None/none

(continues)

TABLE 26.5 Selected Nutrient Composition (Per 100 G Powder) and Sources of Medical Foods for Patients with Disorders of Amino Acid and Fatty Acid Metabolism   (continued)

Disorder/ Medical Foods	Modified Nutrient(s) (mg/100 g, source)	Protein Equivalent[a] (g/100 g, source)	Fat (g/100 g, source)	Carbohydrate (g/100 g, source)	Energy (kcal/100 g)	Linoleic Acid/ α-Linolenic Acid (mg/100 g)	Minerals/ Vitamins Not Added
Nutricia North America[g]							
MMA/PA Anamix Early Years	MET 0, VAL 0	13.5 Amino acids	23 Refined vegetable oils	53 Corn syrup solids	473	NA	None
MMA/PA Anamix Next	MET 0, VAL 0	28 Amino acids	12.5 Refined vegetable oils	41 Corn syrup solids	377	NA	None
XMTVI Maxamum	MET 0, VAL 0	40.0 Amino acids[c]	<1.0	34.0 Sugar, corn syrup solids	305	0/0	None/none
Vitaflo US LLC[h]							
MMA/PA Express	MET 0, ILE 0	60 Amino acids	0.2	13.7	297	NA	None
MMA/PA Cooler (130 ml pouch)	MET 0, ILE 0	11.5 Amino acids	1.3	5.4	79	NA	None
MMA/PA Gel	MET 0, VAL 0	42.0 Amino acids[c]	<0.5	43 Sugar, starch, dried glucose syrup	338	0/0	None
Glutaric aciduria type I *Abbott nutrition[b]*							
Glutarex-1	LYS 0, TRP 0	15.0 Amino acids[c]	High oleic safflower, coconut, soy oils	Corn syrup solids	480	3500/350	NA
Glutarex-2	LYS 0, TRP 0, L-carnitine 1800, Taurine 50	30.0 Amino acids[c]	14.0 High oleic safflower, coconut, soy oils	35.0 Corn syrup solids	410	2200/225	None/none
Mead Johnson Nutritionals[f]							
GA	LYS 0, TRP 0	15.1 Amino acids[c]	26 Vegetable oils	52 Corn syrup solids	500	4000	None

Nutricia North America[g]							
GA 1 Anamix Early Years	LYS 0, TRP 0	13.5	23 Refined vegetable oils	53 Corn syrup solids	473	NA	None
Glutarade Essential GA1	LYS 0, TRP 0	25	13 Canola oil	45 Sugar, modified cornstarch	385	NA	None
Glutarade GA 1 Amino Acid Blend	LYS 0, TRP 0	81	0	0	324	NA	None
Glutarade GA1 Junior	LYS 0, TRP 0	10	10 Canola oil	69 Corn syrup solids, modified food starch	46	NA	None
Vitaflo US LLC[h]							
GA Gel (per packet)	LYS 0, TRP 0	10 Amino acids[c]	<1	10.3	81	NA	None
GA Express (per packet)	LYS 0, TRP 0	15 Amino acids	<1	<1	74	NA	None
Urea cycle enzyme defects							
Abbott nutrition[b]							
Cyclinex-1	Non-essential amino acid-free	7.5 Amino acids	24 High oleic safflower oil	57 Corn syrup solids	480	3900/375	None
Cyclinex-2	Non-essential amino acid-free, L-carnitine 370, Taurine 60	15.0 Amino acids[c]	17.0 High oleic safflower, coconut, soy oils	45.0 Corn syrup solids	440	2800/275	None/none
Mead Johnson Nutritionals[f]							
WND®1	Non-essential amino acid-free	6.5 Amino acids[c]	26 Vegetable oils	60 Corn syrup solids	500	4000	None
WND®2	Non-essential amino acid-free, L-carnitine added, Taurine added	8.2 Amino acids[c]	10.2 Soy oil	71.0 Corn syrup solids, sugar, modified cornstarch	410	5500/ND	None/none

(continues)

TABLE 26.5 Selected Nutrient Composition (Per 100 G Powder) and Sources of Medical Foods for Patients with Disorders of Amino Acid and Fatty Acid Metabolism *(continued)*

Disorder/ Medical Foods	Modified Nutrient(s) (mg/100 g, source)	Protein Equivalent[a] (g/100 g, source)	Fat (g/100 g, source)	Carbohydrate (g/100 g, source)	Energy (kcal/100 g)	Linoleic Acid/ α-Linolenic Acid (mg/100 g)	Minerals/ Vitamins Not Added
Nutricia North America[g]							
UCD Anamix Junior	Non-essential amino acid-free	12 Amino acids	17 Refined vegetable oils	46 Corn syrup solids	385	NA	None
Fatty acid oxidation defects *Mead Johnson nutritionals*[f]							
Pregestimil Lipil	Medium-chain fatty acids	14.0 Casein hydrolysate, L-amino acids[c]	28 MCT, corn oil	51 Corn syrup solids	500	4700/NA	None
Enfaport (per 100 ml)	MCT	3.6	5.6 MCT	10.2	~100	NA	None
Nutricia North America[g]							
Monogen®	Medium-chain fatty acids	11.4 Whey protein concentrate, L-amino acids[c]	11.8 MCT	68 Corn syrup solids	424	NA	None
Vitaflo US LLC[h]							
Lipistart	Medium-chain fatty acids	13.7 Whey protein isolate, sodium caseinate	20.6 MCT	55	450	NA	None

a. g protein equivalent = g nitrogen 3 6.25.
b. Abbott Nutrition, 625 Cleveland Avenue, Columbus, OH 43215; 800-551-5838.
c. Cambrooke Foods, Two Central Street, Framingham, MA 01701; 866-456-9776.
d. Mead Johnson Nutritionals, 2400 W Lloyd Expressway, Evansville, IN 47721; 800-457-3550.
e. Nutricia North America, PO Box 117, Gaithersburg, MD 20884; 800-365-7354.
f. Vitaflo US LLC, 123 East Neck Road, Huntington, NY 11743; 888-848-2356.
Values listed, although accurate at time of publication, are subject to change. The most current information may be obtained by referring to product labels.
Abbreviations: ND, no data; NA, not available.
Data from Data supplied by each company.

toxic amino acid is 14 to 20 times the upper limit of the normal reference range, after 2 to 3 days of no intake of the amino acid, it should be introduced with the lowest recommended amount for age. Frequent monitoring of plasma concentrations of amino acids and other analytes, nutrient intake, and growth can verify the adequacy of intake.[38]

When specific amino acids require restriction, after diagnosis or during illness, patients may require a total deletion for 1 to 3 days or until the plasma concentration reaches the upper limit of the reference range is the best approach to initiating therapy. Longer term deletion or overrestriction may precipitate deficiency of the amino acid(s). The most limiting nutrient determines growth rate in all disorders, and overrestriction of an amino acid, nitrogen (N), or energy will result in further intolerance of the toxic nutrient. Results of amino acid and N deficiencies are described in **TABLE 26.6**. Each patient's nutrition prescription must be individualized to fit specific needs.

TABLE 26.6 Results of Amino Acid and Nitrogen Deficiencies

Amino Acid	Manifestations of Deficiency
Arginine	Elevated blood ammonia Elevated urinary orotic acid Generalized skin lesions Poor wound healing Retarded growth
Carnitine	Fatty myopathy Cardiomyopathy Depressed liver function Neurologic dysfunction Defective fatty acid oxidation Hypoglycemia Hypertriacylglycerolemia
Citrulline	Elevated blood ammonia
Cysteine	Impaired nitrogen balance Impaired sulfur balance Decreased tissue glutathione Hypotaurinemia
Isoleucine	Weight loss or no weight gain Redness of buccal mucosa Fissures at corners of mouth Tremors of extremities Decreased plasma cholesterol Decreased plasma isoleucine
	Elevations in plasma lysine, phenylalanine, serine, tyrosine, and valine Skin desquamation, if prolonged
Leucine	Loss of appetite Weight loss or poor weight gain Decreased plasma leucine Increased plasma isoleucine, methionine, serine, threonine, and valine
Lysine	Weight loss or poor weight gain Impaired nitrogen balance
Methionine	Decreased plasma methionine Increased plasma phenylalanine, proline, serine, threonine, and tyrosine Decreased plasma cholesterol Poor weight gain Loss of appetite
Phenylalanine	Weight loss or poor weight gain Impaired nitrogen balance Aminoaciduria Decreased serum globulins Decreased plasma phenylalanine Mental retardation Anemia
Taurine	Impaired visual function Impaired biliary secretion
Threonine	Arrested weight gain Glossitis and reddening of the buccal mucosa Decreased plasma globulin Decreased plasma threonine
Tryptophan	Weight loss or no weight gain Impaired nitrogen retention Decreased plasma cholesterol
Tyrosine	Impaired nitrogen retention Catecholamine deficiency Thyroxine deficiency
Valine	Poor appetite, drowsiness Excess irritability and crying Weight loss or decrease in weight gain Decreased plasma albumin
Nitrogen	No or decreased weight gain Impaired nitrogen retention

Food	Amount	PHE (mg)	TYR (mg)	Protein (g)	Energy (kcal)
Phenex-1 powder	79 g	0	1185	11.9	379
Prophree powder[a]	6 g	0	0	0	30
Total		0	1185	11.9	409
Per kg body weight		0	348	3.5	120

Add water to make 620 mL (21 fl oz).
[a]510 kcal/100 g powder.

FIGURE 26.1 PKU Case Formula Calculation Example 1

After establishing a diagnosis of classical PKU, a prescription must be given for the nutrition management of the patient. For the neonate who weighs 3.4 kg and has an initial blood PHE concentration of 1600 μmol/L with a blood tyrosine (TYR) concentration of 50 μmol/L, the initial prescription may be as follows for the first 3 days:

PHE, mg $\quad 0 \times 3.4$ kg $= 0$ mg/day

TYR, mg $\quad 348 \times 3.4$ kg $= 1183$ mg/day

Protein, g $\quad 3.5 \times 3.4$ kg $= 11.9$ g/day

Energy, kcal 120×3.4 kg $= 408$ kcal/day

Plan the diet by first determining which medical food will be used (see **FIGURE 26.1**).

PHE must be added to the diet to prevent its deficiency as blood/plasma PHE concentration declines.

PHE, mg $\quad 35 \times 3.4$ kg $\; = 119$ mg/day

TYR, mg $\quad 304 \times 3.4$ kg $= 1034$ mg/day

Protein, g $\quad 3.5 \times 3.4$ kg $\; = 11.9$ g/day

Energy, kcal 120×3.4 kg $= 408$ kcal/day

First add whole protein infant formula to supply the required PHE. Similac Advance with Iron powder contains 465 mg PHE, 10.8 g protein, and 521 kcal per 100 g powder. To determine the amount of Similac powder to add, divide 119 g by the 465 mg PHE and multiply by 100; this yields 26 g. To determine the remaining protein to give as medical food, subtract the 2.8 g protein in 26 g Similac powder from 11.9 g to get 9.1 g. Phenex-1 contains 1500 mg TYR, 15 g protein, and 480 kcal per 100 g powder. Divide 9.1 g protein by 15.0 to get 60.6 g powder. Round to 61 g. Multiply 480 kcal per 100 g by 0.61 g to obtain 293 kcal. Remaining energy, if any is required, is determined by adding 135 kcal of Similac with 293 kcal of Phenex-1. This yields 428 kcal. No further energy is required. **FIGURE 26.2** shows the nutrient breakdown of this recipe.

Nutrition therapy of the patient with classical MSUD should be introduced with the first suspicion of disease in order to prevent severe illness. The 3.4 kg child should be offered a BCAA-free medical food for the first 2–3 days of therapy. **FIGURE 26.3** shows the nutrient breakdown of

Food	Amount	PHE (mg)	TYR (mg)	Protein (g)	Energy (kcal)
Similac Advance with Iron powder	26 g	121	117	2.8	135
Phenex-1 powder	61 g	0	915	9.1	293
Total		121	1032	11.9	422
Per kg body weight		36	304	3.5	124

Add water to yield 628 mL (21 fluid ounces).

FIGURE 26.2 PKU Case Formula Calculation Example 2

Food	Amount	Protein (g)	Energy (kcal)
Ketonex-1 powder	79 g	11.9	379
Prophree powder[a]	20 g	—	100
Total		11.9	478
Per kg body weight		3.5	140

Add water to yield 710 mL (24 oz).
a. 510 kcal/100 g powder

FIGURE 26.3 MSUD Case Formula Calculation Example 1

this recipe. A prescription that includes protein and at least 140 kcal/kg should be written:

$$\text{Protein, g} \quad 3.5 \times 3.4 \text{ kg} = 11.9 \text{ g}$$
$$\text{Energy, kcal} \quad 140 \times 3.4 \text{ kg} = 476 \text{ kcal}$$

The three BCAAs must be added to the diet to prevent deficiency, and ILE must be added on or before day four to prevent skin desquamation. The amount of LEU added at this time may be less than when the

plasma concentration has reached the treatment range. The amount of VAL added may be the full prescription depending on the plasma concentration.

$$\text{ILE, mg} \quad 60 \times 3.4 \text{ kg} = 204 \text{ mg}$$
$$\text{LEU, mg} \quad 75 \times 3.4 \text{ kg} = 255 \text{ mg}$$
$$\text{VAL, mg} \quad 70 \times 3.4 \text{ kg} = 238 \text{ mg}$$
$$\text{Protein, g} \quad 3.5 \times 3.4 \text{ kg} = 11.9 \text{ g}$$
$$\text{Energy, kcal} \quad 140 \times 3.4 \text{ kg} = 476 \text{ kcal}$$

Fill the LEU prescription with Similac Advance with Iron powder, which contains 575 mg ILE, 1080 mg LEU, and 640 mg VAL per 100 g powder.

All other patients with IEMs have nutrient requirements that may differ widely. Thus, the diet prescription must be individualized to support normal growth of each patient. **FIGURE 26.4** shows the nutrient breakdown of this recipe.

Protein requirements of infants and children with IEMs are normal if liver or renal function is not compromised. However, the form in which the protein is administered must be altered in order to restrict specific amino acids. Consequently, medical foods formulated from free amino acids must be used with small amounts of intact protein to provide amino acid and N requirements. Because N retention from free amino acid mixes differs from that of amino acids derived from intact protein as reviewed by Acosta[55], recommended protein intakes of infants and children with inborn errors of amino acid metabolism are 125–150%

Food	Amount	ILE (mg)	LEU (mg)	VAL (mg)	Protein (g)	Energy (kcal)
Similac Advance with Iron powder	24 g	138	259	154	2.6	125
Ketonex-1 powder	62 g	0	0	0	9.3	298
ILE solution[a]	6.6 mL	66	0	0	0	0
VAL solution[a]	8.4 mL	0	0	84	0	0
Prophree powder[b]	10 g	0	0	0	0	51
Total		204	259	238	11.9	474
Per kg body weight		60	76	70	3.5	140

[a] 10 mg/mL
[b] 510 kcal/100 g powder
Add water to make 650 mL (22 fl oz). As plasma LEU concentration decreases a greater amount of Similac may be added to help maintain plasma ILE, LEU, and VAL in the treatment range and to support normal growth.

FIGURE 26.4 MSUD Case Formula Calculation Example 2

greater than DRIs.[1] Other factors may also contribute to the need by patients with inherited amino acid disorders for greater protein intakes than recommended for normal persons, as reported by Loots et al.[56] Conjugation of PHE in the liver and later excretion in the urine of the compounds produced was reported by Moldave and Meister.[57] **TABLE 26.7** describes urinary loss of some of these conjugates, but plasma concentrations at which these losses occur are not provided, nor is their total daily loss given. Medical food and intact protein should be given four to six times daily to enhance nitrogen retention.[58–60] According to Arnold et al,[61] plasma transthyretin concentrations are positively correlated with linear growth, with concentrations of at least 200 mg/L resulting in the greatest height for age. Acosta and Yannicelli[62] found similar correlations in 2- to 13-year-old children with PKU. Yannicelli et al.[63] reported poor linear growth in children with methylmalonic or propionic acidemia who

failed to ingest adequate protein and energy. In fact, protein intake as recommended by Acosta leads to excellent growth with greater restricted amino acid tolerance than when RDA for protein is provided.

Fat intakes and the essential fatty acids, linoleic and α-linolenic, should meet RDAs,[1] except in mitochondrial fatty acid oxidation defects. Acosta et al.[72] found no essential fatty acid deficiency in patients with PKU undergoing nutrition therapy, except in those ingesting fat-free medical foods.

Energy intakes of infants and children with inborn errors of metabolism must be adequate to help support normal rates of growth. Provision of apparently adequate amino acids and N without sufficient energy will lead to growth failure. Pratt and associates[73] suggested that energy requirements are greater than normal when L-amino acids supply the protein equivalent. Maintaining adequate energy intake is essential for normal growth and development and to prevent catabolism.

TABLE 26.7 Urinary Loss of Some Conjugated Amino Acids by Patients with Various IEMs

Inborn Error	Amino Acid Conjugate
β-ketothiolase	β-methylglutaconic acid (ILE)
Branched-chain ketoaciduria (MSUD)	Acetylleucine (LEU), acetylisoleucine (ILE), acetylvaline (VAL), lactylleucine (LEU), lactyl-isoleucine (ILE), lactylvaline (VAL), β-hydroxy-isovaleryl conjugates of GLY, ILE, LEU, VAL
Isovaleric acidemia	Isovalerylalanine (LEU, ALA), isovalerylasparagine, (LEU, ASPNH$_2$), isovaleric-β-D-glucuronide (LEU), isovalerylglycine, isovalerylglutamic acid (LEU, GLY, GLU), isovalerylhistidine (LEU, HIS), isovaleryllysine (LEU, LYS), isovaleryltryptophan (LEU, TRP), β-hydroxy isovaleric acid (LEU), acetyltryptophan (TRP)
Methylmalonic acidemia	β-methylglutaconic acid (ILE)
Phenylketonuria	Phenylalanine (PHE), phenylacetylglutamine (PHE, GLUNH$_2$), phenyllactic acid (PHE), phenylpyruvic acid (PHE), acetylphenylalanine (PHE).
Propionic acidemia	β-methylglutaconic acid (ILE)
Tyrosinemia	Acetylphenylalanine (PHE), acetyltyrosine (TYR)

Abbreviations: ASPNH2, asparagine; GLU, glutamate; GLUNH2, glutamine; GLY, glycine; HIS, histidine; ILE, isoleucine; LEU, leucine; LYS, lysine; PHE, phenylalanine; TRP, tryptophan; TYR, tyrosine.

Data from Loots DT, Mienie LJ, Erasmus E. Amino-acid depletion induced by abnormal amino-acid conjugation and protein restriction in isovaleric acidemia. *Eur J Clin Nutr.* 2007;61:1323–1327.[56]

Dorland L, Duran M, Wadman SK, Niederwieser A, Bruinvis L, Ketting D. Isovaleryl-glucuronide, a new urinary metabolite in isovaleric acidemia. Identification problems due to rearrangement reactions. *Clin Chim Acta.*1983;134(1–2):77–83.[64]

Duran M, Bruinvis L, Ketting D, Karmerling JP, Wadman SK, Schutgens RB. The identification of (E)-2-methylglutaconic acid, a new isoleucine metabolite in the urine of patients with beta-ketothiolase deficiency, propionic acidaemia and methylmalonic acidaemia. *Biomed Mass Spectrom.*1982;9:1–5.[65]

Hagenfeldt L, Naglo AS. New conjugated urinary metabolites in intermediate type maple syrup urine disease. *Clin Chim Acta.* 1987;169:77–83.[66]

Jellum E, Horn L, Thoresen O, Krittingen EA, Stokke O. Urinary excretion of N-acetyl amino acids in patients with some inborn errors of amino acid metabolism. *Scand J Clin Lab Invest Suppl.* 1986;184:21–26.[67]

Lehnert W. N-isovalerylalanine and N-isovalerylsarcosine: two new minor metabolites in isovaleric acidemia. *Clin Chim Acta.* 1983;134(1–2):207–212.[68]

Lehnert W, Werle E. Elevated excretion of N-acetylated branched-chain amino acids in maple syrup urine disease. *Clin Chim Acta.* 1986;172:123–126.[69]

Loots DT, Erasmus E, Mienie LJ. Identification of 19 new metabolites by abnormal amino acid conjugation in isovaleric acidemia. *Clin Chem.* 2005;5:1510–1512.[70]

Woolf LI. Excretion of conjugated phenylacetic acid in phenylketonuria. *Biochem J.* 1951;49:ix–x.[71]

If RDA[1] for energy cannot be achieved through oral feeds, nasogastric, gastrostomy, or parenteral feeds must be employed. Mathematical formulas for calculating protein and energy requirements for the child with a metabolic disorder ingesting an elemental food with failure to thrive can be found in other sources.[11] Amino acid solutions designed for specific metabolic defects may be obtained from Apria Healthcare (http://apria.com/home/) if parenteral alimentation is required. Care must be taken to prevent overweight or obesity because weight loss results in elevated plasma amino acid concentrations. Fluid intake should be 1.5 mL/kcal for infants and 1.0 mL/kcal for children. Most adults will ingest adequate fluid.

Major, trace, and ultratrace mineral and vitamin intakes should exceed RDA for age.[1,74–77] If the medical food mixture fails to supply ≥ 100% of requirements for infants and children, appropriate supplements should be given. In patients with PKU, plasma phenylalanine concentrations > 480 μmol/L may lead to loss of bone matrix[62,63,75–77] in spite of adequate calcium, phosphorous, and vitamin D intakes. All organic acidemias, unless well controlled, will result in bone mineral loss.[78] Alexander et al.[37] reported poor absorption of a number of minerals when free amino acids were the primary protein source. Acosta and Yannicelli[62] and Pasquali et al.[77] reported increased bone collagen loss with age in children with PKU as plasma PHE increased, compared with normal children. Nutrient intakes of calcium, phosphorus, and vitamin D met or exceeded RDA for age, and concentrations of plasma calcium, phosphorus, and serum vitamin D were adequate.

▶ Urea Cycle Disorders

Eight enzyme defects have been reported in the urea cycle resulting in elevated concentrations of blood ammonia.[41,42] Four of the defects are suspected by elevated concentrations of blood **arginine** (ARG) or **citrulline** (CIT) on newborn screening (see Table 26.1). Consequently, differential diagnosis is essential for appropriate therapy.

The urea cycle normally contributes large amounts of ARG to the body ARG pool. When the urea cycle is nonfunctional, ARG becomes an essential amino acid.[2,41] Consequently, L-ARG must be administered in all disorders of the urea cycle except arginase deficiency. In **ornithine transcarbamylase** (OTC) deficiency, L-CIT may be given in place of or with L-ARG. When administered in adequate amounts, these amino acids also enhance waste N excretion.[42] L-ARG, when given orally, should be in the base form because the hydrochloride form will cause acidosis.

Protein restriction resulting in nitrogen restriction is the primary approach to preventing elevated blood ammonia in all except **citrin deficiency** (CIT II), which requires a high protein, low carbohydrate diet.[43] Citrin is an aspartate-glutamate carrier. Protein quality is determined by its essential amino acid content and completion of digestion. Protein synthesis and N utilization are more efficient when all amino acids are present in appropriate amounts at the same time. Severe restriction of intact protein leads to inadequate intake of several essential and conditionally essential amino acids, as well as minerals and vitamins. Because of this, medical foods consisting of essential and conditionally essential amino acids, minerals, and vitamins have been devised. Carnitine, cystine, taurine, and tyrosine may not be synthesized in adequate amounts when liver parenchymal cells are damaged. Thus, any medical food used for therapy of urea cycle disorders should contain carnitine, cystine, taurine, and tyrosine. Overrestriction of an essential amino acid or N leads to decreased protein synthesis or body protein catabolism and increased blood ammonia concentration. To provide adequate amounts of essential amino acids in the protein-restricted diet, from one-half to two-thirds of the protein prescription should be supplied by medical food,[38] as long as growth is proceeding. During the prepubertal growth spurt, greater amounts of protein may be required than previously needed. Maintenance of anabolism is essential to prevent hyperammonemia.

The protein quality of medical foods must be evaluated based on their amino acid, mineral, and vitamin content because intact protein sources, such as dairy products, meat, fish and other seafood, and poultry normally supply large amounts of minerals and vitamins. Intracellular minerals are important for protein synthesis. Medical foods devised for patients with urea cycle disorders must supply all minerals and vitamins not contributed by the small quantities of low-protein breads/cereals, fruits, fats, and vegetables the patient may ingest. Acosta et al.[44] reported that adequate intakes of protein and energy for 6 months in 17 patients resulted in a change in anthropometric z-scores of length from −1.2 to −0.8 ($p = 0.04$), a head circumference change from −1.0 to −0.68 ($p = 0.22$), and a weight change from −0.9 to −0.4 ($p = 0.01$). Plasma albumin concentration increased from 34 g/L at baseline to 38 g/L at 6 months. Mean protein intake in infants 0 < 6 months of age was 70% of **Food and Agriculture Organization** (FAO) recommendations and 62% in 6 < 12-month-old infants. Linear growth increased without an increase in plasma ammonia concentrations.

Because protein intake is severely restricted in urea cycle enzyme defects in all except CIT II, energy (kcal) intake should be increased to prevent use of muscle protein for energy purposes, thereby preventing catabolism of body protein. The best energy-to-protein ratio is unknown in these disorders; however, obesity should be avoided. Energy is the first requirement of the body, and inadequate energy intake for protein synthesis and other needs will lead to elevated blood ammonia concentration.[2]

Waste N excretion is enhanced through treatment with sodium benzoate, sodium phenylacetate, or sodium phenylbutyrate. Sodium benzoate is conjugated with glycine primarily in hepatic and renal cell mitochondria to form hippurate, which is cleared by the kidney.[57] Sodium phenylacetate conjugates with glutamine in kidney and liver cells to form phenylacetylglutamine, which is excreted by the kidney.[79,80] Phenylacetic acid conjugates with taurine in the kidney.[79] Glycine is readily made from serine. Tetrahydrofolate is required for this reaction to occur. Glycine also can be synthesized from glutamate. **Pyridoxal phosphate** (PLP) and an aldolase are required for this set of reactions. Because several coenzymes are required to maintain serine, **nicotinamide-adenine dinucleotide** (NAD), PLP, and glycine pools and the use of CoA in synthesis of hippurate, folate, pantothenate, pyridoxine, and niacin should be administered at greater than RDAs[1] for age when sodium benzoate is given therapeutically. Because dietary intake of potassium is often low and use of drugs to enhance waste N loss can lead to its urinary excretion, frequent monitoring of plasma potassium (K1) concentration is essential to maintain it within the normal range.[41] Daily supplements of KCl may be required because very low plasma K1 concentration can lead to death.

▶ Galactosemia

Galactosemias have been screened for in the United States for almost as long as PKU. Three forms of galactosemia have been reported: galactokinase deficiency, galactose-4-epimerase deficiency, and galactose-1-phosphate uridyl transferase (GALT)[21] deficiency.

Deletion of galactose in all forms of galactosemia must be accompanied by adequate intakes of protein, energy, minerals, and vitamins. Galactose binds with phosphate in patients with GALT deficiencies. This intracellular sequestering of phosphorus in combination with excess urinary phosphate loss (Fanconi syndrome) suggests the need for phosphorus intake greater than the RDA.[1] Inadequate calcium intake coupled with hypogonadism results in depressed bone mineral density in patients with galactosemia.[81,82] When GALT-deficient prepubertal patients were given 750 mg calcium, 1.0 mg vitamin K_1, and 10 mcg vitamin D_3 daily for 2 years, in addition to their galactose-restricted diet, a significant increase in bone mineral content of the spine occurred.[45]

Therapy of galactosemia due to GALT deficiency, although lifesaving in the infant, has resulted in less than optimum outcomes. Poor outcomes may be the result of small but significant intakes of naturally occurring galactose in fruits, vegetables, grains, legumes (dried beans and peas), and other foods.[46] On the other hand, in vivo synthesis of galactose[83,84] may be responsible for long-term complications in patients with gene mutations resulting in no enzyme activity. Defective tissue galactosylation of proteins, carbohydrates, and lipids, which is depressed by elevated concentrations of erythrocyte galactose-1-phosphate in the patient, may contribute.[85,86]

Infant formula powders made from soy protein isolate without added lactose contain significantly less galactose than do liquid soy protein isolate formulas, formulas for lactase deficiency, or formulas made from hydrolyzed casein, due to the added carrageenan.[21] Milk products, including all soft cheeses and some hard cheeses, and organ meats must be eliminated. Careful label reading for the presence of lactose, casein, or whey and examination of all drug ingredients should be practiced before suggesting the use of any food or drug.[21] Lactobionic acid, found in Neocalglucon, should not be used in patients with galactosemia due to the presence of galactose.[87]

Rates of decline in erythrocyte galactose-1-phosphate differ in infants with differing genotypes. Infants with a genotype of Q188R/Q188R, all receiving the same diet management, had an erythrocyte galactose-1-phosphate of 4.9 mg/dL at 5 to 8 months of age, and patients with a genotype of Q188R/other had a concentration of 3.3 mg/dL at the same age. Patients with a genotype of other/other had an erythrocyte galactose-1-phosphate of 2.5 mg/dL when in the same age range.[88] Using the breath test to measure galactose oxidation also indicates differences in utilization of galactose in patients by genotype.[89] Whether to eliminate more than milk from the diet of adults with GALT deficiency is not known, but is now being discussed by some medical geneticists.

▶ Inborn Errors of Fatty Acid Oxidation

Fatty acids are a primary fuel for the body when fasting is prolonged, and are a direct source of fuel for heart and skeletal muscle. Ketones such as acetoacetate and β-hydroxybutyric acid, obtained during hepatic fat metabolism, are an important energy source for the brain and other tissues.[90] Fat restriction in long-chain and very-long-chain fatty acid oxidation defects; replacement of most fat with MCT; addition of the docosahexaenoic acid precursor, α-linolenic acid, with the use of canola, soy, walnut, or flaxseed oils[13]; avoidance of fasting; glucose therapy as needed; and uncooked cornstarch have improved outcomes. Patients with a defect in medium- or short-chain fatty acid oxidation require avoidance of fasting and of MCT oil, the addition of glucose for hypoglycemia, and uncooked cornstarch as needed. The recommendation for fat is 30–35% of energy for children and adults.

Patients with VLCAD, LCHAD, TFP, or CPT 2 deficiency require about 10% of energy as long-chain fats and about 20% of energy as MCT. With this restriction of long-chain fats, absorption of fat-soluble vitamins, especially vitamin E, may prove difficult. Thus, supplementation with a water-miscible form of vitamin E should be considered if plasma α-tocopherol concentrations are below reference range when frequently analyzed. Ingested vitamins A and D should remain in normal ranges.[55] MCT mixed with juice given before exercise to patients with LCHAD, LCAD, or TFP lowered muscle pain and the incidence of rhabdomyolysis more than in patients given only juice.[13]

Genetic Metabolic Dietitians International has developed resources for helping to manage patients with VLCAD or MCAD deficiency. These nutrition guidelines are available at http://www.gmdi.org/Resources /NutritionGuidelines/VLCADGuidelines/ and http:// www.gmdi.org.

Protein intake at much greater than the DRIs may be beneficial in helping to control hypoglycemia and in preventing the obesity that occurs in patients fed high-carbohydrate diets. Patients with LCHAD or TFP deficiency fed 30% of energy as protein[13] had higher resting energy expenditure and lower energy intake while on the high protein diet than on a diet containing only 11% of energy as protein. Patients with medium- and short-chain

fatty acid oxidation defects may benefit with up to 20% of energy as protein to help control hypoglycemia.

Malonyl-CoA decarboxylase is present in high amounts in human heart and skeletal muscle, and the liver, kidney, and pancreas.[47,91] Malonyl-CoA decarboxylase deficiency results in variable clinical symptoms including hypoglycemia, hypotonia, cardiomyopathy, developmental delay, acidosis, seizures, and elevated urinary malonic acid.[92,93] Moderate long-chain fat restriction, MCT, and L-carnitine supplementation with frequent feedings appear to be beneficial.[93,94]

▶ Conclusion

Overall, inborn errors of metabolism are a very diverse group of disorders affecting amino acid, fat, and carbohydrate metabolism. Nutrition management for individuals with these disorders requires specialized knowledge of biochemical processes, the pathophysiology of organ systems, as well as the science and application of nutrition, growth, and development. These patients require individualized plans to meet the specific nutrient needs based on the genetic disorder while taking into consideration the biochemical factors. Nutrient requirements need to be adjusted to meet specialized needs in patients with IEMs.

Study Questions

1. How are the majority of inborn errors of metabolism identified?
2. What is the goal range for blood phenylalanine levels in patients with PKU?
3. Identify several metabolic formulas appropriate to use with a newly diagnosed infant with PKU.
4. What is the recommended treatment dose range for PKU patients taking Kuvan?
5. What amino acids are restricted with Maple Syrup Urine disease (MSUD)?
6. In most metabolic disorders are total energy needs increased?
7. In which group of metabolic disorders is the overall total protein/kg/day restricted?

References

1. Otten JJ, Hellwig JP, Meyers LD. *Dietary Reference Intakes: The Essential Guide to Nutrient Requirements.* Washington, DC: National Academies Press; 2006.
2. Elsas LJ, Acosta PB. Inherited metabolic disease: amino acids, organic acids, and galactose. In: Ross AC, Caballero B, Cousins RJ, Tucker KL, Ziegler TR eds. *Modern Nutrition in Health and Disease,* 11th ed. Philadelphia, PA: Lippincott Williams & Wilkins; 2012:909–959.
3. Goldblum OM, Brusilow SW, Maldonado YA, Farmer ER. Neonatal citrullinemia associated with cutaneous manifestations and arginine deficiency. *J Am Acad Dermatol.* 1986;14:321–326.
4. Borum PR, Bennett SG. Carnitine as an essential nutrient. *J Am Coll Nutr.* 1986;5:177–182.
5. Sansaricq C, Garg S, Norton PM, Phansalkar SV, Snyderman SE. Cystine deficiency during diet therapy of homocystinemia. *Acta Paediatr Scand.* 1975;64:215–218.
6. Laidlaw SA, Kopple JD. Newer concepts of the indispensable amino acids. *Am J Clin Nutr.* 1987;46:593–605.
7. Blau N, Thony B, Cotton RGH, Hyland K. Disorders of tetrahydrobiopterin and related biogenic amines. In: Scriver CR, Beaudet AL, Sly WS, Valle D, eds. *The Metabolic and Molecular Bases of Inherited Disease,* 8th ed. New York, NY: McGraw-Hill; 2001:1725–1776.
8. Acosta PB. Nutrition support for inborn errors. In: Samour PQ, King K, eds. *Handbook of Pediatric Nutrition,* 3rd ed. Boston, MA: Jones & Bartlett Publishers; 2005:239–286.

9. Frazier DM. Newborn screening by mass spectrometry. In: Acosta PB, ed. *Nutrition Management of Patients with Inherited Metabolic Disorders.* Sudbury, MA: Jones & Bartlett Publishers; 2010:21–65.

10. American College of Medical Genetics. Newborn screening: toward a uniform screening panel and system. *Genet Med.* 2006;8(suppl1):1S–252S.

11. Acosta PB. *Nutrition Management of Patients with Inherited Metabolic Disorders.* Sudbury, MA: Jones & Bartlett Publishers; 2010.

12. Chace DH, Lim T, Hansen CR, Adam BW, Hannon WH. Quantification of malonylcarnitine in dried blood spots by use of MS/MS varies by stable isotope internal standard composition. *Clin Chim Acta.* 2009;402(1–2):14–18.

13. Gillingham MB. Nutrition management of patients with inherited disorders of mitochondrial fatty acid oxidation. In: Acosta PB, ed. *Nutrition Management of Patients with Inherited Metabolic Disorders.* Sudbury, MA: Jones & Bartlett Publishers; 2010:369–403.

14. Korman SH. Inborn errors of isoleucine degradation. *Mol Genet Metab.* 2006;89:289–299.

15. Matalon KM. Introduction to genetics and genetics of inherited metabolic disorders. In: Acosta PB, ed. *Nutrition Management of Patients with Inherited Metabolic Disorders.* Sudbury, MA: Jones and Bartlett Publishers; 2010:1–19.

16. Miinalainen IJ, Schmitz W, Huotari A, et al. Mitochondrial 2, 4-dienoyl-CoA reductase deficiency in mice results in severe hypoglycemia with stress intolerance and unimpaired ketogenesis. *PLoS Genet.* 2009;5:e1000543.

17. Molven A, Matre GE, Duran M, et al. Familial hyperinsulinemia and hypoglycemia caused by a defect in the SCHAD enzyme of mitochondrial fatty acid oxidation. *Diabetes.* 2004;53:221–227.

18. Sim KG, Wiley V, Carpenter K, et al. Carnitine palmitoyltransferase I deficiency in neonate identified by dried blood spot free carnitine and acylcarnitine profile. *J Inherit Metab Dis.* 2001;24:51–59.

19. Acosta PB, Matalon KM. Nutrition management of patients with inherited disorders of aromatic amino acids. In: Acosta PB, ed. *Nutrition Management of Patients with Inherited Metabolic Disorders.* Sudbury, MA: Jones & Bartlett Publishers; 2010:119–174.

20. Marriage B. Nutrition management of patients with inherited disorders of branched-chain amino acid metabolism. In: Acosta PB, ed. *Nutrition Management of Patients with Inherited Metabolic Disorders.* Sudbury, MA: Jones & Bartlett Publishers; 2010:175–236.

21. Acosta PB. Nutrition management of patients with inherited disorders of galactose metabolism. In: Acosta PB, ed. *Nutrition Management of Patients with Inherited Metabolic Disorders.* Sudbury, MA: Jones & Bartlett Publishers; 2010:343–367.

22. van Calcar S. Nutrition management of patients with inherited disorders of sulfur amino acid metabolism. In: Acosta PB, ed. *Nutrition Management of Patients with Inherited Metabolic Disorders.* Sudbury, MA: Jones & Bartlett Publishers; 2010:237–281.

23. Yannicelli S. Nutrition management of patients with inherited disorders of organic acid metabolism. In: Acosta PB, ed. *Nutrition Management of Patients with Inherited Metabolic Disorders.* Sudbury, MA: Jones & Bartlett Publishers; 2010:283–341.

24. Blau N, Koch R, Matalon R, Stevens RC. Five years of synergistic scientific effort on phenylketonuria therapeutic development and molecular understanding. *Mol Genet Metab.* 2005;86:S1.

25. Rosenblatt DS, Fenton W. Inherited disorders of folate and cobalamin transport and metabolism. In: Scriver CR, Beaudet AL, Sly WS, Valle D, eds. *The Metabolic and Molecular Bases of Inherited Disease,* 8th ed. New York, NY: McGraw-Hill; 2001:3897–3934.

26. Bonkowsky HL, Magnussen CR, Collins AR, Doherty JM, Hess RA, Tschudy DP. Comparative effects of glycerol and dextrose on porphyrin precursor excretion in acute intermittent porphyria. *Metabolism.* 1976;25:405–414.

27. Langenbeck U, Burgard P, Wendel U, Lindner M, Zschocke J. Metabolic phenotypes of phenylketonuria. Kinetic and molecular evaluation of the Blaskovics protein loading test. *J Inherit Metab Dis.* 2009;32:506–513.

28. Blaskovics ME, Schaeffler GE, Hack S. Phenylalaninaemia. Differential diagnosis. *Arch Dis Child.* 1974;49:835–843.

29. Blaskovics ME. Diagnostic considerations in phenylalaninemic subjects before and after dietary therapy. *Ir Med J.* 1976;69:410–414.

30. Bremer JH. Transitory hyperphenylalaninemia. In: Bickel H, Hudson FP, Woolf LI, eds. *Phenylketonuria and Some Other Inborn Errors of Amino Acid Metabolism.* Stuttgart: Georg Thieme Verlag; 1971:93–97.

31. Gjetting T, Petersen M, Guldberg P, Guttler F. Missense mutations in the N-terminal domain of human phenylalanine hy-droxylase interfere with binding of regulatory phenylalanine. *Am J Hum Genet.* 2001;68:1353–1360.

32. Wolf B. Disorders of biotin metabolism. In: Scriver CR, Beaudet AL, Sly WS, Valle D, eds. *The Metabolic and Molecular Bases of Inherited Disease,* 8th ed. New York, NY: McGraw-Hill; 2001:3935–3962.

33. Sarkissian CN, Gamez A, Wang L, et al. Preclinical evaluation of multiple species of PEGylated recombinant phenylalanine ammonia lyase for the treatment of phenylketonuria. *Proc Natl Acad Sci U S A.* 2008;105:20894–20899.

34. Zinnanti WJ, Lazovic J, Griffin K, et al. Dual mechanism of brain injury and novel treatment strategy in maple syrup urine disease. *Brain.* 2009;132:903–918.

35. Matalon R, Michals-Matalon K, Bhatia G, et al. Double blind placebo control trial of large neutral amino acids in treatment of PKU: effect on blood phenylalanine. *J Inherit Metab Dis.* 2007;30:153–158.

36. Rudman D, Feller A. Evidence for deficiencies of conditionally essential nutrients during total parenteral nutrition. *J Am Coll Nutr.* 1986;5:101–106.

37. Alexander JW, Clayton BE, Delves HT. Mineral and trace-metal balances in children receiving normal and synthetic diets. *Q J Med.* 1974;169:80–111.

38. Acosta PB, Yannicelli S. *Nutrition Support Protocols,* 4th ed. Columbus, OH: Ross Products Division, Abbott Laboratories; 2001.

39. Guttler F, Olesen ES, Wamberg E. Diurnal variations of serum phenylalanine in phenylketonuric children on low phenylalanine diet. *Am J Clin Nutr.* 1969;22:1568–1570.

40. Gropper SS, Acosta PB. Effect of simultaneous ingestion of L-amino acids and whole protein on plasma amino acid and urea nitrogen concentrations in humans. *J Parenter Enteral Nutr.* 1991;15:48–53.

41. Singh RH. Nutritional management of patients with urea cycle disorders. *J Inherit Metab Dis.* 2007;30:880–887.

42. Brusilow S, Horwich A. Urea cycle enzymes. In: Scriver CR, Beaudet AL, Sly WS, Valle D, eds. *The Metabolic and Molecular Bases of Inherited Disease,* 8th ed. New York, NY: McGraw-Hill; 2001:1909–1963.

43. Dimmock D, Kobayashi K, Iijima M, et al. Citrin deficiency: a novel cause of failure to thrive that responds to a high-protein, low-carbohydrate diet. *Pediatr.* 2007;119:e773–e777.

44. Acosta PB, Yannicelli S, Ryan AS, et al. Nutritional therapy improves growth and protein status of children with a urea cycle enzyme defect. *Mol Genet Metab.* 2005;86: 448–455.

45. Panis B, Vermeer C, van Kroonenburgh MJ, et al. Effect of calcium, vitamins K_1 and D_3 on bone in galactosemia. *Bone.* 2006;39:1123–1129.

46. Acosta PB, Gross KC. Hidden sources of galactose in the environment. *Eur J Pediatr.* 1995;154:S87–S92.

47. Sacksteder KA, Morrell JC, Wanders RJ, Matalon R, Gould SJ. MCD encodes peroxisomal and cytoplasmic forms of malonyl-CoA decarboxylase and is mutated in malonyl-CoA decarboxylase deficiency. *J Biol Chem.* 1999;274:24461–24468.

48. Anderson HC, Marble M, Shapiro E. Long-term outcome in treated combined methylmalonic acidemia and homocystinuria. *Genet Med.* 1999;1:146–150.

49. Carrillo-Carrasco J, Sloan J, Valle D, Hamosh A, Venditti CP. Hydroxocobalimin dose escalation improves metabolic control in cblC. *J Inherit Metab Dis.* 2009;52:728–731.

50. Huemer M, Simma B, Fowler B, Suormala T, Bodamer OA, Sass JO. Prenatal and postnatal treatment in cobalamin C defect. *J Pediatr.* 2005;147:469–472.

51. Urbon Artero A, Aldona Gomez J, Reig Del Moral C, Nieto Conde C, Merinero Cortes B. Neonatal onset methylmalonic aciduria and clinical improvement with betaine therapy. *An Esp Pediatr.* 2002;56:337–341.

52. Singh RH. Nutrition management of patients with inherited disorders of urea cycle enzymes. In: Acosta PB, ed. *Nutrition Management of Patients with Inherited Metabolic Disorders.* Sudbury, MA: Jones and Bartlett Publishers; 2010:405–429.

53. Smith DL, Bodamer OA. Practical management of combined methylmalonic aciduria and homocystinuria. *J Child Neurol.* 2002;17:353–356.

54. Spiekerkoetter U, Lindner M, Santer R, et al. Treatment recommendations in long-chain fatty acid oxidation defects: consensus from a workshop. *J Inherit Metab Dis.* 2009;32:498–505.

55. Acosta PB. Evaluation of nutrition status. In: Acosta PB, ed. *Nutrition Management of Patients with Inherited Metabolic Disorders.* Sudbury, MA: Jones & Bartlett Publishers; 2010:67–98.

56. Loots DT, Mienie LJ, Erasmus E. Amino-acid depletion induced by abnormal amino-acid conjugation and protein restriction in isovaleric acidemia. *Eur J Clin Nutr.* 2007;61:1323–1327.

57. Moldave K, Meister A. Synthesis of phenylacetylglutamine by human tissue. *J Biol Chem.* 1957;229:463–476.

58. Dangin M, Boirie Y, Garcia-Rodenas C, et al. The digestion rate of protein is an independent regulating factor of postprandial protein retention. *Am J Physiol Endocrinol Metab.* 2001;280:E340–E348.

59. Herrmann ME, Brosicke HG, Keller M, Monch E, Helge H. Dependence of the utilization of a phenylalanine-free amino acid mixture on different amounts of single dose ingested. A case report. *Eur J Pediatr.* 1994;153:501–503.

60. Schoeffer A, Herrmann ME, Brosicke HG, Moench E. Effect of dosage and timing of amino acid mixtures on nitrogen retention in patients with phenylketonuria. *J Nutr Med.* 1994;4:415–418.

61. Arnold GL, Vladutiu CJ, Kirby RS, Blakely EM, Deluca JM. Protein insufficiency and linear growth restriction in phenylketonuria. *J Pediatr.* 2002;141:243–246.

62. Acosta PB, Yannicelli S. Nutrient intake and biochemical status of children with phenylketonuria undergoing nutrition management. Unpublished data. Columbus, OH: Ross Products Division, Abbott Laboratories; 2003.

63. Yannicelli S, Acosta PB, Velazquez A, et al. Improved growth and nutrition status in children with methylmalonic or propionic acidemia fed an elemental medical food. *Mol Genet Metab.* 2003;80:181–188.

64. Dorland L, Duran M, Wadman SK, Niederwieser A, Bruinvis L, Ketting D. Isovaleryl-glucuronide, a new urinary metabolite in isovaleric acidemia. Identification problems due to rearrangement reactions. *Clin Chim Acta.* 1983;134(1–2):77–83.

65. Duran M, Bruinvis L, Ketting D, Karmerling JP, Wadman SK, Schutgens RB. The identification of (E)-2-methylglutaconic acid, a new isoleucine metabolite in the urine of patients with beta-ketothiolase deficiency, propionic acidaemia and methylmalonic acidaemia. *Biomed Mass Spectrom.* 1982;9:1–5.

66. Hagenfeldt L, Naglo AS. New conjugated urinary metabolites in intermediate type maple syrup urine disease. *Clin Chim Acta.* 1987;169:77–83.

67. Jellum E, Horn L, Thoresen O, Krittingen EA, Stokke O. Urinary excretion of N-acetyl amino acids in patients with some inborn errors of amino acid metabolism. *Scand J Clin Lab Invest Suppl.* 1986;184:21–26.

68. Lehnert W. N-isovalerylalanine and N-isovalerylsarcosine: two new minor metabolites in isovaleric acidemia. *Clin Chim Acta.* 1983;134(1–2):207–212.

69. Lehnert W, Werle E. Elevated excretion of N-acetylated branched-chain amino acids in maple syrup urine disease. *Clin Chim Acta.* 1986;172:123–126.

70. Loots DT, Erasmus E, Mienie LJ. Identification of 19 new metabolites by abnormal amino acid conjugation in isovaleric acidemia. *Clin Chem.* 2005;5:1510–1512.

71. Woolf LI. Excretion of conjugated phenylacetic acid in phenylketonuria. *Biochem J.* 1951;49:ix–x.

72. Acosta PB, Yannicelli S, Singh R, et al. Intake and blood levels of fatty acids in treated patients with phenylketonuria. *J Pediatr Gastroenterol Nutr.* 2001;33:253–259.

73. Pratt EL, Snyderman SE, Cheung MW, et al. The threonine requirement of the normal infant. *J Nutr.* 1955;56:231–251.

74. Acosta PB, Yannicelli S, Singh RH, Elsas LJ, Mofidi S, Steiner RD. Iron status of children with phenylketonuria undergoing nutrition therapy assessed by transferrin receptors. *Genet Med.* 2004;6:96–101.

75. Yannicelli S, Medeiros DM. Elevated plasma phenylalanine concentrations may adversely affect bone status of phenylketonuric mice. *J Inherit Metab Dis.* 2002;25: 347–361.

76. Acosta PB, Yannicelli S. Plasma micronutrient concentrations in infants undergoing therapy for phenylketonuria. *Biol Trace Elem Res.* 1999;67:75–84.

77. Pasquali M, Singh R, Kennedy MJ, et al. Pyridinium cross-links: a parameter of bone matrix turnover in phenylketonuria. *Book of Abstracts*, 5th Meeting of the International Society for Neonatal Screening, June 26–29, 2002. Genoa, Italy.

78. Bushinsky DA. Acid-base imbalance and the skeleton. *Eur J Nutr*. 2001;40:238–244.

79. Ambrose AM, Powder FW, Sherwin CP. Further studies on the detoxification of phenylacetic acid. *J Biol Chem*. 1933;101:669–675.

80. James MO, Smith RL, Williams RT, Reidenberg M. The conjugation of phenylacetic acid in man, sub-human primates and some non-primate species. *Proc R Soc Lond B Biol Sci*. 1972;182:25–35.

81. Kaufman FR, Loro ML, Azen C, Wenz E, Gilsanz V. Effect of hypogonadism and deficient calcium intake on bone density in patients with galactosemia. *J Pediatr*. 1993;123:365–370.

82. Rubio-Gozalbo ME, Hamming S, van Kroonenburgh MJ, Bakker JA, Vermeer C, Forget PP. Bone mineral density in patients with classic galactosaemia. *Arch Dis Child*. 2002;87:57–60.

83. Berry GT, Moate PJ, Reynolds RA, et al. The rate of de novo galactose synthesis in patients with galactose-1-phosphate uridyltransferase deficiency. *Mol Genet Metab*. 2004;81:22–30.

84. Schadewaldt P, Kamalanathan L, Hammen HW, Wendel U. Age dependence of endogenous galactose formation in Q188R homozygous galactosemic patients. *Mol Genet Metab*. 2004;81:31–44.

85. Charlwood J, Clayton P, Keir G, Mian N, Winchester B. Defective galactosylation of serum transferrin in galactosemia. *Glycobiology*. 1998;8:351–357.

86. Lai K, Langley SD, Khwaja FW, Schmitt EW, Elsas LJ. GALT deficiency causes UDP-hexose deficit in human galactosemic cells. *Glycobiology*. 2003;13:285–294.

87. Harju M. Lactobionic acid as a substrate of β-galactosidases. *Milchwissenschaft*. 1990;45:411–415.

88. Singh RH, Kennedy MJ, Jonas CR, Dembure P, Elsas LJ. Whole body oxidation and galactosemia genotype: prognosis for galactose tolerance in the first year of life. *J Inherit Metab Dis*. 2003;26:123A.

89. Berry GT, Singh RH, Mazur AT, et al. Galactose breath testing distinguishes variant and severe galactose-1-phosphate uridyltransferase genotypes. *Pediatr Res*. 2000;48:323–328.

90. Roe CR, Ding J. Mitochondrial fatty acid oxidation disorders. In: Scriver CR, Beaudet AL, Sly WS, Valle D, eds. *The Metabolic and Molecular Bases of Inherited Disease*, 8th ed. New York, NY: McGraw-Hill; 2001:2297–2326.

91. Saggerson D. Malonyl-CoA, a key signaling molecule in mammalian cells. *Annu Rev Nutr*. 2008;28:253–272.

92. Ficicioglu C, Chrisant MR, Payan I, Chace DH. Cardiomyopathy and hypotonia in a 5-month-old infant with malonyl-CoA decarboxylase deficiency: potential for preclinical diagnosis with expanded newborn screening. *Pediatr Cardiol*. 2005;26:881–883.

93. Salomons GS, Jakobs C, Pope LL, et al. Clinical, enzymatic and molecular characterization of nine new patients with malonyl-coenzyme A decarboxylase deficiency. *J Inherit Metab Dis*. 2007;30:23–28.

94. Yano S, Sweetman L, Thorburn DR, Mofidi S, Williams JC. A new case of malonyl coenzyme A decarboxylase deficiency presenting with cardiomyopathy. *Eur J Pediatr*. 1997;156:382–383.

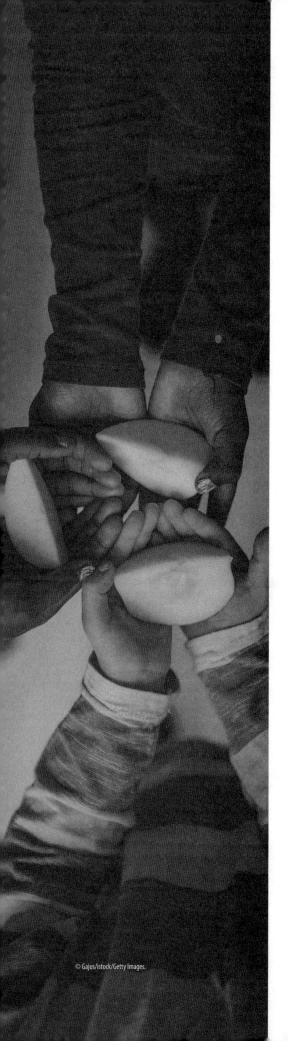

SECTION VII
Emerging Practice

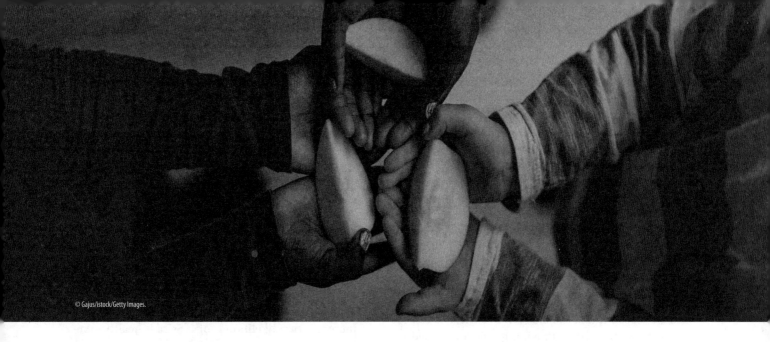

© Gajus/istock/Getty Images.

CHAPTER 27

Measuring Outcomes

Susan L. Goolsby and Susan Konek

LEARNING OBJECTIVES

- Describe the advances in quality in healthcare and more specifically in dietetics.
- Define outcomes related to quality improvement in healthcare and dietetics.
- Identify terms, tools, and resources for conducting quality improvement research.
- Develop quality improvement research in one's own dietetic healthcare setting.

▶ Introduction

The history of quality improvement in healthcare dates back as early as the 19th century when obstetrician, Ignaz Semmelweis, promoted hand washing as a way to decrease the rate of infection. In the early 1900's, Ernest Codman, a surgeon, was one of the first to propose the theory of outcomes research which he termed the "End Result" system. The idea was simple, "that *every* hospital should follow *every* patient it treats, long enough to determine whether or not the treatment has been successful, and then to inquire, 'If not, why not?' with a view to preventing similar failures in the future".[1] In modern medicine, specifically in the last fifty years some of the **quality improvement** (QI) movements have included studies that examined processes in healthcare that could be improved for better patient outcomes.

The National Academy of Medicine, formerly known as the Institute of Medicine (IOM), defines quality as "the degree to which health services for individuals and populations increase the likelihood of desired health outcomes and are consistent with current professional knowledge."[2] In 2010, the Patient Protection and Affordable Care Act mandated that evidence-based practice guidelines become an integral component of the national health care quality strategy with the goal of providing affordable care that leads to healthier communities. Evidence-based practice guidelines are essential for delivering quality care that is safe, effective, efficient, personalized, timely, and equitable.[3] The **World Health Organization** (WHO) defines an outcome measure as a "change in the health of an individual, group of people, or population that is attributable to an intervention or series of interventions."

http://www.who.int/healthpromotion/about/HPR%20 Glossary%201998.pdf.[4] The **Institute for Healthcare Improvement** (IHI) has stated the goal of measuring outcomes is to 1) improve the patient experience of care, 2) improve the health of populations and 3) reduce the cost of healthcare (the Triple Aim of healthcare). Healthcare organizations are trying to achieve the Triple Aim measure outcomes to determine the interventions that could improve care, identify variations of care, and to obtain evidence about interventions that work best for different types of patients and their circumstances.[5] Quality can be improved without measuring outcomes but *change* cannot be proven to improve outcomes if they are not measured. Likewise, QI strategies, just like medical interventions, need to rest on a strong evidence base. Providing evidence-based practice requires the study of outcomes.

"The **Academy of Nutrition and Dietetics** (Academy), the leading professional organization for **registered dietitian nutritionists** (RDNs) and **registered diet technicians** (DTRs), leads the way for Quality Management and Improvement in food and nutrition."[6] In the last fifteen years, several advancements have been made by the Academy starting with the development of the **Nutrition Care Process** (NCP), a standardized care process and language specific to the dietetics profession. In 2014, the Quality Management Committee of the Academy developed four Standards of Excellence in Nutrition and Dietetics for Organization Self-Assessment and Quality Improvement: Quality of Leadership, Quality of Organization, Quality of Practice and Quality of Outcomes. The Standards of Excellence is a self-assessment and quality improvement tool for the organization to demonstrate RDN contributions to quality patient care and provide outcomes to leadership. A critical aspect of healthcare QI is that it is the responsibility of the entire organization. Every person is responsible for continually examining the processes in their environment and striving to improve the processes hence the term "continuous process improvement, aka QI. RDNs can demonstrate their value to their institution and their field by becoming actively involved in QI and making evidence-based decisions in their professional practice. For the most part, Academy tools discussed in this chapter are available for non-members, including students, on the Academy website at www.eatright.org.

This chapter will provide the nutrition clinician an overview of the large topic of outcomes measurement as a means to improve the care of patients and clients in the pediatric setting.

Although not specific for pediatric nutrition, all models and tools described are appropriate to pediatric nutrition improvement in all practice settings.

▶ Quality Terms Defined

Food and Nutrition Practitioners are increasingly engaging in quality improvement throughout their practice settings. Many are implementing quality measures in their facilities and/or conducting quality improvement and performance measurement activities. The Academy definitions and resources, described below, provide insight into QI for all practice segments of food, nutrition, and dietetics including: health care, education and research, business and industry, and community nutrition, and public health:

- **Quality healthcare** is the degree to which health services for individuals and populations increase the likelihood of desired health outcomes and are consistent with current professional knowledge.[7]
- **Quality Improvement (QI)** consists of systematic and continuous actions that lead to measurable improvement in services and/or the status of targeted individuals or groups.[8]
- **Quality Management** is a systematic process with identified leadership, accountability and dedicated resources for the purpose of meeting or exceeding established professional standards. The Academy monitors the quality of nutrition services and provides guidelines for safe, effective, patient-focused care.
- **Project Scope** should be the dimensions for which the project will cover. As a general rule, scope should start small and cover an area within the control of the work group.
- **Outcomes Measurement** is the single measurement, generally higher level that will inform the success of the current state or process.
- **Process Measurements** are the 2 to 4 subprocesses which feed into and drive the outcomes measurement.

A complete list of quality related terms and their definitions can be accessed at the Academy website at http://www.eatrightpro.org/~/media/eatrightpro%.[9]

▶ Nutrition Practice Quality Improvement Approaches and Models

This section will provide a brief look at quality resources, models and tools that can be used by food and nutrition professionals in the development of their outcomes measurement programs.

The National Academy of Medicine has played a major role in guiding healthcare organizations in their efforts to improve safety. In 1999, the IOM in Washington, DC, USA, released *To Err Is Human: Building a Safer Health System*, a descriptive report of the patient safety crisis in the United States. In 2001, IOM followed up with *Crossing the Quality Chasm: A New Health System for the 21st Century*, which was a detailed look at the huge divide between good health care and the health care that people actually receive. The report pointed to the need for tremendous change in order to "cross the chasm" and provide safer healthcare for all.

The *6 Aims of Improving Health Care Quality* is a look at the other side of the chasm, one that provides clear direction on the components of these goals. **TABLE 27.1**

TABLE 27.1 6 Aims of Improving Health Care Quality: Application Examples

Aim	Description	Application Examples
Safe	Avoid injuries to patients from the care that is intended to help them.	■ Patients receive the same care on the weekend as they do during the week. ■ Patients are visited and assessed face-to-face. ■ RDNs follow Nutrition Care Process and deliver evidence-based nutritional care. ■ Use proper handwashing techniques ■ Make care seamless when transferring a patient from one staff member to the next ■ RDN Order writing privileges to decrease mistakes of incorrect formulas ordered by physicians
Timely	Reduce waits for both the recipients and providers of care.	■ Staffing is appropriate to ensure patients are assessed and monitored for best outcomes. ■ Round with the medical team and utilize a mobile computer to document nutritional findings/decisions in the electronic medical record. ■ RDN order writing privileges to decrease time patient waits for diet/formula orders to be implemented.
Efficient	Avoid waste, including waste of equipment, supplies, ideas, and energy.	■ Apply standards of care consistently, with no variation in the process. ■ Develop time saving tools (quick links to spreadsheets that calculate energy needs or z-scores, for example)
Effective	Provide care based on scientific knowledge to all those who could benefit and refrain from providing care to those not likely to benefit (avoid overuse, underuse, and misuse).	■ Provide evidence-based nutrition interventions to all who can benefit, utilizing the tools provided (Nutrition Care Manual, Evidence-Analysis Library (EAL))
Equitable	Provide care that does not vary in quality because of personal characteristics such as gender, ethnicity, geographic location, and socioeconomic status.	■ Become educated on the value of differences to achieve cultural competence.
Patient-centered	Provide care that is respectful of and responsive to individual patient preferences, needs, and values and ensure that patient values guide all clinical decisions.	■ Study patient outcomes ■ Lead the development and implementation of strategies for improving care of patients at the bedside

Modified from Hakel-Smith, N. Quality management and improvement. In: J.A. Grim and S.R. Roberts, eds. *The Clinical Nutrition Manager's Handbook*. Chicago, IL: Cathy Iammartino;2014:91–114.[10]

lists a description and examples of each of the Aims for improving health care quality.

Evidence-based practice is an approach to health care wherein health practitioners use the best evidence possible, i.e., the most appropriate information available, to make decisions for individuals, groups, and populations. Evidence-based practice incorporates successful strategies that improve client outcomes and are derived from various sources of evidence including research, national guidelines, policies, consensus statements, systematic analysis of clinical experience, quality improvement data, specialized knowledge and the skills of experts.

If a particular area of pediatric nutrition is not supported by strong evidence, the solution is to initiate practice based research and measure outcomes. **Practice-based Research** is an original investigation undertaken in order to gain new knowledge partly by means of practice and the outcomes of that practice.

Quality Improvement Models

There are many different models for improvement that can be utilized in the healthcare setting, including:

1. The Model for Improvement
2. FOCUS-PDCA
3. Six-Sigma DMAIC
4. Six-Sigma DFSS
5. Seven-Step problem-solving
6. Lean Improvement.

These improvement models are frequently used in the healthcare setting; others can be found by searching the literature. Even more numerous are the tools that can be used in each model. Organizational leaders have found that within an organization, it is important to use a common method for conducting all quality improvement projects. For the sake of space and simplicity, this chapter will describe the models commonly utilized in healthcare.

The Model for Improvement

The model for improvement is based on three important questions:

1. What are we trying to improve?
2. How will we know if the change we make is an improvement?
3. What change can we make that will result in an improvement?

These questions drive the improvement and the Plan-Do-Study-Act (PDSA) cycle which is a powerful vehicle for testing, learning, implementing, and disseminating change. PDSA cycles can help a team plan for, carry out, and learn from small tests of change. Starting

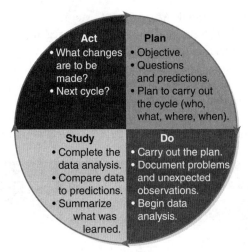

Langley GL, Moen R, Nolan KM, Nolan TW, Norman CL, Provost LP. *The Improvement Guide: A Practical Approach to Enhancing Organizational Performance.* 2nd ed. San Francisco, CA: Jossey-Bass Publishers;2009.[11]

FIGURE 27.1 PDSA Cycle

small and using the PDSA model helps minimize and mitigate common risks associated with problematic or failed implementation of changes.[11]

FIGURE 27.1 illustrates the iterative process of the PDSA framework.

FOCUS-PDCA

FOCUS-PDCA is a variation of The Model for Improvement. This model is designed for both process improvement and problem solving. The name is derived from the steps of the model:

1. **F**ind a process to improve
2. **O**rganize a team that knows the process
3. **C**larify the current process
4. **U**nderstand the causes of process variation
5. **S**elect the process improvement
6. **P**lan improvement, data collection
7. **D**o improvement, data collection, data analysis
8. **C**heck data for process improvement, customer outcome, lessons learned
9. **A**ct to hold the change

Six-Sigma DMAIC and DFSS

Six-Sigma methodology was developed in the late 1980s by Motorola as a **Total Quality Management** (TQM) program to reduce variation: https://www.sixsigmaonline.org/.[12] *DMAIC* (define-measure-analyze-improve-control) is a basic framework of the Six Sigma methodology. Definitions of the five steps are:

1. **Define** process improvement goals
2. **Measure** the current process to develop baseline data
3. **Analyze** to verify cause and effect of relevant factors

4. Improve the process and transition to standard processes
5. Control to ensure that any variances are corrected before they result in defects

DFSS stands for "Design for Six Sigma" and there are many variations on these five to six step approaches. The version chosen to use depends on the process that is being measured.

- DMADV: Define, Measure, Analyze, Design, Verify
- DMCDOV: Define, Measure, Characterize, Design, Optimize, Verify
- DMEDI: Define, Measure, Explore, Develop, Implements

Seven-Step Problem-Solving Process

The Seven-Step Problem-Solving Process morphed from Toyota's "Practical Problem-Solving Process" This model provides a structured basis to help deliver outcomes and solutions to the problem. The steps include:

1. Define project purpose and scope
2. Define the current situation
3. Cause Analysis
4. Solutions
5. Results
6. Standardization
7. Future plans

Lean Improvement

The Lean approach is adapted from **Toyota's Production System** (TPS) and focuses on continuously reducing waste in operations, products, and services. Running a Lean organization means more value is created for patients or clients with fewer resources. The characteristics of a lean organization and supply chain are described in *Lean Thinking*, by Womack and Jones. They recommend that a leader who is beginning a project to transform their department or organization to a lean one should think about three issues to help guide the change:

- **Purpose**: What customer (patient/client) problems will the leader solve to achieve his own purpose of prospering/succeeding?
- **Process**: How will the leader assess each major process to make sure each step is valuable, capable, available, adequate, and flexible?
- **People**: How can the leader ensure that every important process has someone responsible for continually evaluating it in terms of business purpose and lean process? How can every person involved in the process be actively engaged in completing it correctly and continually improving it?[13]

Quality Improvement Tools
Team Charter

Change is never easy and as the scope of an improvement effort expands, the team should have a written aim that answers the question, "What are we trying to accomplish?" The team charter is a document that is developed together by the work group; it clarifies team direction while establishing boundaries. It is created early, during the formation of the team.

The team charter has two purposes. First, it serves as a source for the team members to illustrate the focus and direction of the team. Second, it educates others (for example, the organizational leaders and other work groups), on the direction of the team. More can be found on developing a team charter with an example of a charter at this link: www.teamlti.com/charter/page0/files/Charter6.pdf.[14]

Diagrams

An important strategy for improving a process is to understand how the current process works. Diagrams are a good way to chart the existing process and brainstorm how a new process might fit into the organization.

The ***Fishbone Diagram (Cause & Effect)*** tool can be used to map the process and brainstorm factors that could change in order to produce a better outcome (see **FIGURE 27.2**). This diagram is used to collect and organize current knowledge about potential causes of problems or variation. The tool is useful in PDSA Cycle for developing changes for discovering, organizing, and summarizing a group's knowledge about causes contributing to a problem.[11]

A ***Driver Diagram*** is another approach to describing theories of improvement (see **FIGURE 27.3**). It is a tool to help organize theories and ideas when asking, "What change can we make that will result in improvement?" The initial driver diagram lays out the descriptive theory of improved outcomes that can be tested. The diagram should be updated throughout an improvement project as progress is made and theories are tested.[11]

Interrelationship diagrams show cause-and-effect relationships, and help analyze the natural links between different aspects of a complex situation (see **FIGURE 27.4**).

"An interrelationship diagram:

- Encourages team members to think in multiple directions rather than linearly
- Explores the cause and effect relationships among all the issues, including the most controversial
- Allows key issues to emerge naturally rather than to be forced by a dominant or powerful team member
- Systematically surfaces the basic assumptions and reasons for disagreements among team members
- Allows a team to identify root cause(s) even when credible data does not exist"[16]

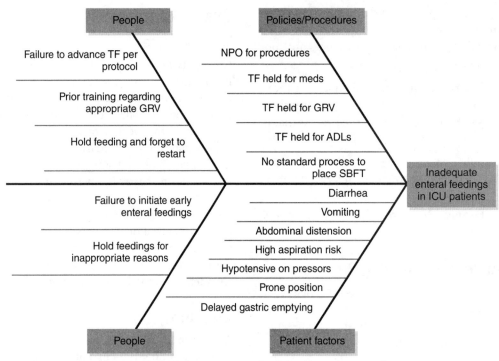

Data from Hakel-Smith, N. Quality management and improvement. In: J.A. Grim and S.R. Roberts, eds. *The Clinical Nutrition Manager's Handbook*. Chicago, IL: Cathy Iammartino;2014:91–114.[10] Roberts S, Grim J. Cause and effect diagram. In: *ICU Enteral Feedings*. ABC Baylor Quality Improvement Presentation. Baylor Health Care System; 2009.[15]

FIGURE 27.2 Fishbone Diagram

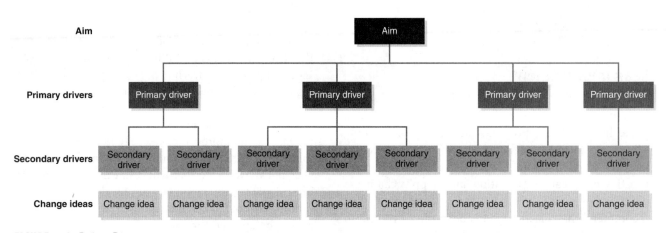

FIGURE 27.3 Driver Diagram

▶ Academy and Commission on Dietetics Registration (CDR) Resources for Completing QI/Outcomes Research

An important member benefit of the Academy of Nutrition and Dietetics is access to position and practice papers, the Nutrition Care Manual, continuing education, networking and list serves, and the Evidence Analysis Library. When a member of the Academy has a practice-based question, they can start the search with the Academy website to determine if there is a ready answer to the question and determine the strength of the evidence to support that answer.

Compiled resources from Academy of Nutrition and Dietetics and Commission on Dietetic Registration

▶ Key Points about Outcomes Research

Outcomes research is an investigation that measures the result of an intervention provided to a patient, client or community and it is different from other types of

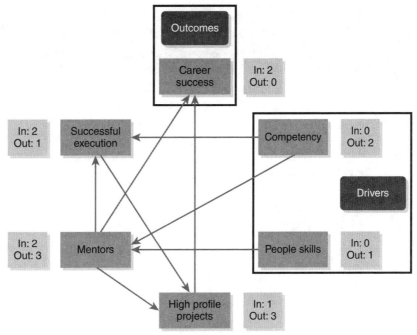

FIGURE 27.4 Interrelationship Diagram[17]

TABLE 27.2 Description of the Academy and CDR Resources for Completing QI/Outcomes Research

Resource	Description with Link
Quality Management/QI	Collected by the Quality Leader Alliance of the Academy's Quality Management Committee http://www.eatrightpro.org/resources/practice/quality-management/quality-improvement[18]
Evidence Analysis Library®	Launched in 2004; Online resource contains systematic reviews and evidence-based nutrition practice guidelines for registered dietitian nutritionists and other members of the health care team http://www.andeal.org[19]
ANDHII (Academy of Nutrition and Dietetics Health Informatics Infrastructure)	A unique web application platform with tools to help registered dietitian nutritionists provide the highest-quality care for patients and clients, track outcomes of their interventions, conduct research in important areas of nutrition science and contribute to a national quality registry. Provides dietetics practitioners with tools to track and report outcomes. Guides dietetics practitioners through each step of the Nutrition Care Process, collecting impact data that can be used in public policy and quality improvement research. http://www.andhii.org[20]
Standards of Excellence for Organization Self-Assessment and Quality Improvement	A tool to measure and evaluate an organization's programs, services, and initiatives that identify and distinguish the RDN brand as the professional expert in food and nutrition. Standards of Excellence criteria apply to all practice segments of nutrition and dietetics: health care, education and research, business and industry, and community nutrition and public health. Academy Standards of Excellence in Nutrition and Dietetics for Organization Self-Assessment and Quality Improvement[21]

(continues)

TABLE 27.2 Description of the Academy and CDR Resources for Completing QI/Outcomes Research *(continued)*

Resource	Description with Link
Dietetics Practice-based Research Network (DPBRN)	Conducts, supports, promotes and advocates for practice-based research that answers questions important to dietetics practice. DPBRN members are RDNs who share a common interest in improving patient care through practice-based research or designing research projects that draw from the knowledge and understanding of practicing clinicians. Network members work in a variety of practice settings and specialties and include practitioners, researchers and students A. Links to webinars from the Dietetics Practice-based Research Network (DPBRN): http://www.eatrightpro.org/resource/research/projects-tools-and-initiatives/dpbrn/dpbrn-projects[22] B. Link to general resources for developing a research project, conducting a literature search, a webinar on Quality Improvement research and other research-related topics: http://www.eatrightpro.org/resource/research/projects-tools-and-initiatives/dpbrn/steps-to-developing-a-research-project-resources-to-help[23] C. Tools and resources for utilizing secondary datasets to enhance your own quality improvement project: https://www.eatrightpro.org/resource/research/projects-tools-and-initiatives/dpbrn/academy-datasets[24]

research because of its purpose. Data collected in outcomes studies include the desired outcomes as well as other variables which may be related to the intervention or outcome. Measures of the intervention must be specific to ensure that it is that intervention that produces the outcomes. Outcomes measures must also be defined specifically before collecting data. Possible confounding variables that should be measured include differences in care providers, differing patient characteristics such as age, gender, socio-economic status, and type or severity of illness. **TABLE 27.3** describes specific nutrition-related outcome measures based on general outcomes indicators.

▶ How to Get Started with an Outcomes Research Project

Whichever methods or tools are utilized, selecting a quality improvement project must be meaningful for the individuals/team conducting the project. A good place to start for ideas for an outcomes research study is the EAL list of Grade V questions. The EAL was completed in May of 2015 and there were nearly 6,000 research articles reviewed with over a thousand conclusion statements made. However, there were over 250 Grade V conclusion statements indicating that there is not enough evidence available to support or refute the conclusion. This indicates that more research is needed. The following link gives directions on how to find the Grade V questions which are listed by topic area: https://www.andeal.org/grade-v.[26] An individual identifies a possible concern

or problem that affects the patient population that they work with on a regular basis and decides to investigate the cause for the concern by asking questions. This is the beginning of a QI project. The individual may want to go back to the 6 Aims of Improving Healthcare Quality illustrated in Table 27.1 to determine which of the aims coincides with the problem. For example, are there many patients on your health care team that are undernourished yet not receiving the diagnosis of malnutrition? More than one of the aims could be involved in this missed diagnosis scenario:

1. Safe: the patient may develop other life-threatening complications, or their condition may deteriorate from the delay in intervention caused by the lack of diagnosing malnutrition.
2. Timely: if malnutrition is not recognized, aggressive nutritional intervention may be delayed.
3. Effective: the patient may not receive nutritional care for malnutrition if it is not diagnosed. What does this mean for your patient? What does this mean for your healthcare institution? The lack of the identification and documentation of malnutrition may relate to both efficiency and effectiveness in healthcare.

After selecting a question of interest, a thorough literature review of the subject should be conducted to identify recent work that has been published in the subject area. This will also help with further narrowing and defining the research question.

TABLE 27.3 Dietetics Specific Outcomes Measures

Outcomes Indicator	Outcomes to Measure
Morbidity	Episodes of hyper or hypoglycemia, kidney failure, acute diarrhea, malnutrition, osteopenia, osteoporosis
Physiologic	Hemoglobin A1c %, cholesterol level, Triglycerides, weight gain, energy intake, Protein intake, pressure ulcer stage
Behavioral	Healthy food choices, self-monitoring, correctly counting carbohydrates
Knowledge	Knowledge of disease, diet, risk factors
Financial	Cost for special formula, reimbursement for diagnosis, staffing cost, cost for family to travel for nutrition counseling
Functional status (physical, mental or social)	Self-feeding, swallowing, body image, anxiety about NG tube feeds, eating behaviors among family or peers, lost school days
General health and well-being	Growth and development, health status after diet change
Disease specific quality of life (QoL)	Diabetes, Eating Disorder, or CF QoL
Caregiver Outcomes	Caregiver burden after dietary intervention

Modified from Adair CE. Getting Your Measures Right in Dietetic Outcomes Research. The Canadian Foundation for Dietetic Research. Available at: https://www.cfdr.ca/CMSTemplates/CFDRWebsite/Templates/dloads/CFDR_research_resource_CAdair.pdf. Accessed October 17, 2017.[25]

Ask the following questions: What is the population you want to study? What is the nutrition intervention used with this population? What outcome do you want to investigate in terms of clinical effectiveness? Use this simple template to get started:

In patients with _____ (patient population), what is the impact of _____ (intervention) compared with _____ (comparison group) on _____ (outcome)?

Remember that the comparison group may be patients who do not receive the intervention. In the malnutrition example, 1) the patient population are those with severe malnutrition, 2) the intervention is whatever the standard intervention is for those diagnosed with severe malnutrition, 3) the comparison group are the patients with malnutrition who are not diagnosed, and 4) the outcome measured could be weight gain, BMI z-score, MAMC, resolution of micronutrient deficiencies, or it could be a financial outcome like reimbursement for malnutrition. A good outcomes research question or topic should be specific as to *what* intervention will be provided and what outcomes are expected, *who* the study population is and *where* they are located. Further

define your research question by asking the following questions:

1. What is the intervention? (Ex: peri-operative feeding protocol, 0.5 gm/kg extra Protein for patients at risk for developing pressure ulcers, monitoring for malnutrition)

2. What is the outcome? (Ex: Improved recovery time from surgery, prevention of pressure ulcers, increased reimbursement for malnutrition diagnosis)

3. Who is the population to which the results can be generalized? (Ex: Adolescent trauma patients, School age children with cerebral palsy and profound developmental disorders, Pediatric acute care hospital patients)

4. Where are the outcomes to be collected? (Ex: Acute care surgical center, Long-term pediatric care facility, Acute care pediatric hospital)

Once an idea for a QI/Outcomes project has been established, the project aim should be defined, and the status quo determined. The **Institution's Review Board** (IRB) should be consulted in order to determine whether or not the project needs approval. Most outcomes research will receive an expedited review if one is needed at all. The project team should also be formed. Who to include on the team is an important aspect of any QI project because having the right people can support the success of the program. Include a representative from any area that might be affected by the potential change in practice—other RDNs, nurses, a physician champion and someone from the facility's administration.

Now that approaches, modules and tools for developing a QI project have been described, two examples are presented to put these methods and resources into action.

▶ Conclusion

Questions from patients, clients, and other stakeholders are continuously being generated; however, the information needs of practitioners are not being met. Due to limitations of time, information resources, search skills, and funding, many questions go unanswered. The solution to this problem lies in the willingness of every practitioner to conduct quality improvement projects and outcomes research.

For dietitians to remain competitive within the health care, education, and business arenas, they **must** incorporate evidence-based practice into their day-to-day activities and decisions. Evidence-based practice enhances credibility with other healthcare team members and will help dietitians be more effective and efficient in their practice. Evidence-based practice can help to standardize practice. Outcomes data can be collected and analyzed in order to continue to improve the quality and effectiveness of practice.

Outcomes research feeds quality improvement which in turn leads to evidence-based practice.

🔍 CASE STUDIES

Case Study #1

Sara, an RDN at a large pediatric teaching hospital read a recently published A.S.P.E.N. publication titled, "New Pediatric Malnutrition Etiology-Related Malnutrition Definitions" which outlined guidelines for diagnosing malnutrition in infants and children.[27] Sara noted that she and her colleagues, while assessing their patients and identifying many of the markers of malnutrition, were not using that diagnosis, therefore, neither were the physicians with whom they were working. Sara completed a more in-depth literature search on pediatric malnutrition and learned that there were steps in the process of diagnosing malnutrition that she and her co-workers were missing. Sara saw not only a gap in care of her patients, but also a missed opportunity for reimbursement for this care.

Sara took action and began a retrospective review of all pediatric in-patients 3 months and older (excluding the ICUs and any infants who were not at least 3 months adjusted for gestational age) at her hospital in the past year in order to determine the scope of the perceived problem. She knew she had to establish the status quo in order to measure any change that a proposed process change might make. In her review of inpatients, she found that only 10 percent of the patients who were positive for malnutrition, using the ASPEN criteria, received that diagnosis. Sara concluded that increasing the diagnosis of malnutrition would make a good process improvement project because it had the potential to improve patient outcomes and improve reimbursement to the hospital.

TABLE 27.4 Project Charter Table

Project Charter/DMAIC Worksheet

Project Name: Malnutrition Documentation

Problem Statement:
Only 10% (114) in-patients in the past year were diagnosed with malnutrition while 90% (>1000) of patients with BMI or Wt/Lt z-scores indicating malnutrition were not given that diagnosis.

Opportunity/Primary Aim:
Increased documentation of malnutrition improves patient outcomes in several key areas including: decreased hospital acquired infections; decreased fall-risk; decreased hospital acquired wounds and improved wound healing.

Secondary Aim:
Increased documentation of malnutrition could increase revenue through higher acuity room charges.

Team Members:
BF, ICU RDN
AO, General Team RDN and eating disorder specialist
SB, Process Improvement RN
CR, Discharge Planner
VO, DTR
RP and DJ, IT specialists
CS and SB, RN coding specialist
LW, RN educator

Project Owner: Sara, RDN
Facilitator: MG, Outpatient RDN

Project Sponsor:
JD, Sr. VP for Safety and Patient Care

Champions:
Project: DK, Director of QI
Physician: JV, Medical Director for Department of Clinical Nutrition and Gastroenterology

SMART Goal(s)

Increase documentation of malnutrition and its comorbidities by 50% by April 30, 2014.

Process Measurement(s)
- Education on malnutrition documentation and coding.
- Documentation of malnutrition and its comorbidities.

Balancing Measurement(s)
- Revenue from documentation of malnutrition
- Coding of malnutrition

Outcomes Measurement(s)
Percent of appropriately diagnosed patients related to malnutrition and its comorbidities.

Project Boundary & Scope:
This project will include patients diagnosed with malnutrition, malnourished patients without a diagnosis of malnutrition, and patients with co-morbities of malnutrition. Any patient without the presence or diagnosis of malnutrition will not be included.

Define	Measure	Analyze	Improve	Control
Start Date: 8/15/2012	Start Date: 10/3/2012	Start Date: 10/31/2012	Start Date:	Start Date:
End Date: 9/30/2012	End Date: 11/30/2012	End Date: 12/15/2012	End Date:	End Date:
_X_ Finalize Team _X_ Clarify Problem Statement _X_ Identify Project Scope _X_ Define SMART Goals	_X_ Flowchart the Process ___ Fishbone Diagram _X_ Develop Data Collection Plan _X_ Define baseline data	___ Analyze data ___ Identify Root Causes of Variation ___ Develop Key Driver Diagram ___ Brainstorm Tests of Change	___ Prioritize Test of Change ___ Plan Test of Change ___ Implement Test of Change ___ Document on Run Chart Test of Change	___ Identify ways to Sustain the new process and create reliability ___ Establish ongoing monitoring plan

Sara next decided who to get involved on her process improvement team. She developed a Problem Statement and Aims to help describe the project to those she wanted on her team, then began recruiting the team. The team members met and wrote a Team Charter and decided on the Project Scope.

During the first meeting with the team, Sara utilized a Fishbone Diagram to brainstorm the process of diagnosing malnutrition. The team discovered important breakdowns in the process. One was the RDNs' lack of formal training in

(continues)

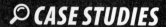

pediatric-specific nutrition focused physical exam (NFPE) and the second was the lack of knowledge throughout the hospital concerning the benefits of properly diagnosing a patient who has malnutrition. By diagramming every aspect of the process of diagnosing malnutrition, the team was able to initiate the first "Do" in the PDSA cycle.

With Sara's team it began with a flow-sheet diagram to discover the process for obtaining anthropometric measurements on patients in this hospital. The process improvement continued with expansion of the education and data collection to other units of the hospital. This process improvement project could also lead to a patient outcomes study determining if properly diagnosing malnutrition did indeed improve related patient outcomes, such as shorter hospital stays, decreased readmission rate, decreased pressure ulcers or shorter pressure ulcer healing time. This example shows the benefits of quality improvement—it is never ending and the cycles are continuous.

Discussion Questions

1. How do you suppose the next P in the PDSA cycle began?
2. What is the next step that Sara should take in planning this improvement project?
3. So far Sara only has anecdotal information to base her theory. What is the next step in a PIP?

Case Study #2

Paula, an RDN, works at AFK, a Pediatric **Long-term care** (LTC) facility for profoundly disabled children. There are 58 residents ranging in age from 9-months to 20-years. She has noticed that many of the children develop osteopenia or osteoporosis despite receiving adequate (DRI) calcium in their enteral feeds. She wants to know if the children would have better bone density z-scores if she were to increase the Calcium plus Vitamin D supplementation to 1.5 times the DRI. She determines that the status quo is that 40 percent of the residents currently have bone density z-scores less than negative 1 (indicating osteopenia) or less than negative 2.4 (indicating osteoporosis). Residents receive **dual-energy x-ray absorptiometry** (DEXA) or bone densitometry annually. Her research question is: In residents at AFK, what is the impact of 1.5 times DRI supplementation of Calcium and Vitamin D?

Paula involves AFK administrators and the Director of Nursing for support of the project. She decides to consult with DPBRN to assist with her study design and analysis. She also determines that she would like to utilize ANDHII for data collection purposes. Academy staff for DPBRN help Paula refine her question to make it more specific to just one diagnosis—Cerebral Palsy, and to exclude residents who are on steroid therapy. They discussed further limiting the inclusion criteria to exclude residents on certain medications especially epilepsy drugs with side effects that include reduced bone density. Paula decided that she would like to include the residents on these medications but to control for it in the data analysis. She also wanted to include only non-weight bearing for ambulation children since these children were the most likely to have abnormal bone density studies. Further, she excluded children who had not had a DEXA performed in the past six months.

After conducting a thorough literature review and consulting the EAL, Paula found very little related literature and no strong evidence to either support or disprove her theory that extra supplementation will improve bone density in children with Cerebral Palsy. What Paula did know and was reinforced in literature is that Calcium carbonate is not well absorbed when given to a person on a **Proton Pump Inhibitor** (PPI) which most of the AFK residents are given. She determined that the best supplement for this population would be calcium citrate and Vitamin D_3.

Study Aim

Improve bone density by at least 10% per year until resident's bone-density z-score measures as normal.

Research Question

Does calcium citrate plus vitamin D liquid supplementation of 150% DRI improve bone density z-score in non-weight-bearing for ambulation children ages 6 to 18 living at AFK who are diagnosed with Cerebral Palsy, and either osteopenia or osteoporosis?

Outcomes Measure

Bone density z-score

By utilizing the services of the DPBRN, Paula was able to receive expert assistance in refining her project. She received training on ANDHII and was not required to obtain IRB approval for the study because "ANDHII has been designed to work within the regulations and guidance issued by the <u>Office for Civil Rights</u> and <u>Office for Human Research Protections</u> so that the data collected would not be Protected Health Information and the collection process would not constitute Human Subjects Research. As a result, using ANDHII in accordance with regulations and its End User License Agreement for the collection of de-identified data regarding routine care would not require HIPAA Authorizations, Business Associate Agreements, or local Institutional Review."[21]

In Paula's clinical judgement, all the residents of AFK could benefit from extra supplementation so she decided to expand the supplementation program to all regardless of their inclusion in the outcomes project. She could do this because she was not comparing two groups, but investigating the outcomes of the supplementation on one group.

Paula's calcium and vitamin D supplementation outcomes research is not completed but she is able to use ANDHII to create graphs and spreadsheets to display changes in the resident's outcomes as the study progresses. She was pleased with how easily she was able to turn a problem into a possible solution to optimize her client's nutritional health by collecting outcomes data.

Discussion Questions

1. How could Paula further refine her question?
2. What bothers you or what problems have you identified in your own practice setting?
3. What other outcomes research could possibly result from Paula's study?
4. What resources are available to all Academy members for nutritional outcomes research or quality improvement projects?

Review Questions

1. What makes outcomes research different from other types of research?

2. What are the 6 Aims of Improving Healthcare Quality?

3. Evidence-based practice....
   A. Is an approach to health care where health practitioners use the best evidence possible to make decisions.
   B. Incorporates successful strategies that improve client outcomes.
   C. Is derived from various sources including research, national guidelines, policies, consensus statements and systematic analysis of clinical experience.
   D. All of the above.

4. What is one tool that RDNs and DTRs have available to them that contains evidence-based practice guidelines?

5. Which of the following questions is NOT part of the basis for The Model for Improvement?

A. What change can we make that will result in an improvement?
B. How can the healthcare system increase reimbursement?
C. What are we trying to improve?
D. How will we know if the change we make is an improvement?

6. What is another name for the Fishbone Diagram? And what is its purpose?

7. What is a unique web application platform available to RDNs and DTRs to track outcome of their interventions?

8. How might an RDN establish a question for an outcomes research project?
A. Find something about their patient population or process that bothers them and study it.
B. Look at the EAL list of Grade 5 questions.
C. Read literature to see what improvement projects or outcomes studies are being done in other similar work settings.
D. All of the above

References

1. Band R. Ernest Amory Codman, MD, 1869–1940. *Clin Orthop Relat Res.* 2009;467(11):2763–2765.
2. Committee on Quality Health Care in America, Institute of Medicine. *Crossing the quality chasm: A New Health System for the 21st Century.* Washington, DC: National Academy Press;2001.
3. Agency for Healthcare Research and Quality. *About the National Quality Strategy.* Washington, DC: Dept. of Health and Human Services;2011.
4. Nutbeam, D. Health promotion glossary. World Health Organization. Available at: http://www.who.int/health promotion/about/HPR%20Glossary%201998.pdf. Accessed September 9, 2017.
5. The IHI Triple Aim. Institute for health improvement. Available at: http://www.ihi.org/Engage/Initiatives/TripleAim /Pages/default.aspx. Accessed September 9, 2017.
6. Price JA, Kent S, Cox SA, McCauley SM, Parekh J, Klein C. Using academy standards of excellence in nutrition

and dietetics for organization self-assessment and quality improvement. J Acad Nutr Diet. 2014;114(8):1277–1292.

7. National Quality Forum. Why quality? Available at: http://www.qualityforum.org/Home.aspx. Accessed August 23, 2017

8. HRSA Quality Toolkit. Health resources and services administration. Available at: http://www.hrsa.gov/quality/toolbox/methodology/quality improvement/index.html. Accessed August 23, 2017.

9. Academy of Nutrition and Dietetics. Measures definition. Available at: http://www.eatrightpro.org/~/media/eatrightpro%20files/practice/quality%20management/measures_definitions.ashx. Accessed July 20, 2017.

10. Hakel-Smith, N. Quality management and improvement. In: Grim JA, Roberts SR, eds. *The Clinical Nutrition Manager's Handbook*. Chicago, IL: Cathy Iammartino; 2014:91–114.

11. Langley GL, Moen R, Nolan KM, Nolan TW, Norman CL, Provost LP. *The Improvement Guide: A Practical Approach to Enhancing Organizational Performance*. 2nd ed. San Francisco, CA: Jossey-Bass Publishers;2009.

12. Six Sigma Online. Available at: https://www.sixsigmaonline.org/. Accessed August 23, 2017.

13. Lean Enterprise Institute. Available at: https://www.lean.org/. Accessed October 17, 2017

14. Team Charter. Learning Technologies, Inc. Available at: www.teamlti.com/charter/page0/files/Charter6.pdf. Accessed October 23, 2017.

15. Roberts S, Grim J. Cause and effect diagram. In: *ICU Enteral Feedings*. ABC Baylor Quality Improvement Presentation. Baylor Health Care System; 2009.

16. Minnesota Department of Health. What is an interrelationship digraph? Available at: http://www.health.state.mn.us/divs/opi/qi/toolbox/interrelationshipdigraph.html. Accessed October 17, 2017.

17. Six Sigma. Six Sigma study guide. Available at: http://sixsigmastudyguide.com/wp-content/uploads/2014/12/interrelatinship-diagraph.jpg. Accessed October 17, 2017.

18. Academy of Nutrition and Dietetics. Quality management. Available at: http://www.eatrightpro.org/resources/practice/quality-management/quality-improvement. Accessed July 23, 2017.

19. Academy of Nutrition and Dietetics. Evidence analysis library. Available at: http://www.andeal.org. Accessed July 23, 2017.

20. Murphy W. Academy of Nutrition and Dietetics Health Informatics Infrastructure (ANDHII). Available at: http://www.andhii.org. Accessed July 23, 2017.

21. Academy of Nutrition and Dietetics. Academy standards of excellence in nutrition and dietetics for organization self-assessment and quality improvement. Available at: http://www.eatrightpro.org/SSO/Journal.aspx?redir=article/S2212-2672(14)00451-1/fulltext. Accessed August 20, 2017.

22. Academy of Nutrition and Dietetics. DPBRN projects. Available at: http://www.eatrightpro.org/resource/research/projects-tools-and-initiatives/dpbrn/dpbrn-projects. Accessed July 23, 2017.

23. Academy of Nutrition and Dietetics. Steps to developing a research project: resources to help. Availabe at: http://www.eatrightpro.org/resource/research/projects-tools-and-initiatives/dpbrn/steps-to-developing-a-research-project-resources-to-help. Accessed September 9, 2017.

24. Academy of Nutrition and Dietetics. Academy datasets. Available at: https://www.eatrightpro.org/resource/research/projects-tools-and-initiatives/dpbrn/academy-datasets. Accessed May, 2017.

25. Adair C.E. Getting your measures right in dietetic outcomes research. The Canadian Foundation for Dietetic Research. Available at: https://www.cfdr.ca/CMSTemplates/CFDRWebsite/Templates/dloads/CFDR_research_resource_CAdair.pdf. Accessed October 17, 2017.

26. Academy of Nutrition and Dietetics. Research gaps: additional research needed! Available at: https://www.andeal.org/grade-v. Accessed July, 2017.

27. American Society for Parenteral and Enteral Nutrition. A.S.P.E.N. releases new pediatric malnutrition etiology-related malnutrition definitions. Available at: https://www.nutritioncare.org/Press_Room/2013/A_S_P_E_N_Releases_New_Pediatric_Malnutrition_Etiology-Related_Malnutrition_Definitions/. Accessed June, 2013.

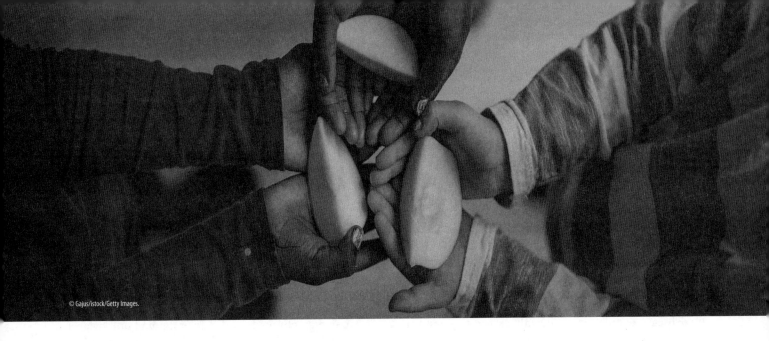

© Gajus/istock/Getty Images.

CHAPTER 28

Integrative Medicine and Nutrition

Jennifer Panganiban, Andrea Gilbaugh, Ama Tettey-Fio, and Maria Mascarenhas

LEARNING OBJECTIVES

- To define Complementary and Alternative Medicine, Integrative Health, and Nutrition
- To identify the different types of diets used in Integrative Nutrition
- To identify the indications for use of these specialized diets
- To recognize the possible nutritional deficiencies when using these diets
- To be aware of the different herbal therapies available

▶ Introduction

Complementary and Alternative Medicine (CAM) is an umbrella term encompassing a broad range of modalities, healing philosophies, and approaches. If a non-mainstream practice is used together with conventional medicine, it is considered *complementary* and if it is used in place of conventional medicine it is considered *alternative*.[1] CAM is often classified into one of five domains: 1) whole medical systems, 2) mind-body medicine, 3) biologically-based practices, 4) manipulative and body based practices, and 5) energy medicine. Whole medical systems represent the theories and practices of traditional Chinese medicine, Ayurveda medicine, and homeopathy. Mind-body interventions involve modalities such as prayer and meditation, and are meant to facilitate the connection between the mind and body. Herbal products, dietary supplements and diets comprise the category of biologically based therapies. Body-based practices employ human touch to manipulate the physical body, such as massage or craniosacral therapy. Finally, energy therapies, such as tai chi and reiki, harness the body's energy fields to promote health and healing. These classification entities encompass a wide range of diverse therapies and may have disparate, but interrelated, therapeutic targets.

Recently, in the United States, the National Center for Complementary and Integrative Health has moved towards a two subgroup classification system: mind and body practices or natural products. Furthermore, identifying that most Americans use non-mainstream practices in conjunction with, not as an alternative to conventional treatments has led to the development of the term integrative medicine or health. **Integrative health** (IH) refers to incorporating and integrating complementary approaches into mainstream healthcare practices for disease management and prevention.

The use of CAM or IH practices is quite common. The National Survey Data in the United States suggest 33.2% of adults and 11.6% of children used complementary health approaches.[2] Rates of IH use in chronic pediatric disease populations frequently exceed those in the general population. Complementary health approaches in the pediatric population were most commonly used for neck and back pain (8.9%), musculoskeletal conditions other than neck and back pain (6.0%), and head or chest colds (5.1%). It is worth noting that although anxiety and stress were the fourth most common conditions, the specific approaches used to treat anxiety and stress are among the lowest risk and are the most effective. Such approaches include biofeedback, yoga, and mindfulness.[3]

In this chapter we explore the interest, utilization, and efficacy of using biologically based therapies, specifically integrative nutrition for the adjuvant treatment of common diseases seen in pediatrics.

▶ Integrative Nutrition

Nutrition is a central component of integrative medicine. In using a holistic approach to treating patients, practitioners of integrative medicine address diet as a determinant of health and use the many beneficial properties of food in the treatment plan. Specific dietary interventions have been prescribed in the following pediatric diseases and are outlined below.

Elimination, Restricted, Oligoantigenic or Few Foods Diet

Elimination diets strive to reduce or eradicate symptoms of disease by eliminating commonly sensitizing food allergens and antigens. Oligoantigenic diets are extensive elimination diets, which remove all but a limited number of foods that are less commonly consumed with low allergenic potential. The elimination is typically followed by a challenge phase whereby individual foods are reintroduced in the diet. This diet has been used to treat **Eosinophilic Esophagitis** (EoE), Migraines, and ADHD in the pediatric population.

The most common elimination diet is the **Six Food Elimination Diet** (SFED), which excludes milk, egg, wheat, soy, fish/shellfish, and peanuts/tree nuts from the diet in children and adults with EoE. Multiple studies have been performed in pediatrics demonstrating up to 74% clinical and histologic remission with the use of the SFED in EoE.[4] A recent prospective, 8 week multi-center study of seventy-eight patients looked at a **Four Food Elimination Diet** (FFED) which excludes only milk, egg, wheat, and soy. This was also highly effective in eradicating clinical, endoscopic, and histologic signs of EoE in 64% of patients when used in combination with a proton pump inhibitor. The most common identified food trigger in this study was cow's milk (85%) followed more distantly by egg, wheat and soy (19–35%).[5]

Using an elimination diet for migraine prophylaxis is generally discouraged by neurologists, and there is a dearth of research on the topic. A small double-blind elimination trial performed in 88 children showed that an oligoantigenic diet consisting of lamb, chicken, rice, potato, apple, banana, brassica, vitamin supplements, and water induced migraine remission in 93% of subjects.[6–8]

A 2009 randomized control study of children with ADHD found that when compared with a routine diet, a restricted diet resulted in a statistically significant improvement in behavior ratings for 70% of children. These children no longer met the DSM-IV criteria for ADHD.[9]

Elimination diets have a specific role in certain disease entities but this must be used cautiously given these diets are difficult to implement and sustain and pose an increased risk for nutritional deficiencies. Thus these patients must be followed closely.

Histamine-free Diet

Histamine intolerance (HI) is created when there is a buildup of excess histamine in the body.[10–13] Excess histamine can be created when there is an abnormality in histamine metabolism, such as a deficiency of **diamine oxidase** (DAO), a main enzyme involved in histamine metabolism within the gastrointestinal tract. Histamine can build up when it is released from intracellular vesicles in response to an allergen.[11] It can also be ingested in excess. Dietary therapy for HI includes avoiding foods high in histamine. These include oily fish, tomatoes, eggplant, alcoholic beverages, cured meats, fermented foods, chocolate, vanilla, fruit, vegetables, eggs, and aged cheeses.[10–13]

Since DAO is found in the GI tract, gastrointestinal symptoms such as abdominal pain, diarrhea, and vomiting are usually the primary manifestations of HI.[10–12] However, involvement of the central nervous system, skin, reproductive organs, and cardiovascular system has also been noted.[12] Common non-GI manifestations include headache, skin rash, dysmenorrhea and tachycardia.[12]

A small sample observational study demonstrated a reduction in chronic abdominal pain in 88% of patients who underwent a 4-week histamine free diet.[10] A low histamine diet may be nutritionally adequate if whole food groups are not eliminated.

Ketogenic Diet/Modified Atkins Diet

The **Ketogenic diet** (KD) is high in fat, restrictive in protein, and very low in carbohydrates. The most commonly used KDs use a fat: non-fat ratio of 4:1 or 3:1.[14–17] Other variants include the **modified Atkins diet** (MAD) and the **low glycemic index treatment** (LGIT). Both MADs and LGITs restrict carbohydrate intake while encouraging a daily fat caloric intake of 60–70%.[14,18,19] Since KDs restrict carbohydrate intake, they induce the body to metabolize fat rather than glucose.[14–17,20] As a result, plasma levels of ketones, rather than glucose, rise after meals. This is known as a ketogenic metabolism. The mechanism by which the KD works is not well understood, but decreased availability of glucose for glycolysis is thought to play a role.[14,20] KDs have been used to treat neurological conditions, specifically epilepsy.[14,16,20–22]

A Cochrane review of 427 children and adolescents with epilepsy showed that 55% of those adhering to a 4:1 ketogenic diet for 3 months experienced no seizures[16], and 85% of patients experienced a reduction of seizure activity. Additionally, a systematic review showed a greater than 50% improvement of the frequency of infantile spasms within 6 months on a ketogenic diet.[17]

Dietary counseling is important for patients on KD therapy. In addition to reduced dietary options, palatability may be a concern in the pediatric population. While initial lipid panel values may fluctuate, they tend to stabilize or even improve with time; high-density lipoprotein values have been found to increase while triglyceride values decrease.[12] Some patients may exhibit symptoms of KD intolerance, including headaches, acidosis, constipation, and hypoglycemia. Such patients may benefit from dietary ratio adjustment in order to adjust ketone levels, or the use of citrate or sodium bicarbonate.[14] Patients on a ketogenic diet require close monitoring with a dietitian in order to assess for micronutrient deficiencies and ensure adequate growth and development.

Gluten and Casein Free Diets

A **Gluten-free diet** (GFD) has become increasingly well known in recent years. This diet eliminates all gluten-containing grains specifically wheat, barley, and rye. Oats are usually tolerated as long as there is no cross contamination with any gluten containing products.[23,24] By facilitating intestinal mucosal healing, the GFD is an integral part of treating celiac disease and nonceliac gluten sensitivity.[25,26]

A retrospective study evaluating 227 children with **celiac disease** (CD) placed on a GFD for at least 24 months found a significant improvement in gastrointestinal symptoms (bloating, diarrhea, weight loss, and abdominal pain) in 81–90% of their subjects and 100% improvement in extra intestinal manifestations (dermatitis herpetiformis, myalgia, stomatitis, seizures, and delayed puberty).[27] A lifelong GFD is currently the only treatment for celiac disease.

A **Casein-free diet** (CFD) is a diet that excludes the protein casein found in milk and milk products. This is the treatment for cow's milk allergy. Symptoms may involve the gastrointestinal tract, skin, and respiratory system. It has been found that exposure to cow's milk during the first 3 days of life causes a sustained and elevated production of anti-CMP (cow milk protein), and children who are exclusively formula fed do not have such antibodies.[28–31] One study found that having a higher IgG antibody concentration to alpha casein might predict a longer duration of cow milk allergy.[28]

Both gluten and casein-free diets have also been linked to a possible improvement in **autism spectrum disorders** (ASD).[32,33] Symptoms of ASD reported to improve with using these diets include 'communication' as measured by the Autism Diagnostic Observation Schedule and 'social interaction' by the Gilliam Autism Rating Scale, as well as 'autistic traits', 'communication' and 'social contact' by a Danish scale of autism. Despite reported improvements, there is not enough evidence at this time to support using these diets in ASD.

Children placed on a gluten free diet are at risk for certain nutritional deficiencies. This includes inadequate intake of fiber, iron, B vitamins, and minerals. In the US, most refined wheat flour is enriched with B vitamins and iron after processing. However, refined gluten free grains may not be enriched. Intake of nutrient dense foods high in vitamins and minerals, especially plant-based foods, should be encouraged. Casein restricted diets may result in less than recommended intake of calcium if not supplemented through other sources. These children should be assessed on an individual basis with consideration for calories, fat, protein, calcium, and vitamin D intake. It is important for patients who are adhering to GFD or CFD to follow up long term with their primary provider and dietitian to avoid these deficiencies and ensure efficacy of the diet.

The Feingold Diet

The Feingold Diet, also known as the K-P or Kaiser-Permanente Diet, was introduced in the 1970s as a treatment for hyperactive children. Dr. Feingold hypothesized that eliminating foods that contain artificial food colors/flavors and naturally occurring salicylates would reduce hyperactivity. Subsequently, Dr. Feingold advocated restricting preservatives and allowed the intake of salicylates in those without significant salicylate sensitivity. Dr. Feingold initially reported that he observed positive response to the diet in 30–50% of children.[34] Many studies soon followed to test this hypothesis. In 1983, an initial meta-analysis including 23 studies concluded Feingold's diet modifications were not validated as an effective intervention for hyperactivity.[35]

Feingold's list in the 1982 paper of high salicylate foods includes almonds, apples (and cider, vinegar), apricots, berries, cloves, cucumbers, pickles, currants, grapes, raisins, wine, nectarines, oranges, peaches, plums or prunes, tangerines, green peppers, tomatoes, tea, coffee, and wintergreen oil.[36]

A double blind placebo control study performed in England in 2007, found increased hyperactive behavior in the healthy children who received a beverage containing artificial color or the preservative sodium benzoate, or both.[37] The results of this study warranted enough concern in the EU, that the European Parliament announced in 2008 that food containing six synthetic food colors (three are approved by the **US Food and Drug Administration** (FDA): FD&C Red No. 40, Yellow No. 5, and Yellow No. 6[38,39]) must be labeled with "may have an adverse effect on activity and attention in children"[40]; the FDA did not agree on the need for a label warning.

More recent versions of the diet eliminate only artificial food additives and or dyes.[41] The effect of food additives and food allergy on hyperactivity and behavior remains controversial. Several meta-analyses and systematic reviews much later concluded that in some children, synthetic food colors have a small but significant effect on ADHD symptoms.[42-44] Authors later focused on higher quality studies, but discrepancies between parent and teacher/observer ratings were found[42] and now these older studies may be outdated.[45]

The amount of artificial food color certified in 2010 had reportedly increased fivefold per capita from 1950, with beverages contributing largely to intake, as well as candy, cereals, and other foods.[46] A small subset of children may be more sensitive to food colors and preservatives, which could be discussed with families who ask providers about the need to eliminate these.

Low FODMAP Diet

The low FODMAP diet is now a well-known restriction diet for **irritable bowel syndrome** (IBS), but the acronym was initially introduced in a hypothesis related to the development of Crohn's disease.[47,48] **Fermentable oligosaccharides, disaccharides, monosaccharides, and polyols** (FODMAPs) are short chain carbohydrates and sugar alcohols that are poorly absorbed in the small intestine and rapidly fermented in the colon. Oligosaccharides include **fruto-oligosaccharides** (FOS), **galacto-oligosaccharides** (GOS), fructans, raffinose, inulin; simple sugars include fructose (in excess of glucose) and lactose; examples of polyols are the sugar alcohols: sorbitol, mannitol and xylitol.[49] The low FODMAP diet includes a number of food restrictions, which are liberalized per personal tolerance or if failed response to the diet after a 4-6 week restriction period.[50]

In a cross-over RCT completed in 33 children with IBS, 7 to 17 years of age, patients on a low FODMAP diet reported fewer episodes and decreased severity of abdominal pain compared with a usual diet over 2 days[51]; the benefit of a longer intervention time has been questioned, as in adults the maximum response has been reported to be 7 days.[52] In adults with IBS, the available evidence supports the efficacy of a low FODMAP diet for treating functional gastrointestinal symptoms such as bloating and abdominal pain[53], although there has been criticism regarding the quality of much of the research.[54]

A recent Cochrane review concluded that in children with IBS, the evidence is inadequate to support recommending a low FODMAPs diet or a fructose restricted diet.[55] Concerns for using the low FODMAP diet may include inappropriate use in a child with feeding difficulty, the risk of nutritional inadequacy, and influence on disordered eating patterns.[53, 56] The unknown long-term effects on the gut microbiota have also been discussed.[57] Restricted diets in children warrant caution. Involving a specialized dietitian for assessing the diet and education may allow for adjustments of potentially high or excessive intake of FODMAP foods without considering the full restrictions of the low FODMAP diet.[58]

Mediterranean Diet

The **Mediterranean diet** (MD) is a group of traditional eating patterns from people living around the Mediterranean sea; some characteristics, such as an emphasis on a plant based diet and minimal intake of processed foods, are shared with other dietary patterns associated with health promotion[59], and are in contrast to the energy dense "Western" dietary pattern which has been described as nutrient poor.[60]

The MD is described as rich in fruits, vegetables, legumes, cereal grains, nuts, seeds, often includes fish or other seafood, includes moderate intake of dairy, moderate alcohol consumption (typically wine at meals), low consumption of red meat, and olive oil is the main source of added fat.[61] The healthy characteristics of the diet are that it is high in fiber, high in antioxidants and polyphenols, includes intake of low glycemic index carbohydrates, monounsaturated fats, and an improved omega 6: omega 3 ratio compared with the Western Diet.[62] Extra virgin olive oil is high in the monounsaturated fat oleic acid, but also is high in many polyphenols; one of the phenolic compounds of interest, found in virgin olive oil, oleocanthal, has shown anti-inflammatory activity in vitro and has been described as a naturally occurring NSAID.[63]

In adults, the eating pattern has been associated with decreased cardiovascular events, neurodegenerative disease, metabolic syndrome, obesity, incidence of some cancers, as well as overall mortality[64-68], and healthy dietary patterns, such as the traditional MD may decrease depression risk.[69] An inflammatory component is associated with all of these diseases[69-70], which may be influenced by components of the MD, the overall dietary pattern, as well as lifestyle.

The MD pattern has been described as an example of an "anti-inflammatory" diet[71]; biomarkers of inflammation including **C-reactive protein** (CRP) and others, have been found to be favorable in intervention studies comparing the MD to the "Western-type" and meat based diets.[72,73] Individual foods and nutrients within the diet have also been investigated for influence on inflammatory markers. In children and adolescents, markers of inflammation and oxidative stress have been found to be inversely related to fruit and vegetable intake (potato fries and juice excluded), which may be important for chronic disease prevention into adulthood.[74,75]

In Pediatrics, the MD has been associated with a protective effect on asthma/wheezing symptoms as demonstrated in observational studies.[76,77] Maternal adherence to the MD and protective effect on asthma/wheeze in offspring has been described[78] but not concluded in other studies controlling for lifestyle factors such as maternal education level.[79,80] If cardiovascular risk begins in childhood, a healthy diet early in life may be an important part of disease prevention; adherence to the MD in children has been associated with an inverse relationship to arterial stiffness, an improved lipid profile, and decreased values for carotid intima-media thickness, which may be relevant for decreased risk of cardiovascular disease.[81-85] It has been observed that analyzing associations from the available research may be difficult, since study results may be influenced by the incidence of inaccurate reporting of foods by study participants.[86]

A study completed by 42 children and adolescents in Mexico showed a Mediterranean style diet for 16 weeks had benefits on fasting glucose, lipid profiles, and BMI (without weight loss) in obese children with at least one metabolic syndrome component.[87] In the Black Sea region of Turkey, low adherence to the MD was found in ~70% of 106 overweight or obese children with **Non-alcoholic fatty Liver disease** (NAFLD) using the KIDMED index.[88] In a study in Italy with 243 obese children with NAFLD, they also found low KIDMED scores were significantly higher in patients with NAFLD; poor adherence was associated with higher CRP, higher fasting insulin, as well as increased steatosis and fibrosis when biopsy was performed.[89] The MD pattern has been inversely associated with childhood obesity in 8 European countries.[90] The Mediterranean diet is an example of an eating pattern associated with

health promotion; randomized control trials would help to better understand positive associations.

Botanical Therapies

These are plants with special properties that have been used as food, flavoring for food, and medicinally. They may have positive health benefits as seen in this section.

Chamomile is an herb native to Europe in the Asteraceae/Compositae or daisy family; the flowering tops produced by the chamomile plant have been used medicinally for thousands of years.[91] German Chamomile (Matricaria recutita or Matricaria chamomilla) and Roman Chamomile (Chamaemelum nobile) are two common varieties used. Chamomile is used topically, as an inhalant, in personal care products, as well as orally in teas, tinctures, capsules, and as a mouthwash; traditionally, chamomile has been used for such conditions as those related to inflammation of the skin, wound healing, digestive aliments, certain types of pain, fever, and for calming effects.[92]

More information is available for German chamomile which may have sedative effects, possible effects on osteoblast activity, as well as antibacterial, anti-viral, anti-fungal, anti-inflammatory, anti-ulcer, and anti-spasmodic effects.[93,94] The essential oil from German chamomile is high in alpha-bisabolol and contains related sesquiterpenes such as chamazulene, which contributes to the blue color of the oil when freshly distilled. The flower heads contain coumarins, mucilage, and flavonoids, such as quercetin and apigenin.[95,96]

Chamomile has been reported to improve symptoms in infants with colic, in multi-ingredient products with fennel[97,98]; however, fennel alone may improve symptoms[99] and overall the evidence is assessed as low quality.[100] In Germany, a specific product containing apple pectin and German chamomile (Diarrhoesan) was used in two trials in children aged 6 months to 6 years as an adjuvant treatment for acute diarrhea, and was reported to reduce the duration of acute diarrhea as well as improve symptom relief.[101,102] However, pectin alone may have benefit.[103]

In the US chamomile has GRAS status (generally recognized as safe for human consumption), and is likely safe in children, although it may cause allergic reaction in a small percentage of people, with higher risk in those sensitive to plants in the Asteraceae/Compositae family, such as ragweed, chrysanthemums, marigolds, and daisy.[93,104]

Cranberries are produced by an evergreen shrub native to North America that grows in wetlands or bogs. The berries and leaves of the cranberry plant have been used medicinally for bladder and stomach ailments, for wounds and other conditions.[105] Cranberries (Vaccinium macrocarpon) contain organic acids (quinic, citric, malic, other), which contribute to the astringent taste, flavonoids including anthocyanidins, flavanols such as catechins and **proanthocyanidins** (PAC) (including

A-type PAC, less common in other fruit), flavonols such as quercetin, and the raw berries contain significant vitamin C.[106,107] Flavonoids may interfere with bacterial adhesion to the urinary epithelium, and cranberry may contain active constituents with antibacterial activity, but the actual concentration in the urine is unclear.[108] A-type PAC has specifically shown anti-adhesion properties in vitro.[109]

In a randomized control trial including 40 children 5–18 years of age, with a history of at least 2 positive urine cultures in the previous year, 2ml/kg of a juice standardized to 37% PAC was provided for 1 year, and a 65% reduction risk of a **urinary tract infection** (UTI) was reported in the treatment group compared with placebo.[110] In a double-blind randomized placebo-controlled trial completed by 255 children, intake of cranberry juice made from diluted concentrate at 5 ml/kg/day (up to 300 ml/day) for 6 months did not appear to significantly decrease the number of children experiencing at least 1 UTI recurrence, but did reduce additional UTI recurrences by 43% compared with placebo (a drink that did not contain fruit).[111] In a recent meta-analysis, authors concluded that cranberry intake was associated with a significant decrease in the incidence of UTIs in children 2–17 years.[112] Previous reviews have differed for studies included and conclusions regarding the efficacy of cranberry for prevention of UTIs.[113,114] There is no evidence that cranberry is effective for treating UTI and more evidence is needed to determine if its use provides benefit for other conditions.

Cranberry juice appears safe for most children. There is contradictory evidence about interactions with medications metabolized by CYP2C9, monitoring may be in indicated in patients receiving drugs such as warfarin.[108] Some evidence suggests that cranberry juice, cranberry/lingonberry concentrate, and cranberry juice with standardized PAC content may benefit children with recurrent UTIs (without deformities of the urinary tract), but further quality studies are recommended. Optimal dose and formulation are unclear, palatability may be an issue, and it is generally recommended to limit daily juice intake. In younger children (avoid in infants), the AAP recommends limiting juice to a maximum of 4 oz/day.[115]

Echinacea is a flowering plant native to North America in the Asteraceae/Compositae family; the roots and aerial parts of the plant have been used in teas, juice, extracts, capsules, tablets, and topically; nine species are known, the most commonly used medicinally are Echinacea purpurea or Echinacea angustifolia; Echinacea pallida has also been used.[116,117] Echinacea species vary in amounts of active components and have been commonly confused in the past.[118] Echinacea contains alkamides, caffeic acid derivatives, polysaccharides, and other constituents, which may contribute to antibacterial,

antifungal, antiviral, anti-inflammatory, antioxidant, immunologic, and wound healing effects.[117]

Echinacea has been used for preventing and treating the common cold, however the research is conflicting for efficacy. A 2014 Cochrane review of 24 studies noted the difficulty in comparing research with significantly different Echinacea preparations, including different species and parts of the plant; benefit was not concluded for treating colds, but a possible weak benefit was noted over placebo for reduction in frequency.[119] The pediatric study included in the review was a randomized, double blind placebo-controlled trial evaluating 407 children, 2–11 years of age. In the analysis, participants received either Echinacea purpurea (aerial parts of the plant) 7.5 or 10 ml/day or placebo for up to 10 days with each **upper respiratory infection** (URI) and up to 3 URIs over a 4 month period. Echinacea purpurea at this dose was not reported to be effective in treating URI symptoms, and rash was reported to occur 7% with echinacea compared to 3% with placebo.[120]

A low incidence of adverse reactions have been reported, the most common of those reported are gastrointestinal symptoms and rashes; in rare cases allergic and immunostimulant effects have been severe, and one case report describes acute liver failure in a 2 year old.[117,121] Echinacea use has been cautioned against in children less than 12 years of age, and its use is contraindicated in children less than 1 year of age.[122,123]

Black Elderberry is a dark purple/black berry produced by the European or Black elder plant (Sambucus nigra); this is one of many elderberry species, found in Europe as well as parts of Asia, Africa, and North America.[124] The fruit has been used to make wine, as well as foods including pies, jams, and syrups. Various parts of the plant have been used in traditional medicine, and different pharmacological activity has been reported for the flowers.[125] Elderberries contain flavonoids including anthocyanidins, quercetin, rutin, isoquercetin, as well as tannins, essential oil, vitamins A, C, and other micronutrients.[126,127] A cyanogenic glycoside in the leaves, stems, unripe, or uncooked fruit can cause nausea, vomiting, and diarrhea.[128] Processing or cooking affects the content of elderberry phenolics and cyanogenic glycosides.[129] Active constituents are thought to have antiviral, immune-modulating, and possible anti-inflammatory actions. In a few trials, elderberry extracts appeared to be effective in reducing influenza duration or symptoms if taken in the first 24–48 hr;[130,131] this may be due to inhibition by flavonoids of viral attachment to host cells.[132] No adverse reactions were noted in trials with short-term use of a specific elderberry extract product in adults or children >5 years of age, however, safety documentation is not available otherwise in children.[133] Use has been cautioned if a patient has a history of autoimmune disease or is taking immunosuppressants, due to theoretical interactions.[124]

Ginger (Zingiber officinale) is a flowering tropical plant that has been used medicinally since ancient times. The branched fragrant rhizome (the underground stem, sometimes referred to as "ginger root") is used widely as a culinary spice as well as a fragrance in non-food products.[134] Active constituents vary between fresh and dry forms of ginger and include gingerols, gingerdiones, shogaols, paradols, volatile oils, and others.[135] Components of ginger may have anti-inflammatory, antiemetic, analgesic, antitussive and other properties, although, when the whole rhizome is used, not all pharmacological effects may occur.[136]

Many studies, albeit mainly in adults, have investigated ginger as an antiemetic, or anti-inflammatory, and/or analgesic in specific conditions. There is some evidence ginger may reduce pain in teenage girls, and adults, with dysmenorrhea.[137] In a placebo-controlled randomized trial including girls 15–18 years of age, 250 mg ginger powder given three times per day for 4 days starting the day before menstruation improved pain significantly compared with placebo.[138]

There is conflicting evidence for using ginger for chemotherapy-induced nausea and vomiting, although ginger powder provided in divided doses (1 or 2 gm/day, based on weight) in addition to standard antiemetic medication seemed to reduce the severity of acute and delayed nausea and vomiting in a double blind, randomized trial in older children and young adults receiving chemotherapy with cisplatin/doxorubicin.[139] Short term use at the doses provided in the clinical trials is seemingly safe for older children and young adults, and ginger, when used in food as a spice, has GRAS status from the FDA;[140] higher doses of ginger may increase the risk of side effects such as abdominal discomfort, and there is a theoretical interaction with antiplatelet drugs or anticoagulant drugs such as warfarin.[136]

Milk thistle (Silybum marianum) produces large spiny flowers; the plant is a member of the Asteraceae/Compositae family and grows in many parts of the world.[141] Milk thistle seeds have been used medicinally, the flower and leaves have been consumed as a vegetable, and the roasted seeds have been used as a coffee substitute.[142] Extract from the seeds contains silymarin, a mixture of flavonolignans including silibinin (silybin A and B), and has shown antioxidant, anti-inflammatory, antiviral, hepatoprotective, renal protective, and anti-cancer effects. Silymarin seems to be able to inhibit the proliferation of certain cancer cells, stabilize hepatocyte membranes, activate enzymes in detoxification pathways; silymarin, silibinin, and silybin have shown the ability to stimulate enzymes involved in liver cell regeneration.[142]

The use of milk thistle for liver related dysfunction dates back to ancient times.[143] Milk thistle has also been used intravenously (silibinin) in Europe for Amanita (death cap) mushroom poisoning, topically for skin issues, and orally for a number of other aliments.[142,143]

Use of milk thistle in clinical studies in adults has provided mixed results, and lack of quality trials is noted.[142,144] In a randomized, double-blind, placebo controlled trial including children with ALL and chemotherapy associated hepatoxicity, participants that received a specialized milk thistle product containing standardized silibinin with phosphatidylcholine (to improve bioavailability) for 28 days, had significantly lower **aspartate aminotransferase** (AST) at 56 days but not at 28 days;[145] the supplement was thought to be tolerated, and did not appear to compromise the chemotherapy.

Adverse reactions reported include occasional gastrointestinal distress, headache and allergic reactions.[142] Although clinical trials do not provide a significant safety profile in children, milk thistle has long been use as a food.[146]

Peppermint (Mentha x piperita) is a perennial herb in the mint family grown throughout Europe, North America, also found in Africa.[147] Mint was used thousands of years ago as a digestive aid and for cough and cold,[148] with records of use noted in ancient Greece, Rome, and Egypt.[149] Peppermint is used in food and beverages, as a flavoring or scent in many non-food products, in aromatherapy to reduce stress and improve cognitive function, as well as topically and orally for anti-inflammatory, analgesic, antispasmodic, and other effects.[150] Peppermint oil is the essential oil extracted from the above ground parts of the plant; it is composed of a mixture of compounds, primarily menthol (at least 44% in pharmaceutical grade peppermint oil) and menthone; peppermint oil also contains <1–4% pugelone, a chemical concerning for toxic effects, is less if the oil is made with mature leaves.[146,150] Menthol is thought to be responsible for the antispasmodic effects seen in IBS, by blocking the calcium channels that effect motility.[150]

Some evidence suggests topical peppermint oil may help relieve tension headaches, may be possibly effective when used for barium-enema colonic spasm, or in patients undergoing endoscopy, and several studies have shown enteric-coated peppermint oil may improve IBS symptoms.[150] A few studies have investigated the use of enteric-coated peppermint oil in children. A trial completed by 88 children 4–13 years of age with functional abdominal pain, included a treatment arm with enteric coated peppermint 187 or 374 mg (upper end used for patients over 45 kg) 30 minutes before meals, three times daily; compared with placebo (folic acid), the peppermint oil decreased pain duration, frequency as well as severity of pain, and compared to a probiotic/prebiotic supplement, decreased pain duration and severity; no side effects were reported.[151]

Adverse effects reported with the use of peppermint oil include allergic reactions, perianal burning (enteric-coated form), abdominal pain, vomiting, chemical burns with large amounts of pure oil, and heartburn, which may be ameliorated by using enteric-coated capsules unless these are taken with antacids.[150] Peppermint oil should not be used topically on infants or young children around the nasal area or chest due to risk of bronchospasm and possible respiratory arrest. Additionally, is not recommended with cholelithiasis or cholecystitis.[148,152] Enteric-coated peppermint may be safe under medical supervision in older children;[150,152] use in infants and young children is not recommended.[148]

Curcumin is the active yellow pigment of the spice, turmeric. It is an herb belonging to the ginger family native to India and Southeast Asia. Curcumin is commonly used in Indian traditional cuisine and medicine. It has been found to have anti-inflammatory, anti-oxidant, and anti-tumor effects. Curcumin activity includes suppressing interleukin-1 (IL-1) and tumor necrosis factor alpha (TNF α), two main cytokines that play an important role in the regulation of inflammatory responses. Curcumin has been used to treat both **ulcerative colitis** (UC) and **Crohn's disease** (CD) although studies have been mainly performed in adults.

A 2012 Cochrane review found curcumin is a safe and effective therapy for maintenance of remission in quiescent UC when given as adjunctive therapy along with mesalamine or sulfasalazine. A multicenter randomized double blind Japanese study, evaluated eighty-nine patients who were randomized to receive either curcumin (1 g twice daily) or placebo, in addition to sulfasalazine or mesalamine, for 6 months. The relapse rate was significantly lower in the curcumin group, 4.7% compared with placebo 20.5%, $p = 0.04$.[153] This was reinforced by a multi-center double blind randomized control trial, which evaluated 50 patients with active mild-moderate UC on 5-ASA who did not respond to 2 weeks of max 5-ASA oral and topical therapy. Patients were randomly assigned to curcumin 3g/d (n = 26) or placebo (n = 24) × 4 weeks. Clinical response (reduction of ≥3 points in **simple clinical colitis activity index** (SCCAI)) was achieved by 17 patients (65.3%) in the curcumin group vs. 3 patients (12.5%) in the placebo group ($p < 0.001$). Endoscopic remission was observed in 8 of the 22 patients evaluated in the curcumin group (38%), compared with 0 of 16 patients evaluated in the placebo group.[154] Curcumin has been also evaluated in Crohn's disease. A pilot study of five patients demonstrated that intake of 360 mg of curcumin three times a day could help decrease inflammatory markers and clinical symptoms.[155] A pediatric tolerability study was performed in 11 patients with mild UC or CD. Three patients had a decrease in their clinical symptoms scores and none had a relapse or worsening of symptoms.[156] Side effects of curcumin use include dyspepsia, diarrhea, distension, reflux, gassiness, nausea, and vomiting. It also has been found to interact with anti-coagulants, hypoglycemic medications and iron, as well as increase sulfasalazine

levels. Thus this must be discontinued at least 2 weeks before any surgery.

▶ Additional Biologic Therapies

Omega 3 polyunsaturated fatty acids (n-3 PUFAs) H4 are a type of **polyunsaturated fatty acid** (PUFA) found in fish and fish oil, nuts, and seeds. Examples include **alpha-linolenic acid** (ALA) **docosahexanenoic acid** (DHA) and **eicosapentaenoic acid** (EPA). EPA is the most common storage form of fatty acids and converts to DHA as needed.[157] It has been found to have anti-inflammatory and immunomodulatory properties. Fatty fish such as salmon and tuna are rich in omega 3 **free fatty acids** (FFA). Omega 3's have been used in the context of treating ADHD, allergy and asthma in children.

It has been shown that there is an association between n-3 PUFA supplementation and reduction of ADHD symptoms.[157,158] A recent meta-analysis of randomized, double-blind, placebo-controlled studies in subjects aged 4–17 with ADHD showed that per parental report DHA supplementation significantly improved both overall behavioral symptoms, inattention, and hyperactivity.[157] DHA supplementation also had an effect on scores using the Conner's cognition subscale and the Conner's DSM-IV inattention subscale.[157] The same meta-analysis found that total ADHD score and inattention were improved with EPA supplementation.

Cohort studies have shown that infants and children who consumed fish experienced a reduction in allergies.[159-162] Studies have also shown that infants and children of lactating or pregnant women who were supplemented with DHA experienced less asthma and allergy symptoms.[159-164] Although supplementing with fish oil to increase consumption of n-3 PUFAs can be beneficial, it is recommended that young children limit fish intake due to concerns of higher mercury seen in fish such as tuna. An alternative is ALA, which is found in nuts and seeds. Using Omega 3 FFA is generally safe but side effects may include a fishy after taste, nausea, diarrhea, and heartburn. Fish oil can have additive anticoagulant/antiplatelet effects and interact with NSAIDS and may potentiate some of the adverse effects of glucocorticoids.

Pre/probiotics

Prebiotics are nondigestible food ingredients that promote the growth of limited strains of (probiotic) bacteria in the human body, e.g., fructo-oligosaccharides, galacto oligosaccharides, and gluco- and xylo-oligosaccharides. Probiotics are live microorganisms capable of surviving and inducing a beneficial effect in the host. Diet influences the composition of the gut microbiome, likely inducing an effect on the functional capacity of the gut;

studies have found that in the pediatric population diet dictates which bacteria flourish in the gut.[165] Differences in diet can be attributed to both cultural and regional preferences. The combination of probiotics, prebiotics and dietary interventions can eventually induce a shift in the gut microbiome but this may take months to years to induce such a change.[165] In addition to improving microbiome diversity it is surmised that probiotics stimulate the immune system, triggering healing in the gut. Pre and Probiotics have been used for gastrointestinal conditions such as necrotizing enterocolitis, clostridium difficile, and inflammatory bowel disease.[166]

It has been demonstrated that the gut microbiome of infants who develop **necrotizing enterocolitis** (NEC) has more gamma Proteobacteria than those who do not develop NEC.[167,168] In addition to breast milk consumption, probiotics have reduced the development of severe NEC as well as all-cause mortality in premature infants.[167,169–172] Probiotics have also been shown to treat recurrent C. difficile,[165,169–175] which has been associated with limited microbial diversity in the gut.[165,176] Meta analyses have shown that administration of lactobacillus GG in the pediatric population reduced antibiotic-associated diarrhea by 60%.[167,177,178] Studies have shown that probiotics including lactobacillus GG have alleviated symptoms and shortened disease course in patients with bacterial or viral gastroenteritis, although these results were not always replicable.[165,167,179,180]

As dietary supplements, pre- and probiotics have the potential to transform the gut microbiome and reduce symptoms of disease. However, more definitive studies are needed to prove the efficacy of probiotic administration in reducing gastrointestinal symptoms, as studies utilize different probiotics and use different treatment protocols. As with any biologically based approach to health, in infants and children growth should be monitored to determine supplement efficacy and ensure normal development.

▶ Monitoring Growth

An important consideration when using a dietary approach to health in the pediatric population is maintaining appropriate growth for age. Depending on the diet used, micro and/or macronutrient deficiencies could develop, impeding appropriate growth and development. Therefore, it is important to ensure families participate in regular follow up visits with both their primary provider and dietitian.

▶ Conclusion

Nutrition and diet are important components of health promotion and therapy. Research is ongoing. We are learning more about the role of nutrition in health and disease prevention with validation of what different cultures have known for centuries. Despite these proposed dietary approaches to illness, higher quality studies, specifically in pediatrics are needed before widespread implementation. Maintaining a cursory level of understanding and awareness of the different Integrative health modalities, including knowledge of efficacy, indications, contraindications, and possible nutritional deficiencies are essential to ensure patient safety. This will facilitate an open practitioner-client relationship and support the practitioner's ability to educate their patients and families about the power of food. Developing healthy eating habits in childhood will lay down the foundation for good health later on in life. Knowing this, Integrative health and nutrition hold much promise for the future.

🔍 CASE STUDY

History

AA is a 12 year old F presenting to clinic with a history of abdominal pain, diarrhea, and gassiness that has been occurring for the past year. Abdominal pain is generalized in nature and occurs mostly during school days and seems to worsen during high periods of stress. This is associated with diarrhea, which may vary from 4–10 times per day, usually watery, non-foul smelling with no mucus or blood seen in the stool. Diarrhea increases with food intake but the family has not been able to identify which types of foods make it worse. The family also notes that AA seems to have issues with intermittent abdominal distention and excessive gassiness. They have attempted restricting lactose in the diet with no improvement of symptoms. They have also tried restricting gluten from the diet with minimal success. Due to current symptoms AA has been limiting her overall intake, with noted weight loss, due to fear of having these symptoms at school. AA is currently taking a proton pump inhibitor, an antispasmodic and probiotic with only minimal improvement in symptoms. Denies bullying at school but mom reports AA is a high achiever and seems to have an anxious personality. Denies family history of IBD, celiac, or thyroid disease in the family. Denies any recent travel or sick contacts. Is not taking any medications except as stated above. She has missed many days in school and this has been making her even more anxious. Family is now interested in a low FODMAPS diet that has been mentioned by their GI provider.

(continues)

⌕ CASE STUDY

Work Up Included

- CBC with diff, thyroid studies, CMP, inflammatory markers, celiac panel- normal
- Infectious stool studies and fecal calprotectin- normal
- Low vitamin 25-OH
- Abdominal ultrasound- normal
- Physical Examination: normal except for minimal subcutaneous stores with normal muscle mass

Diagnosis Per MD

Irritable bowel syndrome–diarrhea type
Assessment:
Age: 12 years
Sex: Female
Weight: 35 kg
Length: 152 cm
Weight for age z-score: −0.97
Length for age z-score: 0.03
BMI z-score: −1.48
Weight gain velocity percentage of the norm: 0% (weight loss of 2 kg in the past 3 months); length appears to be tracking.
Estimated nutrient intake: 1200 kcal, 50 grams protein
Estimated nutrient needs:
Energy: low energy/activity noted
RDA: TEE: 1645 kcal
DRI: TEE: 1844 kcal (using PA 1.16)
Schofield: BMR = 1200 × activity factor 1.5 = 1800 kcal
WHO: REE 1173 × activity factor 1.5 = 1760 kcal
Protein:
RDA: 1 gm/kg/day
DRI: 0.95 gm/kg/day
Percentage of nutrient intake of estimated needs: Energy intake based on DRI = 65% (additional kcal may be required for catch-up). Protein intake based on DRI = 150%.

Nutrition Diagnosis

Mild malnutrition related to suspected decreased calorie intake in the setting of GI symptoms and what appears to be restricted oral intake as evidenced by 5% weight loss from usual body weight in 3 months and based on BMI z-score > −1.0 – 1.99

Discussion

Diet was reviewed and notable for including several foods considered as high FODMAPs including fruits such as apples and pears, vegetables such as cauliflower and broccoli, fruit juice in smoothies (2 cups daily), honey daily, beans, dairy including milk and other, and wheat. Patient avoids eating fast food, greasy foods or sweets and is interested in eating "healthier". Previous attempt to restrict gluten and dairy was not reported to result in a significant improvement in symptoms. Diet history notable for skipping meals during school for fear of GI symptoms, limiting portions, and restrictions as above.

As the use of a low FODMAPs diet in children is not a standard of care for IBS treatment, it would be warranted to discuss concerns with further restriction. If the family would like to try FODMAPs restrictions, under the care of a GI provider, the restricted diet should be monitored for nutritional adequacy and appropriate liberalization or discontinuation if failed response.

Low vitamin D level noted, with supplementation started 1 month ago as recommended by MD, plan noted to recheck level at GI follow-up.

Intervention

Discussed patient with the GI provider before the visit, who thought that it was appropriate to try to limit FODMAP intake without recommending the full restrictions of the low FODMAPs diet. High FODMAPs foods were identified in the diet history. Discussed with the family recommendations to eliminate the apple juice, choose lower FODMAPs fruits/vegetables (provided examples), limit intake of honey, consider switch to lactose free milk and continue to include yogurt in diet, and limit intake of beans for one month. At the GI follow-up visit, discuss restrictions and clinical concerns with provider.

Encouraged patient to avoid skipping meals and increase portions as able; discussed nutrient dense (high calorie) foods to include in diet.

Monitoring and Evaluation

Weight gain velocity- monitor for nutritional adequacy per concern for weight and BMI decrease. Plan per GI provider for follow-up 1 month.

Questions

1. Other than micronutrient deficiencies, what other concerns are there for restricted diets in children, especially for this patient?
2. What would you recommend for calorie intake?
3. What would be an appropriate goal for weight gain?

References

1. U.S. Department of Health & Human Services, National Institutes of Health. Complementary, alternative, or integrative health: what's in a name? Available at: https://nccih.nih.gov/sites/nccam.nih.gov/files/Whats_In_A_Name_06-16-2016/pdf.
2. National Institutes of Health, National Center for Complementary and Integrative Health. What Complementary and Integrative Approaches do Americans Use? https://nccih.nih.gov/research/statistics/NHIS/2012/key-findings.
3. Black LI, Clarke TC, Barnes PM, et al. Use of complementary health approaches among children aged 4–17 years in the United States: National Health Interview Survey, 2007–2012. *Nat Health Stat Report*. 2015;10(78):1–19.
4. Kagalwalla AF, Sentongo TA, Ritz S, et al. Effect of six-food elimination diet on clinical and histologic outcomes in eosinophilic esophagitis. *Clin Gastroenterol Hepatol*. 2006; 4:1097–1102.
5. Kagalwalla A, Wechsler JB, Amsden K et al. Efficacy of a 4-food elimination diet for children with Eosinophilic Esophagitis. Clin Gastroenterol Hepatol. 2017; 15(11):1698–1707.
6. Egger J, Carter CM, Wilson J, Turner MW, Soothill JF. Is migraine food allergy? A double-blind controlled trial of oligoantigenic diet treatment. Lancet. 1983; 2:865–869.
7. Egger J, Carter CM, Soothill JF, Wilson J. Oligoantigenic diet treatment of children with epilepsy and migraine. *J Pediatr*. 1989;114:51–58.
8. Millichap J, Lee MM. The diet factor in pediatric and adolescent migraine. Pediatr Neurol. 28(1):9–15.
9. Pelsser LM et al. A randomized controlled trial on the effects of food on ADHD. Eur *Child Adolesc Psychiatry*. 2009;18(1):12–19.
10. Hoffmann KM, Gruber E, Deutschmann A, Jahnel J, Hauer AC. Histamine intolerance in children with chronic abdominal pain. *Archives of Disease in Childhood*. 2014;98(10):832–833.
11. Kovacova-Hanuskova E, Buday T, Gavliakova S, Plevkova J. Histamine, histamine intoxication and intolerance. *Allergologia et Immunopathologia*. 2015;43(5): 498–506.
12. Rosell-Camps A, Zibetti S, Pérez-Esteban G, Vila-Vidal M, Ferrés-Ramis L, García-Teresa-García E. Histamine intolerance as a cause of chronic digestive complaints in pediatric patients. Revista Española de Enfermedades Digestivas. 2013;105(4): 201–207.
13. Visciano P, Schirone M, Tofalo R, Suzzi, G. Histamine poisoning and control measures in fish and fishery products. *Frontiers in Microbiology*. 2014; 5. doi:10.3389/fmicb.2014.0050.
14. Roehl K, Sewak S L. Practice Paper of the Academy of Nutrition and Dietetics: Classic and Modified Ketogenic Diets for Treatment of Epilepsy. *J Acad Nutr Diet*. 2017;117(8): 1279–292.
15. Neal EG, Chaffe H, Schwartz RH, et al. The ketogenic diet for the treatment of childhood epilepsy: A randomized controlled trial. *Lancet Neurol*. 2008;7(6):500–506.
16. Martin K, Jackson CF, Levy RG, Cooper PN. Ketogenic diet and other dietary treatments for epilepsy. *Cochrane Database Syst Rev*. 2016; 2:CD001903.
17. Prezioso G, Carlone G, Zaccara G, Verrotti A. Efficacy of ketogenic diet for infantile spasms: A systematic review. *Acta Neurologica Scandinavica*. 2017;137(1): 4–11.
18. Cervenka MC, Kossoff EH. Dietary treatment of intractable epilepsy. *Continuum (Minneap, Minn)*. 2013;19 (3 Epilepsy):756–766.
19. Klein P, Janousek J, Barber A, Weissberger R. Ketogenic diet treatment in adults with refractory epilepsy. *Epilepsy Behav*. 2010;19(4):575–579.
20. Bough KJ, Rho JM. Anticonvulsant mechanisms of the ketogenic diet. *Epilepsia*. 2007;48(1):43–58.
21. Ma W, Berg J, Yellen G. Ketogenic diet metabolites reduce firing in central neurons by opening KATP channels. *J Neurosci*. 2007;27(14):3618–3625.
22. Yudkoff M, Daikhin Y, Nissim I, et al. Response of brain amino acid metabolism to ketosis. *Neurochem Int*. 2005;47(1–2):119–128.
23. Rubio-Tapia A, Hill ID, Kelly CP, Calderwood AH, Murray JA, American College of Gastroenterology. ACG clinical guidelines: diagnosis and management of celiac disease. *Am J Gastroenterol*. 2013;108(5):656–676.
24. Sey MS, Par tt J, Gregor J. Prospective study of clinical and histological safety of pure and uncontaminated Canadian oats in the management of celiac disease. *J Parenter Enteral Nutr*. 2011;35:459–464.

25. Markku, M. Celiac disease treatment: gluten-free diet and beyond. *J Pediatr Gastroenterol Nutr.* 2014; 59: 15–1.

26. Leonard M, Sapone A. et al. Celiac disease and nonceliac gluten sensitivity. JAMA .2017;318(7):647–656.

27. Sansotta N, Amirikian K, Guandalini S, Jericho H. Celiac disease symptom resolution: effectiveness of the gluten free diet. J Pediatr Gastroenterol Nutr. 2018;66(1):48–52.

28. Hidvegi, E, Cserhati E, Kereki E, Arato A. et al. Serum immunoglobulin E, IgA, and IgG antibodies to different cow's milk proteins in children with cow's milk allergy: Association with prognosis and clinical manifestations. *Pediatr Allergy Immunol.* 2002; 13:255–261.

29. Keller KM, Burgin-Wolf A, Lippold R, Lentze MJ. Quality assurance in diagnostics: Are there normal values for IgG-antibodies to cow's milk proteins? *Klin Paediatr.* 1999:211:384–388.

30. Juvonen P, Mansson M, Kjellman NI, Bjorksten B, Jakobsson I. Development of immunoglobulin G and immunoglobulin E antibodies to cow's milk proteins and ovalbumin after a temporary neonatal exposure to hydrolyzed and whole cow's milk proteins. *Pediatr Allergy Immunol.* 1999; 10:191–198.

31. Saarinen KM, Juntunen-Backman K, Jarvenpaa AL, et al. Supplementary feeding in maternity hospitals and the risk of cow's milk allergy: A prospective study of 6209 infants. *J Allergy Clin Immunol.* 1999;104:457–461.

32. Piwowarczyk A, Horvath A, Lukasik J, Pisula E, Szajewska H. Gluten- and casein-free diet and autism spectrum disorders in children: a systematic review. *Eur J Nutr.* 2017;57(2):433–440.

33. Mari-Bauset S Zazpe I, Mari-Sanchis A, Llopis-Gonzalez A, Morales Suarez-Varela M.,. Evidence of the gluten-free and casein-free diet in autism spectrum disorders: a systematic review. *J Child Neurol.* 2014;29(12):1718–1727.

34. Feingold BF. Hyperkinesis and learning disabilities linked to artificial food flavors and colors. *Am J Nurs.* 1975;75(5):797–803.

35. Kavale KA, Forness SR. Hyperactivity and diet treatment: a meta-analysis of the Feingold hypothesis. *J Learn Disabil.* 1983;16(6):324–30.

36. Feingold BF. The role of diet in behaviour. *Ecol Dis.* 1982; 1:153–165.

37. McCann D, Barrett A, Cooper A, et al. Food additives and hyperactive behavior in 3-year-old and 8/9-year-old children in the community: a randomized, double-blinded, placebo-controlled trial. *Lancet.* 2007;370:1560–156.

38. Lehto S, Buchweitz M, Klimm A, et al. Comparison of food colour regulations in the EU and the U.S.: a review of current provisions. *Food Addit Contam.* 2017;34(3):335–355.

39. U.S. Food and Drug Administration. Color Additives. 2017 Available at: https://www.fda.gov/ForIndustry/ColorAdditives.

40. European Parliament [news release]. Modernising the rules on food additives and labelling of azo dyes. July 8, 2008. Available at: http://www.europarl.europa.eu/sides/getDoc.do?type=IM-PRESS&reference=20080707IPR33563&language=EN. Accessed November 10, 2017.

41. Kanarek RB. Artificial food dyes and attention deficit hyperactivity disorder. *Nutr Rev.* 2011;69:385–391.

42. Schab DW, Trinh NT. Do artificial food colours promote hyperactivity in children with hyperactive syndromes? A meta-analysis of double-blind placebo-controlled trials. *J Dev Behav Pediatr.* 2004;25:423–434.

43. Nigg JT, Lewis K, Edinger T, Falk M. Meta-analysis of attention-deficit/hyperactivity disorder or attention-deficit/hyperactivity disorder symptoms, restriction diet, and synthetic food color additives. *J Am Acad Child Adolesc Psych.* 2012;51(1):86–97.

44. Rojas NL, Chan E. Old and new controversies in the alternative treatment of attention-deficit hyperactivity disorder. *Ment Retard Dev Disabil Res Rev.* 2005; 11: 116–130.

45. Nigg JT, Holton K. Restriction and elimination diets in ADHD treatment. *Child Adolesc Psychiatr Clin N Am.* 2014;23(4):937–953.

46. Stevens LJ, Burgess JR, Stochelski MA, Kuczek T. Amounts of artificial food dyes and added sugars in foods and sweets commonly consumed by children. *Clin. Pediatr.* 2015;54:309–321.

47. Gibson P, Shepherd SJ. Personal view: Food for thought—Western lifestyle and susceptibility to Crohn's disease. The FODMAP hypothesis. *Aliment Pharmacol Ther.* 2005; 21:1399–1409.

48. Gibson, PR. History of the low FODMAP diet. *J Gastroenterol Hepatol.* 2017;32:5–7.

49. Spiller R. How do FODMAPS work? *J Gastroenterol Hepatol.* 2017;32 (suppl 1):36–39.

50. Barrett, JS. How to institute the low-FODMAP diet. *J Gastroenterol Hepatol.* 2017; 32:8–10.

51. Chumpitazi BP, Cope JL, Hollister EB, et al. Randomised clinical trial: gut microbiome biomarkers are associated with clinical response to a low FODMAP Diet in children with Irritable Bowel Syndrome. *Alimentary Pharmacol Ther.* 2015;42(4):418–427.

52. Hill P, Muir JG, Gibson PR. Controversies and recent developments of the Low-FODMAP Diet. *Gastroenterol & Hepatol.* 2017; 13(1):36–45.

53. Marsh A, Eslick E.M, Eslick G.D. Does a diet low in FODMAPs reduce symptoms associated with functional gastrointestinal disorders? A comprehensive systematic review and meta-analysis. *Eur. J. Nutr.* 2016;55:897–906.

54. Gibson PR. The evidence base for efficacy of the low FODMAP diet in irritable bowel syndrome: is it ready for prime time as a first-line therapy? *J. Gastroenterol. Hepatol.* 2017;32:32–35.

55. Newlove-Delgado TV, Martin AE, Abbott RA et al. Dietary interventions for recurrent abdominal pain in childhood. *Cochrane Database Syst Rev.* 2017;23(3): CD010972.

56. Wilson K, Hill RJ. The role of food intolerance in functional gastrointestinal disorders in children. *Aust Fam Physician.* 2014.;43(10):686–689.

57. Staudacher HM, Whelan K. The low FODMAP diet: recent advances in understanding its mechanisms and efficacy in IBS. *Gut.* 2017;66:1517–1515.

58. Iacovou M. Adapting the low FODMAP diet to special populations: infants and children. *J Gastroenterol Hepatol.* 2017;32(suppl1):43–45

59. Willcox DC, Scapagnini G, Willcox BJ. Healthy aging diets other than the Mediterranean: a focus on the Okinawan diet. *Mech Ageing Dev.* 2014;136:148–162.

60. Cordain L, Eaton SB, Sebastian A, et al. Origins and evolution of the Western diet: health implications for the 21st century. *Am J Clin Nutr.* 2005;81:341–354.

61. Bach-Faig A, Berry EM, Lairon D, et al. Mediterranean diet pyramid today. Science and cultural updates. *Public Health Nutr.* 2011;14:2274–2284.

62. Katz DL, Meller S. Can we say what diet is best for health? *Annu Rev Public Health.* 2014;35(1):83–103.

63. Parkinson L, Keast R. Oleocanthal. A phenolic derived from virgin olive oil: a review of the beneficial effects on Inflammatory Disease. *Int J Mol Sci.* 2014;15(7):12323–12334.

64. Seguí-Gómez M, de la Fuente C, Vázquez Z, de Irala J, Martinez-Gonzalez MA. Cohort profile: the 'Seguimiento Universidad de Navarra' (SUN) study. *Int J Epidemiol.* 2006;35:1417–1422.

65. Rumawas ME, Meigs JB, Dwyer JT, McKeown NM, Jacques PF. Mediterranean-style dietary pattern, reduced risk of metabolic syndrome traits, and incidence in the Framingham Offspring Cohort. *Am J Clin Nutr.* 2009;90(6):1608–1614.

66. Esposito K, Marfella R, Ciotola M, et al. Effects of a Meditereanean-style diet on endothelial dysfunction and markers of vascular inflammation in the metabolic syndrome. *J Am Med Assoc.* 2004;292(12):1440–1446.

67. Kastorini CM, Milionis HJ, Esposito K, Giugliano D, Goudevenos JA, Panagiotakos DB. The effect of mediterranean diet on metabolic syndrome and its components: A meta-analysis of 50 studies and 534,906 individuals. *J Am Coll Cardiol.* 2011;57(11):1299–1313.

68. Sofi F, Cesari F, Abbate R, Gensini GF, Casini A. Adherence to Mediterranean diet and health status: meta-analysis. BMJ. 2008;337:a1344.

69. Opie RS, Itsiopoulos C, Parletta N, Sanchez-Villegas A, Akbaraly TN, Ruusunen A, et al. Dietary recommendations for the prevention of depression. *Nutr. Neurosci.* 2017;20:161–171.

70. Calder PC, Albers R, Antoine JM, et al. Inflammatory disease processes and interactions with nutrition. *Br. J. Nutr.* 2009;101:S1–S45.

71. Galland L. Diet and inflammation. *Nutr Clin Pract.* 2010;25(6):634–640.

72. Barbaresko J, Koch M, Schulze MB, Nothlings U. Dietary pattern analysis and biomarkers of low-grade inflammation: a systematic literature review. *Nutr. Rev.* 2013;71:511–527.

73. Nigro E, Scudiero O, Monaco ML, et al. New insight into adiponectin role in obesity and obesity-related diseases. *BioMed Res Int.* 2014;2014:658913.

74. Holt EM, Steffen LM, Moran A, Basu S, Steinberger J, Ross J A, et al. Fruit and vegetable consumption and its relation to markers of inflammation and oxidative stress in adolescents. *J. Am. Diet. Assoc.* 2009;109:414–421.

75. Qureshi MM, Singer MR, Moore LL. A cross-sectional study of food group intake and C-reactive protein among children. *Nutr & Metab.* 2009; 6:40.

76. Papamichael M, Itsiopoulos C, Susanto N, Erbas, B. Does adherence to the Mediterranean dietary pattern reduce asthma symptoms in children? a systematic review of observational studies. *Public Health Nutrition.* 2017;20(15): 2722–2734.

77. Castro-Rodriguez JA, Garcia-Marcos L. What are the effects of a Mediterranean Diet on Allergies and Asthma in Children? *Frontiers in Pediatr.* 2017;5:72.

78. Chatzi L, Torrent M, Romieu I, et al. Mediterranean diet in pregnancy is protective for wheeze and atopy in childhood. *Thorax.* 2008;63:507–513.

79. Shaheen SO, Northstone K, Newson RB, Emmett PM, Sherriff A, Henderson AJ Dietary patterns in pregnancy and respiratory and atopic outcomes in childhood. *Thorax.* 2009;64(5):411–417.

80. Nguyen AN, Elbert NJ, Pasmans SGMA, et al. Diet quality throughout early life in relation to allergic sensitization and atopic diseases in childhood. *Nutrients.* 2017;9(8):841.

81. Giannini C, Diesse L, D'Adamo E et al. Influence of the Mediterranean diet on carotid intima-media thickness in hypercholesterolaemic children: a 12-month intervention study. *Nutr Metab Cardiovasc Dis.* 2014;24:75–82.

82. Lydakis C, Stefanaki E, Stefanaki S, Thalassinos E, Kavousanaki M, Lydaki D. Correlation of blood pressure, obesity, and adherence to the Mediterranean diet with indices of arterial stiffness in children. *Eur J Pediatr.* 2012;171:1373–1382.

83. Stoner L, Weatherall M, Skidmore P, et al. Cardiometabolic risk variables in preadolescent children: a factor analysis. *JAHA.* 2017;6(10).

84. Berenson GS. Cardiovascular risk begins in childhood. *Am J Prev Med.* 2009;37(1):S1–2.

85. Esposito K, Marfella R, Ciotola M, et al. Effects of a Meditereanean-style diet on endothelial dysfunction and markers of vascular inflammation in the metabolic syndrome. *J Am Med Assoc.* 2004; 292(12):1440–1446.

86. Funtikova AN, Navarro E, Bawaked RA, Fíto M, Schröder H. Impact of diet on cardiometabolic health in children and adolescents. *Nutr J.* 2015;14:118.

87. Velázquez-López L, Santiago-Díaz G, Nava-Hernández J, Muñoz-Torres AV, Medina-Bravo P, Torres-Tamayo M. Mediterranean-style diet reduces metabolic syndrome components in obese children and adolescents with obesity. *BMC Pediatr.* 2014;14:175.

88. Cakir M., Akbulut UE, Okten A. Association between adherence to the mediterranean diet and presence of nonalcoholic fatty liver disease in children. *Child Obes.* 2016;12:279–285.

89. Della Corte C, et al. Good adherence to the Mediterranean diet reduces the risk for NASH and diabetes in pediatric patients with obesity: The results of an Italian Study. *Nutr.* 2017;39:8–14.

90. Tognon G., Moreno LA, Mouratidou T, et al. Adherence to a Mediterranean-like dietary pattern in children from eight European countries. The IDEFICS study. *Int. J. Obes.* 2014;38:108–114.

91. Singh O, Khanam Z, Misra N, Srivastava MK. Chamomile (Matricaria chamomilla L.): An overview. *Pharmacogn Rev.* 2011;5(9):82–95.

92. Srivastava JK, Shankar E, Gupta S. Chamomile: A herbal medicine of the past with bright future. *Mol Med Report.* 2010;3(6):895–901.

93. Natural Medicines. German chamomile [Monograph]. Available at: https://naturalmedicines-therapeuticsresearch-com. Accessed December 4, 2107.

94. Natural Medicines. Roman chamomile [Monograph]. Available at: https://naturalmedicines-therapeuticsresearch-com. Accessed December 4, 2107.

95. Matricaria chamomilla (German chamomile). Monograph. *Altern Med Rev.* 2008.; 13(1):58–62.

96. WHO. Flos Chamomillae. WHO monographs on selected medicinal plants - Volume 1. Available at: http://apps.who.int/medicinedocs/pdf/s2200e/s2200e.pdf. 1999:86–93.

97. Weizman Z, Alkrinawi S, Goldfarb D, et al. Efficacy of herbal tea preparation in infantile colic. *J Pediatr.* 1993;122(4):650–652.

98. Savino F, Cresi F, Castagno E, et al. A randomized double-blind placebo-controlled trial of a standardized extract

of Matricariae recutita, Foeniculum vulgare and Melissa officinalis (ColiMil) in the treatment of breastfed colicky infants. *Phytother Res*.2005;19:335–340.

99. Alexandrovich I, Rakovitskaya O, Kolmo E, Sidorova T, Shushunov S. The effect of fennel (Foeniculum vulgare) seed oil emulsion in infantile colic: a randomized, placebo-controlled study. *Altern Ther Health Med*. 2003; 9(4):58–61.

100. Biagioli E, Tarasco V, Lingua C, Moja L, Savino F. Pain-relieving agents for infantile colic. *Cochrane Database Syst Rev*. 2016;9:CD009999.

101. Becker B, Kuhn U, Hardewig-Budny B. Double-blind, randomized evaluation of clinical efficacy and tolerability of an apple pectin-chamomile extract in children with unspecific diarrhea. Arzneimittelforschung. 2006;56(6):387–393.

102. De la Motte S, Bose-O'Reilly S, Heinisch M, Harrison F. Double-blind comparison of an apple pectin-chamomile extract preparation with placebo in children with diarrhea. *Arzneimittelforschung*. 1997;47(11):1247–1249.

103. Rabbani GH, Teka T, Zaman B, et al. Clinical studies in persistent diarrhea: dietary management with green banana or pectin in Bangladeshi children. *Gastroenterol*. 2001; 121:554–560.

104. Gardiner P. Complementary, holistic, and integrative medicine: chamomile. Pediatr Rev. 2007;28(4).

105. National Center for Complementary and Alternative Medicine. Available at: https://nccih.nih.gov/health/cranberry. Accessed December 4, 2017.

106. Klein MA. Cranberry. In: Coates PM, Betz JM, Blackman MR, et al., eds. *Encyclopedia of Dietary Supplements*. 2nd ed. New York, NY: Informa Healthcare; 2010:193–201.

107. Gu L, Kelm MA, Hammerstone JF, et al. Concentrations of proanthocyanidins in common foods and estimations of normal consumption. *J Nutr*. 2004;134:613–617.

108. Natural Medicines. Cranberry [Monograph]. Available at: https://naturalmedicines-therapeuticsresearch-com. Accessed December 4, 2107.

109. Howell AB, Reed JD, Krueger CG, Winterbottom R, Cunningham DG, Leahy M. A-type cranberry proanthocyanidins and uropathogenic bacterial anti-adhesion activity. *Phytochemistry*. 2005; 66(18):2281–2291.

110. Afshar K, Stothers L, Scott H, MacNeily AE. Cranberry juice for the prevention of pediatric urinary tract infection: a randomized controlled trial. *J Urol*. 2012;188:1584–1587.

111. Salo J, Uhari M, Helminen M, et al. Cranberry juice for the prevention of recurrences of Urinary Tract Infections in Children: A Randomized Placebo-Controlled Trial. *Clin Infect Dis*. 2012;54(3): 340–346.

112. Luís Â, Domingues F, Pereira L. Can cranberries contribute to reduce the incidence of urinary tract infections? A systematic review with meta-analysis and trial sequential analysis of clinical trials. *J Urol*. 2017;198(3):614–621.

113. Jepson RG, Williams G, Craig JC. Cranberries for preventing urinary tract infections. *Cochrane Database Syst Rev*. 2012;(10):CD001321.

114. Wang CH, Fang CC, Chen NC, et al. Cranberry-containing products for prevention of Urinary Tract Infections in susceptible populations: a Systematic Review and Meta-analysis of Randomized Controlled Trials. *Arch Intern Med*. 2012;172(13):988–996.

115. Heyman M, Abrams SA. Fruit Juice in Infants, Children, and Adolescents: Current Recommendations. Section on Gastroenterology, Hepatology, and Nutrition, Committee on Nutrition. *Pediatr*. 2017;139(6): doi:10.1542/peds. 2017-0967.

116. National Center for Complementary and Alternative Medicine. Available at: https://nccih.nih.gov/health/echinacea /ataglance.htm. Accessed December 4, 2017.

117. Natural Medicines Echinacea [Monograph]. Available at: https://naturalmedicines-therapeuticsresearch-com. Accessed December 4, 2107.

118. Speroni E, Govoni P, Guizzardi S, et al. Anti-inflammatory and cicatrizing activity of Echinacea pallida Nutt. root extract. *J Ethnopharmacol*. 2002;79:265–272.

119. Karsch-Völk M, Barrett B, Kiefer D, Bauer R, Ardjomand-Woelkart K, Linde K. Echinacea for preventing and treating the common cold. *Cochrane Database Syst Rev*. 2014;2:CD000530.

120. Taylor JA, et al. Efficacy and safety of Echinacea in treating upper respiratory tract infections in children: a randomized controlled trial. *JAMA*. 2003;290:2824–2830.

121. Lawrenson JA, Walls T, Day AS. Echinacea-induced acute liver failure in a child. *J Paediatr Child Health*. 2014;50(10):841.

122. European Medicines Agency. Community Herbal Monograph on Echinacea purpurea L. Committee on Herbal Medicinal Products (HMPC). London, England: 2015; Contract No: EMA/HMPC/48704/2014.

123. Bauer R, Woelkart K. Echineaca. In: Coates PM, Betz JM, Blackman MR, et al., eds. *Encyclopedia of Dietary Supplements*. 2nd ed. New York, NY: Informa Healthcare; 2010: 226–234.

124. Natural Medicines. Elderberry [Monograph]. Available at: https://naturalmedicines-therapeuticsresearch-com. Accessed December 1, 2107.

125. WHO.WHO monographs on selected medicinal plants - Volume 2. Available at: http://apps.who.int/medicinedocs /en/d/Js4927e/26.html. Accessed December 2, 2017.

126. Alt Med Review. Sambucus nigra (Elderberry) [Monograph] Available at: http://www.altmedrev.com/publications/10/1/51.pdf. Accessed Dec 2, 2017.

127. USDA. Agricultural Research Service. USDA National Nutrient Database for Standard Reference. Food Search. Available at: https://ndb.nal.usda.gov/ndb/foods/show/2200. Accessed December 2, 2017.

128. National Center for Complementary and Alternative Medicine website. Available at: https://nccih.nih.gov/health /euroelder. Accessed December 2, 2017.

129. Senica M, Stampar F, Veberic R, Mikulic-Petkovsek M. Processed elderberry (Sambucus nigra L.) products: a beneficial or harmful food alternative? *Food Sci Technol*. 2016;72:182–188.

130. Zakay-Rones Z, Varsano N, Zlotnik M, et al. Inhibition of several strains of influenza virus in vitro and reduction of symptoms by an elderberry extract (Sambucus nigra L.) during an outbreak of influenza B Panama. *J Altern Comp Med*. 1995;1:361–369.

131. Zakay-Rones Z, Thom E, Wollan T, Wadstein J. Randomized study of the efficacy and safety of oral elderberry extract in the treatment of influenza A and B virus infections. *J Inter Med Res* (2004)32:132–140.

132. Roschek B, Jr, Fink RC, McMichael MD, Li D, Alberte RS. Elderberry flavonoids bind to prevent H1N1 infection in vitro. *Phytochem*. 2009;70:1255–1261.

133. European Medicines Agency. Community Herbal Monograph on Assessment report on 10. Sambucus nigra L.,

fructus. Committee on Herbal Medicinal Products (HMPC). London, England: 2015; Contract No.: EMA/HMPC/44208/2012.

134. National Center for Complementary and Alternative Medicine. Available at: http://nccih.nih.gov/health/ginger. Accessed December 2, 2017.

135. European Medicines Agency Final assessment report on Zingiber officinale Roscoe, rhizoma. Available at: http://www.ema.europa.eu/docs/en_GB/document_library/Herbal_-_HMPC_assessment_report/2012/06/WC500128140.pdf. Accessed December 2, 2017.

136. Natural Medicines.Ginger [Monograph]. Available at: https://naturalmedicines-therapeuticsresearch-com. Accessed November 10, 2017.

137. Daily JW, Zhang X, Kim da S, et al. Efficacy of ginger for alleviating the symptoms of Primary Dysmenorrhea: a systematic review and meta-analysis of Randomized Clinical Trials. *Pain Med.* 2015;16(12):2243–2255.

138. Kashefi F, Khajehei M, Tabatabaeichehr M, Alavinia M, Asili J. Comparison of the effect of ginger and zinc sulfate on primary dysmenorrhea: a placebo-controlled randomized trial. *Pain Manag Nurs.* 2014;15(4):826–833.

139. Pillai AK, Sharma KK, Gupta YK, et al. Anti-emetic effect of ginger powder versus placebo as an add-on therapy in children and young adults receiving high emetogenic chemotherapy. *Pediatr Blood Cancer.* 2011;56:234–238.

140. Food and Drug Administration. CFR - Substances generally recognized as safe under the Code of Federal Regulations Title 21. Available at: https://www.accessdata.fda.gov/scripts/cdrh/cfdocs/cfcfr/CFRSearch.cfm?fr=182.10. Accessed November 10, 2017.

141. WHO monograph. Fructus Silybi Mariae. WHO monographs on selected medicinal plants - Volume 2. Available at: http://apps.who.int/medicinedocs/pdfs/4927e/s4927e.pdf. 1999:300–316.

142. Natural Medicines. Milk Thistle [Monograph]. Available at: https://naturalmedicines-therapeuticsresearch-com. Accessed November 10, 2017.

143. Ladas E, Kroll DJ, Kelly KM. Milk Thistle. In: Coates PM, Betz JM, Blackman MR, et al., eds. *Encyclopedia of Dietary Supplements.* 2nd ed. New York, NY: Informa Healthcare; 2010:550–561.

144. Rambaldi A, Jacobs BP, Gluud C. Milk thistle for alcoholic and/or hepatitis B or C virus liver diseases. *Cochrane Database of Syst Rev.* 2007(4): CD003620.

145. Ladas EJ, Kroll DJ, Oberlies NH, et al. A randomized, controlled, double-blind, pilot study of milk thistle for the treatment of hepatotoxicity in childhood acute lymphoblastic leukemia (ALL) *Cancer.* 2010;116:506–513.

146. Bahmani M, Shirzad, H, Rafieian S, Rafieian-Kopaei M, Silybum marianum: Beyond hepatoprotection. *J. Evid Based Complement Altern Med.* 2015;20:292–301.

147. Johns OR. Essence of peppermint, a history of the medicine and its bottle. *Hist Archaeol.* 1981;15(2):1–57.

148. Kligler B, Chaudhary S. Peppermint oil. *Am Fam Phy.* 2007;75(7):1027–1030.

149. National Center for Complementary and Alternative Medicine. Herbs at a glance: Peppermint oil. Available at: https://nccih.nih.gov/health/peppermintoil. Accessed December 2, 2017.

150. Natural Medicines. Peppermint [Monograph]. Available at: https://naturalmedicines-therapeuticsresearch-com. Accessed November 10, 2017.

151. Asgarshirazi M, Shariat M, Dalili H. Comparison of the effects of pH-Dependent Peppermint Oil and Synbiotic Lactol (Bacillus coagulans + Fructooligosaccharides) on Childhood Functional Abdominal Pain: A Randomized Placebo-Controlled Study. *Iran Red Crescent Med J.* 2015;25;17(4).

152. Charrois TL1, Hrudey J, Gardiner P, Vohra S. Peppermint oil. *Pediatr Rev.* 2006;27(7):e49–e51.

153. Omer B, Krebs S, Omer H, Noor TO. Steroid-sparing effect of wormwood (Artemisia absinthium) in Crohn's disease: A double-blind placebo-controlled study. *Phytomedicine.* 2007;14:87–95.

154. Krebs S, Omer T N, Omer B. Wormwood (Artemisia absinthium) suppresses tumour necrosis factor alpha and accelerates healing in patients with Crohn's disease - A controlled clinical trial. *Phytomedicine.* 2010;17:305–309.

155. Ren J, Tao Q, Wang X, Wang Z, Li J. Efficacy of T2 in active Crohn's disease: a prospective study report. *Dig Dis Sci.* 2007;52:1790–1797.

156. Tao Q, Ren JA, Ji ZL, Li JS, Wang XB, Jiang XH. [Maintenance effect of polyglycosides of Tripterygium wilfordii on remission in postoperative Crohn disease]. *Zhonghua Wei Chang Wai Ke Za Zhi.* 2009;12:491–493.

157. Chang J, Su K, Mondelli V, Pariante CM. Omega-3 polyunsaturated fatty acids in youths with attention deficit hyperactivity disorder: a systematic review and meta-analysis of clinical trials and biological studies. *Neuropsychopharmacol.* 2017;43(3):534–545.

158. Chang JP, Jiling L, Huang YT, Lu YJ, Su KP. Delay aversion, temporal processing, and N-3 fatty acids intake in children with attention- deficit/hyperactivity disorder (ADHD). *Clin Psychol.* 2016;4:1094–1103.

159. Muley P, Shah M, Muley A. Omega-3 fatty acids supplementation in children to prevent asthma: is it worthy?- a systematic review and meta-analysis. *J Allergy.* 2015; Article ID 312052, 7 pages. Available at: http://dx.doi.org/10.1155/2015/312052.

160. Hodge L, Salome CM, PeatJK, Haby MM, Xuan W, Woolcock AJ. Consumption of oily fish and childhood asthma risk. *Med J Australia.* 1996;164(3):137–140.

161. Andreasyan K, Ponsonby AL, Dwyer T, et al., A differing pattern of association between dietary fish and allergen-specific subgroups of atopy, *Allergy.* 2005;60(5):671–677.

162. Dunder T, Kuikka L, Turtinen J, Räsänen L, Uhari M. Diet, serum fatty acids, and atopic diseases in childhood. *Allergy: Eur J Allergy Clin Immunol.* 2001;56(5)425–428.

163. Romieu I, Torrent M Garcia-Esteban R, et al., Maternal fish intake during pregnancy and atopy and asthma in infancy. *Clin Exp Allergy.*, 2007;37(4):518–525.

164. Salam MT, Li YF, Langholz B, Gilliland FD. Maternal fish consumption during pregnancy and risk of early childhood asthma. *J Asthma.* 2005;42(6):513–518.

165. Versalovich J. The human microbiome and probiotics: implications for pediatrics. *Ann Nutr Metab.* 2013;63 (suppl 2):42–52.

166. Lenfestey MW, Neu J. Probiotics in newborns and children. *Pediatr Clin North Am.* 2017; 64(6):1271–1289.

167. Michail S, Sylvester F, et al. Clinical efficacy of probiotics: review of the evidence with focus on children. *J Pediatr Gastroenterol Nutr.* 2006; 43:550–557.

168. Mai V, Young CM, Ukhanova M, et al. Fecal microbiota in pre-mature infants prior to necrotizing enterocolitis. *PLoS One.* 2011;6:e20647.

169. Gorbach SL, Chang TW, Goldin B: Successful treatment of relapsing *Clostridium difficile* colitis with *Lactobacillus* GG. *Lancet.* 1987;2:1519.

170. Gorbach SL. Probiotics and gastrointestinal health. *Am J Gastroenterol.* 2000; 95(suppl 1):S2–S4.

171. Alfaleh K, Anabrees J, Bassler D, Al-Kharfi T. Probiotics for prevention of necrotizing enterocolitis in preterm infants. *Cochrane Database Syst Rev.* 2011;3:CD005496.

172. Mihatsch WA, Braegger CP, Decsi T, et al. Critical systematic review of the level of evidence for routine use of probiotics for reduction of mortality and prevention of necrotizing enterocolitis and sepsis in preterm infants. *Clin Nutr.* 2012;31:6–15.

173. Guandalini S. Probiotics for prevention and treatment of diarrhea. *J Clin Gastroenterol.* 2011;45(suppl): S149–S153.

174. Preidis GA, Versalovic J. Targeting the human microbiome with antibiotics, probiotics, and prebiotics: gastroenterology enters the metagenomics era. *Gastroenterol.* 2009; 136:2015–2031.

175. Goldenberg JZ, Ma SS, Saxton JD, et al. Probiotics for the prevention of *Clostridium difficile*-associated diarrhea in adults and children. *Cochrane Database Syst Rev.* 2013; 5:CD006095.

176. Chang JY, Antonopoulos DA, Kalra A, et al. Decreased diversity of the fecal microbiome in recurrent *Clostridium difficile*-associated diarrhea. *J Infect Dis.* 2008;197:435– 438.

177. Cremonini F, Di Caro S, Nista EC, et al. Meta-analysis: the effect of probiotic administration on antibiotic-associated diarrhoea. *Aliment Pharmacol Ther.* 2002;16(8):1461–1467.

178. D'Souza AL, et al. Probiotics in prevention of antibiotic associated diarrhoea: meta-analysis. *BMJ.* 2002;324:1361.

179. Szajewska H, et al. Efficacy of Lactobacillus GG in prevention of nosocomial diarrhea in infants. *J Pediatr.* 2001;138:361Y5.

180. Saavedra JM, Bauman NA, Oung I, Perman JA, Yolken RH. Feeding of Bifidobacterium bifidum and Streptococcus thermophilus to infants in hospital for prevention of diarrhoea and shedding of rotavirus. *Lancet.* 1994;344(8929):1046–1049.

Index

Note: Page numbers followed by *f* indicate figures; page numbers followed by *t* indicate tables.